# BRITISH NATIONAL FORMULARY

Number 23
(March 1992)

British Medical Association
and
Royal Pharmaceutical Society of Great Britain

Copies may be obtained through any bookseller or, in any case of difficulty, direct from the publishers:

British Medical Association
Tavistock Square
London WC1H 9JP, England

The Pharmaceutical Press
Royal Pharmaceutical Society of Great Britain
1 Lambeth High Street
London SE1 7JN, England

ISBN: 0 85369 253 X. ISSN: 0260–535X

Typeset in Great Britain by Page Bros, Norwich, Norfolk NR6 6SA and printed and bound by The Bath Press, Bath, Avon BA2 3BL.

# Joint Formulary Committee
# 1991–92

*Chairman*

C. F. George, BSc, MD, FRCP, FFPM

*Deputy Chairman*

C. R. Hitchings, BPharm, MSc, FRPharmS, MCPP

*Committee Members*

Alison Blenkinsopp, PhD,
BPharm, MRPharmS

P. E. Green, BSc, MSc, LLM,
MRPharmS

K. H. Jones, MD, MB, BCh

P. A. Leech, MRCS, LRCP,
DMJ(clin)

F. P. Marsh, MA, MB, BChir,
FRCP

G. M. Mitchell, KStJ, MB, ChB,
FRPharmS

Jane Richards, MB BS, MRCS,
LRCP, FRCGP,
D(Obst)RCOG, DCH

P. C. Waller, MD, MRCP
(alternate to K. H. Jones)

N. L. Wood, BPharm,
MRPharmS

*Joint Secretaries*

Natalie-Jane Macdonald, MB, ChB, MRCP

A. Wade, BPharm, MPhil, FRPharmS

*Executive Editor*

Anne B. Prasad, FRPharmS

*Senior Assistant Editor*

Sheenagh M. Townsend-Smith, BSc, DipLib

*Assistant Editors*

A. G. Desson, BPharm, MSc, MRPharmS (until Nov. 1991)

D. K. Mehta, BPharm, MSc, MRPharmS

Anjana Patel, BPharm, MSc, PhD, MRPharmS

*Editorial Assistants*

Pamela M. Mason, BSc, MSc, PhD, MRPharmS

*Executive Secretary*

Susan M. Thomas, BSc(Econ), MA

# Contents

## APPENDIXES AND INDEXES

# Arrangement of Information

**Guidance on prescribing**
This part includes information on prescription writing, prescribing for children and elderly patients, and prescribing in terminal care. Information is also given on adverse reactions, controlled drugs, and dependence.

**Emergency treatment of poisoning**
The main intention of this chapter is to provide information on the management of acute poisoning when first seen in the home, although aspects of hospital-based treatment are mentioned.

**Classified notes on drugs and preparations**
The main text consists of classified notes on drugs and preparations used in the treatment of diseases and conditions. These notes are divided into 15 chapters, each of which is related to a particular system of the human body or to another main subject. Each chapter is then divided into sections which begin with appropriate *notes for prescribers*. These notes are intended to provide information to doctors, pharmacists, nurses etc. to facilitate the selection of suitable treatment. The notes are followed by details of relevant drugs and preparations.

DRUGS appear under pharmacopoeial or other non-proprietary titles. When there is an *appropriate current monograph* (Medicines Act 1968, Section 65) preference is given to a name at the head of that monograph; otherwise a British Approved Name, if available, is used. If there is an acknowledged reference drug, information on it is usually given first; otherwise the drugs are arranged alphabetically.

PREPARATIONS usually follow immediately after the drug which is their main ingredient. They are printed in text-sized type but those considered by the Committee to be less suitable for prescribing are described in smaller type. Small type is also used for the entries describing foods for special diets, stoma and urinary appliances, and wound management products. Preparations are included under a non-proprietary title only if:
(a) they are marketed under such a title,
(b) they are not otherwise prescribable under the NHS, or
(c) they may be prepared extemporaneously.
If proprietary preparations are of a distinctive colour this is stated, but flavour is not usually mentioned.
In the case of compound preparations the indications, cautions, contra-indications, side-effects, and drug interactions of all constituents should be taken into account in prescribing; usually the ingredients should be looked up separately.

PREPARATIONS NOT AVAILABLE FOR NHS PRESCRIPTION. The symbol NHS has been placed against those preparations included in the BNF that are not prescribable under the NHS. Those prescribable only for specific disorders have a foot-note specifying the condition(s) for which the preparation remains available. Prescribers are reminded that some preparations which are not *prescribable* by brand name under the NHS may nevertheless be *dispensed* using the brand name in question providing that the prescription has been written in the form of an appropriate non-proprietary name.

PRESCRIPTION-ONLY MEDICINES. The symbol PoM has been placed against those preparations that are available only on medical or dental prescription. For more detailed information see *Medicines, Ethics and Practice*, No. 7, London, Pharmaceutical Press, 1991 (and subsequent editions as available). The symbol CD indicates that the preparation is subject to the prescription requirements of the Misuse of Drugs Act. For regulations governing prescriptions for such preparations see pages 7–9.

PRICES (see p. 1) have been calculated whenever possible from the basic cost used in pricing NHS prescriptions dispensed in August 1991, see p. 1 for further details.

**Appendixes and indexes**
The appendixes include information on interactions, liver disease, renal impairment, pregnancy, breast-feeding, intravenous additives, borderline substances, and cautionary and advisory labels for dispensed medicines. Where relevant they are designed for use in association with the main body of the text.
    The Dental Practitioners' List is also included in this section. The indexes consist of the Index of Manufacturers and the Main Index.

# Preface

The present format of the British National Formulary was introduced in February 1981. Information is included on most products available to prescribers in the United Kingdom. The product entries, are preceded by relevant notes to help in the choice of appropriate treatment.

Basic net prices are included to provide better indications of relative cost. Where there is a choice of suitable preparations for a particular disease or condition the relative cost may be used in making a selection. It should be emphasised, however, that cost-effective prescribing must take into account other factors (such as dose frequency and duration of treatment) that affect the total cost. The use of more expensive drugs is justified if it will result in better treatment of the patient or a reduction of the length of an illness or the time spent in hospital.

The BNF is intended to be a pocket book for rapid reference and so cannot contain all the information necessary for prescribing and dispensing. It should be supplemented as necessary from specialised publications. Manufacturers' data sheets prepared in accordance with the Medicines (Data Sheet) Regulations 1972 are available for most proprietary medicines and these should also be consulted. Less detail is given in the chapters on malignant disease and immunosuppression, and anaesthesia, as it is expected that those undertaking treatment will have specialised knowledge and will consult specialist literature. Supplementary information may be available from local drug information services.

The Joint Formulary Committee acknowledges the help of individuals and organisations that provided information or advised on specific matters. The principal contributors for this edition were J. M. Aitken, S. P. Allison, D. G. Arkell, R. S. Atkinson, C. G. Barnes, L. Beeley, R. H. Behrens, I. Burgess, C. M. Castleden, D. A. Chamberlain, B. T. Colvin, C. Diamond, R. Dinwiddie, A. J. Duxbury, H. M. Elliston, A. M. Geddes, A. H. Ghodse, J. Guillebaud, C. H. Hawkes, A. V. Hoffbrand, M. J. S. Langman, P. N. Leigh, R. Levinsky, R. Marks, M. W. McNicol, G. M. Mead, M. R. Moore, D. J. Oliver, L. E. Ramsay, P. A. Routledge, R. S. Sawers, M. C. Sheppard, S. D. Shorvon, M. Tarr, A. Tattersfield, G. R. Thompson, V. R. Tindall, M. D. Vickers, D. G. Waller, D. A. Warrell, P. Watkins, K. Watson, G. B. Wyatt. The Committee also wishes to express its thanks to correspondents in the pharmaceutical industry who provided information and made numerous comments on points of detail, to colleagues who have advised members of the committee and the editorial staff on specific matters, to R. Jackson for valuable advice on appliances, to D. Seyoum for valuable editorial assistance during his 6 months as holder of the 1991 BNF Scholarship, to S. A. Shah for assistance with proofreading, and to J. Holmes and T. M. Roberts for clerical assistance. Finally, the Committee would like to thank those doctors, pharmacists, nurses, and others who sent comments and suggestions.

Comments and constructive criticism will be welcome, and should be sent to:
Executive Editor,
British National Formulary,
c/o Royal Pharmaceutical Society of Great Britain,
1 Lambeth High Street,
London SE1 7JN.

# Changes

The BNF is revised twice yearly and numerous changes are made between issues. All copies of BNF No. 22 (September 1991) should therefore be withdrawn and replaced by BNF No. 23 (March 1992). Significant changes have been made in the following sections for BNF No. 23:

Snake bites, p. 22
Colostomy and ileostomy appliances (section 1.8)
ACE inhibitors (section 2.5.5)
Oxygen concentrators (section 3.6)
Phenytoin equivalence (section 4.8.1)
Drugs used in parkinsonism (section 4.9)
Malaria [treatment] (section 5.4.1)
Drugs for strongyloidiasis (section 5.5.8)

Drugs for genito-urinary disorders (section 7.4)
Appliances for urinary disorders (section 7.5)
Vitamin D (section 9.6.4)
Preparations for warts and calluses (section 13.7)
Elastic hosiery (section 13.13.10)
Appendix 3 [reorganisation]
Appendix 7 [indications amended]
Appendix 8 [cautionary label changes]

## Dose Changes

*Preparations affected by changes in dose statements introduced into BNF No. 23:*

*Afrazine*, p. 382
Antiseptic mouth preparations [more details], pp. 385–6
Aprotinin, p. 102
Atenolol [hypertension], pp. 71–3
*Betadine* mouthwash, p. 386
Bethanechol, p. 288
*Biogastrone*, p. 35
Cefsulodin, p. 205
Cefuroxime [child], p. 206
Chloramphenicol, p. 214
Cholera vaccine, p. 436
Cholestyramine [hyperlipidaemia], p. 103
Clemastine [child], p. 121
Cromoglycate [nasal spray], p. 381
Diltiazem [elderly], p. 88

*Hormonin*, p. 262
Ivermectin, p. 242
Nabilone, p. 164
Netilmicin, p. 212
Omeprazole, p. 35
Ondansetron, p. 165
*Premarin* tablets, p. 263
Promethazine hydrochloride [child], pp. 123, 135, 165
Propofol, p. 450
*Pyrogastrone*, p. 35
Ranitidine [duodenal ulcer], p. 33
Sulphinpyrazone, p. 361
Tobramycin, p. 212
Typhoid vaccine, p. 443
Vancomycin [rate of infusion], p. 216

## Classification Changes

| | |
|---|---|
| 1.7.2 | *Anacal* now in 1.7.1 |
| 1.8.1 | no longer exists |
| 1.8.2 | no longer exists |
| 3.4 | Antihistamines, hyposensitisation, and allergic emergencies [title change] |
| 5.1.14 | HA–1A now in 14.5 |
| 6.1.6 | Diagnostic and monitoring agents for diabetes mellitus [title change and reorganisation] |
| 6.5 and 6.7 | Reclassification and reorganisation |
| 7.1 | Drugs used in obstetrics [title change]; ductus arteriosus now 7.1.1.1 |

| | |
|---|---|
| 7.1.2 | now Mifepristone |
| 7.1.3 | now Myometrial relaxants |
| 7.5 | Appliances for urinary disorders [new section] |
| 9.1.1.1 | *Forceval* now in 9.6.7 |
| 13.1 and 13.2 | Reclassification and reorganisation; flexible collodion now in 13.10.5 |
| 13.13.8 | *Varihesive* now in 1.8 |
| 13.13.10 | Elastic hosiery [new section] |
| 15.1.4.1 | Anxiolytics and neuroleptics [formerly in 15.1.4.2] |
| 15.1.4.2 | Non-opioid analgesics |
| 15.1.4.3 | Opioid analgesics [formerly in 15.1.4.1] |

# New Preparations

*New monographs*

## CEFODIZIME (BNF section 5.1.2)

*Indications:* see under Dose
*Cautions; Contra-indications; Side-effects:* see under Cefaclor
*Dose:* by intramuscular or intravenous injection or by intravenous infusion, lower respiratory-tract infection (including pneumonia and bronchopneumonia), 1 g every 12 hours
Upper and lower urinary-tract infections (including acute and chronic pyelonephritis and cystitis), 1 g every 12 hours *or* 2 g daily (as a single dose); single doses over 1 g intravenous route only

▼ PoM **Timecef**® (Roussel)
*Injection*, powder for reconstitution, cefodizime (as disodium salt), net price 1-g vial = £11.32
Electrolytes: Na⁺ 3.18 mmol/g

## LAMOTRIGINE (BNF section 4.8.1)

*Indications:* adjunctive treatment of partial seizures and secondarily generalised tonic-clonic seizures not satisfactorily controlled with other antiepileptics
*Cautions:* closely monitor (including hepatic, renal and clotting parameters) if rash, fever, influenza-like symptoms, drowsiness, or worsening of seizure control develops, especially in first month of treatment (although causal relationship not established lamotrigine given with other antiepileptics has been associated with rapidly progressive illness with status epilepticus, multi-organ dysfunction and disseminated intravascular coagulation); avoid abrupt withdrawal (taper off over 2 weeks); pregnancy and breast-feeding; **interactions:** Appendix 1 (lamotrigine)
*Contra-indications:* hepatic or renal impairment
*Side-effects:* rashes (rarely angioedema and Stevens-Johnson syndrome); diplopia, blurred vision, dizziness, drowsiness, headache, unsteadiness, tiredness, gastro-intestinal disturbances, irritability, aggression; see also Cautions
*Dose:* with existing antiepileptic therapy, initially 50 mg twice daily (50 mg once daily in patients taking sodium valproate) for 14 days; usual maintenance 200–400 mg daily (100–200 mg daily in patients taking sodium valproate) in 2 divided doses
CHILD under 12 years and ELDERLY, not yet recommended

▼ PoM **Lamictal**® (Wellcome)
*Tablets*, both yellow, lamotrigine 50 mg, net price 56-tab pack = £32.64; 100 mg, 56-tab pack = £56.32

*Existing monographs*

PoM **Didronel PMO**® (Norwich Eaton)
*Tablets*, 14 white, disodium etidronate 400 mg; 76 pink, effervescent, calcium carbonate 1.25 g (Cacit®). Net price per pack = £40.20. Label: 10 patient information leaflet, C, food and calcium. BNF section 6.6.2
*Dose:* established vertebral osteoporosis (90-day cycles) 1 etidronate daily for 14 days, then 1 calcium daily for 76 days

**Diprobath**® (Schering-Plough)
*Bath additive*, isopropyl myristate 39%, light liquid paraffin 46%. Net price 500 mL = £8.55. BNF section 13.2.1.1
*Additives:* none as listed in section 13.1
Add 25 mL/bath (infants 10 mL)

PoM **Minocin MR**® (Lederle)
*Capsules*, m/r, yellow/brown (enclosing yellow and orange pellets), minocycline hydrochloride 100 mg. Net price 49-cap pack = £27.68. Label: 6, 25. BNF section 5.1.3
*Dose:* acne, 1 capsule daily

PoM **Nifensar XL**® (Rhône-Poulenc Rorer)
*Tablets*, m/r, yellow, nifedipine 20 mg. Net price 28-tab pack = £7.56. Label: 21, 25. BNF section 2.6.2
*Dose:* mild to moderate hypertension, initially 40 mg once daily (initially 20 mg in elderly or if previously treated with nifedipine, or in renal impairment); usual maintenance dose 20–40 mg daily; max. 100 mg daily

**Nitro-Dur**® (Schering-Plough)
*Dressing '0.1 mg/h'*, self-adhesive, releasing glyceryl trinitrate approx. 2.5 mg/24 hours when in contact with skin. Net price 28 = £16.14. Counselling, see administration below. BNF section 2.6.1
*Dressing '0.2 mg/h'*, self-adhesive, releasing glyceryl trinitrate approx. 5 mg/24 hours when in contact with skin. Net price 28 = £17.92. Counselling, see administration below.
*Dressing '0.4 mg/h'*, self-adhesive, releasing glyceryl trinitrate approx. 10 mg/24 hours when in contact with skin. Net price 28 = £19.84. Counselling, see administration below.
*Dressing '0.6 mg/h'*, self-adhesive, releasing glyceryl trinitrate approx. 15 mg/24 hours. Net price 28 = £21.83. Counselling, see administration below.
ADMINISTRATION: prophylaxis of angina, apply one '0.2 mg/h' dressing to chest or outer upper arm; replace every 24 hours, siting replacement dressing on different area; adjust dose according to response

## New Preparations (*continued*)

### Preparations included in appropriate sections of BNF No. 23

Adenocor, p. 65
AeroBec inhalers,
    pp. 117–18
Alvedon, p. 167
AmBisome, p. 228
Amoxil Fiztab, p. 199
Calpol Extra, p. 169
Capozide LS, p. 82
Celectol, p. 73
Climaval, p. 262
Diflucan suspension, p. 228
Flemoxin, p. 200
Flexin-25, p. 352

Flexin-LS, p. 352
Flixonase, p. 381
Glytrin, p. 85
Halfan, p. 236
Imigran, p. 177
Kytril, p. 163
Laboprin DL [replaces
    Laboprin], p. 167
Loceryl, p. 415
Molipaxin CR, p. 155
Napratec, p. 353
Naprosyn EC, p. 353
Norgalax, p. 42

Noroxin, p. 368
Nuvelle, p. 262
Oruvail, p. 365
Pharmorubicin solution,
    p. 306
Pulmicort Respules, p. 118
Retrovir syrup, p. 231
Rhinolast, p. 380
Savlon Dry, p. 423
Sinemet CR, p. 186
SRM-Rhotard, p. 172
Synarel, p. 274
Teflox, p. 226

Toradol, p. 455
Tri-Minulet, p. 285
Ucerax, p. 139
Unasyn, p. 200
Vicks Ultra Chloraseptic,
    p. 386
Voltarol 75 mg SR, p. 350
Zantac effervescent tablets,
    p. 33
Zinnat sachets and
    suspension, p. 206
Zithromax, p. 213

*Note.* Rimifon injection, Ro-A-Vit injection, and Synkavit tablets remain available

# Discontinued Preparations

### Preparations discontinued during the compilation of BNF No. 23

Achromycin syrup
Actidil
Afrazine nasal drops
Alexitol tablets
Antepar elixir
Antraderm Forte
Bactrim intravenous
    infusion
Banocide
Bronchodil tablets
Chloraseptic throat spray
Cologel
Congesteze syrup
Disadine DP

Distaquaine V-K syrup
Esbatal
Eudemine tablets
Finalgon
Formulix
Framycort
Framygen
Hypercal-B
Keflin
Kerecid
Laboprin [replaced by
    Laboprin DL]
Lotussin
Malinal

Mantadine
Megaclor
Micturin
Min-I-Mix
    Methylprednisolone
Minims Castor Oil
Miol
Moditen Enanthate
Monistat
Mucogel tablets
Navidrex-K
Neo-Naclex-K
Niferex tablets
Omnopon-Scopolamine

Panmycin syrup
Parahypon
Provera suspension
Serpasil
Serpasil-Esidrex
Sodium Amytal tablets
Solprin
Stiedex LPN
Tachyrol
Urisal
Valium suppositories
X-Prep
Zadstat infusion

*Note.* Product licences for triazolam preparations (including Halcion®) have been suspended.

---

### Oral syringes

From 1 April 1992, when fractional doses are prescribed, *oral liquid medicines* will **no longer** be diluted to a 5-mL dose (or multiple thereof). Instead the pharmacist will supply an **oral syringe**. The oral syringe will be marked in 0.5 mL divisions from 1 to 5 mL to measure doses of less than 5 mL. The 5-mL spoon will continue in use for doses of 5 mL (or multiple thereof). The oral syringe will be provided with an adaptor and an instruction leaflet.

# Drug Information Services

Information on any aspect of drug therapy can be obtained, free of charge, from Regional and District Drug Information Services. Details regarding the *local* services provided within your Region can be obtained by telephoning the following numbers.

*England*

| | | |
|---|---|---|
| Birmingham | 021-311 1974 | Direct Line |
| | *or* 021-378 2211 | Extn 2296/2297 |
| Bristol | 0272 282867 | Direct Line |
| Guildford | 0483 504312 | Direct Line |
| Ipswich | 0473 704430 | Direct Line |
| | *or* 0473 704431 | Direct Line |
| Leeds | 0532 430715 | Direct Line |
| Leicester | 0533 555779 | Direct Line |
| Liverpool | 051-236 4620 | Extn 2126/2127/2128 |
| London (Guy's Hospital) | 071-955 5000 | Extn 3594/5892 |
| | *or* 071-378 0023 | Direct Line |
| London (London Hospital) | 071-377 7487 | Direct Line |
| | *or* 071-377 7488 | Direct Line |
| London (Northwick Park) | 081-869 3973 | Direct Line |
| Manchester | 061-225 2063 | Direct Line |
| | *or* 061-276 6270 | Direct Line |
| Newcastle | 091-232 1525 | Direct Line |
| Oxford | 0865 221808 | Direct Line |
| | *or* 0865 221836 | Direct Line |
| Southampton | 0703 796908 | Direct Line |
| | *or* 0703 796909 | Direct Line |

*Northern Ireland*

| | | |
|---|---|---|
| Belfast | 0232 248095 | Direct Line |
| Londonderry | 0504 45171 | Extn 3262 |

*Scotland*

| | | |
|---|---|---|
| Aberdeen | 0224 681818 | Extn 52316 |
| Dundee | 0382 60111 | Extn 2351 |
| Edinburgh | 031-229 2477 | Extn 2094/2416/2443 |
| | *or* 031-229 3901 | Direct Line |
| Glasgow | 041-552 4726 | Direct Line |
| Inverness | 0463 234151 | Extn 288 |
| | *or* 0463 220157 | Direct Line |

*Wales*

| | | |
|---|---|---|
| Cardiff | 0222 742979 | Direct Line |

---

**Poisons Information Services**

| | |
|---|---|
| Belfast | 0232 240503 |
| Birmingham | 021-554 3801 |
| Cardiff | 0222 709901 |
| Dublin | 0001 379964 *or* 0001 379966 |
| Edinburgh | 031-229 2477 |
| | 031-228 2441 (Viewdata) |
| Leeds | 0532 430715 *or* 0532 432799 |
| London | 071-635 9191 *or* 071-955 5095 |
| Newcastle | 091-232 5131 |

*Note.* Some of these centres also advise on laboratory analytical services which may be of help in the diagnosis and management of a small number of cases.

# Guidance on Prescribing

## Prices in the BNF

Basic **net prices** have been introduced into the BNF in order to provide better indications of relative cost. Whenever possible they have been calculated from the basic cost used in pricing NHS prescriptions dispensed in August 1991; unless an original pack is available these prices are based on the largest pack size of the preparation in use in community pharmacies. The price for an extemporaneously prepared preparation has been omitted where the net cost of the ingredients used to make it would give a misleadingly low impression of the final price.

The unit of 20 is still sometimes used as a basis for comparison, but where suitable original packs are available these are priced instead.

Gross prices vary as follows:
1. Costs to the NHS are greater than the net prices quoted and include professional fees and overhead allowances;
2. Private prescription charges are calculated on a separate basis;
3. Over-the-counter sales are at retail price, as opposed to basic net price, and include VAT.

**BNF prices are NOT, therefore, suitable for quoting to patients seeking private prescriptions or contemplating over-the-counter purchases.**
A fuller explanation of costs to the NHS may be obtained from the Drug Tariff.
It should be noted that separate Drug Tariffs are operative in England and Wales, Scotland, and Northern Ireland. Prices in the different tariffs may vary.

## PACT and SPA
PACT (Prescribing Analysis and Costs) and SPA (Scottish Prescribing Analysis) automatically provide general practitioners with information about their prescribing. The information is sent on a quarterly basis direct from the Prescription Pricing Authority. It is available at three levels of complexity:
*Level 1 reports* compare practice prescribing with that of the local Family Health Services Authority (FHSA) or Health Board (in Scotland) and national averages—they are produced once a quarter for each general practitioner;
*Level 2 reports* are produced for general practitioners with above average costs—they can also be requested;
*Level 3 reports* are available only on request—they are effectively a list of all items prescribed by the general practitioner, grouped into the BNF therapeutic categories, giving detailed cost information. These reports are termed level 2 in Scotland since the intermediate level is not produced.

# General Guidance

Medicines should be prescribed only when they are essential, and in all cases the benefit of administering the medicine should be considered in relation to the risk involved. This is particularly important during pregnancy where the risk to both mother and fetus must be considered (for further details see Prescribing in Pregnancy, Appendix 4).

ABBREVIATION OF TITLES. In general, titles of drugs and preparations should be written *in full*. Unofficial abbreviations should not be used as they may be misinterpreted; obsolete titles, such as Mist. Expect. and Mist. Tussis should not be used.

NON-PROPRIETARY TITLES. Where non-proprietary ('generic') titles are given, they should be used in prescribing. This will enable any suitable product to be dispensed, thereby saving delay to the patient and sometimes expense to the health service. The only exception is where bioavailability problems are so important that the patient should always receive the same brand; in such cases, the brand name or the manufacturer should be stated. Non-proprietary titles should **not** be invented for the purposes of prescribing generically since this can lead to confusion (see also Compound Names, p. 5).

Titles used as headings for monographs may be used freely in Great Britain and Northern Ireland but in other countries may be subject to restriction.

Many of the non-proprietary titles used in this book are titles of monographs in the European Pharmacopoeia, British Pharmacopoeia or British Pharmaceutical Codex 1973. In such cases the preparations must comply with the standard (if any) in the appropriate publication, as required by the Medicines Act (section 65).

PROPRIETARY TITLES. Names followed by the symbol® are or have been used as proprietary names in the United Kingdom. These names may in general be applied only to products supplied by the owners of the trade marks.

DOSES. The doses stated in the BNF are intended for general guidance and represent, unless otherwise stated, the usual range of doses that are generally regarded as being suitable for adults; unless otherwise indicated the quantities are those generally suitable for administration on one occasion.

ORAL SYRINGES. From 1 April 1992, when fractional doses are prescribed, *oral liquid medicines* will **no longer** be diluted to a 5-mL dose (or multiple thereof). Instead the pharmacist will supply an **oral syringe**. The oral syringe will be marked in 0.5 mL divisions from 1 to 5 mL to measure doses of less than 5 mL. The 5-mL spoon will continue in use for doses of 5 mL (or multiple thereof). The oral syringe will be provided with an adaptor and an instruction leaflet.

STRENGTHS AND QUANTITIES. The strength or quantity to be contained in capsules, lozenges, tablets, etc. should be stated by the prescriber.

If a pharmacist receives an incomplete prescription for a systemically administered preparation other than a prescription for a controlled drug and considers it would not be appropriate for the patient to return to the doctor, the following procedures will apply:

(a) an attempt must always be made to contact the prescriber to ascertain the intention;

(b) if the attempt is successful the pharmacist must, where practicable, subsequently arrange for details of quantity, strength where applicable, and dosage to be inserted by the prescriber on the incomplete form;

(c) where, although the prescriber has been contacted, it has not proved possible to obtain the written intention regarding an incomplete prescription, the pharmacist may endorse the form 'p.c.' (prescriber contacted) and add details of the quantity and strength where applicable of the preparation supplied, and of the dose indicated. The endorsement should be initialled and dated by the pharmacist;

(d) where the prescriber cannot be contacted and the pharmacist has sufficient information to make a professional judgment the preparation may be dispensed. If the quantity is missing the pharmacist may supply sufficient to complete up to 5 days' treatment; except that where a combination pack (i.e. a proprietary pack containing more than one medicinal product) or oral contraceptive is prescribed by name only, the smallest pack shall be dispensed. In all cases the prescription must be endorsed 'p.n.c.' (prescriber not contacted) the quantity, the dose, and the strength (where applicable) of the preparation supplied must be indicated, and the endorsement must be initialled and dated;

(e) if the pharmacist has any doubt about exercising discretion, an incomplete prescription must be referred back to the prescriber.

ADDITIVES. Oral liquid preparations in the BNF that do not contain *fructose*, *glucose* or *sucrose* are labelled "sugar-free".

Where the presence of *gluten* or of *tartrazine* is specified on a data sheet this is indicated in the BNF against the preparation in question; not all data sheets provide details of additives therefore if it is essential to know whether a preparation is free of gluten or of tartrazine the manufacturer should be contacted.

Information is provided on *preservatives* in eye-drops.

Information is provided on *selected additives* in skin preparations (for details see section 13.1).

EXTEMPORANEOUS PREPARATION. The BP direction that a preparation must be *freshly prepared* indicates that it must be made not more than 24 hours before it is issued for use. The direction that a preparation should be *recently prepared* indicates that deterioration is likely if the preparation is stored for longer than about 4 weeks at 15° to 25°.

APPLIANCES AND CHEMICAL REAGENTS. A limited selection of appliances (including elastic hosiery, and trusses) and chemical reagents is available for prescribing by general medical practitioners in the NHS; details of these are now included in BNF.

DRUGS AND DRIVING. Prescribers should advise patients if treatment is likely to affect their ability to drive motor vehicles. This applies particularly to drugs with sedative effects and patients should be warned that these effects are increased by alcohol. See also Appendix 8.

NOTICE CONCERNING PATENTS. In the BNF certain drugs have been included notwithstanding the existence of actual or potential patent rights. In so far as such substances are protected by Letters Patent, their inclusion in this Formulary neither conveys, nor implies, licence to manufacture.

HEALTH AND SAFETY. When handling chemical or biological materials particular attention should be given to the possibility of allergy, fire, explosion, radiation, or poisoning. Some substances, including corticosteroids, antibiotics, phenothiazines, and many cytotoxics, are irritant or very potent and should be handled with caution. Contact with the skin and inhalation of dust should be avoided.

SAFETY IN THE HOME. Patients must be warned to keep all medicines out of the reach of children. All solid dose oral medicines should be dispensed either in reclosable *child-resistant containers* complying with the British Standard or in unit packaging of strip or blister type unless:
(i) they are in manufacturers' original packs so designed that transfer to a reclosable child-resistant container would be a retrograde or unnecessary procedure;
(ii) the patient is elderly or handicapped and would have difficulty in opening a child-resistant container;
(iii) the patient specifically requests otherwise.
  In cases (ii) and (iii) the pharmacist should make a particular point of advising that the medicines be kept well out of the reach of children.
  All patients should be advised to dispose of *unwanted medicines* by flushing them down a WC or returning them to a supplier for destruction.

NAME OF MEDICINE. The name of the medicine should appear on the label unless the prescriber indicates otherwise.
1. Subject to the conditions of paragraphs 4 and 6 below, the name of the prescribed medicine is stated on the label unless the prescriber deletes the letters 'NP' which appear on NHS prescription forms.
2. The strength is also stated on the label in the case of tablets, capsules, and similar preparations that are available in different strengths.
3. If it is the wish of the prescriber that a description such as 'The Sedative Tablets' should appear on the label, the prescriber should write the desired description on the prescription form.
4. The arrangement will extend to approved names, proprietary names or titles given in the BP, BPC, BNF, or DPF. The arrangement does not apply when a prescription is written so that several ingredients are given.
5. The name written on the label is that used by the prescriber on the prescription.
6. If more than one item is prescribed on one form and the prescriber does not delete the letters 'NP', each dispensed medicine is named on the label, subject to the conditions given above in paragraph 4. If the prescriber wants only selected items on such a prescription to be so labelled this should be indicated by deleting the letters 'NP' on the form and writing 'NP' alongside the medicines to be labelled.
7. When a prescription is written other than on an NHS prescription form the name of the prescribed preparation will be stated on the label of the dispensed medicine unless the prescriber indicates otherwise.
8. The Council of the Royal Pharmaceutical Society advises that the labels of dispensed medicines should indicate the total quantity of the product dispensed in the container to which the label refers. This requirement applies equally to solid, liquid, internal, and external preparations. If a product is dispensed in more than one container, the reference should be to the amount in each container.

SCOPE OF THE BNF. The BNF is intended for the guidance of medical practitioners, pharmacists, dentists, nurses, and other workers who have the necessary training and experience to interpret the information it provides. It is intended as a reference book for the pocket, and should be supplemented by a study of more detailed publications when required.

---

**Security and validity of prescriptions**

The Councils of the British Medical Association and the Royal Pharmaceutical Society have issued a joint statement on the security and validity of prescriptions.

In particular, prescription forms should:
(i) not be left unattended at reception desks;
(ii) not be left in a car where they may be visible; and
(iii) when not in use, be kept in a locked drawer within the surgery and at home.

Where there is any doubt about the authenticity of a prescription, the pharmacist should contact the prescriber. If this is done by telephone, the number should be obtained from the directory rather than relying on the prescription form information, which may be false.

# Prescription Writing

> The following recommendations are acceptable for **prescription-only medicines** (PoM). For items marked **CD** see Controlled Drugs and Drug Dependence p. 7.

Prescriptions should be written legibly in ink or otherwise as to be indelible[1], should be dated, should state the full name and address of the patient, and should be signed in ink by the prescriber[2]. The age of the patient should preferably be stated, and is a legal requirement in the case of prescription-only medicines for children under 12 years of age.

In general practice the following should be noted:

(a) For solids, quantities of 1 gram or more should be written as 1 g etc.

Quantities less than 1 gram should be written in milligrams, e.g. 500 mg, not 0.5 g.

Quantities less than 1 mg should be written in micrograms, e.g. 100 micrograms, not 0.1 mg.

When decimals are unavoidable a zero should be written in front of the decimal point where there is no other figure, e.g. 0.5 mL, not .5 mL.

Use of the decimal point is acceptable to express a range, e.g. 0.5 to 1 g.

(b) 'Micrograms' and 'nanograms' should **not** be abbreviated. Similarly 'units' should **not** be abbreviated.

(c) The term 'millilitre' (ml or mL)[3] is used in medicine and pharmacy, and cubic centimetre, c.c., or cm³ should not be used.

(d) Dose and dose frequency should be stated; in the case of preparations to be taken 'as required' a **minimum dose interval** should be specified.

For oral liquid preparations of the *linctus* or *elixir* type and for *preparations for children*, doses should preferably be stated in terms of 5-mL spoonfuls.

For *mixtures for adults*, doses should preferably be stated in 10-mL quantities; unless the prescription states otherwise, the patient will be directed to take the dose with water.

When doses other than 5 or 10 mL are prescribed the dose-volume will be provided by means of an **oral syringe**, see p. 2 (except for preparations intended to be measured with a pipette).

Suitable quantities:

Elixirs, Linctuses, and Paediatric
   Mixtures (5-mL dose), 50, 100, or 150 mL
Adult Mixtures (10-mL dose), 200 or 300 mL
Ear Drops, Eye-drops, and Nasal Drops,
   10 mL (or the manufacturer's pack)
Eye Lotions, Gargles, and Mouth-washes, 200 mL
Liniments, 100 mL

(e) For suitable quantities of dermatological preparations, see section 13.1.

(f) The names of drugs and preparations should be written clearly and **not** abbreviated, using approved titles **only**.

(g) The symbol 'NP' on NHS forms should be deleted if it is required that the name of the preparation should not appear on the label. For full details see p. 3.

(h) The quantity to be supplied may be stated by indicating the number of days of treatment required in the box provided on NHS forms. In most cases the exact amount will be supplied. This does not apply to items directed to be used as required; if the dose and frequency are not given the quantity to be supplied should be stated.

When several items are ordered on one form the box can be marked with the number of days of treatment providing the quantity is added for any item for which the amount cannot be calculated.

(i) Although directions should preferably be in **English without abbreviation**, it is recognised that some Latin abbreviations are used (for details see Inside Back Cover).

(j) A prescription for a preparation that has been withdrawn or needs to be specially imported for a named patient should be handwritten. The name of the preparation should be endorsed with the prescriber's signature and the letters 'WD' (withdrawn or specially-imported drug); there may be considerable delay in obtaining a withdrawn medicine.

1. It is permissible to issue carbon copies of NHS prescriptions as long as they are signed in ink.
2. Computer-generated facsimile signatures do not meet the legal requirement.
3. The use of capital 'L' in mL is a printing convention throughout the BNF; both mL and ml are recognised abbreviations for SI units.

# Computer-issued Prescriptions

For computer-issued prescriptions the following recommendations of the Joint Computing Group of the General Medical Services Committee and the Royal College of General Practitioners should also be noted:

1. The computer must print out the date[1], the patient's surname, one forename, other initials, and address, and may also print out the patient's title. The age of children under 12 years must be printed in the box available; a facility may exist to print out the age of older children and adults as well.

2. The doctor's name[2] must be printed at the bottom of the prescription form; this will be the name of the doctor responsible for the prescription (who will normally sign it). The doctor's surgery address, reference number, and Family Health Services Authority (FHSA)[3] are also necessary. In addition, the surgery telephone number should be printed.

3. When prescriptions are to be signed by trainees, assistants, locums, or deputising doctors, the name of the doctor printed at the bottom of the form must still be that of the responsible principal. To avoid difficulties for the pharmacist checking the prescription, the name of the signing doctor may be printed in the signature box, to be signed over on prescribing.

4. Names of medicines must come from a dictionary held in the computer memory, to provide a check on the spelling and ensure that the name is written in full. The computer can be programmed to recognise both the non-proprietary and the proprietary name of a particular drug and to print out the preferred choice, but must not print out both names. For medicines not in the dictionary, separate checking mechanisms are required—the user must be warned that no check was possible and the entire prescription must be entered in the lexicon.

5. The dictionary may contain information on the usual doses, formulations, and (where relevant) pack sizes to produce standard predetermined prescriptions for common preparations, and to provide a check on the validity of an individual prescription on entry.

6. The prescription must be printed in English without abbreviation; information may be entered or stored in abbreviated form. The dose must be in numbers, the frequency in words, and the quantity in numbers in brackets, thus: 40 mg four times daily (112).

It must also be possible to prescribe by indicating the length of treatment required, see (h) above.

7. The BNF recommendations should be followed as in (a), (b), (c), (d), and (e) above.

8. Checks may be incorporated to ensure that all the information required for dispensing a particular drug has been filled in. Instructions such as 'as directed' should be avoided. For the instruction 'when required' the maximum daily dose should normally be specified.

9. Numbers and codes used in the system for organising and retrieving data must never appear on the form.

## Compound names.

Generic names of compound preparations which appear in the BNF are those approved by the British Pharmacopoeia Commission; whenever possible they reflect the names of the active ingredients.

Prescribers should avoid creating their own compound names for the purposes of generic prescribing; such names do not have an approved definition and can be misinterpreted.

Special care should be taken to avoid errors when prescribing compound preparations; in particular the hyphen in the prefix 'co-' should be retained.

10. Supplementary warnings or advice should be written in full, should not interfere with the clarity of the prescription itself, and should be in line with any warnings or advice in the BNF; numerical codes should not be used.

11. A mechanism (such as printing a series of non-specific characters) may be incorporated to cancel out unused space, or wording such as 'no more items on this prescription' may be added after the last item. Otherwise the doctor should delete the space manually.

12. To avoid forgery the computer may print on the form the number of items to be dispensed (somewhere separate from the box for the pharmacist). The number of items per form need be limited only by the ability of the printer to produce clear and well-demarcated instructions with sufficient space for each item and a spacer line before each fresh item.

13. Handwritten alterations should only be made in exceptional circumstances—it is preferable to print out a new prescription. Any alterations that are made must be written in the doctor's own handwriting and countersigned.

14. Prescriptions for controlled drugs cannot be produced by a printer[4]. If there is a record of such a prescription in the computer, it must not be printed. Instead the computer may print out a blank form with the doctor's name[1] and other details printed at the bottom.

15. The strip of paper on the side of the FP10[5](Comp) may be used for various purposes but care should be taken to avoid including confidential information. It may be advisable for the patient's name to appear at the top, but this should be preceded by 'confidential'.

16. In rural dispensing practices prescription requests (or details of medicines dispensed) will normally be entered in one surgery. The prescriptions (or dispensed medicines) may then need to be delivered to another surgery or location; if possible the computer should hold up to 10 alternatives.

---

1. The exemption for own handwriting regulations for phenobarbitone does not apply to the date; a computer-generated date need not be deleted but the date must also be added by the prescriber.
2. Except in Scotland where it does not appear.
3. Health Board in Scotland.
4. Except in the case of phenobarbitone (but see also footnote 1) or where the prescriber has been exempted from handwriting requirements, for details see Controlled Drugs and Drug Dependence p. 7.
5. GP10 in Scotland.

# Emergency Supply of PoM at Patient's Request[1]

The Medicines (Products Other Than Veterinary Drugs) (Prescription Only) Order 1983, as amended, allows exemptions from the Prescription Only requirements for emergency supply to be made by a person lawfully conducting a retail pharmacy business provided:

(a) that the pharmacist has interviewed the person requesting the prescription-only medicine and is satisfied:
(i) that there is immediate need for the prescription-only medicine and that it is impracticable in the circumstances to obtain a prescription without undue delay;
(ii) that treatment with the prescription-only medicine has on a previous occasion been prescribed by a doctor[2] for the person requesting it;
(iii) as to the dose which it would be appropriate for the person to take;

(b) that no greater quantity shall be supplied than will provide five days' treatment except when the prescription-only medicine is:
(i) an ointment, cream, or preparation for the relief of asthma in an aerosol dispenser when the smallest pack can be supplied;
(ii) an oral contraceptive when a full cycle may be supplied;
(iii) an antibiotic in liquid form for oral administration when the smallest quantity that will provide a full course of treatment can be supplied;

(c) that an entry shall be made in the prescription book stating:
(i) the date of supply;
(ii) the name, quantity and, where appropriate, the pharmaceutical form and strength;
(iii) the name and address of the patient;
(iv) the nature of the emergency;

(d) that the container or package must be labelled to show:
(i) the date of supply;
(ii) the name, quantity and, where appropriate, the pharmaceutical form and strength;
(iii) the name of the patient;
(iv) the name and address of the pharmacy;
(v) the words 'Emergency supply'.

(e) that the prescription-only medicine is not a substance specifically excluded from the emergency supply provision, and does not contain a Controlled Drug specified in schedules 1, 2, or 3 to the Misuse of Drugs Regulations 1985 except for phenobarbitone or phenobarbitone sodium for the treatment of epilepsy: for details see *Medicines, Ethics and Practice*, No. 7, London, Pharmaceutical Press, 1991 (and subsequent editions as available).

ROYAL PHARMACEUTICAL SOCIETY'S GUIDELINES
(1) The pharmacist should consider the medical consequences, if any, of **not** supplying.
(2) The pharmacist should identify the patient by means of documentary evidence and/or personal knowledge.
(3) The doctor who prescribed on a previous occasion should be identified and contacted, if possible.
(4) The patient should be asked whether the doctor has stopped the treatment.
(5) The patient should be asked whether any other medicine is being taken at the same time to check drug interactions.
(6) An emergency supply should not be made if the item requested was prescribed previously more than six months prior to the request. Variations may be made in the case of illnesses that occur infrequently, e.g. hay fever, asthma attack, or migraine.
(7) Consideration should be given to providing less than five days' supply if this is justified.
(8) Labelling should be clear and legible and there should be some suitable identification of emergency supply entries in the prescription book.

---

1. For emergency supply at the request of a doctor see *Medicines, Ethics and Practice*, No. 7, London, Pharmaceutical Press, 1991 (and subsequent editions as available).
2. The doctor must be a UK-registered doctor.

---

> **Plasma concentrations** in the BNF are expressed in mass units per litre (e.g. mg/litre). The approximate equivalent in terms of amount of substance units (e.g. micromol/litre) is given in brackets.

# Approximate Conversions and Units

| lb | kg | stones | kg | mL | fl. oz |
|----|------|--------|-------|------|--------|
| 1 | 0.45 | 1 | 6.35 | 50 | 1.8 |
| 2 | 0.91 | 2 | 12.70 | 100 | 3.5 |
| 3 | 1.36 | 3 | 19.05 | 150 | 5.3 |
| 4 | 1.81 | 4 | 25.40 | 200 | 7.0 |
| 5 | 2.27 | 5 | 31.75 | 500 | 17.6 |
| 6 | 2.72 | 6 | 38.10 | 1000 | 35.2 |
| 7 | 3.18 | 7 | 44.45 | | |
| 8 | 3.63 | 8 | 50.80 | | |
| 9 | 4.08 | 9 | 57.15 | | |
| 10 | 4.54 | 10 | 63.50 | | |
| 11 | 4.99 | 11 | 69.85 | | |
| 12 | 5.44 | 12 | 76.20 | | |
| 13 | 5.90 | 13 | 82.55 | | |
| 14 | 6.35 | 14 | 88.90 | | |
| | | 15 | 95.25 | | |

**Mass**
| | |
|---|---|
| 1 kilogram (kg) | = 1000 grams (g) |
| 1 gram (g) | = 1000 milligrams (mg) |
| 1 milligram (mg) | = 1000 micrograms |
| 1 microgram | = 1000 nanograms |
| 1 nanogram | = 1000 picograms |

**Volume**
| | |
|---|---|
| 1 litre | = 1000 millilitres (mL) |
| 1 millilitre | = 1000 microlitres |
| 1 pint | $\approx$ 568 mL |

**Other units**
| | |
|---|---|
| 1 kilocalorie (kcal) | = 4186.8 joules (J) |
| 1000 kilocalories (kcal) | = 4.1868 megajoules (MJ) |
| 1 megajoule (MJ) | = 238.8 kilocalories (kcal) |
| 1 millimetre of mercury (mmHg) | = 133.3 pascals (Pa) |
| 1 kilopascal (kPa) | = 7.5 mmHg (pressure) |

# Controlled Drugs and Drug Dependence

PRESCRIPTIONS. Preparations which are subject to the prescription requirements of the Misuse of Drugs Regulations 1985, i.e. preparations specified in schedules 2 and 3, are distinguished throughout the BNF by the symbol **CD** (Controlled Drugs). The principal legal requirements relating to medical prescriptions are listed below.

Prescriptions ordering Controlled Drugs subject to prescription requirements must be *signed* and *dated*[1] by the prescriber and specify the prescriber's *address*. The prescription must always state *in the prescriber's own handwriting*[2] in ink or otherwise so as to be indelible:

1. The name and address of the patient;
2. In the case of a preparation, the form[3] and where appropriate the strength of the preparation;
3. The total quantity of the preparation, or the number of dose units, *in both words and figures;*
4. The dose.

A prescription may order a Controlled Drug to be dispensed by instalments; the amount of the instalments and the intervals to be observed must be specified.[4] Prescriptions ordering 'repeats' on the same form are **not** permitted.

It is an offence for a doctor to issue an incomplete prescription and a pharmacist is **not** allowed to dispense a Controlled Drug unless all the information required by law is given on the prescription. Failure to comply with the regulations concerning the writing of prescriptions will result in inconvenience to patients and delay in supplying the necessary medicine.

DEPENDENCE AND MISUSE. The prevalence of drug dependence and misuse in Great Britain, particularly amongst young people, continues to give cause for concern to teachers, social workers, and the police, as well as doctors.

The most serious drugs of addiction are **diamorphine** (heroin), **morphine**, and the **synthetic opioids**; illicit **cocaine** is now also a problem.

Despite marked reduction in the prescribing of **amphetamines** there is concern that abuse of illicitly produced amphetamine and related compounds is widespread.

The principal **barbiturates** are now Controlled Drugs, but phenobarbitone and phenobarbitone sodium or a preparation containing either of these are exempt from the handwriting requirement (**important:** the exemption does **not** apply to the date; a computer-generated date need not be deleted but the date must also be added by the prescriber). Moreover, for the treatment of epilepsy phenobarbitone and phenobarbitone sodium are available under the emergency supply regulations (p. 6).

**Cannabis** (Indian hemp) has no approved medicinal use and cannot be prescribed by doctors (except under licence from the Home Secretary). Its use is illegal but has become widespread in certain sections of society. Cannabis is a mild hallucinogen seldom accompanied by a desire to increase the dose; withdrawal symptoms are unusual. **Lysergide** (lysergic acid diethylamide, LSD) is a much more potent hallucinogen; its use can lead to severe psychotic states in which life may be at risk.

---

1. A prescription is valid for 13 weeks from the date stated thereon.
2. Unless the prescriber has been specifically exempted from this requirement or unless the prescription contains no controlled drug other than phenobarbitone or phenobarbitone sodium or a preparation containing either of these. The exemption does **not** apply to the date; a computer-generated date need not be deleted but the date must also be added by the prescriber.
3. The dosage form (e.g. tablets) must be included on a Controlled Drugs prescription irrespective of whether it is implicit in the proprietary name (e.g. Tenuate Dospan®) or of whether only one form is available.
4. A special form, FP10(HP)(ad), in Scotland HBP(A), is available to doctors in NHS drug treatment centres for prescribing cocaine, dextromoramide, diamorphine, dipipanone, methadone, morphine, or pethidine by instalments for addicts. In Scotland general practitioners can prescribe by instalments on form GP10. In England and Wales forms FP10 and FP10(HP) are not suitable for this purpose but form FP10(MDA) is available. **Important:** in all cases a special licence is necessary to prescribe cocaine, diamorphine, or dipipanone for addicts except for treatment of organic disease or injury, for details see p. 9.

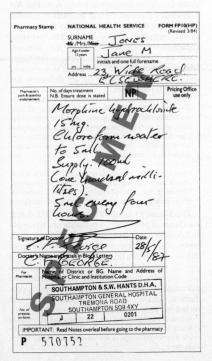

PRESCRIBING DRUGS LIKELY TO CAUSE DEPEN-
DENCE OR MISUSE. The prescriber has three main
responsibilities:

1. To avoid creating dependence by introducing
drugs to patients without sufficient reason. In this
context, the proper use of the morphine-like drugs
is well understood. The dangers of other controlled drugs are less clear because recognition of
dependence is not easy and its effects, and those
of withdrawal, are less obvious. Perhaps the most
notable result of uninhibited prescribing is that a
very large number of patients in the country take
tablets which do them neither much good nor
much harm, but are committed to them indefinitely because they cannot readily be stopped.

2. To see that the patient does not gradually
increase the dose of a drug, given for good medical
reasons, to the point where dependence becomes
more likely. This tendency is seen especially with
hypnotics and anxiolytics (for CSM advice see
section 4.1). The prescriber should keep a close
eye on the amount prescribed to prevent patients
from accumulating stocks that would enable them
to arrange their own dosage or even that of their
families and friends. A minimal amount should
be prescribed in the first instance, or when seeing
a new patient for the first time.

3. To avoid being used as an unwitting source of
supply for addicts. Methods include visiting more
than one doctor, fabricating stories, and forging
prescriptions. A doctor should therefore be wary
of prescribing for strangers and may be able to
get information about suspected opioid addicts
from the Home Office (for details see p. 9).

Patients under temporary care should be given
only small supplies of drugs unless they present
an unequivocal letter from their own doctors.
Doctors should also remember that their own
patients may be doing a collecting round with
other doctors, especially in hospitals. It is sensible
to decrease dosages steadily or to issue weekly or
even daily prescriptions for small amounts if it is
apparent that dependence is occurring.

The stealing and misuse of prescription forms
could be minimised by the following precautions:

(a) do not leave unattended if called away from the consulting room or at reception desks; do not leave in a
car where they may be visible; when not in use, keep
in a locked drawer within the surgery and at home;

(b) draw a diagonal line across the blank part of the form
under the prescription;

(c) write the quantity in words and figures when prescribing drugs prone to abuse; this is obligatory for
controlled drugs (see Prescriptions, above);

(d) alterations are best avoided but if any are made they
should be clear and unambiguous; add initials against
altered items;

(e) if prescriptions are left for collection they should be
left in a safe place in a sealed envelope.

TRAVELLING ABROAD. Prescribed drugs listed in
schedules 4 and 5 to the Misuse of Drugs Regulations 1985 are not subject to import or export
licensing but doctors are advised that patients
travelling abroad may only carry 15 days' supply
of any schedule 2 or 3 prescribed controlled drug
without a licence. If especially high doses are
prescribed, however, or if prescriptions are for a
longer period, an import or export licence may
be required. Licences are issued by the Home

Secretary, Home Office, Drugs Branch, Queen
Anne's Gate, London SW1H 9AT, telephone
071-273 3806.

There is no standard application form but applications must be supported by a letter from a
doctor giving details of:

the patient's name and current address;

the quantities of drugs to be carried;

the strength and form in which the drugs will be
dispensed;

the dates of travel to and from the United Kingdom.

Ten days should be allowed for processing the
application.

Individual doctors who wish to take Controlled
Drugs abroad while accompanying patients, may
similarly be issued with licences. Licences are
not normally issued to doctors who wish to take
Controlled Drugs abroad solely in case a family
emergency should arise.

These import/export licences for named individuals do not have any legal status outside the
UK and are only issued to comply with the Misuse
of Drugs Act and facilitate passage through UK
Customs control. For clearance in the country to
be visited it would be necessary to approach that
country's embassy or High Commission in the
UK.

# The Misuse of Drugs Act, 1971

This Act was passed in 1971 to provide more
flexible and more comprehensive control over the
misuse of drugs of all kinds than was possible
under the earlier Dangerous Drugs Act. The Act
as amended prohibits certain activities in relation
to 'Controlled Drugs', in particular their manufacture, supply, and possession. The penalties
applicable to offences involving the different
drugs are graded broadly according to the *harm-
fulness attributable to a drug when it is misused*
and for this purpose the drugs are defined in the
following three classes:

Class A includes: alfentanil, cocaine, dextromoramide,
diamorphine (heroin), dipipanone, lysergide (LSD),
methadone, morphine, opium, pethidine, phencycli-
dine, and class B substances when prepared for injection

Class B includes: oral amphetamines, barbiturates, cannabis, cannabis resin, codeine, ethylmorphine, glutethimide, pentazocine, phenmetrazine, and
pholcodine

Class C includes: certain drugs related to the amphetamines such as benzphetamine and chlorphentermine,
buprenorphine, diethylpropion, mazindol, meprobamate, pemoline, pipradrol, and most benzodiazepines

The Misuse of Drugs Regulations 1985 define
the classes of person who are authorised to supply
and possess controlled drugs while acting in their
professional capacities and lay down the conditions under which these activities may be carried
out. In the regulations drugs are divided into
five schedules each specifying the requirements
governing such activities as import, export, production, supply, possession, prescribing, and
record keeping which apply to them.

Schedule 1 includes drugs such as cannabis and lysergide
which are not used medicinally. Possession and supply
are prohibited except in accordance with Home Office
authority.

**Schedule 2** includes drugs such as diamorphine (heroin), morphine, pethidine, quinalbarbitone, glutethimide, amphetamine, and cocaine and are subject to the full controlled drug requirements relating to prescriptions, safe custody, the need to keep registers, etc. (unless exempted in schedule 5).

**Schedule 3** includes the barbiturates (except quinalbarbitone, now schedule 2), buprenorphine, diethylpropion, mazindol, meprobamate, pentazocine, and phentermine. They are subject to the special prescription requirements (except for phenobarbitone, see p. 7) but not to the safe custody requirements (except for buprenorphine and diethylpropion) nor to the need to keep registers (although there are requirements for the retention of invoices for 2 years).

**Schedule 4** includes 34 benzodiazepines and pemoline which are subject to minimal control. In particular, controlled drug prescription requirements do not apply and they are not subject to safe custody.

**Schedule 5** includes those preparations which, because of their strength, are exempt from virtually all Controlled Drug requirements other than retention of invoices for two years.

## Notification of Addicts

The Misuse of Drugs (Notification of and Supply to Addicts) Regulations 1973 require that any doctor who attends a person who the doctor considers or has reasonable grounds to suspect, is addicted to any drug shall, within seven days of the attendance, furnish in writing particulars of that person to:

Chief Medical Officer,
Home Office, Drugs Branch,
Queen Anne's Gate, London SW1H 9AT.

The drugs commonly in use to which the Regulations apply are:

| | |
|---|---|
| Cocaine | Methadone |
| Dextromoramide | Morphine |
| Diamorphine | Opium |
| Dipipanone | Oxycodone |
| Hydrocodone | Pethidine |
| Hydromorphone | Phenazocine |
| Levorphanol | Piritramide |

*Note.* Dipipanone is only legally available as Diconal® Tablets. These have been much misused by opiate addicts in recent years; only medical practitioners with a special licence may now prescribe them for addicts to treat addiction. Doctors and others should be suspicious of young people who ask for them, especially as temporary residents.

Particulars[1] to be notified to the Chief Medical Officer are:

Name and address
Sex
Date of birth
National Health Service number
Date of attendance
Name of drugs of addiction
Whether patient injects any drug (whether or not notifiable)

Notification must be confirmed annually in writing if the patient is still being treated by the practitioner. Notified information is incorporated in an Index of Addicts which is maintained in the Home Office and information from this is available on a confidential basis to doctors; in fact, it is good medical practice to check all new cases of addiction or suspected addiction with the Index before prescribing or supplying controlled drugs since this is a safeguard against addicts obtaining supplies simultaneously from two or more doctors. Enquiries can be made either in writing to the Chief Medical Officer or, preferably, by telephoning 071-273 2213. To keep notified information confidential, such enquiries are normally answered by means of a return telephone call. The reply will come from lay staff who are not qualified to give guidance on the clinical handling of cases; a recorded telephone service is available for out-of-office hours.

The preceding paragraph applies only to medical practitioners in England, Scotland, and Wales. In Northern Ireland notification should be sent to:

Chief Medical Officer,
Department of Health and Social Services,
Dundonald House,
Belfast BT4 3SF.
Enquiries should also be made to that Department, telephone 0232 650111 extension 229.

## Prescribing of diamorphine (heroin), dipipanone, and cocaine for addicts

The Misuse of Drugs (Notification of and Supply to Addicts) Regulations 1973 also provide that only medical practitioners who hold a special licence issued by the Home Secretary may prescribe diamorphine, dipipanone (Diconal®), or cocaine for addicts; other practitioners must refer any addict who requires these drugs to a treatment centre. Whenever possible the addict will be introduced by a member of staff from the treatment centre to a pharmacist whose agreement has been obtained and whose pharmacy is conveniently sited for the patient. Prescriptions for weekly supplies will be sent to the pharmacy by post and will be dispensed on a daily basis as indicated by the doctor. If any alterations of the arrangements are requested by the addict, the portion of the prescription affected must be represcribed and not merely altered. *General practitioners and other doctors may still prescribe diamorphine, dipipanone, and cocaine for patients (including addicts) for relief of pain due to organic disease or injury without a special licence.*

For prescription-writing guidelines, see p. 7.

---

1. Only the particulars of which the doctor has knowledge need be notified immediately; the remainder may be notified at a later date. General practitioners and hospital doctors may now obtain notification forms from their Regional Health Authority Database Administrator; private doctors, police surgeons, and prison medical officers may obtain form HSA2/1(rev) for notification from their Family Health Services Authority (FHSA).

# Adverse Reactions to Drugs

Any drug may produce unwanted or unexpected adverse reactions. Detection and recording of these is of vital importance. Doctors are urged to help by reporting adverse reactions to:

CSM
Freepost
London SW8 5BR
(071-273 3000)

Yellow prepaid lettercards for reporting are available from the above address or by dialling 100 and asking for 'CSM Freefone'; also, forms are bound in this book (inside back cover).

A 24-hour Freefone service is now available to all parts of the United Kingdom, for doctors seeking advice and information on adverse reactions; it may be obtained by dialling 100 and asking for 'CSM Freefone'. Outside office hours a telephone-answering machine will take messages.

The following regional centres also collect data:

| | |
|---|---|
| CSM Mersey | CSM Northern |
| Freepost | Freepost 1085 |
| Liverpool L3 3AB | Newcastle upon Tyne |
| (051-236 4620 Extn 2126) | NE1 1BR |
| | (091-232 1525 Direct Line) |
| CSM Wales | CSM West Midlands |
| Freepost | Freepost |
| Cardiff CF4 1ZZ | Birmingham B15 1BR |
| (0222 759541 Direct Line) | (021-627 2179 Direct Line) |

Suspected adverse reactions to *any* therapeutic agent should be reported, including drugs, blood products, vaccines, X-ray contrast media, dental or surgical materials, intra-uterine devices, and contact lens fluids.

### ADROIT

Adverse Drug Reactions On-line Information Tracking (ADROIT) has now been introduced to facilitate the monitoring of adverse drug reactions.

NEWER DRUGS. These are indicated by the sign ▼. Doctors are asked to report *all* suspected reactions (i.e. any adverse or any unexpected event, however minor, which could conceivably be attributed to the drug). Reports should be made despite uncertainty about a causal relationship, irrespective of whether the reaction is well recognized, and even if other drugs have been given concurrently.

ESTABLISHED DRUGS. Doctors are asked to report *all* serious suspected reactions, including those that are fatal, life-threatening, disabling, incapacitating, or which result in or prolong hospitalisation; they should be reported even if the effect is well recognised.

Examples include anaphylaxis, blood disorders, endocrine disturbances, effects on fertility, haemorrhage from any site, renal impairment, jaundice, ophthalmic disorders, severe CNS effects, severe skin reactions, reactions in pregnant women, and any drug interactions. Reports of serious adverse reactions are required to enable risk/benefit ratios to be compared with other drugs of a similar class. For established drugs doctors are asked not to report well-known, relatively minor side-effects, such as dry mouth with tricyclic antidepressants, constipation with opioids, or nausea with digoxin.

### Special problems

*Delayed drug effects.* Some reactions (e.g. cancers, chloroquine retinopathy, and retroperitoneal fibrosis) may become manifest months or years after exposure. Any suspicion of such an association should be reported.

*The elderly.* Doctors are asked to be particularly alert to adverse reactions in the elderly.

*Congenital abnormalities.* When an infant is born with a congenital abnormality or there is a malformed aborted fetus doctors are asked to consider whether this might be an adverse reaction to a drug and to report all drugs (including self-medication) taken during pregnancy.

*Vaccines.* Doctors are asked to report all suspected reactions to both new and established vaccines. The balance between risks and benefits needs to be kept under continuous review.

### Prevention of adverse reactions

Adverse reactions may be prevented as follows:
1. Never use any drug unless there is a good indication. If the patient is pregnant do not use a drug unless the need for it is imperative.
2. It is very important to recognise allergy and idiosyncrasy as causes of adverse drug reactions. Ask if the patient had previous reactions.
3. Ask if the patient is already taking other drugs *including self-medication*; remember that interactions may occur.
4. Age and hepatic or renal disease may alter the metabolism or excretion of drugs, so that much smaller doses may need to be prescribed. Pharmacogenetic factors may also be responsible for variations in the rate of metabolism, notably of isoniazid and the tricyclic antidepressants.
5. Prescribe as few drugs as possible and give very clear instructions to the elderly or any patient likely to misunderstand complicated instructions.
6. When possible use a familiar drug. With a new drug particularly alert for adverse reactions or unexpected events.
7. If serious adverse reactions are liable to occur warn the patient.

---

**Defective Medicines**

During the manufacture or distribution of a medicine an error or accident may occur whereby the finished product does not conform to its specification. While such a defect may impair the therapeutic effect of the product and could adversely affect the health of a patient, it should **not** be confused with an Adverse Drug Reaction where the product conforms to its specification.

The Defect Medicines Report Centre operates a 24-hour service to assist with the investigation of problems arising from licensed medicinal products thought to be defective, and to co-ordinate any necessary protective action. Reports on suspect defective medicinal products should include the brand or the non-proprietary name, the name of the manufacturer or supplier, the strength and dosage form of the product, the product licence number, the batch number or numbers of the product, the nature of the defect, and an account of any action already taken in consequence. The Centre can be contacted at:

The Defect Medicines Report Centre
Medicines Control Agency
Room 1801, Market Towers
1 Nine Elms Lane
London SW8 5NQ
071-273 0574 (weekdays 8.30 am–5.30 pm)
*or* 071-210 5368 or 5371 (any other time)

times daily. Hyoscine hydrobromide may also be helpful, given sublingually at a dose of 300 micrograms 3 times daily as Kwells® (Nicholas) tablets, or as a continuous subcutaneous infusion of 0.6–2.4 mg over 24 hours using a syringe driver.

*Gastric distension pain* due to pressure on the stomach may be helped by a preparation incorporating an antacid with an antiflatulent (see section 1.1.1.1) and by domperidone 10 mg 3 times daily before meals.

HEADACHE. See under Raised Intracranial Pressure, below.

MUSCLE SPASM. The pain of muscle spasm can be helped by a muscle relaxant such as diazepam 5–10 mg daily or baclofen 5–10 mg 3 times daily.

NERVE PAIN. Pain due to *nerve compression* may be reduced by a corticosteroid such as dexamethasone 8 mg daily, which reduces oedema around the tumour, thus reducing compression.

Dysaesthetic or stabbing pain resulting from *nerve irritation* may be reduced by amitriptyline 25–75 mg at night, or by carbamazepine 200 mg 3 times daily.

## MISCELLANEOUS CONDITIONS

RAISED INTRACRANIAL PRESSURE. Headache due to raised intracranial pressure often responds to a high dose of a corticosteroid, such as dexamethasone 16 mg daily for 4 to 5 days, subsequently reduced to 4 to 6 mg daily if possible.

INTRACTABLE COUGH. Intractable cough may be relieved by moist inhalations or may require regular administration of an oral morphine hydrochloride solution in an initial dose of 5 mg every 4 hours. Methadone linctus should be avoided as it has a long duration of action and tends to accumulate.

DYSPNOEA. Dyspnoea may be relieved by regular oral morphine hydrochloride solution in carefully titrated doses, starting at 5 mg every 4 hours. Diazepam 5–10 mg daily may be helpful; a corticosteroid, such as dexamethasone 4 to 8 mg daily, may also be helpful if there is bronchospasm or partial obstruction.

EXCESSIVE RESPIRATORY SECRETION. Excessive respiratory secretion (death rattle) may be reduced by subcutaneous injection of hyoscine hydrobromide 400 to 600 micrograms every 4 to 8 hours.

RESTLESSNESS AND CONFUSION. Restlessness and confusion may require treatment with haloperidol 1 to 3 mg by mouth every 8 hours. Chlorpromazine 25–50 mg by mouth every 8 hours is an alternative, but causes more sedation. Methotrimeprazine is also used occasionally for restlessness.

HICCUP. Hiccup due to gastric distension may be helped by a preparation incorporating an antacid with an antiflatulent (see section 1.1.1.1). If this fails, metoclopramide 10 mg every 6 to 8 hours by mouth or by intramuscular injection can be added;

if this also fails, chlorpromazine 10 to 25 mg every 6 to 8 hours can be tried.

ANOREXIA. Anorexia may be helped by prednisolone 15 to 30 mg daily or dexamethasone 2 to 4 mg daily.

CONSTIPATION. Constipation is a very common cause of distress and should be prevented if possible by the regular administration of laxatives; a faecal softener with a peristaltic stimulant (e.g. co-danthramer), or lactulose solution with a senna preparation should be used (see sections 1.6.2 and 1.6.3).

FUNGATING GROWTH. Fungating growth may be treated by cleansing with a mixture of 1 part of 4% povidone-iodine skin cleanser solution and 4 parts of liquid paraffin. Oral administration of metronidazole (see section 5.1.11) may eradicate the anaerobic bacteria responsible for the odour of fungating tumours; topical application (see section 13.10.1.2) is also used but may increase the likelihood of resistance.

CAPILLARY BLEEDING. Capillary bleeding may be reduced by applying gauze soaked in adrenaline solution (1 in 1000).

DRY MOUTH. Dry mouth may be due to candidiasis which can be treated by nystatin oral suspension or pastilles, amphotericin lozenges, or miconazole oral gel after food; alternatively, fluconazole can be given by mouth (see section 5.2). Dry mouth can also be a side-effect of morphine.

PRURITUS. Pruritus, even when associated with obstructive jaundice, often responds to simple measures such as emollients. In the case of obstructive jaundice, further measures include administration of cholestyramine or an anabolic steroid, such as stanozolol 5–10 mg daily; antihistamines can be helpful (see section 3.4.1).

CONVULSIONS. Patients with cerebral tumours or uraemia may be susceptible to convulsions. Prophylactic treatment with phenytoin or carbamazepine (see section 4.8.1) should be considered. When oral medication is no longer possible, diazepam as suppositories 10–20 mg every 4 to 8 hours (see section 4.8.2), or phenobarbitone by injection 50–200 mg twice daily is continued as prophylaxis.

DYSPHAGIA. A corticosteroid such as dexamethasone 8 mg daily may help, temporarily, if there is an obstruction due to tumour. See also under Dry Mouth.

INSOMNIA. Patients with advanced cancer may not sleep because of discomfort, cramps, night sweats, joint stiffness, or fear. There should be appropriate treatment of these problems before hypnotics are used. Benzodiazepines, such as temazepam, may be useful (see section 4.1.1).

NAUSEA AND VOMITING. Nausea and vomiting are very common in patients with advanced cancer. The cause should be diagnosed before treatment with anti-emetics (see section 4.6) is started.

HYPERCALCAEMIA. See section 9.5.1.2.

# Prescribing for the Elderly

Old people, especially the very old, require special care and consideration from prescribers.

Elderly patients are apt to receive multiple drugs for their multiple diseases. This greatly increases the risk of drug interactions as well as other adverse reactions. Moreover, symptoms such as headache, sleeplessness, and lightheadedness which may be associated with social stress, as in widowhood, loneliness, and family dispersal can lead to further prescribing, especially of psychotropics. The use of drugs in such cases can at best be a poor substitute for effective social measures and at worst pose a serious threat from adverse reactions.

In very old subjects, manifestations of normal ageing may be mistaken for disease and lead to inappropriate prescribing. For example, drugs such as prochlorperazine are commonly misprescribed for giddiness due to age-related loss of postural stability. Not only is such treatment ineffective but the patient may experience serious side-effects such as drug-induced parkinsonism, postural hypotension, and mental confusion.

Self-medication with over-the-counter products or with drugs prescribed for a previous illness (or even for another person) may be an added complication. Discussion with relatives and a home visit may be needed to establish exactly what is being taken.

The ageing nervous system shows increased *susceptibility* to many commonly used drugs, such as opioid analgesics, benzodiazepines, and antiparkinsonian drugs, all of which must be used with caution.

PHARMACOKINETICS. While drug distribution and metabolism may be significantly altered, the most important effect of age is reduction in renal clearance, frequently aggravated by the effects of prostatism, nephrosclerosis, or chronic urinary tract infection. Many aged patients thus possess only limited reserves of renal function, excrete drugs slowly, and are highly susceptible to nephrotoxic drugs. Acute illness may lead to rapid reduction in renal clearance, especially if accompanied by dehydration. Hence, a patient stabilised on a drug with a narrow margin between the therapeutic and the toxic dose (e.g. digoxin) may rapidly develop adverse effects in the aftermath of a myocardial infarction or a respiratory tract infection.

The net result of pharmacokinetic changes is that tissue concentrations are commonly increased by over 50%, and aged and debilitated patients may show even larger changes.

COMMON ADVERSE REACTIONS. Adverse reactions often present in the elderly in a vague and non-specific fashion. *Mental confusion* is often the presenting symptom (caused by almost any of the commonly used drugs). Other common manifestations are *constipation* (with antimuscarinics and many tranquillisers) and postural *hypotension* and *falls* (with diuretics and many psychotropics).

Many hypnotics with long half-lives have serious hangover effects of drowsiness, unsteady gait, and even slurred speech and confusion. Those with short half-lives should be used but they too can present problems (see section 4.1.1). Short courses of hypnotics are occasionally useful for helping a patient through an acute illness or some other crisis but every effort must be made to avoid dependence.

Diuretics are overprescribed in old age and should not be used on a long-term basis to treat simple gravitational oedema which will usually respond to increased movement, raising the legs, and support stockings. A few days of diuretic treatment may speed the clearing of the oedema but it should rarely need continued drug therapy.

Other drugs which commonly cause adverse reactions are antiparkinsonian drugs, antihypertensives, psychotropics, and digoxin; the usual maintenance dose of digoxin in very old patients is 125 micrograms daily (62.5 micrograms is often inadequate, and toxicity is common in those given 250 micrograms).

Drug-induced blood disorders are much more common in the elderly. Therefore drugs with a tendency to cause bone marrow depression (e.g. co-trimoxazole, mianserin) should be avoided unless there is no acceptable alternative.

Bleeding associated with aspirin and other NSAIDs is more common in the elderly, and the outcome tends to be more serious.

The elderly generally require a lower maintenance dose of warfarin than younger adults; once again, the outcome of bleeding tends to be more serious.

GUIDELINES. First one must always pose the question of whether a drug is indicated at all.

It is a sensible policy to prescribe from a limited range of drugs and to be thoroughly familiar with their effects in the elderly.

Dosage should generally be substantially lower than for younger patients and it is common to start with about 50% of the adult dose. Some drugs (e.g. chlorpropamide) should be avoided altogether.

Review repeat prescriptions regularly. It may be possible to stop the drug (e.g. digoxin can often be withdrawn) or it may be necessary to reduce the dose to match diminishing renal function.

Simplify regimens. Elderly patients cannot normally cope with more than three different drugs and, ideally, these should not be given more than twice daily. In particular, regimens which call for a confusing array of dosage intervals should be avoided.

Write full instructions on every prescription (*including* repeat prescriptions) so that containers can be properly labelled with full directions. Avoid imprecisions like 'as directed'. Child-resistant containers may be unsuitable.

Instruct patients what to do when drugs run out, and also how to dispose of any that are no longer necessary.

If these guidelines are followed most elderly people will cope adequately with their own medicines. If not then it is essential to enrol the help of a third party, usually a relative but sometimes a home help, neighbour, or a sheltered-housing warden.

# Emergency Treatment of Poisoning

| Poisons Information Services | |
|---|---|
| Belfast | 0232 240503 |
| Birmingham | 021-554 3801 |
| Cardiff | 0222 709901 |
| Dublin | 0001 379964 |
| | *or* 0001 379966 |
| Edinburgh | 031-229 2477 |
| | 031-228 2441 |
| | (Viewdata) |
| Leeds | 0532 430715 |
| | *or* 0532 432799 |
| London | 071-635 9191 |
| | *or* 071-955 5095 |
| Newcastle | 091-232 5131 |

*Note.* Some of these centres also advise on laboratory analytical services which may be of help in the diagnosis and management of a small number of cases.

**CONSULT POISONS INFORMATION CENTRES DAY AND NIGHT**

These notes deal with the initial management of acute poisoning in the home; brief mention only is given of hospital-based treatment. The notes are only guidelines and it is strongly recommended that **poisons information services** (see previous page) be consulted in cases where there is doubt about the degree of risk or about appropriate management.

HOSPITAL ADMISSION. All patients who show features of poisoning should generally be admitted to hospital. Patients who have taken poisons with delayed actions should also be admitted, even if they appear well; delayed-action poisons include aspirin, iron, paracetamol, tricyclic antidepressants, co-phenotrope (diphenoxylate with atropine, *Lomotil®*), and paraquat, also modified-release capsules or tablets. A note should be sent of what is known and what treatment has been given.

It is often impossible to establish with certainty the identity of the poison and the size of the dose. Fortunately this is not usually important because only a few poisons (such as opioids, paracetamol, and iron) have specific antidotes and few patients require active removal of the poison. Most patients must be treated symptomatically. Nevertheless, knowledge of the type of poisoning does help in anticipating the course of events. Patients' reports may be of little help, as they may be confused or may only be able to say that they have taken an undefined amount, possibly of mixed drugs. Parents may think a child has taken something which could be poisonous and may exaggerate or underplay the risks out of anxiety or guilt. Sometimes symptoms are due to an illness such as appendicitis. Accidents can arise from a number of domestic and industrial products (the contents of which are not generally known).

> The **poisons information services** (see p. 15) will provide advice on all aspects of poisoning day and night.

# General care

## RESPIRATION

Respiration is often impaired in unconscious patients. An obstructed airway requires immediate attention. Pull the tongue forward, remove dentures and oral secretions, hold the jaw forward, insert an oropharyngeal airway if one is available, and turn the patient semiprone. The risk of inhaling vomit is minimised with the patient positioned semiprone and head down.

Most poisons that impair consciousness also depress respiration. Assisted ventilation by mouth-to-mouth or Ambu bag inflation may be needed. Oxygen is not a substitute for adequate ventilation, though it should be given in the highest concentration possible in poisoning with carbon monoxide and irritant gases.

**Respiratory stimulants** do not help and are **potentially dangerous**.

## BLOOD PRESSURE

Hypotension is common in severe poisoning with central nervous system depressants. A systolic blood pressure of less than 70 mmHg may lead to irreversible brain damage or renal tubular necrosis. The patient should be carried head downwards on a stretcher and nursed in this position in the ambulance. Oxygen should be given to correct hypoxia and an intravenous infusion should be set up if at all practicable. Vasopressor drugs should be **not** be used.

Fluid depletion without hypotension is common after prolonged coma and after aspirin poisoning due to vomiting, sweating, and hyperpnoea.

## HEART

Cardiac conduction defects and arrhythmias may occur in acute poisoning, notably with tricyclic antidepressants. Arrhythmias often respond to correction of underlying hypoxia or acidosis. Ventricular arrhythmias that have been confirmed by emergency ECG and which are causing serious hypotension may require treatment with lignocaine 50–100 mg by slow intravenous injection. Supraventricular arrhythmias are seldom life-threatening and drug treatment is best withheld until the patient reaches hospital.

## BODY TEMPERATURE

Hypothermia may develop in patients of any age who have been deeply unconscious for some hours particularly following overdose with barbiturates or phenothiazines. It may be missed unless temperature is measured rectally using a low-reading rectal thermometer. It is best treated by wrapping the patient in blankets to conserve body heat. Hot-water bottles are of little value and may cause burns.

## CONVULSIONS

Single short-lived convulsions do not require treatment. Diazepam, up to 10 mg by slow intravenous injection, preferably in emulsion form, should be given if convulsions are protracted or recur frequently; it should not be given intramuscularly.

> CONSULT POISONS INFORMATION CENTRES DAY AND NIGHT—see p. 15

# Removal and elimination

## REMOVAL FROM THE STOMACH

The dangers of attempting to empty the stomach have to be balanced against the toxicity of the ingested poison, as assessed by the quantity ingested, the inherent toxicity of the poison, and the time since ingestion. Gastric emptying is clearly unnecessary if the risk of toxicity is small or if the patient presents too late.

Emptying the stomach by **gastric lavage** or **emesis** is of doubtful value if attempted more than 4 hours after ingestion. However, a worthwhile recovery of salicylates can be achieved up to 24 hours after ingestion and of tricyclic antidepressants (which delay gastric emptying) up to 8 hours after ingestion. The chief danger of gastric aspiration and lavage is inhalation of stomach contents, and it should **not** be attempted in drowsy or comatose patients unless there is a good enough cough reflex or the airway can be protected by a cuffed endotracheal tube. Stomach tubes should **not** be passed after corrosive poisoning.

Petroleum products are more dangerous in the lungs than in the stomach and therefore removal from the stomach is **not** advised because of the risk of inhalation.

On balance gastric lavage is seldom practicable or desirable before the patient reaches hospital.

Emesis induced by using **ipecacuanha** (Paediatric Ipecacuanha Emetic Mixture BP) is favoured in children and is also effective in adults. It may be given safely in the home providing that the patient is fully conscious and that the poison ingested is neither a corrosive nor a petroleum distillate.

Salt solutions, copper sulphate, apomorphine, and mustard are dangerous and should **not** be used.

## IPECACUANHA

*Indications:* induction of emesis in selected patients, see notes above
*Cautions:* avoid in poisoning with corrosive compounds or petroleum products (risk of aspiration); shock; history of convulsions; cardiovascular disease
*Side-effects:* excessive vomiting and mucosal damage; cardiac effects if absorbed
*Dose:* see under preparation below

**Ipecacuanha Emetic Mixture, Paediatric** (BP)
Paediatric Ipecacuanha Emetic
Note. Paediatric Ipecacuanha Emetic Mixture is equivalent in strength to Ipecac Syrup USP
*Mixture,* ipecacuanha liquid extract 0.7 mL, hydrochloric acid 0.025 mL, glycerol 1 mL, syrup to 10 mL
*Dose:* ADULT 30 mL; CHILD 6–18 months 10 mL, older children 15 mL; the dose is followed by a tumblerful of water and repeated after 20 minutes if necessary

## PREVENTION OF ABSORPTION

Given by mouth, **activated charcoal** can bind many poisons in the stomach, thereby *reducing their absorption*, but it is only effective if given within 1–2 hours of ingestion. It is safe and is particularly useful for the prevention of absorption of poisons which are toxic in small amounts, e.g. antidepressants.

For the use of charcoal in active elimination techniques, see below.

**Carbomix®** (Penn)
*Powder,* activated charcoal. Net price 50-g bottle = £10.93
*Dose:* reduction of absorption, 50 g; CHILD, 25 g (50 g in severe poisoning)
Active elimination, see below
**Medicoal®** (Torbet)
*Granules,* effervescent, activated charcoal 5 g/sachet. Net price 5-sachet pack = £3.28; 30-sachet pack = £16.50
*Caution:* povidone (present as suspending agent) may cause pneumonitis after aspiration
*Dose:* Dose excluded because product not recommended

## ACTIVE ELIMINATION TECHNIQUES

Repeated doses of **activated charcoal** by mouth *enhance the elimination* of some drugs after they have been absorbed; repeated doses are given after overdosage with:

| | |
|---|---|
| Aspirin | Phenobarbitone |
| Carbamazepine | and other barbiturates |
| Dapsone | Phenytoin |
| Digitoxin | Quinine |
| Digoxin | Theophylline |

The usual adult dose of activated charcoal is 50 g initially then 25 g every 4 hours.

Other techniques intended to enhance the elimination of poisons after absorption are only practicable in hospital and are only suitable for a small number of severely poisoned patients. Moreover, they only apply to a limited number of poisons. Examples include:
Forced alkaline diuresis for salicylates and phenobarbitone
Haemodialysis for salicylates, phenobarbitone, methyl alcohol (methanol), ethylene glycol, and lithium
Haemoperfusion for medium- and short-acting barbiturates, chloral hydrate, meprobamate, and theophylline.

# Specific drugs

## ALCOHOL

Acute intoxication with alcohol (ethanol) is common in adults but also occurs in children. The features include ataxia, dysarthria, nystagmus, and drowsiness, which may progress to coma, with hypotension and acidosis. Aspiration of vomit is a special hazard and hypoglycaemia may occur in children and some adults. Patients are managed supportively with particular attention to maintaining a clear airway and measures to reduce the risk of aspiration of gastric contents. The blood glucose is measured and glucose given if indicated.

## ANALGESICS (NON-OPIOID)

ASPIRIN. Absorption of aspirin and other salicylates may be delayed, especially if enteric-coated tablets have been taken; blood concentrations taken within the first 6 hours may therefore be misleadingly low.

The chief features of poisoning are hyperventilation, tinnitus, deafness, vasodilatation, and sweating. Coma is uncommon but indicates very severe poisoning. The associated acid-base disturbances are complex.

Gastric emptying is carried out in all cases; a worthwhile recovery of salicylates can be achieved up to 24 hours after ingestion.

Treatment must be in hospital where plasma salicylate, pH, and electrolytes can be measured. Fluid losses are replaced and forced alkaline diuresis is considered when the plasma-salicylate concentration is greater than

500 mg/litre (3.6 mmol/litre) in adults or
300 mg/litre (2.2 mmol/litre) in children.

NSAIDs. Mefenamic acid is the most significant member of this group encountered in overdosage. Convulsions are the only important feature of toxicity and are treated with diazepam.

Ibuprofen may cause nausea, vomiting, and tinnitus, but more serious toxicity is very uncommon. Gastric emptying is indicated if more than 10 tablets have been ingested within the preceding 4 hours, followed by symptomatic measures.

PARACETAMOL. As little as 10–15 g (20–30 tablets) of paracetamol may cause severe hepatocellular necrosis and, less frequently, renal tubular necrosis. Nausea and vomiting, the only early features of poisoning, usually settle within 24 hours. Persistence beyond this time, often associated with the onset of right subcostal pain and tenderness, usually indicates development of hepatic necrosis. Liver damage is maximal 3–4 days after ingestion and may lead to encephalopathy, haemorrhage, hypoglycaemia, cerebral oedema, and death.

Therefore, despite a lack of significant early symptoms, patients who have taken an overdose of paracetamol should be transferred to hospital urgently.

Gastric emptying is carried out if the overdose was taken within 4 hours of admission.

Antidotes such as **acetylcysteine** and **methionine** protect the liver if given within 10–12 hours of ingestion; acetylcysteine may also be effective up to and beyond 15 hours but expert advice is **essential.**

Patients at risk of liver damage and therefore requiring treatment can be identified from a single measurement of the plasma-paracetamol concentration, related to the time from ingestion, provided this time interval is not less than 4 hours; earlier samples may be misleading. The concentration is compared against a reference line joining plots of 200 mg/litre (1.32 mmol/litre) at 4 hours and 30 mg/litre (0.2 mmol/litre) at 15 hours, on a semi-logarithmic graph. Those whose concentrations are above that line are treated either with acetylcysteine intravenously or with methionine by mouth. Patients on enzyme-inducing drugs (e.g. carbamazepine, phenobarbitone, phenytoin, rifampicin, and alcohol) may develop toxicity at **lower** plasma-paracetamol concentrations; they should be treated with acetylcysteine if their plasma-paracetamol concentrations are 50% or more of the standard reference line.

In remote areas, emesis should be induced if the patient presents within 4 hours of the overdose.

Methionine (2.5 g) should be given by mouth once vomiting has occurred; it is seldom practicable to give acetylcysteine outside hospital. Once the patient reaches hospital the need to continue treatment with the antidote will be assessed from the plasma-paracetamol concentration (related to the time from ingestion).

See also Co-proxamol, under Analgesics (opioid).

## ACETYLCYSTEINE
*Indications:* paracetamol overdosage (see notes above)
*Cautions:* asthma
*Side-effects:* rashes, anaphylaxis
*Dose: by intravenous infusion,* in glucose intravenous infusion 5%, initially 150 mg/kg in 200 mL over 15 minutes, followed by 50 mg/kg in 500 mL over 4 hours, then 100 mg/kg in 1000 mL over 16 hours

PoM **Parvolex**® (DF)
*Injection,* acetylcysteine 200 mg/mL. Net price course of 12 amps of 10 mL = £31.75

## METHIONINE
*Indications:* paracetamol overdosage, see notes above
*Dose: by mouth,* 2.5 g initially, followed by 3 further doses of 2.5 g every 4 hours

**Methionine Tablets** (Evans), DL-methionine 250 mg. Net price course of 40 tabs = £7.52

## ANALGESICS (OPIOID)

Opioids (narcotic analgesics) cause varying degrees of coma, respiratory depression, and pinpoint pupils. The specific antidote **naloxone** is indicated if there is coma or bradypnoea. Since naloxone is short-acting repeated injections are necessary according to the respiratory rate and depth of coma. Alternatively, it may be given by continuous intravenous infusion, the rate of administration being adjusted according to response.

CO-PROXAMOL. Combinations of dextropropoxyphene and paracetamol (co-proxamol) are frequently taken in overdosage. The initial features are those of acute opioid overdosage with coma, respiratory depression, and pinpoint pupils. Patients may die of acute cardiovascular collapse before reaching hospital (particularly if alcohol has also been consumed) unless adequately resuscitated or given **naloxone** as antidote to the dextropropoxyphene. Paracetamol hepatotoxicity may develop later and should be anticipated and treated as indicated above.

## NALOXONE HYDROCHLORIDE
*Indications:* overdosage with opioids; for postoperative respiratory depression, see section 15.1.7
*Cautions:* physical dependence on opioids; cardiac irritability; naloxone is short-acting, see notes above
*Dose: by intravenous injection,* 0.8–2 mg repeated at intervals of 2–3 minutes to a max. of 10 mg if respiratory function does not improve (then question diagnosis); CHILD 10 micrograms/kg; subsequent dose of 100 micrograms/kg if no response

*By subcutaneous or intramuscular injection*, as intravenous injection but only if intravenous route not feasible (onset of action slower)
*By continuous intravenous infusion*, 2 mg diluted in 500 mL intravenous infusion solution at a rate adjusted according to the response

PoM **Naloxone** (Non-proprietary)
*Injection,* naloxone hydrochloride 400 micrograms/ mL. Net price 1-mL amp = £4.92
PoM **Min-I-Jet®  Naloxone** (IMS)
*Injection,* naloxone hydrochloride 400 micrograms/ mL. Net price 1-mL disposable syringe = £5.17; 2-mL disposable syringe = £9.66
PoM **Narcan®** (Du Pont)
*Injection,* naloxone hydrochloride 400 micrograms/ mL, net price 1-mL amp = £4.92, 1-mL disposable syringe = £5.44; 1 mg/mL, 2-mL amp = £22.00
**Neonatal preparations** —see section 15.1.7

## ANTIDEPRESSANTS

Tricyclic and related antidepressants cause dry mouth, coma of varying degree, hypotension, hypothermia, hyperreflexia, extensor plantar responses, convulsions, respiratory failure, cardiac conduction defects, and arrhythmias. Dilated pupils and urinary retention also occur. Metabolic acidosis may complicate severe poisoning; delirium with confusion, agitation, and visual and auditory hallucinations, is common during recovery.

Symptomatic treatment and activated charcoal by mouth may reasonably be given in the home before transfer but hospital admission is strongly advised, and supportive measures to ensure a patent airway and adequate ventilation during transfer are mandatory. Intravenous diazepam may be required for control of convulsions (preferably in emulsion form). Although arrhythmias are worrying, the use of anti-arrhythmic drugs is best avoided. Diazepam given by mouth is usually adequate to sedate delirious patients but large doses may be required.

## HYPNOTICS AND ANXIOLYTICS

BARBITURATES. These cause drowsiness, coma, respiratory depression, hypotension, and hypothermia. The duration and depth of cerebral depression vary greatly with the drug, the dose, and the tolerance of the patient. The severity of poisoning is often greater with a large dose of barbiturate hypnotics than with the longer-acting phenobarbitone. The majority of patients survive with supportive measures alone. Forced alkaline diuresis may be considered in severe phenobarbitone poisoning. Charcoal haemoperfusion is the treatment of choice for the small minority of patients with very severe barbiturate poisoning who fail to improve, or who deteriorate despite good supportive care.

BENZODIAZEPINES. Benzodiazepines taken alone cause drowsiness, ataxia, dysarthria, and occasionally minor and short-lived depression of consciousness. They potentiate the effects of other central nervous system depressants taken concomitantly. Flumazenil, a benzodiazepine

antagonist, may be used in the *differential diagnosis* of unclear cases of multiple drug overdose but expert advice is **essential**.

## IRON SALTS

Iron poisoning is commonest in childhood and is usually accidental. The symptoms are nausea, vomiting, abdominal pain, diarrhoea, haematemesis, and rectal bleeding. Hypotension, coma, and hepatocellular necrosis occur later. Mortality is reduced with intensive and specific therapy with **desferrioxamine**, which chelates iron. The stomach should be emptied at once, preferably by inducing vomiting as this is quickest. Gastric lavage in hospital should follow as soon as possible, leaving a solution of 5–10 g of desferrioxamine mesylate in 50–100 mL water in the stomach. The serum-iron concentration is measured as an emergency and parenteral desferrioxamine given to chelate absorbed iron in excess of the expected iron binding capacity.

### DESFERRIOXAMINE MESYLATE
*Indications:* removal of iron from the body in poisoning; for use in chronic iron overload, see section 9.1.3
*Cautions:* avoid prochlorperazine
*Side-effects:* pain at site of intramuscular injection, anaphylactic reactions, and hypotension when given too rapidly by intravenous injection
*Dose: by mouth* after gastric lavage, see notes above
*By intramuscular injection,* 1–2 g in 10–20 mL of water for injections every 3–12 hours; max. 6 g in 24 hours
*By continuous intravenous infusion,* up to 15 mg/kg/hour; max. 80 mg/kg in 24 hours

PoM **Desferal®** (Ciba)
*Injection,* powder for reconstitution, desferrioxamine mesylate. Net price 500-mg vial = £2.53

## LITHIUM

Most cases of lithium intoxication occur as a complication of long-term therapy and are caused by reduced excretion of the drug due to a variety of factors including dehydration, deterioration of renal function, infections, and co-administration of diuretics (or other drugs that interact). Acute deliberate overdoses may also occur with delayed onset of symptoms (12 hours or more) due to slow entry of lithium into the tissues and continuing absorption from modified-release formulations.

The early clinical features are non-specific and may include apathy and restlessness which could be confused with mental changes due to the patient's depressive illness. Vomiting, diarrhoea, ataxia, weakness, dysarthria, muscle twitching, and tremor may follow. Severe poisoning is associated with convulsions, coma, renal failure, electrolyte imbalance, dehydration, and hypotension.

Therapeutic lithium concentrations are within the range of 0.4–1.0 mmol/litre; concentrations in excess of 2.0 mmol/litre are usually associated with serious toxicity and such cases may need treatment with forced diuresis or dialysis (if there is renal failure). In acute overdosage much higher serum concentrations may be present without features of toxicity and measures to increase urine production are usually all that are necessary. Otherwise treatment is supportive with special regard to electrolyte balance, renal function, and control of convulsions.

## PHENOTHIAZINES AND RELATED DRUGS

Phenothiazines cause less depression of consciousness and respiration than other sedatives. Hypotension, hypothermia, sinus tachycardia, and arrhythmias (particularly with thioridazine) may complicate poisoning. Dystonic reactions can occur with therapeutic doses, (particularly with prochlorperazine and trifluoperazine) and convulsions may occur in severe cases. Drugs to control arrhythmias and convulsions may be needed. Dystonic reactions are rapidly abolished by injection of drugs such as benztropine or procyclidine (see section 4.9.2).

## STIMULANTS

AMPHETAMINES. These cause wakefulness, excessive activity, paranoia, hallucinations, and hypertension followed by exhaustion, convulsions, hyperthermia, and coma. The early stages can be controlled by chlorpromazine and, if necessary, beta-blockers. Later, tepid sponging, anticonvulsants, and artificial respiration may be needed. Amphetamine excretion can be increased by forced acid diuresis but this is seldom necessary.

COCAINE. Cocaine can be smoked, sniffed, or injected. It stimulates the central nervous system causing agitation, dilated pupils, tachycardia, hypertension, hallucinations, hypertonia, and hyperreflexia. Convulsions, coma and metabolic acidosis may develop in the worst cases. Sedation, with intravenous diazepam, may be all that is necessary but intravenous propranolol may be indicated for severe intoxication.

## THEOPHYLLINE

Theophylline and related drugs are often prescribed as modified-release formulations and toxicity may therefore be delayed. They cause vomiting (which may be severe and intractable), agitation, restlessness, dilated pupils, and sinus tachycardia. More serious effects are haematemesis, convulsions, and supraventricular and ventricular arrhythmias. Profound hypokalaemia may develop rapidly.

The stomach should be emptied as early as possible. Elimination of theophylline may be enhanced by repeated doses of activated charcoal by mouth (see also under Active Elimination Techniques). Hypokalaemia is corrected by intravenous infusion of potassium chloride and may be so severe as to require 60 mmol/hour (high doses under ECG monitoring). Convulsions should be controlled by intravenous administration of diazepam (emulsion preferred). Sedation with chlor-

promazine or diazepam may be necessary in agitated patients. Providing the patient is **not** an asthmatic, extreme tachycardia, hypokalaemia, and hyperglycaemia may be reversed by intravenous administration of propranolol (see section 2.4).

# Other poisons

CONSULT POISONS INFORMATION CENTRES
DAY AND NIGHT—see p. 15

## CYANIDES

Cyanide antidotes include dicobalt edetate, given alone, and sodium nitrite, followed by sodium thiosulphate. These antidotes are held for emergency use in hospitals as well as in centres where cyanide poisoning is a risk such as factories and laboratories.

### DICOBALT EDETATE

*Indications:* acute poisoning with cyanides
*Cautions:* owing to toxicity to be used only when patient tending to lose, or has lost, consciousness; not to be used as a precautionary measure
*Side-effects:* transient hypotension, tachycardia, and vomiting
*Dose:* by intravenous injection, 300 mg (20 mL) over 1 minute, followed by 50 mL of glucose intravenous infusion 50%, both repeated once or twice if necessary

PoM **Kelocyanor®** (Lipha)
*Injection,* dicobalt edetate 300 mg/20 mL. Net price 20-mL amp = £2.66

### SODIUM NITRITE

*Indications:* poisoning with cyanides in conjunction with sodium thiosulphate
*Side-effects:* flushing and headache due to vasodilatation

PoM **Sodium Nitrite Injection**
*Injection,* sodium nitrite 3% (30 mg/mL) in water for injections
*Dose:* 10 mL by intravenous injection over 3 minutes, followed by 25 mL of sodium thiosulphate injection 50%, by intravenous injection over 10 minutes
Available from Martindale, Penn, etc. (special order)

### SODIUM THIOSULPHATE

*Indications:* poisoning with cyanides in conjunction with sodium nitrite

PoM **Sodium Thiosulphate Injection**
*Injection,* sodium thiosulphate 50% (500 mg/mL) in water for injections
*Dose:* see above under Sodium Nitrite Injection
Available from Martindale, Penn, etc. (special order)

## HEAVY METALS

Heavy metal antidotes include dimercaprol, penicillamine, and sodium calciumedetate.

### DIMERCAPROL
(BAL)
*Indications:* poisoning by antimony, arsenic, bismuth, gold, mercury, thallium; adjunct (with sodium calciumedetate) in lead poisoning
*Cautions:* hypertension
*Contra-indications:* not indicated for iron or cadmium poisoning; severe hepatic impairment
*Side-effects:* hypertension, tachycardia, malaise, nausea, vomiting, lachrymation, sweating, burning sensation (mouth and eyes), constriction of throat and chest, headache, muscle spasm, abdominal pain, tingling of extremities; pyrexia in children; pain on injection
*Dose: by intramuscular injection*, 2.5–3 mg/kg every 4 hours for 2 days, 2–4 times on the 3rd day, then 1–2 times daily for 10 days or until recovery

PoM **Dimercaprol Injection** (Boots), dimercaprol 50 mg/mL. Net price 2-mL amp = 70p

### PENICILLAMINE
*Indications:* poisoning by certain toxic metal ions, particularly by copper and lead
*Cautions; Contra-indications; Side-effects:* see section 10.1.3
*Dose:* 1–2 g daily in divided doses before food until urinary lead is stabilised at less than 500 micrograms/day; CHILD 20 mg/kg daily

**Preparations**
See section 10.1.3

### SODIUM CALCIUMEDETATE
*Indications:* poisoning by heavy metals, especially lead
*Cautions:* renal impairment
*Side-effects:* nausea, cramp; in overdosage renal damage
*Dose: by intravenous infusion*, adults and children, up to 40 mg/kg twice daily in sodium chloride intravenous infusion 0.9% or glucose intravenous infusion 5% for up to 5 days, repeated if necessary after 48 hours

PoM **Ledclair**® (Sinclair)
*Injection*, sodium calciumedetate 200 mg/mL. Net price 5-mL amp = £3.43

## NOXIOUS GASES

CARBON MONOXIDE. Carbon monoxide poisoning is now usually due to inhalation of smoke, car exhaust, or fumes caused by blocked flues or incomplete combustion of fuel gases in confined spaces. Its toxic effects are entirely due to hypoxia.

Immediate treatment is essential. The person should be removed into the fresh air, the airway cleared, and **oxygen** 100% administered as soon as available. Artificial respiration should be given as necessary and continued until adequate spontaneous breathing starts, or stopped only after persistent and efficient treatment of cardiac arrest

has failed. Admission to hospital is desirable because complications may arise after a delay of hours or days. Cerebral oedema should be anticipated in severe poisoning and is treated with an intravenous infusion of mannitol (see section 2.2.5). Referral for hyperbaric oxygen treatment should be discussed with the poisons information services if the victim is or has been unconscious or has a blood carboxyhaemoglobin concentration of more than 40%.

SULPHUR DIOXIDE, CHLORINE, PHOSGENE, AMMONIA. The immediate effect of all except phosgene is coughing and choking. Pulmonary oedema, with severe breathlessness and cyanosis may develop suddenly up to 36 hours after exposure. Death may occur. Patients are kept under observation and those who develop pulmonary oedema are given corticosteroids and oxygen. Assisted ventilation may be necessary in the most serious cases.

## PESTICIDES

PARAQUAT. Concentrated liquid paraquat preparations (e.g. Gramoxone®), available to farmers and horticulturists, contain 10–20% paraquat and are extremely toxic. Granular preparations, for garden use, contain only 2.5% paraquat and have caused few deaths.

Paraquat has local and systemic effects. Splashes in the eyes irritate and ulcerate the cornea and conjunctiva. Copious washing of the eye and instillation of antibacterial eye-drops, should aid healing but it may be a long process. Skin irritation, blistering, and ulceration can occur from prolonged contact both with the concentrated and dilute forms. Inhalation of spray, mist, or dust containing paraquat may cause nose bleeding and sore throat but not systemic toxicity.

Ingestion of concentrated paraquat solutions is followed by nausea, vomiting, and diarrhoea. Painful ulceration of the tongue, lips, and fauces may appear after 36 to 48 hours together with renal failure. Some days later there may be dyspnoea with pulmonary fibrosis due to proliferative alveolitis and bronchiolitis.

Treatment should be started immediately. The single most useful measure is oral administration of either **Fuller's earth** or **bentonite** to adsorb paraquat and reduce absorption. The stomach is then emptied by careful gastric lavage and 300 mL of a suspension containing 30 g of Fuller's earth and 15 g of magnesium sulphate should be left in the stomach. Further quantities of 300 mL of a 30% Fuller's earth suspension are given after 2 and after 4 hours; magnesium sulphate or mannitol is given as required to produce diarrhoea and empty the gut. Some authorities prefer regimens employing 15% Fuller's earth suspensions. Intravenous fluids and analgesics are given as necessary. Oxygen therapy should be avoided if possible since this may exacerbate damage to the lungs. Measures to enhance elimination of absorbed paraquat are probably valueless but should be discussed with the poisons information services who will also give guidance on predicting the likely outcome from plasma concentrations. Paraquat absorption can be confirmed by a simple qualitative urine test.

ORGANOPHOSPHORUS INSECTICIDES. Organophosphorus insecticides are usually supplied as powders or dissolved in organic solvents. All are absorbed through the bronchi and intact skin as well as through the gut and inhibit cholinesterase activity thereby prolonging and intensifying the effects of acetylcholine. Toxicity between different compounds varies considerably, and onset may be delayed after skin exposure.

Anxiety, restlessness, dizziness, headache, miosis, nausea, hypersalivation, vomiting, abdominal colic, diarrhoea, bradycardia, and sweating are common. Muscle weakness and fasciculation may develop and progress to generalised flaccid paralysis including the ocular and respiratory muscles. Convulsions, coma, pulmonary oedema with copious bronchial secretions, hypoxia, and arrhythmias occur in severe cases. Hyperglycaemia and glycosuria without ketonuria may also be present.

Further absorption should be prevented by emptying the stomach, removing the patient to fresh air, or removing soiled clothing and washing contaminated skin. In severe poisoning it is vital to ensure a clear airway, frequent removal of bronchial secretions, and adequate ventilation and oxygenation. **Atropine** will reverse the muscarinic effects of acetylcholine and is given in a dose of 2 mg as atropine sulphate injection (intramuscularly or intravenously according to the severity of poisoning) every 20 to 30 minutes until the skin becomes flushed and dry, the pupils dilate, and tachycardia develops.

**Pralidoxime mesylate** (P2S), a cholinesterase reactivator, is indicated, as an adjunct to atropine, in moderate or severe poisoning but is only effective if given within 24 hours. It may be obtained from designated centres, the names of which are held by the poisons information services (see p. 15). A dose of 1 g by intramuscular injection or, diluted with 10–15 mL water for injections, by slow intravenous injection should produce improvement in muscle power within 30 minutes but repeated doses or, in severe cases, an intravenous infusion of up to 500 mg/hour may be required.

## PRALIDOXIME MESYLATE

*Indications:* adjunct to atropine in the treatment of organophosphorus poisoning
*Cautions:* renal impairment, myasthenia gravis
*Contra-indications:* poisoning due to carbamates and to organophosphorus compounds without anticholinesterase activity
*Side-effects:* drowsiness, dizziness, disturbances of vision, nausea, tachycardia, headache, hyperventilation, and muscular weakness
*Dose: by intramuscular injection,* 1 g initially followed by 1–2 further doses if necessary; in very severe poisoning the initial dose can be doubled; usual max. 12 g in 24 hours
*By slow intravenous injection* (diluted to 10–15 mL with water for injections and given over 5–10 minutes) 1 g initially followed by 1–2 further doses if necessary; in very severe poisoning the initial

dose can be doubled; usual max. 12 g in 24 hours
CHILD 20–60 mg/kg as required depending on severity of poisoning and response

**PoM Pralidoxime Mesylate Injection,** pralidoxime mesylate 200 mg/mL. Available as 5-mL amps (from designated centres)

## SNAKE AND INSECT BITES

SNAKE BITE. Acute poisoning due to venomous snakes is rare in the United Kingdom and the only indigenous venomous snake is the adder. The bite may cause local and systemic effects. Local effects include pain, swelling, and 'tender enlargement of regional lymph nodes. Systemic effects include early transient hypotension with syncope, angioedema, abdominal colic, diarrhoea, and vomiting, with later persistent or recurrent hypotension, ECG abnormalities, spontaneous systemic bleeding, coagulopathy, acute respiratory distress syndrome, and acute renal failure. There is a small risk of fatal envenoming especially in children and the elderly.

Indications for antivenom treatment include systemic envenoming, especially hypotension (see above), polymorphonuclear leucocytosis and local envenoming if, after bites on the hand or foot, swelling extends beyond the wrist or ankle within 4 hours of the bite. Two ampoules of **Zagreb antivenom** (Regent) are diluted with 2–3 volumes of sodium chloride intravenous infusion 0.9% and given by slow intravenous injection (not more than 1 mL of antivenom per minute) or by intravenous infusion. The **same dose** should be used for **adults** and **children**. The dose can be repeated in 1–2 hours if there is no clinical improvement. Adrenaline injection must be immediately to hand for treatment of anaphylactic antivenom reactions (for full details see section 3.4.3).

Antivenom is available for certain foreign snakes and spiders. Information on identification, management, and supply, telephone:

| | |
|---|---|
| Liverpool | 051-708 9393 |
| Liverpool (Walton Hospital Pharmacy) (supply only) | 051-525 3611 |
| London | 071-635 9191 |
| Oxford | (0865) 220968 or (0865) 60871 |

INSECT BITES. Stings from ants, wasps, bees, and hornets cause local pain and swelling but seldom cause severe toxicity. If the bite is in the mouth or on the tongue marked swelling may cause respiratory distress. The stings from these insects are usually treated by cleansing the area, applying a cooling lotion (such as a calamine preparation), and giving an antihistamine by mouth. Bee stings should be removed by scraping them off with a finger nail or knife before cleansing the area. Anaphylactic reactions require treatment with **adrenaline**. Inhalation of adrenaline (Medihaler-epi®, see section 3.4.3) is sufficient for mild attacks and is convenient for patients at risk to carry. A dose of 0.5–1 mL of adrenaline injection 1 in 1000 (1 mg/mL) should be given intramuscularly in more severe cases (for full details see section 3.4.3).

# Classified Notes on Drugs and Preparations

# 1: Drugs acting on the
# GASTRO-INTESTINAL SYSTEM

The drugs and preparations in this chapter are described under the following sections:

**1.1** Antacids
**1.2** Antispasmodics and other drugs altering gut motility
**1.3** Ulcer-healing drugs
**1.4** Antidiarrhoeal drugs
**1.5** Treatment of chronic diarrhoeas
**1.6** Laxatives
**1.7** Preparations for haemorrhoids
**1.8** Stoma care
**1.9** Drugs affecting intestinal secretions

## 1.1 Antacids

**1.1.1** Aluminium- and magnesium-containing
**1.1.2** Sodium bicarbonate
**1.1.3** Calcium- and bismuth-containing

Antacids are still useful for treating gastro-intestinal disease; they can often relieve symptoms in both *ulcer* and *non-ulcer dyspepsia*, and in *reflux oesophagitis*. They are best given when symptoms occur or are expected, usually between meals and at bedtime, four or more times daily; additional doses may be required up to once an hour. Conventional doses e.g. 10 mL three or four times daily of liquid magnesium–aluminium antacids promote ulcer healing, possibly less well than antisecretory agents (section 1.3); proof of a relationship between healing and neutralising capacity is lacking. Liquid preparations are more effective than solids.

INTERACTIONS. Antacids should not be taken at the same time as other drugs as they may impair their absorption. Antacids may also damage enteric coatings designed to prevent dissolution in the stomach.

### 1.1.1 Aluminium- and magnesium-containing antacids

**Aluminium-** and **magnesium-containing** antacids, such as magnesium carbonate, hydroxide and trisilicate, and aluminium glycinate and hydroxide, being relatively insoluble in water, are long-acting if retained in the stomach. They are suitable for most antacid purposes. Magnesium-containing antacids tend to be laxative whereas aluminium-containing antacids may be constipating. Aluminium accumulation does not appear to be a risk if renal function is normal (see also appendix 3).

Compound preparations have no clear advantages over simpler preparations: neutralising capacity may be the same.

Complexes, such as **hydrotalcite** and **magaldrate**, confer no special advantage.

> **Low Na⁺**
> The words low Na⁺ added after some preparations indicate a sodium content of less than 1 mmol per tablet or 10-mL dose.

## ALUMINIUM HYDROXIDE

*Indications:* dyspepsia; for use in hyperphosphataemia, see section 9.5.2.2
*Cautions:* see notes above; porphyria, see section 9.8.2; **interactions:** Appendix 1 (antacids and adsorbents)
*Contra-indications:* hypophosphataemia

Aluminium-only preparations
**Aluminium Hydroxide** (Non-proprietary)
*Tablets,* dried aluminium hydroxide 500 mg. Net price 20 = 29p
*Dose:* 1–2 tablets chewed 4 times daily and at bedtime or as required
*Mixture* (gel), about 4% w/w Al₂O₃ in water, with a peppermint flavour. Net price 200 mL = 36p
*Dose:* antacid, 5–10 mL 4 times daily between meals and at bedtime or as required; CHILD 6–12 years, up to 5 mL 3 times daily
*Note.* The brand name NHS Aludrox® (Charwell) is used for aluminium hydroxide mixture; net price 200 mL = 77p. For NHS Aludrox® tablets see preparations with magnesium, below.

**Alu-Cap®** (3M)
*Capsules,* green/red, dried aluminium hydroxide 475 mg (low Na⁺). Net price 120-cap pack = £3.84
*Dose:* antacid, 1 capsule 4 times daily and at bedtime

With magnesium
NHS **Aludrox®** (Charwell)
*Tablets,* aluminium hydroxide-magnesium carbonate co-dried gel 282 mg, magnesium hydroxide 85 mg. Net price 60 = £1.69
*Dose:* 1 or 2 tablets chewed 4 times daily between meals and at bedtime when required

NHS **Dijex®** (Crookes)
*Tablets,* pink, aluminium hydroxide-magnesium carbonate co-dried gel 400 mg (low Na⁺). Net price 30 = 63p
*Dose:* 1–2 tablets chewed every 2–4 hours when required
*Liquid,* aluminium hydroxide mixture 98%, magnesium hydroxide 1.7%. Net price 200 mL = £1.24
*Dose:* 5–10 mL every 2–4 hours when required

NHS **Gastrils®** (Jackson)
*Pastilles,* green (mint-flavoured) or yellow (fruit-flavoured), s/c, aluminium hydroxide-magnesium carbonate co-dried gel 500 mg. Net price 40 g = 61p
*Dose:* 1–2 pastilles sucked when required; CHILD 1 pastille 3 times daily

NHS **Gelusil®** (W-L)
*Tablets,* dried aluminium hydroxide 250 mg, magnesium trisilicate 500 mg (low Na⁺). Net price 50 = £1.76
*Dose:* 1–2 tablets chewed or sucked after meals or when required; CHILD half adult dose

---

**Maalox®** (Rhône-Poulenc Rorer)
*Tablets*, dried aluminium hydroxide 400 mg, magnesium hydroxide 400 mg (low Na⁺). Net price 20 = 28p
*Dose:* 1–2 tablets chewed 20 minutes–1 hour after meals and at bedtime or when required
*Suspension*, sugar-free, dried aluminium hydroxide 220 mg, magnesium hydroxide 195 mg/5 mL (low Na⁺). Net price 100 mL = 39p; 20 × 10-mL sachets = 78p
*Dose:* 10–20 mL 20 minutes–1 hour after meals and at bedtime or when required

**Maalox TC®** (Rhône-Poulenc Rorer)
*Tablets*, dried aluminium hydroxide 600 mg, magnesium hydroxide 300 mg (low Na⁺). Net price 100 = £3.60
*Suspension*, sugar-free, dried aluminium hydroxide 600 mg, magnesium hydroxide 300 mg/5 mL (low Na⁺). Net price 500 mL = £3.60
*Dose:* antacid, 1–2 tablets chewed or 5–10 mL suspension 4 times daily 20 minutes–1 hour after meals and at bedtime or as required; duodenal ulcer, 3 tablets or 15 mL suspension 4 times daily (treatment) *or* twice daily (prevention of recurrence)

**Mucogel®** (Pharmax)
*Suspension*, sugar-free, dried aluminium hydroxide 220 mg, magnesium hydroxide 195 mg/5 mL (low Na⁺). Net price 500 mL = £1.96
*Dose:* 10–20 mL 3 times daily, 20 minutes–1 hour after meals, and at bedtime or when required

---

## MAGNESIUM CARBONATE

*Indications:* dyspepsia
*Cautions:* renal impairment; see also notes above; **interactions:** Appendix 1 (antacids and adsorbents)
*Contra-indications:* hypophosphataemia
*Side-effects:* diarrhoea; belching due to liberated carbon dioxide

**Aromatic Magnesium Carbonate Mixture** (BP) (Aromatic Magnesium Carbonate Oral Suspension)
*Oral suspension*, light magnesium carbonate 3%, sodium bicarbonate 5%, in a suitable vehicle containing aromatic cardamom tincture. Extemporaneous preparations should be recently prepared according to the following formula: light magnesium carbonate 300 mg, sodium bicarbonate 500 mg, aromatic cardamom tincture 0.3 mL, double-strength chloroform water 5 mL, water to 10 mL. Contains about 6 mmol Na⁺/10 mL. Net price 200 mL = 30p
*Dose:* 10 mL 3 times daily in water

For compound preparations with aluminium, see under Aluminium Hydroxide (previous page)

---

## MAGNESIUM TRISILICATE

*Indications:* dyspepsia
*Cautions; Contra-indications:* see under Magnesium Carbonate
*Side-effects:* diarrhoea

**Magnesium Trisilicate Tablets, Compound** (BP)
*Tablets*, magnesium trisilicate 250 mg, dried aluminium hydroxide 120 mg. Net price 20 = 20p
*Dose:* 1–2 tablets chewed when required

**Magnesium Trisilicate Mixture** (BP) (Magnesium Trisilicate Oral Suspension)
*Oral suspension*, 5% each of magnesium trisilicate, light magnesium carbonate, and sodium bicarbonate in a suitable vehicle with a peppermint flavour. Extemporaneous preparations should be recently prepared according to the following formula: magnesium trisilicate 500 mg, light magnesium carbonate 500 mg, sodium bicarbonate 500 mg, concentrated peppermint emulsion 0.25 mL, double-strength chloroform water 5 mL, water to 10 mL. Contains about 6 mmol Na⁺/10 mL. Net price 200 mL = 22p
*Dose:* 10 mL 3 times daily in water

**Magnesium Trisilicate Oral Powder, Compound** (BP)
*Oral powder*, magnesium trisilicate 250 mg, chalk 250 mg, heavy magnesium carbonate 250 mg, sodium bicarbonate 250 mg/g. Contains about 3 mmol Na⁺/g. Net price 20 g = 16p. Label: 13
*Dose:* 1–5 g in liquid when required

For compound preparations with aluminium, see under Aluminium Hydroxide (previous page)

---

### ALUMINIUM-MAGNESIUM COMPLEXES

## HYDROTALCITE

Aluminium magnesium carbonate hydroxide hydrate
*Indications:* dyspepsia
*Cautions:* see notes above; **interactions:** Appendix 1 (antacids and adsorbents)

**Hydrotalcite** (Non-proprietary)
*Tablets*, hydrotalcite 500 mg. Net price 56 = 81p
*Dose:* 2 tablets chewed between meals and at bedtime; CHILD 6–12 years 1 tablet
*Suspension*, hydrotalcite 500 mg/5 mL. Net price 500-mL pack = £1.95
*Dose:* 10 mL between meals and at bedtime; CHILD 6–12 years 5 mL
*Note.* The brand name NHS Altacite® (Roussel) is used for hydrotalcite suspension and tablets; see section 1.1.1.1 for Altacite Plus® preparations.

## MAGALDRATE

A synthetic combination of aluminium and magnesium hydroxides and sulphuric acid
*Indications:* dyspepsia
*Cautions:* see notes above; **interactions:** Appendix 1 (antacids and adsorbents)

**Magaldrate** (Non-proprietary)
*Suspension*, magaldrate 800 mg/5 mL. Net price 100 mL = 38p
*Dose:* 5–10 mL after meals and at bedtime; CHILD 6–12 years 2.5–5 mL
*Note.* The brand name NHS Dynese® (Galen) is used for magaldrate suspension; it is sugar-free and low Na⁺.

---

## 1.1.1.1    Aluminium- and magnesium-containing antacids with additional ingredients

Activated dimethicone (simethicone), given alone or added to an antacid as an antifoaming agent to relieve flatulence, is of uncertain value. Alginates added as protectants against *reflux oesophagitis* may be useful, but surface anaesthetics (e.g. oxethazaine) added to improve symptom relief are of doubtful efficacy. The amount of additional ingredient or antacid in individual preparations varies widely, as does their sodium content, so that preparations may not be freely interchangeable.

Preparations containing activated dimethicone with an antacid may be useful for the relief of hiccup in terminal care.

**NHS Actonorm®** (Wallace Mfg)
*Gel*, dried aluminium hydroxide 220 mg, activated dimethicone 25 mg, magnesium hydroxide 200 mg/5 mL (low Na$^+$). Net price 200 mL = £1.70
*Dose:* 5–20 mL when required

**Algicon®** (Rhône-Poulenc Rorer)
*Tablets*, aluminium hydroxide-magnesium carbonate co-dried gel 360 mg, magnesium alginate 500 mg, magnesium carbonate 320 mg, potassium bicarbonate 100 mg, sucrose 1.5 g (low Na$^+$). Net price 60 = £2.40
*Dose:* 1–2 tablets 4 times daily (chewed after meals and at bedtime)
*Suspension*, yellow, aluminium hydroxide-magnesium carbonate co-dried gel 140 mg, magnesium alginate 250 mg, magnesium carbonate 175 mg, potassium bicarbonate 50 mg/5 mL (low Na$^+$). Net price 500 mL = £2.60
*Dose:* 10–20 mL 4 times daily (after meals and at bedtime)

**Altacite Plus®** (Roussel)
**NHS** *Tablets*, co-simalcite 250/500 (activated dimethicone 250 mg, hydrotalcite 500 mg) (low Na$^+$). Net price 20 = £1.05
*Dose:* 2 tablets chewed between meals and at bedtime when required; CHILD 8–12 years 1 tablet
*Suspension*, sugar-free, co-simalcite 125/500 (activated dimethicone 125 mg, hydrotalcite 500 mg)/5 mL (low Na$^+$). Net price 500 mL = £1.85
*Dose:* 10 mL between meals and at bedtime when required; CHILD 8–12 years 5 mL

**Asilone®** (Boots)
**NHS** *Tablets*, dried aluminium hydroxide 500 mg, activated dimethicone 270 mg (low Na$^+$). Net price 30-tab pack = £1.54
*Dose:* 1–2 tablets chewed or sucked before meals and at bedtime
*Suspension*, sugar-free, dried aluminium hydroxide 420 mg, activated dimethicone 135 mg, light magnesium oxide 70 mg/5 mL (low Na$^+$). Net price 500 mL = £1.95
*Dose:* 5–10 mL before meals and at bedtime

*Note.* Asilone® Liquid is the same formula as Asilone® Suspension but is in a 200-mL pack (net price £1.13)

**NHS Carbellon®** (Torbet)
*Tablets*, black, activated charcoal 100 mg, magnesium hydroxide 100 mg, peppermint oil 0.003 mL. Net price 50-tab pack = £1.20
*Dose:* 2–4 tablets chewed 3 times daily; CHILD 6–12 years 2 tablets 3 times daily

**Diovol®** (Pharmax)
*Suspension*, sugar-free, aluminium hydroxide 200 mg, dimethicone 25 mg, magnesium hydroxide 200 mg/5 mL (low Na$^+$). Net price 300 mL = £1.16
*Dose:* 5–10 mL when required

**Gastrocote®** (Boehringer Mannheim)
*Tablets*, alginic acid 200 mg, dried aluminium hydroxide 80 mg, magnesium trisilicate 40 mg, sodium bicarbonate 70 mg. Contains about 1 mmol Na$^+$/tablet. Net price 100 = £3.76
*Dose:* 1–2 tablets chewed 4 times daily (after meals and at bedtime)
*Liquid*, sugar-free, peach-coloured, dried aluminium hydroxide 80 mg, magnesium trisilicate 40 mg, sodium alginate 220 mg, sodium bicarbonate 70 mg/5 mL. Contains 1.8 mmol Na$^+$/5 mL. Net price 500 mL = £2.86
*Dose:* 5–15 mL 4 times daily (after meals and at bedtime)

**Gastron®** (Sanofi Winthrop)
*Tablets*, alginic acid 600 mg, dried aluminium hydroxide 240 mg, magnesium trisilicate 60 mg, sodium bicarbonate 210 mg. Contains about 3 mmol Na$^+$/tablet. Net price 100-tab pack = £4·49
*Dose:* 1–2 tablets chewed 3 times daily after meals and 2 tablets at bedtime

**Gaviscon®** (R&C)
*Tablets*, alginic acid 500 mg, dried aluminium hydroxide 100 mg, magnesium trisilicate 25 mg, sodium bicarbonate 170 mg. Contains 2 mmol Na$^+$/tablet. Net price 60 = £2.25
*Dose:* 1–2 tablets chewed after meals and at bedtime, followed by water; CHILD 1 tablet
*Liquid*, pink, sugar-free, sodium alginate 250 mg, sodium bicarbonate 133.5 mg, calcium carbonate 80 mg/5 mL. Contains about 3 mmol Na$^+$/5 mL. Net price 100 mL = 54p
*Dose:* 10–20 mL after meals and at bedtime; CHILD 5–10 mL

**Infant Gaviscon®** (R&C)
*Oral powder*, sugar-free, sodium alginate 225 mg, magnesium alginate 87.5 mg, dried aluminium hydroxide 112.5 mg with colloidal silica and mannitol/dose (half dual-sachet). Contains 0.92 mmol Na$^+$/dose. Net price 15 dual-sachets (30 doses) = £2.46
*Dose:* INFANT under 4.5 kg 1 dose (half dual-sachet) mixed with feeds (or water in breast-fed infants) when required; over 4.5 kg 2 doses (1 dual-sachet); CHILD 2 doses (1 dual-sachet) in water after each meal
*Note.* Not to be used in premature infants, or where excessive water loss likely (e.g. fever, diarrhoea, vomiting, high room temperature)
IMPORTANT. This is a new formulation; each half of the dual-sachet is identified as 'one dose'. To avoid errors prescribe as 'dual-sachet' with directions in terms of 'dose'

**Infacol®** (Pharmax)
*Liquid*, sugar-free, activated dimethicone 40 mg/mL (low Na+). Net price 50 mL = £1.42. Counselling, use of dropper
*Dose:* gripes, colic or wind pains, INFANT 0.5–1 mL before feeds

**PoM Mucaine®** (Wyeth)
*Suspension*, sugar-free, aluminium hydroxide mixture 4.75 mL, magnesium hydroxide 100 mg, oxethazaine 10 mg/5 mL. Net price 200-mL pack = 76p
*Dose:* 5–10 mL (without fluid) 3–4 times daily (15 minutes before meals and at bedtime or when required)

**Maalox Plus®** (Rhône-Poulenc Rorer)
**NHS** *Tablets*, white/yellow, dried aluminium hydroxide 200 mg, activated dimethicone 25 mg, magnesium hydroxide 200 mg (low Na+). Net price 50 = £1.67
*Dose:* 1–2 tablets chewed 4 times daily after meals and at bedtime or when required
*Suspension*, sugar-free, dried aluminium hydroxide 220 mg, activated dimethicone 25 mg, magnesium hydroxide 195 mg/5 mL (low Na+). Net price 500 mL = £1.95
*Dose:* 5–10 mL 4 times daily (after meals and at bedtime or when required)

**Polycrol®** (Nicholas)
*Tablets*, green/white, aluminium hydroxide-magnesium carbonate co-dried gel 275 mg, activated dimethicone 25 mg, magnesium hydroxide 100 mg (low Na+). Net price 20-tab pack = 46p; 200-tab pack = £2.90
*Dose:* 1–2 tablets chewed between meals and at bedtime or when required; CHILD 5–12 years 1 tablet 2–3 times daily
*Gel*, sugar-free, aluminium hydroxide mixture 4.75 mL, activated dimethicone 25 mg, magnesium hydroxide 100 mg/5 mL (low Na+). Net price 300 mL = £1.16
*Dose:* 5–10 mL between meals and at bedtime or when required; CHILD 5–12 years 5 mL up to six times daily

**Polycrol Forte®** (Nicholas)
*Tablets*, aluminium hydroxide-magnesium carbonate co-dried gel 275 mg, activated dimethicone 250 mg, magnesium hydroxide 100 mg (low Na+). Net price 12-tab pack = 46p; 120-tab pack = £1.74
*Dose:* 1–2 tablets chewed between meals and at bedtime or when required
*Gel*, sugar-free, aluminium hydroxide mixture 4.75 mL, activated dimethicone 125 mg, magnesium hydroxide 100 mg/5 mL (low Na+). Net price 300 mL = £1.16
*Dose:* 5–10 mL between meals and at bedtime or when required; CHILD 5–12 years 5 mL, up to six times daily

**NHS Simeco®** (Wyeth)
*Tablets*, pink/white, aluminium hydroxide–magnesium carbonate co-dried gel 282 mg, activated dimethicone 25 mg, magnesium hydroxide 85 mg. Net price 60-tab pack = £3.15
*Dose:* 2 tablets to be chewed after or between meals and at bedtime
*Suspension*, aluminium hydroxide 215 mg, activated dimethicone 25 mg, magnesium hydroxide 80 mg/5 mL. Net price 200 mL = £1.35
*Dose:* 10 mL after or between meals and at bedtime; CHILD 6–12 years, up to 5 mL 3 times daily

**Topal®** (Innovex)
*Tablets*, alginic acid 200 mg, dried aluminium hydroxide 30 mg, light magnesium carbonate 40 mg with lactose 220 mg, sucrose 880 mg (low Na+). Net price 42 = £1.67
*Dose:* 1–3 tablets chewed 4 times daily (after meals and at bedtime); CHILD half adult dose

**NHS Unigest®** (Unigreg)
*Tablets*, dried aluminium hydroxide 450 mg, dimethicone 400 mg (low Na+). Net price 12 = 98p
*Dose:* 1–2 tablets chewed or sucked after meals and at bedtime or when required

## 1.1.2 Sodium bicarbonate

Sodium bicarbonate, being soluble in water, is rapid-acting, but absorbed bicarbonate can cause alkalosis in excessive doses. Like other carbonate-containing antacids it liberates carbon dioxide which causes belching. Sodium bicarbonate and antacid preparations with a high sodium content, such as magnesium trisilicate mixture, should be avoided in patients on salt-restricted diets (in heart failure, and hepatic and renal impairment).

### SODIUM BICARBONATE
*Indications:* rapid relief of dyspepsia
*Cautions:* renal impairment; patients on a sodium-restricted diet; avoid prolonged use; **interactions:** Appendix 1 (antacids and adsorbents)
*Side-effects:* belching due to liberated carbon dioxide and, with prolonged use, alkalosis

**Sodium Bicarbonate** (BP). Label: 13
*Dose:* 1–5 g in water when required
**Sodium Bicarbonate Tablets, Compound** (BP) (Soda Mint Tablets), sodium bicarbonate 300 mg. Contains about 4 mmol Na+/tab
*Dose:* 2–6 tablets sucked when required

## 1.1.3 Calcium- and bismuth-containing antacids

Bismuth-containing antacids (unless chelates) are best avoided because absorbed bismuth can be neurotoxic, causing encephalopathy; they tend to be constipating. Calcium-containing antacids can induce rebound acid secretion: with modest doses the clinical significance is doubtful, but prolonged high doses also cause hypercalcaemia and alkalosis, and can precipitate the milk alkali syndrome. **Interactions:** Appendix 1 (antacids and adsorbents).

**NHS Nulacin®** (Bencard)
*Tablets*, calcium carbonate 130 mg, heavy magnesium carbonate 30 mg, heavy magnesium oxide 130 mg, magnesium trisilicate 230 mg, with milk solids, dextrins and maltose (low Na+). Net price 25 = 82p
*Additives: include gluten*
*Dose:* 1 tablet chewed or sucked when required between meals and at bedtime; max. 8 tablets daily
**NHS Roter®** (Roterpharma)
*Tablets*, pink, bismuth subnitrate 300 mg, frangula 25 mg, magnesium carbonate 400 mg, sodium bicarbonate 200 mg. Net price 20 = 48p
*Dose:* 1–2 tablets dispersed in warm water 3 times daily after meals

---

## 1.2    Antispasmodics and other drugs altering gut motility

The smooth muscle relaxant properties of anti-muscarinic and other antispasmodic drugs may be useful as adjunctive treatment in *non-ulcer dyspepsia*, in the *irritable bowel syndrome*, and in *diverticular disease*. The gastric antisecretory effects of conventional antimuscarinic drugs are of little practical significance since dosage is limited by atropine-like side-effects. Moreover, they have been superseded by more powerful and specific antisecretory drugs, including the histamine $H_2$-receptor antagonists and the selective antimuscarinic pirenzepine.

The dopamine-receptor antagonists metoclopramide and domperidone have different properties, tending to stimulate transit in the gut.

### ANTIMUSCARINICS

The antimuscarinics (less correctly termed 'anticholinergics') can be divided into atropine and its related alkaloids (including the belladonna alkaloids), and synthetic antimuscarinics. The synthetic antimuscarinics can, in turn, be divided into **tertiary amine** (dicyclomine hydrochloride) and **quaternary ammonium compounds** (ambutonium bromide, mepenzolate bromide, pipenzolate bromide, poldine methylsulphate, and propantheline bromide). The tertiary amine dicyclomine hydrochloride has a much less marked antimuscarinic action than atropine and may also have some direct action on smooth muscle.

Quaternary ammonium compounds are less lipid soluble than atropine and so may be less likely to cross the blood–brain barrier; they are also less well absorbed. Although central atropine-like side-effects, such as confusion, are thereby reduced, peripheral atropine-like side-effects remain common with dry mouth, difficult visual accommodation, hesitant micturition, and constipation at doses which act as gut neuromuscular relaxants or inhibitors of acid secretion. The elderly are particularly susceptible; glaucoma and urinary retention may occur.

Antimuscarinics tend to relax the oesophageal sphincter and should be avoided in patients with symptomatic reflux; all antispasmodics should be avoided in paralytic ileus. Despite these side-effects antimuscarinics are nevertheless useful in some *dyspeptics*, in the *irritable bowel syndrome*, and in *diverticular disease*. A dose at night will delay gastric emptying and prolong the gastric retention of antacids, thus helping to reduce nocturnal acidity; side-effects are also better tolerated then.

The quaternary ammonium compound, **hyoscine butylbromide** is advocated as a gastro-intestinal antispasmodic, but it is poorly absorbed and its action is brief; the injection is a useful antispasmodic in endoscopy and radiology.

## ATROPINE SULPHATE and BELLADONNA ALKALOIDS

*Indications:* see notes above; atropine sulphate, see also section 15.1.3

*Cautions:* elderly; urinary retention, prostatic enlargement, tachycardia, cardiac insufficiency, paralytic ileus, ulcerative colitis, and pyloric stenosis; may aggravate gastro-oesophageal reflux; pregnancy and breast-feeding; **interactions:** Appendix 1 (antimuscarinics)

*Contra-indications:* closed-angle glaucoma

*Side-effects:* dry mouth with difficulty in swallowing and thirst, dilatation of the pupils with loss of accommodation and sensitivity to light, increased intra-ocular pressure, flushing, dry skin, bradycardia followed by tachycardia, palpitations and arrhythmias, difficulty with micturition, and constipation; rarely fever, confusional states and rashes

Compound preparations

**NHS Actonorm®** (Wallace Mfg)
*Powder*, atropine sulphate 100 micrograms, aluminium hydroxide gel 50 mg, calcium carbonate 145 mg, magnesium carbonate 381.4 mg, magnesium trisilicate 50 mg, sodium bicarbonate 373 mg, peppermint oil 500 micrograms/g. Net price 85 g = £1.86. Label: 13
*Dose:* one level 5-mL spoonful (2 g) in liquid 3–4 times daily; elderly, initially 5 mL twice daily

**NHS Alka-Donna®** (Carlton)
*Suspension*, belladonna alkaloids 60 micrograms (calc. as hyoscyamine), aluminium hydroxide mixture 2.15 mL, magnesium trisilicate 342.5 mg/5 mL. Net price 100 mL = 13p
*Dose:* 5–10 mL 3 times daily between meals

**NHS Aluhyde®** (Sinclair)
*Tablets*, scored, belladonna liquid extract 7.8 mg, dried aluminium hydroxide 245 mg, magnesium trisilicate 245 mg. Net price 50-tab pack = £3.43
*Dose:* 2 tablets 3 times daily

**NHS Bellocarb®** (Sinclair)
*Tablets*, beige, scored, belladonna dry extract 10 mg (equivalent to 100 micrograms of hyoscyamine), magnesium carbonate 300 mg, magnesium trisilicate 300 mg. Net price 50-tab pack = £3.43
*Dose:* 1–2 tablets 4 times daily

## AMBUTONIUM BROMIDE

*Indications:* adjunct in gastro-intestinal disorders characterised by smooth muscle spasm

*Cautions; Contra-indications; Side-effects:* see under Atropine Sulphate and notes above

**NHS PoM Aludrox SA®** (Charwell)
*Suspension*, sugar-free, green, ambutonium bromide 2.5 mg, aluminium hydroxide mixture 4.75 mL, magnesium hydroxide 100 mg/5 mL. Net price 100 mL = 38p
*Dose:* 5–10 mL 3–4 times daily between meals and at bedtime

## DICYCLOMINE HYDROCHLORIDE

*Indications:* adjunct in gastro-intestinal disorders characterised by smooth muscle spasm

*Cautions; Contra-indications; Side-effects:* see under Atropine Sulphate; contra-indicated in infants under 6 months

*Dose:* 10–20 mg 3 times daily; CHILD 6–24 months 5–10 mg up to 3–4 times daily, 15 minutes before feeds, 2–12 years 10 mg 3 times daily

PoM **Merbentyl**® (Merrell)
*Tablets*, dicyclomine hydrochloride 10 mg. Net price 20 = 58p
*Syrup*, dicyclomine hydrochloride 10 mg/5 mL. Diluent syrup, life of diluted preparation 14 days. Net price 100 mL = 88p
PoM **Merbentyl 20**® (Merrell)
*Tablets*, dicyclomine hydrochloride 20 mg. Net price 84-tab pack = £4.89

Compound preparations
**Kolanticon**® (Merrell)
*Gel*, sugar-free, dicyclomine hydrochloride 2.5 mg, dried aluminium hydroxide 200 mg, light magnesium oxide 100 mg, activated dimethicone (simethicone USP) 20 mg/5 mL. Net price 200 mL = £1.33; 500 mL = £1.90
*Dose:* 10–20 mL every 4 hours when required

## HYOSCINE BUTYLBROMIDE

*Indications:* adjunct in gastro-intestinal disorders characterised by smooth muscle spasm
*Cautions; Contra-indications; Side-effects:* see under Atropine Sulphate and notes above; avoid in porphyria (see section 9.8.2)
*Dose: by mouth*, 20 mg 4 times daily; CHILD 6–12 years, 10 mg 3 times daily
*By intramuscular or intravenous injection* (acute spasm), 20 mg, repeated after 30 minutes if necessary

PoM **Buscopan**® (Boehringer Ingelheim)
*Tablets*, coated, hyoscine butylbromide 10 mg. Net price 20 = 81p (not recommended, see notes above)
*Injection*, hyoscine butylbromide 20 mg/mL. Net price 1-mL amp = 19p

## MEPENZOLATE BROMIDE

*Indications:* adjunct in gastro-intestinal disorders characterised by smooth muscle spasm
*Cautions; Contra-indications; Side-effects:* see under Atropine Sulphate and notes above
*Dose:* 25–50 mg 3–4 times daily

PoM **Cantil**® (Boehringer Mannheim)
*Tablets*, yellow, scored, mepenzolate bromide 25 mg. Net price 50-tab pack = £2.75
*Additives: include* tartrazine

## PIPENZOLATE BROMIDE

*Indications:* adjunct in gastro-intestinal disorders characterised by smooth muscle spasm
*Cautions; Contra-indications; Side-effects:* see under Atropine Sulphate and notes above
*Dose:* 5 mg 3 times daily and 5–10 mg at night

PoM **Piptal**® (Boehringer Mannheim)
*Tablets*, peach, pipenzolate bromide 5 mg. Net price 50 = £1.14

Compound preparations
PoM **Piptalin**® (Boehringer Mannheim)
*Suspension*, orange, sugar-free, pipenzolate bromide 4 mg, activated dimethicone 40 mg/5 mL. Diluent syrup or water, life of diluted suspension 14 days. Net price 100 mL = £1.11
*Dose:* 10 mL 3–4 times daily before meals; CHILD up to 10 kg 2.5 mL, 10–20 kg 2.5–5 mL, 20–40 kg 5 mL, 3–4 times daily 15 minutes before meals (or feeds)

## POLDINE METHYLSULPHATE

*Indications:* adjunct in gastro-intestinal disorders characterised by smooth muscle spasm
*Cautions; Contra-indications; Side-effects:* see under Atropine Sulphate and notes above
*Dose:* 2–4 mg 4 times daily

PoM **Nacton**® (Bencard)
*Tablets*, scored, poldine methylsulphate 2 mg. Net price 112-tab pack = £1.89
*Tablets forte*, orange, scored, poldine methylsulphate 4 mg. Net price 112-tab pack = £3.61

## PROPANTHELINE BROMIDE

*Indications:* adjunct in gastro-intestinal disorders characterised by smooth muscle spasm; for use in urinary frequency, see section 7.4.2
*Cautions; Contra-indications; Side-effects:* see under Atropine Sulphate and notes above
*Dose:* 15 mg 3 times daily at least 1 hour before meals and 30 mg at night, max. 120 mg daily

PoM **Pro-Banthine**® (Gold Cross)
*Tablets*, pink, s/c, propantheline bromide 15 mg. Net price 100 = £2.34. Label: 23

OTHER ANTISPASMODICS

Alverine citrate, mebeverine hydrochloride, and peppermint oil are believed to be direct relaxants of intestinal smooth muscle and may relieve pain in the *irritable bowel syndrome* and *diverticular disease*. They have no serious adverse effects but, like all antispasmodics, should be avoided in paralytic ileus. Peppermint oil occasionally causes heartburn.

## ALVERINE CITRATE

*Indications:* adjunct in gastro-intestinal disorders characterised by smooth muscle spasm; dysmenorrhoea
*Cautions:* pregnancy
*Contra-indications:* paralytic ileus
*Dose:* 60–120 mg 1–3 times daily; CHILD 8–12 years, 60 mg 3 times daily

**Spasmonal**® (Norgine)
*Capsules*, blue/grey, alverine citrate 60 mg. Net price 20 = £2.24

Compound preparations
**¹Alvercol®** (Norgine)
*Granules*, beige, coated, sterculia 62%, alverine
citrate 0.5%. Net price 500 g = £12.50. Label:
25, 27, counselling, see below
*Dose:* irritable bowel syndrome, 1–2 heaped 5-mL
spoonfuls swallowed without chewing with water once
or twice daily after meals; CHILD 6–12 years, half adult
dose
COUNSELLING. Preparations that swell in contact with
liquid should always be carefully swallowed with water
and should not be taken immediately before going to
bed
1. Formerly Normacol Antispasmodic

## MEBEVERINE HYDROCHLORIDE

*Indications:* adjunct in gastro-intestinal disorders
characterised by smooth muscle spasm
*Cautions:* paralytic ileus; avoid in porphyria (see
section 9.8.2.)

PoM **Colofac®** (Duphar)
*Tablets*, s/c, mebeverine hydrochloride 135 mg.
Net price 20 = £1.67. Label: 22
*Dose:* 1 tablet 3 times daily preferably 20 minutes before
meals
*Liquid*, yellow, sugar-free, mebeverine hydro-
chloride 50 mg (as embonate)/5 mL. Net price
300 mL = £3.50. Label: 22
*Dose:* ADULT and CHILD over 10 years, 15 mL 3 times
daily, preferably 20 minutes before food

Compound preparations
PoM **Colven®** (R&C)
*Granules*, yellowish-brown, effervescent,
ispaghula husk 3.5 g, mebeverine hydrochloride
135 mg/sachet. Contains 6.1 mmol Na⁺/sachet;
caution in renal impairment. Net price 60
sachets = £15.00. Label: 13, 22, counselling,
see below
*Dose:* irritable bowel syndrome, 1 sachet in water morning and night 30 minutes before food; an additional
sachet may also be taken before the midday meal if
necessary
COUNSELLING. Preparations that swell in contact with
liquid should always be carefully swallowed with water
and should not be taken immediately before going to
bed

## PEPPERMINT OIL

*Indications:* relief of abdominal colic and distension, particularly in irritable bowel syndrome
*Cautions:* ulcerative colitis, paralytic ileus, rarely
sensitivity to menthol
*Side-effects:* heartburn, rarely, allergy
LOCAL IRRITATION. Capsules should not be broken or
chewed because this would release peppermint oil causing irritation of mouth or oesophagus

**Colpermin®** (Tillotts)
*Capsules*, e/c, light blue/dark blue, green band,
peppermint oil 0.2 mL. Net price 100-cap
pack = £12.76. Label: 5, 22, 25
*Dose:* 1–2 capsules, swallowed whole with water, 3 times
daily before meals for up to 2–3 months if necessary

**Mintec®** (Innovex)
*Capsules*, e/c, green/ivory, peppermint oil
0.2 mL. Net price 100-cap pack = £12.80.
Label: 5, 22, 25
*Dose:* 1–2 capsules, swallowed whole with water, 3 times
daily before meals for up to 2–3 months if necessary

## MOTILITY STIMULANTS

**Metoclopramide** and **domperidone** are dopamine
antagonists which stimulate gastric emptying and
small intestinal transit, and enhance the strength
of oesophageal sphincter contraction. Metoclopramide is used in some patients with *non-
ulcer dyspepsia*, for speeding the transit of barium
during intestinal follow-through examination, and
as accessory treatment for *oesophageal reflux*.
Both metoclopramide and domperidone are useful in nonspecific or cytotoxic-induced *nausea and
vomiting* (see section 4.6).

Metoclopramide and, occasionally, domperidone induce extrapyramidal reactions with facial
and skeletal muscle spasms and oculogyric crises.
These are more common in the young (especially
girls and young women) and the very old, usually
occur shortly after starting treatment, and subside
within 24 hours of stopping the drug. Injection of
an antiparkinsonian agent such as procyclidine
(see section 4.9.2) will abort attacks. Other side-
effects include gynaecomastia and galactorrhoea;
diarrhoea can occur. Dosage of both should be
reduced in renal impairment and both should be
avoided immediately after abdominal surgery.

**Cisapride** is a newly introduced motility stimulant believed to promote release of acetylcholine
in the gut wall; it does not have dopamine-antag-
onist properties. It is of use in treating *oesophageal reflux and gastric stasis* and in the short-
term management of *non-ulcer dyspepsia*.

## CISAPRIDE

*Indications:* see under dose
*Cautions:* halve dose initially in hepatic and renal
impairment; elderly; **interactions:** Appendix 1
(cisapride)
*Contra-indications:* where gastro-intestinal
stimulation dangerous; pregnancy
*Side-effects:* abdominal cramps and diarrhoea,
occasional headaches and lightheadedness;
convulsions and extrapyramidal effects
reported
*Dose:* ADULT and CHILD over 12 years
Symptoms and mucosal lesions associated with
gastro-oesophageal reflux, 10 mg 3–4 times
daily; 12-week course recommended
Symptoms of impaired gastric motility secondary to disturbed and delayed gastric emptying
associated with diabetes, systemic sclerosis and
autonomic neuropathy, 10 mg 3–4 times daily
initially for 6 weeks (but longer treatment may
be necessary)
Symptoms of dyspepsia (peptic ulcer or other
lesions excluded), 10 mg 3 times daily (usual
course 4 weeks)
COUNSELLING. Advise patient to take 15–30 minutes
before meals and at bedtime (to control night symptoms)

PoM **Alimix**® (Cilag)
*Tablets*, scored, cisapride (as monohydrate) 10 mg, net price 120-tab pack = £38.57.
Counselling, administration, see above
PoM **Prepulsid**® (Janssen)
*Tablets*, scored, cisapride (as monohydrate) 10 mg, net price 112-tab pack = £36.00.
Counselling, administration, see above

## DOMPERIDONE
See section 4.6

## METOCLOPRAMIDE HYDROCHLORIDE
*Indications:* see notes above; for use in nausea and vomiting, see section 4.6
PATIENTS UNDER 20 YEARS. Use restricted to severe intractable vomiting of known cause, vomiting of radiotherapy and cytotoxics, aid to gastro-intestinal intubation, pre-medication
*Cautions; Side-effects; Dose:* see notes above and section 4.6

**Preparations:** see section 4.6

### 1.2.1 Compound antispasmodic preparations
These preparations should be avoided, especially where they contain barbiturates. Sedatives should only be used in gastro-intestinal disease on their own individual merits.

NHS **CD Alka-Donna-P**® (Carlton)
*Tablets*, belladonna dry extract 8 mg, phenobarbitone 8 mg, dried aluminium hydroxide 250 mg, magnesium trisilicate 500 mg. Net price 20 = 7p
*Dose:* 1–2 tablets sucked before meals when required
NHS **APP Stomach Tablets**® (Consolidated)
*Tablets*, homatropine methylbromide 1.5 mg, aluminium hydroxide gel 15 mg, bismuth carbonate 12.5 mg, calcium carbonate 183 mg, magnesium carbonate 180 mg, magnesium trisilicate 108 mg. Net price 20 = 27p
*Dose:* 1–2 tablets 3–4 times daily after meals
NHS **APP Stomach Powder**® (Consolidated)
*Powder*, homatropine methylbromide 1 mg, aluminium hydroxide gel 30 mg, bismuth carbonate 20 mg, calcium carbonate 379 mg, magnesium carbonate 370 mg, magnesium trisilicate 200 mg/g. Net price 100 g = 95p.
Label: 13
*Dose:* 5-mL spoonful in liquid 3–4 times daily

## 1.3 Ulcer-healing drugs

Peptic ulceration commonly involves the stomach, duodenum, and lower oesophagus; after gastric surgery it involves the gastro-enterostomy stoma.
General measures, including stopping smoking and taking **antacids**, promote healing as do the use of a wide variety of antisecretory and other treatments. **H₂-receptor antagonists** (cimetidine, famotidine, nizatidine, ranitidine) are all very effective in *gastric and duodenal ulcer* and to a lesser extent in *oesophageal disease*. Relapse is common when treatment ceases, and can be managed by further short courses of treatment or by maintenance H₂-receptor antagonist therapy. **Pirenzepine** (a selective antimuscarinic) and **misoprostol** (a prostaglandin analogue) also inhibit acid secretion; **bismuth chelate** and **sucralfate** act by as yet poorly understood means. **Carbenox-**

olone, a liquorice derivative, causes fluid retention too commonly for routine use; a **deglycyrrhinised liquorice** preparation is of doubtful efficacy. The proton pump inhibitor **omeprazole** is an effective treatment for *gastric and duodenal ulcers* and particularly for *erosive oesophagitis*.
Associated infection with *Helicobacter pylori* can be suppressed temporarily by bismuth chelate; it may possibly be suppressed permanently when antibiotics (amoxycillin or tetracycline, with metronidazole) are given at the same time, but antibiotic-associated colitis is an important risk and metronidazole resistance to *H. pylori* is easily acquired.
*NSAID-associated peptic ulceration* can be treated with the conventional range of drugs. Short-term treatment in patients taking NSAIDs may prevent the development of peptic ulcers but has not been shown to prevent complications of bleeding or perforation.

### 1.3.1 H₂-receptor antagonists
All H₂-receptor antagonists heal *gastric and duodenal ulcers* by reducing gastric acid output as a result of H₂-receptor blockade; like cimetidine and ranitidine, the newer ones (famotidine and nizatidine) can also be expected to relieve *peptic oesophagitis* and, in high doses, to reduce gastric acid output in the *Zollinger–Ellison syndrome*.
Maintenance treatment with half doses prevents *ulcer relapse*, but does not modify the natural course of the disease when treatment has ceased; it is probably best given in courses of 4–6 weeks with further short courses if symptoms recur. Maintenance treatment is best suited to those with frequent severe recurrences and to the elderly who suffer ulcer complications.
Treatment of *undiagnosed dyspepsia* may be acceptable in younger patients but is undesirable in older people because the diagnosis of gastric cancer may be delayed.
Therapy can promote healing of NSAID-associated ulcers but there is no proof that the ulcer complications are prevented.
Clear proof that treatment is beneficial in *haematemesis* and *melaena* is lacking, but prophylactic use reduces the frequency of bleeding from gastroduodenal erosions in *hepatic coma*, and possibly in other conditions requiring *intensive care*. Treatment also reduces the frequency of *acid aspiration* in obstetric patients at delivery (Mendelson's syndrome).

SIDE-EFFECTS. H₂-receptor antagonists are well tolerated and side-effects are uncommon with few significant differences between available drugs. Dizziness, somnolence or fatigue, and rash have occasionally been reported with all of them, and there are rare reports of headache, liver dysfunction, and blood disorders. Other rare reports include bradycardia or AV block, confusion, interstitial nephritis (cimetidine), and urticaria and angioedema. Cimetidine is also associated with occasional gynaecomastia and rare reports of impotence and myalgia. Causal relationships of other reports, such as pancreatitis, are unclear.

INTERACTIONS. Cimetidine retards oxidative hepatic drug metabolism by binding to microsomal cytochrome P450. It should be avoided in patients stabilised on warfarin, phenytoin, and theophylline (or aminophylline), but other interactions (see **Appendix 1**) may be of less clinical relevance. Famotidine, nizatidine, and ranitidine do not share the drug metabolism inhibitory properties of cimetidine.

## CIMETIDINE

*Indications:* benign gastric and duodenal ulceration, stomal ulcer, reflux oesophagitis, Zollinger-Ellison syndrome, other conditions where gastric acid reduction is beneficial (see notes above and section 1.9.4)

*Cautions:* see notes above; renal and hepatic impairment (reduce dose); pregnancy and breast-feeding. Avoid intravenous injection in high dosage (may rarely cause arrhythmias) and in cardiovascular impairment; **interactions:** Appendix 1 (histamine $H_2$-antagonists) and notes above

*Side-effects:* altered bowel habit, dizziness, rash, tiredness; reversible confusional states, reversible liver damage, headache; rarely, decreased blood counts, muscle or joint pain, bradycardia and AV block; interstitial nephritis and acute pancreatitis reported; gynaecomastia is also an occasional problem with cimetidine but usually only in high dosage (see also notes above)

*Dose: by mouth*, 400 mg twice daily (with breakfast and at night) *or* 800 mg as a single daily dose at night (benign gastric and duodenal ulceration). Doses should be taken for at least 4 weeks (6 weeks in gastric ulceration, 8 weeks in NSAID-associated ulceration); when necessary the dose may be increased to 400 mg 4 times daily or rarely (e.g. as in stress ulceration) to a max. of 2.4 g daily in divided doses; CHILD 20–30 mg/kg daily in divided doses

Maintenance, 400 mg at night *or* 400 mg morning and night

Reflux oesophagitis, 400 mg 4 times daily for 4–8 weeks, Zollinger-Ellison syndrome, 400 mg 4 times daily or occasionally more

Gastric acid reduction (prophylaxis of acid aspiration; do not use syrup), obstetrics 400 mg at start of labour, then up to 400 mg every 4 hours if required (max. of 2.4 g daily); surgical procedures 400 mg 90–120 minutes before induction of general anaesthesia

Short-bowel syndrome, 400 mg twice daily (with breakfast and at bedtime) adjusted according to response

To reduce degradation of pancreatic enzyme supplements, 0.8–1.6 g daily in 4 divided doses according to response 1–1½ hours before meals

*By intramuscular injection*, 200 mg every 4–6 hours; max. 2.4 g daily

*By slow intravenous injection*, 200 mg given over at least 2 minutes; may be repeated every 4–6 hours; if a larger dose is needed or there is cardiovascular impairment, the dose should be diluted and given over at least 10 minutes (infusion is preferable); max. 2.4 g daily

*By intravenous infusion*, 400 mg in 100 mL of sodium chloride 0.9% intravenous infusion infused over ½–1 hour (may be repeated every 4–6 hours) *or* by continuous infusion at an average rate of 50–100 mg/hour over 24 hours, max. 2.4 g daily; CHILD, *by intramuscular injection or slow intravenous injection or infusion*, 20–30 mg/kg daily in divided doses

PoM **Cimetidine** (Non-proprietary)
*Tablets*, cimetidine 200 mg, net price 120-tab pack = £17.64; 400 mg, 60-tab pack = £18.59; 800 mg, 30-tab pack = £17.72
Available from APS (200 mg, 400 mg), Ashbourne (Peptimax® 200 mg, 400 mg, 800 mg), Cox (200 mg, 400 mg, 800 mg), Kerfoot (200 mg, 400 mg, 800 mg)

PoM **Dyspamet®** (Bridge)
*Chewtab®* (chewable tablets), sugar-free, cimetidine 200 mg. Net price 120-tab pack = £16.73. Counselling, chew thoroughly
*Suspension*, sugar-free, cimetidine 200 mg/5 mL. Contains sorbitol 2.79 g/5 mL. Net price 600 mL = £21.89

PoM **Tagamet®** (SK&F)
*Tablets*, all green, f/c, cimetidine 200 mg, net price 120-tab pack = £17.80; 400 mg, 60-tab pack = £20.56; 800 mg, 30-tab pack = £20.56
*Effervescent tablets*, sugar-free, cimetidine 400 mg. Contains 7.7 mmol Na⁺/tablet. Net price 60-tab pack = £18.69. Label: 13
*Syrup*, orange, cimetidine 200 mg/5 mL. Net price 600 mL = £25.90
*Injection*, cimetidine 100 mg/mL. Net price 2-mL amp = 30p
*Intravenous infusion*, cimetidine 4 mg/mL in sodium chloride intravenous infusion 0.9%. Net price 100-mL infusion bag = £1.86

Cimetidine with alginate
PoM **Algitec®** (SK&F)
*Chewtab®* (chewable tablets), off-white, cimetidine 200 mg, alginic acid 500 mg. Contains 2.05 mmol Na⁺/tablet. Net price 120-tab pack = £22.49. Counselling, chew thoroughly
*Suspension*, cimetidine 100 mg, sodium alginate 250 mg/5 mL. Contains 1.43 mmol Na⁺/5 mL. Net price 600 mL = £15.41
*Dose:* gastro-oesophageal reflux disease, 1 tablet chewed or 10 mL suspension 4 times daily (after meals and at bedtime), increased if necessary to 2 tablets or 20 mL suspension 4 times daily; to be taken for 4–8 weeks

## FAMOTIDINE

*Indications:* see under Dose
*Cautions:* see under Cimetidine; does not inhibit hepatic microsomal drug metabolism
*Side-effects:* see under Cimetidine
*Dose:* benign gastric and duodenal ulceration, treatment, 40 mg at night for 4–8 weeks; maintenance, 20 mg at night

Gastro-oesophageal reflux disease, 20 mg twice daily for 6–12 weeks

Zollinger–Ellison syndrome, 20 mg every 6 hours (higher dose in those who have previously been receiving another $H_2$-antagonist)

PoM **Pepcid**® (Morson)
*Tablets*, famotidine 20 mg (beige), net price 28-tab pack = £14.00; 40 mg (brown), 28-tab pack = £26.60

## NIZATIDINE

*Indications:* see under Dose
*Cautions:* see under Cimetidine; does not inhibit hepatic microsomal drug metabolism
*Side-effects:* see under Cimetidine; sweating also reported; rare reports of gynaecomastia
*Dose:* benign gastric and duodenal ulceration, treatment, 300 mg at night *or* 150 mg twice daily for 4–8 weeks; maintenance, 150 mg at night for up to 1 year
Gastro-oesophageal reflux disease, 150–300 mg twice daily for up to 12 weeks

PoM **Axid**® (Lilly)
*Capsules*, nizatidine 150 mg (pale yellow/dark yellow), net price 28-cap pack = £14.11; 300 mg (pale yellow/brown), 28-cap pack = £27.05

## RANITIDINE

*Indications:* benign gastric and duodenal ulceration, stomal ulcer, reflux oesophagitis, Zollinger–Ellison syndrome, other conditions where reduction of gastric acidity is beneficial (see notes above and section 1.9.4)
*Cautions:* see under Cimetidine; does not significantly inhibit hepatic microsomal drug metabolism
*Side-effects:* see under Cimetidine; rare reports of breast swelling and tenderness in men
*Dose: by mouth*, 150 mg twice daily (morning and night), or for patients with gastric and duodenal ulceration 300 mg as a single daily dose at night, for 4 to 8 weeks, up to 6 weeks in chronic episodic dyspepsia, and up to 8 weeks in reflux oesophagitis and NSAID-associated ulceration in duodenal ulcer 300 mg can be given twice daily for 4 weeks to achieve a higher healing rate
Zollinger–Ellison syndrome, 150 mg 3 times daily increased if necessary to up to 6 g daily in divided doses
Maintenance, 150 mg at night
CHILD 8–18 years up to 150 mg twice daily
Gastric acid reduction (prophylaxis of acid aspiration) in obstetrics, *by mouth*, 150 mg at onset of labour, then every 6 hours; surgical procedures, *by intramuscular or slow intravenous injection*, 50 mg 45–60 minutes before induction (intravenous injection diluted to 20 mL and given over at least 2 minutes), or *by mouth*, 150 mg 2 hours before induction, and also, when possible on the preceding evening
*By intramuscular injection*, 50 mg every 6–8 hours
*By slow intravenous injection*, 50 mg diluted to 20 mL and given over at least 2 minutes; may be repeated every 6–8 hours

*By intravenous infusion*, 25 mg/hour for 2 hours; may be repeated every 6–8 hours
*or*, for prophylaxis of stress ulceration, following initial slow intravenous injection of 50 mg (as above) by *continuous infusion*, 125–250 micrograms/kg per hour

PoM **Zantac**® (Glaxo)
*Tablets*, f/c, ranitidine (as hydrochloride) 150 mg, net price 60-tab pack = £29.76; 300 mg, 30-tab pack = £27.43
*Dispersible tablets*, f/c, scored, sugar-free, ranitidine 150 mg (as hydrochloride). Net price 60-tab pack = £31.25. Label: 13
*Effervescent tablets*, pale yellow, ranitidine (as hydrochloride) 150 mg (contains 14.3 mmol Na⁺/tablet), net price 60-tab pack = £31.25; 300 mg (contains 20.8 mmol Na⁺/tablet), 30-tab pack = £31.25. Label: 13
*Syrup*, sugar-free, ranitidine (as hydrochloride) 75 mg/5 mL. Net price 300 mL = £22.32
*Injection*, ranitidine 25 mg (as hydrochloride)/mL. Net price 2-mL amp = 64p

### 1.3.2 Selective antimuscarinics

**Pirenzepine** is a selective antimuscarinic drug which inhibits gastric acid and pepsin secretion with fewer peripheral side-effects than the drugs in section 1.2. As it does not cross the blood-brain barrier it is unlikely to have central effects. It is as effective as $H_2$-receptor antagonists in healing *gastric and duodenal ulcers* and may also be useful in maintenance treatment. It has also been used in conjunction with $H_2$-receptor antagonists in resistant cases.

## PIRENZEPINE

*Indications:* benign gastric and duodenal ulceration
*Side-effects:* occasionally dry mouth and visual disturbances; agranulocytosis and thrombocytopenia have been reported
*Dose:* 50 mg twice daily, increased if necessary to a max. of 150 mg daily in 3 divided doses, for 4–6 weeks, or in resistant cases for up to 3 months. Doses should preferably be taken 30 minutes before meals

PoM **Gastrozepin**® (Boots)
*Tablets*, scored, pirenzepine hydrochloride, equivalent to anhydrous pirenzepine hydrochloride, 50 mg. Net price 60 = £24.60. Label: 22

### 1.3.3 Chelates and complexes

**Tripotassium dicitratobismuthate** is a bismuth chelate effective in healing *gastric and duodenal ulcers*. It may act by a direct toxic effect on gastric *Helicobacter (Campylobacter) pylori*, or by stimulating mucosal prostaglandin or bicarbonate secretion. The healing tends to be longer lasting but relapse still occurs. The bismuth content is low but absorption has been reported; encephalopathy (described with older high-dose bismuth

---

preparations) has not been reported. As the elixir, which has a pungent ammoniacal odour, is likely to adhere to food rather than to the surface of the ulcer, patients should be advised to avoid food, antacids, and large quantities of milk when taking doses. Tablets are as effective as the liquid and more palatable.

Sucralfate is another effective treatment for *gastric and duodenal ulcers* and may act by protecting the mucosa from acid-pepsin attack. It is a complex of aluminium hydroxide and sulphated sucrose but has minimal antacid properties.

## BISMUTH CHELATE

*Indications:* benign gastric and duodenal ulceration
*Cautions:* avoid in severe renal impairment; see also notes above; **interactions:** Appendix 1 (bismuth chelate)
*Side-effects:* may darken tongue and blacken faeces; nausea and vomiting reported

### De-Nol® (Brocades)
*Liquid*, red, tripotassium dicitratobismuthate 120 mg/5 mL. Net price 560 mL = £14.65. Counselling, see below
*Dose:* adults, 10 mL twice daily *or* 5 mL 4 times daily; taken for 28 days, followed by further 28 days if necessary; maintenance not indicated but course may be repeated after interval of 1 month; CHILDREN, no longer recommended
COUNSELLING. Each dose to be diluted with 15 mL of water; twice daily dosage to be taken 30 minutes before breakfast and main evening meal; four times daily dosage to be taken as follows: one dose 30 minutes before breakfast, midday meal and main evening meal, and one dose 2 hours after main evening meal; milk should not be drunk by itself during treatment but small quantities may be taken in tea or coffee or on cereal; antacids should not be taken half an hour before or after a dose; may darken tongue and blacken faeces

### De-Noltab® (Brocades)
*Tablets*, white, tripotassium dicitratobismuthate 120 mg. Net price 112-tab pack = £20.98. Counselling, see below
*Dose:* adults 2 tablets twice daily *or* 1 tablet 4 times daily; taken for 28 days followed by further 28 days if necessary; maintenance not indicated but course may be repeated after interval of 1 month; CHILD, not recommended
COUNSELLING. Each dose to be swallowed with a tumblerful of water then as above under De-Nol

## SUCRALFATE

*Indications:* benign gastric and duodenal ulceration; chronic gastritis
*Cautions:* renal disease; **interactions:** Appendix 1 (sucralfate)
*Side-effects:* constipation; diarrhoea, nausea, indigestion, dry mouth, rash, pruritus, back pain, dizziness, insomnia, and vertigo; also gastric discomfort reported

*Dose:* 2 g twice daily (on rising and at bedtime) *or* 1 g 4 times daily 1 hour before meals and at bedtime, taken for up to 6 weeks or in resistant cases 12 weeks; max. 8 g daily
Prophylaxis of stress ulceration (suspension), 1 g 6 times daily (max. 8 g daily)
COUNSELLING. Tablets may be dispersed in 10–15 mL of water; antacids should not be taken half an hour before or after a dose

### PoM Antepsin® (Wyeth)
*Tablets*, scored, sucralfate 1 g. Net price 20 = £2.50. Label: 5, counselling, see dose above
*Suspension*, sucralfate, 1 g/5 mL. Net price 560 mL = £14.00. Label: 5, counselling, antacids

## 1.3.4   Prostaglandin analogues

Misoprostol, a synthetic analogue of prostaglandin $E_1$ (alprostadil) inhibits gastric acid secretion promoting *gastric and duodenal ulcer* healing. It can protect against *NSAID-associated gastric ulcers* but not dyspepsia.

## MISOPROSTOL

*Indications:* see notes above and under Dose
*Cautions:* conditions where hypotension might precipitate severe complications (e.g. cerebrovascular disease, cardiovascular disease)
*Contra-indications:* pregnancy or planning pregnancy (increases uterine tone)
*Side-effects:* diarrhoea (may be severe, reduced by giving single doses not exceeding 200 micrograms and by avoiding magnesium-containing antacids); also reported: abdominal pain, dyspepsia, flatulence, nausea and vomiting, abnormal vaginal bleeding (including intermenstrual bleeding, menorrhagia, and postmenopausal bleeding)
*Dose:* benign gastric and duodenal ulceration and NSAID-associated ulceration, 800 micrograms daily (in 2–4 divided doses) with breakfast (or main meals) and at bedtime; treatment should be continued for at least 4 weeks and may be continued for up to 8 weeks if required
Prophylaxis of NSAID-induced gastric ulcer, 200 micrograms 2–4 times daily according to condition of patient

### PoM Cytotec® (Searle)
*Tablets*, scored, misoprostol 200 micrograms. Net price 56-tab pack = £13.00; 112-tab pack = £26.00

With naproxen
Section 10.1.1.

## 1.3.5   Proton pump inhibitors

Omeprazole inhibits gastric acid by blocking the hydrogen-potassium adenosine triphosphatase enzyme system (the 'proton pump') of the gastric parietal cell. It is an effective treatment for *gastric and duodenal ulcers* and particularly for *erosive oesophagitis*.

## OMEPRAZOLE

*Indications:* see under Dose

*Cautions:* exclude malignancy; avoid in pregnancy and breast-feeding; **interactions:** Appendix 1 (omeprazole)

*Side-effects:* diarrhoea, headache (both may be severe); also nausea, constipation, and flatulence; skin reactions (some serious), photosensitivity reported

*Dose:* benign gastric and duodenal ulcers (including those complicating NSAID therapy) 20 mg daily for 4 weeks in duodenal ulceration or 8 weeks in gastric ulceration; in severe cases increase to 40 mg daily; long-term use not recommended

Zollinger–Ellison syndrome, initially 60 mg once daily; usual range 20–120 mg daily (above 80 mg in 2 divided doses)

Healing of reflux oesophagitis, 20 mg daily for 4 weeks, followed by a further 4–8 weeks if not fully healed; 40 mg daily has been given for 8 weeks in reflux oesophagitis refractory to other treatment; may be continued at 20 mg daily

▼ PoM **Losec**® (Astra)

*Capsules,* pink/brown, enclosing e/c granules, omeprazole 20 mg, net price 28-cap pack = £36.36 (also 5-cap pack, hosp. only). Label: 25

### 1.3.6   Other ulcer-healing drugs

**Carbenoxolone**, a synthetic derivative of glycyrrhizinic acid (a constituent of liquorice) is effective in *gastric ulcer*; it is also effective in *duodenal ulcer* if released at the site of the lesion. However, side-effects (commonly sodium and water retention and occasionally hypokalaemia) may cause or exacerbate hypertension, oedema, cardiac failure, and muscle weakness. For these reasons other drugs are preferred; if used regular monitoring of weight, blood pressure, and electrolytes is advisable during treatment. Carbenoxolone may act by protecting the mucosal barrier from acid–pepsin attack and increasing mucosal mucin production.

**Deglycyrrhizinised liquorice** is free from the above side-effects but is of doubtful efficacy.

### CARBENOXOLONE SODIUM

*Indications:* benign gastric and duodenal ulceration in young and middle-aged patients

*Cautions:* cardiac disease, hypertension, impaired hepatic and renal function; elderly (see under preparations); not recommended in children. See also notes above. Potassium supplements and thiazides may be necessary; **interactions:** Appendix 1 (carbenoxolone)

*Contra-indications:* hypokalaemia, pregnancy; avoid use with spironolactone and amiloride

*Side-effects:* sodium and water retention leading to oedema, alkalosis, hypertension, hypokalaemia

PoM **Biogastrone**® (Sanofi Winthrop)

*Tablets,* scored, carbenoxolone sodium 50 mg. Net price 100-tab pack = £22.77. Label: 21

*Dose:* for gastric ulceration, 2 tablets 3 times daily after meals for 1 week, then 1 tablet 3 times daily for 6–12 weeks; not recommended under 16 years or over 65 years

Compound preparation

PoM **Pyrogastrone**® (Sanofi Winthrop)

*Tablets,* chewable, carbenoxolone sodium 20 mg, alginic acid 600 mg, dried aluminium hydroxide 240 mg, magnesium trisilicate 60 mg, sodium bicarbonate 210 mg (Na⁺ 2.6 mmol/tablet). Net price 100-tab pack = £25.49. Label: 21, 24

*Liquid,* carbenoxolone sodium 10 mg, dried aluminium hydroxide 150 mg (Na⁺ 0.85 mmol, K⁺ 1.5 mmol)/5 mL when reconstituted with water. Net price 500 mL = £12.71. Label: 21

*Dose:* for oesophageal inflammation and ulceration, 1 tablet, chewed, 3 times daily after meals, and 2 at night, for 6–12 weeks or 10 mL liquid 3 times daily after meals and 20 mL at night, for 6–12 weeks; not recommended for children or for adults over 75 years

### LIQUORICE, DEGLYCYRRHIZINISED

*Indications:* benign gastric and duodenal ulceration

**Caved-S**® (Tillotts)

*Tablets,* brown, deglycyrrhizinised liquorice 380 mg, aluminium hydroxide mixture 100 mg, bismuth subnitrate 100 mg, magnesium carbonate 200 mg, sodium bicarbonate 100 mg. Net price 20 = £1.25. Label: 24

*Dose:* benign gastric and duodenal ulceration, treatment, 2 tablets chewed 3 times daily (for duodenal ulceration increased if necessary to 6 times daily); maintenance, 1 tablet chewed 3 times daily (gastric ulceration), 2 tablets chewed 3 times daily (duodenal ulceration); CHILD no longer recommended

*Note.* Caved-S® tablets now contain bismuth subnitrate; long-term use should be avoided, see also section 1.1.3

**Rabro**® (Sinclair)

*Tablets,* brown, deglycyrrhizinised liquorice 400 mg, calcium carbonate 500 mg, frangula 25 mg, magnesium oxide 100 mg. Net price 20 = £1.22. Label: 21, 24

*Dose:* 1–2 tablets chewed and swallowed with liquid 3 times daily after meals for 1–2 months

## 1.4   Antidiarrhoeal drugs

1.4.1   Adsorbents and bulk-forming drugs

1.4.2   Antimotility drugs

The **first line** of treatment in acute diarrhoea, as in gastro-enteritis, is prevention or treatment of fluid and electrolyte depletion. This is particularly important in infants and in frail and elderly patients. Clinical signs of severe dehydration require immediate admission to hospital and urgent replacement of fluid and electrolytes. For details of **oral rehydration therapy** and of preparations available, see section 9.2.1.2.

Antidiarrhoeal drugs are of secondary value in the treatment of diarrhoea, may have undesirable side-effects, and may distract from giving fluids.

Antispasmodics (section 1.2) are occasionally of value in treating abdominal cramp associated with diarrhoea but they should not be used for primary treatment. Antispasmodics and antiemetics should be **avoided** in young children with gastro-enteritis as they are rarely effective and have troublesome side-effects.

Antibiotics and sulphonamides are generally unnecessary in simple gastro-enteritis, even when a bacterial cause is suspected, because the complaint will usually resolve quickly without such treatment, and infective diarrhoeas in the UK are often caused by viral infections. Systemic bacterial infection does, however, need appropriate systemic treatment. **Erythromycin** (see section 5.1.5) or **ciprofloxacin** (see section 5.1.12) can be used for treating enteritis caused by *Campylobacter* spp. For drugs for shigellosis and salmonellosis, see section 5.1, table 1. The general use of sulphonamides in treating diarrhoea of travellers is inadvisable because of the risks of rash and agranulocytosis.

Poorly absorbed drugs such as dihydrostreptomycin, neomycin, and sulphaguanidine should be **avoided** altogether in gastro-intestinal infection. They prolong rather than shorten the time taken to control diarrhoea by causing masked bacterial diarrhoea, carrier states, or pseudomembranous colitis. Clioquinol should be avoided as it is neurotoxic; both it and lactobacillus preparations are valueless.

## 1.4.1  Adsorbents and bulk-forming drugs

Adsorbents such as kaolin are **not** recommended for *acute diarrhoeas*. Bulk-forming drugs, such as ispaghula, methylcellulose, and sterculia (see section 1.6.1) are useful in controlling faecal consistency in ileostomy and colostomy, and in controlling diarrhoea associated with diverticular disease.

### KAOLIN, LIGHT
*Indications:* diarrhoea but see notes above
*Cautions:* **interactions:** Appendix 1 (antacids and adsorbents)

**Kaolin Mixture** (BP)
(Kaolin Oral Suspension)
*Oral suspension,* light kaolin or light kaolin (natural) 20%, and 5% each of light magnesium carbonate and sodium bicarbonate in a suitable vehicle with a peppermint flavour. Extemporaneous preparations should be prepared according to the following formula: light kaolin or light kaolin (natural) 2 g, light magnesium carbonate 500 mg, sodium bicarbonate 500 mg, concentrated peppermint emulsion 0.25 mL, double-strength chloroform water 5 mL, water to 10 mL. It should be recently prepared, unless the kaolin has been sterilised. Net price 200 mL = 57p
*Dose:* 10–20 mL every 4 hours
**Kaopectate**® (Upjohn)
*Mixture,* sugar-free, kaolin 1.03 g/5 mL. Diluent water, life of diluted mixture 14 days. Net price 100 mL = 94p
*Dose:* 10–30 mL every 4 hours; CHILD not recommended therefore no dose stated
**KLN**® (Ashe)
*Mixture,* kaolin 1.15 g, pectin 57.5 mg, sodium citrate 17.25 mg/5 mL. Net price 100 mL = £1.12
*Dose:* CHILD not recommended therefore no dose stated

## 1.4.2  Antimotility drugs

In *acute diarrhoeas* antimotility drugs have a very limited role as adjuncts to fluid and electrolyte replacement (see section 9.2.1.2); they are **not** recommended for acute diarrhoeas in young children.

For comments on their role in *chronic diarrhoeas* see section 1.5.

## CODEINE PHOSPHATE
*Indications:* see notes above
*Cautions; Contra-indications; Side-effects:* see section 4.7.2; not recommended for children; tolerance and dependence may occur with prolonged use; **interactions:** Appendix 1 (opioid analgesics)
*Dose:* see under Preparations below

PoM **Codeine Phosphate Tablets,** codeine phosphate 15 mg, net price 20 = 38p; 30 mg, 20 = 39p; 60 mg, 20 = £1.24. Label: 2
*Dose:* 30 mg 3–4 times daily (range 15–60 mg); CHILD not recommended
*Note.* Travellers needing to take codeine phosphate tablets abroad may require a doctor's letter explaining why they are necessary.

PoM **Diarrest**® (Galen)
*Liquid,* yellow, codeine phosphate 5 mg, dicyclomine hydrochloride 2.5 mg, potassium chloride 40 mg, sodium chloride 50 mg, sodium citrate 50 mg/5 mL. For diarrhoea, vomiting, and cramp. Net price 200 mL = £3.34
*Dose:* 20 mL 4 times daily with water; CHILD 4–5 years 5 mL, 6–9 years 10 mL, 10–13 years 15 mL but see cautions and notes above

**Kaodene**® (Boots)
*Mixture,* codeine phosphate 10 mg, light kaolin 3 g/10 mL. Net price 250 mL = 98p
*Dose:* 20 mL 3–4 times daily; CHILD over 5 years 10 mL but see cautions and notes above

## CO-PHENOTROPE
A mixture of diphenoxylate hydrochloride and atropine sulphate in the mass proportions 100 parts to 1 part respectively
*Indications:* adjunct to rehydration in acute diarrhoea (but see notes above); chronic mild ulcerative colitis
*Cautions; Contra-indications; Side-effects:* see notes above and under Codeine Phosphate; young children are particularly susceptible to OVERDOSAGE and symptoms may be delayed so that observation is needed for at least 48 hours after ingestion; in addition the presence of sub-clinical doses of atropine may give rise to the side-effects of atropine in susceptible individuals or in overdosage

PoM **Lomotil**® (Gold Cross)
*Tablets,* co-phenotrope 2.5/0.025 (diphenoxylate hydrochloride 2.5 mg, atropine sulphate 25 micrograms). Net price 20 = £1.96
*Dose:* initially 4 tablets, followed by 2 tablets every 6 hours until diarrhoea controlled; CHILD 4–8 years 1 tablet 3 times daily, 9–12 years 1 tablet 4 times daily, 13–16 years 2 tablets 3 times daily, but see also notes above

*Liquid,* red, sugar-free, co-phenotrope 2.5/0.025 (diphenoxylate hydrochloride 2.5 mg, atropine sulphate 25 micrograms)/5 mL. Diluent glycerol, life of diluted preparation 14 days. Net price 100 mL = £3.73
*Dose:* initially 20 mL, followed by 10 mL every 6 hours until diarrhoea controlled; CHILD 4–8 years 5 mL 3 times daily, 9–12 years 5 mL 4 times daily, 13–16 years 10 mL 3 times daily, but see also notes above
*Note.* Co-phenotrope 2.5/0.025 tablets are also available from Mepra-pharm (Diarphen®)

---

## LOPERAMIDE HYDROCHLORIDE

*Indications:* adjunct to rehydration in acute diarrhoea in adults and children over 4 years (but see notes above); chronic diarrhoea in adults only

*Cautions; Contra-indications:* see notes above and under Codeine Phosphate (except dependence)

*Side-effects:* abdominal cramps and skin reactions, including urticaria reported; paralytic ileus and abdominal bloating also reported

*Dose:* acute diarrhoea, 4 mg initially followed by 2 mg after each loose stool for up to 5 days; usual dose 6–8 mg daily; max. 16 mg daily; CHILD 4–8 years 1 mg 4 times daily for up to *3 days only*, 9–12 years 2 mg 4 times daily for up to 5 days

Chronic diarrhoea in adults, initially, 4–8 mg daily in divided doses, subsequently adjusted according to response and given in 2 divided doses for maintenance

PoM[1] **Loperamide** (Non-proprietary)
*Capsules,* loperamide hydrochloride 2 mg. Net price 30 = £2.10

PoM[1] **Imodium®** (Janssen)
*Capsules,* green/grey, loperamide hydrochloride 2 mg. Net price 30 = £2.17
*Syrup,* red, sugar-free, loperamide hydrochloride 1 mg/5 mL. Diluent water, life of diluted preparation 14 days. Net price 100 mL = £1.90
1. Loperamide can be sold to the public, for adults and children over 12 years, provided it is licensed and labelled for the treatment of acute diarrhoea; proprietary brands (Arret® capsules and adult syrup and Diocalm Ultra® capsules) are on sale to the public

## MORPHINE

*Indications:* see notes above

*Cautions; Contra-indications; Side-effects:* see notes above and under Codeine Phosphate, sedation and the risk of dependence are greater

**Kaolin and Morphine Mixture** (BP)
(Kaolin and Morphine Oral Suspension)
*Oral suspension,* light kaolin or light kaolin (natural) 20%, sodium bicarbonate 5%, and chloroform and morphine tincture 4% in a suitable vehicle. Extemporaneous preparations should be prepared according to the following formula: light kaolin or light kaolin (natural) 2 g, sodium bicarbonate 500 mg, chloroform and morphine tincture 0.4 mL, water to 10 mL. It should be recently prepared, unless the kaolin has been sterilised. Contains 550 to 800 micrograms of anhydrous morphine/10 mL.
*Dose:* 10 mL every 4 hours in water

# 1.5   Treatment of chronic diarrhoeas

Once tumours are ruled out individual complaints need specific treatment including dietary manipulation as well as drug treatment and the maintenance of a liberal fluid intake.

IRRITABLE BOWEL SYNDROME. This can present with pain, constipation, or diarrhoea, all of which may benefit from a high-fibre diet with bran or other agents which increase stool bulk (section 1.6.1) if necessary. In some patients there may be important psychological aggravating factors which respond to reassurance. Antidiarrhoeal drugs such as **loperamide** may sometimes be necessary but prolonged use may aggravate the condition (section 1.4.2). Opioids such as codeine are better avoided because of the risk of dependence. Antispasmodics (section 1.2) may relieve the pain.

MALABSORPTION SYNDROMES. Individual conditions need specific treatment and also general nutritional consideration. Thus coeliac disease (gluten enteropathy) usually needs a gluten-free diet (Appendix 7) and pancreatic insufficiency needs pancreatin supplements (section 1.9.4).

ULCERATIVE COLITIS. For *acute attacks* topical **corticosteroid** treatment such as prednisolone enemas or suppositories for localised rectal disease will induce remission; foam preparations are especially useful where patients have difficulty retaining liquid enemas. More extensive disease requires oral corticosteroid treatment and severe extensive or fulminant disease needs hospital admission and intravenous corticosteroid administration.

**Sulphasalazine,** a chemical combination of sulphapyridine and 5-aminosalicylic acid ('5-ASA') is useful in mild symptomatic disease requiring oral treatment; it is also available as suppositories for rectal disease. Activity resides in the 5-aminosalicylic acid moiety; sulphapyridine acts only as a carrier to the colonic site of action (but it still causes side-effects). Newer alternatives include **mesalazine** (5-aminosalicylic acid itself, in a modified-release tablet) and **olsalazine** (2 molecules of 5-aminosalicylic acid bonded together, separating in the lower bowel). The sulphonamide-related side-effects of suphasalazine (rashes, blood disorders, azoospermia, and lupoid syndromes) are lacking from mesalazine and olsalazine, but they retain side-effect profiles associated with the 5-aminosalicylic acid moiety (watery diarrhoea, salicylate hypersensitivity, and interstitial nephritis).

Corticosteroids are unsuitable for *maintenance treatment* because of side-effects. Sulphasalazine, mesalazine, and olsalazine all have value in preventing relapse and choice is related in part to their different side-effects. In resistant cases **azathioprine** (see section 8.2.1), 2 mg/kg daily, given under close supervision may be helpful.

Laxatives are required to facilitate bowel movement when proctitis is present but a high-fibre diet and bulk-forming drugs such as **methylcellulose** are more useful in adjusting faecal consistency (section 1.6.1).

Antimotility drugs such as codeine and loperamide should not be used in severe colitis as they can precipitate paralytic ileus and megacolon. They have limited value in mild disease: treatment of the inflammation is more logical. For similar reasons antispasmodics should **not** be used in ulcerative colitis.

CROHN'S DISEASE. Treatment particularly of colonic disease is similar to that for ulcerative colitis. In small bowel disease **sulphasalazine** is of doubtful value. **Oral corticosteroids** (e.g. prednisolone) suppress inflammation, and **metronidazole** may be beneficial possibly through antibacterial activity. Other antibacterials should be given if specifically indicated and for managing bacterial overgrowth in the small bowel.

In both colitis and Crohn's disease general nutritional care and appropriate supplements are essential.

**Cholestyramine** and **aluminium hydroxide mixture** (section 1.1.1), bind unabsorbed bile salts and provide symptomatic relief of diarrhoea following ileal disease or resection, in bacterial colonisation of the small bowel, and in postvagotomy diarrhoea.

PSEUDOMEMBRANOUS COLITIS. This is due to colonisation of the colon with *Clostridium difficile* which may develop after antibiotic therapy. It is usually of acute onset, but may run a chronic course; it is a particular hazard of clindamycin and lincomycin but few antibiotics are free of this side-effect. Oral **vancomycin** (see section 5.1.7) or **metronidazole** (see section 5.1.11) are used as specific treatment; vancomycin may be preferred for very sick patients.

DIVERTICULAR DISEASE. This is treated with a high-fibre diet, **bran supplements**, and **bulk-forming drugs**. Antispasmodics may provide symptomatic relief when colic is a problem (section 1.2). **Antibiotics** should be used only when the diverticula in the intestinal wall become infected. **Antidiarrhoeal** drugs which slow intestinal motility, for example codeine, diphenoxylate, and loperamide could possibly exacerbate the symptoms of diverticular disease and are **contra-indicated**.

## AMINOSALICYLATES

### SULPHASALAZINE
*Indications:* induction and maintenance of remission in ulcerative colitis; treatment of active Crohn's disease (for use in rheumatoid arthritis see section 10.1.3)
*Cautions:* pregnancy; hepatic and renal disease; G6PD deficiency (including breast-feeding of affected infants); slow acetylator status; withdraw treatment if blood disorders, hypersensitivity reactions, or other serious disorders occur; upper gastro-intestinal side-effects become common with doses over 4 g daily; blood counts, liver-function tests, and rheumatoid arthritis, see section 10.1.3
*Contra-indications:* salicylate and sulphonamide hypersensitivity; porphyria (see section 9.8.2)
*Side-effects:* nausea, vomiting, epigastric discomfort, headache, rashes; *occasionally:* fever, minor haematological abnormalities such as Heinz-body anaemia, reversible neutropenia, folate deficiency; reversible azoospermia; *rarely:* pancreatitis, hepatitis, exacerbation of colitis, thrombocytopenia, agranulocytosis, Stevens–Johnson syndrome, neurotoxicity, photosensitisation, lupus erythematosus-like syndrome, and pneumonitis; proteinuria, crystalluria, haematuria, and nephrotic syndrome; urine may be coloured orange; some soft contact lenses may be stained
*Dose: by mouth,* acute attack 1–2 g 4 times daily (but see **cautions**) until remission occurs (if necessary corticosteroids may also be given), reducing to a maintenance dose of 500 mg 4 times daily; CHILD over 2 years, acute attack 40–60 mg/kg daily, maintenance dose 20–30 mg/kg daily
*By rectum,* in suppositories, alone or in conjunction with oral treatment 0.5–1 g morning and night after a bowel movement. As an enema, 3 g at night, retained for at least 1 hour

**PoM Salazopyrin®** (Kabi Pharmacia)
*Tablets,* orange-brown, scored, sulphasalazine 500 mg. Net price 20 = £1.41. Label: 14, counselling, lenses see above
*EN-tablets®* (= tablets e/c), yellow, f/c, sulphasalazine 500 mg. Net price 125-tab pack = £12.75. Label: 5, 14, 25, counselling, lenses see above
*Suspension,* yellow, sulphasalazine 250 mg/5 mL. Net price 473 mL = £15.95. Label: 14, counselling, lenses see above
*Suppositories,* brown, sulphasalazine 500 mg. Net price 10 = £2.95; 50 = £14.02. Label: 14, counselling, lenses see above
*Retention enema,* sulphasalazine 3 g in 100-mL single-dose disposable packs fitted with a nozzle. Net price 7 × 100 mL = £12.75. Label: 14, counselling, lenses see above

## MESALAZINE
*Indications:* maintenance of remission in ulcerative colitis and treatment of mild to moderate exacerbations
*Cautions:* elderly; pregnancy and breast-feeding
*Contra-indications:* salicylate hypersensitivity; renal impairment (nephrotoxic)
*Side-effects:* nausea, diarrhoea, and abdominal pain; headache; exacerbation of symptoms of colitis; rarely reversible pancreatitis, hepatitis, and interstitial nephritis; leucopenia, neutropenia, and thrombocytopenia reported; reversible myocarditis also reported
*Dose: by mouth,* 1.2–2.4 g daily in divided doses
*By rectum,* see under preparations

**PoM Asacol®** (SK&F)
*Tablets,* red, coated with an acrylic-based resin, mesalazine 400 mg. Net price 120-tab pack = £34.30. Label: 25
*Suppositories,* mesalazine 250 mg, net price 20 = £6.50; 100 mg, 10 = £6.50
*Dose:* 3–6 suppositories of 250 mg (max. 3 suppositories of 500 mg) daily in divided doses, with last dose at bedtime

PoM **Pentasa**® (Nordic)

*Tablets*, m/r, enclosing coated granules, mesalazine 250 mg. Net price 200-tab pack = £32.28. Label: 25

*Dose:* maintenance of remission 2 tablets 3 times daily

*Retention enema*, mesalazine 1 g in 100-mL single-dose bottle. Net price 7 × 100 mL = £19.45.

*Dose:* 100 mL enema at bedtime

## OLSALAZINE SODIUM

*Indications:* treatment of acute mild ulcerative colitis and maintenance of remission

*Cautions:* elderly; pregnancy and breast-feeding

*Contra-indications:* salicylate hypersensitivity; renal impairment

*Side-effects:* diarrhoea, abdominal cramps, headache, nausea, dyspepsia, arthralgia, and rash; rarely reversible pancreatitis

*Dose:* acute attack, 1 g daily in divided doses increased if necessary over 1 week to max. 3 g daily (max. single dose 1 g)

Maintenance, 500 mg twice daily

PoM **Dipentum**® (Kabi Pharmacia)

*Capsules*, brown, olsalazine sodium 250 mg. Net price 20 = £4.78. Label: 21

ANION-EXCHANGE RESINS

## CHOLESTYRAMINE

*Indications:* diarrhoea associated with Crohn's disease, ileal resection, vagotomy, diabetic vagal neuropathy, and radiation; pruritus in liver disease, and hypercholesterolaemia, see section 2.12

*Cautions; Contra-indications; Side-effects:* see section 2.12

*Dose:* diarrhoea, 12–24 g daily mixed with water, in single or divided doses, subsequently adjusted as required; max. 36 g daily

COUNSELLING. Other drugs should be taken at least 1 hour before or 4–6 hours after cholestyramine to reduce possible interference with absorption

**Preparations:** section 2.12

CORTICOSTEROIDS

## HYDROCORTISONE

*Indications:* inflammation associated with colitis, proctitis

*Cautions; Contra-indications; Side-effects:* systemic absorption may occur, see section 6.3.3; prolonged use should be avoided; avoid use of enemas and rectal foams in obstruction, bowel perforation, and extensive fistulas; contra-indicated in untreated infection

*Dose:* rectal, see under Preparations

PoM **Hydrocortisone Suppositories,** hydrocortisone or hydrocortisone acetate 25 mg in theobroma oil or other suitable basis. Net price 10 = £3.59

*Dose:* proctitis, 1 suppository inserted night and morning after a bowel movement

PoM **Colifoam**® (Stafford-Miller)

*Foam* in aerosol pack, hydrocortisone acetate 10%. Net price 25 g (= 14 applications) with applicator = £7.25

*Dose:* initially 1 metered application (125 mg hydrocortisone acetate) inserted into the rectum once or twice daily for 2–3 weeks, then once on alternate days

## PREDNISOLONE

*Indications:* induction and maintenance of remission in ulcerative colitis, and Crohn's disease; other indications, see section 6.3.3

*Cautions; Contra-indications; Side-effects:* see under Hydrocortisone and section 6.3.3

*Dose: by mouth*, initial dose 40 mg daily, in single or divided doses, until remission occurs, followed by reducing doses

*By rectum*, see under Preparations

PoM **Predenema**® (Pharmax)

*Retention enema*, prednisolone 20 mg (as sodium metasulphobenzoate) in 100-mL single-dose disposable pack. Net price 10 (standard tube) = £7.72, 7 (long tube) = £9.26

*Dose:* initially 1 enema at bedtime for 2–4 weeks, extending course if good response obtained

PoM **Predfoam**® (Pharmax)

*Foam* in aerosol pack, prednisolone 20 mg (as metasulphobenzoate sodium)/metered application. Net price 25 g (14 applications) with disposable applicators = £7.25

*Dose:* 1 metered application (containing 20 mg prednisolone) inserted into the rectum once or twice daily for 2 weeks, continued for further 2 weeks if good response

PoM **Predsol**® (Glaxo)

*Retention enema*, prednisolone 20 mg (as sodium phosphate) in 100-mL single-dose disposable packs fitted with a nozzle. Net price 7 = £5.24

*Dose:* initially 1 enema at bedtime for 2–4 weeks, extending course if good response obtained

*Suppositories*, prednisolone 5 mg (as sodium phosphate). Net price 10 = £1.00

*Dose:* proctitis and rectal complications of Crohn's disease, 1 suppository inserted night and morning after a bowel movement

CROMOGLYCATE

## SODIUM CROMOGLYCATE

*Indications:* food allergy (in conjunction with dietary restriction)

*Side-effects:* occasional nausea, rashes, and joint pain

*Dose:* 200 mg 4 times daily before meals; CHILD 2–14 years 100 mg; capsules may be swallowed whole or the contents dissolved in hot water and diluted with cold water before taking. May be increased if necessary after 2–3 weeks to a max. of 40 mg/kg daily and then reduced according to the response

PoM **Nalcrom**® (Fisons)

*Capsules*, sodium cromoglycate 100 mg. Net price 100 = £13.73. Label: 22, counselling, see dose above

## 1.6   Laxatives

**1.6.1** Bulk-forming drugs
**1.6.2** Stimulant laxatives
**1.6.3** Faecal softeners
**1.6.4** Osmotic laxatives

Misconceptions about bowel habits have led to excessive laxative use. Abuse may lead to hypokalaemia and an atonic non-functioning colon. Simple constipation is usually relieved by increasing the intake of dietary fibre. The use of laxatives in children is undesirable and the introduction of fruit purée into the diet may be sufficient to regulate bowel action. In infants constipation is often remedied by adjustment of the diet.

Laxatives should generally be **avoided** except where straining will exacerbate a condition (such as angina) or increase the risk of rectal bleeding as in haemorrhoids. Laxatives are also of value in *drug-induced constipation*, for the expulsion of *parasites* after anthelmintic treatment, and to clear the alimentary tract before *surgery and radiological procedures*.

The laxatives that follow have been divided into 4 main groups (sections 1.6.1–1.6.4). This simple classification disguises the fact that some laxatives have a complex action.

## 1.6.1   Bulk-forming drugs

These relieve constipation by increasing faecal mass which stimulates peristalsis, but patients should be told that the full effect may take some days to develop. They are useful in the management of patients with *colostomy*, *ileostomy*, *haemorrhoids*, *anal fissure*, *chronic diarrhoea associated with diverticular disease*, *irritable bowel syndrome*, and *ulcerative colitis* (section 1.5). Adequate fluid intake must be maintained to avoid intestinal obstruction. Unprocessed wheat **bran**, taken with food or fruit juice, is a most effective bulk-forming preparation. Finely ground bran, though more palatable, has poorer water-retaining properties, but can be taken as bran bread or biscuits in appropriately increased quantities. Oat bran is also used.

**Methylcellulose**, **ispaghula**, and **sterculia** are useful in patients who cannot tolerate bran. Methylcellulose also acts as a faecal softener.

### BRAN

*Indications:* see notes above
*Cautions; Contra-indications; Side-effects:* see under Ispaghula Husk. Calcium and iron absorption may be impaired. Avoid in gluten enteropathies and coeliac disease
*Dose:* see preparations below
COUNSELLING. Preparations that swell in contact with liquid should always be carefully swallowed with water and should not be taken immediately before going to bed

**NHS Fybranta**® (Norgine)
*Tablets*, brown, bran 2 g. Net price 20 = 46p. Label: 24, 27, counselling, see above
*Dose:* 1–3 tablets chewed and swallowed with water 3–4 times daily, preferably with meals

**NHS Proctofibe**® (Roussel)
*Tablets*, beige, f/c, fibrous grain extract 375 mg, fibrous citrus extract 94 mg. Net price 20 = 56p. Counselling, see above
*Dose:* adults and children over 3 years 4–12 tablets daily in divided doses swallowed with plenty of water *or* crushed and dispersed in water

**Trifyba**® (Sanofi)
*Powder*, wheat fibre 80%. Net price 56 sachets containing 3.5 g = £3.36. Counselling, see below
*Dose:* 1 sachet 2–3 times daily added to food; CHILD half to one sachet 1–2 times daily added to food
COUNSELLING. At least one glass of water or other liquid should be drunk with the meal

### ISPAGHULA HUSK

*Indications:* see notes above
*Cautions:* adequate fluid intake should be maintained to avoid intestinal obstruction
*Contra-indications:* intestinal obstruction, colonic atony, faecal impaction
*Side-effects:* flatulence, abdominal distension
*Dose:* see preparations below
COUNSELLING. Preparations that swell in contact with liquid should always be carefully swallowed with water and should not be taken immediately before going to bed

**Fybogel**® (R&C)
*Granules*, buff or orange, effervescent, sugar- and gluten-free, ispaghula husk 3.5 g/sachet. Net price 60 sachets (plain or orange flavoured) = £4.24. Label: 13, counselling, see above
*Note.* Contains potassium approx. 7 mmol/sachet
*Dose:* 1 sachet in water twice daily preferably after meals; CHILD ½–1 level 5-mL spoonful

**Isogel**® (Charwell)
*Granules*, pink, sugar-free, ispaghula husk 90%. Net price 200 g = £1.51. Label: 13, counselling, see above
*Dose:* constipation, 2 teaspoonfuls in water once or twice daily, preferably at mealtimes; CHILD 1 teaspoonful
Diarrhoea (section 1.4.1), 1 teaspoonful 3 times daily

**Metamucil**® (Proctor & Gamble)
*Powder*, buff, ispaghula husk 49%, gluten-free. Net price 200 g = 80p. Label: 13, counselling, see above
*Dose:* one 5-mL spoonful 1–3 times daily in 150 mL water; CHILD 6–12 years 2.5–5 mL

**Regulan**® (Proctor & Gamble)
*Powder*, beige, effervescent, ispaghula husk 3.6 g/6.4-g sachet (gluten-free). Net price 30 sachets = £2.12. Label: 13, counselling, see above
*Note.* Contains potassium 6.4 mmol/sachet
*Dose:* 1 sachet in 150 mL water 1–3 times daily; CHILD 6–12 years 2.5–5 mL

## METHYLCELLULOSE

*Indications:* see notes above
*Cautions; Contra-indications; Side-effects:* see under Ispaghula Husk
*Dose:* see preparations below

COUNSELLING. Preparations that swell in contact with liquid should always be carefully swallowed with water and should not be taken immediately before going to bed

### Celevac® (Boehringer Ingelheim)

*Tablets,* pink, methylcellulose '450' 500 mg. Net price 112-tab pack = 93p. Counselling, see above and dose

*Dose:* 3–6 tablets twice daily. In constipation the dose should be taken with at least 300 mL of water. In diarrhoea, ileostomy, and colostomy control, minimise liquid intake for 30 minutes before and after the dose

## STERCULIA

*Indications:* see notes above
*Cautions; Contra-indications; Side-effects:* see under Ispaghula Husk

COUNSELLING. Preparations that swell in contact with liquid should always be carefully swallowed with water and should not be taken immediately before going to bed

### ¹Normacol® (Norgine)

*Granules,* coated, sterculia 62%. Net price 100 g = £1.13; 60 × 7-g sachets = £4.77. Label: 25, 27, counselling, see above

*Dose:* 1–2 heaped 5-mL spoonfuls, or the contents of 1–2 sachets, washed down without chewing with plenty of liquid once or twice daily after meals; CHILD 6–12 years half adult dose
1. formerly Normacol Special

### ²Normacol Plus® (Norgine)

*Granules,* brown, coated, sterculia 62%, frangula (standardised) 8%. Net price 200 g = £2.43; 10 × 7-g sachets = 96p; 60 sachets = £5.11. Label: 25, 27, counselling, see above

*Dose:* constipation and after haemorrhoidectomy, 1–2 heaped 5-mL spoonfuls or the contents of 1–2 sachets washed down without chewing with plenty of liquid once or twice daily after meals
2. formerly Normacol Standard

### 1.6.2  Stimulant laxatives

The recognised stimulant laxatives include **bisacodyl** and members of the **anthraquinone** group, e.g. senna. **Docusate** sodium probably acts both as a stimulant and as a softening agent. **Danthron** has limited indications (see below) because *rodent* studies indicate potential carcinogenic risk. Powerful stimulants such as **cascara** and **castor oil** are obsolete.

Stimulant laxatives increase intestinal motility and often cause abdominal cramp. They should not be used in intestinal obstruction, and prolonged use can precipitate the onset of an atonic non-functioning colon and hypokalaemia. They should preferably be avoided in children.

**Glycerol** suppositories act as a rectal stimulant by virtue of the mildly irritant action of glycerol.

Soft soap is a more severe irritant; the use of soft soap enema should be **avoided**, expecially in pregnancy, as it may inflame the colonic mucosa.

The **parasympathomimetics** bethanechol, distigmine, neostigmine, and pyridostigmine (see sections 7.4.1 and 10.2.1) enhance parasympathetic activity in the gut and increase intestinal motility. They are rarely used for their gastrointestinal effects. Organic obstruction of the gut must first be excluded and they should be used with caution in bowel anastomosis.

Oxyphenisatin is indicated for diagnostic procedures or surgery only, since it causes hepatitis in chronic use.

## BISACODYL

*Indications:* see under Dose; tablets act in 10–12 hours; suppositories act in 20–60 minutes
*Cautions; Contra-indications; Side-effects:* see notes on stimulant laxatives; tablets, griping; suppositories, local irritation
*Dose: by mouth* for constipation, 5–10 mg at night; occasionally necessary to increase to 15–20 mg; CHILD 5 mg
*By rectum* in suppositories for constipation, 10 mg in the morning; CHILD 5 mg
Before radiological procedures and surgery, 10 mg by mouth at bedtime for 2 days before examination and, if necessary, a 10-mg suppository 1 hour before examination.

### Bisacodyl (Non-proprietary)

*Tablets,* e/c, bisacodyl 5 mg. Net price 20 = 26p. Label: 5, 25
*Suppositories,* bisacodyl 10 mg. Net price 12 = 99p
*Paediatric suppositories,* bisacodyl 5 mg. Net price 12 = 96p
Note. The brand name NHS Dulco-Lax® (Boehringer Ingelheim) is used for bisacodyl tablets, net price 20 = 84p; suppositories, 20 = £2.20; paediatric suppositories, 5 = 65p

## DANTHRON

*Indications:* only for: constipation in geriatric practice; prophylaxis and treatment of analgesic-induced constipation in terminally ill patients of all ages; constipation in cardiac failure and coronary thrombosis (conditions in which bowel movement must be free of strain); acts within 6–12 hours
*Cautions; Contra-indications; Side-effects:* see notes on stimulant laxatives; urine may be coloured red; avoid prolonged contact with skin (as in incontinent patients) since irritation and excoriation may occur; avoid in pregnancy and breast-feeding; *rodent* studies indicate potential carcinogenic risk
*Dose:* see next page

PoM **Co-danthramer** (Non-proprietary)
*Suspension,* co-danthramer 25/200 in 5 mL (danthron 25 mg, poloxamer '188' 200 mg/5 mL). Diluent tragacanth mucilage or syrup, life of diluted suspension 14 days. Label: 14 (urine red)
*Dose:* 5–10 mL; CHILD 2.5–5 mL (restricted indications, see notes above)
*Note.* The brand name NHS Codalax® (Napp) is used for co-danthramer 25/200 in 5 mL suspension, net price 300 mL = £9.32, 1 litre = £26.44
*Strong suspension,* co-danthramer 75/1000 in 5 mL (danthron 75 mg, poloxamer '188' 1 g/5 mL). Diluent as above. Label: 14 (urine red)
*Dose:* 2.5–5 mL (restricted indications, see notes above)
*Note.* The brand name NHS Codalax Forte® (Napp) is used for co-danthramer 75/1000 in 5 mL suspension, net price 300 mL = £14.00, 1 litre = £39.66

PoM **Co-danthrusate** (Non-proprietary)
*Capsules,* co-danthrusate 50/60 (danthron 50 mg, docusate sodium 60 mg). Label: 14 (urine red)
*Dose:* 1–3 capsules, usually at bedtime; CHILD 6–12 years 1 capsule
*Note.* The brand name NHS Normax® (Evans) is used for co-danthrusate 50/60 capsules, net price 63-cap pack = £9.20

## DOCUSATE SODIUM
(Dioctyl Sodium Sulphosuccinate)
*Indications:* constipation (oral preparations act within 1–2 days); adjunct in abdominal radiological procedures
*Cautions; Contra-indications; Side-effects:* see notes on stimulant laxatives; also rectal preparations not indicated if haemorrhoids or anal fissure
*Dose: by mouth,* constipation, up to 500 mg daily in divided doses; initial doses should be large and gradually reduced; CHILD over 6 months 12.5–25 mg 3 times daily
With barium meal, 400 mg

**Dioctyl®** (Medo)
*Tablets,* yellow, f/c, docusate sodium 100 mg. Net price 30-tab pack = 83p
*Oral solution 1%,* sugar-free, docusate sodium 50 mg/5 mL. Net price 300-mL pack = £2.25
*Paediatric oral solution,* sugar-free, docusate sodium 12.5 mg/5 mL. Net price 125-mL pack = 73p

Rectal preparations
**Fletchers' Enemette®** (Pharmax)
*Enema,* docusate sodium 90 mg, glycerol 3.78 g, macrogol 2.25 g, sorbic acid 5 mg/5 mL. Net price 5-mL unit = 31p
*Dose:* ADULT and CHILD over 3 years, 5-mL unit when required
**Norgalax Micro-enema®** (Norgine)
*Enema,* docusate sodium 120 mg in 10-g single-dose disposable packs. Net price 10-g unit = 66p
*Dose:* ADULT and CHILD over 12 years, 10-g unit

## GLYCEROL
(Glycerin)
*Indications:* constipation

**Glycerol Suppositories** (BP)
(Glycerin Suppositories)
*Suppositories,* gelatin 140 mg, glycerol 700 mg, purified water to 1 g. Net price 12 = 44p (infant), 49p (child), 54p (adult)
*Dose:* 1 suppository moistened with water before use. The usual sizes are for *infants* small (1-g mould), *children* medium (2-g mould), *adults* large (4-g mould)

## OXYPHENISATIN
*Indications:* see under Dose
*Cautions; Contra-indications; Side-effects:* see notes on stimulant laxatives; avoid repeated use owing to liver toxicity

**Veripaque®** (Sterling-Winthrop)
*Enema,* powder for reconstitution, oxyphenisatin 50 mg in 3 g. Net price 1 vial = £1.90
*Dose:* by rectum before diagnostic procedures or surgery, oxyphenisatin 50 mg dissolved in 2 litres of water given over 5–8 minutes
Adjuvant to barium enema, oxyphenisatin 50 mg mixed thoroughly with 2 litres of barium sulphate enema

## SENNA
*Indications:* constipation; bowel evacuation before abdominal radiological procedures, endoscopy, and surgery; acts in 8–12 hours
*Cautions; Contra-indications; Side-effects:* see notes on stimulant laxatives

**Senna Tablets,** total sennosides 7.5 mg. Net price 20 = 30p
*Dose:* 2–4 tablets, usually at night; initial dose should be low then gradually increased; CHILD over 6 years, half adult dose
*Note.* The brand name NHS Senokot® (see below) is used for Senna tablets
¹**Manevac®** (Galen)
*Granules,* coated, senna fruit 12.4%, ispaghula 54.2%. Net price 250 g = £2.99. Label: 25, 27, counselling, see Ispaghula Husk
*Dose:* 1–2 level 5-mL spoonfuls with water or warm drink after supper and, if necessary, before breakfast *or* every 6 hours in resistant cases for 1–3 days; CHILD 5–12 years 1 level 5-mL spoonful daily
1. Formerly Agiolax®
**Senokot®** (R&C)
NHS *Tablets,* brown, total sennosides (calculated as sennoside B) 7.5 mg. Net price 20 = 30p
*Dose:* 2–4 tablets, usually at bedtime; initial dose should be low then gradually increased; CHILD over 6 years, half adult dose
*Note.* For Senokot tablets on general sale to the public the maximum recommended dose is 2 tablets.
*Granules,* brown, total sennosides (calculated as sennoside B) 15 mg/5 mL or 5.5 mg/g (one 5-mL spoonful = 2.7 g). Net price 100 g = £1.89
*Dose:* 5–10 mL, usually at bedtime; CHILD over 6 years 2.5–5 mL
*Syrup,* brown, total sennosides (calculated as sennoside B) 7.5 mg/5 mL. Net price 100 mL = £1.30
*Dose:* 10–20 mL, usually at bedtime; CHILD 2–6 years 2.5–5 mL, over 6 years 5–10 mL

---

**X-Prep®** (Napp)
Product discontinued

## SODIUM PICOSULPHATE

*Indications:* constipation, bowel evacuation before abdominal radiological procedures, endoscopy, and surgery
*Cautions; Contra-indications; Side-effects:* see notes on stimulant laxatives
*Dose:* see below

**Sodium Picosulphate Elixir,** sodium picosulphate 5 mg/5 mL. Diluent purified water, freshly boiled and cooled, life of diluted elixir 14 days. Acts within 10–14 hours. Net price 100 mL = £1.25
*Dose:* 5–15 mL at night; CHILD 2–5 years 2.5 mL, 5–10 years 2.5–5 mL
*Note.* The brand name NHS Laxoberal® (Windsor) is used for sodium picosulphate elixir 5 mg/5 mL
**Picolax®** (Nordic)
*Oral powder,* sugar-free, sodium picosulphate 10 mg/sachet, with magnesium citrate (for bowel evacuation before radiological procedures, endoscopy, and surgery). Net price 2 sachets = 59p. Label: 10, patient information leaflet, 13, counselling, see below
*Dose:* ADULT and CHILD over 9 years, 1 sachet in water in morning (before 8 a.m.) and a second in afternoon (between 2 and 4 p.m.) of day preceding procedures; CHILD 1–2 years quarter sachet morning and afternoon, 2–4 years half sachet morning and afternoon, 4–9 years 1 sachet morning and half sachet afternoon
Acts within 3 hours of first dose
COUNSELLING. Patients should be warned that heat is generated on addition to water; for this reason the powder should be added initially to 30 mL (2 tablespoonfuls) of water; after 5 minutes (when reaction complete) the solution should be further diluted to 150 mL (about a tumblerful)

## OTHER STIMULANT LAXATIVES

Unstandardised preparations of cascara, frangula, rhubarb, and senna should be **avoided** as their laxative action is unpredictable. Aloes, colocynth, and jalap should be **avoided** as they have a drastic purgative action. Phenolphthalein should be **avoided** as it may cause rashes. Its laxative effects may continue for several days because of enterohepatic recycling; alkaline urine may be coloured pink.

NHS **Alophen®** (W-L)
*Pills,* brown, f/c, aloin 15 mg, phenolphthalein 30 mg. Net price 50 pills = £1.44. Label: 14 (urine pink)
*Dose:* 1–3 pills, usually at bedtime
NHS **Kest®** (Torbet)
*Tablets,* magnesium sulphate 300 mg, phenolphthalein 50 mg. Net price 50 = 94p. Label: 14 (urine pink)
*Dose:* 1 tablet with water at bedtime and 2 tablets in the morning

## 1.6.3 Faecal softeners

Liquid paraffin, the classical lubricant, has disadvantages (see below). Bulk laxatives (section 1.6.1) and non-ionic surfactant 'wetting' agents e.g. docusate sodium (section 1.6.2) also have softening properties. Such drugs are useful for oral administration in the management of haemorrhoids and anal fissure; glycerol suppositories (section 1.6.2) are useful for rectal use.

Enemas containing **arachis oil** lubricate and soften impacted faeces and promote a bowel movement.

---

**CSM recommendations**

Preparations containing liquid paraffin for use as laxatives should no longer be available directly to the public and restrictions should be placed on over-the-counter sales through pharmacies:
pack size be limited to 160 mL;
be indicated only for symptomatic relief of constipation;
be contra-indicated for children under 3 years of age;
prolonged use not advised;
package labels to state 'repeated use is not recommended' and 'consult your doctor if laxatives are needed every day, if you have persistent abdominal pain or have a condition which makes swallowing difficult'.

---

### ARACHIS OIL

*Indications:* see notes above
*Dose:* see below

**Fletchers' Arachis Oil Retention Enema®** (Pharmax)
*Enema,* arachis oil in 130-mL single-dose disposable packs. Net price 130 mL = £1.04
*Dose:* to soften impacted faeces, 130 mL; the enema should be warmed before use

### LIQUID PARAFFIN

*Indications:* constipation but see CSM warning above
*Cautions:* avoid prolonged use
*Side-effects:* anal seepage of paraffin and consequent anal irritation after prolonged use, granulomatous reactions caused by absorption of small quantities of liquid paraffin (especially from the emulsion), lipoid pneumonia, and interference with the absorption of fat-soluble vitamins
*Dose:* 10–30 mL but see CSM warning above

**Liquid Paraffin Oral Emulsion** (BP)
(Liquid Paraffin Emulsion)
*Oral emulsion,* liquid paraffin 5 mL, vanillin 5 mg, chloroform 0.025 mL, benzoic acid solution 0.2 mL, methylcellulose-20 200 mg, saccharin sodium 500 micrograms, water to 10 mL
*Dose:* 10–30 mL at night when required
NHS **Petrolagar®** (Whitehall)
*Emulsion,* sugar-free, liquid paraffin 7%, light liquid paraffin 18%. Net price 100 mL = 54p
*Dose:* 10 mL morning and night or after meals

With phenolphthalein
NHS **Agarol®** (W-L)
*Mixture,* sugar-free, phenolphthalein 66 mg, liquid paraffin 1.6 mL, agar 10 mg/5 mL. Net price 100 mL = 83p. Label: 14 (urine pink)
*Dose:* 5–15 mL, usually at bedtime; CHILD not recommended

---

Prices are **net**, see p. 1

## 1.6.4   Osmotic laxatives

These act by retaining fluid in the bowel by osmosis or by changing the pattern of water distribution in the faeces.

Saline purgatives such as **magnesium hydroxide** are commonly abused but are satisfactory for occasional use; adequate fluid intake should be maintained. **Magnesium salts** are useful where rapid bowel evacuation is required. **Sodium salts** should be avoided as they may give rise to sodium and water retention in susceptible individuals. **Phosphate enemas** are useful in bowel clearance before radiology, endoscopy, and surgery.

**Lactulose** is a semi-synthetic disaccharide which is not absorbed from the gastro-intestinal tract. It produces an osmotic diarrhoea of low faecal pH, and discourages the proliferation of ammonia-producing organisms. It is therefore useful in the treatment of *hepatic encephalopathy*.

## LACTULOSE

*Indications:* constipation (may take up to 48 hours to act), hepatic encephalopathy
*Contra-indications:* galactosaemia, intestinal obstruction
*Side-effects:* flatulence, cramps, and abdominal discomfort
*Dose:* expressed in terms of the elixir containing lactulose 3.35 g/5 mL
Constipation, initially 15 mL twice daily, gradually reduced according to patient's needs; CHILD under 1 year 2.5 mL, 1–5 years 5 mL, 6–12 years 10 mL twice daily, gradually reduced
Hepatic encephalopathy, 30–50 mL 3 times daily, subsequently adjusted to produce 2–3 soft stools daily

**Lactulose** (Non-proprietary)
*Solution*, lactulose 3.35 g/5 mL with other ketoses. Net price 200-mL pack = £1.54
*Note.* The brand name NHS Duphalac® (Duphar) is used for Lactulose solution; net price 200-mL pack = £1.54

## MAGNESIUM SALTS

*Indications; Dose:* see under preparations
*Cautions:* renal impairment (risk of magnesium accumulation); hepatic impairment (see Appendix 2); elderly and debilitated; see also notes above; **interactions:** Appendix 1 (magnesium salts)
*Contra-indications:* acute gastro-intestinal conditions
*Side-effects:* colic

Magnesium citrate
**Citramag**® (Bioglan)
*Powder*, effervescent, providing when dissolved in water magnesium citrate 17.7 g/sachet. Net price 10-sachet pack = £9.70. Label 10, patient information leaflet, 13, counselling, see below
*Dose:* bowel evacuation before radiological examination and surgery, 1 sachet dissolved in 200 mL water and taken at about 8 p.m. on evening before procedure
COUNSELLING. The patient information leaflet advises that hot water is needed to make the solution and that effervescence should be allowed to subside (should be

prepared at 6 p.m. for 8 p.m. dose); high fluid, low residue diet on day before procedure; on day of procedure water only should be taken until completed

Magnesium hydroxide
**Magnesium Hydroxide Mixture** (BP)
(Cream of Magnesia)
An aqueous suspension containing about 8% of hydrated magnesium oxide. Do not store in a cold place
*Dose:* constipation, 25–50 mL when required

Magnesium hydroxide with liquid paraffin (see also CSM recommendations on previous page)
**Liquid Paraffin and Magnesium Hydroxide Emulsion** (BP)
*Oral emulsion*, 25% dispersion of liquid paraffin in an aqueous suspension containing 6% of hydrated magnesium oxide
*Dose:* constipation, 5–20 mL when required

Magnesium sulphate
**Magnesium Sulphate** (Epsom salts). Label: 13, 23
*Dose:* rapid bowel evacuation (acts in 2–4 hours) 5–10 g in a tumblerful of water preferably before breakfast
**Fletchers' Magnesium Sulphate Retention Enema**® (Pharmax)
*Enema*, magnesium sulphate 50%, in 130-mL single-dose disposable packs. Net price 130 mL = 56p (hosp. only)
*Dose:* 130 mL, as an adjunct in neurosurgery to lower cerebrospinal fluid pressure

## PHOSPHATES (RECTAL)

*Indications:* rectal use in constipation; bowel evacuation before abdominal radiological procedures, endoscopy, and surgery
*Cautions:* see notes above
*Contra-indications:* acute gastro-intestinal conditions
*Dose:* see below

¹**Carbalax**® (Pharmax)
*Suppositories*, sodium acid phosphate 1.72 g in an effervescent basis. Net price 12 = £2.30
*Dose:* constipation, 1 suppository, inserted 30 minutes before evacuation is required; moisten with water before use; CHILD, not recommended
1. Formerly Beogex

**Fletchers' Phosphate Enema**® (Pharmax)
*Enema*, sodium acid phosphate 12.8 g, sodium phosphate 10.24 g, purified water, freshly boiled and cooled, to 128 mL (corresponds to Phosphates Enema Formula B). Net price 128 mL with standard tube = 44p, with long rectal tube = 62p
*Dose:* 128 mL; CHILD, over 3 years, reduced according to body weight (under 3 years not recommended)

## SODIUM CITRATE (RECTAL)

*Indications:* rectal use in constipation
*Cautions:* see notes above
*Contra-indications:* acute gastro-intestinal conditions
*Dose:* see below

**Micolette Micro-enema®** (Cusi)
*Enema*, sodium citrate 450 mg, sodium lauryl sulphoacetate 45 mg, glycerol 625 mg, together with citric acid, potassium sorbate, and sorbitol in a viscous solution, in 5-mL single-dose disposable packs with nozzle. Net price 5 mL = 33p
*Dose:* ADULT and CHILD over 3 years, 5–10 mL

**Micralax Micro-enema®** (Evans)
*Enema*, sodium citrate 450 mg, sodium alkyl-sulphoacetate 45 mg, together with glycerol and sorbitol in a viscous solution in 5-mL single-dose disposable packs with nozzle. Net price 5 mL = 45p
*Dose:* ADULT and CHILD over 3 years, 5 mL

**Relaxit Micro-enema®** (Kabi Pharmacia)
*Enema*, sodium citrate 450 mg, sodium lauryl sulphate 75 mg, sorbic acid 5 mg, together with glycerol and sorbitol in a viscous solution in 5-mL single-dose disposable packs with nozzle. Net price 5 mL = 15p
*Dose:* ADULT and CHILD over 3 years, 5 mL

---

## BOWEL CLEANSING SOLUTIONS

Bowel cleansing solutions are used before colonic surgery, colonoscopy, or barium enema to ensure the bowel is free of solid contents. They are **not** treatments for constipation.

*Indications:* see above

*Cautions:* pregnancy; ulcerative colitis; impaired gag reflex; unconscious or semiconscious or possibility of regurgitation or aspiration; prevent absorption of oral medication

*Contra-indications:* gastro-intestinal obstruction, gastric retention, perforated bowel; toxic colitis, toxic megacolon or ileus; weight less than 20 kg

*Side-effects:* nausea, bloating, abdominal cramps (usually transient—reduced by taking more slowly); rarely vomiting, anal irritation; urticaria, rhinorrhoea and dermatitis reported

PoM **Bowel Cleansing Solutions**
*Oral powder*, macrogol 3350 or 4000 (polyethylene glycol 3350 or 4000) 59 g, anhydrous sodium sulphate 5.685 g, sodium bicarbonate 1.685 g, sodium chloride 1.465 g, potassium chloride 743 mg/sachet. Label: 10, counselling
Four sachets when reconstituted with water to 4 litres provides an iso-osmotic solution for bowel cleansing before surgery, colonoscopy or radiological procedures
*Dose: by mouth*, 240 mL (1 tumblerful) of reconstituted solution every 10–15 minutes, or by nasogastric tube 20–30 mL/minute, until 4 litres have been consumed or watery stools are free of solid matter (usually 3 litres). First bowel movement occurs after approximately 1 hour
COUNSELLING. Advise patient to take at least 2 hours after and preferably 3–4 hours after food; more palatable if chilled; do not add flavouring or other ingredients; drink each portion as rapidly as possible
After reconstitution the solution should be kept in a refrigerator and discarded if unused after 48 hours
Available from Norgine (*Klean-Prep®*), net price 4 sachets (to provide 4 litres) = £8.60; and Seward (*Golytely®*), net price 4 sachets (to provide 4 litres) = £4.50.

## 1.7 Preparations for haemorrhoids

1.7.1 Soothing preparations
1.7.2 Compound preparations with corticosteroids
1.7.3 Rectal sclerosants

Anal and perianal pruritus, soreness, and excoriation are best treated by application of bland ointments, suppositories, and dusting-powders (section 1.7.1). These conditions occur commonly in patients suffering from haemorrhoids, fistulas, and proctitis. Careful local toilet as well as adjustment of the diet to avoid hard stools, and bulk-forming materials such as bran (section 1.6.1) and a high residue diet are also helpful. In proctitis these measures may supplement treatment with corticosteroids or sulphasalazine (see section 1.5).

When necessary topical preparations containing **local anaesthetics** (section 1.7.1) or **corticosteroids** (section 1.7.2) are used provided perianal thrush has been excluded. Perianal thrush is best treated with **nystatin** by mouth and by local application (see sections 5.2, 7.2.2, and 13.10.2).

### 1.7.1 Soothing preparations

Bland soothing preparations containing mild astringents such as bismuth subgallate, zinc oxide, and hamamelis may give symptomatic relief in haemorrhoids. Many proprietary preparations also contain lubricants, vasoconstrictors, or mild antiseptics.

Prolonged application of preparations containing **resorcinol** should be **avoided** because it may interfere with thyroid function. Heparinoids are claimed to promote the resorption of local oedema and extravasated blood.

**Local anaesthetics** are used to relieve pain associated with *haemorrhoids*, and *pruritus ani* but good evidence is lacking. Lignocaine ointment (see section 15.2) is used before emptying the bowel to relieve pain associated with *anal fissure*. Alternative local anaesthetics include amethocaine, cinchocaine, and pramoxine, but they are more irritant.

Local anaesthetics should be used for short periods only (no longer than 2 weeks) since they may cause sensitisation of the anal skin.

ADMINISTRATION. Unless otherwise indicated a suppository is usually inserted into the rectum night and morning and after a bowel movement. Rectal ointments and creams are applied night and morning and after a bowel movement, externally or by rectum using a rectal nozzle.
*Note.* Local anaesthetic ointments can be absorbed through the rectal mucosa therefore excessive application should be avoided, particularly in infants and children.

**Bismuth Subgallate Suppositories, Compound,** bismuth subgallate 200 mg, castor oil 60 mg, resorcinol 60 mg, zinc oxide 120 mg, in theobroma oil or other suitable basis. Net price 12 = £1.82

---

**Hamamelis and Zinc Oxide Suppositories.**
Usual strength hamamelis dry extract 200 mg,
zinc oxide 600 mg. Net price 12 = £2.35

**Anacal**® (Panpharma)
*Rectal ointment*, laureth '9' 5%, heparinoid
0.2%. Net price 30 g (with rectal nozzle) =
£3.04
Apply 1–4 times daily
*Suppositories*, laureth '9' 50 mg, a heparinoid
4 mg.
Net price 10 = £1.70
Insert 1 suppository once or twice daily

**Anodesyn**® (Crookes)
*Ointment*, ephedrine hydrochloride 0.25%, lignocaine hydrochloride 0.5%, allantoin 0.5%.
Net price 25 g = £1.16
*Suppositories*, ephedrine hydrochloride 5.1 mg,
lignocaine hydrochloride 10.25 mg, allantoin
10.25 mg. Net price 12 = £1.22

**Anusol**® (W-L)
*Cream*, bismuth oxide 2.14%, Peru balsam
1.8%, zinc oxide 10.75%. Net price 23 g (with
rectal nozzle) = £1.28
*Ointment*, bismuth oxide 0.875%, bismuth
subgallate 2.25%, zinc oxide 10.75%, Peru
balsam 1.875%. Net price 25 g (with rectal
nozzle) = £1.25
*Suppositories*, bismuth oxide 24 mg, bismuth
subgallate 59 mg, Peru balsam 49 mg, zinc oxide
296 mg. Net price 12 = £1.11

## 1.7.2  Compound preparations with corticosteroids

Corticosteroids are often combined with antibiotics, local anaesthetics, and soothing agents.
They are suitable for occasional short-term use
after exclusion of infections, such as herpes
simplex; see section 13.4 for general comments
on topical corticosteroids.

Antibiotics may do little more than encourage
the growth of resistant bacteria and should be
avoided. See section 1.7.1 for comment on local
anaesthetics.

PoM **Anugesic-HC**® (P-D)
*Cream*, benzyl benzoate 1.2%, bismuth oxide
0.875%, hydrocortisone acetate 0.5%, Peru
balsam 1.85%, pramoxine hydrochloride 1%,
zinc oxide 12.35%. Net price 30 g (with rectal
nozzle) = £6.19
Apply night and morning and after a bowel movement;
do not use for longer than 7 days
*Suppositories*, benzyl benzoate 33 mg, bismuth
oxide 24 mg, bismuth subgallate 59 mg, hydrocortisone acetate 5 mg, Peru balsam 49 mg,
pramoxine hydrochloride 27 mg, zinc oxide
296 mg. Net price 12 = £2.64
Insert 1 suppository night and morning and after a
bowel movement; do not use for longer than 7 days

PoM **Anusol-HC**® (P-D)
*Ointment*, benzyl benzoate 1.25%, bismuth oxide
0.875%, bismuth subgallate 2.25%, hydrocortisone
acetate 0.25%, Peru balsam 1.875%, zinc oxide 10.75%.
Net price 30 g (with rectal nozzle) = £5.81
Apply night and morning and after a bowel movement;
do not use for longer than 7 days

*Suppositories*, benzyl benzoate 33 mg, bismuth oxide
24 mg, bismuth subgallate 59 mg, hydrocortisone acetate 10 mg, Peru balsam 49 mg, zinc oxide 296 mg. Net
price 12 = £2.64
*Additives:* include tartrazine lake
Insert 1 suppository night and morning and after a bowel
movement; do not use for longer than 7 days

PoM **Betnovate**® (Glaxo)
*Rectal ointment*, betamethasone valerate 0.05%,
lignocaine hydrochloride 2.5%, phenylephrine
hydrochloride 0.1%. Net price 30 g (with
applicator) = £1.50
Apply 2–3 times daily until inflammation subsides then
once daily, externally or by rectum; do not use for
longer than 7 days

PoM **Proctofoam HC**® (Stafford-Miller)
*Foam* in aerosol pack, hydrocortisone acetate
1%, pramoxine hydrochloride 1%. Net price
24-g pack (approx. 40 applications) with
applicator = £4.83
*Dose:* haemorrhoids and proctitis, 1 applicatorful (4–
6 mg hydrocortisone acetate, 4–6 mg pramoxine hydrochloride) by rectum 2–3 times daily and after a bowel
movement

PoM **Proctosedyl**® (Roussel)
*Ointment*, cinchocaine hydrochloride 0.5%,
hydrocortisone 0.5%. Net price 30 g = £6.65
(with cannula)
Apply morning and night and after a bowel movement,
externally or by rectum
*Suppositories*, cinchocaine hydrochloride 5 mg,
hydrocortisone 5 mg. Net price 12 = £3.00
Insert 1 suppository night and morning and after a bowel
movement

PoM **Scheriproct**® (Schering Health Care)
*Ointment*, cinchocaine hydrochloride 0.5%,
prednisolone hexanoate 0.19%. Net price
30 g = £4.41
Apply twice daily for 5–7 days (3–4 times daily on 1st
day if necessary), then once daily for few days after
symptoms have cleared
*Suppositories*, cinchocaine hydrochloride 1 mg,
prednisolone hexanoate 1.3 mg. Net price 12 =
£2.08
Insert 1 suppository daily after a bowel movement, for
5–7 days (in severe cases initially 2–3 times daily)

PoM **Ultraproct**® (Schering Health Care)
*Ointment*, cinchocaine hydrochloride 0.5%,
fluocortolone hexanoate 0.095%, fluocortolone
pivalate 0.092%. Net price 30 g (with rectal
nozzle) = £1.85
Apply twice daily for 5–7 days (3–4 times daily on 1st
day if necessary), then once daily for few days after
symptoms have cleared
*Suppositories*, cinchocaine hydrochloride 1 mg,
fluocortolone hexanoate 630 micrograms, fluocortolone pivalate 610 micrograms. Net price
12 = £2.15
Insert 1 suppository daily after a bowel movement, for
5–7 days (in severe cases initially 2–3 times daily) then
1 suppository every other day for 1 week

PoM **Uniroid**® (Unigreg)
*Ointment*, cinchocaine hydrochloride 0.5%, hydrocortisone 0.5%, neomycin sulphate 3400 units, polymyxin
B sulphate 6250 units/g. Net price 15 g (with
applicator) = £2.77
Apply 3 times daily, preferably after a bowel movement,
externally or by rectum; do not use for longer than 7
days

---

Abbreviations and symbols, see inside front cover                    Prices are **net**, see p. 1

*Suppositories*, cinchocaine hydrochloride 5 mg, hydrocortisone 5 mg, neomycin sulphate 6800 units, polymyxin B sulphate 12 500 units. Net price 10 = £2.09
Insert 1 suppository 3 times daily, preferably after a bowel movement; do not use for longer than 7 days

PoM **Xyloproct®** (Astra)
*Ointment* (water-miscible), aluminium acetate 3.5%, hydrocortisone acetate 0.275%, lignocaine 5%, zinc oxide 18%. Net price 30 g (with applicator) = £3.48
Apply several times daily
*Suppositories*, aluminium acetate 50 mg, hydrocortisone acetate 5 mg, lignocaine 60 mg, zinc oxide 400 mg. Net price 10 = £1.63
Insert 1 suppository at night and after a bowel movement

### 1.7.3 Rectal sclerosants

**Oily phenol injection** is used to inject haemorrhoids particularly when unprolapsed.

**PHENOL**
*Indications:* see notes above
*Side-effects:* irritation, tissue necrosis

**Oily Phenol Injection**, (BP), phenol 5% in a suitable fixed oil. Net price 2-mL amp = 71p; 5-mL amp = £2.08; 25-mL vial = £5.00
*Dose:* 2–3 mL into the submucosal layer at the base of the pile; several injections may be given at different sites, max. total injected 10 mL at any one time

# 1.8 Stoma care

Prescribing for patients with stoma calls for special care. The following is a brief account of some of the main points to be borne in mind.

*Enteric-coated* and *modified-release* preparations are **unsuitable**, particularly in patients with ileostomies, as there may not be sufficient release of the active ingredient.

*Laxatives*. Enemas and washouts should **not** be prescribed for patients with ileostomies as they may cause rapid and severe dehydration.

Colostomy patients may suffer from constipation and whenever possible should be treated by increasing fluid intake or dietary fibre. **Bulk-forming laxatives** (section 1.6.1) should be tried. If they are insufficient, as small a dose as possible of senna (section 1.6.2) should be used. Preparations such as X-Prep® should be avoided when preparing patients for radiological procedures as they may cause severe dehydration with nausea, vomiting, and griping.

*Antidiarrhoeals*. Drugs such as **loperamide**, **codeine phosphate**, or **co-phenotrope** (diphenoxylate with atropine) are effective. Bulk-forming drugs (section 1.6.1) may be tried but it is often difficult to adjust the dose appropriately.

**Antibiotics** should **not** be given for an episode of acute diarrhoea.

*Antacids*. The tendency to diarrhoea from magnesium salts or constipation from aluminium salts may be increased in these patients.

*Diuretics* should be used with caution in patients with ileostomies as they may become excessively dehydrated and potassium depletion may easily occur. It is usually advisable to use a **potassium-sparing** diuretic (see section 2.2.3).

*Digoxin*. Patients with a stoma are particularly susceptible to hypokalaemia if on digoxin therapy and potassium supplements or a potassium-sparing diuretic may be advisable (for comment see section 9.2.1.1).

*Potassium supplements*. Liquid formulations are preferred to modified-release formulations (see above).

*Analgesics*. Opioid analgesics (see section 4.7.2) may cause troublesome constipation in colostomy patients. When a non-opioid analgesic is required **paracetamol** is usually suitable but anti-inflammatory analgesics may cause gastric irritation and bleeding.

*Iron preparations* may cause loose stools and sore skin in these patients. If this is troublesome and if iron is definitely indicated one of the intramuscular iron preparations (see section 9.1.1.2) should be used. Modified-release preparations should be **avoided** for the reasons given above.

Patients are usually given advice about the use of cleansing agents, protective creams, lotions, deodorants, or sealants whilst in hospital, either by the surgeon or by the health authority stoma care nurses. Voluntary organisations offer help and support to patients with stoma.

### STOMA APPLIANCES AND ASSOCIATED PRODUCTS
For urostomy pouches see section 7.5

### CLOSED POUCHES

Closed pouches are suitable for patients with a **colostomy** and well-formed stools

Body's Care range
**Rubber bags screwcap** (Body's Care)
*Black butyl*, one-piece closed pouch. Net price 1 day pouch = £23.25; 1 night pouch = £27.12
*White rubber*, one-piece closed pouch. Net price 1 day pouch = £12.92; 1 night pouch = £14.89
**Rubber bags spout** (Body's Care)
*Black butyl*, one-piece closed pouch. Net price 1 day pouch or night pouch = £24.35
*White rubber*, one-piece closed pouch. Net price 1 day pouch or night pouch = £11.62

Cambmac range
**Dansac®** (Cambmac)
*Combi Colo F*, one-piece pouch with filter, opaque or clear. Net price 100 pouches (standard pouch: 25, 30, 38, 44, 50, or 63 mm holes; small pouch: 25, 30, or 38 mm holes) = £133.05
*CombiMicro C + S*, one-piece pouch with porous adhesive, filter, skin barrier ring, and fabric backing, opaque or clear. Net price 30 pouches (25, 32, 38, 44, 50, 63 mm or cut-to-fit holes) = £55.75
*Mini Cap*, one-piece pouch with filter, opaque. Net price 50 pouches (30 or 44 mm holes) = £44.30
*Mini Petit C*, one-piece pouch with porous adhesive skin protector, fabric backing, and filter, opaque. Net price 30 pouches (cut-to-fit) = £49.25

*Standard Colo*, one-piece pouch with filter, clear. Net price 100 pouches (22, 30, 32, or 38 mm holes) = £119.50

*Supersquare System*, two-piece pouch with filter, opaque or clear. Net price 100 (standard or small) pouches to fit 50 mm base plate = £115.55; 100 (standard) pouches to fit 80 mm base plate = £146.55

### CliniMed range
**Biopore**® (CliniMed)
One-piece pouch with porous adhesive and filter, white/clear. Net price 50 pouches (25, 30, 35, 40, 45, 50 mm holes) = £58.75

**Biotrol**® (CliniMed)
*Colo S*, one-piece pouch with skin protector adhesive, white. Net price 30 pouches (25, 30, 35, 40, 45, 50, or 60 mm holes) = £54.20

*Elite Closed*, covered one-piece pouch with skin protector adhesive and filter, white or skin-tone. Net price 30 pouches (25, 30, 35, 40, 45, 50, 60, 70 mm or cut-to-fit holes) = £57.35

*Integrale*, one-piece pouch with skin protector adhesive and filter, white. Net price 30 pouches (25, 30, 35, 40, 45, 50, 60, 70 mm or cut-to-fit holes) = £57.35

*Preference Closed*, fabric covered one-piece pouch with skin protector adhesive, porous adhesive collar, and filter, white or skin-tone. Net price 30 pouches (25, 30, 35, 40, 45, 50, 60 mm or cut-to-fit holes) = £53.10

### Coloplast range
**Comfort**® (Coloplast)
*Extra*, one-piece closed pouch. Net price, No. 1 (24 mm hole), 100 pouches = £76.00; No. 2 (30 or 40 mm holes), 100 = £92.00; No. 3, 30 mm hole, 100 = £111.00, 50 mm hole, 100 = £112.00

*Regular*, one-piece closed pouch. Net price, No. 1 (24 mm hole), 100 pouches = £64.00; No. 2 (30 mm hole), 100 = £76.00; No. 3 (30 mm hole), 100 = £91.00; No. 5 (24 mm hole), 100 = £85.00

**Conseal**® **System** (Coloplast)
Two-piece pouch. Net price 30 bags (to fit 40 or 50 mm base plates) = £31.80

**K-Flex**® (Coloplast)
One-piece closed pouch with karaya skin protector and filter. Net price 20 pouches (clear: 10, 30, or 40 mm holes; opaque: 30 or 40 mm holes) = £54.60

**mc2000**® (Coloplast)
One-piece pouch with double seal and filter, opaque or clear. Net price 30 pouches (25, 30, 35, 40, 45, 50, 55, or 60 mm holes) = £60.00

**mc2002**® (Coloplast)
Two-piece pouch with filter, opaque or clear. Net price 30 pouches (to fit 40 or 60 mm base plates) = £33.90

**pc3000**® (Coloplast)
One-piece pouch, opaque or clear. Net price 30 pouches (25, 30, 35, 40, 45, 50, or 55 mm holes; 25 mm can be cut to fit up to 60 mm) = £56.40

### ConvaTec range
**Colodress**® (ConvaTec)
*Colodress*, one-piece closed pouch with textured backing, opaque beige. Net price 30 pouches (19, 32, 38, 45, or 50 mm holes; 19 mm can be cut to fit) = £54.75

*Colodress Plus*, one-piece closed pouch with single-release paper and filter. Net price 30 pouches (opaque or clear: 19, 25, 32, 38, 45, or 50 mm holes; opaque: 64 mm hole; 19 mm can be cut to fit) = £54.75

**Surgicare System**® **2** (ConvaTec)
*System 2*, two-piece closed pouch, white. Net price 30 pouches (to fit 38, 45, 57, or 70 mm flanges) = £27.34

*System 2 Combihesive*, two-piece closed pouch with textured backing, beige. Net price 30 pouches (to fit 38, 45, 57, or 70 mm flanges) = £27.34; with filter, 30 pouches = £28.24; Mini pouches, 20 pouches (to fit 32, 38, 45, or 57 mm flanges) = £15.48

### Hollister range
**Classic** (Hollister)
All with 25, 32, 38, 44, 51, 64, or 76 mm holes

*Adhesive* (series 217), one-piece closed pouch with adhesive and filter, clear. Net price 50 pouches = £53.42

*Karaya seal* (series 716), one-piece closed pouch with karaya skin protector (without filter), must be worn with belt, clear. Net price 30 pouches = £45.44

*Karaya seal with filter* (series 211), one-piece closed pouch with karaya skin protector and filter, must be worn with belt, opaque. Net price 30 pouches = £45.44

*Karaya 5*® *Seal* (series 331 and 332), one-piece closed pouch with porous adhesive, karaya skin protector, and filter, may be worn with belt, opaque or clear. Net price 30 pouches = £55.09

*Microporous adhesive* (series 314), one-piece compact closed pouch with porous adhesive and filter, may be worn with belt, clear. Net price 50 pouches = £57.81

**Premium**® (Hollister)
All with 25, 32, 38, 44, 51, 64, or 76 mm holes

*Karaya 5*® *Seal* (series 355 and 353), one-piece closed pouch with porous adhesive, karaya skin protector and filter, may be worn with belt, opaque or clear. Net price 15 pouches = £27.85

*Synthetic Seal* (series 354 and 356), one-piece closed pouch with porous adhesive, synthetic skin protector seal and filter, opaque or clear. Net price 15 pouches = £29.04

**HolliGard**® (Hollister)
All with 25, 32, 38, 44, 51, 64, or 76 mm holes

*Microporous adhesive* (series 411), one-piece closed pouch with porous adhesive, HolliGard® seal, and filter, may be worn with belt, opaque. Net price 30 pouches = £57.86

*Without adhesive* (series 416), one-piece closed pouch with HolliGard® seal and filter, must be worn with belt, clear. Net price 30 pouches = £52.46

**Guardian**® (Hollister)
All with 38, 51, or 64 mm holes

*Guardian* (series 451 and 450), two-piece closed pouch with filter, opaque or clear. Net price 15 pouches = £13.05

*Guardian mini-pouch* (series 452), two-piece compact closed pouch with filter, opaque. Net price 15 pouches = £13.00

### Leyland range
**Rubber bags** (Leyland)
*White rubber*, one-piece closed pouch with spout outlet. Net price (both 19, 25, or 28 mm holes), 1 day pouch = £10.13; 1 night pouch = £10.93

### Rüsch range
**Ostopore**® (Rüsch)
*Colo AV-opaque*, one-piece closed pouch with adhesive and vent. Net price 30 pouches (25, 32, 38, or 45 mm holes) with 2 belt flanges = £37.20

*Colo KAV-opaque*, one-piece closed pouch with karaya seal skin protector, adhesive, and vent. Net price 30 pouches (25, 32, 38, 45, or 51 mm holes) with 5 belt flanges = £50.70

*Colo KAV-transparent*, one-piece closed pouch with karaya seal skin protector, adhesive, and vent. Net price 30 pouches (32, 38, 45, or 51 mm holes) with 30 belt flanges = £64.50

### Salts range
**NHS Cohflex**® (Salts)
*Closed*, one-piece pouch with single-release paper, wafer, and filter, fabric front and back, opaque. Net price 30 pouches (all may be cut to fit; 30, 40, 50, 60 mm or 10–60 mm cut-to-fit holes) = £57.47

**Eakin**® (Salts)
*Closed*, one-piece pouch, white or clear. 32, 45, or 64 mm holes, net price 20 pouches = £35.25; 90 mm hole, 20 pouches = £44.36

**Kombo**® (Salts)
*Kombo closed*, one-piece pouch with karaya skin protector seal and adhesive, clear. Net price (30, 40. 50, or 60 mm holes), 30 pouches = £50.97; with filter, 30 pouches = £61.98

**Palex**® (Salts)

*BCLF bag* (= pouch), one-piece closed pouch with CL resin seal, porous adhesive, and filter. Net price 30 pouches (25, 32, 38, 44, 51, 64 mm or cut-to-fit holes) = £51.00

*BCLF Petite mini bag* (= pouch), one-piece closed pouch with CL resin seal, porous adhesive, and filter. Net price 30 pouches (25, 32, 38, 44 mm or cut-to-fit holes) = £45.00

**Simplicity 1**® (Salts)

*Closed*, one-piece pouch with porous adhesive, skin protector seal, and filter, fabric front and back. Net price 30 pouches (all may be cut to fit; opaque: 30, 40, 50, or 60 mm holes; opaque or clear: cut-to-fit holes) =£57.47

*Paediatric*, closed one-piece pouch with single-release paper, porous adhesive, clear. Net price 30 pouches (13 mm cut-to-fit hole) = £37.42

**Simplicity 2**® (Salts)

*Closed*, two-piece closed pouch (may also be applied directly to skin). Net price 30 pouches (40, 50, 60, or 70 mm holes, also 30 mm only for direct application to skin) = £28.77

**Solo**® (Salts)

*Solo closed*, one-piece pouch with single-release paper, and adhesive flange, clear. Net price (30, 40, 50, or 60 mm holes), 30 pouches = £16.78; with filter, 30 pouches = £25.34

Shannon range

**Colostomy** (Shannon)

*Appliance*. Net price, 1 appliance (TJS 962) = £15.39

*Day bag* (= pouch). Net price 1 pouch, TJS 948f = £20.27; TJS 948j = £23.19

*Disposable bag* (= pouch). Net price TJS 948g, 100 pouches = £10.04

*Night bag* (= pouch). Net price 1 pouch, TJS 948e = £23.19; TJS 948k = £25.29

*Outfit*. Net price 1 TJS 948A = £68.43, 1 TJS 948NA = £66.27; 1 TJS 948T = £36.29

**Easychange**® (Shannon)

*Appliance*. Net price 1 appliance = £4.06

*Spare bag* (= pouch). Net price 100 pouches = £40.50

**Shannon**

*Disposable bag* (= pouch), closed pouches with plasters. Net price 12 pouches = £5.55

*Elastic necks*. Net price 50 pouches = £20.25

Shaw range

**Hainsworth**® (Shaw)

*Hainsworth bag* (= pouch), one-piece closed pouch. Net price (both 1, 1.25, 1.5, or 2 inch holes), 20 pouches with body mould adhesive = £34.50; 20 pouches with Healwell® adhesive = £18.10

**Shaw** (Shaw)

*Colostomy outfit*, comprising, 4-inch wide elastic belt with groinstrap (26 to 42-inch), 1 flange and 100 colostomy pouches. Net price one NSI 6 outfit with 11 × 6inch pouches = £31.95; one NSI 7 outfit with 12 × 8-inch pouches = £32.60; one NSI 8 outfit with 11 × 6-inch pouches = £34.95

*Double seal*, one-piece closed pouch. Net price 100 11 × 6-inch pouches = £8.25; 100 12 × 8-inch pouches = £9.05

*Stick-on bag* (pouch), one-piece closed pouch with plasters. Net price 10 pouches = £6.90

Simcare range

**Adhesive** (Simcare)

*Stomabag*, one-piece closed pouch with adhesive, opaque. Net price (25, 32, 38, 44, 51, or 64 mm holes), 90 pouches = £105.30; with filter, 90 pouches = £118.35

**Beta**® (Simcare)

*Closed*, two-piece pouch with filter. Net price, 1 kit comprising 30 pouches and 8 Seel-a-peel sheets (100 × 100 mm) = £44.16; 90 spare pouches = £121.57

**Chiron**® (Simcare)

*Clearseal* (= pouch), one-piece closed pouch. Net price 10 305 × 127-mm pouches (22 mm hole) = £12.41

*Closed bag*, one-piece pouch. Net price 10 305 × 127-mm or 230 × 127-mm pouches (38 mm hole) = £12.41

**Chironseal**® (Simcare)

*Closed bag* (= pouch), one-piece closed pouch. Net price 10 305 × 102-, 305 × 127-, 230 × 127-, or 305 × 150-mm pouches (22 or 38 mm holes) = £9.30; 10 305 × 205- or 305 × 255-mm pouches (22 or 38 mm hole) = £10.69

*Reinforced*, one-piece disposable closed pouch. Net price 10 305 × 102-mm (25 or 38 mm holes) or 305 × 127-mm (38 mm hole) pouches = £12.41

**EC1**® (Simcare)

*Colo Classic*, one-piece closed pouch with wafer, comfort backing, and filter, opaque or clear. Net price 30 pouches (25, 32, 38, 44, 51, 64 mm or 15–44 mm cut-to-fit holes) = £58.53

**Omni**® (Simcare)

*Closed*, one-piece pouch with wafer, porous adhesive, filter. Net price 30 pouches (opaque: 25, 32, 38, 44, or 51 mm; opaque or clear: 15–44 mm cut-to-fit holes) = £59.39

**Redifit**® (Simcare)

*Continuation bag* (= pouch), one-piece closed pouch with karaya skin protector, may be worn with belt, opaque. Net price 20 pouches (32, 38, 44, 51, 64, or 75 mm holes) = £59.96

*Non-adhesive bag* (= pouch), one-piece closed pouch, must be worn with belt. Net price 20 pouches with karaya skin protector (opaque: 44 or 51 mm holes; clear: 44, 51, or 64 mm holes) = £59.96; without karaya, 20 pouches (opaque, 38 mm hole) = £45.50

**Rediseal**® (Simcare)

*Small bag* (= pouch), one-piece PVC compact closed pouch, opaque. Net price 10 pouches (38, 44, or 51 mm holes) = £11.71

**Symphony**® (Simcare)

*WC Disposable*, one-piece closed pouch with wafer and filter. Net price 30 pouches (opaque or clear: 25, 32, 38, 44, or 51 mm holes; opaque: 15–44 mm cut-to-fit holes) = £62.16

Simpla range

**Phoenix**® (Simpla)

*Closed*, one-piece closed pouch. Net price (both 32, 40, or 45 mm holes) 100 pouches = £128.06; 100 casual pouches = £119.12

**Sassco**® (Simpla)

*Closed*, one-piece closed pouch. Net price 100 pouches (32, 40, or 45 mm holes) = £124.34

**Simplaseel**® (Simpla)

*Closed*, one-piece pouch. Net price 30 pouches (26, 32, 40, 45, 50 mm or cut-to-fit holes) = £58.63; 30 casual pouches (32, 40, or 45 mm holes) = £54.54

Thackraycare range

**Schacht**® (Thackraycare)

*Colostomy bag* (= pouch), one-piece closed pouch. Net price 100 pouches = £32.30

*Colostomy appliance*. Net price 1 appliance = £27.85

**Slimline**® (Thackraycare)

*Colostomy appliance*. Net price 1 appliance = £30.25

Ward range

**Ward**

*Disposable bag* (= pouch), one-piece closed pouch. Net price 10 24 × 4-inch pouches with 4 × 3-inch plasters = £7.17; 10 12 × 5-inch pouches with 4 × 4-inch plasters = £7.17

*Celluloid colostomy cup*, with sponge or solid rim. Net price 1 (small, medium, or large) cup = £29.75; with belt fitting, 1 cup = £33.95; 1 pouch with mount outlet = £12.36

Welland range

**Welland**® (Welland)

*Colostomy bag* (= pouch), one-piece closed pouch with wafer and filter, opaque or clear. Net price 30 pouches (25, 32, 38, 44, 51, 60 mm or cut-to-fit holes) = £49.35

*Softback colostomy bag*, one-piece closed pouch with wafer, filter, and soft backing, opaque or clear. Net price 30 pouches (25, 32, 38, 44, 51, 60 mm or cut-to-fit holes) = £50.65

## DRAINABLE POUCHES

Drainable pouches are suitable for patients with an **ileostomy** or a **colostomy** with fluid effluent

Body's Care range
**Rubber bags screwcap** (Body's Care)
*Black butyl*, one-piece pouch. Net price 1 day pouch = £20.41; 1 night pouch = £23.81
*White rubber*, one-piece pouch. Net price 1 day pouch = £11.34; 1 night pouch = £13.07
**Rubber bags spout** (Body's Care)
*Black butyl*, one-piece pouch. Net price 1 day or night pouch = £21.55
*White rubber*, one-piece pouch. Net price 1 day pouch = £10.21; 1 night pouch = £10.80

Bullen range
**Lenbul®** (Bullen)
*Day bag* (= pouch), one-piece pouch. Net price 1 pouch with screwcap outlet = £11.56; 1 pouch with screwcap outlet and larger opening = £12.00; 1 pouch with metal strip = £13.87; 1 pouch with tap outlet = £13.93
*Night bag* (= pouch), one-piece pouch. Net price 1 pouch with screwcap outlet = £12.73; 1 pouch with screwcap outlet and larger opening = £13.21; 1 pouch with metal strip = £13.87; 1 pouch with tap outlet = £15.34

Cambmac range
**Dansac®** (Cambmac)
*Combi D + A*, one-piece pouch with adhesive and karaya skin protector, opaque. Net price 30 pouches (19, 22, 25, 32, 38, 50, or 63 mm holes) = £67.10
*Combi Ileo F*, one-piece pouch, opaque. Net price 100 pouches (standard: 22 or 30 mm holes; small: 19 or 25 mm holes) = £147.95
*CombiMicro D + S*, one-piece pouch with porous adhesive, skin barrier ring, and fabric backing. Net price 30 pouches (25, 32, 38, 44, 50, 63 mm or cut-to-fit holes), opaque = £59.35; clear, 30 pouches = £56.00
*Mini Infant*, one-piece pouch with skin barrier ring and fabric backing, clear. Net price 30 pouches (cut-to-fit holes) = £48.60
*Mini Petit D*, one-piece pouch with skin barrier ring and fabric backing, opaque or clear. Net price 30 pouches (cut-to-fit holes) = £51.20
*Supersquare System*, two-piece pouch, opaque or clear. Net price 30 standard or small pouches to fit 50 mm base plate = £33.50; 30 standard pouches to fit 80 mm base plate = £48.40

CliniMed range
**Biotrol®** (CliniMed)
*Elite*, fabric covered one-piece pouch with skin protector adhesive and clamp closure, white or skin-tone. Net price 30 pouches (20, 25, 30, 35, 40, 45, 50, 60, 70 mm or cut-to-fit holes) = £58.75
*Ileo S*, one-piece pouch with skin protector adhesive, white. Net price 30 pouches (20, 25, 30, 35, 40, 45, 50, 60, 70 mm or cut-to-fit holes) = £58.75
*Post-op*, one-piece pouch with skin protector adhesive, for temporary or permanent colostomies or ileostomies, clear. Net price (cut-to-fit holes) small, 30 pouches = £59.40; large, 30 pouches = £83.90
*Preference*, fabric covered one-piece pouch with skin protector adhesive, porous adhesive collar, and fabric backing, skin-tone. Net price 30 pouches (20, 25, 30, 35, 40, 45, 50, 60 mm or cut-to-fit holes) = £58.75

Coloplast range
**Ileo B®** (Coloplast)
One-piece pouch with zinc oxide adhesive, clear or white. Net price 100 pouches (20 mm hole) = £138.00
*Mini*, one-piece compact pouch with zinc oxide adhesive, white. Net price 100 pouches (20 mm hole) = £137.00

**K-Flex®** (Coloplast)
One-piece pouch with karaya skin protector, clear. Net price 30 pouches (10 or 40 mm holes) = £64.20
**mc2000®** (Coloplast)
One-piece pouch with double seal, opaque or clear. Net price 30 pouches (20, 25, 30, 35, 40, 45, 50, 55, 60 mm holes or clear pouch with cut-to-fit hole) = £63.60
*Mini*, one-piece compact pouch, opaque. Net price 30 pouches (20, 25, 30, 35, or 40 mm holes) = £60.00
**mc2002®** (Coloplast)
Two-piece pouch, opaque or clear. Net price 30 pouches (to fit 40 or 60 mm base plates) = £37.50
*Post-op*, two-piece pouch, clear. Net price, to fit 70 mm base plate, 10 bags with clip = £15.30; to fit 100 mm base plate, 10 bags with clip = £20.10
**pc3000®** (Coloplast)
One-piece pouch, opaque or clear. Net price 30 pouches (20, 25, 30, 35, 40, 45, 50, 55, or 60 mm holes; 20 mm can be cut to fit up to 60 mm) = £56.70

ConvaTec range
**Ileodress®** (ConvaTec)
*Ileodress*, one-piece pouch with textured backing. Net price 10 standard pouches with clip (opaque or clear: 19, 38, 45, 50, or 64 mm holes; 19 mm can be cut to fit; opaque only: 25 and 32 mm holes) = £18.64; 10 small pouches with clip, opaque (19, 25, 32, 38, 45, 50, or 64 mm holes; 19 mm can be cut to fit) = £18.25
*Ileodress Plus*, one-piece pouch with single-release paper. Net price 10 standard pouches with clip (opaque or clear: 19, 38, 45, 50, or 64 mm holes; 19 mm can be cut to fit; opaque only: 25 and 32 mm holes) = £18.64
**Little Ones®** (ConvaTec)
*Paediatric*, one-piece pouch. Net price 15 pouches (8 mm cut-to-fit hole) = £25.65
**Surgicare System® 2** (ConvaTec)
*System 2*, two-piece pouches, white. Net price 10 pouches with clip (to fit 32, 38, 45, 57, or 70 mm flanges) = £9.27
*System 2 Combihesive*, two-piece pouches with textured backing. Net price 10 standard or small pouches with clip, beige, (to fit 32, 38, 45, 57, or 70 mm flanges) = £9.35; 10 standard pouches with clip, clear, to fit 45, 57, or 70 mm flanges = £9.35, to fit 100 mm flanges = £16.53

Drew range
**Drew**
*Ileostomy bag* (= pouch), one-piece pouch. Net price 50 D1/1 pouches = £56.65; 50 D1/6 pouches = £40.44

Hollister range
**Classic** (Hollister)
All with 25, 32, 38, 44, 51, 64, or 76 mm holes
*Karaya seal* (series 721), one-piece pouch with karaya skin protector seal, must be worn with belt, clear. Net price 30 pouches with 1 clamp = £56.07
*Karaya 5® transparent*, one-piece pouch with karaya skin protector seal, may be worn with belt. 30- or 40-cm clear pouch with microporous adhesive (series 322 and 327), net price 30 pouches with 1 clamp = £64.35; 30-cm pouches with regular adhesive (series 722) = £64.35
*Karaya 5® opaque*, one-piece pouch with karaya skin protector seal and porous adhesive, may be worn with belt. Net price 30 pouches with 1 clamp, 23-cm pouches (series 313) = £64.35; 30-cm pouches (series 311) = £61.97
**Guardian®** (Hollister)
All with 25, 38, 51, or 64 mm holes
*Guardian* (series 461 and 460), two-piece pouch, opaque or clear. Net price 10 pouches with 1 clamp = £8.70; larger pouch to fit 102-mm flange, 10 pouches (clear) with 1 clamp = £18.85
*Guardian mini-pouch*, two-piece compact pouch, opaque. Net price (series 464), 10 pouches = £8.70; **NHS** with inner film and replaceable filter (series 463), 10 pouches with pack of filters and 1 clamp

NHS *With replaceable filter* (series 462), two-piece pouch with inner film and replaceable filter, clear. 10 pouches with pack of filters and 1 clamp
**Premium®** (Hollister)
*Karaya 5® seal* (series 360), one-piece pouch with porous adhesive and karaya skin protector seal, clear. Net price 15 pouches (25, 32, 38, 44, 51, 64, or 76 mm holes) with 1 clamp = £31.58
*Karaya 5® seal with filter* (series 366), one-piece pouch with porous adhesive, karaya skin protector seal, and replaceable filter, may be worn with belt, clear. Net price 15 pouches (25, 32, 38, 44, 51, or 64 mm holes) with 1 clamp and filter elements = £35.13
*Synthetic seal* (series 364), one-piece pouch with porous adhesive and synthetic skin protector seal, clear. Net price 15 pouches (25, 32, 38, 44, 51, or 64 mm holes) with 1 clamp = £31.58

Leyland range
**Birkbeck®** (Leyland)
*Rubber*, one-piece pouch, black or pink. Net price (both 19, 38, or 54 mm holes), 1 day pouch = £22.63; 1 night pouch = £25.88
*Disposable*, one-piece plastic pouch. Net price 100 pouches = £13.69
**Rubber bags** (Leyland)
*White rubber*, one-piece pouch. Net price, 1 day pouch (38, 44, or 51 mm holes) = £10.13; 1 screwcap pouch (38 mm hole) = £10.93; 1 pouch with vent (38 mm hole) = £12.11
*White rubber child bag* (= pouch), one-piece pouch. Net price (both 19, 25, or 28 mm holes), 1 day pouch = £9.76; 1 night pouch = £11.95
*Latex rubber*, one-piece pouch. Net price 1 day pouch (38, 44, or 51 mm holes) = £11.00; 1 night pouch (19, 25, or 28 mm holes) = £12.15

Rüsch range
**Ostopore®** (Rüsch)
*Ileo KAV-opaque*, one-piece pouch with karaya seal skin protector, adhesive, and vent, opaque. Net price 30 pouches (25, 32, or 38 mm holes) with 30 belt flanges and 10 clips = £56.70
*Mini pouch*, one-piece pouch. Net price 30 pouches (25, 32, 38, 45, or 51 mm holes) = £32.40

Salts range
NHS **Cohflex®** (Salts)
*Drainable*, one-piece pouch with single-release paper, wafer, and fabric front and back. Net price 30 pouches with integral closure clip (opaque: 30, 40, 50, or 60 mm, all may be cut to fit; clear: 10–60 mm cut-to-fit holes) = £59.94
*Paediatric drainable*, one-piece small pouch with single-release paper, wafer, and fabric backing, opaque/clear. Net price 30 pouches with integral closure clip (10–50 mm cut-to-fit holes) = £47.28
**Eakin®** (Salts)
*Drainable*, one-piece pouch, white or clear. Net price 20 small or large pouches (32, 45, or 64 mm holes = £40.74; 20 wide pouches, clear (90 mm hole) = £86.47
*Fistula*, one-piece pouch. Net price 10 large pouches = £98.26; starter, 20 small pouches = £84.73, 20 medium pouches = £110.24
**Light White** (Salts)
*Drainable*, one-piece pouch, white. Net price 30 large, small, or medium pouches (all 25, 32, or 38 mm holes) = £40.73
*Drainable self-adhesive*, one-piece pouch with adhesive, white. Net price 30 pouches (large: 25, 32, 38, or 44 mm holes; small and medium: 25, 32, or 38 mm holes) = £46.21
**Koenig Rutzen® screwcap** (Salts)
All with screwcap outlet
*Black butyl all rubber*, one-piece pouch. Net price 1 large

or small pouch (both 25, 32, 38, 44, or 51 mm holes) = £26.02; with bridge (soft-face Maggie Bag), 1 pouch (large: 25, 32, 38, 44, or 51 mm holes; small: 25, 32, or 38 mm) = £33.54
*Black butyl reinforced*, one-piece pouch. Net price 1 large or small pouch (both 25, 32, or 38 mm holes) = £33.54; with bridge (hard-face Maggie Bag), 1 pouch (large: 25, 32, 38, 44, or 51 mm holes; small: 25, 32, or 38 mm) = £39.09
**Koenig Rutzen® spout** (Salts)
All with spout outlet
*Black butyl all rubber*, one-piece pouch. Net price 1 large or small pouch (both 25, 32, 38, 44, or 51 mm holes) = £18.88; with bridge, 1 pouch (large: 25, 32, 38, 44, or 51 mm holes; small: 25, 32, or 38 mm) = £24.97
*Black butyl reinforced*, one-piece pouch. Net price 1 large or small pouch (25, 32, or 38 mm holes) = £25.38; with bridge, 1 pouch (large: 25, 32, 38, 44, or 51 mm holes; small: 25, 32, or 38 mm) = £31.25
**Kombo®** (Salts)
*Kombo drainable*, one-piece pouch with karaya skin protector seal and adhesive, clear. Net price 30 pouches (30, 40, 50, 60, or 80 mm holes) = £48.82; with filter, 30 pouches = £67.12
**Rubber bags** (Salts)
All must be used with flange
*Black butyl screw*, one-piece bag with screwcap outlet. Net price 1 large or small pouch = £24.73
*Black butyl spout*, one-piece bag with spout outlet. Net price 1 large or small pouch = £17.84
*White screw*, one-piece bag with screwcap outlet. Net price 1 large or small pouch = £8.25
*White spout*, one-piece bag with spout outlet. Net price 1 large or small pouch = £6.99
**Salger®** (Salts)
*Drainable*, one-piece pouch. Net price 10 pouches (40 or 57 mm holes) = £9.51
**Simplicity®** (Salts)
*Drainable*, two-piece pouch, clear. Net price 30 230 × 137-mm pouches (40, 50, or 60 mm holes) = £15.29
*Post-op*, two-piece pouch, clear. Net price 30 300 × 125-mm pouches (40, 50, or 60 mm holes) = £13.28
**Simplicity 1®** (Salts)
*Drainable*, one-piece pouch with porous adhesive and skin protector seal, fabric front and back. Net price 30 pouches with integral closure clip (opaque: 30, 40, 50, or 60 mm, all may be cut to fit; opaque or clear: 10–60 mm cut-to-fit hole) = £59.94
*Paediatric drainable*, one-piece pouch with porous adhesive and skin protector seal, clear. Net price 30 pouches (cut-to-fit hole) = £37.42
*Post-op*, one-piece pouch with single-release paper and wafer, clear. Net price 10 pouches (both cut-to-fit holes), small = £50.65; large = £69.55
**Simplicity 2®** (Salts)
*Drainable*, two-piece pouch (may also be applied directly to skin). Net price 15 pouches (40, 50, 60, or 70 mm holes, also 30 mm only for direct application to skin) = £15.97
*Post-op*, two-piece pouch (may also be applied directly to skin). Net price 30 pouches (40, 50, 60, or 70 mm holes, also 30 mm only for direct application to skin) = £31.53
*Transverse*, two-piece pouch (may also be applied directly to skin). Net price 10 pouches (cut-to-fit hole) = £35.84
**Solo®** (Salts)
*Drainable*, one-piece pouch with single-release paper and adhesive, clear. Net price 30 pouches (30, 40, 50, 60 or 80 mm holes) = £19.93; with filter, 30 pouches = £25.13
NHS **United®** (Salts)
*Soft & Secure drainable*, one-piece pouch, opaque or clear. Net price 10 pouches (38, 45, or 57 mm holes) = £8.47

Shaw range
**Hainsworth®** (Shaw)
*Drainable bag*, one-piece pouch with adhesive. Net price
20 pouches (0.875, 1, 1.25, or 1.5 inch holes) = £34.50
**Rubber bags** (Shaw)
*Black screwcap*, one-piece pouch with screwcap outlet.
Net price (both 19, 38 or 54 mm holes), 1 day pouch =
£19.40; 1 night pouch = £20.65

Simcare range
**Adhesive** (Simcare)
*Stomabag*, one-piece pouch with adhesive, opaque. Net
price 60 pouches (19, 25, 32, 38, 51 mm or cut-to-fit
holes) = £76.99
**Beta®** (Simcare)
*Post-op*, two-piece large capacity pouch. Net price (cut-
to-fit hole), 4 pouches with 1 wire closure = £26.94, 20
pouches with 20 wire closures = £39.34
**Cavendish®** (Simcare)
*Odourproof*, one-piece pouch. Net price (all 25, 32, or
38 mm holes), 10 opaque pouches with non-adhesive
flange = £26.71; 10 opaque pouches with adhesive
flange = £32 17; 10 clear PVC pouches = £26.88
**Chiron® screwcap** (Simcare)
All with screwcap outlet
*Butyl rubber day bag* (= pouch), one-piece pouch, black.
Net price 1 pouch (38, 44, or 51 mm hole) = £27.38
*Butyl rubber night bag* (= pouch), one-piece pouch,
black. Net price 1 pouch (38 or 44 mm holes) = £32.86
*Latex rubber day bag* (= pouch), one-piece pouch. Net
price 1 pouch (38 mm hole) = £13.70
*Latex rubber night bag* (= pouch), one-piece pouch. Net
price 1 pouch (38 mm hole) = £18.14
*White rubber day bag* (= pouch), one-piece pouch. Net
price 1 pouch (38, 44, or 51 mm) = £15.76, child-size
pouch (38 mm hole) = £13.70; body-size outlet, 1 pouch
(38 mm  hole) = £15.76, child-size pouch (38 mm
hole) = £12.46
*White rubber night bag* (= pouch), one-piece pouch. Net
price 1 pouch (38 or 51 mm hole) = £18.14; body-size
outlet, 1 pouch (38 mm hole) = £15.07
**Chiron® spout** (Simcare)
*White rubber bag* (= pouch), one-piece pouch. Net price
1 day pouch (38 mm hole) = £13.55; 1 night pouch
(38 mm hole) = £14.72
**EC1®** (Simcare)
*Ileo classic*, one-piece pouch with wafer and comfort
backing, opaque. Net price 30 pouches with 1 clamp
(19, 25, 32, 38, 44 mm or 10–44 mm cut-to-fit holes) =
£61.31
*Mini classic*, one-piece compact pouch with wafer and
comfort backing, opaque or clear. Net price 30 pouches
with 1 clamp (10–44 mm cut-to-fit holes) = £61.31
*Post-op classic*, one-piece pouch with wafer and comfort
backing, clear. Net price 30 pouches with 1 clamp,
10–64 mm cut-to-fit holes = £63.24; 10–90 mm cut-to-fit
holes = £89.49
**Omni®** (Simcare)
*Drainable*, one-piece pouch with porous adhesive wafer
and replaceable filter. Net price 20 pouches (opaque:
25, 32, 38, 44 mm; opaque or clear: 10–44 mm cut-
to-fit hole) = £40.85; NHS opaque (10–90 mm cut-to-fit
hole) = £48.43
**Redifit®** (Simcare)
*Opaque*, one-piece pouch with karaya skin protector,
may be worn with belt. Net price 20 pouches with 2
closure clips (25, 32, 38, 44, 51, or 64 mm holes) =
£59.97; small outline pouches, 20 pouches with 2 closure
clips (25, 32, or 38 mm) = £59.97
*Clear fronted*, one-piece pouch with karaya skin protector, may be worn with belt. Net price 20 pouches with
2 closure clips (25, 32, 44, 51, or 64 mm holes) = £59.97

Simpla range
**Sassco®** (Simpla)
*Ileostomy bag* (= pouch), one-piece pouch. Net price
100 pouches (26 or 32 mm holes) = £142.75
**Simplaseel®** (Simpla)
*Drainable bag* (= pouch), one-piece pouch, opaque. Net
price 30 pouches (26, 32, 40, 45, or 50 mm holes) =
£59.54
*Post-op drainable bag* (= pouch), one-piece pouch. Net
price 10 pouches = £32.28
*Paediatric drainable bag* (= pouch), one-piece pouch.
Net price 30 pouches = £51.79

Thackraycare range
**Raymed®** (Thackraycare)
*Butyl day bag* (= pouch), one-piece pouch. Net price 1
pouch with screwcap outlet = £22.60; 1 pouch with tap
outlet = £23.75
**Schacht®** (Thackraycare)
*Ileostomy*, one-piece pouches. Net price 50 pouches =
£19.80
**Stomalite® Mk 2 Ileo** (Thackraycare)
*Day bag* (= pouch), one-piece pouch. Net price 5
pouches (1, 1.25, or 1.5 inch holes) = £17.00
*Night bag* (= pouch), one-piece pouch. Net price 5
pouches (1, 1.25, or 1.5 inch holes) = £17.00
**Stomastar®** (Thackraycare)
*Drain*, one-piece pouch. Net price (all 1, 1.25, 1.5, 2,
2.5, or 3 inch holes), 10 adhesive pouches = £14.90; 10
pouches with belt plate = £14.90; 10 adhesive pouches
with belt plate = £17.20

Ward range
**Rubber bags** (Ward)
*Black rubber bag* (= pouch), one-piece pouch with screwcap outlet. Net price (19, 35, or 54 mm hole), 1 day
pouch = £14.94; 1 night pouch = £15.60
*White rubber ileostomy bag* (= pouch) *with flange*, pouch
with St. Mark's flange. Net price 1 pouch = £22.65
*White rubber ileostomy bag* (= pouch), one-piece pouch.
Net price 1 day pouch (screwcap or spout outlet) =
£10.20; 1 night pouch (screwcap or spout outlet) =
£11.49; tap outlet, 1 day pouch = £14.95; 1 night
pouch = £16.64
*White rubber transverse ileostomy bag* (= pouch), one-
piece pouch. Net price 1 pouch = £23.95

Welland range
**Welland®** (Welland)
*Ileostomy bag* (= pouch), one-piece pouch with wafer,
opaque or clear. Net price 30 pouches (25, 32, 38, 44,
51 mm or cut-to-fit holes) = £49.00
*Softback ileostomy bag* (= pouch), one-piece with wafer
and soft backing, opaque or clear. Net price 30 pouches
(25, 32, 38, 44, 51 mm or cut-to-fit holes) = £52.00
*Mini-bag*, one-piece with wafer, clear. Net price (both
cut-to-fit holes), 30 pouches = £48.50; with soft backing,
30 pouches = £50.50
*Oval drainable*, one-piece pouch with wafer, opaque. Net
price (both cut-to-fit holes), 30 pouches = £53.00; with
soft backing, 30 pouches = £55.00
*Oval post-op*, one-piece pouch with wafer, clear. Net
price (both cut-to-fit holes), 30 pouches = £53.00; with
soft backing, 30 pouches = £55.00

# DEODORANT AND ADHESIVE PREPARATIONS AND DEVICES, AND ADHESIVE REMOVERS

### Adhesive preparations
**Aquadry®** (Thackraycare)
*Medical adhesive*. Net price 20 mL (with brush) = £3.25
**Dow Corning DC 355®** (Dow Corning)
*Medical adhesive brushable*. Net price 20-mL bottle (with
brush) = £2.92

---

**Dow Corning B Spray**® (Dow Corning)
*Spray adhesive.* Net price 206-g aerosol spray = £9.64
**Hollister**® (Hollister)
*Medical adhesive spray* (with silicones). Net price 170-g aerosol spray = £11.50
**Latex adhesive solution** (Salt)
Net price per tube = £1.62. Label: 15

**Adhesive devices**
See Drug Tariff for further details
Adhesive discs (3M—Stomaseal®, Salts—Reliaseal®, Simcare)
Adhesive rings, elastic (Simcare); plastic (Shannon); rubber (Shannon)
Adhesive plasters (Bullen, Drew, Leyland, Salts—Transacryl®, Zopla®, Shannon—Easychange® with rings, Shaw, Simcare—Chiron®, Carshalton®, Ward)
Kidney seals (Simcare)

**Adhesive removers**
**Dow Corning Remover**® (Dow Corning)
*Adhesive remover spray.* Net price 227-g aerosol spray = £7.59
**Hollister**® (Hollister)
*Adhesive remover spray.* Net price 170-g spray = £9.63
**Salts 'SPR' Plaster Remover (Rezolve**®) (Salts)
*Adhesive remover spray.* Net price 70-g aerosol spray = £2.41. Label: 15

**Deodorants**
Atmocol® is used as a deodorising spray when emptying the appliance. The other deodorants listed are placed in the appliance.

**Atmocol**® (Thackraycare)
*Aerosol deodorant.* Net price 1 unit (400 sprays) = £1.90
**Chironair Odour Control Liquid**® (Simcare)
*Deodorant solution.* Net price 113 g = £4.79
**Colostomy Plus**® (Shannon)
*Deodorant.* Net price 1 unit = £2.46
**Dor**® (Simpla)
*Deodorant solution.* Net price 7 mL = £1.48
**Forest Breeze**® (Shaw)
*Deodorant.* Net price 1 unit = £2.73
**Limone**® (CliniMed)
*Deodorant spray.* Net price 50 mL = £3.60
**Nilodor**® (Cussons)
*Deodorant solution.* Net price (with dropper) 7.5 mL = £1.60; 15 mL = £2.82
**Ostobon**® (Coloplast)
*Deodorant powder.* Net price 22 g = £3.23
**Saltair No-Roma**® (Salts)
*Deodorant solution.* Net price 30 mL = £1.93; 300 mL = £6.28
**Stomogel**® (Thackraycare)
*Deodorant gel.* Net price 50 g = £2.60
**Sween**® (Bullen & Smears)
*Deodorant.* Net price 15 mL = £3.55
**Translet Plus One**® (Rüsch)
*Deodorant solution for men.* Net price 7 mL = £2.64
**Translet Plus Two**® (Rüsch)
*Deodorant solution for women.* Net price 7 mL = £2.64

## BELTS, CLOSURES, COVERS

See Drug Tariff for further details
**Bag closures**
Clamps (Clinimed—Biotrol®, Hollister, Simcare—Carshalton®, Simpla)
Clips (ConvaTec, Drew, Salts, Shaw, Thackraycare)
Rings (Shaw)
Tape (Shannon)

**Bag covers** (Body's Care, Bullen, Clinimed—Biotrol®, Coloplast—Ileo B®, Uro®, ConvaTec—Surgicare® System 2, Drew, Hollister, North West Ostomy, Rüsch—Ostopore®, Salts—Eakin®, Shaw, Simcare—Redifit®, Symphony®, Simpla, Steeper, Welland)
**Belts** (Body's Care, Bullen, Cambmac—Dansac®, Clinimed—Biotrol®, Coloplast—K Flex®, ConvaTec, Drew, Ellis, Hollister, Leyland)

## FILTERS, BRIDGES, FLANGES

See Drug Tariff for further details
**Filters and Bridges** (Clinimed—Biotrol®, Coloplast—Filtrodor®, Maclet®, ConvaTec, Cuxson, Hollister, Salt, Simcare)
**Flanges** various sizes (Body's Care, Bullen—Lenbul®, Drew, Leyland, Salts—Salger®, Shannon, Shaw, Simcare—Chiron®, Redifit®, Thackraycare—Schacht®, Slimline®, Ward)

## IRRIGATION AND WASHOUT APPLIANCES

See Drug Tariff for further details
**Irrigation and washout appliances** (Astra, Cambmac, Clinimed—Biotrol®, Coloplast, Hollister, Ward)

## PRESSURE PLATES, SHIELDS

See Drug Tariff for further details
**Pressure plates** (Body's Care, Coloplast, Drew, Salts, Shannon, Simcare, Thackraycare)
**Shields** (Body's Care—St. Mark's Shield, Salts)

## SKIN PROTECTIVES, FILLERS, CLEANSERS

**Skin protectives, fillers, and cleansers**
**Bullen Karaya Gum Powder**® (Bullen)
*Powder.* Net price 70 g = £4.14
**Chiron**® (Simcare)
*Barrier cream* (with antiseptic). Net price 52 g = £4.12
**CliniShield Barrier Wipes**® (CliniMed)
*Barrier wipes.* Net price 50 = £9.80
**Comfeel**® (Coloplast)
*Barrier cream.* Net price 60 g = £3.14
*Protective film.* Net price 30 sachets = £7.50; applicator = £3.47
**Derma-gard**® (Simcare)
*Protective skin wipes.* Net price 50 = £12.07
**Hollister**® (Hollister)
*Karaya paste.* Net price 128 g = £5.70
  Do not apply to severely excoriated skin
*Karaya powder.* Net price 71 g = £6.77
*Skin gel.* Net price 28 g = £4.95. Label: 15
  Do not apply to severely excoriated skin
**Orabase**® (ConvaTec)
*Paste,* see section 12.3.1
**Orahesive**® (ConvaTec)
*Powder* (with adherent properties), see section 12.3.1
**Saltair**® (Salts)
*Karaya gum powder.* Net price per puffer pack = £3.63
*Ostomy cleansing soap* (soap spirit). Net price 110-mL = £2.18
*Skin prep wipes.* Net price 50 = £12.14
**Simcare**® (Simcare)
*Karaya gel.* Net price 35 g = £4.94
*Karaya gum powder.* Net price 100 g = £5.81
*Karaya gum sheet.* Net price 1 = £5.82
**Simpla**® (Simpla)
*Gel.* Net price 35 g = £5.23

**Stomahesive**® (ConvaTec)
*Paste*. Net price 60 g = £5.41. For filling and sealing skin creases
**Stomobar**® (Thackraycare)
*Barrier cream*. Net price 20 g = £1.90
**Stomosol**® (Thackraycare)
*Deodorising antiseptic liquid*. Dilute before use. Net price 200 mL = £4.12
**Translet**® (Rüsch)
*Barrier cream*. Net price 51 g = £2.64
*Wipes*. Net price 30 = £4.99
**United Skin Barrier Paste**® (Salt)
*Paste*. Net price 70 g = £5.46
**Varihesive**® (ConvaTec)
*Wafers*, gelatin 20%, pectin 20%, polyisobutylene 40%, carmellose sodium 20%. Net price 5 wafers (10 × 10 cm) = £7.40

## STOMA CAPS AND DRESSINGS

See Drug Tariff for further details
**Stoma caps and dressings** (Bullen, Coloplast—Colocap®, ConvaTec—Colodress®, Hollister, Salts—Simplicity®, Simcare, Steeper)

## TUBING

See Drug Tariff for further details
**Tubing** (Hollister, Salt, Simcare, Steeper)

# 1.9   Drugs affecting intestinal secretions

1.9.1 Drugs acting on the gall bladder
1.9.2 Drugs which increase gastric acidity
1.9.3 Aprotinin
1.9.4 Pancreatin

## 1.9.1   Drugs acting on the gall bladder

The bile acids **chenodeoxycholic** or **ursodeoxycholic acid** are used in selected patients to dissolve cholesterol gallstones as an alternative to surgery. They are only suitable for patients who have mild symptoms, unimpaired gall bladder function, and small or medium sized radiolucent stones; they are not suitable for radio-opaque stones, which are unlikely to be dissolved. Patients should preferably be supervised in hospital because radiological monitoring is required. Long-term prophylaxis may be needed after complete dissolution of the gallstones has been confirmed (preferably with cholecystograms and ultrasound on two separate occasions) as gallstones may recur in up to 25% of patients within one year of stopping treatment.

**Dehydrocholic acid** is used to improve biliary drainage by stimulating the secretion of thin watery bile. It is given after surgery of the biliary tract to flush the common duct and drainage tube and wash away small calculi obstructing flow through the common bile duct but its value has not been established.

A **terpene** mixture (Rowachol®) also raises biliary cholesterol solubility. It is less effective than the bile acids but may be a useful adjunct.

## CHENODEOXYCHOLIC ACID

*Indications; Cautions:* see notes above
*Contra-indications:* do not use when stones are radio-opaque, in pregnancy, in non-functioning gall bladders, in chronic liver disease, and inflammatory diseases of the small intestine and colon
*Side-effects:* diarrhoea particularly initially with high dosage (reduce dose for few days), pruritus, minor hepatic abnormalities and transient rise in serum transaminases
*Dose:* 10–15 mg/kg daily as a single dose at bedtime *or* in divided doses for 3–24 months, depending on size of stone; treatment is continued for 3 months after stones dissolve

PoM **Chendol**® (CP)
*Capsules*, orange/white, chenodeoxycholic acid 125 mg. Net price 224-cap pack = £48.50
*Tablets*, orange, f/c, scored, chenodeoxycholic acid 250 mg. Net price 112-tab pack = £47.50
PoM **Chenofalk**® (Thames)
*Capsules*, chenodeoxycholic acid 250 mg. Net price 60 = £18.00
*Additives: include* gluten

## DEHYDROCHOLIC ACID

*Indications:* see notes above
*Contra-indications:* complete mechanical biliary obstruction and occlusive hepatitis, chronic liver disease
*Dose:* 250–750 mg, 3 times daily
Cholecystography, 500–750 mg every 4 hours for 12 hours before and after the examination

**Dehydrocholic Acid** (Non-proprietary)
*Tablets*, dehydrocholic acid 250 mg. Net price 20 = £7.17

## URSODEOXYCHOLIC ACID

*Indications; Cautions; Contra-indications:* see under Chenodeoxycholic Acid
*Side-effects:* see under Chenodeoxycholic Acid; diarrhoea occurs rarely; liver changes have not been reported
*Dose:* 8–12 mg/kg (obese patients up to 15 mg/kg) daily as a single dose at bedtime or in divided doses, for up to 2 years; treatment is continued for 3–4 months after stones dissolve

PoM **Destolit**® (Merrell)
*Tablets*, scored, ursodeoxycholic acid 150 mg. Net price 60 = £19.40. Label: 21
PoM **Ursofalk**® (Thames)
*Capsules*, ursodeoxycholic acid 250 mg. Net price 60 = £31.50. Label: 21
*Additives: include* gluten

## OTHER PREPARATIONS FOR BILIARY DISORDERS

PoM **Rowachol**® (Monmouth)
*Capsules*, green, e/c, borneol 5 mg, camphene 5 mg, cineole 2 mg, menthol 32 mg, menthone 6 mg, pinene 17 mg in olive oil. Net price 50-cap pack = £7.54. Label: 22
*Dose:* 1–2 capsules 3 times daily before food
**Interactions:** Appendix 1 (*Rowachol*®)

## 1.9.2 Drugs which increase gastric acidity

Muripsin® is used in achlorhydria and hypochlorhydria but is of uncertain value; it replaced dilute hydrochloric acid.

**Muripsin®** (Norgine)
*Tablets*, orange, f/c, glutamic acid hydrochloride 500 mg: 1 tablet ≈ 1 mL dilute hydrochloric acid. Net price 50 = £5.28. Label: 21
*Dose:* 1–2 tablets with meals

## 1.9.3 Aprotinin

Now in section 2.11.

## 1.9.4 Pancreatin

Supplements of pancreatin are given by mouth to compensate for reduced or absent exocrine secretion in cystic fibrosis, and following pancreatectomy, total gastrectomy, or chronic pancreatitis. They assist the digestion of starch, fat, and protein.

Pancreatin is inactivated by gastric acid therefore pancreatin preparations are best taken with food ( or immediately before or after food). Gastric acid secretion may be reduced by giving cimetidine or ranitidine an hour beforehand (section 1.3). Concurrent use of antacids also reduces gastric acidity. The newer enteric-coated preparations such as Creon®, Nutrizym GR®, and Pancrease® deliver a higher enzyme concentration in the duodenum (providing the granules are swallowed whole without chewing).

Since pancreatin is also inactivated by heat, excessive heat should be avoided if preparations are mixed with liquids or food; the resulting mixtures should not be kept for more than one hour.

Dosage is adjusted according to size, number, and consistency of stools, so that the patient thrives; extra allowance may be needed if snacks are taken between meals.

Pancreatin may irritate the skin around mouth and anus, particularly if preparations are retained in the mouth or dosage is excessive. Hypersensitivity reactions occur occasionally and may affect those handling the powder.

For reference to acetylcysteine in cystic fibrosis, see Acetylcysteine Granules (section 3.7).

### PANCREATIN
*Indications; Cautions; Side-effects:* see above
*Dose:* see below

**Cotazym®** (Organon)
*Capsules*, green, pancreatin, providing minimum of: protease 450 units, lipase 13 000 units, amylase 9000 units. Net price 56-cap pack = £1.86. Counselling, see dose
*Dose:* 6 capsules daily in divided doses; contents sprinkled on food

**Creon®** (Duphar)
*Capsules*, brown/yellow, enclosing buff-coloured e/c granules of pancreatin, providing: protease 210 units, lipase 8000 units, amylase 9000 units. Net price 100 = £13.33.
*Dose:* initially 1–2 capsules with meals either taken whole or contents mixed with fluid or soft food (then swallowed immediately without chewing); usual range 5–15 capsules daily

**Nutrizym® GR** (Merck)
*Capsules*, green/orange, enclosing e/c pellets of pancreatin, providing minimum of: protease 650 units, lipase 10 000 units, amylase 10 000 units. Net price 100 = £12.52. Counselling, see dose
*Dose:* 1–2 capsules with meals swallowed whole or contents sprinkled on soft food (then swallowed immediately without chewing); dosage may be increased in severe cases

**Pancrease®** (Cilag)
*Capsules*, enclosing e/c beads of pancreatin, providing minimum of: protease 330 units, lipase 5000 units, amylase 2900 units. Net price 100 = £17.07. Counselling, see dose
*Dose:* 1–2 (occasionally 3) capsules during each meal and 1 capsule with snacks swallowed whole or contents sprinkled on liquid or soft food (then swallowed immediately without chewing)

**Pancrex®** (Paines & Byrne)
*Granules*, pancreatin, providing minimum of: protease 300 units, lipase 5000 units, amylase 4000 units/g. Net price 100 g = £7.15, 500 g = £28.61. Label: 25, counselling, see dose
*Dose:* 5–10 g 4 times daily with meals washed down or mixed with liquid

**Pancrex V®** (Paines & Byrne)
*Capsules*, pancreatin, providing minimum of: protease 430 units, lipase 8000 units, amylase 9000 units. Net price 100 = £4.29. Counselling, see dose
*Dose:* up to 1 year 1–2 capsules mixed with feeds; adults and children over 1 year 2–6 capsules 4 times daily with meals, swallowed whole or sprinkled on food
*Capsules '125'*, pancreatin, providing minimum of: protease 160 units, lipase 2950 units, amylase 3300 units. Net price 50 = £1.63. Counselling, see dose
*Dose:* NEONATE 1–2 capsules with feeds
*Tablets*, e/c, s/c, pancreatin, providing minimum of: protease 110 units, lipase 1900 units, amylase 1700 units. Net price 100 = £1.43. Label: 5, 25, counselling, see dose
*Dose:* 5–15 tablets 4 times daily before meals
*Tablets forte*, e/c, s/c, pancreatin, providing minimum of: protease 330 units, lipase 5600 units, amylase 5000 units. Net price 100 = £3.72. Label: 5, 25, counselling, see dose
*Dose:* 6–10 tablets 4 times daily before meals
*Powder*, pancreatin, providing minimum of: protease 1400 units, lipase 25 000 units, amylase 30 000 units/g. Net price 100 g = £9.75, 250 g = £20.76. Counselling, see dose
*Dose:* 0.5–2 g 4 times daily washed down or mixed with liquid

## 2: Drugs used in the treatment of diseases of the
# CARDIOVASCULAR SYSTEM

## 2.1   Positive inotropic drugs

2.1.1  Cardiac glycosides
2.1.2  Phosphodiesterase inhibitors

Positive inotropic drugs increase the force of contraction of the myocardium; for sympathomimetics with inotropic activity see section 2.7.1.

### 2.1.1   Cardiac glycosides

The principal actions of the cardiac glycosides are an increase in the force of myocardial contraction and a reduction in the conductivity of the heart. They are most useful in the treatment of *supraventricular tachycardias*, especially for controlling ventricular response in atrial fibrillation. *Heart failure* may also be improved, even in patients in sinus rhythm, because of changes in the availability of intracellular calcium; this action is relatively unimportant, however, compared with effects that can be achieved with diuretics and vasodilators. Except when needed to maintain satisfactory rhythm, cardiac glycosides can often be withdrawn from patients with heart failure that is well controlled, without clinical deterioration. In the elderly who are particularly susceptible to digitalis toxicity, cardiac glycosides should be used with special care in the management of heart failure without atrial fibrillation.

Loss of appetite, nausea, and vomiting are common toxic effects; sinus bradycardia, atrioventricular block, ventricular extrasystoles, and sometimes ventricular tachycardia or atrial tachycardia with block also occur—especially in the presence of underlying conducting system defects or myocardial disease. These unwanted effects depend both on the plasma concentrations of the drugs and on the sensitivity of the conducting system or myocardium, which is often increased in heart disease. Thus, no one plasma concentration can indicate toxicity reliably but the likelihood increases progressively through the range 1.5 to 3 micrograms/litre for digoxin; higher steady-state concentrations must certainly be avoided. Measurements of plasma concentration are not necessary, however, unless problems occur during maintenance treatment. Hypokalaemia predisposes to toxicity, therefore diuretics used with digoxin should either be potassium sparing or should be given with potassium supplements.

Renal function is the most important determinant of digoxin dosage, whereas elimination of digitoxin depends on metabolism by the liver. Toxicity can often be managed by discontinuing therapy and correcting hypokalaemia if appropriate; serious manifestations require urgent specialist management. Digoxin-specific antibody fragments are available for reversal of life-threatening overdosage (see next page).

**Digoxin** is the glycoside most commonly used. In patients with *mild failure* a loading dose is not required, and a satisfactory plasma concentration can be achieved over a period of about a week, using a dose of 125 to 250 micrograms twice a day which may then be reduced having special regard to renal function. Because it has a long half-life maintenance doses need only be given once daily (but higher doses should be divided to avoid nausea). For management of *atrial fibrillation* the maintenance dose can usually be governed by ventricular response which should not be allowed to fall below 60 beats per minute except in special and recognised circumstances, e.g. with the concomitant administration of beta-blockers.

When *very rapid control* is needed, digoxin may be given intravenously in a digitalising dose of 0.75 to 1 mg, preferably as an infusion (suggested volume 50 mL) over two or more hours, followed by normal maintenance therapy. The intramuscular route is not recommended, except when other methods of administration are not available.

**Lanatoside C** is less well absorbed than digoxin. Most is converted to digoxin after ingestion. The maintenance dose is about twice that of digoxin, and depends in part on renal function.

**Digitoxin** has a long half-life and maintenance doses, again, need only be given once daily.

CHILDREN. The dose is based on body-weight; they require a relatively larger dose of digoxin than adults.

### DIGOXIN

*Indications:* heart failure, supraventricular arrhythmias (particularly atrial fibrillation)
*Cautions:* recent infarction, hypothyroidism; reduce dose in the elderly and in renal impairment; avoid hypokalaemia; **interactions:** Appendix 1 (cardiac glycosides)
*Contra-indications:* supraventricular arrhythmias caused by Wolff-Parkinson-White syndrome
*Side-effects:* anorexia, nausea, vomiting, diarrhoea, abdominal pain; visual disturbances, headache, fatigue, drowsiness, confusion, delirium, hallucinations; arrhythmias, heart block; see also notes above

---

*Dose: by mouth*, rapid digitalisation, 1–1.5 mg in divided doses over 24 hours; less urgent digitalisation,  250–500 micrograms  daily (higher dose divided)

Maintenance,  62.5–500  micrograms  daily (higher dose divided) according to renal function and, in atrial fibrillation, on heart-rate response; usual range, 125–250 micrograms daily (elderly 125 micrograms)

For intravenous doses, see notes above

*Note.* For plasma concentration monitoring blood should ideally be taken at least 6 hours after a dose

PoM **Digoxin** (Non-proprietary)
*Tablets*, digoxin 62.5 micrograms, net price 20 = 9p; 125 micrograms, 20 = 6p; 250 micrograms, 20 = 9p
*Injection*,  digoxin  250 micrograms/mL,  see Lanoxin®
*Paediatric injection*, digoxin 100 micrograms/mL (hosp. only, available from Boots)

PoM **Lanoxin**® (Wellcome)
*Tablets*, digoxin 125 micrograms, net price 20 = 32p; 250 micrograms (scored), 20 = 28p
*Injection*, digoxin 250 micrograms/mL. Net price 2-mL amp = 65p

PoM **Lanoxin-PG**® (Wellcome)
*Tablets*, blue, digoxin 62.5 micrograms. Net price 20 = 32p
*Elixir*, yellow, digoxin 50 micrograms/mL. Do not dilute, measure with pipette. Net price 60 mL = £5.23. Counselling, use of pipette

## DIGITOXIN
*Indications:*  heart  failure,  supraventricular arrhythmias (particularly atrial fibrillation)
*Cautions; Contra-indications; Side-effects:* see under Digoxin
*Dose:* maintenance, 50–200 micrograms daily

PoM **Digitoxin** (Evans)
*Tablets*, digitoxin 100 micrograms, net price 20 = 43p

## LANATOSIDE C
*Indications:*  heart  failure,  supraventricular arrhythmias (particularly atrial fibrillation)
*Cautions; Contra-indications; Side-effects:* see under Digoxin
*Dose:* slow digitalisation 1.5–2 mg daily for 3–5 days; maintenance 0.25–1 mg daily

PoM **Cedilanid**® (Sandoz)
*Tablets*, scored, lanatoside C 250 micrograms. Net price 20 = 30p

## DIGOXIN-SPECIFIC ANTIBODY

PoM **Digibind**® (Wellcome)
*Injection*, powder for preparation of infusion, digoxin-specific antibody fragments (F(ab)) 40 mg. Net price per vial = £87.44
For reversal of life-threatening manifestations of intoxication by digoxin; although designed specifically to treat digoxin overdose has successfully reversed digitoxin overdose

## 2.1.2  Phosphodiesterase inhibitors
Enoximone and milrinone are selective phosphodiesterase inhibitors which exert most of their effect on the myocardium. Sustained haemodynamic benefit has been observed after administration, but as yet there is no conclusive evidence of any beneficial effect on survival.

## ENOXIMONE
*Indications:* congestive heart failure where cardiac output reduced and filling pressures increased
*Cautions:* heart failure associated with hypertrophic cardiomyopathy, stenotic or obstructive valvular disease or other outlet obstruction; monitor blood pressure, heart rate, ECG, central venous pressure, fluid and electrolyte status, platelet count, hepatic enzymes; reduce dose in renal impairment; avoid extravasation
*Side-effects:* ectopic beats; less frequently ventricular  tachycardia  or  supraventricular arrhythmias (more likely in patients with pre-existing arrhythmias); hypotension; also headache,  insomnia,  nausea  and  vomiting, diarrhoea; occasionally, chills, oliguria, fever, urinary retention; upper and lower limb pain
*Dose: by slow intravenous injection* (rate not exceeding 12.5 mg/minute), diluted before use, initially 0.5–1 mg/kg, then 500 micrograms/kg every 30 minutes until satisfactory response or total of 3 mg/kg given; maintenance, initial dose of up to 3 mg/kg may be repeated every 3–6 hours as required
*By intravenous infusion*, initially 90 micrograms/kg/minute over 10–30 minutes, followed by continuous or intermittent infusion of 5–20 micrograms/kg/minute
Total dose over 24 hours should not normally exceed 24 mg/kg

PoM **Perfan**® (Merrell)
*Injection*, enoximone 5 mg/mL. For dilution before use. Net price 20-mL amp = £15.40
*Note.* Plastic apparatus should be used; crystal formation if glass used

## MILRINONE
*Indications:* short-term treatment of severe congestive heart failure unresponsive to conventional  maintenance  therapy  (not immediately after myocardial infarction); acute heart failure, including low output states, following heart surgery
*Cautions; Side-effects:* see under Enoximone; also correct hypokalaemia, monitor renal function, chest pain reported
*Dose: by slow intravenous injection* (over 10 minutes), 50 micrograms/kg followed by *intravenous infusion* at a rate of 375–750 nanograms/kg/minute, usually for up to 12 hours following surgery or for 48–72 hours in congestive heart failure; max. daily dose 1.13 mg/kg

▼ PoM **Primacor**® (Sanofi Winthrop)
*Injection,* milrinone (as lactate) 1 mg/mL. For dilution before use. Net price 10-mL amp = £16.22

## 2.2   Diuretics

**2.2.1** Thiazides and related diuretics
**2.2.2** Loop diuretics
**2.2.3** Potassium-sparing diuretics
**2.2.4** Potassium-sparing diuretics with other diuretics
**2.2.5** Osmotic diuretics
**2.2.6** Mercurial diuretics
**2.2.7** Carbonic anhydrase inhibitors
**2.2.8** Diuretics with potassium

**Thiazides** (section 2.2.1) are used to relieve oedema due to *heart failure* and, in lower doses, to reduce *blood pressure.*

**Loop diuretics** (section 2.2.2) are used in pulmonary oedema due to *left ventricular failure* and in patients with *longstanding heart failure* who no longer respond to thiazides.

**Combination diuretic therapy** may be effective in patients with oedema resistant to treatment with one diuretic. For example, a loop diuretic may be combined with a potassium-sparing diuretic (section 2.2.3).

The combination of a thiazide with spironolactone is of value in *less severe heart failure* when hypokalaemia is difficult to counter or when any degree of hypokalaemia should be avoided, as in patients with a continuing tendency to life-threatening ventricular arrhythmias.

THE ELDERLY. Diuretics are overprescribed in old age and the elderly are particularly susceptible to many of their side-effects. They should not be used on a long-term basis to treat simple gravitational oedema (which will usually respond to increased movement, raising the legs, and support stockings).

POTASSIUM LOSS. Hypokalaemia may occur with both thiazide and loop diuretics. It is dangerous in severe coronary artery disease and in patients also being treated with cardiac glycosides. Often the use of potassium-sparing diuretics (section 2.2.3) avoids the need to take potassium supplements.

In hepatic failure hypokalaemia caused by diuretics can precipitate encephalopathy, particularly in alcoholic cirrhosis; diuretics may also increase the risk of hypomagnesaemia in alcoholic cirrhosis, leading to arrhythmias.

Potassium supplements are seldom necessary when thiazides are used in the routine treatment of hypertension. For further comment see section 9.2.1.1.

### 2.2.1   Thiazides and related diuretics

Thiazides and related compounds are moderately potent diuretics; they inhibit sodium reabsorption at the beginning of the distal convoluted tubule. They act within 1 to 2 hours of oral administration and most have a duration of action of 12 to 24 hours; they are usually administered early in the day so that the diuresis does not interfere with sleep.

In the management of *hypertension* a low dose of a thiazide, e.g. bendrofluazide 2.5 mg daily, produces a maximal or near-maximal blood pressure lowering effect, with very little biochemical disturbance. Higher doses cause more marked changes in plasma potassium, uric acid, glucose, and lipids, with no advantage in blood pressure control, and should not be used. Optimum doses for the control of *heart failure* may be larger, and long-term effects are of less importance.

**Bendrofluazide** is widely used for mild or moderate heart failure when the patient is not desperately ill and severe pulmonary oedema is not present. It is also used for hypertension—alone in the treatment of mild hypertension or with other drugs in more severe hypertension.

**Chlorthalidone,** a thiazide-related compound, has a longer duration of action than the thiazides and may be given on alternate days to control oedema. It is also useful if acute retention is liable to be precipitated by a more rapid diuresis or if patients dislike the altered pattern of micturition promoted by diuretics.

Other thiazides do not offer any significant advantage over those mentioned above, and newer ones are more expensive than the longer-established thiazides.

**Metolazone** is particularly effective when combined with a loop diuretic (even in renal failure); profound diuresis may occur therefore the patient should be monitored carefully.

**Xipamide** resembles chlorthalidone structurally, and is more potent than the other thiazides.

**Indapamide** is also chemically related to chlorthalidone. It is claimed to lower blood pressure with less metabolic disturbance, particularly less aggravation of diabetes mellitus.

### BENDROFLUAZIDE

*Indications:* oedema, hypertension
*Cautions:* may cause hypokalaemia, aggravates diabetes and gout; pregnancy (see also Appendix 4) and breast-feeding; renal and hepatic impairment (avoid if severe, see Appendixes 2 and 3); see also notes above; **interactions:** Appendix 1 (diuretics)
*Contra-indications:* hypercalcaemia, severe renal and hepatic impairment, Addison's disease, porphyria (see section 9.8.2)
*Side-effects:* impotence (reversible on withdrawal of treatment), hypokalaemia (see also notes above), hypomagnesaemia, hyponatraemia, hypercalcaemia, hypochloraemic alkalosis, hyperuricaemia, gout, hyperglycaemia, and increases in plasma cholesterol concentration; less commonly rashes, photo-

sensitivity, neutropenia, and thrombocytopenia (when given in late pregnancy neonatal thrombocytopenia has been reported)
*Dose:* oedema, initially 5–10 mg in the morning, daily *or* on alternate days; maintenance 2.5–10 mg 1–3 times weekly
Hypertension, 2.5 mg in the morning; higher doses rarely necessary (see notes above)

PoM **Bendrofluazide** (Non-proprietary)
*Tablets*, bendrofluazide 2.5 mg, net price 20 = 14p; 5 mg, 20 = 5p
Available from APS, Berk (Berkozide®), Boots (Aprinox®), Cox, DF (Neo-NaClex®, 5 mg only), Evans, Kerfoot, Leo (Centyl®)

## BENZTHIAZIDE
*Cautions; Contra-indications; Side-effects:* see under Bendrofluazide

**Preparation**
Ingredient of Dytide® (section 2.2.4)

## CHLOROTHIAZIDE
*Indications:* oedema, hypertension
*Cautions; Contra-indications; Side-effects:* see under Bendrofluazide
*Dose:* oedema, initially 0.5–1 g 1–2 times daily; maintenance 0.5–1 g daily, on alternate days, or less frequently
Hypertension, 0.5–1 g daily in single or divided doses

PoM **Saluric®** (MSD)
*Tablets*, scored, chlorothiazide 500 mg. Net price 20 = 38p

## CHLORTHALIDONE
*Indications:* oedema, hypertension; diabetes insipidus (see section 6.5.2)
*Cautions; Contra-indications; Side-effects:* see under Bendrofluazide
*Dose:* oedema, initially 50 mg in the morning *or* 100–200 mg on alternate days, reduced for maintenance if possible
Hypertension, 25 mg, increased to 50 mg if necessary, in the morning

PoM **Hygroton®** (Geigy)
*Tablets*, yellow, scored, chlorthalidone 50 mg, net price 20 = 82p

## CLOPAMIDE
*Cautions; Contra-indications; Side-effects:* see under Bendrofluazide

**Preparation**
Ingredient of Viskaldix® (see under Pindolol, section 2.4)

## CYCLOPENTHIAZIDE
*Indications:* oedema, hypertension
*Cautions; Contra-indications; Side-effects:* see under Bendrofluazide

*Dose:* oedema, initially 0.5–1 mg in the morning; maintenance 500 micrograms on alternate days
Hypertension, 250–500 micrograms in the morning
Max. 1.5 mg daily

PoM **Navidrex®** (Ciba)
*Tablets*, scored, cyclopenthiazide 500 micrograms. Net price 20 = 35p
*Additives: include* gluten

## HYDROCHLOROTHIAZIDE
*Indications:* oedema, hypertension
*Cautions; Contra-indications; Side-effects:* see under Bendrofluazide
*Dose:* oedema, initially 50–100 mg daily; maintenance 25–50 mg on alternate days
Hypertension, 25 mg daily, can be increased to 50–100 mg daily if necessary

PoM **Esidrex®** (Ciba)
*Tablets*, both scored, hydrochlorothiazide 25 mg, net price 20 = 57p; 50 mg, 20 = £1.05
*Additives: include* gluten
PoM **HydroSaluric®** (MSD)
*Tablets*, both scored, hydrochlorothiazide 25 mg, net price 20 = 29p; 50 mg, 20 = 54p

## HYDROFLUMETHIAZIDE
*Indications:* oedema, hypertension
*Cautions; Contra-indications; Side-effects:* see under Bendrofluazide
*Dose:* oedema, initially 50–200 mg in the morning; maintenance 25–50 mg on alternate days
Hypertension, 25–50 mg daily

PoM **Hydrenox®** (Boots)
*Tablets*, hydroflumethiazide 50 mg. Net price 20 = 38p

## INDAPAMIDE
*Indications:* hypertension
*Cautions:* renal impairment (stop if deterioration); monitor plasma potassium and urate concentrations in elderly, hyperaldosteronism, gout, or with concomitant cardiac glycosides; hyperparathyroidism (discontinue if hypercalcaemia); pregnancy and breast-feeding; **interactions:** Appendix 1 (diuretics)
*Contra-indications:* recent cerebrovascular accident, severe hepatic impairment
*Side-effects:* hypokalaemia, headache, dizziness, fatigue, muscular cramps, nausea, anorexia, diarrhoea, constipation, dyspepsia, rashes (erythema multiforme, epidermal necrolysis reported); rarely orthostatic hypotension, metabolic alkalosis, hyperglycaemia, increased plasma urate concentrations, paraesthesia, photosensitivity, impotence, renal impairment, reversible acute myopia; diuresis with doses above 2.5 mg daily
*Dose:* 2.5 mg daily in the morning

---

PoM **Natrilix**® (Servier)
*Tablets*, pink, s/c, indapamide 2.5 mg. Net price
30-tab pack = £5.96, 60-tab pack = £11.72

## MEFRUSIDE
*Indications:* oedema, hypertension
*Cautions; Contra-indications; Side-effects:* see
under Bendrofluazide
*Dose:* initially 25–50 mg in the morning,
increased to 75–100 mg for oedema; maintenance 25 mg daily *or* on alternate days

PoM **Baycaron**® (Bayer)
*Tablets*, scored, mefruside 25 mg. Net price 20 =
£1.41

## METHYCLOTHIAZIDE
*Indications:* oedema, hypertension
*Cautions; Contra-indications; Side-effects:* see
under Bendrofluazide
*Dose:* 2.5–5 mg in the morning, increased to
10 mg daily if required

PoM **Enduron**® (Abbott)
*Tablets*, pink, scored, methyclothiazide 5 mg.
Net price 20 = 41p

## METOLAZONE
*Indications:* oedema, hypertension
*Cautions; Contra-indications; Side-effects:* see
under Bendrofluazide; also profound diuresis
on concomitant administration with frusemide
(monitor patient carefully)
*Dose:* see preparations below

PoM **Metenix 5**® (Hoechst)
*Tablets*, blue, metolazone 5 mg. Net price 20 =
£1.75
*Dose:* oedema, 5–10 mg in the morning,
increased if necessary to 20 mg daily in resistant
oedema, max. 80 mg daily
Hypertension, initially 5 mg in the morning;
maintenance 5 mg on alternate days

Low dose
*Note.* Xuret® brand of metolazone has a much lower
dose than other brands of metolazone. It must therefore
be prescribed by brand name and is not interchangeable
with other brands of metolazone
PoM **Xuret**® (Galen)
*Tablets*, metolazone 500 micrograms. Net price
56-tab pack = £6.08
*Dose:* mild to moderate hypertension, 1 tablet
daily in the morning; increased if necessary to
2 tablets daily

## POLYTHIAZIDE
*Indications:* oedema, hypertension
*Cautions; Contra-indications; Side-effects:* see
under Bendrofluazide
*Dose:* usually 1–4 mg daily; in hypertension 500
micrograms daily may be adequate

PoM **Nephril**® (Pfizer)
*Tablets*, scored, polythiazide 1 mg. Net price 28-
tab pack = 79p

## XIPAMIDE
*Indications:* oedema, hypertension
*Cautions; Contra-indications:* see under Bendrofluazide
*Side-effects:* slight gastro-intestinal disturbances;
mild dizziness
*Dose:* oedema, initially 40 mg in the morning,
increased to 80 mg in resistant cases; maintenance 20 mg in the morning
Hypertension, usual dose 20 mg in the morning
(may be increased to 40 mg if necessary, but not
if other antihypertensive therapy being given)

PoM **Diurexan**® (ASTA Medica)
*Tablets*, scored, xipamide 20 mg. Net price 14-
tab pack = £1.97

## 2.2.2  Loop diuretics
These drugs inhibit resorption from the ascending
loop of Henle in the renal tubule and are powerful
diuretics. Hypokalaemia may develop, and care
is needed to avoid hypotension. If there is an
enlarged prostate, urinary retention may occur;
this is less likely if small doses and less potent
diuretics are used initially.

**Frusemide** and **bumetanide** are similar in
activity; both act within 1 hour of oral administration and diuresis is complete within 6 hours
so that, if necessary, they can be given twice in
one day without interfering with sleep. Following
intravenous administration they have a peak effect
within 30 minutes. The degree of diuresis associated with these drugs is dose related. In patients
with impaired renal function very large doses may
occasionally be needed; in such doses both drugs
can cause deafness and bumetanide can cause
myalgia.

**Ethacrynic acid** has a similar onset and duration
of action. Gastro-intestinal side-effects are more
severe and deafness may occur in patients with
renal failure, especially when it is given
intravenously.

**Piretanide** is the newest member of this group;
it has properties similar to those of frusemide and
bumetanide, but is promoted for the treatment of
hypertension.

## FRUSEMIDE
*Indications:* oedema, oliguria due to renal failure
*Cautions:* pregnancy (see also Appendix 4); may
cause hypokalaemia and hyponatraemia; aggravates diabetes mellitus and gout; liver failure,
prostatic enlargement; **interactions:** Appendix
1 (diuretics)
*Contra-indications:* precomatose states associated with liver cirrhosis; porphyria (see section
9.8.2)
*Side-effects:* hyponatraemia, hypokalaemia (see
also section 2.2), hypochloraemic alkalosis,
increased calcium excretion, hypotension; less
commonly nausea, gastro-intestinal disturbances, hyperuricaemia and gout; hyperglycaemia (less common than with thiazides);

temporary increase in plasma cholesterol and triglyceride concentrations; rarely rashes and bone marrow depression (withdraw treatment), pancreatitis (with large parenteral doses), tinnitus and deafness (usually with large parenteral doses and rapid administration and in renal impairment)

*Dose: by mouth*, oedema, initially 40 mg in the morning; maintenance 20 mg daily *or* 40 mg on alternate days, increased in resistant oedema to 80 mg daily; CHILD 1–3 mg/kg daily

Oliguria, initially 250 mg daily; if necessary larger doses, increasing in steps of 250 mg, may be given every 4–6 hours to a max. of a single dose of 2 g (rarely used)

*By intramuscular injection or slow intravenous injection* (rate not exceeding 4 mg/minute), initially 20–50 mg; CHILD 0.5–1.5 mg/kg to a max. daily dose of 20 mg

*By intravenous infusion* (by syringe pump if necessary), in oliguria, initially 250 mg over 1 hour (rate not exceeding 4 mg/minute), if satisfactory urine output not obtained in the subsequent hour further 500 mg over 2 hours, then if no satisfactory response within subsequent hour, further 1 g over 4 hours, if no response obtained dialysis probably required; effective dose (up to 1 g) can be repeated every 24 hours

PoM **Frusemide** (Non-proprietary)
*Tablets*, frusemide 20 mg, net price 20 = 29p; 40 mg, 20 = 8p; 500 mg, 20 = £6.00
Available from APS (20 mg, 40 mg, 500 mg), Ashbourne (Frumax® 40 mg), Berk (Dryptal® 40 mg, 500 mg), CP (Rusyde® 20 mg, 40 mg), Evans (20 mg, 40 mg), Kerfoot (20 mg, 40 mg)
*Oral solutions*, sugar-free, frusemide 1 mg/mL available as Lasix® paediatric liquid; frusemide 4, 8, and 10 mg/mL available from RP Drugs (special order)
*Injection*, frusemide 10 mg/mL, net price 2-mL amp = 27p

PoM **Lasix**® (Hoechst)
*Tablets*, all scored, frusemide 20 mg, net price 28-tab pack = 84p; 40 mg, 28-tab pack = £1.22; 500 mg (yellow), 20 = £11.74
*Paediatric liquid*, sugar-free, frusemide 1 mg/mL when reconstituted with purified water, freshly boiled and cooled, net price 150 mL = £1.13
*Injection*, frusemide 10 mg/mL, net price 2-mL amp = 26p; 5-mL amp = 54p; 25-mL amp = £2.27
*Note.* Large volume frusemide injections also available from David Bull, IMS (Min-I-Jet®)

## BUMETANIDE
*Indications:* oedema, oliguria due to renal failure
*Cautions; Contra-indications:* see under Frusemide (but has been used in porphyria, see section 9.8.2)
*Side-effects:* see under Frusemide; also myalgia
*Dose: by mouth*, 1 mg in the morning, repeated after 6–8 hours if necessary; severe cases, increased up to 5 mg or more daily
ELDERLY, 500 micrograms daily may be sufficient

*By intravenous injection*, 1–2 mg, repeated after 20 minutes; when *intramuscular injection* considered necessary, 1 mg initially then adjusted according to response
*By intravenous infusion*, 2–5 mg over 30–60 minutes

PoM **Burinex**® (Leo)
*Tablets*, both scored, bumetanide 1 mg, net price 20 = £1.14; 5 mg, 20 = £8.01
*Liquid*, green, sugar-free, bumetanide 1 mg/ 5 mL. Net price 150 mL = £3.41
*Injection*, bumetanide 500 micrograms/mL. Net price 2-mL amp = 41p; 4-mL amp = 71p; 10-mL amp = £1.49

## ETHACRYNIC ACID
*Indications:* oedema, oliguria due to renal failure
*Cautions; Contra-indications; Side-effects:* see under Frusemide and notes above; gastro-intestinal disturbances more severe; also pain on injection
*Dose: by mouth*, initially 50 mg daily after breakfast; effective initial range of 50–150 mg daily (max. 400 mg) can often be reduced for maintenance and given on alternate days (daily doses above 50 mg divided)
*By slow intravenous injection or infusion*, 50 mg, increased to 100 mg if necessary

PoM **Edecrin**® (MSD)
*Tablets*, scored, ethacrynic acid 50 mg. Net price 20 = 75p. Label: 21
*Injection*, powder for reconstitution, ethacrynic acid (as sodium salt). Net price 50-mg vial = £1.05

## PIRETANIDE
*Indications:* hypertension
*Cautions:* causes hypokalaemia, monitor plasma electrolytes in hepatic and renal impairment; prostatism; **interactions:** Appendix 1 (diuretics)
*Contra-indications:* severe electrolyte imbalance, hypovolaemia
*Side-effects:* rarely nausea, vomiting, diarrhoea, rashes; myalgia after high doses
*Dose:* 6–12 mg in the morning with food

PoM **Arelix**® (Hoechst)
*Capsules*, m/r, green/orange, enclosing yellow pellets, piretanide 6 mg. Net price 28-cap pack = £3.70. Label: 21

## 2.2.3  Potassium-sparing diuretics
**Amiloride** and **triamterene** on their own are weak diuretics. They cause retention of potassium and are therefore used as an alternative to giving potassium supplements with thiazide or loop diuretics. (See section 2.2.4 for compound preparations with thiazides or loop diuretics.)

**Spironolactone** is also a potassium-sparing diuretic, and potentiates thiazide or loop diuretics by antagonising aldosterone. It is of value in the treatment of the oedema of cirrhosis of the liver and is effective in oedema of heart failure, particularly when congestion has caused hepatic engorgement.

Spironolactone is also used in primary hyper-aldosteronism (Conn's syndrome).

**Potassium canrenoate** has similar uses to spironolactone, but can be given parenterally. It is metabolised to canrenone, which is also a metabolite of spironolactone.

Potassium supplements must **not** be given with potassium-sparing diuretics.

## AMILORIDE HYDROCHLORIDE

*Indications:* oedema, potassium conservation with thiazide and loop diuretics

*Cautions:* pregnancy; diabetes mellitus; elderly; **interactions:** Appendix 1 (diuretics)

*Contra-indications:* hyperkalaemia, renal failure

*Side-effects:* include gastro-intestinal disturbances, dry mouth, rashes, confusion, orthostatic hypotension, hyperkalaemia, hyponatraemia

*Dose:* alone, initially 10 mg daily *or* 5 mg twice daily, adjusted according to response; max. 20 mg daily

With other diuretics, congestive heart failure and hypertension, initially 5–10 mg daily

Cirrhosis with ascites, initially 5 mg daily

PoM **Amiloride** (Non-proprietary)

*Tablets,* amiloride hydrochloride 5 mg, net price 20 = £1.36

Available from APS, Ashbourne (Amilospare®), Berk (Berkamil®), Cox, Evans, Kerfoot

*Oral solution,* sugar-free, amiloride hydrochloride 5 mg/5 mL available from RP Drugs (special order)

PoM **Midamor**® (Morson)

*Tablets,* yellow, amiloride hydrochloride 5 mg. Net price 20 = £1.46

## TRIAMTERENE

*Indications:* oedema, potassium conservation with thiazide and loop diuretics

*Cautions; Contra-indications:* see under Amiloride Hydrochloride; monitor plasma urea and potassium, particularly in the elderly and in renal impairment; also may cause blue fluorescence of urine

*Side-effects:* include gastro-intestinal disturbances, dry mouth, rashes; slight decrease in blood pressure, hyperkalaemia; photosensitivity and blood disorders also reported; triamterene found in kidney stones

*Dose:* initially 150–250 mg daily, reducing to alternate days after 1 week; taken in divided doses after breakfast and lunch; lower initial dose when given with other diuretics

COUNSELLING. Urine may look slightly blue in some lights

PoM **Dytac**® (Bridge)

*Capsules,* maroon, triamterene 50 mg. Net price 30-cap pack = £1.94. Label: 14 (see above), 21

## ALDOSTERONE ANTAGONISTS

## POTASSIUM CANRENOATE

*Indications:* oedema associated with secondary aldosteronism, liver failure, chronic decompensated heart disease

*Cautions; Contra-indications:* see under Spironolactone; also contra-indicated in hyponatraemia

*Side-effects:* nausea and vomiting, particularly after high doses; hyperkalaemia, especially in renal impairment; pain and irritation at injection site

*Dose:* by slow intravenous injection or intravenous infusion, 200–400 mg daily (exceptionally 800 mg)

PoM **Spiroctan-M**® (Boehringer Mannheim)

*Injection,* potassium canrenoate 20 mg/mL. Net price 10-mL amp = 72p

## SPIRONOLACTONE

*Indications:* oedema and ascites in cirrhosis of the liver, malignant ascites, nephrotic syndrome, congestive heart failure; primary aldosteronism

*Cautions:* potential human metabolic products carcinogenic in *rodents*; elderly; hepatic and renal impairment (avoid if severe); **interactions:** Appendix 1 (diuretics)

*Contra-indications:* hyperkalaemia, severe renal impairment; pregnancy and breast-feeding; Addison's disease; porphyria (see section 9.8.2)

*Side-effects:* gastro-intestinal disturbances, gynaecomastia; hyperkalaemia

*Dose:* 100–200 mg daily, increased to 400 mg if required; CHILD 3 mg/kg daily in divided doses

PoM **Spironolactone** (Non-proprietary)

*Tablets,* spironolactone 25 mg, net price 20 = 54p; 50 mg, 20 = £2.40; 100 mg, 20 = £2.20

Available from APS, Ashbourne (Spirospare®), Berk (Spirolone®), Cox, Evans, Kerfoot, Lagap (Laractone®)

*Oral suspensions,* sugar-free, spironolactone 5, 10, 25, and 50 mg/5 mL available from RP Drugs (special order)

PoM **Aldactone**® (Searle)

*Tablets,* all f/c, spironolactone 25 mg (buff), net price 20 = £1.80; 50 mg (off-white), 20 = £3.59; 100 mg (buff), 20 = £7.18

PoM **Spiroctan**® (Boehringer Mannheim)

*Tablets,* both s/c, spironolactone 25 mg (blue, contains tartrazine), net price 20 = £1.48; 50 mg (green), 20 = £2.84

*Capsules,* green, spironolactone 100 mg. Net price 28-cap pack = £7.75

## 2.2.4    Potassium-sparing diuretics with other diuretics

Although it is preferable to prescribe thiazides and potassium-sparing diuretics separately, the use of fixed combinations may be justified if compliance is a problem. For **interactions,** see Appendix 1 (diuretics).

## Amiloride with thiazides

**PoM Co-amilozide** (Non-proprietary)

*Tablets*, co-amilozide 5/50 (amiloride hydrochloride 5 mg, hydrochlorothiazide 50 mg). Net price 20 = £1.34

Available from Abbott (Normetic®), APS, Ashbourne (Amilmaxco 5/50®), Cox, Kerfoot, Norton (Amilco®), Schwarz (Hypertane 50®), Shire (Vasetic®)

*Dose:* 1–2 tablets, increased if necessary to max. of 4, daily

*Tablets*, co-amilozide 2.5/25 available as Moduret 25®

**PoM Moduret 25®** (Morson)

*Tablets*, off-white, co-amilozide 2.5/25 (amiloride hydrochloride 2.5 mg, hydrochlorothiazide 25 mg). Net price 28-tab pack = £2.08

*Dose:* 1–4 tablets, increased if necessary to a max. of 8, daily

**PoM Moduretic®** (Du Pont)

*Tablets*, peach, scored, co-amilozide 5/50 (amiloride hydrochloride 5 mg, hydrochlorothiazide 50 mg). Net price 30 = £2.70

*Dose:* 1–2 tablets, increased if necessary to a max. of 4, daily

*Oral solution*, co-amilozide 5/50 (amiloride hydrochloride 5 mg, hydrochlorothiazide 50 mg/5 mL). Do not dilute. Net price 200 mL = £4.95

*Dose:* as for tablets above (5 mL = 1 tablet)

**PoM Navispare®** (Ciba)

*Tablets*, f/c, orange, amiloride 2.5 mg, cyclopenthiazide 250 micrograms. Net price 28-tab pack = £1.79

*Dose:* 1–2 tablets in the morning

## Amiloride with loop diuretics

**PoM Burinex A®** (Leo)

*Tablets*, ivory, scored, amiloride hydrochloride 5 mg, bumetanide 1 mg. Net price 28-tab pack = £3.28

*Dose:* 1–2 tablets daily

**PoM Frumil®** (Rhône-Poulenc Rorer)

*LS tablets,* orange, co-amilofruse 2.5/20 (amiloride hydrochloride 2.5 mg, frusemide 20 mg). Net price 28-tab pack = £3.25, 56-tab pack = £6.37

*Dose:* 1 tablet in the morning

*Tablets*, orange, scored, co-amilofruse 5/40 (amiloride hydrochloride 5 mg, frusemide 40 mg). Net price 28-tab pack = £3.97, 56-tab pack = £7.77

*Dose:* 1–2 tablets in the morning

*Forte tablets,* orange, scored, co-amilofruse 10/80 (amiloride hydrochloride 10 mg, frusemide 80 mg). Net price 28-tab pack = £7.38, 56-tab pack = £14.47

*Dose:* 1 tablet daily in the morning

**PoM Lasoride®** (Hoechst)

*Tablets*, yellow, co-amilofruse 5/40 (amiloride hydrochloride 5 mg, frusemide 40 mg). Net price 28-tab pack = £3.33

*Dose:* 1–2 tablets in the morning

## Triamterene with thiazides

COUNSELLING. Urine may look slightly blue in some lights

**PoM Dyazide®** (SK&F)

*Tablets*, peach, scored, triamterene 50 mg, hydrochlorothiazide 25 mg. Net price 30-tab pack = £2.41. Label: 14 (see above), 21

*Dose:* hypertension, 1 tablet daily after breakfast; oedema, 2 tablets daily (1 after breakfast and 1 after midday meal) increased to 3 daily if necessary (2 after breakfast and 1 after midday meal); usual maintenance, 1 daily or 2 on alternate days; max. 4 daily

*Note.* Tablets containing triamterene 50 mg and hydrochlorothiazide 25 mg are also available from Ashbourne (TriamaxCo®), Norton (Triamco®)

**PoM Dytide®** (Bridge)

*Capsules*, clear/maroon, triamterene 50 mg, benzthiazide 25 mg. Net price 30-cap pack = £2.08. Label: 14 (see above), 21

*Dose:* oedema, initially 3 capsules daily (2 after breakfast and 1 after midday meal) for 1 week then 1 or 2 on alternate days

**PoM Kalspare®** (Cusi)

*LS tablets*, peach, f/c, triamterene 50 mg, chlorthalidone 25 mg. Net price 28-tab pack = £2.95. Label: 14 (see above), 21

*Dose:* 1–2 tablets in the morning

*Tablets*, orange, f/c, scored, triamterene 50 mg, chlorthalidone 50 mg. Net price 28-tab pack = £3.27. Label: 14 (see above), 21

*Dose:* 1–2 tablets in the morning

## Triamterene with loop diuretics

COUNSELLING. Urine may look slightly blue in some lights

**PoM Frusene®** (Fisons)

*Tablets*, yellow, scored, triamterene 50 mg, frusemide 40 mg. Net price 56-tab pack = £4.90. Label: 14 (see above), 21

*Dose:* 1–2 tablets daily

## Spironolactone with thiazides

**PoM Aldactide 25®** (Gold Cross)

*Tablets*, buff, f/c, co-flumactone 25/25 (hydroflumethiazide 25 mg, spironolactone 25 mg). Net price 20 = £3.07

*Dose:* congestive heart failure, initially 4 tablets daily; range 1–8 daily

**PoM Aldactide 50®** (Gold Cross)

*Tablets*, buff, f/c, co-flumactone 50/50 (hydroflumethiazide 50 mg, spironolactone 50 mg). Net price 20 = £5.79

*Dose:* congestive heart failure, initially 2 tablets daily; range 1–4 daily

## Spironolactone with loop diuretics

**PoM Lasilactone®** (Hoechst)

*Capsules*, blue/white, spironolactone 50 mg, frusemide 20 mg. Net price 28-cap pack = £5.04

*Dose:* resistant oedema, 1–4 capsules daily

## 2.2.5 Osmotic diuretics

Osmotic diuretics are rarely used in heart failure as they may acutely expand the blood volume. **Mannitol** is used in cerebral oedema—a typical dose is 1 g/kg as a 20% solution given by rapid intravenous infusion.

## MANNITOL

*Indications:* see notes above
*Cautions:* extravasation causes inflammation and thrombophlebitis
*Contra-indications:* congestive cardiac failure, pulmonary oedema
*Side-effects:* chills, fever
*Dose: by intravenous infusion,* diuresis, 50–200 g over 24 hours, preceded by a test dose of 200 mg/kg by slow intravenous injection
Cerebral oedema, see notes above

PoM **Mannitol** (Non-proprietary)
*Intravenous infusion,* mannitol 10%, 20%, and 25%
   Available from Baxter (10% and 20%) and IMS (Min-I-Jet® Mannitol 25%)

### 2.2.6 Mercurial diuretics

They are effective diuretics but are now little used because of their nephrotoxicity. Mersalyl **must** be given by intramuscular injection; intravenous use may cause severe hypotension and sudden death.

## MERSALYL

*Indications:* oedema unresponsive to other diuretics
*Cautions:* recent myocardial infarction, treatment with cardiac glycosides, frequent extrasystoles
*Contra-indications:* renal impairment; pregnancy; porphyria (see section 9.8.2)
*Side-effects:* gastro-intestinal disturbances, allergic reactions

PoM **Mersalyl Injection,** mersalyl sodium 100 mg, theophylline 50 mg/mL
*Dose:* by deep intramuscular injection, 0.5–2 mL

### 2.2.7   Carbonic anhydrase inhibitors

Acetazolamide and dichlorphenamide are weak diuretics, and are little used for their diuretic effect. They inhibit the formation of aqueous fluid, and are used in glaucoma (see section 11.6). Although acetazolamide is used as a prophylactic measure for mountain sickness it is not a substitute for acclimatisation.

### 2.2.8   Diuretics with potassium

Many patients on diuretics do not need potassium supplements (see section 9.2.1.1). For many of those who do, the amount of potassium ion in combined preparations may not be enough, and for this reason their use is to be discouraged.
   Diuretics with potassium and potassium-sparing diuretics should **not** usually be given together.

COUNSELLING. Modified-release potassium tablets should be swallowed whole with plenty of fluid during meals while sitting or standing

PoM **Burinex K**® (Leo)
*Tablets,* bumetanide 500 micrograms, potassium 7.7 mmol for modified release. Net price 20 = 85p. Label: 25, 27, counselling, see above
PoM **Centyl K**® (Leo)
*Tablets,* green, bendrofluazide 2.5 mg, potassium 7.7 mmol for modified release. Net price 20 = 58p. Label: 25, 27, counselling, see above

PoM **Diumide-K Continus**® (ASTA Medica)
*Tablets,* f/c, white/orange, frusemide 40 mg, potassium 8 mmol for modified release. Net price 30-tab pack = £2.35. Label: 25, 27, counselling, see above
PoM **Hygroton-K**® (Geigy)
*Tablets,* red, s/c, chlorthalidone 25 mg, potassium 6.7 mmol for modified release. Net price 20 = 48p. Label: 25, 27, counselling, see above
   *Additives: include* gluten and azo dyes
PoM **Lasikal**® (Hoechst)
*Tablets,* white/yellow, f/c, frusemide 20 mg, potassium 10 mmol for modified release. Net price 20 = £1.09. Label: 25, 27, counselling, see above
PoM **Lasix + K**® (Hoechst)
*Calendar pack,* 30 white scored tablets, frusemide 40 mg; 60 m/r yellow tablets, potassium chloride (potassium 10 mmol). Net price = £3.05. Label: 25, 27, counselling, see above
PoM **Neo-NaClex-K**® (DF)
   Product discontinued

## 2.3   Anti-arrhythmic drugs

2.3.1 Management of arrhythmias
2.3.2 Drugs for arrhythmias

### 2.3.1   Management of arrhythmias

Management of an arrhythmia, apart from the treatment of associated heart failure, requires precise diagnosis of the type of arrhythmia, and electrocardiography is essential.
*Ectopic beats.* If spontaneous with a normal heart, these rarely require treatment beyond reassurance. If they are particularly troublesome, beta-blockers are sometimes effective and may be safer than other suppressant drugs.
*Atrial fibrillation.* The ventricular rate can be controlled with digoxin (section 2.1.1).
*Atrial flutter.* The ventricular rate can often be controlled with digoxin. Reversion to sinus rhythm (if indicated) is best achieved by appropriately synchronised d.c. shock, rather than by drug therapy. If the arrhythmia is long-standing a period of treatment with anticoagulants should be considered before cardioversion to avoid the complication of emboli.
*Paroxysmal supraventricular tachycardia.* In most patients this remits spontaneously or can be returned to sinus rhythm by reflex vagal stimulation with respiratory manoeuvres, prompt squatting, or pressure over one carotid sinus (**important:** pressure over carotid sinus should be restricted to monitored patients, it can be dangerous in recent ischaemia, digitalis toxicity, or the elderly).
   If vagal stimulation fails, digitalisation or intravenous administration of a beta-blocker may be effective. Intravenous administration of verapamil is useful for patients without myocardial or valvular disease (**important:** never in patients recently treated with beta-blockers, see section 2.3.2). For arrhythmias that are poorly tolerated, synchronised d.c. shock usually provides rapid relief.

---

In cases of paroxysmal supraventricular tachycardia with block, digitalis toxicity should be suspected. In addition to stopping administration of the cardiac glycoside and giving potassium supplements, intravenous administration of a beta-blocker or phenytoin may be useful. Specific digoxin antibody is available if the toxicity is considered life-threatening (section 2.1.1).

*Acute arrhythmias after myocardial infarction.* It is best to do nothing in patients with a paroxysmal tachycardia or rapid irregularity of the pulse until an ECG record is obtainable. If the condition of the patient is such that death due to the arrhythmia seems possible 100 mg of lignocaine should be given intravenously. Bradycardia, particularly if complicated by hypotension, should be treated with atropine sulphate, given intravenously in an initial dose of 300 micrograms, increasing to 1 mg if necessary.

*Ventricular tachycardia.* Drug treatment is used both for the treatment of ventricular tachycardia and for prophylaxis of recurrent attacks that merit suppression. Ventricular tachycardia requires treatment most commonly in the acute stage of myocardial infarction, but the likelihood of this and other life-threatening arrhythmias diminishes sharply over the first 24 hours after the attack, especially in patients without heart failure or shock. Lignocaine is the preferred drug for emergency use. Other drugs are best administered under specialist supervision. Very rapid ventricular tachycardia causes profound circulatory collapse and should be treated urgently with d.c. shock.

## 2.3.2  Drugs for arrhythmias

Anti-arrhythmic drugs can be classified clinically into those that act on supraventricular arrhythmias (e.g. verapamil), those that act on both supraventricular and ventricular arrhythmias (e.g. quinidine), and those that act on ventricular arrhythmias (e.g. lignocaine).

They can also be classified according to their effects on the electrical behaviour of myocardial cells during activity (termed 'action potential'):

| | |
|---|---|
| Class Ia, b, c | Membrane stabilising drugs (e.g. quinidine, lignocaine, flecainide respectively) |
| Class II | Beta-blockers |
| Class III | Amiodarone, Bretylium, and Sotalol (also Class II) |
| Class IV | Calcium-channel blockers (includes verapamil but not the nifedipine group) |

This latter classification (the Vaughan Williams classification) is of less clinical significance.

CAUTIONS. The negative inotropic effects of anti-arrhythmic drugs tend to be additive therefore special care should be taken if two or more are used, especially in impaired myocardial function. Most or all drugs that are effective in countering arrhythmias can also provoke them in some circumstances; moreover, hypokalaemia enhances the arrhythmogenic (pro-arrhythmic) effect of many drugs.

## SUPRAVENTRICULAR ARRHYTHMIAS

Oral administration of a **cardiac glycoside** (such as digoxin, section 2.1.1) is the treatment of choice in slowing ventricular response in cases of atrial fibrillation and atrial flutter. Intravenous digoxin, preferably infused slowly, is occasionally required if the ventricular rate needs rapid control. Ouabain acts more quickly but may be difficult to obtain since it is not on the UK market.

**Verapamil** (section 2.6.2) is usually effective for supraventricular tachycardias. An initial intravenous dose may be followed by oral treatment; hypotension may occur with larger doses. It should not be used for tachyarrhythmias where the QRS complex is wide (i.e. broad complex) unless a supraventricular origin has been established beyond reasonable doubt. It is also contraindicated in atrial fibrillation with pre-excitation (e.g. Wolff-Parkinson-White syndrome). It should not be used in children with arrhythmias without specialist advice; some supraventricular arrhythmias in childhood can be accelerated by verapamil with dangerous consequences.

> **Verapamil** should not be injected into patients recently treated with **beta-blockers** because of the risk of hypotension and asystole. It has been suggested that when verapamil injection has been given first, an interval of 30 minutes before giving a beta-blocker is sufficient but this too is open to doubt.
>
> It may even be hazardous to give verapamil and a beta-blocker together by mouth (should only be contemplated if myocardial function well preserved).

## ADENOSINE

*Indications:* rapid reversion to sinus rhythm of paroxysmal supraventricular tachycardias, including those associated with accessory pathways (e.g. Wolff-Parkinson-White syndrome); aid to diagnosis of broad or narrow complex supraventricular tachycardias

*Cautions:* atrial fibrillation or flutter with accessory pathway (increased conduction down anomalous pathway may develop); asthma; *interactions:* Appendix 1 (adenosine)

*Contra-indications:* second- or third-degree atrioventricular block and sick sinus syndrome (unless pacemaker fitted)

*Side-effects:* include transient facial flush, dyspnoea, choking sensation, nausea, lightheadedness; severe bradycardia reported (requiring temporary pacing); ECG may show transient rhythm disturbances

*Dose:* by rapid intravenous injection, 3 mg over 2 seconds with cardiac monitoring; if necesary followed by 6 mg after 1–2 minutes, and then by 12 mg after a further 1–2 minutes

▼ PoM **Adenocor**® (Sanofi Winthrop)
*Injection*, adenosine 3 mg/mL in physiological saline. Net price 2-mL vial = £4.15 (hosp. only)

## CARDIAC GLYCOSIDES
Section 2.1.1

## VERAPAMIL
Section 2.6.2

### SUPRAVENTRICULAR AND VENTRICULAR ARRHYTHMIAS

**Amiodarone** is used in the treatment of tachycardia associated with the Wolff-Parkinson-White syndrome. It may only be used for the treatment of other arrhythmias when other drugs are ineffective or contra-indicated and should be initiated only under hospital or specialist supervision. These include paroxysmal supraventricular, nodal and ventricular tachycardias, atrial fibrillation and flutter, and ventricular fibrillation. Since amiodarone has a very long half-life it only needs to be given once daily (but high doses may cause nausea unless divided). It may be given by intravenous infusion as well as by mouth, and has the advantage of causing little or no myocardial depression. Unlike oral amiodarone, intravenous amiodarone may act relatively rapidly.

Most patients taking amiodarone develop corneal microdeposits (reversible on withdrawal of treatment); these rarely interfere with vision, but drivers may be dazzled by headlights at night. Because of the possibility of phototoxic reactions, patients should be advised to shield the skin from light and to use a wide-spectrum sunscreen such as RoC Total Sunblock® (section 13.8.1) to protect against both long ultraviolet and visible light.

Amiodarone contains iodine and can cause disorders of thyroid function; both hypothyroidism and hyperthyroidism may occur. Thyroid function tests which rely on plasma concentrations of thyroxine alone, rather than on both thyroxine and triiodothyronine, may be spuriously elevated, but where doubt exists amiodarone should be withdrawn. Monitoring of tri-iodothyronine (T3) concentrations about every six months may give early warning of amiodarone-related thyrotoxicosis (which can be very refractory to treatment).

Pneumonitis should always be suspected if new or progressive shortness of breath or cough develops. Fresh neurological symptoms should raise the possibility of peripheral neuropathy (although this is rare).

**Beta-blockers** (section 2.4) act as anti-arrhythmic drugs principally by attenuating the effects of the sympathetic system on automaticity and conductivity within the heart. Some have additional anti-arrhythmic effects. They may be used in conjunction with digoxin to control the ventricular response in atrial fibrillation, especially in patients with thyrotoxicosis. Beta-blockers are also useful in the management of supraventricular tachycardias.

Evidence is now available that at least some **beta-blockers** (such as metoprolol) can reduce the incidence of life-threatening arrhythmias in the acute stage of myocardial infarction.

**Disopyramide** may be given by intravenous injection to control arrhythmias after myocardial infarction (including those not responding to lignocaine), but it impairs cardiac contractility. Oral administration of disopyramide is useful but it has an antimuscarinic effect which limits its use in patients with glaucoma or prostatic hypertrophy.

**Flecainide** is a newer drug in the same general class as lignocaine. It may be of value for serious symptomatic ventricular arrhythmias. It may also be indicated for junctional re-entry tachycardias. Preliminary results with paroxysmal atrial fibrillation are promising.

**Procainamide** can be given by intravenous injection to control ventricular arrhythmias, but prolonged oral use can cause a syndrome resembling systemic lupus erythematosus.

**Quinidine** may be effective in suppressing supraventricular and ventricular arrhythmias. It may itself precipitate rhythm disorders, and is best used on specialist advice; it can cause hypersensitivity reactions and gastro-intestinal upsets.

## AMIODARONE HYDROCHLORIDE
*Indications:* see notes above (should be initiated in hospital)
*Cautions:* liver-function and thyroid-function tests required in long-term therapy; interferes with tests of thyroid function; heart failure; renal impairment; elderly; severe bradycardia and conduction disturbances in excessive dosage; intravenous use may cause moderate and transient fall in blood pressure (circulatory collapse precipitated by rapid administration or overdosage); **interactions:** Appendix 1 (amiodarone)
*Contra-indications:* sinus bradycardia, sino-atrial heart block; unless pacemaker fitted avoid in severe conduction disturbances or sinus node disease; avoid intravenous use in severe respiratory failure, circulatory collapse, severe arterial hypotension, congestive heart failure; thyroid dysfunction; pregnancy and breast-feeding; iodine sensitivity; porphyria (see section 9.8.2)
*Side-effects:* reversible corneal microdeposits (sometimes with night glare), rarely impaired vision due to optic neuritis; peripheral neuropathy and myopathy (usually reversible on withdrawal), bradycardia and conduction disturbances (see Cautions); phototoxicity and rarely persistent slate-grey skin discoloration (see also notes above); hypothyroidism, hyperthyroidism, diffuse pulmonary alveolitis and fibrosis, hepatitis; rarely nausea, vomiting, metallic taste, tremor, nightmares, vertigo, headache, sleeplessness, fatigue, benign raised intracranial pressure, epididymitis; ataxia, rashes (including exfoliative dermatitis), vasculitis, blood disorders, increased prothrombin time reported; anaphylaxis on rapid injection, also bronchospasm or apnoea in respiratory failure
*Dose: by mouth*, 200 mg 3 times daily for 1 week reduced to 200 mg twice daily for a further week; maintenance, usually 200 mg daily or the minimum required to control the arrhythmia

---

*By intravenous infusion* via caval catheter, 5 mg/kg over 20–120 minutes with ECG monitoring; max. 1.2 g in 24 hours

PoM **Cordarone X**® (Sanofi Winthrop)
*Tablets*, both scored, amiodarone hydrochloride 100 mg, net price 28-tab pack = £5.13; 200 mg, 28-tab pack = £8.40. Label: 11
*Injection*, amiodarone hydrochloride 50 mg/mL. Net price 3-mL amp = £1.54. For dilution and use as an infusion

## DISOPYRAMIDE
*Indications:* ventricular arrhythmias, especially after myocardial infarction; supraventricular arrhythmias
*Cautions:* glaucoma; heart failure (avoid if severe); prostatic enlargement; hepatic and renal impairment; elderly; pregnancy; **interactions:** Appendix 1 (disopyramide)
*Contra-indications:* second- and third-degree heart block and sinus node dysfunction (unless pacemaker fitted); cardiogenic shock; severe uncompensated heart failure
*Side-effects:* myocardial depression, hypotension, atrioventricular block; antimuscarinic effects include dry mouth, blurred vision, urinary retention
*Dose: by mouth*, 300–800 mg daily in divided doses
*By slow intravenous injection*, 2 mg/kg over at least 5 minutes to a max. of 150 mg, with ECG monitoring, followed immediately *either* by 200 mg *by mouth*, then 200 mg every 8 hours for 24 hours *or* 400 micrograms/kg/hour *by intravenous infusion*; max. 300 mg in first hour and 800 mg daily

PoM **Disopyramide** (Non-proprietary)
*Capsules*, disopyramide 100 mg, net price 20 = £1.60; 150 mg, 20 = £2.68
Available from APS, Kerfoot (100 mg), Monmouth (Isomide® 100 mg)
PoM **Rythmodan**® (Roussel)
*Capsules*, disopyramide 100 mg (green/beige), net price 84-cap pack = £7.52; 150 mg, 84-cap pack = £11.27
*Injection*, disopyramide 10 mg (as phosphate)/mL, net price 5-mL amp = 70p

Modified release
PoM **Dirythmin SA**® (Astra)
*Durules*® (= tablets, m/r), f/c, disopyramide 150 mg (as phosphate). Net price 20 = £2.53. Label: 25
*Dose:* 300 mg every 12 hours; max. 900 mg daily
PoM **Rythmodan Retard**® (Roussel)
*Tablets*, m/r, scored, f/c, disopyramide 250 mg (as phosphate). Net price 56-tab pack = £16.24. Label: 25
*Dose:* 250–375 mg every 12 hours
Note. Modified-release capsules containing disopyramide 250 mg (as phosphate) also available from Monmouth (Isomide® CR)

## FLECAINIDE ACETATE
*Indications:* (should be initiated in hopital) *tablets and injection:* AV nodal reciprocating tachycardia, Wolff-Parkinson-White syndrome and similar conditions with accessory pathway and anterograde or retrograde conduction; *tablets only:* symptomatic sustained ventricular tachycardia, premature ventricular contractions and/or non-sustained ventricular tachycardia causing disabling symptoms in patients resistant to or intolerant of other therapy; *injection only:* ventricular tachyarrhythmias resistant to other treatment
*Cautions:* patients with pacemakers (especially those who may be pacemaker dependent because stimulation threshold may rise appreciably); avoid in sino-atrial disorders or second-degree or greater AV block unless pacing rescue available; elderly; reduce dose in hepatic and renal impairment; pregnancy (toxicity in *animal* studies); **interactions:** Appendix 1 (flecainide)
*Contra-indications:* heart failure; history of myocardial infarction and either asymptomatic ventricular ectopics or asymptomatic non-sustained ventricular tachycardia
*Side-effects:* dizziness, visual disturbances (corneal deposits reported); arrhythmogenic (proarrhythmic) effect; rarely nausea and vomiting; reversible increases in liver enzymes, jaundice; ataxia, sensory neuropathy, pulmonary fibrosis, pneumonitis also reported
*Dose: by mouth*, 100 mg twice daily; max. 400 mg daily, reduced after 3–5 days if possible; elderly 100 mg twice daily, reduced after 1 week if possible
*By slow intravenous injection*, 2 mg/kg over 10–30 minutes, max. 150 mg, with ECG monitoring; followed if required by *infusion* at a rate of 1.5 mg/kg/hour for 1 hour, subsequently reduced to 100–250 micrograms/kg/hour for up to 24 hours; max. cumulative dose in first 24 hours, 600 mg; transfer to *oral* treatment, as above

PoM **Tambocor**® (3M)
*Tablets*, scored, flecainide acetate 100 mg. Net price 60-tab pack = £19.98
*Injection*, flecainide acetate 10 mg/mL. Net price 15-mL amp = £4.25

## PROCAINAMIDE HYDROCHLORIDE
*Indications:* ventricular arrhythmias, especially after myocardial infarction; atrial tachycardia
*Cautions:* elderly; hepatic and renal impairment, asthma, myasthenia gravis; **interactions:** Appendix 1 (procainamide)
*Contra-indications:* heart block, heart failure, hypotension
*Side-effects:* nausea, diarrhoea, rashes, fever, myocardial depression, heart failure, lupus erythematosus-like syndrome, agranulocytosis after prolonged treatment

*Dose: by mouth*, ventricular arrhythmias, up to 50 mg/kg daily in divided doses, preferably controlled by measurement of plasma concentration (dosage intervals can range from 3–6 hours); atrial arrhythmias, higher doses may be required

*By slow intravenous injection*, rate not exceeding 50 mg/minute, 100 mg with ECG monitoring, repeated at 5-minute intervals until arrhythmia controlled; max. 1 g

*By intravenous infusion*, 500–600 mg over 25–30 minutes with ECG monitoring, followed by maintenance at rate of 2–6 mg/minute, then if necessary oral treatment as above, starting 3–4 hours after infusion

PoM **Pronestyl**® (Squibb)
*Tablets*, scored, procainamide hydrochloride 250 mg. Net price 20 = 94p
*Injection*, procainamide hydrochloride 100 mg/mL. Net price 10-mL vial = £1.90

Modified release
PoM **Procainamide Durules**® (Astra)
*Tablets*, m/r, yellow, procainamide hydrochloride 500 mg. Net price 20 = £1.46. Label: 25
*Dose:* 1–1.5 g every 8 hours

## QUINIDINE

*Indications:* suppression of supraventricular tachycardias and ventricular arrhythmias (see notes above)
*Cautions:* 200-mg test dose to detect hypersensitivity reactions; **interactions:** Appendix 1 (quinidine)
*Contra-indications:* heart block
*Side-effects:* see under Procainamide Hydrochloride; also ventricular arrhythmias, thrombocytopenia, haemolytic anaemia; rarely granulomatous hepatitis; also cinchonism (see Quinine, section 5.4.1) with tinnitus, visual disturbances, headache, hot and flushed skin, confusion, vertigo, vomiting, and abdominal pain
*Dose: by mouth*, quinidine sulphate 200–400 mg 3–4 times daily
*Note.* Quinidine sulphate 200 mg ≡ quinidine bisulphate 250 mg

PoM **Quinidine Sulphate** (Non-proprietary)
*Tablets*, quinidine sulphate 200 mg, net price 20 = £1.31; 300 mg, 20 = £1.76

Modified release
PoM **Kiditard**® (Delandale)
*Capsules*, m/r, blue, quinidine bisulphate 250 mg. Net price 20 = £2.43. Label: 25
*Dose:* 500 mg every 12 hours, adjusted as required
PoM **Kinidin Durules**® (Astra)
*Tablets*, m/r, f/c, quinidine bisulphate 250 mg. Net price 20 = £2.15. Label: 25
*Dose:* 500 mg every 12 hours, adjusted as required

## VENTRICULAR ARRHYTHMIAS

**Bretylium** is only used as an anti-arrhythmic drug in resuscitation. It is given both intramuscularly and intravenously but can cause severe hypotension, particularly after intravenous administration; nausea and vomiting can occur with either route. The intravenous route should only be used in emergency when there is doubt about absorption because of inadequate circulation.

**Lignocaine** is relatively safe when used by slow intravenous injection and should be considered first for emergency use. Though effective in suppressing ventricular tachycardia and reducing the risk of ventricular fibrillation following myocardial infarction, it has not been shown convincingly to reduce mortality when used prophylactically in this condition. In patients with cardiac or hepatic failure doses may need to be reduced to avoid convulsions, depression of the central nervous system, or depression of the cardiovascular system.

**Mexiletine** may be given as a slow intravenous injection if lignocaine is ineffective; it has a similar action. Adverse cardiovascular and central nervous system effects may limit the dose tolerated; nausea and vomiting may prevent an effective dose being given by mouth.

**Phenytoin** by slow intravenous injection is sometimes useful in ventricular arrhythmias particularly those caused by cardiac glycosides.

**Propafenone** is a newer drug for the prophylaxis and treatment of ventricular arrhythmias and is undergoing evaluation in some supraventricular arrhythmias. For CSM advice on avoidance in obstructive airways disease, see next page.

**Tocainide** is an analogue of lignocaine; because of a high incidence of blood disorders its use is limited to treatment of life-threatening symptomatic ventricular tachyarrhythmias associated with severely compromised left ventricular function in patients who do not respond to other therapy or for whom other therapy is contraindicated.

## BRETYLIUM TOSYLATE
*Indications:* ventricular arrhythmias resistant to other treatment
*Cautions:* do not give noradrenaline or other sympathomimetic amines; may exacerbate ventricular arrhythmias due to cardiac glycosides; **interactions:** Appendix 1 (bretylium)
*Contra-indications:* phaeochromocytoma
*Side-effects:* hypotension, nausea and vomiting
*Dose: by intramuscular injection*, 5 mg/kg repeated after 6–8 hours if necessary
*By slow intravenous injection*, 5–10 mg/kg over 8–10 minutes with blood pressure and ECG monitoring; may be repeated after 1–2 hours to a total dosage of 30 mg/kg (initial dose being diluted to 10 mg/mL in glucose 5% or sodium chloride intravenous infusion)
Maintenance 5–10 mg/kg *by intramuscular injection* every 6–8 hours *or* 1–2 mg/minute *by intravenous infusion*

PoM **Bretylate**® (Wellcome)
*Injection*, bretylium tosylate 50 mg/mL. Net price 10-mL amp = £19.81

PoM **Min-I-Jet**® **Bretylium Tosylate** (IMS)
*Injection*, bretylium tosylate 50 mg/mL. Net price 10-mL disposable syringe = £25.16

## LIGNOCAINE HYDROCHLORIDE

*Indications:* ventricular arrhythmias, especially after myocardial infarction

*Cautions:* lower doses in congestive cardiac failure, in hepatic failure, and following cardiac surgery; **interactions:** Appendix 1 (lignocaine)

*Contra-indications:* sino-atrial disorders, all grades of atrioventricular block, severe myocardial depression; porphyria (see 9.8.2)

*Side-effects:* confusion, convulsions

*Dose: by intravenous injection*, in patients without gross circulatory impairment, 100 mg as a bolus over a few minutes, followed by *infusion* of 2–4 mg/minute

PoM **Lignocaine in Glucose Injection**, lignocaine hydrochloride 0.1% (1 mg/mL) and 0.2% (2 mg/mL) in glucose intravenous infusion 5%. 500-mL containers
Available from Baxter

PoM **Min-I-Jet**® **Lignocaine** (IMS)
*Injection*, lignocaine hydrochloride 1% (10 mg/mL), net price 10-mL syringe = £2.97; 2% (20 mg/mL), 5-mL syringe = £2.71

PoM **Select-A-Jet**® **Lignocaine** (IMS)
*Injection*, lignocaine hydrochloride 20% (200 mg/mL). To be diluted before use. Net price 5-mL vial = £4.06

PoM **Xylocard**® (Astra)
*Injection 100 mg*, lignocaine hydrochloride (anhydrous) 20 mg/mL. Net price 5-mL syringe = £1.65

*Intravenous infusion*, lignocaine hydrochloride (anhydrous) 200 mg/mL. To be diluted before use. Net price 5-mL syringe (1 g) = £2.01; 10-mL syringe (2 g) = £2.35

## MEXILETINE HYDROCHLORIDE

*Indications:* ventricular arrhythmias, especially after myocardial infarction

*Cautions:* hepatic impairment; close monitoring on initiation of therapy (including ECG, blood pressure, etc.); **interactions:** Appendix 1 (mexiletine)

*Contra-indications:* bradycardia, heart block

*Side-effects:* bradycardia, hypotension, confusion, convulsions, psychiatric disorders, dysarthria, nystagmus, tremor; jaundice, hepatitis, and blood disorders reported

*Dose: by mouth*, initial dose 400 mg (may be increased to 600 mg if opioid analgesics also given), followed after 2 hours by 200–250 mg 3–4 times daily

*By intravenous injection*, 100–250 mg at a rate of 25 mg/minute with ECG monitoring followed by *infusion* of 250 mg as a 0.1% solution over 1 hour, 125 mg/hour for 2 hours, then 500 micrograms/minute

PoM **Mexitil**® (Boehringer Ingelheim)
*Capsules*, mexiletine hydrochloride 50 mg (purple/red), net price 20 = 91p; 200 mg (red), 20 = £2.18

*Injection*, mexiletine hydrochloride 25 mg/mL. Net price 10-mL amp = £1.36

Modified release
PoM **Mexitil PL**® (Boehringer Ingelheim)
*Perlongets*® (= capsules, m/r, each enclosing 5 miniature tablets), turquoise/scarlet, mexiletine hydrochloride 360 mg. Net price 56-cap pack = £10.98. Label: 25
*Dose:* 1 capsule twice daily

## PHENYTOIN SODIUM

*Indications:* arrhythmias, see notes above; for use in epilepsy, see section 4.8.1

*Cautions; Contra-indications; Side-effects:* see section 4.8.2

*Dose:* arrhythmias, *by intravenous injection* via caval catheter, 3.5–5 mg/kg at a rate not exceeding 50 mg/minute, with blood pressure and ECG monitoring; repeat once if necessary

**Preparations**
See section 4.8.2

## PROPAFENONE HYDROCHLORIDE

*Indications:* ventricular arrhythmias

*Cautions:* heart failure; hepatic and renal impairment; elderly; pacemaker patients; pregnancy; CSM advises great caution in obstructive airways disease owing to beta-blocking activity (contra-indicated if severe); **interactions:** Appendix 1 (propafenone)

*Contra-indications:* uncontrolled congestive heart failure, cardiogenic shock (except arrhythmia induced), severe bradycardia, uncontrolled electrolyte disturbances, severe obstructive pulmonary disease, marked hypotension; myasthenia gravis; unless adequately paced avoid in sinus node dysfunction, atrial conduction defects, second degree or greater atrioventricular block, bundle branch block or distal block

*Side-effects:* constipation, blurred vision, dry mouth (due to antimuscarinic action); dizziness, nausea and vomiting, fatigue, bitter taste, diarrhoea, headache, and allergic skin reactions reported; postural hypotension, particularly in elderly; bradycardia, sino-atrial, atrioventricular, or intraventricular blocks; arrhythmogenic (pro-arrhythmic) effect; rarely cholestasis, blood disorders, lupus syndrome, seizures

*Dose:* 70 kg and over, initially 150 mg 3 times daily after food under direct hospital supervision with ECG monitoring and blood pressure control, increased at intervals of at least 3 days to 300 mg twice daily and, if necessary, to max. 300 mg 3 times daily; under 70 kg, reduce dose ELDERLY may respond to lower doses

PoM **Arythmol**® (Knoll)
*Tablets*, both f/c, propafenone hydrochloride
150 mg, net price 90-tab pack = £19.98; 300 mg
(scored), 60-tab pack = £19.98. Label: 21, 25

## TOCAINIDE HYDROCHLORIDE

*Indications:* ventricular arrhythmias (restricted
use—see notes above)
*Cautions:* weekly blood counts essential for first
12 weeks, then monthly; severe hepatic or renal
impairment, uncompensated heart failure,
pregnancy (toxicity in *animal* studies); **interactions:** Appendix 1 (tocainide)
*Contra-indications:* see under Lignocaine
Hydrochloride
*Side-effects:* CNS effects including tremor, dizziness, convulsions, paraesthesia; gastro-intestinal effects including nausea and vomiting;
bradycardia and hypotension after injection;
rash and fever; lupus erythematosus-like syndrome, fibrosing alveolitis, agranulocytosis,
aplastic anaemia, and thrombocytopenia—see
also notes above; psychiatric disorders reported
*Dose:* chronic arrhythmias, *by mouth*, 1.2 g daily
in 3 divided doses; max. 2.4 g daily
Acute treatment, *by slow intravenous injection
or infusion*, 500–750 mg over 15–30 minutes
with ECG monitoring, followed immediately
by 800 mg by mouth.
Maintenance, *by mouth*, 1.2 g daily in 3 divided
doses

PoM **Tonocard**® (Astra)
*Tablets*, yellow, f/c, tocainide hydrochloride
400 mg, net price 20 = £3.35
*Injection*, tocainide hydrochloride  50 mg/mL.
Net price 15-mL vial = £5.80

# 2.4   Beta-adrenoceptor blocking drugs

Beta-adrenoceptor    blocking    drugs    (beta-
blockers) block the beta-adrenoreceptors in the
heart, peripheral vasculature, bronchi, pancreas,
and liver.

Many beta-blockers are now available and in
general they are all equally effective. There are,
however, differences between them which may
affect choice in treating particular diseases or
individual patients.

Intrinsic sympathomimetic activity (ISA, partial agonist activity) represents the capacity of
beta-blockers to stimulate as well as to block
adrenergic receptors. Oxprenolol, pindolol, and
acebutolol have intrinsic sympathomimetic
activity; they tend to cause less bradycardia than
the other beta-blockers and may also cause less
coldness of the extremities.

Some beta-blockers are lipid soluble and some
are water soluble. Atenolol, nadolol, and sotalol
are the most water-soluble; they are less likely to
enter the brain, and may therefore cause less sleep
disturbance and nightmares. Water-soluble beta-
blockers are excreted by the kidneys; they

accumulate in renal impairment and dosage
reduction is therefore often necessary.

Some beta-blockers have a relatively short duration of action and have to be given twice or three
times daily. Many of these are, however, available
in modified-release formulations so that in general
it is not necessary to give beta-blockers more
often than once daily for hypertension. For angina
twice-daily treatment may sometimes be needed
even with a modified-release formulation.

All beta-blockers slow the heart and may induce
myocardial depression and precipitate heart
failure. They should not therefore be given to
patients who have incipient cardiac failure or
those with second- or third-degree heart block.
Sotalol may prolong the QT interval, and has
occasionally caused life-threatening ventricular
arrhythmias. Particular care should be taken to
avoid hypokalaemia in patients taking sotalol.

Beta-blockers may precipitate asthma and this
effect can be dangerous. Some, such as atenolol,
betaxolol, bisoprolol, metoprolol, and (to a lesser
extent) acebutolol, have less effect on the $beta_2$
(bronchial) receptors and are, therefore, relatively cardioselective, but they are not cardio-
specific. They have a lesser effect on airways
resistance but are not free of this side-effect.
Patients who have a tendency towards obstructive
airways disease must be treated with great caution
and may require to take increased doses of their
$beta_2$-stimulants (e.g. salbutamol) to overcome
the effect of blockade of the bronchial adrenoceptors.

> **CSM advice.** Beta-blockers, even those with
> apparent cardioselectivity, should not be used
> in patients with asthma or a history of obstruc-
> tive airways disease, unless no alternative
> treatment is available. In such cases the risk
> of inducing bronchospasm should be appreci-
> ated and appropriate precautions taken.

Beta-blockers may occasionally aggravate
intermittent claudication.

Beta-blockers can lead to a small deterioration
of glucose tolerance in diabetics; they also interfere with metabolic and autonomic responses to
hypoglycaemia. Their use is not contra-indicated
in diabetics, but cardioselective beta-blockers
may be preferable and they should be avoided
altogether in those with frequent episodes of
hypoglycaemia.

**Labetalol** combines alpha- and beta-receptor
blocking activity. The alpha-blocking activity in
the peripheral vessels lowers peripheral resistance
but there is no evidence that labetalol has an
important advantage over other beta-blockers as
regards reduction of blood pressure.

### HYPERTENSION

Beta-blockers are effective antihypertensive
drugs but their mode of action is not understood;
they reduce cardiac output, alter baroceptor reflex
sensitivity, and block peripheral adrenoceptors.

Some beta-blockers depress plasma renin secretion. It is possible that a central effect may also explain their mode of action. Blood pressure can usually be controlled with relatively few side-effects. In general the dose of beta-blocker does not have to be as high as originally thought. The maximum dose of oxprenolol and propranolol necessary is probably 320 mg daily. Atenolol can usually be given in a dose of 50 mg daily and it is no longer considered necessary to increase to 100 mg.

Combined thiazide/beta-blocker preparations may help compliance but combined preparations should only be used when blood pressure is not adequately controlled by a thiazide or a beta-blocker alone. Beta-blockers reduce, but do not abolish, the tendency for diuretics to cause hypokalaemia.

Beta-blockers can be used to control the pulse rate in patients with *phaeochromocytoma*. However, they should never be used alone as beta-blockade without concurrent alpha-blockade may lead to a hypertensive crisis. For this reason phenoxybenzamine should always be used together with the beta-blocker.

## ANGINA

Beta-blockers improve exercise tolerance and relieve symptoms in patients with angina; this effect is caused by their reduction of cardiac work. As with hypertension there is no good evidence of the superiority of any one drug, although occasionally a patient will respond better to one beta-blocker than to another. There is some evidence that sudden withdrawal may cause an exacerbation of angina therefore gradual reduction of dose is preferable when beta-blockers are to be stopped. There is a risk of precipitating heart failure when beta-blockers and verapamil are used together in established ischaemic heart disease (**important**: see section 2.3.2).

## MYOCARDIAL INFARCTION

Several studies have shown that some beta-blockers can cause a reduction in the recurrence rate of myocardial infarction. However, pre-existing heart failure, hypotension, bradyarrhythmias, and obstructive airways disease render this group of drugs unsuitable in some patients who have recovered from a myocardial infarction. Atenolol and metoprolol may reduce early mortality after intravenous and subsequent oral administration in the acute phase, while timolol and propranolol have protective value when started in the early convalescent phase. The evidence relating to other beta-blockers is less convincing; some have not been tested in trials of secondary protection. It is also not known whether the protective effect of beta-blockers continues after two years; it is possible that sudden cessation may cause a rebound worsening of myocardial ischaemia.

## ARRHYTHMIAS

Beta-blockers are used to control supraventricular tachycardia following myocardial infarction, see above.

## THYROTOXICOSIS

Beta-blockers are used in pre-operative preparation for thyroidectomy. Administration of propranolol can reverse clinical features of thyrotoxicosis within 4 days. Routine tests of increased thyroid function remain unaltered. The thyroid gland is rendered less vascular thus making surgery easier (see section 6.2.2).

## OTHER USES

Beta-blockers have been used to alleviate some symptoms of anxiety; probably patients with palpitations, tremor, and tachycardia respond best. (See also sections 4.1.2 and 4.9.3.) Beta-blockers are also used in the prophylaxis of migraine (see section 4.7.4.2). Beta-blockers are used topically in the management of glaucoma (see section 11.6).

## PROPRANOLOL HYDROCHLORIDE

*Indications:* see under Dose
*Cautions:* late pregnancy and breast-feeding (see also Appendices 4 and 5); avoid abrupt withdrawal in angina; reduce oral dose of propranolol in liver disease; liver function deteriorates in portal hypertension; reduce initial dose in renal impairment; diabetes; myasthenia gravis; see also notes above; **interactions:** Appendix 1 (beta-blockers), **important:** verapamil interaction, see also section 2.3.2
*Contra-indications:* asthma or history of obstructive airways disease (see CSM advice on previous page), uncontrolled heart failure, sick sinus syndrome, second or third degree heart block, cardiogenic shock
*Side-effects:* bradycardia, heart failure, bronchospasm, peripheral vasoconstriction, gastrointestinal disturbances, fatigue, sleep disturbances; rare reports of rashes and dry eyes (reversible on withdrawal)
*Dose: by mouth*, hypertension, initially 80 mg twice daily, increased at weekly intervals as required; maintenance 160–320 mg daily
Portal hypertension, initially 40 mg twice daily, increased to 80 mg twice daily according to heart-rate; max. 160 mg twice daily
Phaeochromocytoma (only with an alpha-blocker), 60 mg daily for 3 days before surgery; 30 mg daily in patients unsuitable for surgery
Angina, initially 40 mg 2–3 times daily; maintenance 120–240 mg daily
Arrhythmias, hypertrophic obstructive cardiomyopathy, anxiety tachycardia, and thyrotoxicosis, 10–40 mg 3–4 times daily

Anxiety with symptoms such as palpitations, sweating, tremor, 40 mg twice daily, increased to 3 times daily if necessary

Prophylaxis after infarction, 40 mg 4 times daily for 2–3 days, then 80 mg twice daily, beginning 5 to 21 days after infarction

Migraine prophylaxis and essential tremor, initially 40 mg 2–3 times daily; maintenance 80–160 mg daily

*By intravenous injection*, arrhythmias and thyrotoxic crisis, 1 mg over 1 minute; if necessary repeat at 2-minute intervals; max. 10 mg (5 mg in anaesthesia)

*Note.* Excessive bradycardia can be countered with intravenous injection of atropine sulphate 0.6–2.4 mg in divided doses of 600 micrograms

PoM **Propranolol** (Non-proprietary)

*Tablets*, propranolol hydrochloride 10 mg, net price 20 = 5p; 40 mg, 20 = 8p; 80 mg, 20 = 15p; 160 mg, 20 = 26p. Label: 8

Available from APS (Apsolol®), Ashbourne (Propanix®), Berk (Berkolol®), Cox, CP (Cardinol®), DDSA (Angilol®), Evans, Kerfoot

*Oral suspensions*, propranolol hydrochloride 5 mg/5 mL and 50 mg/5 mL available from RP Drugs (special order)

PoM **Inderal**® (ICI)

*Tablets*, all pink, f/c, propranolol hydrochloride 10 mg, net price 20 = 18p; 40 mg, 20 = 50p; 80 mg, 20 = 81p. Label: 8

*Injection*, propranolol hydrochloride 1 mg/mL, net price 1-mL amp = 22p

Modified release

PoM **Half-Inderal LA**® (ICI)

*Capsules*, m/r, lavender/pink, propranolol hydrochloride 80 mg. Net price 28-cap pack = £5.04. Label: 8, 25

PoM **Inderal-LA**® (ICI)

*Capsules*, m/r, lavender/pink, propranolol hydrochloride 160 mg. Net price 28-cap pack = £6.92. Label: 8, 25

*Note.* Modified-release capsules containing propranolol hydrochloride 160 mg also available from Ashbourne (Propanix®), CP (Sloprolol®), Lagap (Bedranol SR®), Monmouth (Betadur CR®)

With diuretic

PoM **Inderetic**® (ICI)

*Capsules*, propranolol hydrochloride 80 mg, bendrofluazide 2.5 mg. Net price 20 = £2.02. Label: 8

*Dose:* hypertension, 1 capsule twice daily

PoM **Inderex**® (ICI)

*Capsules*, pink/grey, propranolol hydrochloride 160 mg (m/r), bendrofluazide 5 mg. Net price 28-cap pack = £7.73. Label: 8, 25

*Dose:* hypertension, 1 capsule daily

## ACEBUTOLOL

*Indications:* see under Dose

*Cautions; Contra-indications; Side-effects:* see under Propranolol Hydrochloride

*Dose:* hypertension, initially 400 mg once daily *or* 200 mg twice daily, increased after 2 weeks to 400 mg twice daily if necessary

Angina, initially 400 mg once daily *or* 200 mg twice daily; 300 mg 3 times daily in severe angina; up to 1.2 g daily has been used

Arrhythmias, 0.4–1.2 g daily in 2–3 divided doses

PoM **Sectral**® (Rhône-Poulenc Rorer)

*Capsules*, acebutolol (as hydrochloride) 100 mg (buff/white), net price 84-cap pack = £7.14; 200 mg (buff/pink), 56-cap pack = £9.16. Label: 8

*Tablets*, f/c, acebutolol 400 mg (as hydrochloride). Net price 28-tab pack = £8.88. Label: 8

With diuretic

PoM **Secadrex**® (Rhône-Poulenc Rorer)

*Tablets*, f/c, acebutolol 200 mg (as hydrochloride), hydrochlorothiazide 12.5 mg. Net price 28-tab pack = £8.39. Label: 8

*Dose:* hypertension, 1 tablet daily, increased to 2 daily as a single dose if necessary

## ATENOLOL

*Indications:* see under Dose

*Cautions; Contra-indications; Side-effects:* see under Propranolol Hydrochloride; reduce dose in renal impairment (25-mg tablets available)

*Dose: by mouth*,

Hypertension, 50 mg daily (higher doses no longer considered necessary)

Angina, 100 mg daily in 1 or 2 doses

Arrhythmias, 50–100 mg daily

*By intravenous injection*, arrhythmias, 2.5 mg at a rate of 1 mg/minute, repeated at 5-minute intervals to a max. of 10 mg

*Note.* Excessive bradycardia can be countered with intravenous injection of atropine sulphate 0.6–2.4 mg in divided doses of 600 micrograms

*By intravenous infusion*, arrhythmias, 150 micrograms/kg over 20 minutes, repeated every 12 hours if required

Early intervention within 12 hours of infarction, 5–10 mg *by slow intravenous injection*, then *by mouth* 50 mg after 15 minutes, 50 mg after 12 hours, then 100 mg daily

PoM **Atenolol** (Non-proprietary)

*Tablets*, atenolol 50 mg, net price 28-tab pack = £4.81; 100 mg, 28-tab pack = £6.80. Label: 8

Available from APS, Ashbourne (Atenix®), Berk (Antipressan®), Cox, CP (Totamol®), Evans, Kerfoot, Shire (Vasaten®)

PoM **Tenormin**® (Stuart)

*'25' tablets*, f/c, atenolol 25 mg. Net price 28-tab pack = £4.31. Label: 8

*LS tablets*, orange, f/c, scored, atenolol 50 mg. Net price 28-tab pack = £5.49. Label: 8

*Tablets*, orange, f/c, scored, atenolol 100 mg. Net price 28-tab pack = £6.98. Label: 8

*Syrup*, sugar-free, atenolol 25 mg/5 mL. Net price 300 mL = £8.35. Label: 8

*Injection*, atenolol 500 micrograms/mL. Net price 10-mL amp = 90p (hosp. only)

**With diuretic**

PoM **Co-tenidone** (Non-proprietary)
*Tablets*, co-tenidone 50/12.5 (atenolol 50 mg, chlorthalidone 12.5 mg), net price 28-tab pack = £5.27; co-tenidone 100/25 (atenolol 100 mg, chlorthalidone 25 mg), 28-tab pack = £7.50. Label: 8
Available from Ashbourne (AtenixCo®), Kerfoot
*Dose:* hypertension, 1 tablet daily (but see also under Dose above)

PoM **Kalten**® (Stuart)
*Capsules*, red/ivory, atenolol 50 mg, co-amilozide 2.5/25 (anhydrous amiloride hydrochloride 2.5 mg, hydrochlorothiazide 25 mg). Net price 28-cap pack = £7.49. Label: 8
*Dose:* hypertension, 1 capsule daily

PoM **Tenoret 50**® (Stuart)
*Tablets*, brown, f/c, co-tenidone 50/12.5 (atenolol 50 mg, chlorthalidone 12.5 mg). Net price 28-tab pack = £5.85. Label: 8
*Dose:* hypertension, 1 tablet daily

PoM **Tenoretic**® (Stuart)
*Tablets*, brown, f/c, co-tenidone 100/25 (atenolol 100 mg, chlorthalidone 25 mg). Net price 28-tab pack = £8.33. Label: 8
*Dose:* hypertension, 1 tablet daily (but see also under Dose above)

**With calcium-channel blocker**
*Note.* Only indicated when calcium-channel blocker or beta-blocker alone proves inadequate

PoM **Beta-Adalat**® (Bayer)
*Capsules*, reddish-brown, atenolol 50 mg, nifedipine 20 mg (m/r). Net price 28-cap pack = £10.90. Label: 8, 25
*Dose:* hypertension, 1 capsule daily, increased if necessary to twice daily; elderly, 1 daily
Angina, 1 capsule twice daily

PoM **Tenif**® (Stuart)
*Capsules*, reddish-brown, atenolol 50 mg, nifedipine 20 mg (m/r). Net price 28-cap pack = £10.90. Label: 8, 25
*Dose:* hypertension, 1 capsule daily, increased if necessary to twice daily; elderly, 1 daily
Angina, 1 capsule twice daily

## BETAXOLOL HYDROCHLORIDE

*Indications:* hypertension
*Cautions; Contra-indications; Side-effects:* see under Propranolol Hydrochloride; reduce dose in renal impairment
*Dose:* 20 mg daily (elderly patients 10 mg), increased to 40 mg if required

PoM **Kerlone**® (Lorex)
*Tablets*, f/c, scored, betaxolol hydrochloride 20 mg. Net price 28-tab pack = £7.70. Label: 8

## BISOPROLOL FUMARATE

*Indications:* hypertension, angina
*Cautions; Contra-indications; Side-effects:* see under Propranolol Hydrochloride; reduce dose in hepatic and renal impairment

*Dose:* usual dose 10 mg daily (5 mg may be adequate in some patients); max. recommended dose 20 mg daily

PoM **Emcor**® (Merck)
*LS Tablets*, yellow, f/c, scored, bisoprolol fumarate 5 mg. Net price 28-tab pack = £7.98. Label: 8
*Tablets*, orange, f/c, scored, bisoprolol fumarate 10 mg. Net price 28-tab pack = £8.96. Label: 8

PoM **Monocor**® (Cyanamid)
*Tablets*, both f/c, bisoprolol fumarate 5 mg (pink), net price 28-tab pack = £7.98; 10 mg, 28-tab pack = £8.96. Label: 8

## CARTEOLOL HYDROCHLORIDE

*Indications:* angina
*Cautions; Contra-indications; Side-effects:* see under Propranolol Hydrochloride
*Dose:* 10 mg daily; if necessary increased gradually to 30 mg daily

PoM **Cartrol**® (Sanofi Winthrop)
*Tablets*, carteolol hydrochloride 10 mg. Net price 28-tab pack = £5.60. Label: 8

## CELIPROLOL HYDROCHLORIDE

*Indications:* mild to moderate hypertension
*Cautions:* pregnancy, breast-feeding; avoid abrupt withdrawal; hepatic and renal impairment (avoid if severe); **interactions**: Appendix 1 (beta-blockers)
*Contra-indications:* as for Propranolol Hydrochloride; also severe renal impairment
*Side-effects:* headache, dizziness, fatigue, nausea and somnolence; rarely bradycardia
*Dose:* 200 mg once daily in the morning, increased to 400 mg once daily if necessary

▼ PoM **Celectol**® (Rhône-Poulenc Rorer)
*Tablets*, f/c, yellow, scored, celiprolol hydrochloride 200 mg. Net price 28-tab pack = £9.80. Label: 22

## LABETALOL HYDROCHLORIDE

*Indications:* hypertension (including hypertension in pregnancy, hypertension with angina, and hypertension following acute myocardial infarction); hypertensive crisis (but see section 2.5); controlled hypotension in surgery
*Cautions:* late pregnancy, breast-feeding; avoid abrupt withdrawal; stop and do not restart if liver damage occurs; interferes with laboratory tests for catecholamines; **interactions**: Appendix 1 (beta-blockers)
*Contra-indications:* as for Propranolol Hydrochloride; also liver disease
*Side-effects:* postural hypotension (avoid upright position during and for 3 hours after intravenous administration), tiredness, weakness, headache, rashes, scalp tingling, difficulty in micturition, epigastric pain, nausea, vomiting; liver damage (see Cautions); rarely lichenoid rash

*Dose: by mouth*, initially 100 mg (50 mg in elderly) twice daily with food, increased at intervals of 14 days to usual dose of 200 mg twice daily; up to 800 mg daily in 2 divided doses (3–4 divided doses if higher); max. 2.4 g daily

*By intravenous injection*, 50 mg over at least 1 minute, repeated after 5 minutes if necessary; max. 200 mg

Note. Excessive bradycardia can be countered with intravenous injection of atropine sulphate 0.6–2.4 mg in divided doses of 600 micrograms

*By intravenous infusion*, 2 mg/minute; usual range 50–200 mg, higher doses in phaeochromocytoma

Hypertension of pregnancy, 20 mg/hour, doubled every 30 minutes; usual max. 160 mg/hour

Hypertension following infarction, 15 mg/hour, gradually increased to max. 120 mg/hour

**PoM Labetalol Hydrochloride** (Non-proprietary)
*Tablets*, all f/c, labetalol hydrochloride 100 mg, net price 20 = £1.43; 200 mg, 20 = £2.27; 400 mg, 20 = £3.58. Label: 8, 21
Available from APS, Cox, Evans, Kerfoot, Lagap (Labrocol®)

**PoM Trandate®** (DF)
*Tablets*, all orange, f/c, labetalol hydrochloride 50 mg, net price 56-tab pack = £5.05; 100 mg, 56-tab pack = £5.56; 200 mg, 56-tab pack = £9.02; 400 mg, 20 = £4.26. Label: 8, 21
*Injection*, labetalol hydrochloride 5 mg/mL. Net price 20-mL amp = £2.83

## METOPROLOL TARTRATE

*Indications:* see under Dose
*Cautions; Contra-indications; Side-effects:* see under Propranolol Hydrochloride; reduce dose in hepatic and renal impairment
*Dose: by mouth*, hypertension, initially 100 mg daily, maintenance 100–400 mg daily in 1–2 doses
Angina, 50–100 mg 2–3 times daily
Arrhythmias, usually 50 mg 2–3 times daily; up to 300 mg daily in divided doses if necessary
Migraine prophylaxis, 100–200 mg daily in divided doses
Thyrotoxicosis, 50 mg 4 times daily
*By intravenous injection*, arrhythmias, up to 5 mg at rate 1–2 mg/minute, repeated after 5 minutes if necessary, total dose 10–15 mg
Note. Excessive bradycardia can be countered with intravenous injection of atropine sulphate 0.6–2.4 mg in divided doses of 600 micrograms
In surgery, 2–4 mg *by slow intravenous injection* at induction or to control arrhythmias developing during anaesthesia; 2-mg doses may be repeated to a max. of 10 mg
Early intervention within 12 hours of infarction, 5 mg *by intravenous injection* every 2 minutes to a max. of 15 mg, followed after 15 minutes by 50 mg *by mouth* every 6 hours for 48 hours; maintenance 200 mg daily

**PoM Metoprolol Tartrate** (Non-proprietary)
*Tablets*, metoprolol tartrate 50 mg, net price 20 = 94p; 100 mg, 20 = £1.75. Label: 8
Available from APS, Ashbourne (Mepranix®), Cox, Kerfoot

**PoM Betaloc®** (Astra)
*Tablets*, both scored, metoprolol tartrate 50 mg, net price 20 = 92p, 56-tab pack = £2.90; 100 mg, 20 = £1.71. Label: 8
*Injection*, metoprolol tartrate 1 mg/mL. Net price 5-mL amp = 45p

**PoM Lopresor®** (Geigy)
*Tablets*, both f/c, scored, metoprolol tartrate 50 mg (pink), net price 56-tab pack = £3.26; 100 mg (blue), 56-tab pack = £6.06. Label: 8

Modified release
**PoM Betaloc-SA®** (Astra)
*Durules®* (= tablets, m/r), metoprolol tartrate 200 mg. Net price 28-tab pack = £6.51. Label: 8, 25
*Dose:* 200–400 mg daily

**PoM Lopresor SR®** (Geigy)
*Tablets*, m/r, yellow, f/c, metoprolol tartrate 200 mg. Net price 28-tab pack = £7.42. Label: 8, 25
*Dose:* 200–400 mg daily

With diuretic
**PoM Co-Betaloc®** (Astra)
*Tablets*, scored, metoprolol tartrate 100 mg, hydrochlorothiazide 12.5 mg. Net price 28-tab pack = £6.65. Label: 8
*Dose:* hypertension, 1–3 tablets daily in single or divided doses

**PoM Co-Betaloc SA®** (Astra)
*Tablets*, yellow, f/c, metoprolol tartrate 200 mg (m/r), hydrochlorothiazide 25 mg. Net price 28-tab pack = £8.20. Label: 8, 25
*Dose:* hypertension, 1 tablet daily

**PoM Lopresoretic®** (Geigy)
*Tablets*, f/c, scored, metoprolol tartrate 100 mg, chlorthalidone 12.5 mg. Net price 56-tab pack = £7.47. Label: 8
*Dose:* hypertension, 1–2 tablets in the morning; max. 3–4 daily in single or divided doses

## NADOLOL

*Indications:* see under Dose
*Cautions; Contra-indications; Side-effects:* see under Propranolol Hydrochloride; reduce dose in renal impairment
*Dose:* hypertension, 80 mg daily, increased at weekly intervals if required; max. 240 mg daily
Angina, 40 mg daily, increased at weekly intervals if required; usual max. 160 mg daily
Arrhythmias, initially 40 mg daily, increased to 160 mg if required; reduce to 40 mg if bradycardia occurs
Migraine prophylaxis, initially 40 mg daily, increased by 40 mg at weekly intervals; usual maintenance dose 80–160 mg daily
Thyrotoxicosis, 80–160 mg daily

PoM **Corgard**® (Squibb)
*Tablets*, both blue, nadolol 40 mg, net price 28-tab pack = £5.22; 80 mg, 28-tab pack = £7.55. Label: 8

**With diuretic**
PoM **Corgaretic 40**® (Squibb)
*Tablets*, scored, nadolol 40 mg, bendrofluazide 5 mg. Net price 28-tab pack = £6.07. Label: 8
*Dose:* hypertension, 1–2 tablets daily
PoM **Corgaretic 80**® (Squibb)
*Tablets*, scored, nadolol 80 mg, bendrofluazide 5 mg. Net price 28-tab pack = £8.69. Label: 8
*Dose:* hypertension, 1–2 tablets daily

## OXPRENOLOL HYDROCHLORIDE
*Indications:* see under Dose
*Cautions; Contra-indications; Side-effects:* see under Propranolol Hydrochloride
*Dose:* hypertension, initially 80 mg twice daily, increased as required at weekly intervals; max. 480 mg daily
Angina, 40–160 mg 3 times daily
Arrhythmias, initially 20–40 mg 3 times daily, increased as necessary
Anxiety symptoms (short-term use), initially 40 mg twice daily, increased if necessary to 160 mg daily in divided doses

PoM **Oxprenolol** (Non-proprietary)
*Tablets*, all coated, oxprenolol hydrochloride 20 mg, net price 20 = 30p; 40 mg, 20 = 43p; 80 mg, 20 = 71p; 160 mg, 20 = £1.38. Label: 8
Available from APS (Apsolox®, 80-mg tablets contain tartrazine), Cox, Evans, Kerfoot
PoM **Trasicor**® (Ciba)
*Tablets*, all f/c, oxprenolol hydrochloride 20 mg (contain gluten), net price 20 = 58p; 40 mg (contain gluten), 20 = 96p; 80 mg (beige), 56-tab pack = £4.10; 160 mg (orange), 56-tab pack = £7.38. Label: 8

Modified release
PoM **Slow-Trasicor**® (Ciba)
*Tablets*, m/r, f/c, oxprenolol hydrochloride 160 mg. Net price 28-tab pack = £6.50. Label: 8, 25
*Dose:* 160–480 mg daily
Note. Modified-release tablets containing oxprenolol hydrochloride 160 mg also available from Ashbourne (Oxyprenix®)

**With diuretic**
PoM **Trasidrex**® (Ciba)
*Tablets*, red, s/c, co-prenozide 160/0.25 (oxprenolol hydrochloride 160 mg (m/r), cyclopenthiazide 250 micrograms). Net price 28-tab pack = £6.73. Label: 8
*Dose:* hypertension, 1 tablet daily, increased to 2 daily as a single dose if necessary

## PENBUTOLOL SULPHATE
*Indications:* hypertension
*Cautions; Contra-indications; Side-effects:* see under Propranolol Hydrochloride
*Dose:* see below

**With diuretic**
PoM **Lasipressin**® (Hoechst)
*Tablets*, yellow-white, f/c, scored, penbutolol sulphate 40 mg, frusemide 20 mg. Net price 30-tab pack = £8.49. Label: 8
*Dose:* hypertension, 1 tablet daily, increased to twice daily if necessary

## PINDOLOL
*Indications:* see under Dose
*Cautions; Contra-indications; Side-effects:* see under Propranolol Hydrochloride; reduce dose in renal impairment
*Dose:* hypertension, initially 5 mg 2–3 times daily *or* 15 mg once daily, increased as required at weekly intervals; max. 45 mg daily
Angina, 2.5–5 mg up to 3 times daily

PoM **Visken**® (Sandoz)
*Tablets*, both scored, pindolol 5 mg, net price 100-tab pack = £7.46; 15 mg, 30-tab pack = £6.71. Label: 8

**With diuretic**
PoM **Viskaldix**® (Sandoz)
*Tablets*, scored, pindolol 10 mg, clopamide 5 mg. Net price 28-tab pack = £5.72. Label: 8
*Dose:* hypertension, 1 tablet daily in the morning, increased to 2 daily if necessary; max. 3 daily

## SOTALOL HYDROCHLORIDE
*Indications:* see under Dose
*Cautions; Contra-indications; Side-effects:* see under Propranolol Hydrochloride; reduce dose in renal impairment; occasionally causes atypical ventricular arrhythmias (torsade de pointes)—special need to avoid hypokalaemia if given with thiazide or loop diuretic (also stop if severe or persistent diarrhoea etc.)
*Dose: by mouth*, hypertension and angina, initially 80 mg twice daily *or* 160 mg once daily; maintenance 160 mg daily, increased to 400–600 mg daily if necessary
Arrhythmias, 120–240 mg daily in single or divided doses
Thyrotoxicosis, 120–240 mg daily in single or divided doses
Prophylaxis after infarction, 320 mg daily, starting 5–14 days after infarction
*By slow intravenous injection*, arrhythmias, 20–60 mg over 2–3 minutes with ECG monitoring, repeated if necessary with 10-minute intervals between injections; up to 100 mg over 3 minutes or longer
Note. Excessive bradycardia can be countered with intravenous injection of atropine sulphate 0.6–2.4 mg in divided doses of 600 micrograms

---

PoM **Beta-Cardone**® (DF)

*Tablets*, all scored, sotalol hydrochloride 40 mg (green), net price 20 = 79p; 80 mg (pink), 20 = £1.17; 200 mg, 30-tab pack = £4.15. Label: 8

PoM **Sotacor**® (Bristol-Myers)

*Tablets*, sotalol hydrochloride 80 mg (pink), net price 28-tab pack = £2.05; 160 mg (blue), 28-tab pack = £4.05. Label: 8

*Injection*, sotalol hydrochloride 10 mg/mL. Net price 4-mL amp = £1.76

With diuretic

*Note.* Increased risk of hypokalaemia if combined with thiazide or loop diuretic (see Cautions above)

PoM **Sotazide**® (Bristol-Myers)

*Tablets*, blue, sotalol hydrochloride 160 mg, hydrochlorothiazide 25 mg. Net price 28-tab pack = £7.12. Label: 8

*Dose:* hypertension, 1 tablet daily, increased to 2 daily if necessary

PoM **Tolerzide**® (Bristol-Myers)

*Tablets*, lilac, sotalol hydrochloride 80 mg, hydrochlorothiazide 12.5 mg. Net price 28-tab pack = £4.05. Label: 8

*Dose:* hypertension, 1 tablet daily

---

## TIMOLOL MALEATE

*Indications:* see under Dose

*Cautions; Contra-indications; Side-effects:* see under Propranolol Hydrochloride

*Dose:* hypertension, initially 5 mg twice daily *or* 10 mg once daily; max. 60 mg daily

Angina, initially 5 mg 2–3 times daily, maintenance 15–45 mg daily

Prophylaxis after infarction, initially 5 mg twice daily, increased after 2 days to 10 mg twice daily, starting 7 to 28 days after infarction

Migraine prophylaxis, 10–20 mg daily

PoM **Betim**® (Leo)

*Tablets*, scored, timolol maleate 10 mg. Net price 20 = £1.75. Label: 8

PoM **Blocadren**® (MSD)

*Tablets*, blue, scored, timolol maleate 10 mg. Net price 20 = £2.12. Label: 8

With diuretic

PoM **Moducren**® (Morson)

*Tablets*, blue, scored, timolol maleate 10 mg, co-amilozide 2.5/25 (amiloride hydrochloride 2.5 mg, hydrochlorothiazide 25 mg). Net price 28-tab pack = £8.00. Label: 8

*Dose:* hypertension, 1–2 tablets daily as a single dose

PoM **Prestim**® (Leo)

*Tablets*, scored, timolol maleate 10 mg, bendrofluazide 2.5 mg. Net price 20 = £2.79. Label: 8

*Dose:* hypertension, 1–2 tablets daily; max. 4 daily

PoM **Prestim Forte**® (Leo)

*Tablets*, scored, timolol maleate 20 mg, bendrofluazide 5 mg. Net price 20 = £5.88. Label: 8

*Dose:* hypertension, ½–2 tablets daily in single or divided doses

## 2.5   Antihypertensive therapy

2.5.1 Vasodilator antihypertensive drugs
2.5.2 Centrally acting antihypertensive drugs
2.5.3 Adrenergic neurone blocking drugs
2.5.4 Alpha-adrenoceptor blocking drugs
2.5.5 Angiotensin-converting enzyme inhibitors
2.5.6 Ganglion blocking drugs
2.5.7 Tyrosine hydroxylase inhibitors

Antihypertensive therapy has improved the outlook for patients with high blood pressure by decreasing the frequency of stroke, heart failure, and renal failure. The recommendations of the British Hypertension Society are that, in general, patients whose diastolic pressure averages 110 mmHg or higher when measured on three separate occasions, or 100 to 109 mmHg when measured repeatedly over 4 to 6 months, should receive antihypertensive therapy. Below that level the benefits of therapy are unproven. The usual aim should be to reduce the diastolic blood pressure preferably to below 90 mmHg and certainly below 100 mmHg. The quality of control of blood pressure at follow-up is an important predictor of outcome, and efficient long-term care is necessary.

*Malignant* (or accelerated) hypertension or very severe hypertension (diastolic blood pressure >140 mmHg) requires urgent treatment in hospital but is not an indication for parenteral antihypertensive therapy. Normally treatment should be by mouth with a beta-blocker (atenolol or labetalol) or a calcium-channel blocker (nifedipine). Within the first 24 hours the diastolic blood pressure should be reduced to 100–110 mmHg. Over the next two or three days blood pressure should be normalised by using beta-blockers, calcium-channel blockers, diuretics, vasodilators, or angiotensin-converting enzyme inhibitors. Very rapid falls in blood pressure can cause reduced cerebral perfusion leading to cerebral infarction and blindness, a reduction in renal perfusion causing a deterioration in renal function, and myocardial ischaemia. Parenteral antihypertensive drugs are, therefore, hardly ever necessary.

On the rare occasions when a parenteral antihypertensive is necessary, sodium nitroprusside by infusion is the drug of choice.

In moderate to severe hypertension (diastolic blood pressure >110 mmHg) or in patients with vascular complications, antihypertensive drugs are best added 'stepwise' until control has been achieved; an attempt can then be made to 'step down' treatment under supervision. In mild uncomplicated hypertension (diastolic blood pressure <110 mmHg), drugs may be substituted rather than added. The strategy for reducing blood pressure is probably best as follows:

1. *Non-drug treatment*—obesity, high alcohol intake, and high salt intake may elevate blood pressure and these should be corrected.

2. *Diuretic therapy*—any thiazide will be effective, e.g. bendrofluazide 2.5 mg/day (section 2.2.1).

---

The optimum dose of a thiazide used to treat hypertension is the lowest possible dose; higher doses do not have a major additional anti-hypertensive effect, but do cause more metabolic side-effects. Potassium supplements are seldom necessary but plasma potassium concentration should be checked 3 to 4 weeks after starting treatment. Potassium-sparing diuretics (amiloride or triamterene) are usually not necessary in the routine treatment of hypertension, unless hypokalaemia develops.

3. *Beta-adrenoceptor blocking drugs* (section 2.4) should be used in combination with a thiazide where they are not effective alone.

4(a). *Calcium-channel        blockers*—calcium-channel blockers such as nifedipine, nicardipine, and verapamil have antihypertensive efficacy broadly similar to that of thiazides or beta-blockers. Minor side-effects are more common, and their safety during long-term treatment is less well established; they should therefore be considered for hypertension only when thiazides and beta-blockers are contra-indicated, not tolerated, or fail to control blood pressure. There are important differences     between     verapamil     and dihydropyridine calcium-channel blockers such as nifedipine and nicardipine (see section 2.6.2).

4(b). *ACE inhibitors* (section 2.5.5)—all ACE inhibitors may cause a precipitate drop in blood pressure in patients with renal impairment and/or receiving diuretic therapy; they should be given in low initial doses and where possible diuretic therapy should be omitted for a few days before starting. About 20% of women and 10% of men receiving an ACE inhibitor develop a persistent dry cough.

5. *Other     drugs*—Vasodilators     (hydralazine, minoxidil, diazoxide), alpha-adrenoceptor blocking drugs (prazosin, terazosin, doxazosin), and centrally acting drugs (methyldopa, reserpine) are generally reserved for patients whose blood pressure is not controlled by, or who have contra-indications to, the drugs already mentioned.

SYSTOLIC HYPERTENSION. High systolic blood pressure carries a poor prognosis. This may be because the height of the systolic blood pressure reflects evidence of end-organ damage caused by the hypertension itself. The quality of control of systolic blood pressure may have some importance in determining the outcome in patients with antihypertensive treatment.

HYPERTENSION IN PREGNANCY. It is important to control blood pressure in pregnancy. High blood pressure may be due to pre-existing essential hypertension or to pre-eclampsia. Oral methyldopa is safe in pregnancy. Beta-blockers are effective and safe in the third trimester but may cause intra-uterine growth retardation when used from earlier in pregnancy. Hydralazine by mouth is useful as second-line therapy; intravenous injection can be used to control hypertensive crises associated with *eclampsia*.

HYPERTENSION IN THE ELDERLY. There is evidence that treating hypertension in patients up to the age of 80 years is worthwhile provided treatment is carefully supervised. Little or no benefit has been shown in those over 80.

## 2.5.1   Vasodilator antihypertensive drugs

These are potent drugs, especially when used in combination with a beta-blocker and a thiazide.

**Diazoxide** is diabetogenic and is not used by mouth, except in very severe hypertension; it can be used by intravenous injection in hypertensive emergencies.

**Hydralazine** given by mouth is a useful adjunct to other treatment, but when used alone causes tachycardia and fluid retention. Side-effects can be few if the dose is kept below 100 mg daily, but systemic lupus erythematosus should be suspected if there is unexplained weight loss, arthritis, or any other unexplained ill health.

**Sodium nitroprusside** is given by intravenous infusion to control severe hypertensive crises.

**Minoxidil** should be reserved for the treatment of severe hypertension resistant to other drugs. Vasodilatation is accompanied by increased cardiac output and tachycardia and the patients develop fluid retention. For this reason a beta-blocker and a diuretic (usually frusemide, in high dosage) are mandatory. Hypertrichosis is troublesome and renders this drug unsuitable for women.

**Prazosin** and **terazosin** (section 2.5.4) have alpha-blocking and vasodilator properties.

### DIAZOXIDE
*Indications:* acute treatment of severe hypertension associated with renal disease (but see section 2.5)
*Cautions:* ischaemic heart disease, pregnancy, labour, impaired renal function; **interactions:** Appendix 1 (diazoxide)
*Side-effects:* tachycardia, hyperglycaemia, sodium and water retention
*Dose: by rapid intravenous injection* (less than 30 seconds), 1–3 mg/kg to max. single dose of 150 mg (see below); may be repeated after 5–15 minutes if required
*Note.* Single doses of 300 mg have been associated with angina and with myocardial and cerebral infarction

PoM **Eudemine**® (A&H)
*Injection*, diazoxide 15 mg/mL. Net price 20-mL amp = £2.70

### HYDRALAZINE HYDROCHLORIDE
*Indications:* moderate to severe hypertension, with beta-blocker and thiazide; hypertensive crisis (but see section 2.5)
*Cautions:* reduce initial dose in renal impairment; coronary artery disease (may provoke angina, avoid after myocardial infarction until stabilised), cerebrovascular disease; over-rapid blood pressure reduction is occasionally encountered even with low parenteral doses; pregnancy,     breast-feeding;     **interactions:** Appendix 1 (hydralazine)

*Contra-indications:* idiopathic systemic lupus erythematosus, severe tachycardia, high output heart failure, myocardial insufficiency due to mechanical obstruction, cor pulmonale, dissecting aortic aneurysm; porphyria (see section 9.8.2)

*Side-effects:* tachycardia, fluid retention, nausea, and vomiting; headache; systemic lupus erythematosus-like syndrome after long-term therapy with over 100 mg daily (or less in women) (see also notes above); rarely rashes, fever, changes in blood count, peripheral neuritis

*Dose: by mouth,* 25 mg twice daily, increased to a max. of 50 mg twice daily (see notes above)
*By slow intravenous injection,* 5–10 mg over 20 minutes; may be repeated after 20–30 minutes (see Cautions)
*By intravenous infusion,* initially 200–300 micrograms/minute; maintenance usually 50–150 micrograms/minute

PoM **Hydralazine** (Non-proprietary)
*Tablets,* hydralazine hydrochloride 25 mg, net price 20 = 27p; 50 mg, 20 = 55p
PoM **Apresoline**® (Ciba)
*Tablets,* both s/c, hydralazine hydrochloride 25 mg (yellow), net price 20 = 36p; 50 mg (violet), 20 = 70p
*Additives:* include gluten
*Injection,* powder for reconstitution, hydralazine hydrochloride. Net price 20-mg amp = 32p

## MINOXIDIL

*Indications:* severe hypertension, in addition to a diuretic and a beta-blocker
*Cautions:* see notes above; angina; after myocardial infarction (until stabilised); lower doses in dialysis patients; pregnancy; **interactions:** Appendix 1 (minoxidil)
*Contra-indications:* phaeochromocytoma; porphyria (see section 9.8.2)
*Side-effects:* sodium and water retention; weight gain, peripheral oedema, tachycardia, hypertrichosis; reversible rise in creatinine and blood urea nitrogen; occasionally, gastro-intestinal disturbances, breast tenderness, rashes
*Dose:* initially 5 mg daily, in 1–2 doses, increased by 5–10 mg every 3 or more days; max. usually 50 mg daily

PoM **Loniten**® (Upjohn)
*Tablets,* all scored, minoxidil 2.5 mg, net price 20 = £2.47; 5 mg, 20 = £4.40; 10 mg, 20 = £8.52

## SODIUM NITROPRUSSIDE

*Indications:* hypertensive crisis (but see section 2.5); controlled hypotension in surgery; acute or chronic heart failure
*Cautions:* hypothyroidism, severe renal impairment, impaired cerebral circulation, elderly; monitor plasma-cyanide concentration; **interactions:** Appendix 1 (nitroprusside)
*Contra-indications:* severe hepatic impairment; vitamin B$_{12}$ deficiency; Leber's optic atrophy; compensatory hypertension

*Side-effects:* headache, dizziness, nausea, retching, abdominal pain, perspiration, palpitations, apprehension, retrosternal discomfort—reduce infusion rate
*Dose:* hypertensive crisis, in patients not already receiving antihypertensives, *by intravenous infusion,* 0.3–1 micrograms/kg/minute initially, then adjusted; usual range 0.5–6 micrograms/kg/minute (20–400 micrograms/minute); max. 8 micrograms/kg/minute; lower doses for patients already being treated with antihypertensives
Lower doses should also be employed for controlled hypotension in surgery (max. 1.5 micrograms/kg/minute)
Heart failure, *by intravenous infusion,* initially 10–15 micrograms/minute, increased every 5–10 minutes as necessary; usual range 10–200 micrograms/minute; max. 280 micrograms/minute (4 micrograms/kg/minute)

PoM **Sodium Nitroprusside** (Non-proprietary)
*Intravenous solution,* sodium nitroprusside 10 mg/mL. For dilution and use as an infusion. Net price 5-mL vial = £3.65
Available from David Bull, CP
PoM **Nipride**® (Roche)
*Infusion,* sodium nitroprusside 50-mg amp (with solvent for reconstitution). Net price = £4.00

## 2.5.2  Centrally acting antihypertensive drugs

This group includes methyldopa and clonidine and is largely falling from use.

**Methyldopa,** however, has the advantage of being safe in asthmatics, in heart failure, and in pregnancy. Side-effects are minimised if the daily dose is kept below 1 g.

Clonidine has the disadvantage that sudden withdrawal may cause a hypertensive crisis.

Reserpine and rauwolfia are no longer used in Britain.

## CLONIDINE HYDROCHLORIDE

*Indications:* hypertension (for use in migraine, see section 4.7.4.2)
*Cautions:* must be withdrawn gradually to avoid hypertensive crisis; Raynaud's syndrome or other occlusive peripheral vascular disease; history of depression; avoid in porphyria (see section 9.8.2); **interactions:** Appendix 1 (clonidine)
DRIVING. Drowsiness may affect performance of skilled tasks (e.g. driving); effects of alcohol may be enhanced
*Side-effects:* dry mouth, sedation, depression, fluid retention, bradycardia, Raynaud's phenomenon, headache, dizziness, euphoria, nocturnal unrest, rash, nausea, constipation, rarely impotence
*Dose: by mouth,* 50–100 micrograms 3 times daily, increased every second or third day; max. daily dose usually 1.2 mg
*By slow intravenous injection,* 150–300 micrograms; max. 750 micrograms in 24 hours

PoM **Catapres**® (Boehringer Ingelheim)
*Tablets*, both scored, clonidine hydrochloride 100 micrograms, net price 84-tab pack = £5.39; 300 micrograms, 84-tab pack = £12.56. Label: 3, 8
*Injection*, clonidine hydrochloride 150 micrograms/mL. Net price 1-mL amp = 27p
PoM **Dixarit**® (migraine), see section 4.7.4.2

Modified release
PoM **Catapres**® **Perlongets** (Boehringer Ingelheim)
*Capsules*, m/r, red/yellow, clonidine hydrochloride 250 micrograms. Net price 56-cap pack = £12.74. Label: 3, 8, 25
*Dose:* usually 1 capsule in the evening; 2–3 capsules daily (1 morning and 1–2 evening) if necessary

## METHYLDOPA
*Indications:* hypertension, in conjunction with diuretic; hypertensive crisis when immediate effect not necessary
*Cautions:* positive direct Coombs' test in up to 20% of patients (may affect blood cross-matching); interference with laboratory tests; reduce initial dose in renal impairment; blood counts and liver-function tests advised; **interactions:** Appendix 1 (methyldopa)
DRIVING. Drowsiness may affect performance of skilled tasks (e.g. driving); effects of alcohol may be enhanced
*Contra-indications:* history of depression, active liver disease, phaeochromocytoma; porphyria (see section 9.8.2)
*Side-effects:* dry mouth, sedation, depression, drowsiness, diarrhoea, fluid retention, failure of ejaculation, liver damage, haemolytic anaemia, systemic lupus erythematosus-like syndrome, parkinsonism, rashes, nasal stuffiness
*Dose: by mouth*, 250 mg 2–3 times daily, gradually increased at intervals of 2 or more days; max. daily dose 3 g
ELDERLY 125 mg twice daily initially, gradually increased; max. daily dose 2 g
*By intravenous infusion*, methyldopate hydrochloride 250–500 mg, repeated after 6 hours if required

PoM **Methyldopa** (Non-proprietary)
*Tablets*, coated, methyldopa (anhydrous) 125 mg, net price 20 = 43p; 250 mg, 20 = 68p; 500 mg, 20 = £1.38. Label: 3, 8
PoM **Aldomet**® (MSD)
*Tablets*, all yellow, f/c, methyldopa (anhydrous) 125 mg, net price 20 = 77p; 250 mg, 20 = £1.19; 500 mg, 20 = £2.34. Label: 3, 8
*Suspension*, methyldopa 250 mg/5 mL. Do not dilute. Net price 200 mL = £3.96. Label: 3, 8
*Injection*, methyldopate hydrochloride 50 mg/mL. Net price 5-mL amp = £2.31
PoM **Dopamet**® (Berk)
*Tablets*, all yellow, f/c, methyldopa (anhydrous) 125 mg, net price 20 = 43p; 250 mg, 20 = 73p; 500 mg, 20 = £1.46. Label: 3, 8
*Additives: include tartrazine*

With diuretic
PoM **Hydromet**® (MSD)
*Tablets*, pink, f/c, methyldopa (anhydrous) 250 mg, hydrochlorothiazide 15 mg. Net price 20 = £1.52. Label: 3, 8

## RAUWOLFIA ALKALOIDS
*Indications:* hypertension
*Cautions:* heart failure, arteriosclerosis, pregnancy, breast-feeding; **interactions:** Appendix 1 (rauwolfia alkaloids)
*Contra-indications:* history of depression, phaeochromocytoma, peptic ulcer, Parkinson's disease, ulcerative colitis, thyrotoxicosis, renal impairment, epilepsy
*Side-effects:* include dry mouth, nasal congestion, sedation, depression, postural hypotension, bradycardia, fluid retention

PoM **Hypercal**® (Carlton)
*Tablets*, rauwolfia alkaloids 2 mg. Net price 20 = 10p. Label: 3

## 2.5.3 Adrenergic neurone blocking drugs
These drugs prevent the release of noradrenaline from postganglionic adrenergic neurones. Guanethidine also depletes the nerve endings of noradrenaline. These drugs do not control supine blood pressure and may cause postural hypotension. For this reason they have largely fallen from use, but they may be necessary in combination with other therapy in resistant hypertension.

## GUANETHIDINE MONOSULPHATE
*Indications:* moderate to severe hypertension that has failed to respond adequately to other antihypertensives, in conjunction with a diuretic or a vasodilator antihypertensive
*Cautions:* postural hypotension may cause falls in elderly; coronary or cerebral arteriosclerosis, asthma, history of peptic ulceration; pregnancy; **interactions:** Appendix 1 (adrenergic neurone blockers)
*Contra-indications:* phaeochromocytoma, renal failure, heart failure
*Side-effects:* postural hypotension, failure of ejaculation, fluid retention, nasal congestion, headache, diarrhoea, drowsiness
*Dose: by mouth*, 10 mg daily, increased by 10 mg at weekly intervals; usual daily dose 25–50 mg
*By intramuscular injection*, 10–20 mg, repeated after 3 hours if required

PoM **Ismelin**® (Ciba)
*Tablets*, guanethidine monosulphate 10 mg, net price 20 = 46p; 25 mg (pink), 20 = £1.03
*Additives: include gluten*
*Injection*, guanethidine monosulphate 10 mg/mL. Net price 1-mL amp = 23p

## BETHANIDINE SULPHATE
*Indications; Cautions; Contra-indications; Side-effects:* see under Guanethidine Monosulphate (except diarrhoea)
*Dose:* 10 mg (elderly 5 mg) 3 times daily after food, increased by 5 mg at intervals; max. daily dose 200 mg

PoM **Bendogen**® (Lagap)
*Tablets*, scored, bethanidine sulphate 10 mg, net price 20 = £1.20. Label: 21

## DEBRISOQUINE

*Indications; Cautions; Contra-indications; Side-effects:* see under Guanethidine Monosulphate (except diarrhoea)
*Dose:* 10 mg 1–2 times daily, increased by 10 mg every 3 days; usual range 20–60 mg daily (120 mg or higher in severe hypertension)

PoM **Declinax®** (Roche)
*Tablets*, both scored, debrisoquine (as sulphate) 10 mg, net price 20 = 77p; 20 mg (blue), 20 = £1.12

### 2.5.4   Alpha-adrenoceptor blocking drugs

**Prazosin** has post-synaptic alpha-blocking and vasodilator properties and rarely causes tachycardia. It may, however, cause a rapid reduction in blood pressure after the first dose and should be introduced with caution. **Doxazosin** and **terazosin** have properties similar to those of prazosin.

**Phenoxybenzamine** and **indoramin** are alphablockers which are effective agents, but have many side-effects. Phenoxybenzamine is used with a beta-blocker in the short-term management of severe hypertensive episodes associated with phaeochromocytoma; it is also used in the management of severe shock unresponsive to conventional therapy.

**Phentolamine** is used rarely as a suppression test for phaeochromocytoma.

PROSTATIC HYPERTROPHY. Both prazosin and indoramin are also indicated for prostatic hypertrophy (see below and also section 7.4.1).

## DOXAZOSIN

*Indications:* hypertension, if necessary in conjunction with thiazide or beta-blocker
*Cautions:* care with initial dose (postural hypotension); **interactions:** Appendix 1 (alphablockers)
*Side-effects:* postural hypotension (rarely associated with fainting); dizziness, vertigo, headache, fatigue, asthenia, oedema
*Dose:* 1 mg daily, increased after 1–2 weeks to 2 mg daily, and thereafter to 4 mg daily, if necessary; max. 16 mg daily

PoM **Cardura®** (Invicta)
*Tablets*, doxazosin (as mesylate) 1 mg, net price 28-tab pack = £9.60; 2 mg, 28-tab pack = £12.80; 4 mg, 28-tab pack = £16.00

## INDORAMIN

*Indications:* see preparations below
*Cautions:* avoid alcohol (enhances rate and extent of absorption); control incipient heart failure with diuretics and digoxin; hepatic or renal impairment; elderly patients; Parkinson's disease; epilepsy (convulsions in *animal* studies); history of depression; **interactions:** Appendix 1 (alpha-blockers)
DRIVING. Drowsiness may affect performance of skilled tasks (e.g. driving); effects of alcohol may be enhanced
*Contra-indications:* established heart failure; patients receiving MAOIs

*Side-effects:* sedation; also dizziness, depression, failure of ejaculation, dry mouth, nasal congestion, extrapyramidal effects, weight gain
*Dose:* see preparations below

PoM **Baratol®** (Wyeth)
*Tablets*, both f/c, indoramin (as hydrochloride) 25 mg (blue), net price 20 = £2.15; 50 mg (green, scored), 20 = £3.80. Label: 2
*Dose:* hypertension, usually in conjunction with thiazide or beta-blocker, initially 25 mg twice daily, increased by 25–50 mg daily at intervals of 2 weeks; max. daily dose 200 mg in 2–3 divided doses

Prostatic hypertrophy
PoM **Doralese®** (Bencard)
*Tablets*, yellow, f/c, indoramin 20 mg. Net price 60-tab pack = £8.40. Label: 2
*Dose:* benign prostatic hypertrophy, 20 mg twice daily; increased if necessary by 20 mg every 2 weeks to max. 100 mg daily in divided doses; ELDERLY, 20 mg at night may be adequate
*Note.* Not licensed for treatment of hypertension

## PHENOXYBENZAMINE HYDROCHLORIDE

*Indications:* phaeochromocytoma (see notes above)
*Cautions:* elderly patients; congestive heart failure; severe or ischaemic heart disease (avoid for 3–4 weeks after myocardial infarction), marked arteriosclerosis (avoid if history of cerebrovascular accident); renal impairment; carcinogenic in *animals*; pregnancy; avoid in porphyria (see section 9.8.2); avoid infusion in hypovolaemia; avoid extravasation (irritant to tissues)
*Side-effects:* postural hypotension with dizziness and marked compensatory tachycardia, lassitude, nasal congestion, miosis, inhibition of ejaculation; rarely gastro-intestinal disturbances; decreased sweating and dry mouth after intravenous infusion; idiosyncratic profound hypotension within few minutes of starting infusion
*Dose: by mouth*, phaeochromocytoma, 10 mg daily, increased by 10 mg daily; usual dose 1–2 mg/kg daily in 2 divided doses

PoM **Dibenyline®** (SK&F)
*Capsules*, red/white, phenoxybenzamine hydrochloride 10 mg. Net price 30-cap pack = £3.19
*Injection concentrate*, phenoxybenzamine hydrochloride 50 mg/mL. To be diluted before use. 2-mL amp (hosp. only)
*Dose: by intravenous infusion* (preferably through large vein;, phaeochromocytoma and adjunct in severe shock, 1 mg/kg daily in 200 mL physiological saline over at least 2 hours; do not repeat within 24 hours (intensive care facilities needed)
CAUTION. Owing to risk of contact sensitisation doctors, nurses, and other health workers should avoid contamination of hands

## PHENTOLAMINE MESYLATE

*Indications:* hypertensive crises due to phaeo-chromocytoma or interaction of foods with MAOIs, diagnosis of phaeochromocytoma; clonidine withdrawal; acute left ventricular failure

*Cautions:* monitor blood pressure (avoid in hypotension), heart rate

*Side-effects:* hypotension, tachycardia, dizziness; nausea, diarrhoea, nasal congestion

*Dose: by intravenous injection,* 5–10 mg repeated if necessary

*By intravenous infusion,* 5–60 mg over 10–30 minutes at a rate of 0.2–2 mg/minute

PoM **Rogitine**® (Ciba)

*Injection*, phentolamine mesylate 10 mg/mL. Net price 1-mL amp = 27p

## PRAZOSIN HYDROCHLORIDE

*Indications:* see under Dose

*Cautions:* first dose may cause collapse due to hypotension (therefore should be taken on retiring to bed); elderly; reduce initial dose in renal impairment; **interactions:** Appendix 1 (alpha-blockers)

*Side-effects:* postural hypotension, drowsiness, weakness, dizziness, headache, lack of energy, nausea, palpitations; urinary frequency, incontinence reported

*Dose:* hypertension, 500 micrograms 2–3 times daily, the initial dose on retiring to bed at night (to avoid collapse, see Cautions); increased to 1 mg 2–3 times daily after 3–7 days; further increased if necessary to max. 20 mg daily

Congestive heart failure, 500 micrograms 2–4 times daily (initial dose at bedtime, see above), increasing to 4 mg daily in divided doses; maintenance 4–20 mg daily (but rarely used)

Raynaud's syndrome, initially 500 micrograms twice daily (initial dose at bedtime, see above); maintenance 1–2 mg twice daily

Benign prostatic hypertrophy, initially 500 micrograms twice daily for 3–7 days (initial dose at bedtime, see above), dose subsequently adjusted according to response; usual maintenance (and max.) 2 mg twice daily

PoM **Hypovase**® (Invicta)

*Tablets*, prazosin hydrochloride 500 micrograms, net price 56-tab pack = £2.41; 1 mg (orange, scored), 56-tab pack = £3.10; 2 mg (scored), 56-tab pack = £4.21; 5 mg (scored), 56-tab pack = £9.07; starter pack of 8 × 500-microgram tabs and 32 × 1-mg tabs = £2.90. Label: 3, counselling, see dose above

## TERAZOSIN

*Indications:* mild to moderate hypertension

*Cautions:* first dose may cause collapse due to hypotension (within 30–90 minutes, therefore should be taken on retiring to bed) (may also occur with rapid dose increase); **interactions:** Appendix 1 (alpha-blockers)

*Side-effects:* dizziness, lack of energy, peripheral oedema; urinary frequency reported

*Dose:* 1 mg at bedtime (compliance with bedtime dose important to avoid collapse, see Cautions); dose doubled after 7 days if necessary; usual maintenance dose 2–10 mg daily; more than 20 mg daily rarely improves efficacy

PoM **Hytrin**® (Abbott)

*Tablets*, terazosin (as hydrochloride) 2 mg (yellow), net price 28-tab pack = £12.32; 5 mg (tan), 28-tab pack = £18.54; 10 mg (blue), 28-tab pack = £26.10; starter pack of 7 × 1-mg tabs and 21 × 2-mg tabs = £12.95. Label: 3, counselling, see dose above

## 2.5.5 Angiotensin-converting enzyme inhibitors

(ACE inhibitors)

Angiotensin-converting enzyme inhibitors inhibit the conversion of angiotensin I to angiotensin II. They are effective and generally well tolerated, but experience is limited as regards long-term use.

They should therefore be considered for *hypertension* only when thiazides and beta-blockers are contra-indicated, not tolerated, or fail to control blood pressure. All may cause very rapid falls of blood pressure in some patients. Therefore where possible diuretic therapy should be stopped for a few days before initiating therapy and the first dose should preferably be given at bedtime.

ACE inhibitors have a valuable role in *heart failure* when used as an adjunct to diuretics and, where appropriate, digoxin. They have been shown to improve the prognosis substantially, and in this respect are superior to regimens such as modified-release nitrates with hydralazine. Introduction of an ACE inhibitor should be considered when heart failure is not completely controlled by frusemide 80 mg daily (or an equivalent dose of another loop diuretic). To avoid dangerous hyperkalaemia, any potassium-sparing diuretic should be omitted from the diuretic regimen before introducing an ACE inhibitor, changing to the loop diuretic alone; potassium supplements should also be discontinued. Profound first-dose hypotension is common (and potentially serious) when ACE inhibitors are introduced to patients with heart failure receiving loop diuretics. Temporary withdrawal of the loop diuretic reduces the risk, but may cause severe rebound pulmonary oedema. The ACE inhibitor should therefore be started at very low dosage (e.g. captopril 6.25 mg), with the patient recumbent and under close supervision, and with facilities available to treat profound hypotension. Treatment should therefore generally be initiated under hospital supervision.

RENAL IMPAIRMENT. ACE inhibitors occasionally cause impairment of renal function which may progress and become severe. At particular risk are those with pre-existing renal disease or impairment, the elderly, and those with bilateral renal artery stenosis (or stenosis of the artery supplying a single functioning kidney). Concomitant treatment with NSAIDs increases the risk of renal damage, and potassium-sparing diuretics or use of potassium-containing salt substitutes increase the risk of hyperkalaemia. Renal function and electrolytes should be checked before starting an ACE inhibitor, and monitored during treatment.

ACE inhibitors should be used with **particular caution** in patients with peripheral vascular disease or generalised atherosclerosis, as such patients may have clinically silent renovascular disease.

COMBINATION PRODUCTS. A number of products incorporating an ACE inhibitor with a thiazide diuretic are now available. Use of these combination products should be reserved for patients whose blood pressure has not responded to a thiazide diuretic or an ACE inhibitor alone (see also comments above).

## CAPTOPRIL

*Indications:* mild to moderate essential hypertension alone or with thiazide therapy and severe hypertension resistant to other treatment (but see cautions and notes above); congestive heart failure (adjunct)

*Cautions:* diuretics (**important:** see notes above); first doses may cause hypotension especially in patients taking diuretics, on a low-sodium diet, on dialysis, or dehydrated; monitor renal function before and during treatment; reduce dose or **avoid** in renal impairment (white cell counts and urinary protein estimations needed); see also notes above; **interactions:** Appendix 1 (ACE inhibitors)

*Contra-indications:* hypersensitivity to ACE inhibitors; known or suspected renovascular disease, aortic stenosis or outflow tract obstruction; pregnancy; porphyria (see section 9.8.2)

*Side-effects:* persistent dry cough, throat discomfort, voice changes; loss of taste, sore mouth, abdominal pain, rash, angioedema, hypotension (see Cautions); proteinuria, thrombocytopenia, neutropenia, agranulocytosis, hyperkalaemia (all more common in renal impairment); increases in liver enzymes, liver damage, and cholestatic jaundice reported; renal impairment, see notes above

*Dose:* hypertension, used alone, initially 12.5 mg twice daily; if used in addition to diuretic (see notes), in elderly, or in renal impairment, initially 6.25 mg twice daily (first dose at bedtime); usual maintenance dose 25 mg twice daily; max. 50 mg twice daily (rarely 3 times daily in severe hypertension)

Heart failure (adjunct), initially 6.25–12.5 mg under close hospital supervision; usual maintenance dose 25 mg 2–3 times daily

PoM **Capoten**® (Squibb)

*Tablets,* captopril 12.5 mg (scored), net price 100 = £18.86; 25 mg, 56-tab pack = £12.03, 90-

tab pack = £19.34; 50 mg (scored), 56-tab pack = £20.50, 90-tab pack = £32.95 (also available as Acepril®)

With diuretic
*Note.* For mild to moderate hypertension in patients stabilised on the individual components in the same proportions
PoM **Capozide**® (Squibb)

*LS tablets,* scored, captopril 25 mg, hydrochlorothiazide 12.5 mg. Net price 28-tab pack = £11.25

*Tablets,* scored, captopril 50 mg, hydrochlorothiazide 25 mg. Net price 28-tab pack = £16.07 (also available as Acezide®)

## CILAZAPRIL

*Indications:* essential hypertension where standard therapy ineffective or inappropriate because of adverse effects (but see cautions and notes above)

*Cautions; Contra-indications:* see under Captopril and notes above

*Side-effects:* see under Enalapril

*Dose:* initially, 1 mg once daily; usual range 2.5–5 mg once daily; if used in addition to diuretic (see notes) or in elderly, initially 500 micrograms once daily; if patient also has congestive heart failure, initially 500 micrograms once daily under close hospital supervision
*Note.* If possible discontinue diuretic for 2–3 days beforehand (see also notes above)

▼ PoM **Vascace**® (Roche)

*Tablets,* all f/c, cilazapril 250 micrograms (pink), net price 28-tab pack = £3.87; 500 micrograms (white), 28-tab pack = £4.10; 1 mg (yellow), 28-tab pack = £7.06; 2.5 mg (pink), 28-tab pack = £10.67.

## ENALAPRIL MALEATE

*Indications:* all grades of essential hypertension (but see cautions and notes above); congestive heart failure (adjunct)

*Cautions; Contra-indications:* see under Captopril and notes above

*Side-effects:* persistent dry cough, throat discomfort, voice changes; dizziness, headache, fatigue, weakness, hypotension (see Cautions), change of taste, nausea, diarrhoea, muscle cramps, rash, and angioedema; renal impairment, see notes above

*Dose:* hypertension, used alone, initially 5 mg daily; if used in addition to diuretic (see notes), in elderly patients, or in renal impairment, initially 2.5 mg daily; usual maintenance dose 10–20 mg daily; max. 40 mg daily

Heart failure (adjunct), initially 2.5 mg daily under close hospital supervision; usual maintenance 10–20 mg daily

PoM **Innovace**® (MSD)

*Tablets,* enalapril maleate 2.5 mg, net price 50 = £10.00; 5 mg (scored), 28-tab pack = £7.86, 50 = £14.03; 10 mg (red), 28-tab pack = £11.03, 50 = £19.69; 20 mg (peach), 28-tab pack = £13.10, 50 = £23.40

With diuretic
*Note.* For mild to moderate hypertension in patients stabilised on the individual components in the same proportions
PoM **Innozide**® (MSD)
*Tablets*, yellow, scored, enalapril maleate 20 mg,
hydrochlorothiazide 12.5 mg. Net price 28-tab
pack = £14.56

## FOSINOPRIL
*Indications:* essential hypertension where standard therapy ineffective or inappropriate
because of adverse effects (but see cautions and
notes above)
*Cautions; Contra-indications:* see under Captopril and notes above
*Side-effects:* see under Enalapril; upper respiratory symptoms; palpitations, chest pain,
paraesthesia, pruritus, pancreatitis also
reported
*Dose:* initially 10 mg daily; usual maintenance
20 mg daily; max. 40 mg daily
*Note.* If used in addition to diuretic, discontinue diuretic
several days before and resume after about 4 weeks
if blood pressure inadequately controlled (if diuretic
therapy cannot be stopped careful medical supervision
for several hours)

▼ PoM **Staril**® (Squibb)
*Tablets*, fosinopril sodium 10 mg, net price 28-
tab pack = £12.04; 20 mg, 28-tab pack = £21.00

## LISINOPRIL
*Indications:* all grades of essential hypertension
(but see cautions and notes above); congestive
heart failure (adjunct)
*Cautions; Contra-indications:* see under Captopril and notes above
*Side-effects:* see under Enalapril; palpitations
also reported
*Dose:* hypertension, initially 2.5 mg daily; usual
maintenance dose 10–20 mg daily; max. 40 mg
daily
*Note.* In hypertension discontinue diuretic for 2–3 days
beforehand and resume later if required (see also notes
above)
Heart failure (adjunct), initially 2.5 mg daily
under close hospital supervision; usual maintenance dose 5–20 mg daily

PoM **Carace**® (Morson)
*Tablets*, lisinopril 2.5 mg (blue), net price 50 =
£15.30; 5 mg (scored), 28-tab pack = £10.14;
10 mg (yellow, scored), 28-tab pack = £12.13;
20 mg (orange, scored), 28-tab pack = £20.30
PoM **Zestril**® (ICI)
*Tablets*, lisinopril (as dihydrate) 2.5 mg, net price
28-tab pack = £7.84; 5 mg (pink, scored), 28-
tab pack = £9.83; 10 mg (pink), 28-tab pack =
£12.13; 20 mg (red), 28-tab pack = £20.96

With diuretic
*Note.* For mild to moderate hypertension in patients stabilised on the individual components in the same proportions
PoM **Carace Plus**® (Morson)
*Tablets*, yellow, scored, lisinopril 20 mg, hydrochlorothiazide 12.5 mg. Net price 28-tab pack =
£17.36, 56-tab pack = £34.72

PoM **Zestoretic**® (ICI)
*Tablets*, lisinopril 20 mg, hydrochlorothiazide
12.5 mg. Net price 28-tab pack = £17.36

## PERINDOPRIL
*Indications:* essential hypertension where standard therapy is ineffective or inappropriate
because of adverse effects (but see cautions and
notes above); congestive heart failure (adjunct)
*Cautions; Contra-indications:* see under Captopril and notes above
*Side-effects:* see under Enalapril; abdominal
pain, mood and sleep disturbances also
reported
*Dose:* hypertension, initially 2 mg daily; usual
maintenance dose 4–8 mg once daily; max. 8 mg
daily
*Note.* In hypertension discontinue diuretic 3 days
beforehand and resume later if required (see also notes
above)
Heart failure (adjunct), initial dose 2 mg in the
morning under close hospital supervision; usual
maintenance 4 mg daily

▼ PoM **Coversyl**® (Servier)
*Tablets*, perindopril tert-butylamine 2 mg, net
price 30-tab pack = £9.45; 4 mg (scored), 30-
tab pack = £13.00. Label: 22

## QUINAPRIL
*Indications:* all grades of essential hypertension
where standard therapy ineffective or inappropriate because of adverse effects (but see
cautions and notes above); congestive heart
failure (adjunct)
*Cautions; Contra-indications:* see under Captopril and notes above
*Side-effects:* see under Enalapril; rhinitis, sinusitis, pharyngitis, dyspepsia, abdominal pain,
back pain, vomiting, chest pain, insomnia, paraesthesia, nervousness also reported
*Dose:* hypertension, initially 5 mg daily; with a
diuretic, in elderly, or in renal impairment
initially 2.5 mg daily; usual maintenance dose
20–40 mg daily in single or 2 divided doses; up
to 80 mg daily has been given
Heart failure (adjunct), initial dose 2.5 mg
under close hospital supervision; usual maintenance 10–20 mg daily in 2 divided doses; max.
40 mg daily

PoM **Accupro**® (P-D)
*Tablets*, all brown, f/c, quinapril 5 mg, net price
28-tab pack = £9.82; 10 mg, 28-tab pack =
£10.07; 20 mg, 28-tab pack = £10.32

## RAMIPRIL
*Indications:* mild to moderate essential hypertension where standard therapy ineffective or
inappropriate because of adverse effects (but
see cautions and notes above)
*Cautions; Contra-indications:* see under Captopril and notes above

Prices are **net**, see p. 1

*Side-effects:* see under Enalapril; also abdominal pain, vomiting; increases in blood urea nitrogen and serum creatinine (particularly in renal impairment)

*Dose:* initially 1.25 mg daily, increased at intervals of 1–2 weeks; usual range 2.5–5 mg daily; max. 10 mg daily

Note. Discontinue diuretic for 2–3 days beforehand and resume later if required (see also notes above)

▼ PoM **Tritace**® (Astra, Hoechst)
*Capsules,* ramipril 1.25 mg (yellow/white), net price 28-cap pack = £5.44; 2.5 mg (orange/white), 28-cap pack = £7.70; 5 mg (red/white), 28-cap pack = £9.79

### 2.5.6   Ganglion-blocking drugs

**Trimetaphan** is used to provide controlled hypotension in surgery.

### TRIMETAPHAN CAMSYLATE

*Indications:* see notes above

*Cautions:* hepatic or renal impairment, diabetes mellitus, elderly, cerebral or coronary vascular disease, adrenal insufficiency, Addison's disease, CNS degenerative disease

*Contra-indications:* severe arteriosclerosis, severe cardiac disease, pyloric stenosis, pregnancy

*Side-effects:* tachycardia and respiratory depression (particularly with muscle relaxants); constipation, increased intra-ocular pressure, pupillary dilatation

*Dose: by intravenous infusion*, 3–4 mg/minute initially, then adjusted according to response

PoM **Arfonad**® (Roche)
*Injection*, trimetaphan camsylate 50 mg/mL. Net price 5-mL amp = £3.12. For dilution and use as an infusion

### 2.5.7   Tyrosine hydroxylase inhibitor

**Metirosine** inhibits the enzyme tyrosine hydroxylase, and hence the synthesis of catecholamines. It is used in the pre-operative management of phaeochromocytoma, and long term in patients unsuitable for surgery; an alpha-adrenoceptor blocking drug (e.g. phenoxybenzamine) may also be required. Metirosine should **not** be used to treat essential hypertension.

### METIROSINE

*Indications:* see notes above

*Cautions:* maintain high fluid intake and adequate blood volume; may impair ability to drive or operate machinery; **interactions:** Appendix 1 (metirosine)

*Side-effects:* sedation; extrapyramidal symptoms; diarrhoea (may be severe); hypersensitivity reactions

*Dose:* initially 250 mg 4 times daily, increased to max. of 4 g daily in divided doses; doses of 2–3 g daily should be given for 5–7 days before surgery

PoM **Demser**® (MSD)
*Capsules,* blue, metirosine 250 mg (hosp. only). Label: 2

## 2.6   Nitrates and other vasodilators, and calcium-channel blockers

2.6.1  Nitrates
2.6.2  Calcium-channel blockers
2.6.3  Peripheral vasodilators
2.6.4  Cerebral vasodilators

Most patients with *angina pectoris* are treated with beta-blockers (section 2.4) or calcium-channel blockers (section 2.6.2). However, short-acting nitrates (section 2.6.1) retain an important role both for prophylactic use before exertion and for chest pain occurring at rest. Nitrates are sometimes used as sole therapy, especially in elderly patients with infrequent symptoms.

Vasodilators are known to act in *heart failure* either by:

arteriolar dilatation which reduces both peripheral vascular resistance and left ventricular pressure at systole and results in improved cardiac output, *or*

venous dilatation which results in dilatation of capacitance vessels, increase of venous pooling, and diminution of venous return to the heart (decreasing left ventricular end-diastolic pressure).

For a comment on the role of ACE inhibitors in heart failure, see section 2.5.5.

### 2.6.1   Nitrates

*Sublingual* **glyceryl trinitrate** is one of the most effective drugs for providing rapid symptomatic relief of angina, but its effect lasts only for 20 to 30 minutes. Though a potent coronary vasodilator, its principal benefit follows from a reduction in venous return which reduces left ventricular work. Unwanted effects such as flushing, headache, and postural hypotension may limit therapy, especially when angina is severe or when patients are unusually sensitive to the effects of nitrates. The 300-microgram tablet is often appropriate when glyceryl trinitrate is first used and tolerance to the unwanted effects has not developed. Duration of action may be prolonged by *modified-release* preparations. The *aerosol spray* provides an alternative method of rapid relief of symptoms for those who find difficulty in dissolving sublingual preparations. The *percutaneous* preparations may be useful in the prophylaxis of angina for patients who suffer attacks at rest, especially at night.

**Isosorbide dinitrate** is active *sublingually* and is a more stable preparation for those who only require nitrates infrequently. It is also effective by mouth for prophylaxis; although the effect is slower in onset, it may persist for several hours. Duration of action of up to 12 hours is claimed for *modified-release* preparations. The activity of isosorbide dinitrate may depend on the production of active metabolites, the most important of which is isosorbide mononitrate. **Isosorbide mononitrate** itself is also available for angina prophylaxis, though the advantages over isosorbide dinitrate have not yet been firmly established.

Glyceryl trinitrate or isosorbide dinitrate may be tried by *intravenous injection* when the sublingual form is ineffective in patients with chest pain due to myocardial infarction or severe ischaemia. Intravenous injections are also useful in the treatment of acute left ventricular failure.

TOLERANCE. Some patients on long-acting or transdermal nitrates rapidly develop tolerance (with reduced therapeutic effects). Reduction of blood-nitrate concentrations to low levels for 4 to 8 hours each day usually maintains effectiveness in such patients. If tolerance is suspected after the use of transdermal patches they should be removed for several consecutive hours in each 24 hours; in the case of modified-release tablets of isosorbide dinitrate (and conventional formulations of isosorbide mononitrate), the second of the two daily doses can be given after about 8 hours rather than after 12 hours. Conventional formulations of isosorbide mononitrate should not usually be given more than twice daily unless small doses are used; modified-release formulations of isosorbide mononitrate should only be given once daily.

## GLYCERYL TRINITRATE

*Indications:* prophylaxis and treatment of angina; left ventricular failure
*Cautions:* hypotensive conditions (avoid intravenous); tolerance (see notes above); **interactions:** Appendix 1 (glyceryl trinitrate)
*Contra-indications:* marked anaemia, head trauma, cerebral haemorrhage, closed-angle glaucoma
*Side-effects:* throbbing headache, flushing, dizziness, postural hypotension, tachycardia
*Dose:* sublingually, 0.3–1 mg, repeated as required
By *mouth*, 2.6–6.4 mg as modified-release tablets, 2–3 times daily
By *intravenous infusion*, 10–200 micrograms/minute

Short-acting tablets and sprays
**Glyceryl Trinitrate** (Non-proprietary)
*Tablets*, glyceryl trinitrate 300 micrograms, net price 100 = £1.05; 500 micrograms, 100 = 44p; 600 micrograms, 100 = 67p. Label: 16
Note. Glyceryl trinitrate tablets should be supplied in glass containers of not more than 100 tablets, closed with a foil-lined cap, and containing no cotton wool wadding; they should be discarded after 8 weeks in use
**Coro-Nitro Spray®** (Boehringer Mannheim)
*Aerosol spray*, glyceryl trinitrate 400 micrograms/metered dose. Net price 200-dose unit = £3.36
*Dose:* treatment or prophylaxis of angina, spray 1–2 doses under tongue and then close mouth
Caution: flammable

**Glytrin Spray®** (Sanofi Winthrop)
*Aerosol spray*, glyceryl trinitrate 400 micrograms/metered dose. Net price 200-dose unit = £3.28. Label: 10 patient information leaflet
*Dose:* treatment or prophylaxis of angina, spray 1–2 doses under tongue and then close mouth
Note. No need to shake canister
Caution: flammable
**GTN 300 mcg** (Martindale)
*Tablets*, glyceryl trinitrate 300 micrograms. Net price 100 = £1.18. Label: 16
**Nitrolingual Spray®** (Lipha)
*Aerosol spray*, glyceryl trinitrate 400 micrograms/metered dose. Net price 200-dose unit = £4.36
*Dose:* treatment or prophylaxis of angina, spray 1–2 doses under tongue and then close mouth
Note. No need to shake canister
Caution: flammable

Modified-release tablets
**Nitrocontin Continus®** (ASTA Medica)
*Tablets*, m/r, both pink, glyceryl trinitrate 2.6 mg, net price 20 = 67p; 6.4 mg, 20 = 88p. Label: 25
**Suscard®** (Pharmax)
*Buccal tablets*, m/r, glyceryl trinitrate 1 mg, net price 20 = £1.95; 2 mg, 20 = £2.91; 3 mg, 20 = £4.08; 5 mg, 20 = £5.72. Counselling, see administration below
*Dose:* treatment of angina, 2 mg as required (1 mg in sensitive patients), increased to 3 mg if necessary; prophylaxis 1–3 mg 3 times daily; 5 mg in severe angina
Congestive heart failure, 5 mg 3 times daily, increased to 10 mg 3 times daily in severe cases
Acute heart failure, 5 mg repeated until symptoms abate
ADMINISTRATION. Tablets are placed between upper lip and gum, and left to dissolve
**Sustac®** (Pharmax)
*Tablets*, m/r, all pink, glyceryl trinitrate 2.6 mg, net price 20 = £1.21; 6.4 mg, 20 = £1.74; 10 mg, 20 = £2.43. Label: 25
*Dose:* severe angina, 10 mg 3 times daily

Parenteral preparations
Note. Glass or polyethylene apparatus is preferable; loss of potency will occur if PVC is used
PoM **Glyceryl Trinitrate** (Non-proprietary)
*Injection*, glyceryl trinitrate 5 mg/mL. To be diluted before use. Net price 5-mL amp = £6.00; 10-mL amp = £12.00
Available from David Bull
PoM **Nitrocine®** (Schwarz)
*Injection*, glyceryl trinitrate 1 mg/mL. To be diluted before use or given undiluted with syringe pump. Net price 10-mL amp = £9.45; 50-mL bottle = £22.15
PoM **Nitronal®** (Lipha)
*Injection*, glyceryl trinitrate 1 mg/mL. To be diluted before use or given undiluted with syringe pump. Net price 5-mL vial = £2.20; 50-mL vial = £18.00

PoM **Tridil**® (Du Pont)

*Injection*, to be diluted before use, glyceryl tri-nitrate 500 micrograms/mL, net price 10-mL amp = £4.50; 5 mg/mL, 10-mL amp = £21.88, 10-mL amp with polyethylene giving set = £24.98

Transdermal preparations

**Deponit**® (Schwarz)

'*5*' *dressing*, self-adhesive, transparent, releasing glyceryl trinitrate approx. 5 mg/24 hours when in contact with skin. Net price 30 = £19.25. Label: 10 patient information leaflet, counselling, see administration below

'*10*' *dressing*, self-adhesive, transparent, releasing glyceryl trinitrate approx. 10 mg/24 hours when in contact with skin. Net price 30 = £21.19. Label: 10 patient information leaflet, counselling, see administration below

ADMINISTRATION: prophylaxis of angina, apply one '5' or one '10' dressing to lateral chest wall; replace every 24 hours, siting replacement dressing on different area; see also notes above

**Percutol**® (Cusi)

*Ointment*, glyceryl trinitrate 2%. Net price 30 g = £6.14. Counselling, see administration below

ADMINISTRATION: prophylaxis of angina, ½–2 inches of ointment measured on to Applirule, which is applied to body (usually chest, arm, or thigh) without rubbing in, and secured with a dressing; repeat every 3–4 hours or as required

*Note.* 1 inch of ointment contains glyceryl trinitrate 16.64 mg

**Transiderm-Nitro**® (Geigy)

'*5*' *dressing*, self-adhesive, pink, releasing glyceryl trinitrate approx. 5 mg/24 hours when in contact with skin. Net price 30 = £15.95. Label: 10 patient information leaflet, counselling, see administration below

'*10*' *dressing*, self-adhesive, pink, releasing glyceryl trinitrate approx. 10 mg/24 hours when in contact with skin. Net price 30 = £17.54. Label: 10 patient information leaflet, counselling, see administration below

ADMINISTRATION: prophylaxis of angina, apply one '5' or one '10' dressing to lateral chest wall; replace every 24 hours, siting replacement dressing on different area; max. two '10' dressings daily; see also notes above

Prophylaxis of phlebitis and extravasation ('5' dressing only), see literature

## ISOSORBIDE DINITRATE

*Indications:* prophylaxis and treatment of angina; left ventricular failure

*Cautions; Contra-indications; Side-effects:* see under Glyceryl Trinitrate

*Dose: sublingually*, 5–10 mg

*By mouth*, daily in divided doses, angina 30–120 mg, left ventricular failure 40–160 mg, up to 240 mg if required

*By intravenous infusion*, 2–10 mg/hour

Short-acting tablets

**Isosorbide Dinitrate** (Non-proprietary)

*Tablets*, isosorbide dinitrate 10 mg, net price 20 = 30p; 20 mg, 20 = 70p

**Cedocard**® (Tillotts)

*Cedocard-5 tablets* (sublingual), scored, isosorbide dinitrate 5 mg. Net price 20 = 46p

*Cedocard-10 tablets*, pink, scored, isosorbide dinitrate 10 mg. Net price 20 = 38p

*Cedocard-20 tablets*, blue, scored, isosorbide dinitrate 20 mg. Net price 20 = 73p

*Cedocard-40 tablets*, green, scored, isosorbide dinitrate 40 mg. Net price 20 = £1.51

**Isordil**® (Wyeth)

*Tablets* (sublingual), pink, isosorbide dinitrate 5 mg. Net price 20 = 23p. Label: 26

*Tablets*, both scored, isosorbide dinitrate 10 mg, net price 20 = 23p; 30 mg, 20 = 54p

**Sorbichew**® (Stuart)

*Tablets* (chewable), green, scored, isosorbide dinitrate 20 mg. Net price 20 = 31p. Label: 24

**Sorbitrate**® (Stuart)

*Tablets*, both scored, isosorbide dinitrate 10 mg (yellow), net price 20 = 29p; 20 mg (blue), 20 = 43p

**Vascardin**® (Nicholas)

*Tablets*, scored, isosorbide dinitrate 10 mg (as diluted isosorbide dinitrate), net price 20 = 28p

Modified-release preparations

**Cedocard Retard**® (Tillotts)

*Retard-20 tablets*, m/r, yellow, scored, isosorbide dinitrate 20 mg. Net price 20 = £2.05. Label: 25

*Dose:* prophylaxis of angina, 1 tablet every 12 hours

*Retard-40 tablets*, m/r, orange-red, scored, isosorbide dinitrate 40 mg. Net price 60-tab pack = £11.37. Label: 25

*Dose:* prophylaxis of angina, 1–2 tablets every 12 hours

**Isoket Retard**® (Schwarz)

*Retard-20 tablets*, m/r, yellow, scored, isosorbide dinitrate 20 mg. Net price 50-tab pack = £3.24. Label: 25

*Retard-40 tablets*, m/r, orange, scored, isosorbide dinitrate 40 mg. Net price 50-tab pack = £7.99. Label: 25

*Dose:* prophylaxis of angina, 20–40 mg every 12 hours

**Isordil Tembids**® (Wyeth)

*Capsules*, m/r, blue/clear, isosorbide dinitrate 40 mg. Net price 20 = £1.28. Label: 25

*Dose:* prophylaxis of angina, 1 capsule 2–3 times daily

**Soni-Slo**® (Lipha)

*Capsules*, m/r, pink/clear, enclosing off-white pellets, isosorbide dinitrate 20 mg. Net price 20 = £1.19. Label: 25

*Capsules*, m/r, red/clear, enclosing off-white pellets, isosorbide dinitrate 40 mg. Net price 20 = £1.40. Label: 25

*Dose:* prophylaxis of angina, 40–120 mg daily in divided doses

**Sorbid SA**® (Stuart)

*Sorbid-20 SA capsules*, m/r, red/yellow, isosorbide dinitrate 20 mg. Net price 56-cap pack = £3.59. Label: 25

*Dose:* prophylaxis of angina, 1–2 capsules twice daily

*Sorbid-40 SA capsules*, m/r, red/clear, iso-sorbide dinitrate 40 mg. Net price 56-cap pack = £5.13. Label: 25
*Dose:* prophylaxis of angina, 1–2 capsules twice daily

Parenteral preparations
PoM **Cedocard IV**® (Tillotts)
*Injection*, isosorbide dinitrate 1 mg/mL. To be diluted before use. Net price 10-mL amp = £4.33; 50-mL infusion bottle = £21.50; 100-mL infusion bottle = £29.69
Note. Glass or polyethylene infusion apparatus is preferable; loss of potency if PVC used

PoM **Isoket**® (Schwarz)
*Injection 0.05%*, isosorbide dinitrate 500 micrograms/mL. To be diluted before use or given undiluted with syringe pump. Net price 50-mL bottle = £11.50
*Injection 0.1%*, isosorbide dinitrate 1 mg/mL. To be diluted before use. Net price 10-mL amp = £4.33; 50-mL bottle = £21.50; 100-mL bottle = £29.69
Note. Glass or polyethylene infusion apparatus is preferable; loss of potency if PVC used

## ISOSORBIDE MONONITRATE

*Indications:* prophylaxis and treatment of angina; adjunct in congestive heart failure
*Cautions; Contra-indications; Side-effects:* see under Glyceryl Trinitrate
*Dose:* initially 20 mg 2–3 times daily *or* 40 mg twice daily (10 mg twice daily in those who have not previously received nitrates); up to 120 mg daily in divided doses if required

**Isosorbide Mononitrate** (Non-proprietary)
*Tablets*, isosorbide mononitrate 10 mg, net price 20 = £1.10; 20 mg, 20 = £1.40; 40 mg, 20 = £2.82. Label: 25
**Elantan**® (Schwarz)
*Elantan 10 tablets*, scored, isosorbide mono-nitrate 10 mg. Net price 50-tab pack 2= £3.33. Label: 25
PoM *Elantan 20 tablets*, scored, isosorbide mono-nitrate 20 mg. Net price 50-tab pack = £4.34. Label: 25
PoM *Elantan 40 tablets*, scored, isosorbide mono-nitrate 40 mg. Net price 50-tab pack = £7.07. Label: 25
**Ismo**® (Boehringer Mannheim)
*Ismo 10 tablets*, isosorbide mononitrate 10 mg. Net price 20 = £1.16. Label: 25
*Ismo 20 tablets*, isosorbide mononitrate 20 mg. Net price 60-tab pack = £5.10. Label: 25
*Starter pack*, 8 tablets, isosorbide mononitrate 10 mg; 60 tablets, scored, isosorbide mono-nitrate 20 mg. Net price = £5.52. Label: 25
*Ismo 40 tablets*, isosorbide mononitrate 40 mg. Net price 20 = £2.79. Label: 25
**Isotrate**® (Bioglan)
*Tablets*, isosorbide mononitrate 20 mg. Net price 60-tab pack = £4.20. Label: 25
**Monit**® (Stuart)
*Tablets*, scored, isosorbide mononitrate 20 mg. Net price 56-tab pack = £4.78. Label: 25

**Monit LS**® (Stuart)
*Tablets*, isosorbide mononitrate 10 mg. Net price 56-tab pack = £3.74. Label: 25
**Mono-Cedocard**® (Tillotts)
*Mono-Cedocard 10 tablets*, orange, scored, iso-sorbide mononitrate 10 mg. Net price 60-tab pack = £3.77. Label: 25
*Mono-Cedocard 20 tablets*, scored, isosorbide mononitrate 20 mg. Net price 20 = £2.06. Label: 25
*Mono-Cedocard 40 tablets*, scored, isosorbide mononitrate 40 mg. Net price 60-tab pack = £9.35. Label: 25

Modified release
**Elantan LA50**® (Schwarz)
*Capsules*, m/r, pink/dark pink, enclosing white micropellets, isosorbide mononitrate 50 mg. Net price 28-cap pack = £11.30. Label: 25
*Dose:* prophylaxis of angina, 1 capsule daily in the morning
PoM **Imdur**® (Astra)
*Durules*® (= tablets m/r), yellow, f/c, scored, isosorbide mononitrate 60 mg. Net price 28-tab pack = £11.43. Label: 25
*Dose:* prophylaxis of angina, 1 tablet in the morning (half a tablet if headache occurs), increased to 2 tablets if required
**Ismo Retard**® (Boehringer Mannheim)
*Tablets*, m/r, s/c, isosorbide mononitrate 40 mg. Net price 28-tab pack = £10.50. Label: 25
*Dose:* prophylaxis of angina, 1 tablet daily in the morning
¹**MCR-50**® (Tillotts)
*Capsules*, m/r, containing white micropellets, isosorbide mononitrate 50 mg. Net price 28-cap pack = £11.37. Label: 25
*Dose:* prophylaxis of angina, 1 capsule in the morning, increased to 2 capsules if required
1. Full product name Mono Cedocard Retard-50
**Monit SR**® (Stuart)
*Tablets*, m/r, s/c, isosorbide mononitrate 40 mg. Net price 28-tab pack = £10.50. Label: 25
*Dose:* prophylaxis of angina, 1 tablet daily in the morning

## PENTAERYTHRITOL TETRANITRATE

*Indications:* prophylaxis of angina
*Cautions; Contra-indications; Side-effects:* see under Glyceryl Trinitrate
*Dose:* see below

**Cardiacap**® (Consolidated)
*Capsules*, m/r, blue/yellow, pentaerythritol tetranitrate 30 mg. Net price 30-cap pack = £1.55. Label: 25
*Dose:* prophylaxis of angina, 30 mg every 12 hours
**Mycardol**® (Sanofi Winthrop)
*Tablets*, scored, pentaerythritol tetranitrate 30 mg. Net price 20 = 89p. Label: 22
*Dose:* 2 tablets 3–4 times daily

## 2.6.2  Calcium-channel blockers

Calcium-channel blockers (less correctly called 'calcium-antagonists') interfere with the inward displacement of calcium ions through the slow channels of active cell membranes. They influence the myocardial cells, the cells within the specialised conducting system of the heart, and the cells of vascular smooth muscle. Thus, myocardial contractility may be reduced, the formation and propagation of electrical impulses within the heart may be depressed, and coronary or systemic vascular tone may be diminished. They should usually be avoided in heart failure because they may further depress cardiac function and cause clinically significant deterioration.

Calcium-channel blockers differ in their predeliction for the various possible sites of action therefore their therapeutic effects are disparate, with much greater variation than those of beta-blockers. There are important differences between verapamil and the dihydropyridine calcium-channel blockers, nifedipine, nicardipine and isradipine.

**Verapamil** is used for the treatment of *angina, hypertension,* and *arrhythmias* (section 2.3.2). It reduces cardiac output, slows the heart rate, and may impair atrioventricular conduction. It may precipitate heart failure, exacerbate conduction disorders, and cause hypotension at high doses and should **not** be used with beta-blockers (see section 2.3.2). Constipation is the most common side-effect.

**Nifedipine** relaxes vascular smooth muscle and dilates coronary and peripheral arteries. It has more influence on vessels and less on the myocardium than does verapamil, and unlike verapamil has no anti-arrhythmic activity. It rarely precipitates heart failure because any negative inotropic effect is offset by a reduction in left ventricular work. **Nicardipine** has similar effects to those of nifedipine and may produce less reduction of myocardial contractility. **Amlodipine** and **felodipine** also resemble nifedipine and nicardipine in their effects and do not reduce myocardial contractility. They have a longer duration of action and can be given once daily. Nifedipine, nicardipine, and amlodipine are used for the treatment of angina or hypertension. All are valuable in forms of *angina associated with coronary vasospasm;* they are useful as adjuncts to beta-blockers for patients with severe symptoms, and as alternative treatment for those who are intolerant of beta-blockers. Side-effects associated with vasodilatation such as flushing and headache (which become less obtrusive after a few days), and ankle swelling (which does not respond to diuretics) are common.

**Isradipine** has similar effects to those of nifedipine and nicardipine; it is only indicated for *hypertension.*

**Nimodipine** is related to nifedipine but the smooth muscle relaxant effect preferentially acts on cerebral arteries. Its use if confined to prevention of *vascular spasm following subarachnoid haemorrhage.*

**Diltiazem** is effective in most forms of *angina;* the longer-acting formulation is also used for *hypertension.* It may be used in patients for whom beta-blockers are contra-indicated or ineffective. It has a less negative inotropic effect than verapamil and significant myocardial depression occurs rarely. Nevertheless because of the risk of bradycardia it should be used with caution in association with beta-blockers.

WITHDRAWAL. There is some evidence that sudden withdrawal of calcium-channel blockers may be associated with an exacerbation of angina.

---

## AMLODIPINE BESYLATE

*Indications:* hypertension, prophylaxis of angina
*Cautions:* pregnancy; hepatic impairment; **interactions:** Appendix 1 (calcium-channel blockers)
*Side-effects:* headache, oedema, fatigue, nausea, flushing, dizziness
*Dose:* hypertension or angina, initially 5 mg once daily; max. 10 mg daily

---

▼ PoM **Istin**® (Pfizer)
*Tablets,* amlodipine (as besylate) 5 mg. Net price 28-tab  pack = £11.85;  10 mg,  28-tab  pack = £17.70

---

## DILTIAZEM HYDROCHLORIDE

*Indications:* prophylaxis and treatment of angina; hypertension (longer-acting formulation)
*Cautions:* reduce dose in hepatic and renal impairment; heart failure or significantly impaired left ventricular function, mild bradycardia (avoid if severe), first degree AV block, or prolonged PR interval; **interactions:** Appendix 1 (calcium-channel blockers)
*Contra-indications:* severe bradycardia, second- or third-degree heart block (unless pacemaker fitted), sick sinus syndrome; pregnancy (toxicity in *animal* studies); left ventricular failure; porphyria (see section 9.8.2)
*Side-effects:* bradycardia, sino-atrial block, atrioventricular block, hypotension, malaise, headache, hot flushes, gastro-intestinal disturbances, ankle oedema; rarely rashes (toxic erythema reported); hepatitis and depression reported
*Dose:* angina, 60 mg 3 times daily (elderly initially twice daily); increased if necessary to 360 mg daily (max. 480 mg daily)
Longer-acting formulations, see opposite

PoM **Diltiazem** (Non-proprietary)
*Tablets,* m/r, diltiazem hydrochloride 60 mg. Net price 100 = £15.00. Label: 25
Available from APS, Ashbourne (Angiozem®), Cox, Kerfoot, Thames (Britiazim®)
PoM **Adizem-60**® (Napp)
*Tablets,* m/r, f/c, diltiazem hydrochloride 60 mg. Net price 100-tab pack = £15.77. Label: 25
PoM **Tildiem**® (Lorex)
*Tablets,* m/r, off-white, diltiazem hydrochloride 60 mg. Net price 100 = £15.00. Label: 25

---

Longer acting

PoM **Adizem-SR**® (Napp)

*Tablets,* m/r, f/c, diltiazem hydrochloride 120 mg. Net price 56-tab pack = £18.60. Label: 25

*Dose:* prophylaxis of angina, 1 tablet twice daily; max. 2 twice daily

*Note.* Not appropriate for the elderly or those with hepatic or renal impairment

PoM **Tildiem Retard**® (Lorex)

*Tablets,* m/r, diltiazem hydrochloride 90 mg, net price 56-tab pack = £11.34; 120 mg, 56-tab pack = £12.60. Label: 25

*Dose:* mild to moderate hypertension, initially 120 mg twice daily (elderly once daily); up to 360 mg daily may be required (elderly 240 mg daily)

Angina, initially 120 mg twice daily (elderly, dose form not appropriate for initial dose titration); up to 480 mg daily in divided doses may be required (elderly up to 240 mg daily)

## FELODIPINE

*Indications:* hypertension

*Cautions:* withdraw if ischaemic pain occurs; hepatic impairment; breast-feeding; **interactions:** Appendix 1 (calcium-channel blockers)

*Contra-indications:* pregnancy

*Side-effects:* flushing, headache, palpitations, dizziness, fatigue, gravitational oedema, rash and pruritus, gum hyperplasia

*Dose:* initially 5 mg daily in the morning; usual maintenance 5–10 mg once daily; doses above 20 mg daily rarely needed

▼ PoM **Plendil**® (Astra)

*Tablets*, both m/r, f/c, felodipine 5 mg, net price 28-tab pack = £8.12; 10 mg, 28-tab pack = £10.92. Label: 25

## ISRADIPINE

*Indications:* hypertension

*Cautions:* tight aortic stenosis, sick sinus syndrome (if pacemaker not fitted); reduce dose in hepatic or renal impairment; pregnancy (may prolong labour); **interactions:** Appendix 1 (calcium-channel blockers)

*Side-effects:* headache, flushing, dizziness, tachycardia and palpitations, localised peripheral oedema; hypotension uncommon; rarely weight gain, fatigue, abdominal discomfort, rashes

*Dose:* 2.5 mg twice daily (1.25 mg twice daily in elderly, hepatic or renal impairment); increased if necessary after 3–4 weeks to 5 mg twice daily (exceptionally up to 10 mg twice daily); maintenance 2.5 or 5 mg once daily may be sufficient

▼ PoM **Prescal**® (Ciba)

*Tablets*, yellow, scored, isradipine 2.5 mg. Net price 56-tab pack = £11.39

## NICARDIPINE HYDROCHLORIDE

*Indications:* prophylaxis and treatment of angina; mild to moderate hypertension

*Cautions:* withdraw if ischaemic pain occurs or existing pain worsens within 30 minutes of initiating treatment or increasing dose; congestive heart failure; heart failure or significantly impaired left ventricular function; elderly; hepatic or renal impairment; **interactions:** Appendix 1 (calcium-channel blockers)

*Contra-indications:* advanced aortic stenosis; pregnancy

*Side-effects:* dizziness, headache, peripheral oedema, flushing, palpitations, nausea; also gastrointestinal disturbances, drowsiness, insomnia, tinnitus, hypotension, rashes, salivation, frequency of micturition

*Dose:* initially 20 mg 3 times daily, increased to 30 mg 3 times daily (usual range 60–120 mg daily); patients with hypertension controlled on 20–30 mg 3 times daily can be given 30–40 mg twice daily

PoM **Cardene**® (Syntex)

*Capsules*, nicardipine hydrochloride 20 mg (blue/white), net price 20 = £3.04; 30 mg (blue/pale blue), 56-cap pack = £9.89

## NIFEDIPINE

*Indications:* prophylaxis and treatment of angina; hypertension; Raynaud's phenomenon

*Cautions:* withdraw if ischaemic pain occurs or existing pain worsens shortly after initiating treatment; heart failure or significantly impaired left ventricular function; severe hypotension; reduce dose in hepatic impairment; diabetes mellitus; may inhibit labour; breast-feeding; **interactions:** Appendix 1 (calcium-channel blockers)

*Contra-indications:* cardiogenic shock; pregnancy (toxicity in *animal* studies); porphyria (see section 9.8.2)

*Side-effects:* headache, flushing, dizziness, lethargy; also gravitational oedema, rash, nausea, increased frequency of micturition, eye pain, gum hyperplasia; depression reported

*Dose:* see preparations below

PoM **Adalat**® (Bayer)

*Capsules*, both orange, nifedipine 5 mg, net price 20 = £1.63; 10 mg, 20 = £2.44. Label: 21, counselling, see dose

*Dose:* angina and Raynaud's phenomenon, initially 10 mg (elderly 5 mg) 3 times daily with or after food; usual maintenance 5–20 mg 3 times daily; for immediate effect in angina bite into capsule and retain liquid in mouth or swallow (evidence points to more rapid action if contents swallowed)

*Note.* Nifedipine capsules also available from APS, Ashbourne (Angiopine®), Eastern (Calcilat®), Evans, Kerfoot

---

PoM **Adalat**® **IC** (Bayer)
*Coronary injection*, nifedipine 100 micrograms/mL. Net price 2-mL pre-filled syringe = £7.43
*Note.* Use polyethylene catheters only
*Dose:* for treatment of coronary spasm during coronary angiography and balloon angioplasty, 100–200 micrograms via coronary catheter over 90–120 seconds (with monitoring of blood pressure and pulse); reduce dose in severe stenosis; lasts 15 minutes; do not exceed total of six 200-microgram injections in 3 hours

Modified release
PoM **Adalat**® **Retard** (Bayer)
*Retard 10 tablets*, m/r, pink, nifedipine 10 mg. Net price 56-tab pack = £8.34. Label: 21, 25
*Retard 20 tablets*, m/r, pink, nifedipine 20 mg. Net price 20 = £3.86. Label: 21, 25
*Dose:* hypertension and angina prophylaxis, 20 mg twice daily with or after food (initial titration 10 mg twice daily); usual maintenance 10–40 mg twice daily

PoM **Coracten**® (Evans)
*Capsules*, m/r, brown/red, enclosing yellow pellets, nifedipine 20 mg. Net price 20 = £3.01. Label: 25
*Dose:* hypertension and angina prophylaxis, 1 capsule every 12 hours; increased if necessary to 2 capsules every 12 hours

With atenolol
Section 2.4

# NIMODIPINE
**Indications:** prevention and treatment of ischaemic neurological deficits following subarachnoid haemorrhage
**Cautions:** cerebral oedema or severely raised intracranial pressure; avoid concomitant administration of nimodipine tablets and infusion, other calcium-channel blockers, or beta-blockers; impaired renal function or nephrotoxic drugs; pregnancy; **interactions:** Appendix 1 (calcium-channel blockers)
**Side-effects:** hypotension, variation in heart-rate, flushing, headache, gastro-intestinal disorders, nausea, and feeling of warmth; transient increase in liver enzymes after intravenous administration
*Dose:* prevention, *by mouth*, 60 mg every 4 hours (total daily dose 360 mg), starting within 4 days of subarachnoid haemorrhage and continued for 21 days
Treatment, *by intravenous infusion* via central catheter, 1 mg/hour initially, increased after 2 hours to 2 mg/hour, providing no severe decrease in blood pressure; patients with unstable blood pressure or weighing less than 70 kg, 500 micrograms/hour initially or less if necessary; treatment should start as soon as possible and should continue for at least 5 days (max. 14 days); in the event of surgical intervention during treatment continue for at least 5 days after

PoM **Nimotop**® (Bayer)
*Tablets*, yellow, f/c, nimodipine 30 mg. Net price 100-tab pack = £35.30
*Intravenous infusion*, nimodipine 200 micrograms/mL; also contains ethanol 20% and macrogol '400' 17%. Net price 50-mL vial (with polyethylene infusion catheter) = £13.24; 250-mL bottle = £66.20
*Note.* Polyethylene, or polypropylene apparatus should be used; PVC should be avoided

# VERAPAMIL HYDROCHLORIDE
**Indications:** see under Dose
**Cautions:** first-degree heart block; acute phase of myocardial infarction (avoid if bradycardia, hypotension, left ventricular failure); patients taking beta-blockers (**important:** see section 2.3.2—both oral and intravenous routes); reduce dose in hepatic impairment; children, specialist advice only (see section 2.3.2); pregnancy and breast-feeding; **interactions:** Appendix 1 (calcium-channel blockers)
**Contra-indications:** hypotension, bradycardia, second- and third-degree heart block, sick sinus syndrome, cardiogenic shock, sino-atrial block; history of heart failure or significantly impaired left ventricular function, even if controlled by therapy; atrial flutter or fibrillation complicating Wolff-Parkinson-White syndrome; porphyria (see section 9.8.2)
**Side-effects:** constipation; less commonly nausea, vomiting, flushing, headache, dizziness, fatigue, ankle oedema; rarely reversible impairment of liver function; rarely gynaecomastia and gingival hyperplasia after long-term treatment; after intravenous administration, hypotension, bradycardia, heart block, ventricular fibrillation, and asystole
*Dose: by mouth*, supraventricular arrhythmias, 40–120 mg 3 times daily
Angina, 80–120 mg 3 times daily
Hypertension, 240–480 mg daily in 2–3 divided doses
*By slow intravenous injection* over 2 minutes (3 minutes in elderly), 5–10 mg (preferably with ECG monitoring); in paroxysmal tachyarrhythmias a further 5 mg after 5–10 minutes if required

PoM **Verapamil** (Non-proprietary)
*Tablets*, coated, verapamil hydrochloride 40 mg, net price 20 = 89p; 80 mg, 20 = £1.78; 120 mg, 20 = £2.72; 160 mg, 20 = £3.28
PoM **Berkatens**® (Berk)
*Tablets*, all yellow, f/c, verapamil hydrochloride 40 mg, net price 20 = 90p; 80 mg, 20 = £1.80; 120 mg, 20 = £2.59; 160 mg, 20 = £3.27
PoM **Cordilox**® (Abbott)
*Tablets*, all yellow, f/c, verapamil hydrochloride 40 mg, net price 20 = 89p; 80 mg, 20 = £1.78; 120 mg, 20 = £2.72; 160 mg, 56-tab pack = £13.10
*Injection*, verapamil hydrochloride 2.5 mg/mL, net price 2-mL amp = £1.11

**PoM Securon®** (Knoll)
*Tablets*, f/c, verapamil hydrochloride 40 mg, net price 100 = £4.69; 80 mg, 100 = £9.38; 120 mg, 56-tab pack = £7.87, 100 = £14.05; 160 mg, 56-tab pack = £10.49, 100 = £18.73
*Injection*, verapamil hydrochloride 2.5 mg/mL. Net price 2-mL syringe = £1.11

Modified release
**PoM Securon SR®** (Knoll)
*Tablets*, m/r, pale green, f/c, verapamil hydrochloride 240 mg. Net price 28-tab pack = £10.92. Label: 25
*Dose:* hypertension, 1 tablet daily, increased to twice daily if necessary (new patients, initial dose ½ tablet); angina, 1 tablet twice daily (may sometimes be reduced to once daily)
**PoM Univer®** (Rhône-Poulenc Rorer)
*Capsules*, all m/r, verapamil hydrochloride 120 mg (yellow/dark blue), net price 28-cap pack = £7.00; 180 mg (yellow), 56-cap pack = £16.92; 240 mg (yellow/dark blue), 28-cap pack = £11.42. Label: 25
*Dose:* hypertension, 240 mg daily, max. 480 mg daily (new patients, initial dose 120 mg); angina, 360 mg daily, max. 480 mg daily

---

## 2.6.3 Peripheral vasodilators and related drugs

Most serious peripheral disorders, such as *intermittent claudication*, are now known to be due to occlusion of vessels, either by spasm or sclerotic plaques; use of vasodilators may increase blood flow at rest, but no controlled studies have shown any improvement in walking distance or sustained increase in muscle blood flow during exercise. Rest pain is rarely affected.

Management of *Raynaud's syndrome* includes avoidance of exposure to cold and stopping smoking. More severe symptoms may require vasodilator treatment, which is most often successful in primary Raynaud's syndrome. Nifedipine (section 2.6.2), prazosin (section 2.5.4) and thymoxamine have all been shown to be beneficial; cyclandelate, naftidrofuryl, nicotinic acid derivatives, and oxpentifylline are not established as being effective.

CHILBLAINS. Vasodilator therapy is not established as being effective for chilblains (see section 13.14).

## CINNARIZINE
*Indications:* peripheral vascular disease, Raynaud's syndrome
*Cautions; Side-effects:* see section 4.6
*Dose:* initially, 75 mg 3 times daily; maintenance, 75 mg 2–3 times daily

**Stugeron Forte®** (Janssen)
*Capsules*, orange/ivory, cinnarizine 75 mg. Net price 20 = £1.61. Label: 2
**Stugeron®** see section 4.6

## NICOTINIC ACID DERIVATIVES
*Indications:* peripheral vascular disease (for hyperlipidaemia, see section 2.12)
*Side-effects:* flushing, dizziness, nausea, vomiting, hypotension (more frequent with nicotinic acid than derivatives); occasional diabetogenic effect reported with nicotinic acid and nicotinyl alcohol

**Bradilan®** see section 2.12
**Hexopal®** (Sanofi Winthrop)
*Tablets*, scored, inositol nicotinate 500 mg. Net price 20 = £4.17
*Dose:* 1 g 3 times daily, increased to 4 g daily if required
*Tablets forte*, scored, inositol nicotinate 750 mg. Net price 112-tab pack = £34.89
*Dose:* 1.5 g twice daily
*Suspension*, sugar-free, inositol nicotinate 1 g/5 mL. Net price 300 mL = £21.39
*Dose:* as for tablets (above)
**Ronicol®** (Roche)
*Tablets*, scored, nicotinyl alcohol 25 mg (as tartrate). Net price 20 = 37p
*Dose:* 25–50 mg 4 times daily
*Timespan®* (= tablets m/r), red, s/c, nicotinyl alcohol 150 mg (as tartrate). Net price 20 = £1.58. Label: 25
*Dose:* 150–300 mg twice daily

## OXPENTIFYLLINE
*Indications:* peripheral vascular disease
*Cautions:* hypotension, coronary artery disease; avoid in porphyria (see section 9.8.2)
*Side-effects:* gastro-intestinal disturbances, dizziness, headache; rarely flushing, tachycardia
*Dose:* 400 mg 2–3 times daily

**PoM Trental®** (Hoechst)
*Tablets*, m/r, pink, s/c, oxpentifylline 400 mg. Net price 90-tab pack = £17.24. Label: 21, 25

## THYMOXAMINE
*Indications:* primary Raynaud's syndrome (short-term treatment)
*Cautions:* diabetes mellitus
*Side-effects:* nausea, diarrhoea, flushing, headache, dizziness
*Dose:* initially 40 mg 4 times daily, increased to 80 mg 4 times daily if poor initial response; discontinue after 2 weeks if no response

**PoM Opilon®** (P-D)
*Tablets*, yellow, f/c, thymoxamine 40 mg (as hydrochloride). Net price 120-tab pack = £27.48. Label: 21

## OTHER PREPARATION USED IN PERIPHERAL VASCULAR DISEASE

Rutosides (oxerutins, Paroven®) are not vasodilators and are not generally regarded as effective preparations as capillary sealants or for the treatment of cramps.

**Paroven®** (Zyma)
*Capsules*, yellow, oxerutins 250 mg. Net price 20 = £2.34. Label: 21. For relief of symptoms of oedema associated with chronic venous insufficiency

---

### 2.6.4   Cerebral vasodilators

These drugs are claimed to improve mental function. Some improvements in performance of psychological tests have been reported but the drugs have not been shown clinically to be of much benefit in dementia.

## CO-DERGOCRINE MESYLATE

A mixture in equal proportions of dihydroergocornine mesylate, dihydroergocristine mesylate, and (in the ratio 2:1) α- and β-dihydroergocryptine mesylates

*Indications:* adjunct in elderly patients with mild to moderate dementia

*Cautions:* severe bradycardia

*Side-effects:* gastro-intestinal disturbances, flushing, headache, rash, nasal congestion; postural hypotension in hypertensive patients

*Dose:* 1.5 mg 3 times daily *or* 4.5 mg once daily

PoM **Hydergine**® (Sandoz)

*Tablets*, co-dergocrine mesylate 1.5 mg (scored), net price 20 = £2.21; 4.5 mg, 28-tab pack = £11.06. Label: 22

## CYCLANDELATE

*Indications:* cerebral and peripheral vascular disease

*Contra-indications:* acute phase of cerebrovascular accident and myocardial infarction

*Side-effects:* nausea, flushing, dizziness with high doses

*Dose:* 1.2–1.6 g daily in 2–4 divided doses

**Cyclobral**® (Norgine)

*Capsules*, pink/brown, cyclandelate 400 mg. Net price 20 = £2.36

**Cyclospasmol**® (Brocades)

*Capsules*, pink/grey, cyclandelate 400 mg. Net price 20 = £2.40

*Tablets*, pink, s/c, cyclandelate 400 mg. Net price 112-tab pack = £15.91

*Suspension*, cyclandelate 400 mg/5 mL when reconstituted with freshly boiled and cooled purified water. Net price 450-mL pack = £11.87

## NAFTIDROFURYL OXALATE

*Indications:* cerebral and peripheral vascular disease

*Contra-indications:* parenteral administration in atrioventricular block

*Side-effects:* nausea, epigastric pain, rash

*Dose:* see below

PoM **Praxilene**® (Lipha)

*Capsules*, pink, naftidrofuryl oxalate 100 mg. Net price 84-cap pack = £8.60. Label: 25, 27

*Dose:* peripheral vascular disease, 100–200 mg 3 times daily; cerebral vascular disease, 100 mg 3 times daily

*Injection forte*, naftidrofuryl oxalate 20 mg/mL. Net price 10-mL amp = £1.10

*Dose:* peripheral vascular disease only, by intravenous or intra-arterial infusion, 200 mg over at least 90 minutes, twice daily

# 2.7   Sympathomimetics

2.7.1  Inotropic sympathomimetics
2.7.2  Vasoconstrictor sympathomimetics

The properties of sympathomimetics vary according to whether they act on alpha or on beta adrenergic receptors. Adrenaline acts on both alpha and beta receptors and increases both heart rate and contractility (beta$_1$ effects); it can cause peripheral vasodilation (a beta$_2$ effect) or vasoconstriction (an alpha effect).

In *cardiac arrest* adrenaline 1 in 10 000 (1 mg per 10 mL) is recommended in a dose of 10 mL by central intravenous injection. The procedure for cardiopulmonary resuscitation is given in the algorithm (see next page) which reflects the revised recommendations of the Resuscitation Council (UK).

IMPORTANT. For *acute anaphylaxis* use **intramuscular route** (for dose, see p. 124).

## ADRENALINE

*Indications and Dose:* see notes above

*Cautions:* ischaemic heart disease, diabetes mellitus, hyperthyroidism, hypertension; **interactions:** Appendix 1 (sympathomimetics)

*Side-effects:* anxiety, tremor, tachycardia, headache, cold extremities; in overdosage arrhythmias, cerebral haemorrhage, pulmonary oedema

PoM **Adrenaline Injection,** adrenaline 1 in 10000 (adrenaline 100 micrograms/mL as acid tartrate). 10-mL amp.

Available from Martindale and Penn (special order); also from IMS (Min-I-Jet® Adrenaline 3- and 10-mL disposable syringes)

*Note.* Adrenaline Injection BP is 1 in 1000 (adrenaline 1 mg/mL, as acid tartrate), see p. 118

### 2.7.1   Inotropic sympathomimetics

The cardiac stimulants **dobutamine** and **dopamine** act on beta$_1$ receptors in cardiac muscle, and increase contractility with little effect on rate; they are used in cardiogenic shock. Dosage of dopamine is critical since although low doses induce vasodilatation and increase renal perfusion, higher doses (more than 5 micrograms per kg per minute) lead to vasoconstriction and may exacerbate heart failure.

**Xamoterol** also acts on beta$_1$ receptors but being a partial agonist it provokes only a modest stimulatory response at rest. **Important:** for CSM restriction limiting xamoterol to **mild heart failure only**, owing to deterioration in patients with moderate to severe heart failure, see p. 95.

**Dopexamine** acts on beta$_2$ receptors in cardiac muscle to produce its positive inotropic effect; and on peripheral dopamine receptors to increase renal perfusion; it is reported not to induce vasoconstriction.

**Isoprenaline** is less selective and increases both heart rate and contractility; it may prevent Stokes-Adams attacks, but insertion of a pacemaker is preferable.

**Unresponsive**

**No breathing**

**No pulse**

**A**irway — open airway

**B**reathing — rescue breathing

**C**irculation — 2:15 CPR

ARE YOU ALL RIGHT?

**Call for help**
Including
- defibrillator
- airway adjuncts
- oxygen
- emergency kit

**Consider**
- precordial thump in witnessed or monitored arrest

- 2 rescuer CPR 1:5

- and mouth-to-mask ventilation

**ECG**

**Electromechanical dissociation**
QRS without palpable pulse

Adrenaline 1 mg IV

Consider specific therapy
for - hypovolaemia
- pneumothorax
- cardiac tamponade
- pulmonary embolism

Consider calcium chloride (10 ml of 10%)
for - hyperkalaemia
- hypocalcaemia
- calcium antagonists

**Ventricular fibrillation (VF)**

Defibrillate 200 J
Defibrillate 200 J
Defibrillate 360 J
Adrenaline 1 mg IV
Defibrillate 360 J
Lignocaine 100 mg IV
Repeated defibrillations 360 J
Consider
- different paddle positions
- different defibrillator
- other antiarrhythmic drugs

**Apparent asystole**
isoelectric ECG

where VF can be excluded | where VF cannot be excluded

Defibrillate 200 J
Defibrillate 200 J
Defibrillate 360 J

Adrenaline 1 mg IV
Atropine 2 mg IV
Consider pacing
if P waves or any other electrical activity present

**Place paddles** correctly

If flat trace, check switches, connections and gain.

**Give oxygen**

**Secure airway**
Intubate if necessary

**Cannulate large vein**

**Continue CPR**

Continue CPR for up to 2 min. after each drug. Do not interrupt CPR for more than 10 sec., except for defibrillation.
If an I.V. line cannot be established, consider giving double doses of adrenaline, lignocaine or atropine via an endotracheal tube.

PROLONGED RESUSCITATION:
Give 1 mg adrenaline IV every 5 minutes.
Consider 50 mmol sodium bicarbonate (50 ml. of 8.4%) or according to blood gas results.

POST RESUSCITATION CARE
Check
- arterial blood gases
- electrolytes
- chest x-ray
Observe monitor and treat patient in an intensive care area.

The Resuscitation Council (UK)

## DOBUTAMINE HYDROCHLORIDE

*Indications:* inotropic support in infarction, cardiac surgery, cardiomyopathies, septic shock, and cardiogenic shock

*Cautions:* severe hypotension complicating cardiogenic shock

*Side-effects:* tachycardia and marked increase in systolic blood pressure indicate overdosage

*Dose: by intravenous infusion*, 2.5–10 micrograms/kg/minute, adjusted according to response

PoM **Dobutrex**® (Lilly)
*Strong sterile solution*, dobutamine (as hydrochloride) 12.5 mg/mL. For dilution and use as an intravenous infusion. Net price 20-mL vial = £13.92

## DOPAMINE HYDROCHLORIDE

*Indications:* cardiogenic shock in infarction or cardiac surgery

*Cautions:* correct hypovolaemia; low dose in shock due to acute myocardial infarction—see notes above

*Contra-indications:* tachyarrhythmia, phaeochromocytoma

*Side-effects:* nausea and vomiting, peripheral vasoconstriction, hypotension, hypertension, tachycardia

*Dose: by intravenous infusion*, 2–5 micrograms/kg/minute initially (see notes above)

PoM **Dopamine Hydrochloride** (Non-proprietary)
*Strong sterile solution*, dopamine hydrochloride 40 mg/mL, net price 5-mL amp = £4.56; 160 mg/mL, 5-mL amp = £18.29. For dilution and use as an intravenous infusion

PoM **Dopamine Hydrochloride in Dextrose** (Glucose) **Injection** (Abbott)
*Intravenous infusions* (in glucose 5% intravenous infusion), dopamine hydrochloride 800 micrograms/mL, 1.6 mg/mL, and 3.2 mg/mL. 250-mL containers (all hosp. only)

PoM **Intropin**® (Du Pont)
*Strong sterile solution*, dopamine hydrochloride 40 mg/mL, net price 5-mL amp or syringe = £4.80; 160 mg/mL, 5-mL amp = £19.20. For dilution and use as an intravenous infusion

PoM **Select-A-Jet**® **Dopamine** (IMS)
*Strong sterile solution*, dopamine hydrochloride 40 mg/mL. Net price 5-mL vial = £3.88; 10-mL vial = £7.75; 20-mL vial = £11.63. For dilution and use as an intravenous infusion.

## DOPEXAMINE HYDROCHLORIDE

*Indications:* inotropic support and vasodilator in heart failure associated with cardiac surgery

*Cautions:* myocardial infarction, recent angina, hypokalaemia, hyperglycaemia; correct hypovolaemia before starting, monitor blood pressure, pulse, plasma potassium, blood glucose; avoid abrupt withdrawal; **interactions:** Appendix 1 (sympathomimetics)

*Contra-indications:* left ventricular outlet obstruction such as hypertrophic cardiomyopathy or aortic stenosis; phaeochromocytoma, thrombocytopenia

*Side-effects:* increased heart rate (occasionally excessive tachycardia, particularly in atrial fibrillation), ventricular ectopic beats; also reported: nausea, vomiting, anginal pain, tremor

*Dose: by intravenous infusion* via caval catheter, 500 nanograms/kg/minute, may be increased to 1 microgram/kg/minute and further increased up to 6 micrograms/kg/minute in increments of 1 microgram/kg/minute at intervals of 10–15 minutes

▼ PoM **Dopacard**® (Fisons)
*Strong sterile solution,* dopexamine hydrochloride 10 mg/mL (1%). For dilution and use as an intravenous infusion. Net price 5-mL amp = £19.42
*Note.* Contact with metal in infusion apparatus should be minimised

## ISOPRENALINE HYDROCHLORIDE

*Indications:* heart block, severe bradycardia

*Cautions:* ischaemic heart disease, diabetes mellitus, hyperthyroidism; **interactions:** Appendix 1 (sympathomimetics)

*Side-effects:* tachycardia, arrhythmias, hypotension, sweating, tremor, headache

*Dose: by mouth*, 30 mg every 8 hours, then increased; max. daily dose usually 840 mg

*By intravenous infusion*, 0.5–10 micrograms/minute

PoM **Min-I-Jet**® **Isoprenaline** (IMS)
*Injection*, isoprenaline hydrochloride 20 micrograms/mL. Net price 10-mL disposable syringe = £3.23

PoM **Saventrine**® (Pharmax)
*Tablets*, isoprenaline hydrochloride 30 mg. Net price 20 = £1.72

PoM **Saventrine IV**® (Pharmax)
*Strong sterile solution*, isoprenaline hydrochloride 1 mg/mL. For dilution and use as an intravenous infusion. Net price 2-mL amp = 45p

## XAMOTEROL

*Indications:* restricted by CSM to chronic mild heart failure (in patients not breathless at rest but limited by symptoms on exertion)

*Cautions:* withdraw if heart failure deteriorates; cardiac outflow obstruction, arrhythmias (maintain concurrent digoxin in atrial fibrillation), obstructive airways disease (withdraw if worsening, and reverse bronchospasm with inhaled bronchodilator such as salbutamol), reduce dose in renal impairment; pregnancy (toxicity in *animal* studies); **interactions:** Appendix 1 (xamoterol)

---

*Contra-indications:* moderate to severe heart failure; breast-feeding

HEART FAILURE. Patients in whom xamoterol is contraindicated are those:

who are short of breath or fatigued at rest or limited on minimal exercise;

with resting tachycardia (>90 beats per minute) or hypotension (systolic BP<100 mmHg);

with peripheral oedema, raised jugular venous pressure, enlarged liver, or third heart sound;

with (or with history of) acute pulmonary oedema;

who require treatment with frusemide in dose in excess of 40 mg daily (or equivalent);

who require ACE inhibitor treatment

*Side-effects:* gastro-intestinal disturbances, headache, dizziness, bronchospasm, hypotension; also reported: chest pain, palpitations, muscle cramp, rashes

*Dose:* 200 mg daily for 1 week, then 200 mg twice daily

IMPORTANT. Treatment should be started in hospital after full assessment of severity of heart failure by exercise test

PoM **Corwin**® (Stuart)

*Tablets*, yellow, f/c, xamoterol (as fumarate) 200 mg. Net price 56-tab pack = £26.60

## 2.7.2 Vasoconstrictor sympathomimetics

Vasoconstrictors raise blood pressure transiently by constricting peripheral vessels. They are sometimes used as an emergency method of elevating blood pressure. They may also be used in general and spinal anaesthesia to control blood pressure.

The danger of vasoconstrictors is that although they raise blood pressure they do so at the expense of perfusion of vital organs such as the kidney. Further, in many patients with shock the peripheral resistance is already high, and to raise it further is unhelpful. Thus the use of vasoconstrictors in the treatment of shock is to be generally **deprecated**. The use of plasma substitutes, or of inotropic agents such as dopamine or dobutamine is more appropriate (section 2.7.1). Treatment of the underlying condition is obviously important.

## METARAMINOL

*Indications:* acute hypotension

*Cautions; Contra-indications:* see under Noradrenaline Acid Tartrate

*Side-effects:* tachycardia, arrhythmias, reduced renal blood flow

*Dose: by intravenous infusion*, 15–100 mg in 500 mL, adjusted according to response

PoM **Aramine**® (MSD)

*Injection*, metaraminol 10 mg (as tartrate)/mL. Net price 1-mL amp = 48p

## METHOXAMINE HYDROCHLORIDE

*Indications:* hypotension in anaesthesia

*Cautions:* hyperthyroidism; pregnancy; **interactions:** Appendix 1 (sympathomimetics)

*Contra-indications:* severe coronary or cardiovascular disease

*Side-effects:* headache, hypertension, bradycardia

*Dose: by intramuscular injection*, 5–20 mg

*By slow intravenous injection*, 5–10 mg (rate 1 mg/minute)

PoM **Vasoxine**® (Wellcome)

*Injection*, methoxamine hydrochloride 20 mg/mL. Net price 1-mL amp = 52p

## NORADRENALINE ACID TARTRATE

*Indications:* acute hypotension, cardiac arrest

*Cautions:* extravasation at injection site may cause necrosis; **interactions:** Appendix 1 (sympathomimetics)

*Contra-indications:* myocardial infarction, pregnancy

*Side-effects:* headache, palpitations, bradycardia

*Dose: by intravenous infusion*, of a solution containing noradrenaline acid tartrate 8 micrograms/mL (equivalent to noradrenaline base 4 micrograms/mL) at an initial rate of 2 to 3 mL/minute, adjusted according to response

*By rapid intravenous or intracardiac injection*, 0.5 to 0.75 mL of a solution containing noradrenaline acid tartrate 200 micrograms/mL (equivalent to noradrenaline base 100 micrograms/mL)

PoM **Levophed**® (Sanofi Winthrop)

*Strong sterile solution*, noradrenaline acid tartrate 2 mg/mL (equivalent to noradrenaline base 1 mg/mL). For dilution and use as an intravenous infusion. Net price 2-mL amp = 95p; 4-mL amp = £1.39

*Special injection*, noradrenaline acid tartrate 200 micrograms/mL (equivalent to noradrenaline base 100 micrograms/mL). Net price 2-mL amp = 92p

## PHENYLEPHRINE HYDROCHLORIDE

*Indications:* acute hypotension

*Cautions; Contra-indications:* see under Noradrenaline Acid Tartrate; also contra-indicated in severe hypertension and hyperthyroidism

*Side-effects:* hypertension with headache, palpitations, vomiting; tachycardia or reflex bradycardia; tingling and coolness of skin

*Dose: by subcutaneous or intramuscular injection*, 5 mg

*By slow intravenous injection*, 100–500 micrograms

*By intravenous infusion*, 5–20 mg in 500 mL, adjusted according to response

PoM **Phenylephrine Injection 1%** (Boots)

*Injection*, phenylephrine hydrochloride 10 mg/mL. 1-mL amp

## 2.8    Anticoagulants and protamine

2.8.1   Parenteral anticoagulants
2.8.2   Oral anticoagulants
2.8.3   Protamine sulphate

The main use of anticoagulants is to prevent thrombus formation or extension of an existing thrombus in the slower-moving venous side of the circulation, where the thrombus consists of a fibrin web enmeshed with platelets and red cells. They are therefore widely used in the prevention and treatment of *deep-vein thrombosis in the legs*.

Anticoagulants are of less use in preventing thrombus formation in arteries, for in faster-flowing vessels thrombi are composed mainly of platelets with little fibrin. They are used to prevent thrombi forming on *prosthetic heart valves*.

### 2.8.1    Parenteral anticoagulants

**Heparin** is given to initiate anticoagulation and is rapidly effective. As its effects are short-lived it is best given by continuous intravenous infusion; it is preferably not given by intermittent intravenous injection. Oral anticoagulants are started at the same time, and the heparin infusion withdrawn after 3 days.

If oral anticoagulants cannot be given and heparin is continued, its dose is adjusted after determination of the activated partial thromboplastin time.

If haemorrhage occurs it is usually sufficient to withdraw heparin, but if rapid reversal of the effects of heparin is required, protamine sulphate is a specific antidote (section 2.8.3).

For the prophylaxis of thrombosis in patients undergoing heart surgery or renal dialysis full therapeutic doses of heparin are given for the duration of the procedure. Low-dose heparin by subcutaneous injection is widely advocated to prevent postoperative deep-vein thrombosis and pulmonary embolism in 'high risk' patients, i.e. those with obesity, malignant disease, or previous history of thrombosis. Laboratory monitoring is not required with this regimen.

There is evidence that **low molecular weight heparins** are as effective and as safe as unfractionated heparin in the prevention of venous thrombo-embolism. They have a longer duration of action than unfractionated heparin; once-daily dosage means that they are convenient to use.

---

**CSM advice.** Platelet counts should be measured in patients under heparin treatment for longer than 5 days and the treatment should be stopped immediately in those who develop thrombocytopenia.

---

## HEPARIN

*Indications:* treatment of thrombo-embolic disorders such as deep-vein thrombosis and pulmonary embolism; prevention of postoperative thrombosis and thrombo-embolic events in susceptible patients

*Cautions:* pregnancy; **interactions:** Appendix 1 (heparin)

*Contra-indications:* haemophilia and other haemorrhagic disorders, peptic ulcer, cerebral aneurysm, severe hypertension, severe liver disease, recent surgery of eye or nervous system, hypersensitivity to heparin

*Side-effects:* haemorrhage, thrombocytopenia (see CSM advice above), hypersensitivity reactions; osteoporosis after prolonged use, alopecia

*Dose: by intravenous injection*, loading dose of 5000 units followed by continuous *infusion* of 1000–2000 units/hour (approx. 14–28 units/kg/hour) adjusted daily by laboratory monitoring *or* 5000–10 000 units by *intravenous injection* every 4 hours (but *continuous intravenous infusion* preferred, see notes above)

*By subcutaneous injection*, prophylaxis of deep-vein thrombosis, 5000 units 2 hours before surgery, then every 8–12 hours until patient is ambulant; in pregnancy (with monitoring), 10 000 units every 12 hours (important: not intended to cover prevention of prosthetic heart valve thrombosis in pregnancy which calls for separate specialist management)

Treatment of deep-vein thrombosis, initially 10 000–20 000 units every 12 hours *or* 250 units/kg (2500 units/10 kg) every 12 hours, adjusted daily by laboratory monitoring

Note. The above doses do not apply to the low molecular weight heparins (see below)

---

Intravenous preparations

PoM **Heparin Injection** (heparin sodium)
1000 units/mL, net price 1-mL amp = 21p; 5-mL amp = 69p; 5-mL vial = 54p
5000 units/mL, net price 1-mL amp = 33p; 5-mL amp = 98p; 5-mL vial = £1.46
10 000 units/mL, net price 1-mL amp = 45p
25 000 units/mL, net price 1-mL amp = 86p; 5-mL vial = £6.43

PoM **Monoparin®** (CP)
*Injection*, heparin sodium (mucous) 1000 units/mL, net price 1-mL amp = 16p; 5-mL amp = 46p; 10-mL amp = 66p; 5000 units/mL, 1-mL amp = 32p; 5-mL amp = 98p; 25 000 units/mL, 1-mL amp = £1.27

PoM **Multiparin®** (CP)
*Injection*, heparin sodium (mucous) 1000 units/mL, net price 5-mL vial = 45p; 5000 units/mL, 5-mL vial = £1.32; 25 000 units/mL, 5-mL vial = £5.41

---

PoM **Pump-Hep**® (Leo)

*Intravenous infusion*, heparin sodium (mucous) 1000 units/mL. Net price 5-mL amp = 40p; 10-mL amp = 66p; 20-mL amp = 98p

*Dose:* by continuous infusion pump, 20 000–40 000 units daily

PoM **Unihep**® (Leo)

*Injection*, heparin sodium (mucous) 1000 units/mL, net price 1-mL amp = 14p; 5000 units/mL, 1-mL amp = 27p; 10 000 units/mL, 1-mL amp = 45p; 25 000 units/mL, 1-mL amp = £1.07

Subcutaneous preparations

PoM **Heparin Injection** (heparin sodium or heparin calcium)

25 000 units/mL (subcutaneous). Net price 0.2-mL amp = 41p

PoM **Calciparine**® (Sanofi Winthrop)

*Injection* (subcutaneous), heparin calcium 25 000 units/mL. Net price 0.2-mL syringe = 70p; 0.5-mL syringe = £1.50; 0.8-mL amp or syringe = £1.80

PoM **Minihep**® (Leo)

*Injection* (subcutaneous), heparin sodium 25 000 units/mL. Net price 0.2-mL amp = 42p

PoM **Minihep Calcium**® (Leo)

*Injection* (subcutaneous), heparin calcium 25 000 units/mL. Net price 0.2-mL amp = 45p

PoM **Monoparin**® (CP)

*Injection* (subcutaneous), heparin sodium (mucous) 25 000 units/mL. Net price 0.2-mL amp = 37p

PoM **Monoparin Calcium**® (CP)

*Injection* (subcutaneous), heparin calcium 25 000 units/mL. Net price 0.2 mL amp = 52p

PoM **Uniparin**® (CP)

*Injection* (subcutaneous), heparin sodium 25 000 units/mL. Net price 0.2-mL syringe = 60p; 0.4-mL syringe (Uniparin Forte) = £1.30

PoM **Uniparin Calcium**® (CP)

*Injection* (subcutaneous), heparin calcium 25 000 units/mL. Net price 0.2-mL syringe = 60p; 0.5-mL syringe = £1.45

Low molecular weight heparins

▼ PoM **Clexane**® (Rhône-Poulenc Rorer)

*Injection*, enoxaparin (low molecular weight heparin) 100 mg/mL. Net price 0.2-mL syringe (20 mg) = £4.90; 0.4-mL syringe (40 mg) = £8.82

Prophylaxis of deep-vein thrombosis, *by subcutaneous injection, moderate risk*, 20 mg (2000 units) 1–2 hours before surgery then 20 mg (2000 units) every 24 hours for 7–10 days; *high risk*, 40 mg (4000 units) 12 hours before surgery then 40 mg (4000 units) every 24 hours for 7–10 days

Prevention of clotting in extracorporeal circulation (consult data sheet)

▼ PoM **Fragmin**® (Kabi Pharmacia)

*Injection*, dalteparin sodium (low molecular weight heparin) 2500 units/mL, net price 4-mL amp = £5.50; 10000 units/mL, 1-mL amp = £5.50; 12500 units/mL, 0.2-mL syringe = £2.60; 25000 units/mL, 0.2-mL syringe = £3.70

Prophylaxis of deep-vein thrombosis, *by subcutaneous injection, moderate risk*, 2500 units 1–2 hours before surgery for 5 days; *high risk*, 2500 units 1–2 hours before surgery, then 2500 units 12 hours later, then 5000 units every 24 hours for 5 days

Prevention of clotting in extracorporeal circulation (consult data sheet)

Heparin flushes

For maintaining catheter patency sodium chloride injection 0.9% is as effective as heparin flushes for up to 48 hours, and is therefore recommended for cannulas intended to be in place for 48 hours or less. Heparin flushes are recommended for cannulas intended to be in place for longer than 48 hours.

PoM **Hep-Flush**® (Leo)

*Solution*, heparin sodium 100 units/mL. Net price 2-mL amp = 26p; 10-mL vial = £1.30

To maintain patency of catheters, cannulas, etc., 200 units flushed through every 4–8 hours. Not for therapeutic use

PoM **Heplok**® (Leo)

*Solution*, heparin sodium 10 units/mL. Net price 5-mL amp = 30p

To maintain patency of catheters, cannulas, etc., 10–50 units flushed through every 4 hours. Not for therapeutic use

PoM **Hepsal**® (CP)

*Solution*, heparin sodium 10 units/mL. Net price 5-mL amp = 22p

To maintain patency of catheters, cannulas, etc., 50 units flushed through every 4 hours or as required. Not for therapeutic use

---

**Ancrod** reduces plasma fibrinogen by cleavage of fibrin but is not in common use.

## ANCROD

**Indications:** deep-vein thrombosis, prevention of post-operative thrombosis ('named patient' basis only)

**Cautions; Contra-indications; Side-effects:** see under Heparin; resistance may develop; avoid administration with dextrans

**Dose:** by intravenous infusion, 2–3 units/kg over 4–12 hours (usually 6–8 hours), then *by infusion or slow intravenous injection*, 2 units/kg every 12 hours

*By subcutaneous injection*, prophylaxis of deep-vein thrombosis, 280 units immediately after surgery, then 70 units daily for 4 days (fractured femur) or 8 days (hip replacement)

*Note.* The initial infusion must be given slowly, as there is a risk of massive intravascular formation of unstable fibrin. Response can be monitored by observing clot size after the blood has been allowed to stand for about 2 hours, the aim being to predict a dose that produces a 2–3 mm clot. Alternatively, plasma-fibrinogen concentrations can be measured directly.

The major complication of ancrod is haemorrhage, and since it takes 12 to 24 hours for haemostatic fibrinogen concentrations to be restored after stopping administration it may be necessary to give ancrod antivenom (Arvin® Antidote, available from Armour) as an antidote (0.2-mL test dose subcutaneously followed by 0.8 mL intramuscularly, and 30 minutes later 1 mL intravenously). The antivenom may cause anaphylaxis (adrenaline etc. should be available, for details see Allergic Emergencies, section 3.4.3). As an alternative to the antivenom reconstituted freeze-dried fibrinogen may be given, or if this is not available one litre of fresh frozen plasma.

PoM **Arvin**® (Knoll)
*Injection*, ancrod 70 units/mL. 1-mL amp (available only on 'named patient' basis)

**Epoprostenol** (prostacyclin) can be given to inhibit platelet aggregation during renal dialysis either alone or with heparin. Since its half-life is only about 3 minutes it must be given by continuous intravenous infusion. It is a potent vasodilator and therefore its side-effects include flushing, headache, and hypotension.

## EPOPROSTENOL

*Indications:* see notes above
*Cautions:* anticoagulant monitoring required when given with heparin
*Side-effects:* see notes above; also bradycardia, pallor, sweating with higher doses
*Dose:* see manufacturer's literature

PoM **Flolan**® (Wellcome)
*Infusion*, powder for reconstitution, epoprostenol (as sodium salt). Net price 500-microgram vial (with diluent) = £103.86

### 2.8.2   Oral anticoagulants

Oral anticoagulants antagonise the effects of vitamin K, and take at least 36 to 48 hours for the anticoagulant effect to develop; if an immediate effect is required, heparin must be given concomitantly.

The main indication for oral anticoagulant therapy is *deep-vein thrombosis*. Patients with poorly controlled *atrial fibrillation who are at risk of embolisation* should also be treated, as should patients with *mechanical heart valve prostheses*, to prevent emboli developing on the valves; antiplatelet drugs may also be useful in these patients.

Oral anticoagulants should not be used in cerebral thrombosis or peripheral arterial occlusion, but may be of value in patients with *transient brain ischaemic attacks* whether due to carotid or vertebrobasilar arterial disease; if these patients also have severe hypertension anticoagulants are contra-indicated, and antiplatelet drugs are an alternative (section 2.9).

**Warfarin** and other coumarins are the drugs of choice, as they are less likely to cause sensitivity reactions than **phenindione**.

Whenever possible, the base-line prothrombin time should be determined before the initial dose is given.

A typical induction dose of warfarin is 10 mg[1] daily for 2 days (but this should be tailored to individual requirement). The subsequent maintenance dose depends upon the prothrombin time (reported as INR[2]); the currently recommended therapeutic ranges are:

INR 2–2.5 for prophylactic therapy of deep-vein thrombosis including high-risk surgery;
INR 2–3 for prophylactic therapy in hip surgery and fractured femur operations, for treatment of deep-vein thrombosis, pulmonary embolism, and transient ischaemic attacks;
INR 3–4.5 for recurrent deep-vein thrombosis and pulmonary embolism, arterial disease including myocardial infarction, and mechanical prosthetic heart valves.

It is essential that the INR be determined:
daily or on alternate days in early days of treatment, *then*
at longer intervals (depending on response) *then* up to every 8 weeks

The daily maintenance dose[3] of warfarin is usually 3 to 9 mg (taken at the **same time** each day).

The main adverse effect of all oral anti-coagulants is haemorrhage. Omission of dosage with checking of the INR is essential. The following recommendations of the British Society for Haematology are based on the result of the INR and the clinical state:

Life-threatening haemorrhage—immediately give phytomenadione (vitamin K₁) 5 mg by slow intravenous injection and a concentrate of factors II, IX, X (with factor VII concentrate if available). If no concentrate is available, fresh frozen plasma should be infused (approximately 1 litre for an adult) but this may not be effective
Less severe haemorrhage e.g. haematuria and epistaxis—withhold warfarin for one or more days and consider giving phytomenadione (vitamin K₁) 0.5–2 mg[4] by slow intravenous injection
INR 4.5–7 without haemorrhage—withhold warfarin for 1 or 2 days then review
INR > 7 without haemorrhage—withhold warfarin and consider giving phytomenadione (vitamin K₁) 500 micrograms by slow intravenous injection
Unexpected bleeding at therapeutic levels[5]—investigate possibility of underlying cause e.g. unexpected renal or alimentary tract pathology

---

1. Less than 10 mg if base-line prothrombin time prolonged, if liver-function tests abnormal, or if patient in cardiac failure, on parenteral feeding, or over 80 years of age.
2. The International Normalised Ratio (INR) has now replaced the British Ratio (BR).
3. Change in patient's clinical condition, particularly associated with liver disease, intercurrent illness, or drug administration, necessitates more frequent testing. See also **interactions**, Appendix 1 (warfarin). Major changes in diet (especially involving vegetables) may also affect warfarin control.
4. Usually 1 mg adequate and should be given if INR greater than desired.
5. Should always be investigated regardless of INR since even if patients over-anticoagulated bleeding generally has an additional underlying cause.

---

Phytomenadione will take up to 12 hours to act and will prevent oral anticoagulants from acting for several days or even weeks.

PREGNANCY. Oral anticoagulants are weakly teratogenic and should not be given in the first trimester of pregnancy. Women at risk of pregnancy should be warned of this danger. Also, oral anticoagulants cross the placenta with risk of placental or fetal haemorrhage; they should therefore not be given during the last few weeks of pregnancy.

Anticoagulant treatment cards must be carried by patients, and are available from:

DHSS Store
No. 2 Site
Manchester Rd
Heywood
Lancs OL10 2PZ

SHHD (Div IIID)
Room 9
St. Andrew's House
Edinburgh EH1 3DE

Cards giving advice for patients on anticoagulant treatment may be given to patients at the discretion of the doctor or pharmacist.

## WARFARIN SODIUM

*Indications:* prophylaxis of embolisation in rheumatic heart disease and atrial fibrillation; prophylaxis after insertion of prosthetic heart valve; prophylaxis and treatment of venous thrombosis and pulmonary embolism; transient ischaemic attacks

*Cautions:* hepatic or renal disease, recent surgery; **interactions:** Appendix 1 (warfarin)

*Contra-indications:* pregnancy (see notes above), peptic ulcer, severe hypertension, bacterial endocarditis

*Side-effects:* haemorrhage

*Dose:* see notes above

PoM **Marevan**® (DF)
*Tablets,* brown, scored, warfarin sodium 1 mg. Net price 20 = 9p. Label: 10 anticoagulant card
*Tablets,* blue, scored, warfarin sodium 3 mg. Net price 20 = 10p. Label: 10 anticoagulant card
*Tablets,* pink, scored, warfarin sodium 5 mg. Net price 20 = 16p. Label: 10 anticoagulant card

PoM **Warfarin WBP** (Boehringer Ingelheim)
*Tablets,* brown, scored, warfarin sodium 1 mg. Net price 20 = 9p. Label: 10 anticoagulant card
*Tablets,* blue, scored, warfarin sodium 3 mg. Net price 20 = 10p. Label: 10 anticoagulant card
*Tablets,* pink, scored, warfarin sodium 5 mg. Net price 20 = 16p. Label: 10 anticoagulant card

## NICOUMALONE

*Indications:* prophylaxis of embolisation in rheumatic heart disease and atrial fibrillation; prophylaxis after insertion of prosthetic heart valve; prophylaxis and treatment of venous thrombosis and pulmonary embolism; transient ischaemic attacks

*Cautions; Contra-indications; Side-effects:* see under Warfarin Sodium; avoid breast-feeding

*Dose:* 8–12 mg on 1st day; 4–8 mg on 2nd day; maintenance dose usually 1–8 mg daily

PoM **Sinthrome**® (Geigy)
*Tablets,* pink, nicoumalone 1 mg. Net price 20 = 15p. Label: 10 anticoagulant card
*Tablets,* scored, nicoumalone 4 mg. Net price 20 = 31p. Label: 10 anticoagulant card

## PHENINDIONE

*Indications:* prophylaxis of embolisation in rheumatic heart disease and atrial fibrillation; prophylaxis after insertion of prosthetic heart valve; prophylaxis and treatment of venous thrombosis and pulmonary embolism

*Cautions; Contra-indications; Side-effects:* see under Warfarin Sodium; also hypersensitivity reactions including rashes, fever, leucopenia, agranulocytosis, diarrhoea, renal and hepatic damage; urine coloured pink; avoid breast-feeding; **interactions:** Appendix 1 (phenindione)

*Dose:* 200 mg on 1st day; 100 mg on 2nd day; maintenance dose usually 50–150 mg daily

PoM **Dindevan**® (DF)
*Tablets,* phenindione 10 mg, net price 20 = 26p; 25 mg (green), 20 = 36p; 50 mg, 20 = 46p. Label: 10 anticoagulant card, 14 (urine pink)

### 2.8.3 Protamine sulphate

Although protamine sulphate is used to counteract overdosage with heparin, if used in excess it has an anticoagulant effect.

## PROTAMINE SULPHATE

*Indications; Cautions:* see above

*Side-effects:* flushing, hypotension, bradycardia

*Dose: by slow intravenous injection,* 1 mg neutralises 100 units heparin (mucous) or 80 units heparin (lung) when given within 15 minutes; if longer time, less protamine required as heparin rapidly excreted; max. 50 mg

PoM **Protamine Sulphate** (Non-proprietary)
*Injection,* protamine sulphate 10 mg/mL. Net price 5-mL amp = 98p; 10-mL amp = £1.75
Available from CP (Prosulf®)

# 2.9 Antiplatelet drugs

By decreasing platelet aggregation, these drugs may inhibit thrombus formation on the arterial side of the circulation, where thrombi are formed by platelet aggregation and anticoagulants have little effect. Antiplatelet drugs have little effect in venous thromboembolism. **Dipyridamole** is used with anticoagulants to prevent thrombus formation on prosthetic valves.

Encouraging results have been obtained using **aspirin** 300 mg daily for the *secondary* prevention of thrombotic cerebrovascular or cardiovascular disease; studies are still needed to determine whether lower doses (such as 75 mg daily or 300 mg on alternate days) might not be equally (or more) effective. Aspirin has also been shown to reduce mortality when given in a dose of 150 mg daily for a month after myocardial infarction. Low doses of aspirin (such as 75 or 100 mg daily) are also given following bypass surgery. Physicians in the USA have demonstrated that 325 mg on alternate days can have a *primary* preventive action for myocardial infarction but further analysis is awaited before aspirin can be recommended for routine use in primary prevention.

For use of epoprostenol, see section 2.8.1.

## ASPIRIN (antiplatelet)

*Indications:* prophylaxis of cerebrovascular disease or myocardial infarction (see notes above)
*Cautions:* asthma; uncontrolled hypertension; pregnancy; **interactions:** Appendix 1 (aspirin)
*Contra-indications:* children under 12 years and in breast-feeding (Reye's syndrome, see section 4.7.1); active peptic ulceration; haemophilia and other bleeding disorders
*Side-effects:* bronchospasm; gastro-intestinal haemorrhage (occasionally major), also other haemorrhage (e.g. subconjunctival)
*Dose:* see notes above

**Aspirin** (Non-proprietary)
*Dispersible tablets,* aspirin 75 mg, net price 20 = 10p; 300 mg, see section 4.7.1. Label: 13, 21, 32
**Angettes 75**® (Bristol-Myers)
*Tablets,* aspirin 75 mg. Net price 56-tab pack = £1.88. Label: 32
**Nu-Seals Aspirin 300 mg**: see section 4.7.1
**Platet**® (Nicholas)
*Tablets,* effervescent, aspirin 100 mg, net price 30-tab pack = 99p; 300 mg, 30-tab pack = £1.13. Label: 13, 32

## DIPYRIDAMOLE

*Indications:* see notes above
*Cautions:* rapidly worsening angina, aortic stenosis, recent myocardial infarction; may exacerbate migraine, hypotension; **interactions:** Appendix 1 (dipyridamole)
*Side-effects:* nausea, diarrhoea, throbbing headache, hypotension
*Dose: by mouth,* 300–600 mg daily in 3–4 divided doses before food
*By intravenous injection,* diagnostic only, see manufacturer's literature

PoM **Dipyridamole** (Non-proprietary)
*Tablets,* coated, dipyridamole 25 mg, net price 20 = 74p; 100 mg, 20 = £1.89. Label: 22
Available from APS, Ashbourne (Cerebrovase®), Cox, Kerfoot, Shire (Vasyrol®)
PoM **Persantin**® (Boehringer Ingelheim)
*Tablets,* both s/c, dipyridamole 25 mg (orange), net price 84-tab pack = £3.17; 100 mg, 84-tab pack = £8.84. Label: 22
*Injection,* dipyridamole 5 mg/mL. Net price 2-mL amp = 10p

## 2.10    Fibrinolytic drugs

Fibrinolytic drugs act as thrombolytics by activating plasminogen to form plasmin, which degrades fibrin and so breaks up thrombi.

**Streptokinase** is used in the treatment of *life-threatening venous thrombosis,* and in *pulmonary embolism,* but treatment must be started rapidly.

**Urokinase** is currently used for *thrombolysis in the eye* and in *arteriovenous shunts.* It has the advantage of being non-immunogenic.

The value of thrombolytic drugs for the treatment of *myocardial infarction* has recently been established. **Streptokinase, alteplase,** and **anistreplase** have all been shown to reduce mortality when given by the intravenous route; evidence on comparative efficacy is incomplete. The potential for benefit lessens as the delay from the onset of major symptoms increases, but the value of treatment within the first 12 hours is reasonably well established. Knowledge of the role of adjuvant therapy is also incomplete, but in the case of streptokinase the reduction in mortality by aspirin has been shown to be additive whilst immediate heparin is necessary to obtain full efficacy from alteplase. Thrombolytic drugs are indicated for any patient with acute myocardial infarction for whom the benefit is believed to outweigh the risk of treatment. Trials have shown that the benefit is greatest in those with ECG changes that include ST segment elevation and in those with anterior infarction. Patients should not be excluded on account of age alone because mortality in this group is high and the percentage reduction in mortality is the same as in younger patients.

CAUTIONS. Risk of bleeding from venepuncture or invasive procedures, any external chest compression, pregnancy, possibility of pre-existing thrombus as in abdominal aneurysm or enlarged left atrium with atrial fibrillation (risk of dissolution of clot and subsequent embolisation), recent or concurrent anticoagulant therapy.

CONTRA-INDICATIONS. Recent haemorrhage, trauma, or surgery (including dental extraction), coagulation defects, bleeding diatheses, history of cerebrovascular disease especially recent events or with any residual disability, recent symptoms of possible peptic ulceration, heavy vaginal bleeding, severe hypertension, pulmonary disease with cavitation, acute pancreatitis, diabetic retinopathy, severe liver disease, oesophageal varices. In the case of streptokinase or anistreplase, previous allergic reactions to either drug, or therapy with either drug from 5 days to 12 months previously.

SIDE-EFFECTS. Side-effects of thrombolytics are mainly nausea and vomiting and bleeding. Bleeding is usually limited to the site of injection, but intracerebral haemorrhage or bleeding from other sites may occur. Serious bleeding calls for discontinuation of the thrombolytic and may require administration of coagulation factors and antifibrinolytic drugs (aprotinin or tranexamic acid).

Streptokinase and anistreplase may cause allergic reactions and anaphylaxis has been reported (for details of management see Allergic Emergencies, section 3.4.3).

## ALTEPLASE
(rt-PA, tissue-type plasminogen activator)
*Indications:* acute myocardial infarction (see notes above)
*Cautions; Contra-indications; Side-effects:* see notes above
*Dose: by intravenous injection*, 10 mg over 1–2 minutes, followed by *intravenous infusion* of 50 mg over 1 hour, then 40 mg over the subsequent 2 hours (total dose 100 mg over 3 hours); treatment should be initiated within 6 hours; patients weighing less than 67 kg should receive a total dose of 1.5 mg/kg according to the above schedule

PoM **Actilyse**® (Boehringer Ingelheim)
*Injection,* powder for reconstitution, alteplase 20 mg (11.6 mega units)/vial, net price per vial (with diluent and transfer device) = £200.00; 50 mg (29 mega units)/vial, pack of 2 vials (with diluent, transfer device, and infusion bag) = £816.00

## ANISTREPLASE
(APSAC)
*Indications:* acute myocardial infarction (see notes above)
*Cautions; Contra-indications; Side-effects:* see notes above
*Dose: by intravenous injection*, 30 units over 4–5 minutes; treatment should be initiated as soon as possible and preferably within 6 hours

PoM **Eminase**® (Beecham)
*Injection,* powder for reconstitution, anistreplase. Net price 30-unit vial = £495.00

## STREPTOKINASE
*Indications:* deep-vein thrombosis, pulmonary embolism, acute arterial thromboembolism, thrombosed arteriovenous shunts; acute myocardial infarction (see notes above)
*Cautions; Contra-indications; Side-effects:* see notes above
*Dose: by intravenous infusion*, 250 000 units over 30 minutes, then 100 000 units every hour for up to 24–72 hours according to condition (see data sheet)
Myocardial infarction, 1 500 000 units over 60 minutes followed by aspirin 150 mg daily *by mouth* for at least 4 weeks (see data sheet)

PoM **Kabikinase**® (Kabi Pharmacia)
*Injection,* powder for reconstitution, streptokinase; net price 100 000-unit vial = £7.50; 250 000-unit vial = £15.00; 600 000-unit vial = £34.20; 1.5 million-unit vial = £85.00

PoM **Streptase**® (Hoechst)
*Injection,* powder for reconstitution, streptokinase; net price 250 000-unit vial = £15.36; 750 000-unit vial = £40.26; 1.5 million-unit vial = £80.52 (hosp. only)

## UROKINASE
*Indications:* thrombosed arteriovenous shunts and intravenous cannulas; thrombolysis in the eye; deep-vein thrombosis, pulmonary embolism, peripheral vascular occlusion
*Cautions; Contra-indications; Side-effects:* see notes above
*Dose: by instillation into arteriovenous shunt*, 5000–37 500 International units in 2–3 mL sodium chloride intravenous infusion 0.9%
*By intravenous infusion*, 4400 International units/kg over 10 minutes, then 4400 units/kg/hour for 12 hours in pulmonary embolism or 12–24 hours in deep-vein thrombosis; for bolus injection for pulmonary embolism consult data sheet
Peripheral vascular occlusion, consult data sheet
*Intra-ocular administration*, 5000–37 500 International units in 2 mL sodium chloride intravenous infusion 0.9%

PoM **Ukidan**® (Serono)
*Injection,* powder for reconstitution, urokinase; net price 5000 International unit vial = £6.71; 25 000 International unit vial = £23.58; 100 000 International unit vial = £60.00
PoM **Urokinase** (Leo)
*Injection,* powder for reconstitution, urokinase; net price 5 000 International unit vial = £9.75; 25 000 International unit vial = £27.79

# 2.11 Antifibrinolytic drugs and haemostatics

Fibrin dissolution can be impaired by the administration of **tranexamic acid**, which inhibits plasminogen activation and fibrinolysis. It may be useful when haemorrhage cannot be staunched, e.g. in prostatectomy, dental extraction in haemophiliacs, or menorrhagia; it may also be used in hereditary angioedema and in streptokinase overdose.

**Aprotinin** is a proteolytic enzyme inhibitor acting on plasmin and kallidinogenase (kallikrein). It is indicated for patients at high risk of major blood loss during and after open heart surgery with extracorporeal circulation and for patients in whom optimal blood conservation during open heart surgery is an absolute priority; it is also indicated for the treatment of life-threatening haemorrhage due to hyperplasminaemia (occasionally observed during the mobilisation and dissection of malignant tumours, in acute promyelocytic leukaemia, and following thrombolytic therapy).

**Ethamsylate** reduces capillary bleeding in the presence of a normal number of platelets. It does not act by fibrin stabilisation, but probably by correcting abnormal platelet adhesion.

## APROTININ

*Indications:* see notes above
*Side-effects:* occasionally hypersensitivity reactions and localised thrombophlebitis
*Dose: by slow intravenous injection or infusion*
Open heart surgery, loading dose, 2 000 000 units (200 mL) after induction of anaesthesia and before sternotomy, *by slow intravenous injection* initially 50 000 units (5 mL) over several minutes (to detect allergy), remainder *by intravenous infusion* over 20 minutes; maintenance dose, *by intravenous infusion* 500 000 units (50 mL) every hour until end of operation (or early postoperative period in septic endocarditis); pump prime, 2 000 000 units (200 mL) in priming volume of extracorporeal circuit; in septic endocarditis 3 000 000 units (300 mL) added to pump prime
Hyperplasminaemia, *by slow intravenous injection or by infusion* initially, 500 000 units (50 mL) to 1 000 000 units (100 mL) at max. rate 10 mL/min; followed if necessary by 200 000 units (20 mL) every hour until bleeding stops

PoM **Trasylol**® (Bayer)
*Injection,* aprotinin 10 000 kallikrein inactivator units/mL. Net price 50-mL vial = £20.53
*Note.* Aprotinin injection containing 10 000 kallikrein inactivator units/mL also available from Paines & Byrne

## ETHAMSYLATE

*Indications:* see under preparations
*Contra-indications:* porphyria (see section 9.8.2)
*Side-effects:* nausea, headache, rashes
*Dose:* see below

PoM **Dicynene**® (Delandale)
*Tablets,* scored, ethamsylate 500 mg, net price 100-tab pack = £20.12
*Dose:* short-term treatment of blood loss in menorrhagia, 500 mg 4 times daily during menstruation
*Injection,* ethamsylate 125 mg/mL. Net price 2-mL amp = 74p
*Dose:* prophylaxis and treatment of periventricular haemorrhage in low birth-weight infants, by intramuscular or intravenous injection, 12.5 mg/kg every 6 hours
IMPORTANT. The ampoules currently available contain a total of 250 mg in 2 mL volume therefore **small fraction only** required for neonatal use

## TRANEXAMIC ACID

*Indications:* see notes above
*Cautions:* reduce dose in renal impairment; massive haematuria (avoid if risk of ureteric obstruction); regular eye examinations and liver function tests in long-term treatment of hereditary angioedema
*Contra-indications:* thromboembolic disease

*Side-effects:* nausea, vomiting, diarrhoea (reduce dose); giddiness on rapid intravenous injection
*Dose: by mouth*, 1–1.5 g 2–4 times daily
*By slow intravenous injection*, 1 g 3 times daily

PoM **Cyklokapron**® (Kabi Pharmacia)
*Tablets,* f/c, scored, tranexamic acid 500 mg. Net price 60-tab pack = £12.96
*Syrup,* tranexamic acid 500 mg/5 mL. Diluent syrup, life of diluted syrup 14 days. Net price 300 mL = £15.60
*Injection,* tranexamic acid 100 mg/mL. Net price 5-mL amp = £1.35

## BLOOD PRODUCTS

## FACTOR VIII FRACTION, DRIED

(Human Antihaemophilic Fraction, Dried)
A concentrate prepared from pooled plasma from suitable human donors
*Indications:* control of haemorrhage in haemophilia A
*Cautions:* intravascular haemolysis after large or frequently repeated doses in patients with blood groups A, B, or AB
*Side-effects:* allergic reactions including chills, fever; hyperfibrinogenaemia occurred after massive doses with earlier products but less likely since fibrinogen content has now been substantially reduced
Available as: *Dried Factor VIII Fraction, High purity, Heat-treated* (BPL); *Human Antihaemophilic Factor* (SNBTS); *Profilate-SD*® (Alpha); ▼ *Monoclate-P*® (Armour)

## FACTOR VIII INHIBITOR BYPASSING FRACTION

Preparations with factor VIII inhibitor bypassing activity are prepared from human plasma
Human Factor VIII Inhibitor Bypassing Fraction (*Feiba Immuno*, Immuno) is used in patients with factor VIII inhibitors

## FACTOR IX FRACTION, DRIED

Factor IX fraction is prepared from pooled human plasma and may also contain clotting factors II, VII, and X.
*Indications:* congenital factor IX deficiency (haemophilia B)
*Cautions:* risk of thrombosis
*Contra-indications:* disseminated intravascular coagulation
*Side-effects:* allergic reactions, including chills, fever
Available as: *Dried Factor IX Fraction, Heat-Treated* (BPL); *Human Factor IX Concentrate* (SNBTS)

## FRESH FROZEN PLASMA

Fresh frozen plasma is prepared from the supernatant liquid obtained by centrifugation of one donation of whole blood.

*Indications:* to replace coagulation factors or other plasma proteins where their concentration or functional activity is critically reduced, e.g. to reverse warfarin effect

*Cautions:* avoid in circulatory overload; need for compatibility

*Side-effects:* allergic reactions including chills, fever, bronchospasm; adult respiratory distress syndrome

Available from BPL and SNBTS

---

## COLLAGEN COMPRESSES

**Colgen**® Sterile rectangular compress of non-denatured collagen 5 cm × 7 cm, net price each = £4.95; sterile non-denatured collagen powder 0.4 g-vial = £4.95 (Thames)
*Uses:* anti-haemorrhagic and haemostatic

# 2.12   Lipid-lowering drugs

There are a number of common conditions, some familial, in which there are very high plasma concentrations of cholesterol, or triglycerides, or both. There is evidence that therapy which lowers low density lipoprotein (LDL) cholesterol and raises high density lipoprotein (HDL) cholesterol reduces the progression of coronary atherosclerosis and may even induce regression. Lipid-lowering drugs should be reserved for patients in whom severe hyperlipidaemia is inadequately controlled by a modified fat diet. Any drug therapy must be combined with strict adherence to diet, maintenance of near-ideal body weight and, if appropriate, reduction of blood pressure and cessation of smoking.

Severe hyperlipidaemia often requires combinations of lipid-lowering drugs such as an anion-exchange resin with a fibrate, an HMG CoA reductase inhibitor, or nicotinic acid. Combinations of HMG CoA reductase inhibitors with nicotinic acid or a fibrate carry an increased risk of side-effects and should be used with great caution.

---

ANION-EXCHANGE RESINS

**Cholestyramine** and **colestipol** are anion-exchange resins used in the management of hypercholesterolaemia. They act by binding bile acids, preventing their reabsorption; this promotes hepatic conversion of cholesterol into bile acids; the resultant increased LDL-receptor activity of liver cells increases the breakdown of LDL-cholesterol. Thus both compounds effectively reduce LDL-cholesterol but can aggravate hypertriglyceridaemia.

COUNSELLING. Other drugs should be taken at least 1 hour before or 4–6 hours after cholestyramine or colestipol to reduce possible interference with absorption

---

## CHOLESTYRAMINE

*Indications:* hyperlipidaemias, particularly type IIa, in patients who have not responded adequately to diet and other appropriate measures; primary prevention of coronary heart disease in men aged 35–59 years with primary hypercholesterolaemia who have not responded to diet and other appropriate measures; pruritus associated with partial biliary obstruction and primary biliary cirrhosis; diarrhoeal disorders, see section 1.5

*Cautions:* supplements of fat-soluble vitamins and of folic acid may be required with high doses, particularly in children; pregnancy and breast-feeding; **interactions:** Appendix 1 (cholestyramine and colestipol)

*Contra-indications:* complete biliary obstruction

*Side-effects:* nausea and vomiting, constipation or diarrhoea, heartburn, flatulence, abdominal discomfort; on prolonged use, increased bleeding tendency (due to hypoprothrombinaemia associated with vitamin K deficiency)

*Dose:* lipid reduction (after initial introduction over 3–4 weeks) 8–24 g daily in water in single or up to 4 divided doses; up to 36 g daily if necessary

Pruritus, 4–8 g daily in water

PoM **Questran**® (Bristol-Myers)
*Powder*, orange, cholestyramine (anhydrous) 4 g/sachet. Net price 168-sachet pack = £70.21. Label: 13, counselling, avoid other drugs at same time (see notes above)

PoM **Questran A**® (Bristol-Myers)
*Powder*, orange, cholestyramine (anhydrous) 4 g/sachet, with aspartame. Net price 168-sachet pack = £73.72. Label: 13, counselling, avoid other drugs at same time (see notes above)

---

## COLESTIPOL HYDROCHLORIDE

*Indications:* hyperlipidaemias, particularly type IIa, in patients who have not responded adequately to diet and other appropriate measures

*Cautions; Contra-indications; Side-effects:* see under Cholestyramine

*Dose:* 5 g 1–2 times daily in liquid increased if necessary at intervals of 1–2 months to max. of 30 g daily (in single or 2 divided doses)

PoM **Colestid**® (Upjohn)
*Granules*, yellow, colestipol hydrochloride. Net price 30 × 5-g sachets = £12.54. Label: 13, counselling, avoid other drugs at same time (see notes above)

## CLOFIBRATE GROUP

**Clofibrate**, **bezafibrate**, **fenofibrate**, and **gemfibrozil** can be regarded as broad-spectrum lipid-modulating agents in that although their main action is to decrease serum triglycerides they also tend to reduce LDL-cholesterol and to raise HDL-cholesterol.

All can cause a myositis-like syndrome, especially in patients with impaired renal function. In addition, clofibrate predisposes to gallstones by increasing biliary cholesterol excretion; it is therefore only indicated in patients who have had a cholecystectomy.

### BEZAFIBRATE

*Indications:* hyperlipidaemias of types IIa, IIb, III, IV and V in patients who have not responded adequately to diet and other appropriate measures

*Cautions:* renal impairment (avoid if severe); **interactions:** Appendix 1 (clofibrate group)

*Contra-indications:* severe renal or hepatic impairment, hypoalbuminaemia, primary biliary cirrhosis, gall bladder disease, nephrotic syndrome, pregnancy

*Side-effects:* nausea, abdominal discomfort; rarely myositis-like syndrome, pruritus, urticaria, impotence; headache reported

*Dose:* 200 mg 3 times daily with or after food; may be reduced to 200 mg twice daily in hypertriglyceridaemia

PoM **Bezalip®** (Boehringer Mannheim)
*Tablets*, f/c, bezafibrate 200 mg. Net price 20 = £2.11. Label: 21
PoM **Bezalip-Mono®** (Boehringer Mannheim)
*Tablets*, m/r, f/c, bezafibrate 400 mg. Net price 28-tab pack = £8.72. Label: 21, 25
*Dose:* 1 tablet daily in the evening

### CLOFIBRATE

*Indications:* hyperlipidaemias of types IIb, III, IV and V in patients who have not responded adequately to diet and other appropriate measures (but see also notes above)

*Cautions; Contra-indications:* see under Bezafibrate and notes above

*Side-effects:* see under Bezafibrate; also cholesterol cholelithiasis

*Dose:* over 65 kg, 2 g daily (50–65 kg, 1.5 g daily) in 2 or 3 divided doses

PoM **Atromid-S®** (ICI)
*Capsules*, red, clofibrate 500 mg. Net price 100-cap pack = £4.18. Label: 21

### FENOFIBRATE

*Indications:* hyperlipidaemias of types IIa, IIb, III, IV, and V in patients who have not responded adequately to diet and other appropriate measures

*Cautions:* see under Bezafibrate

*Contra-indications:* severe renal or hepatic impairment, existing gall bladder disease, pregnancy

*Side-effects:* see under Bezafibrate

*Dose:* initially 300 mg daily in divided doses with food, adjusted according to response within range 200–400 mg daily; CHILD 5 mg/kg daily

PoM **Lipantil®** (Fournier)
*Capsules*, fenofibrate 100 mg. Net price 84-cap pack = £19.80. Label: 21

### GEMFIBROZIL

*Indications:* hyperlipidaemias of types IIa, IIb, III, IV and V in patients who have not responded adequately to diet and other appropriate measures; primary prevention of coronary heart disease in men aged 40–55 years with hyperlipidaemias that have not responded to diet and other appropriate measures

*Cautions:* lipid profile, blood counts, and liver-function tests before initiating long-term treatment; renal impairment; annual eye examinations; **interactions:** Appendix 1 (clofibrate group)

*Contra-indications:* alcoholism, hepatic impairment, gallstones; pregnancy

*Side-effects:* gastro-intestinal disturbances; pruritus, urticaria, rash, headache, dizziness, blurred vision, painful extremities; rarely myalgia; impotence reported

*Dose:* 1.2 g daily, usually in 2 divided doses; range 0.9–1.5 g daily

PoM **Lopid®** (P-D)
*'300' capsules*, white/maroon, gemfibrozil 300 mg. Net price 100-cap pack = £24.00
*'600' tablets*, f/c, gemfibrozil 600 mg. Net price 56-tab pack = £26.88

## NICOTINIC ACID GROUP

The value of **nicotinic acid** and **nicofuranose** is limited by their side-effects, especially vasodilatation. In doses of 1.5 to 3 g daily they lower both cholesterol and triglyceride concentrations by inhibiting synthesis; they also increase HDL-cholesterol. **Acipimox** seems to have fewer side-effects but may be less effective in its lipid-modulating capabilities

### ACIPIMOX

*Indications:* hyperlipidaemias of types IIa, IIb, and IV in patients who have not responded adequately to diet and other appropriate measures

*Cautions:* renal impairment

*Contra-indications:* peptic ulcer; pregnancy

*Side-effects:* vasodilatation, flushing, itching, rashes, erythema; occasionally, heartburn, epigastric pain, nausea, diarrhoea, headache, malaise

*Dose:* usually 500–750 mg daily in divided doses

PoM **Olbetam®** (Farmitalia Carlo Erba)
*Capsules*, brown/pink, acipimox 250 mg. Net price 100-cap pack = £44.00. Label: 21

---

## NICOFURANOSE

*Indications:* see notes above (for use in peripheral vascular disease, see section 2.6.3)

*Cautions; Side-effects:* see under Nicotinic Acid, but prostaglandin-mediated symptoms less severe

*Dose:* 500 mg 3 times daily, gradually increased if necessary to 1 g 3 times daily

**Bradilan®** (Napp)
*Tablets,* e/c and s/c, nicofuranose 250 mg. Net price 20 = £1.55. Label: 5, 25

## NICOTINIC ACID

*Indications:* see notes above

*Cautions:* diabetes mellitus, gout, liver disease, peptic ulcer

*Contra-indications:* pregnancy, breast-feeding

*Side-effects:* flushing, dizziness, headache, palpitations, pruritus (prostaglandin-mediated symptoms can be reduced by low initial doses taken with meals, or by taking aspirin 300 mg 30 minutes before the dose—needed in only a very small proportion of patients); nausea, vomiting; rarely impaired liver function and rashes

*Dose:* initially 100–200 mg 3 times daily (see above), gradually increased over 2–4 weeks to 1–2 g 3 times daily

**Nicotinic Acid Tablets,** nicotinic acid 50 mg, net price 20 = 13p. Label: 21

---

FISH OILS

A fish-oil preparation (Maxepa®), rich in omega-3 marine triglycerides, is useful in the treatment of severe hypertriglyceridaemia; however, it can sometimes aggravate hypercholesterolaemia.

## OMEGA-3 MARINE TRIGLYCERIDES

*Indications:* reduction of plasma triglycerides in patients with severe hypertriglyceridaemia judged to be at special risk of ischaemic heart disease and/or pancreatitis, in conjunction with dietary and other methods (see notes above)

*Side-effects:* occasional nausea and belching

*Dose:* see under preparations below

**Maxepa®** (DF)
*Capsules,* 1 g (approx. 1.1 mL) concentrated fish oils of composition below. Net price 200-cap pack = £28.57. Label: 21
*Dose:* 5 capsules twice daily with food
*Liquid,* golden-coloured, concentrated fish oils containing, as percentage of total fatty acid composition, eicosapentaenoic acid 18% w/w, docosahexaenoic acid 12% w/w. Vitamin A content less than 100 units/g, vitamin D content less than 10 units/g. Net price 150 mL = £21.43. Label: 21
*Dose:* 5 mL twice daily with food

OTHER DRUGS

**Probucol** decreases both LDL- and HDL-cholesterol; despite the latter effect it appears to promote resolution of xanthomata. Moreover, its antioxidant properties may decrease the atherogenicity of LDL.

**Simvastatin** and **pravastatin** belong to a new class of drugs which competitively inhibit 3-hydroxy-3-methylglutaryl coenzyme A (HMG CoA) reductase, an enzyme that catalyses a step in cholesterol synthesis, especially in the liver. They are more potent than anion-exchange resins in lowering LDL-cholesterol but less effective than the clofibrate group in reducing triglycerides and raising HDL-cholesterol. The main side-effect is reversible myositis, which is rare except in patients also receiving cyclosporin, nicotinic acid, or gemfibrozil (careful monitoring of liver function and creatine phosphokinase should be performed if these drugs are used with an HMG CoA reductase inhibitor).

## PROBUCOL

*Indications:* see notes above

*Cautions:* ECG before treatment in patients with recent myocardial damage, ventricular arrhythmias; avoid pregnancy during and for 6 months after stopping treatment

*Contra-indications:* breast-feeding

*Side-effects:* generally mild and transient and mainly consist of gastro-intestinal effects such as nausea, vomiting, flatulence, diarrhoea, abdominal pain; ventricular arrhythmias and angioedema rarely reported

*Dose:* 500 mg twice daily with food

PoM **Lurselle®** (Merrell)
*Tablets,* scored, probucol 250 mg. Net price 120-tab pack = £13.40. Label: 21

## PRAVASTATIN

*Indications:* primary hypercholesterolaemia (hyperlipidaemia type IIa) in patients intolerant of or not responsive to other therapy

*Cautions; Contra-indications; Side-effects:* as for Simvastatin; **interactions:** Appendix 1 (pravastatin)

*Dose:* usual range 10–40 mg once daily at night, adjusted at intervals of not less than 4 weeks

▼ PoM **Lipostat®** (Squibb)
*Tablets,* both pink, pravastatin sodium 10 mg, net price 28-tab pack = £16.18; 20 mg, 28-tab pack = £31.09

---

## SIMVASTATIN

*Indications:* primary hypercholesterolaemia (hyperlipidaemia type IIa) in patients with cholesterol concentration of 6.5 mmol/litre or greater and resistant to dietary control

*Cautions:* monitor liver function; avoid pregnancy during and for 1 month after treatment; advise patients to report muscle pain; **interactions:** Appendix 1 (simvastatin)

*Contra-indications:* active liver disease; pregnancy (toxicity in *animal* studies) and breastfeeding; porphyria (see section 9.8.2)

*Side-effects:* constipation, flatulence, headache, nausea, dyspepsia, abdominal pain, diarrhoea, fatigue, insomnia, rash, rhabdomyolysis, hepatitis reported; raised creatine phosphokinase concentrations (discontinue if markedly raised or myopathy diagnosed); transient hypotension reported

*Dose:* 10 mg daily at night, adjusted at intervals of not less than 4 weeks; usual range 10–40 mg once daily at night

▼ PoM **Zocor**® (MSD)
*Tablets*, both f/c, simvastatin 10 mg (peach), net price 28-tab pack = £18.29; 20 mg (tan), 28-tab pack = £31.09

# 2.13   Local sclerosants

Ethanolamine oleate and sodium tetradecyl sulphate are used in sclerotherapy of varicose veins, and phenol is used in haemorrhoids (see section 1.7.3).

## ETHANOLAMINE OLEATE

*Indications:* sclerotherapy of varicose veins

*Cautions:* extravasation may cause necrosis of tissues

*Contra-indications:* inability to walk, acute phlebitis, oral contraceptive use, obese legs

*Side-effects:* allergic reactions

PoM **Ethanolamine Oleate Injection,** ethanolamine oleate 5%. Net price 2-mL amp = 70p; 5-mL amp = 65p
*Dose:* by slow injection into empty isolated segment of vein, 2–5 mL divided between 3–4 sites; repeated at weekly intervals

## SODIUM TETRADECYL SULPHATE

*Indications:* sclerotherapy of varicose veins

*Cautions; Contra-indications; Side-effects:* see under Ethanolamine Oleate

PoM **STD**® (STD Pharmaceutical)
*Injection*, sodium tetradecyl sulphate 0.5%, net price 2-mL amp = £1.10; 1%, 2-mL amp = £1.19; 3%, 2-mL amp = £1.28, 5-mL vial = £2.29
*Dose:* by slow injection into empty isolated segment of vein, 0.1–1 mL according to site and condition being treated (consult manufacturer's literature)

---

# 3: Drugs used in the treatment of diseases of the
# RESPIRATORY SYSTEM

In this chapter, drug treatment is described under the following headings:

**3.1** Bronchodilators
**3.2** Corticosteroids
**3.3** Cromoglycate and related therapy
**3.4** Antihistamines, hyposensitisation, and allergic emergencies
**3.5** Respiratory stimulants and surfactants
**3.6** Oxygen
**3.7** Mucolytics
**3.8** Aromatic inhalations
**3.9** Antitussives
**3.10** Systemic nasal decongestants

The initial treatment of exacerbations of chronic bronchitis and bacterial pneumonia is indicated in section 5.1 (Table 1) and the treatment of tuberculosis is discussed in section 5.1.9.

## 3.1 Bronchodilators

**3.1.1** Adrenoceptor stimulants
**3.1.2** Antimuscarinic bronchodilators
**3.1.3** Theophylline
**3.1.4** Compound bronchodilator preparations
**3.1.5** Peak flow meters and inhaler devices

### 3.1.1 Adrenoceptor stimulants (sympathomimetics)

**3.1.1.1** Selective beta$_2$-adrenoceptor stimulants
**3.1.1.2** Other adrenoceptor stimulants

Most *mild to moderate* attacks of asthma respond rapidly to aerosol administration of a selective beta$_2$-adrenoceptor stimulant such as salbutamol or terbutaline (section 3.1.1.1). In *frequently occurring moderate* asthma the introduction of a corticosteroid by inhalation (section 3.2), sodium cromoglycate (section 3.3), or oral theophylline (section 3.1.3) may stabilise the asthma and avoid the use of oral corticosteroids. However in *more severe attacks* a short course of an oral corticosteroid may be necessary to bring the asthma under control (section 3.2).

Treatment of patients with *severe acute asthma* or airways obstruction (see also below) is safer in hospital where oxygen and resuscitation facilities are immediately available.

Patients with *chronic bronchitis* and *emphysema* are often described as having irreversible airways obstruction, but they usually respond partially to the beta$_2$-adrenoceptor stimulant drugs or to the antimuscarinic drug ipratropium (section 3.1.2).

CHOICE OF DRUG. The **selective beta$_2$-adrenoceptor stimulants** (selective beta$_2$-agonists) (section 3.1.1.1) such as salbutamol or terbutaline (preferably given by aerosol inhalation) are the safest and most effective beta-stimulants.

There is some evidence that patients who use beta$_2$-adrenoceptor stimulants on an 'as required' basis show a greater improvement in their asthma than those using them on a regular basis. For patients requiring higher doses of beta$_2$-adrenoceptor stimulants alternative treatment such as an inhaled corticosteroid should be considered.

There are some differences between the various selective beta$_2$-adrenoceptor stimulant drugs. **Salbutamol** and **terbutaline** are available in the widest range of formulations. **Rimiterol** has a shorter duration of action than salbutamol, terbutaline and fenoterol. **Fenoterol** may be less beta$_2$-selective than salbutamol. The dose or frequency of administration of beta$_2$-adrenoceptor stimulants can often be reduced by concurrent treatment with prophylactic drugs such as corticosteroid inhalations (section 3.2) or sodium cromoglycate (section 3.3).

**Salmeterol** is a longer-acting beta$_2$-adrenoceptor stimulant that has recently been introduced for twice daily administration; it is not suitable for the relief of an acute attack (a short-acting beta$_2$-stimulant such as salbutamol should be used). Salmeterol should be added to existing corticosteroid therapy and **not** replace it.

CHOICE OF FORMULATION. The *pressurised aerosol inhaler* is an effective and convenient method of administration for mild to moderate airways obstruction. Aerosol inhalers usually act for about 3 to 5 hours (rimiterol less than the others) but this depends to some extent on the severity of the asthma and on the dose administered. Aerosol inhalation is preferred because it provides relief more rapidly and causes fewer side-effects (such as tremor and nervous tension) than tablets; the drug is delivered directly to the bronchi and is therefore effective in smaller doses.

Patients should be given careful instruction on the use of their pressurised aerosol inhalers and it is important to check that they continue to use them correctly as inadequate technique may be mistaken for drug failure. In particular, it should be emphasised that they must inhale slowly and hold their breath for 10 seconds after inhalation. Most patients can be successfully taught to use pressurised aerosol inhalers but some patients, particularly the elderly, the arthritic, and small children are unable to use them; some patients are unable to synchronise their breathing with the administration of aerosol.

The dose should be stated **explicitly** in terms of the number of inhalations at one time, the frequency, and the maximum number of inhalations allowed in 24 hours. High doses of beta$_2$-stimulants can be dangerous in some patients. Excessive use is usually an indication of inadequately treated asthma. Patients should be advised to seek medical advice when they fail to obtain their usual degree of symptomatic relief as this usually indicates a worsening of the asthma and may require alternative medication. When patients with asthma **are not adequately controlled** with 2 to 4 puffs daily, **addition of a prophylactic drug** such as a corticosteroid inhalation should be considered; this is more convenient for the patient than higher doses of beta$_2$-stimulants and usually provides better overall control.

*Dry powder inhalers* are actuated by the patient's inspiration and hence are of particular value in subjects who cannot use pressurised aerosol inhalers correctly. Some dry powder inhalations occasionally cause coughing.

A variety of spacing devices is now available for use with metered dose inhalers. By providing a space between inhaler and mouth, they reduce the velocity of the aerosol and subsequent impaction on the oropharynx; in addition they allow more time for evaporation of the propellent so that a larger proportion of the particles can be inhaled and deposited in the lungs; also co-ordination of inspiration with actuation of the aerosol is less important. They range from the Bricanyl Spacer® (for terbutaline), a collapsible extended mouthpiece, to larger spacing devices with a one-way valve (Nebuhaler®, Rondo®, Volumatic®). Spacing devices are particularly useful for patients with poor inhalation technique, for children, for patients requiring higher doses, for nocturnal asthma, and for patients prone to develop candidiasis with inhaled corticosteroids.

*Respirator solutions* of salbutamol and terbutaline are increasingly used for the treatment of *acute asthma* both in hospital and in general practice; a respirator solution of fenoterol is also available. They are usually administered over a period of about 15 minutes from a nebuliser, usually driven from an oxygen cylinder in hospital. An electrical compressor is most suitable for domiciliary use but these are costly and not currently prescribable under the NHS. Patients with a severe attack of asthma should have oxygen if possible during nebulisation since beta-adrenoceptor stimulants can cause an increase in arterial hypoxaemia. For patients with *chronic bronchitis and hypercapnia*, however, oxygen can be dangerous, and the nebuliser should be driven by air. The dose prescribed ·by nebuliser is substantially higher than that prescribed by metered dose inhaler. For example, a 2.5-mL Ventolin Nebule® contains 2.5 mg of salbutamol, which is equivalent to 25 puffs from the aerosol inhaler. Patients should therefore be warned that it is dangerous to exceed the stated dose and that if they fail to respond to the usual dose of their respirator solution they should call for help.

*Oral preparations* are available for patients who cannot manage the inhaled route. They are sometimes used for children, though the inhaled route is better and most children can use one or other of the inhalation devices available. They have a slower onset but a slightly more prolonged action than the aerosol inhalers. The *modified-release* preparations may be of value in patients with *nocturnal asthma* as an alternative to the modified-release theophylline preparations (section 3.1.3).

*Intravenous*, and occasionally *subcutaneous*, injections of salbutamol and terbutaline are given for severe acute asthma.

EMERGENCY TREATMENT OF SEVERE ACUTE ASTHMA. Severe asthma can be fatal and **must** be treated promptly and energetically. It is characterised by persistent dyspnoea poorly relieved by bronchodilators, restlessness, exhaustion, a high pulse rate (usually over 110/minute), often pulsus paradoxus of over 10 mmHg, and a very low peak expiratory flow. The respiration is so shallow that wheezing may be absent. Such patients should be given a large dose of a **corticosteroid** (see section 6.3.4)—for adults hydrocortisone 200 mg (preferably as sodium succinate) intravenously or prednisolone 40 mg by mouth, children half these doses. They should also be given a beta$_2$-selective adrenoceptor stimulant such as **salbutamol** or **terbutaline** by nebuliser with oxygen if available.

If there is little response the following additional treatment should be considered: **ipratropium** by nebuliser (section 3.1.2), **aminophylline** by slow intravenous injection, if the patient has not already been receiving theophylline (section 3.1.3), or change of administration of the beta$_2$-selective adrenoceptor stimulant to the intravenous route.

Further treatment of these patients is safer in hospital where resuscitation facilities are immediately available. Treatment should **never** be delayed for investigations, patients should **never** be sedated, and the possibility of a pneumothorax should also be remembered.

If the patient deteriorates despite appropriate pharmacological treatment, intermittent positive pressure ventilation may be needed temporarily.

---

**CSM advice.** Potentially serious hypokalaemia may result from beta$_2$-adrenoceptor stimulant therapy. Particular caution is required in severe asthma, as this effect may be potentiated by concomitant treatment with theophylline and its derivatives, corticosteroids, and diuretics, and by hypoxia. Plasma potassium concentrations should therefore be monitored in severe asthma.

---

CHILDREN. Selective beta$_2$-adrenoceptor stimulants are useful even in children under the age of 18 months. They are most effective by the inhaled route, but an inhalation device may be needed (with the technique carefully checked). They are also effective by mouth. In severe attacks nebulisation using a selective beta$_2$-adrenoceptor stimulant or ipratropium is advisable.

PREGNANCY AND BREAST-FEEDING. It is particularly important that asthma should be well-controlled during pregnancy; where this is achieved asthma has no important effects on pregnancy, labour, or the fetus.

Inhalation has particular advantages as a means of drug administration during pregnancy because the therapeutic action can be achieved without the need for plasma concentrations liable to have a pharmacological effect on the fetus.

---

Severe exacerbations of asthma can have an adverse effect on pregnancy and should be treated promptly with conventional therapy, including oral or parenteral administration of cortico-steroids and nebulisation of a selective beta$_2$-adrenoceptor stimulant; prednisolone is the pre-ferred corticosteroid for oral administration since placental transfer is slower than with some others.

Although theophylline has been given without adverse effects during pregnancy or breast-feed-ing there have been occasional reports of toxicity in the fetus and neonate.

See also under Prescribing in Pregnancy (Appendix 4) and Prescribing during Breast-feed-ing (Appendix 5).

### 3.1.1.1  SELECTIVE BETA$_2$-ADRENOCEPTOR STIMULANTS

## SALBUTAMOL

*Indications:* asthma and other conditions associ-ated with reversible airways obstruction; premature labour, see section 7.1.2

*Cautions:* hyperthyroidism, myocardial insuf-ficiency, arrhythmias, hypertension, pregnancy (but appropriate to use, see notes above), eld-erly patients; intravenous administration to dia-betics (monitor blood glucose; ketoacidosis reported); see also notes above; **interactions:** Appendix 1 (sympathomimetics, beta$_2$)

*Side-effects:* fine tremor (usually hands), nervous tension, headache, peripheral vasodilatation, tachycardia (seldom troublesome when given by aerosol inhalation); hypokalaemia after high doses (**CSM** recommends monitor plasma-pot-assium in severe asthma, see opposite); hyp-ersensitivity reactions including paradoxical bronchospasm, urticaria, and angioedema reported; slight pain on intramuscular injection

*Dose: by mouth,* 4 mg (elderly and sensitive patients initially 2 mg) 3–4 times daily; max. single dose 8 mg (but unlikely to provide much extra benefit or to be tolerated); CHILD under 2 years 100 micrograms/kg 4 times daily; 2–6 years 1–2 mg 3–4 times daily, 6–12 years 2 mg

*By subcutaneous or intramuscular injection,* 500 micrograms, repeated every 4 hours if necessary

*By slow intravenous injection,* 250 micrograms, repeated if necessary

*By intravenous infusion,* initially 5 micrograms/minute, adjusted according to response and heart-rate usually in range 3–20 micrograms/minute, or more if necessary

*By aerosol inhalation,* acute and intermittent episodes of wheezing and asthma, 100–200 mic-rograms (1–2 puffs); CHILD 100 micrograms (1 puff)

Prophylaxis in exercise-induced bronchospasm, 200 micrograms (2 puffs); CHILD 100 mic-rograms (1 puff)

Chronic maintenance therapy, 200 micrograms (2 puffs) 3–4 times daily; CHILD 100 micrograms (1 puff) 3–4 times daily, increased to 200 mic-rograms (2 puffs) if necessary

*By inhalation of a powder* (Rotacaps®, Ven-todisks®), acute and intermittent episodes of wheezing and asthma, 200–400 micrograms; CHILD 200 micrograms

Prophylaxis in exercise-induced bronchospasm (*powder*), 400 micrograms; CHILD 200 mic-rograms

Chronic maintenance therapy (*powder*), 400 micrograms 3–4 times daily; CHILD 200 mic-rograms 3–4 times daily

*Note.* Bioavailability appears to be lower, so rec-ommended doses for dry powder inhalers are twice those in a metered inhaler

*By inhalation of nebulised solution,* chronic bron-chospasm unresponsive to conventional therapy and severe acute asthma, 2.5 mg, repeated up to 4 times daily, increased to 5 mg if necessary; in refractory patients with severe acute asthma up to 10 mg if side-effects permit; CHILD 2.5 mg, increased to 5 mg if required

Oral

**PoM Salbutamol** (Non-proprietary)

*Tablets,* salbutamol (as sulphate) 2 mg, net price 20 = 17p; 4 mg, 20 = 34p

Available from APS, Cox, Evans, Kerfoot, Tillotts (Salbuvent®)

*Syrup,* salbutamol (as sulphate) 2 mg/5 mL, net price 150 mL = 68p

Available from Evans, Tillotts (Salbuvent®)

**PoM Ventolin®** (A&H)

*Tablets,* both pink, scored, salbutamol (as sulphate), 2 mg, net price 20 = 22p; 4 mg, 20 = 43p

*CR Tablets,* modified-release, salbutamol (as sulphate) 4 mg, net price 56-tab pack = £10.00; 8 mg, 56-tab pack = £12.00. Label: 25, 27

*Dose:* 8 mg twice daily; CHILD 3–12 years 4 mg twice daily

*Syrup,* sugar-free, salbutamol 2 mg (as sul-phate)/5 mL. Diluent purified water, freshly boiled and cooled, life of diluted syrup 28 days. Net price 150 mL = 67p

**PoM Volmax®** (DF)

*Tablets,* modified-release, salbutamol (as sulphate) 4 mg, net price 56-tab pack = £10.00; 8 mg, 56-tab pack = £12.00. Label: 25

*Dose:* 8 mg twice daily; CHILD 3–12 years 4 mg twice daily

Parenteral

**PoM Salbuvent®** (Tillotts)

*Injection,* salbutamol (as sulphate) 50 micrograms/mL. Net price 5-mL amp = 57p

*Injection,* salbutamol (as sulphate) 500 micrograms/mL. Net price 1-mL amp = 43p

*Solution for intravenous infusion,* salbutamol (as sulphate) 1 mg/mL. Dilute before use. Net price 5-mL amp = £3.08

---

PoM **Ventolin**® (A&H)

*Injection*, salbutamol 50 micrograms (as sulphate)/mL. Net price 5-mL amp = 57p

*Injection*, salbutamol 500 micrograms (as sulphate)/mL. Net price 1-mL amp = 43p

*Solution for intravenous infusion*, salbutamol 1 mg (as sulphate)/mL. Dilute before use. Net price 5-mL amp = £3.08

Inhalation

COUNSELLING. Advise patients not to exceed prescribed dose and to follow manufacturer's directions

PoM **Salbutamol** (Non-proprietary)

*Aerosol inhalation*, salbutamol 100 micrograms/metered inhalation, net price 200-dose unit = £2.08

Available from APS, Ashbourne (Maxivent®), Cox, Evans, Kent (Kentamol®), Kerfoot, 3M (Aerolin 400®, 400-dose unit; Salbulin®), Tillotts (Salbuvent®)

PoM **Aerolin**® **Autohaler**[1] (3M)

*Aerosol inhalation*, salbutamol 100 micrograms (as sulphate)/metered inhalation. Net price 200-dose breath-actuated unit = £11.00; also 100-dose unit = £5.25 (hosp. only)

[1]replaces *Aerolin Auto*

PoM **Ventodisks**® (A&H)

*Powder for inhalation*, disks containing 8 blisters of salbutamol (as sulphate) 200 micrograms/blister, net price pack of 14 disks with Diskhaler® = £7.11; 14-disk refill = £6.54; 400 micrograms/blister, pack of 14 disks with Diskhaler® = £12.02; 14-disk refill = £11.45

PoM **Ventolin**® (A&H)

*Aerosol inhalation*, salbutamol 100 micrograms/metered inhalation. Net price 200-dose unit = £2.62

*Nebules*® (for use with nebuliser), salbutamol 0.1% (1 mg/mL, as sulphate), net price 2.5 mL (2.5 mg) = 19p; 0.2% (2 mg/mL), 2.5 mL (5 mg) = 38p. May be diluted with physiological saline

*Respirator solution* (for use with a nebuliser or ventilator), salbutamol 0.5% (5 mg/mL, as sulphate). Net price 20 mL = £2.71. May be diluted with physiological saline

*Rotacaps*® (powder for inhalation), salbutamol (as sulphate), 200 micrograms (light-blue/clear), net price 20 = £1.06; 400 micrograms (dark-blue/clear), 20 = £1.79

Note. Capsules containing 200 or 400 micrograms salbutamol (as sulphate) as powder for inhalation also available as Salbutamol Cyclocaps® (Pharbita); only for use with Cyclohaler®

Inhaler devices
See section 3.1.5

## TERBUTALINE SULPHATE

*Indications; Cautions; Side-effects:* see under Salbutamol; premature labour, see section 7.1.2

*Dose:* by mouth, 5 mg 2–3 times daily; CHILD under 3 years 750 micrograms 3 times daily, 3–7 years 0.75–1.5 mg 3 times daily, 7–15 years 1.5–3 mg 3 times daily (as syrup) *or* 2.5 mg 2–3 times daily (as tablets)

*By subcutaneous, intramuscular, or slow intravenous injection*, 250–500 micrograms up to 4 times daily; CHILD 2–15 years 10 micrograms/kg to a max. of 300 micrograms

*By continuous intravenous infusion* as a solution containing 3–5 micrograms/mL, 1.5–5 micrograms/minute for 8–10 hours; reduce dose for children

*By aerosol inhalation*, acute and maintenance treatment, adults and children 250–500 micrograms (1–2 puffs) repeated after 6 hours if necessary; not more than 8 inhalations should be necessary in any 24 hours

*By inhalation of powder* (Turbohaler®), 500 micrograms (1 inhalation) as required; not more than 4 inhalations in any 24 hours

*By inhalation of nebulised solution*, 5–10 mg 2–4 times daily; additional doses may be necessary in severe acute asthma; CHILD, up to 3 years 2 mg, 3–6 years 3 mg; 6–8 years 4 mg, over 8 years 5 mg, 2–4 times daily

Oral and parenteral

PoM **Bricanyl**® (Astra)

*Tablets*, scored, terbutaline sulphate 5 mg. Net price 20 = 71p

*Syrup*, sugar-free, terbutaline sulphate 1.5 mg/5 mL. Diluent water, life of diluted syrup 14 days. Net price 300 mL = £2.24

*Injection*, terbutaline sulphate 500 micrograms/mL. Net price 1-mL amp = 28p; 5-mL amp = £1.30

PoM **Bricanyl SA**® (Astra)

*Tablets*, m/r, terbutaline sulphate 7.5 mg. Net price 20 = £1.59. Label: 25

*Dose:* 7.5 mg twice daily

PoM **Monovent**® (Lagap)

*Syrup*, terbutaline sulphate 1.5 mg/5 mL. Diluent water, life of diluted syrup 14 days. Net price 300 mL = £2.20

Inhalation

COUNSELLING. Advise patients not to exceed prescribed dose and to follow manufacturer's directions; little sensation associated with use of Turbohaler®

*Aerosol inhalation*, terbutaline sulphate 250 micrograms/metered inhalation. Net price 400-dose unit = £5.31; 400-dose unit with Spacer inhaler (collapsible extended mouthpiece) = £7.21; 400-dose refill cannister for use with Nebuhaler or Spacer inhaler = £5.21

*Turbohaler*® (= breath-actuated dry powder inhaler), terbutaline sulphate 500 micrograms/inhalation. Net price 100-dose unit = £8.94

*Respules*® (= single-dose units for nebulisation), terbutaline sulphate 2.5 mg/mL. Net price 20 × 2-mL units = £3.76

*Respirator solution* (for use with a nebuliser or ventilator), terbutaline sulphate 10 mg/mL. Net price 10 mL = £1.35. Before use dilute with sterile physiological saline

Inhaler devices
See section 3.1.5

## FENOTEROL HYDROBROMIDE

*Indications:* reversible airways obstruction

*Cautions; Side-effects:* see under Salbutamol

*Dose:* acute and episodic bronchospasm, *by aerosol inhalation*, 100–200 micrograms (1–2 puffs Berotec '100') 1–3 times daily; not more than 200 micrograms (2 puffs Berotec '100') every 6 hours; max. 800 micrograms daily; CHILD 6–12 years 100 micrograms (1 puff Berotec '100') 1–3 times daily; not more than 200 micrograms (2 puffs Berotec '100') every 6 hours; max. 800 micrograms daily

Persistent bronchospasm not adequately controlled by Berotec '100', *by aerosol inhalation*, 200–400 micrograms (1–2 puffs Berotec '200') 1–3 times daily; not more than 400 micrograms (2 puffs Berotec '200') every 6 hours; max. 1.6 mg daily; CHILD under 16 years, not recommended

*By inhalation of nebulised solution*, 0.5–1.25 mg up to 4 times daily, dilution adjusted to equipment and length of administration; exceptionally 2.5–5 mg may be given under strict medical supervision; CHILD 6–14 years, up to 1 mg 3 times daily

Note. The above doses of fenoterol represent revised recommendations following evidence that fenoterol is effective at doses lower than those recommended previously. The CSM has advised that patients already receiving fenoterol should have their dosage regimens reviewed

PoM **Berotec**® (Boehringer Ingelheim)

COUNSELLING. Advise patients not to exceed prescribed dose and to follow manufacturer's directions

*'100' aerosol inhalation*, fenoterol hydrobromide 100 micrograms/metered inhalation. Net price 200-dose unit = £2.36

*'200' aerosol inhalation*, fenoterol hydrobromide 200 micrograms/metered inhalation. Net price 200-dose unit = £2.78

Note. Only for persistent bronchospasm inadequately controlled by Berotec '100'

*Nebuliser solution*, fenoterol hydrobromide 0.5% (5 mg/mL, 20 drops ≈1 mL). Net price 20 mL (with dropper) = £1.76. For use with nebuliser or ventilator; if dilution is necessary, use only sterile sodium chloride 0.9% solution

## PIRBUTEROL

*Indications:* reversible airways obstruction

*Cautions; Side-effects:* see under Salbutamol

*Dose: by mouth*, 10–15 mg 3–4 times daily

*By aerosol inhalation*, intermittent episodes, prophylaxis in exercise-induced bronchospasm, 200–400 micrograms (1–2 puffs) repeated after 4 hours if necessary; max. 2.4 mg (12 puffs) daily

Chronic maintenance, 400 micrograms (2 puffs) 3–4 times daily or in severe bronchospasm every 4 hours; max. 2.4 mg (12 puffs) daily

PoM **Exirel**® (3M)

*Capsules*, pirbuterol (as hydrochloride) 10 mg (turquoise/olive), net price 20 = 48p; 15 mg (turquoise/beige), 20 = 71p

*Aerosol inhalation*, pirbuterol 200 micrograms (as acetate)/metered inhalation. Net price 200-dose unit = £2.86

COUNSELLING. Advise patients not to exceed prescribed dose and to follow manufacturer's directions

## REPROTEROL HYDROCHLORIDE

*Indications:* reversible airways obstruction

*Cautions; Side-effects:* see under Salbutamol

*Dose: by aerosol inhalation*, intermittent episodes and prophylaxis in exercise-induced bronchospasm, 0.5–1 mg (1–2 puffs) repeated after 3–6 hours if necessary; CHILD 6–12 years 500 micrograms (1 puff)

Chronic maintenance therapy, 1 mg (2 puffs) 3 times daily or in severe bronchospasm every 3–6 hours; CHILD 6–12 years 500 micrograms (1 puff) 3 times daily

PoM **Bronchodil**® (ASTA Medica)

*Aerosol inhalation*, reproterol hydrochloride 500 micrograms/metered inhalation. Net price 400-dose unit = £6.84

COUNSELLING. Advise patients not to exceed prescribed dose and to follow manufacturer's directions

## RIMITEROL HYDROBROMIDE

*Indications:* reversible airways obstruction (particularly when short action required)

*Cautions; Side-effects:* see under Salbutamol

*Dose: by aerosol inhalation*, adults and children 200–600 micrograms (1–3 puffs); should not be repeated in less than 30 minutes; max. 8 doses daily

PoM **Pulmadil**® (3M)

COUNSELLING. Advise patients not to exceed prescribed dose and to follow manufacturer's directions

*Aerosol inhalation*, rimiterol hydrobromide 200 micrograms/metered inhalation. Net price 300-dose unit = £6.32

*Auto aerosol inhalation*, rimiterol hydrobromide 200 micrograms/metered inhalation. Net price 300-dose cartridge in breath-actuated unit = £7.93; replacement cartridge = £6.32

## SALMETEROL

*Indications:* long-term regular treatment of reversible airways obstruction in asthma (including nocturnal and exercise-induced) and chronic bronchitis

Note. CSM has emphasised that salmeterol is not for immediate relief of acute attacks and that existing corticosteroid therapy should not be reduced or withdrawn

*Cautions; Side-effects:* see under Salbutamol and notes above; significant incidence of paradoxical bronchospasm

*Dose: by inhalation*, 50 micrograms (2 puffs or 1 blister) twice daily; up to 100 micrograms (4 puffs or 2 blisters) twice daily in more severe airways obstruction

▼ PoM **Serevent**® (A&H)
*Aerosol inhalation*, salmeterol (as xinafoate (= hydroxynaphthoate)) 25 micrograms/metered inhalation, net price 120-inhalation unit = £28.60
*Powder for inhalation*, disks containing 4 blisters of salmeterol (as xinafoate (= hydroxynaphthoate)) 50 micrograms/blister, net price pack of 14 disks with Diskhaler® = £29.97; 14-disk refill = £29.40

## TULOBUTEROL HYDROCHLORIDE
*Indications:* reversible airways obstruction
*Cautions:* see under Salbutamol; also mild renal impairment (avoid if severe)
*Contra-indications:* moderate to severe renal impairment; acute liver failure, chronic liver disease
*Side-effects:* see under Salbutamol
*Dose:* 2 mg twice daily; increased if necessary to 2 mg 3 times daily; CHILD over 10 years, 1–2 mg twice daily

▼ PoM **Brelomax**® (Abbott)
*Tablets*, scored, tulobuterol hydrochloride 2 mg. Net price 60-tab pack = £13.00

### 3.1.1.2   OTHER ADRENOCEPTOR STIMULANTS

These preparations (including the partially selective orciprenaline) are now regarded as less suitable and less safe for use as bronchodilators than the selective beta$_2$-adrenoceptor stimulants, as they are more likely to cause arrhythmias and other side-effects. They should be avoided whenever possible

   **Adrenaline injection** (1 in 1000) is used in the emergency treatment of acute allergic and anaphylactic reactions (section 3.4.3).

## EPHEDRINE HYDROCHLORIDE
*Indications:* reversible airways obstruction, but see notes above
*Cautions:* hyperthyroidism, diabetes mellitus, ischaemic heart disease, hypertension, renal impairment, elderly; may cause acute retention in prostatic hypertrophy; interaction with MAOIs a disadvantage; **interactions:** Appendix 1 (sympathomimetics)
*Side-effects:* tachycardia, anxiety, restlessness, insomnia common; also tremor, arrhythmias, dry mouth, cold extremities
*Dose:* 3 times daily, 15–60 mg; CHILD 3 times daily, up to 1 year 7.5 mg, 1–5 years 15 mg, 6–12 years 30 mg (not recommended, see above)

PoM [1]**Ephedrine Hydrochloride** (Non-proprietary)
*Tablets*, ephedrine hydrochloride 15 mg, net price 20 = 7p; 30 mg, 20 = 8p; 60 mg, 20 = 28p
*Elixir*, ephedrine hydrochloride 15 mg/5 mL in a suitable flavoured vehicle, containing alcohol 12%. Net price 100 mL = 49p
1. For exemptions see *Medicines, Ethics and Practice*, No. 7, London, Pharmaceutical Press, 1991

**CAM**® (Rybar)
*Mixture*, sugar-free, ephedrine hydrochloride 4 mg/5 mL. Diluent sorbitol solution, life of diluted mixture 28 days. Net price 100 mL = 95p
*Dose:* 20 mL 3–4 times daily; CHILD 3 months–2 years 2.5 mL, 2–4 years 5 mL, 5–12 years 10 mL, 3 times daily (but not recommended, see notes above)

## ISOPRENALINE SULPHATE
*Indications:* reversible airways obstruction, but see notes above
*Cautions; Side-effects:* see under Salbutamol (section 3.1.1.1) and notes above

PoM **Medihaler-iso**® (3M)
*Aerosol inhalation*, isoprenaline sulphate 80 micrograms/metered inhalation. Net price 400-dose vial = £2.73
*Note.* Not recommended therefore no dose stated
PoM **Medihaler-iso Forte**® (3M)
*Aerosol inhalation*, isoprenaline sulphate 400 micrograms/metered inhalation. Net price 400-dose vial = £3.17
*Note.* Not recommended therefore no dose stated

## ORCIPRENALINE SULPHATE
*Indications:* reversible airways obstruction, but see notes above
*Cautions; Side-effects:* see under Salbutamol (section 3.1.1.1) and notes above
*Dose: by mouth*, 20 mg 4 times daily; CHILD up to 1 year 5–10 mg 3 times daily, 1–3 years 5–10 mg 4 times daily, 3–12 years 40–60 mg daily in divided doses (but not recommended, see notes above)
*By aerosol inhalation*, 750–1500 micrograms (1–2 puffs) repeated if necessary after not less than 30 minutes to a max. of 9 mg (12 puffs) daily; CHILD up to 6 years 750 micrograms (1 puff) up to 4 times daily, 6–12 years 750–1500 micrograms (1–2 puffs) up to 4 times daily (but not recommended, see notes above)

PoM **Alupent**® (Boehringer Ingelheim)
*Tablets*, scored, orciprenaline sulphate 20 mg. Net price 112-tab pack = £4.26
*Syrup*, sugar-free, orciprenaline sulphate 10 mg/5 mL. Diluents syrup or sorbitol solution, life of diluted syrup 14 days. Net price 100 mL = 69p
*Aerosol inhalation*, orciprenaline sulphate 750 micrograms/metered inhalation. Net price 300-dose vial with mouthpiece = £3.22; refill vial = £2.66
COUNSELLING. Advise patients not to exceed prescribed dose and to follow manufacturer's directions

## 3.1.2   Antimuscarinic bronchodilators

These drugs have traditionally been regarded as more effective in relieving bronchoconstriction associated with chronic bronchitis. **Ipratropium** may provide some bronchodilation in patients with chronic bronchitis who fail to respond to the selective beta$_2$-adrenoceptor stimulants (section 3.1.1.1). Unlike the older antimuscarinic drugs, side-effects are rare and it does not increase sputum viscosity or affect mucociliary clearance of sputum. The aerosol inhalation has a slower onset of action than that of the beta$_2$-adrenoceptor stimulants, with a maximum effect 30–60 minutes after use; its duration of action is longer than that of beta$_2$-adrenoceptor stimulants following inhalation and bronchodilatation can usually be maintained with treatment three times a day.

Oxitropium has been introduced recently and has a similar duration of action to that of ipratropium

## IPRATROPIUM BROMIDE

*Indications:* reversible airways obstruction, particularly in chronic bronchitis
*Cautions:* glaucoma (standard doses unlikely to be harmful but see also under nebuliser, below); prostatic hypertrophy; pregnancy
*Side-effects:* dry mouth occasionally reported; rarely urinary retention, constipation
*Dose:* see below

PoM **Atrovent**® (Boehringer Ingelheim)
COUNSELLING. Advise patient not to exceed prescribed dose and to follow manufacturer's directions
*Aerosol inhalation,* ipratropium bromide 20 micrograms/metered inhalation. Net price 200-dose unit = £4.21
*Dose: by aerosol inhalation,* 20–40 micrograms (1–2 puffs), in early treatment up to 80 micrograms (4 puffs) at a time, 3–4 times daily; CHILD up to 6 years 20 micrograms (1 puff) 3 times daily, 6–12 years 20–40 micrograms (1–2 puffs) 3 times daily
*Forte aerosol inhalation,* ipratropium bromide 40 micrograms/metered inhalation. Net price 200-dose unit = £4.91
*Dose: by aerosol inhalation* 40 micrograms (1 puff), in early treatment 80 micrograms (2 puffs), 3–4 times daily; CHILD 6–12 years 40 micrograms (1 puff) 3 times daily
*Nebuliser solution,* isotonic, ipratropium bromide 250 micrograms/mL (0.025%); net price 10 × 1-mL unit-dose vials (preservative-free) = £3.20; 10 × 2-mL vials = £3.76. If dilution is necessary use only sterile sodium chloride solution 0.9%
*Dose:* reversible airways obstruction, *by inhalation of nebulised solution,* 100–500 micrograms (0.4–2 mL of a 0.025% solution) up to 4 times daily; CHILD 3–14 years 100–500 micrograms up to 3 times daily. Dilution of solution is adjusted according to equipment and length of administration
Note. Because paradoxical bronchospasm has occurred, first dose should be inhaled under medical supervision.
GLAUCOMA. Acute angle closure glaucoma has been reported in patients given nebulised ipratropium, particularly when used in association with nebulised salbutamol. Special caution is needed and care should be taken to avoid escape from mask to patient's eyes.
PoM **Rinatec**® nasal spray, see section 12.2.2

## OXITROPIUM BROMIDE

*Indications:* reversible airways obstruction, particularly in chronic bronchitis
*Cautions; Side-effects:* see under Ipratropium Bromide; rarely blurring of vision
*Dose: by aerosol inhalation,* 200 micrograms (2 puffs) 2–3 times daily

▼ PoM **Oxivent**® (Boehringer Ingelheim)
*Aerosol inhalation,* oxitropium bromide 100 micrograms/metered inhalation. Net price 200-dose unit = £12.98
COUNSELLING. Advise patient not to exceed prescribed dose and to follow manufacturer's directions

### 3.1.3   Theophylline

Theophylline and its derivatives are used primarily for the relief of bronchospasm. With the introduction of the beta$_2$-adrenoceptor stimulants (section 3.1.1.1), the use of *rapid-release* oral aminophylline and theophylline preparations declined because of the high incidence of side-effects associated with rapid absorption. However, there has been a revival of interest in these drugs since the introduction of *modified-release* preparations which are usually able to produce adequate plasma concentrations for up to 12 hours. These modified-release preparations are all equally effective but due to different pharmacokinetic profiles are not interchangeable without retitration of dosage.

**Theophylline** is metabolised in the liver and there is considerable variation in its half-life in healthy non-smokers, which is even more marked in smokers, in patients with hepatic impairment or heart failure, or if other drugs are taken concurrently. The half-life is *increased* in heart failure, cirrhosis, viral infections, and by drugs such as cimetidine, ciprofloxacin, erythromycin, and oral contraceptives. The half-life is *decreased* in smokers and in heavy drinkers, and by drugs such as phenytoin, carbamazepine, rifampicin, and barbiturates.

These differences in half-life are important because theophylline has a narrow margin between the therapeutic and toxic dose. In most subjects *plasma concentrations* of between 10 and 20 mg/litre are required for satisfactory bronchodilatation. Side-effects can occur with concentrations below 20 mg/litre and are common at concentrations above 30–40 mg/litre.

Theophylline *modified-release* preparations when given as a single dose at night have a useful role in controlling nocturnal asthma and early morning wheezing. They have replaced aminophylline suppositories which cause proctitis and can show an unpredictable response. Recent studies suggest that theophylline may have an additive effect when used in conjunction with small doses of beta$_2$-adrenoceptor stimulants; the combination may increase the risk of side-effects, including arrhythmias.

**Choline theophyllinate** is a modification of theophylline. There is no evidence that it is better tolerated than the modified-release preparations.

**Aminophylline,** a mixture of theophylline with ethylenediamine, is 20 times more soluble than theophylline alone, which is an advantage for the injection but not for the tablets.

The use of aminophylline *injection,* given intravenously, is of established value in the treatment of severe attacks of asthma and is still preferred by many prescribers to intravenous treatment with the selective beta$_2$-adrenoceptor stimulants (section 3.1.1.1). Measurement of *plasma concentrations* may be helpful, and is **essential** if aminophylline is to be given to patients who have been taking oral theophylline preparations, as serious side-effects such as convulsions and arrhythmias can occasionally occur before the appearance of other symptoms of toxicity. For **CSM** advice on hypokalaemia risk, see p. 108.

Aminophylline *suppositories* cause proctitis and show an unpredictable response; they are no longer used. See also under Children (below).

Aminophylline injection was formerly used in the treatment of left ventricular failure but has been superseded by diuretics (see sections 2.2.1 and 2.2.2) and the opioid analgesics (see section 4.7.2) for this purpose. However, it may have a role in patients with heart failure who are also suffering from asthma and bronchitis, where opioids are contra-indicated, though care is needed in using aminophylline in patients with increased myocardial excitability.

CHILDREN. Aminophylline suppositories should **not** be used in children; there have been reports of severe toxicity when adult suppositories have been given to young children. There is no good evidence that theophylline benefits the wheezy infant (unless due to ventilator-induced bronchopulmonary dysplasia); it is indicated for recurrent apnoeic attacks but can be given by mouth.


## THEOPHYLLINE

*Indications:* reversible airways obstruction, severe acute asthma

*Cautions:* see notes above; also liver disease, epilepsy, pregnancy and breast-feeding, cardiac disease, elderly, fever; **CSM** advice on hypokalaemia risk, p. 108; avoid in porphyria (see section 9.8.2); **interactions:** Appendix 1 (theophylline)

*Side-effects:* tachycardia, palpitations, nausea, gastro-intestinal disturbances, headache, insomnia, arrhythmias, and convulsions especially if given rapidly by intravenous injection; overdosage: see Emergency Treatment of Poisoning, p. 20

*Dose:* see below

*Note.* Plasma theophylline concentration for optimum response 10–20 mg/litre (55–110 micromol/litre); narrow margin between therapeutic and toxic dose, see also notes above


**Biophylline®** (Delandale)

*Syrup*, yellow, sugar-free, theophylline hydrate 125 mg (as sodium glycinate)/5 mL. Net price 250 mL = £3.77 (includes 2.5-mL measure). Label: 21

*Dose:* 125–250 mg 3–4 times daily; CHILD 2–6 years 62.5 mg, 7–12 years 62.5–125 mg, 3–4 times daily

PoM **Labophylline®** (LAB)

*Injection*, theophylline 20 mg/mL, lysine 12.2 mg/mL. Net price 10-mL amp = 30p

*Dose:* in patients not previously treated with xanthines, *by slow intravenous injection* (over 20 minutes) initially 200 mg, *or by intravenous infusion* 4 mg/kg; maintenance if required, 500 micrograms/kg/hour for 12 hours, then 400 micrograms/kg/hour; CHILD *by slow intravenous injection* (over 20 minutes) 4 mg/kg initially

**Nuelin®** (3M)

*Tablets*, scored, theophylline 125 mg. Net price 90-tab pack = £3.39. Label: 21

*Dose:* 125 mg 3–4 times daily after food, increased to 250 mg if required; CHILD 7–12 years 62.5–125 mg 3–4 times daily

*Liquid*, brown, theophylline 60 mg (as sodium glycinate)/5 mL. Diluent syrup, life of diluted liquid 14 days. Net price 200 mL = £2.02. Label: 21

*Dose:* 120–240 mg 3–4 times daily after food; CHILD 2–6 years 60–90 mg, 7–12 years 90–120 mg, 3–4 times daily

Modified release

*Note.* The Council of the Royal Pharmaceutical Society of Great Britain advises pharmacists that if a general practitioner prescribes a modified-release, oral theophylline preparation without specifying a brand name, the pharmacist should contact the prescriber and agree the brand to be dispensed. Additionally, it is essential that a patient discharged from hospital should be maintained on the brand on which that patient was stabilised as an in-patient.

**Biophylline®** (Delandale)

*Tablets*, m/r, both scored, theophylline 350 mg, net price 56-tab pack = £5.44; 500 mg, 56-tab pack = £7.44. Label: 25

*Dose:* over 70 kg, 500 mg every 12 hours; under 70 kg and elderly, 350 mg every 12 hours

**Lasma®** (Pharmax)

*Tablets*, m/r, scored, theophylline 300 mg. Net price 20 = £1.94. Label: 25

*Dose:* 300 mg every 12 hours (increased after 1 week to 450 mg every 12 hours in patients over 70 kg); adjust dose by 150-mg increments as required

Total daily dose may be given as single dose at night when nocturnal symptoms predominate (daytime symptoms then controlled with inhaled bronchodilators)

**Nuelin SA®** (3M)

*Tablets*, m/r, theophylline 175 mg. Net price 60-tab pack = £3.13. Label: 25

*Dose:* 175–350 mg every 12 hours; CHILD over 6 years 175 mg every 12 hours

**Nuelin SA 250®** (3M)

*Tablets*, m/r, scored, theophylline 250 mg. Net price 60-tab pack = £4.39. Label: 25

*Dose:* 250–500 mg every 12 hours; CHILD over 6 years 125–250 mg every 12 hours

**Pro-Vent®** (Wellcome)

*Capsules*, m/r, white/clear, theophylline 300 mg. Net price 20 = £2.13. Label: 25

*Dose:* 300 mg every 12 hours, an additional 300 mg may be taken daily (night *or* morning) if plasma concentrations inadequate

---

**Slo-Phyllin®** (Lipha)

*Capsules*, m/r, white/clear, enclosing white pellets, theophylline 60 mg. Net price 56-cap pack = £2.02. Label: 25 *or* counselling, see below

*Capsules*, m/r, brown/clear, enclosing white pellets, theophylline 125 mg. Net price 56-cap pack = £2.55. Label: 25 *or* counselling, see below

*Capsules*, m/r, blue/clear, enclosing white pellets, theophylline 250 mg. Net price 56-cap pack = £3.18. Label: 25 *or* counselling, see below

*Dose:* 250–500 mg every 12 hours; CHILD, every 12 hours, 2–6 years 60–120 mg, 7–12 years 125–250 mg

COUNSELLING. Swallow whole with fluid *or* swallow enclosed granules with soft food (e.g. yoghurt)

**Theo-Dur®** (Astra)

*Tablets*, m/r, both scored, theophylline 200 mg, net price 20 = £1.24; 300 mg, 20 = £1.80. Label: 25

*Dose:* every 12 hours; CHILD up to 35 kg 100 mg, over 35 kg 200 mg, every 12 hours

**Uniphyllin Continus®** (Napp)

*Tablets*, m/r, both scored, theophylline 300 mg, net price 56-tab pack = £5.50; 400 mg, 56-tab pack = £7.51. Label: 25

*Dose:* 200 mg every 12 hours increased after 1 week to 300 mg every 12 hours; over 70 kg 300 mg every 12 hours increased after 1 week to 400 mg every 12 hours

May be appropriate to give larger evening or morning dose to achieve optimum therapeutic effect when symptoms most severe; in patients whose night- or daytime symptoms persist despite other therapy, who are not currently receiving theophylline, total daily requirement may be added as single evening or morning dose

*Paediatric tablets*, m/r, scored, theophylline 200 mg. Net price 56-tab pack = £3.61. Label: 25

*Dose:* CHILD over 5 years, maintenance, 9 mg/kg twice daily

**AMINOPHYLLINE**

*Note:* Aminophylline is a stable mixture or combination of theophylline and ethylenediamine; the ethylenediamine confers greater solubility in water

**Indications:** reversible airways obstruction, severe acute asthma

**Cautions; Side-effects:** see under Theophylline; also allergy to ethylenediamine can cause urticaria, erythema, and exfoliative dermatitis

**Dose:** see below

*Note.* Plasma theophylline concentration for optimum response 10–20 mg/litre (55–110 micromol/litre); narrow margin between therapeutic and toxic dose, see also notes above

**Aminophylline** (Non-proprietary)

*Tablets*, aminophylline 100 mg, net price 20 = 92p. Label: 21

*Dose: by mouth*, 100–300 mg, 3–4 times daily, after food

PoM *Injection*, aminophylline 25 mg/mL, net price 10-mL amp = 61p

Available from Evans, IMS (Min-I-Jet®)

*Dose: by slow intravenous injection* (over 20 minutes), 250–500 mg (5 mg/kg) when necessary; maintenance, if required, in patients not previously treated with theophylline, 500 micrograms/kg/hour *by slow intravenous infusion*

CHILD, *by slow intravenous injection* (over 20 minutes), 5 mg/kg; maintenance, if required, in patients not previously treated with theophylline, 6 months–9 years 1 mg/kg/hour, 10–16 years 800 micrograms/kg/hour *by slow intravenous infusion*

Modified release (see advice on p. 114)

**Pecram®** (Zyma)

*Tablets*, m/r, yellow, aminophylline hydrate 225 mg. Net price 20 = £1.02. Label: 25

*Dose:* 1 tablet twice daily initially, increased if necessary to 2 tablets twice daily (steady-state concentrations usually reached after 3–4 days)

**Phyllocontin Continus®** (Napp)

*Tablets*, m/r, yellow, f/c, aminophylline 225 mg. Net price 60-tab pack = £3.61. Label: 25

*Dose:* 1 tablet twice daily initially, increased after 1 week to 2 tablets twice daily

*Forte tablets*, m/r, yellow, f/c, aminophylline 350 mg. Net price 60-tab pack = £6.00. Label: 25

*Note. Forte* tablets are for smokers and other patients with decreased theophylline half-life (see notes above)

*Paediatric tablets*, m/r, yellow, aminophylline 100 mg. Net price 50-tab pack = £1.94. Label: 25

*Dose:* CHILD over 3 years, 6 mg/kg twice daily initially, increased after 1 week to 12 mg/kg twice daily

*Note.* Modified-release tablets containing aminophylline 225 mg and 350 mg also available from Ashbourne (Amnivent®)

**CHOLINE THEOPHYLLINATE**

**Indications:** reversible airways obstruction

**Cautions; Side-effects:** see under Theophylline

**Dose:** *by mouth*, 100–400 mg 2–4 times daily preferably after food; CHILD, 3 times daily, 3–5 years 62.5–125 mg, 6–12 years 100 mg

*Note.* Plasma theophylline concentration for optimum response 10–20 mg/litre (55–110 micromol/litre); narrow margin between therapeutic and toxic dose, see also notes above

**Choledyl®** (P-D)

*Tablets*, both compression coated, choline theophyllinate 100 mg (pink), net price 20 = 44p; 200 mg (yellow), 20 = 60p

*Syrup*, yellow, choline theophyllinate 62.5 mg/5 mL. Net price 100 mL = £1.29

Modified release (see advice on p. 114)

**Sabidal SR 270®** (Zyma)

*Tablets*, m/r, light yellow, choline theophyllinate 424 mg. Net price 20 = £1.54. Label: 25

*Dose:* 1 tablet twice daily initially, increased after 3 days to 1 in the morning and 2 at night

### 3.1.4   Compound bronchodilator preparations

Most compound bronchodilator preparations have no place in the management of patients with airways obstruction.

In general, patients are best treated with single-ingredient preparations, such as a selective beta$_2$-adrenoceptor stimulant (section 3.1.1.1) or ipratropium bromide (section 3.1.2), so that the dose of each drug can be adjusted. This flexibility is lost with combinations, although those in which both components are effective may occasionally have a role when compliance is a problem.

PoM **Bronchilator**® (Sanofi Winthrop)
*Aerosol inhalation*, isoetharine mesylate 350 micrograms, phenylephrine hydrochloride 70 micrograms/metered dose. Net price 250-dose unit = £11.71
*Dose:* 1–2 puffs repeated after 30 minutes if necessary; max. 8 puffs daily

PoM **Duovent**® (Boehringer Ingelheim)
*Aerosol inhalation*, fenoterol hydrobromide 90 micrograms, ipratropium bromide 36 micrograms/metered inhalation. Net price 200-dose unit with mouthpiece = £5.28 (extension tube also available)
*Dose:* 1–2 puffs 3–4 times daily; CHILD over 6 years 1 puff 3 times daily

PoM **Franol**® (Sanofi Winthrop)
*Tablets*, ephedrine hydrochloride 11 mg, theophylline 120 mg. Net price 100-tab pack = £5.42. Label: 21
*Dose:* 1 tablet 3 times daily; an additional tablet may be taken at bedtime for nocturnal attacks

PoM **Franol Plus**® (Sanofi Winthrop)
*Tablets*, ephedrine sulphate 15 mg, theophylline 120 mg. Net price 20 = £1.50. Label: 21
*Dose:* 1 tablet 3 times daily; an additional tablet may be taken at bedtime for nocturnal attacks

### 3.1.5   Peak flow meters and inhaler devices

Peak flow meters
**Mini-Wright**® (Clement Clarke)
*Peak flow meter*, standard (60 to 800 litres/minute), net price = £6.39, low range (30 to 370 litres/minute) = £6.39, replacement universal mouthpiece = 38p

**Vitalograph**® (Vitalograph)
*Peak flow meter*, standard (50 to 750 litres/minute), net price = £5.99, low range (25 to 280 litres/minute) = £5.99, replacement mouthpiece = 40p

**Wright**® (Ferraris)
*Pocket peak flow meter*, standard (75–800 litres/minute), net price = £5.85, low range (50–400 litres/minute) = £5.85, replacement mouthpiece adult = 38p, paediatric = 38p

Inhaler devices
**Cyclohaler**® (Pharbita)
Breath actuated inhaler for use with Salbutamol Cyclocaps. Net price = 78p

NHS **Haleraid**® (Glaxo)
Device to place over standard inhalers as aid to operation by patients with impaired strength in hands (e.g. with arthritis). Net price = 80p

**Nebuhaler**® (Astra)
*Inhaler*, fitted with plastic cone and one-way valve. For use with Bricanyl and Pulmicort refill canisters. Net price = £4.75

**Rondo**® (Tillotts)
Spacer device for use with Salbuvent. Net price = £2.75

**Rotahaler**® (A&H)
Breath actuated inhaler for use with Rotacaps. Net price = 78p

**Spinhaler**® see section 3.3

**Volumatic**® (A&H)
*Inhaler*, large-volume spacer device. For use with Ventolin, Becotide, Becloforte, and Ventide inhalers. Net price = £2.75

## 3.2   Corticosteroids

Corticosteroids have been used in asthma for many years. In recent years, with the introduction of corticosteroid inhalations, their use has increased and has been extended to the prophylactic treatment of less severe and more chronic asthma, as the side-effects associated with systemic administration (see section 6.3.3) are much reduced.

Corticosteroids are usually of no benefit in patients with chronic bronchitis and emphysema; some patients with asthma, however, may be clinically indistinguishable from those with chronic bronchitis except that they will respond to a trial course of corticosteroids.

The action of corticosteroids is not fully understood but it is probable that they provide relief by reducing bronchial mucosal inflammatory reactions such as oedema and hypersecretion of mucus.

INHALATION. Corticosteroid aerosol inhalations must be used regularly to obtain maximum benefit; alleviation of symptoms usually occurs 3 to 7 days after initiation. **Beclomethasone dipropionate** and **budesonide** appear to be equally effective. *High-dose inhalers* are available for patients who only have a partial response to *standard inhalers*.

The maximum doses for high-dose corticosteroid inhalers are associated with some adrenal suppression (see section 6.3.3), therefore patients on high doses should be given a 'steroid card' and may need corticosteroid cover during an episode of stress (e.g. an operation). Systemic therapy may also be necessary during episodes of infection or increased bronchoconstriction where higher doses are needed and access of inhaled drug to small airways may be reduced; patients may need a reserve supply of tablets.

Corticosteroids are better inhaled using spacing devices (e.g. Nebuhaler® or Volumatic®). These increase airway deposition and reduce oropharyngeal deposition, resulting in a marked reduction in the incidence of candidiasis and reducing systemic absorption (so that there is less adrenal suppression); these devices are bulky, but most patients only need to use them morning and night.

*Dry powder inhalers* (Becotide Rotacaps®) (see section 3.1.1 for description) may be tried in patients who are unable to use the aerosol inhalers.

Beclomethasone dipropionate *suspension for nebulisation* is relatively inefficient because of its poor solubility; only a small amount is nebulised in 15 minutes. A spacing device will allow a larger amount to be administered more effectively and can be used by some children as young as 2 years.

Maximum penetration of inhaled corticosteroid is facilitated if a beta$_2$-adrenoceptor stimulant drug such as salbutamol is inhaled beforehand.

Patients who have been taking long-term oral corticosteroids can often be transferred to inhalation but the transfer must be done slowly, with gradual reduction in dose of oral corticosteroid, and at a time when the asthma is well controlled.

ORAL. *Acute attacks* of asthma should be treated with short courses of oral corticosteroids starting with a high dose, e.g. prednisolone 30 to 40 mg daily for a few days, gradually reduced once the attack has been controlled. Patients whose asthma has deteriorated rapidly usually respond quickly to corticosteroids, which can then be tailed down over a few days; more gradual reduction is necessary in those whose asthma has deteriorated gradually.

For use of corticosteroids in the emergency treatment of *severe acute asthma* see section 3.1.1.

In *chronic continuing asthma*, when the response to other anti-asthma drugs has been relatively small, continued administration of oral corticosteroids may be necessary; in such cases high doses of inhaled corticosteroids should be continued so that oral requirements are reduced to a minimum. Oral corticosteroids should normally be taken as a single dose in the morning to reduce the disturbance to circadian cortisol secretion. Dosage should always be titrated to the lowest dose which controls symptoms. Regular monitored peak flow measurements often help both patient and doctor to adjust the dose optimally. Prednisolone is available as tablets of 1 mg as well as 5 mg, and the smaller tablets may conveniently be used to adjust the maintenance dosage to the minimum necessary.

*Alternate-day* administration has not been very successful in the management of asthma and patients tend to deteriorate during the second 24 hours. If an attempt is made to introduce this pulmonary function should be monitored carefully over the 48 hours.

**Corticotrophin** and **tetracosactrin** (see section 6.5.1) were formerly used instead of the corticosteroids; their value was limited by the variable and unpredictable therapeutic response and the waning of their effect with time.

## BECLOMETHASONE DIPROPIONATE

*Indications:* prophylaxis of asthma especially if not fully controlled by bronchodilators or cromoglycate

*Cautions:* see notes above; also active or quiescent tuberculosis; may need to reinstate systemic therapy during periods of stress or when airways obstruction or mucus prevent drug access to smaller airways

*Side-effects:* hoarseness; candidiasis of mouth or throat, usually only with large doses (reduced by using spacer, see notes above; responds to

antifungal lozenges, see section 12.3.2, without discontinuation of therapy; rinsing the mouth with water after inhalation of a dose may also be helpful)

*Dose:* see preparations below

Standard-dose inhalers

PoM **AeroBec**® (3M)

*Aerosol inhalation*, beclomethasone dipropionate 50 micrograms/metered inhalation, net price 200-inhalation unit = £11.00; 200-inhalation breath-actuated unit (Autohaler®) = £11.00. Label: 8, counselling, dose

*Dose: by aerosol inhalation*, 100 micrograms 3–4 times daily *or* 200 micrograms twice daily (in more severe cases initially 600–800 micrograms daily); CHILD 50–100 micrograms 2–4 times daily

PoM **Becodisks**® (A&H)

*Powder for inhalation*, disks containing 8 blisters of beclomethasone dipropionate 100 micrograms/blister, net price pack of 14 disks with Diskhaler® = £10.99, 14-disk refill = £10.42;

200 micrograms/blister, pack of 14 disks with Diskhaler® = £20.90, 14-disk refill = £20.33;

400 micrograms/blister, pack of 7 disks with Diskhaler® = £20.90, 7-disk refill = £20.33.

Label: 8, counselling, dose

*Dose: by inhalation of powder*, 400 micrograms twice daily *or* 200 micrograms 3–4 times daily; CHILD 100 micrograms 2–4 times daily *or* 200 micrograms twice daily

PoM **Becotide Inhaler**® (A&H)

*Becotide-50 aerosol inhalation*, beclomethasone dipropionate 50 micrograms/metered inhalation. Net price 200-dose unit = £5.56. Label: 8, counselling, dose

*Becotide-100 aerosol inhalation*, beclomethasone dipropionate 100 micrograms/metered inhalation. Net price 200-dose unit = £10.56. Label: 8, counselling, dose

*Becotide-200 aerosol inhalation*, beclomethasone dipropionate 200 micrograms/metered inhalation. Net price 200-dose unit = £20.07. Label: 8, counselling, dose

Note. Becotide-200 not indicated for children

*Dose: by aerosol inhalation*, 200 micrograms twice daily *or* 100 micrograms 3–4 times daily (in more severe cases initially 600–800 micrograms daily); CHILD 50–100 micrograms 2–4 times daily *or* 100–200 micrograms twice daily

PoM **Becotide Rotacaps**® (A&H)

*Rotacaps*®, buff/clear, beclomethasone dipropionate 100 micrograms. Net price 100-cap pack = £7.56. Label: 8, counselling, dose

*Rotacaps*®, brown/clear, beclomethasone dipropionate 200 micrograms. Net price 100-cap pack = £14.35. Label: 8, counselling, dose

*Rotacaps*®, dark brown/clear, beclomethasone dipropionate 400 micrograms. Net price 100-cap pack = £27.27. Label: 8, counselling, dose

*Dose: by inhalation of powder*, 200 micrograms 3–4 times daily or 400 micrograms twice daily; max. 1 mg daily; CHILD 100 micrograms 2–4 times daily *or* 200 micrograms twice daily

PoM **Becotide Suspension for Nebulisation**® (A&H)

*Suspension for nebulisation*, beclomethasone dipropionate 50 micrograms/mL. Net price 10 mL = £2.50. For use with respirator or nebuliser. May be diluted up to 50% with sterile physiological saline

*Dose: by inhalation of nebulised suspension*, CHILD up to 1 year 50 micrograms 2–4 times daily; 1–12 years 100 micrograms 2–4 times daily, adjusted according to response

*Note.* Unsuitable for adults because of large volumes required.

High-dose inhalers

*Note.* High-dose inhalers not indicated for children

PoM **AeroBec Forte**® (3M)

*Aerosol inhalation*, beclomethasone dipropionate 250 micrograms/metered inhalation, net price 200-inhalation unit = £25.10; 200-inhalation breath-actuated unit (Autohaler®) = £25.10. Label: 8, counselling, dose, 10 steroid card

*Dose: by aerosol inhalation*, 250 micrograms 4 times daily *or* 500 micrograms twice daily; if necessary may be increased to 500 micrograms 4 times daily

PoM **Becloforte**® (A&H)

*Aerosol inhalation*, beclomethasone dipropionate 250 micrograms/metered inhalation. Net price 200-dose unit = £23.10; net price Becloforte® VM (2 Becloforte® inhalers with Volumatic®) = £46.20. Label: 8, counselling, dose, 10 steroid card

*Dose: by aerosol inhalation*, 500 micrograms (2 puffs) twice daily *or* 250 micrograms (1 puff) 4 times daily; if necessary may be increased to 500 micrograms 3–4 times daily

Compound preparations

Not recommended, see section 3.3

PoM **Ventide**® (A&H)

*Aerosol inhalation*, beclomethasone dipropionate 50 micrograms, salbutamol 100 micrograms/metered inhalation. Net price 200-dose unit = £8.02. Label: 8, counselling, dose

*Dose:* maintenance, 2 puffs 3–4 times daily; CHILD 1–2 puffs 2–4 times daily

*Paediatric Rotacaps*®, light grey/clear, beclomethasone dipropionate 100 micrograms, salbutamol (as sulphate) 200 micrograms. Net price 100 = £12.59. Label: 8, counselling, dose

*Dose: by inhalation of powder*, 1 Paediatric Rotacap® 2–4 times daily

*Rotacaps*®, dark grey/clear, beclomethasone dipropionate 200 micrograms, salbutamol (as sulphate) 400 micrograms. Net price 100 = £22.83. Label: 8, counselling, dose

*Dose: by inhalation of powder*, 1 Rotacap® 3–4 times daily

Inhaler devices

See section 3.1.5

---

## BUDESONIDE

*Indications; Cautions; Side-effects:* see under Beclomethasone Dipropionate

*Dose:* see preparations

PoM **Pulmicort Inhaler**® (Astra)

*LS aerosol inhalation*, budesonide 50 micrograms/metered inhalation. Net price 200-dose unit with standard or Spacer inhaler = £6.66; 200-dose refill for use with Nebuhaler or Spacer inhaler = £4.66. Label: 8, counselling, dose

*Aerosol inhalation*, budesonide 200 micrograms/metered inhalation. Net price 200-dose unit with standard or Spacer inhaler = £19.00; 200-dose refill for use with Nebuhaler or Spacer inhaler = £17.00; 100-dose unit with standard and Spacer inhaler = £8.16 (hosp. only); 100-dose refill = £8.66 (hosp. only). Label: 8, counselling, dose, 10 steroid card

*Turbohaler*® (= breath-actuated dry powder inhaler), budesonide 200 micrograms/inhalation, net price 100-dose unit = £18.50; 400 micrograms/inhalation, 50-dose unit = £18.50. Label: 8, counselling, dose, 10 steroid card

*Note.* Little sensation associated with use

*Dose: by aerosol inhalation*, 200 micrograms twice daily; may be reduced to not less than 200 micrograms daily; in severe asthma dose may be increased to 1.6 mg daily; CHILD 50–200 micrograms twice daily; in severe asthma may be increased to 400 micrograms twice daily

PoM **Pulmicort Respules**® (Astra)

*Respules*® (= single-dose units for nebulisation), budesonide 250 micrograms/mL, net price 20 × 2-mL unit = £32.00; 500 micrograms/mL, 20 × 2-mL unit = £44.64. May be diluted up to 50% with sterile physiological saline. Label: 8, counselling, dose, 10 steroid card

*Dose: by inhalation of nebulised suspension*, when starting treatment, during periods of severe asthma, and while reducing or discontinuing oral corticosteroids, 1–2 mg twice daily (may be increased further in very severe asthma); CHILD 3 months–12 years, 0.5–1 mg twice daily

Maintenance, usually half above doses

Inhaler devices

See section 3.1.5

## 3.3   Cromoglycate and related therapy

Regular inhalation of sodium cromoglycate can reduce the incidence of attacks of asthma and allow dosage reduction of bronchodilators and oral corticosteroids. In general, prophylaxis with sodium cromoglycate is less effective in adults than prophylaxis with corticosteroid inhalations (see section 3.2) but the fact that in the long term corticosteroid inhalations may be associated with more side-effects needs to be borne in mind. Sodium cromoglycate is of no value in the treatment of acute attacks of asthma.

---

Sodium cromoglycate is of value in the prevention of exercise-induced asthma, a single dose being inhaled half-an-hour beforehand.

The mode of action of sodium cromoglycate is not completely understood but it prevents release of pharmacological mediators of bronchospasm by stabilising mast-cell membranes. It is of particular value in asthma with an allergic basis, but, in practice, it is difficult to predict who will benefit, therefore it is reasonable to try it for a 4-week period in any patient whose asthma is poorly controlled with bronchodilators. Children seem to respond better than adults. Dose frequency is adjusted according to response but is usually 4 times a day initially; this may subsequently be reduced.

If inhalation of the dry powder form of sodium cromoglycate causes bronchospasm a selective beta$_2$-adrenoceptor stimulant such as salbutamol or terbutaline should be inhaled a few minutes beforehand. The nebuliser solution is useful for patients who cannot manage the dry powder inhaler or the aerosol.

**Nedocromil** has a pharmacological action similar to that of sodium cromoglycate.

**Ketotifen** is an antihistamine with an action said to resemble that of sodium cromoglycate. It has not fulfilled its early promise.

## SODIUM CROMOGLYCATE
*Indications:* prophylaxis of asthma
*Side-effects:* coughing, transient bronchospasm, and throat irritation due to inhalation of powder (see also notes above)
*Dose:* see below
COUNSELLING. Regular use is necessary

PoM **Intal**® (Fisons)
*Aerosol inhalation*, sodium cromoglycate 5 mg/metered inhalation. Net price 112-dose unit = £14.52. Label: 8
*Dose: by aerosol inhalation*, adults and children, 10 mg (2 puffs) 4 times daily initially, increased in severe cases or during periods of risk to 6–8 times daily; additional doses may also be taken before exercise; maintenance 5 mg (1 puff) 4 times daily
*Note.* Formerly Intal 5®
*Autohaler*® (= breath-actuated inhaler), sodium cromoglycate 5 mg/metered inhalation. Net price 112-dose unit = £18.99. Label: 8
*Dose:* as for Aerosol inhalation above
*Spincaps*®, yellow/clear, sodium cromoglycate 20 mg. Net price 112-cap pack = £11.59. Label: 8
*Dose: by inhalation of powder*, adults and children, 20 mg 4 times daily, increased in severe cases to 8 times daily
*Spinhaler insufflator*® (for use with Intal and Intal Compound Spincaps). Net price = £1.80
*Nebuliser solution*, sodium cromoglycate 10 mg/mL. Net price 2-mL amp = 25p. For use with power-operated nebuliser
*Dose: by inhalation of nebulised solution*, adults and children, 20 mg 4 times daily, increased in severe cases to 6 times daily

PoM **Intal Compound**® (Fisons)
*Spincaps*®, orange/clear, isoprenaline sulphate 100 micrograms, sodium cromoglycate 20 mg. Net price 112-cap pack = £9.17. Label: 8
*Note.* The compound inhalation of sodium cromoglycate with isoprenaline is not recommended; not only has isoprenaline a less selective action but the inhalation is liable to be used inappropriately for relief of bronchospasm rather than for its prophylactic effect

## KETOTIFEN
*Indications:* see notes above
*Cautions:* previous anti-asthmatic treatment should be continued for a minimum of 2 weeks after initiation of ketotifen treatment; **interactions:** Appendix 1 (antihistamines)
DRIVING. Drowsiness may affect performance of skilled tasks (e.g. driving); effects of alcohol enhanced
*Side-effects:* dry mouth, sedation
*Dose:* 1–2 mg twice daily with food; initial treatment in readily sedated patients 0.5–1 mg at night; CHILD over 2 years 1 mg twice daily

PoM **Zaditen**® (Sandoz)
*Capsules*, ketotifen 1 mg (as hydrogen fumarate). Net price 60-cap pack = £8.35. Label: 2, 8, 21
*Tablets*, off-white, scored, ketotifen 1 mg (as hydrogen fumarate). Net price 60-tab pack = £8.35. Label: 2, 8, 21
*Elixir*, sugar-free, ketotifen 1 mg (as hydrogen fumarate)/5 mL. Net price 150 mL = £4.94. Label: 2, 8, 21

## NEDOCROMIL SODIUM
*Indications:* prophylaxis of asthma
*Side-effects:* see under Sodium Cromoglycate; also headache, nausea (both mild and transient); bitter taste (masked by mint flavour)
*Dose: by aerosol inhalation*, 4 mg (2 puffs) twice daily, increased to 4 times daily if necessary; CHILD under 12 years, not yet recommended

PoM **Tilade Mint**® (Fisons)
*Aerosol inhalation*, nedocromil sodium 2 mg/metered inhalation. Net price 2 × 56-puff mint-flavoured units = £17.76. Label: 8

# 3.4 Antihistamines, hyposensitisation, and allergic emergencies

**3.4.1** Antihistamines
**3.4.2** Hyposensitisation
**3.4.3** Allergic emergencies

For the treatment of asthma see sections 3.1.1 and 3.2. For the treatment of hay fever by nasal application of corticosteroids and prophylaxis with sodium cromoglycate see section 12.2. For eye preparations see section 11.4. For the treatment of allergic skin conditions with topical corticosteroid preparations see section 13.4.

## 3.4.1　Antihistamines

All antihistamines are of potential value in the treatment of *nasal allergies*, particularly seasonal (hay fever), and may be of some value in *vasomotor rhinitis*. They reduce rhinorrhoea and sneezing but are usually less effective for nasal congestion.

Oral antihistamines are also of some value in preventing *urticaria* and are used to treat *allergic rashes, pruritus*, and *insect bites and stings*; they are also used in *drug allergies*. Injections of chlorpheniramine or promethazine are used as an adjunct to adrenaline in the emergency treatment of *angioedema* and *anaphylaxis* (section 3.4.3).

There is no evidence that any one of the older, sedative antihistamines is superior to any other and patients vary widely in their responses. They differ somewhat in duration of action and incidence of side-effects (drowsiness and antimuscarinic effects). Most are relatively short-acting but some, (e.g. promethazine) act for up to 12 hours. They all cause sedation but **promethazine**, **trimeprazine**, and **dimenhydrinate** may be more sedating whereas **chlorpheniramine**, **cyclizine**, and **mequitazine** may be less so.

**Acrivastine**, **astemizole**, **cetirizine**, **loratadine**, and **terfenadine** are newer antihistamines; they are a very major advance over the older antihistamines. They cause less sedation and psychomotor impairment because they only penetrate the blood brain barrier to a slight extent (and for this reason do not alleviate pruritus of non-allergic origin). Astemizole has a relatively slow onset of action and is more appropriate for use on a regular basis than when symptoms occur. The drug interactions described in Appendix 1 apply to a lesser extent to the non-sedative antihistamines, and they do not appear to potentiate the effects of alcohol.

DISADVANTAGES OF ANTIHISTAMINES. With most of the older antihistamines drowsiness is a serious disadvantage; patients should be warned that their ability to drive or operate machinery may be impaired, and that the effects of alcohol may be increased. Other side-effects include headache, psychomotor impairment, antimuscarinic effects such as urinary retention, dry mouth, blurred vision, and gastro-intestinal disturbances; occasional rashes and photosensitivity reactions have been reported; paradoxical stimulation may rarely occur, especially in high dosage or in children. Antihistamines should be used with caution in epilepsy, prostatic hypertrophy, glaucoma, and hepatic disease. Most antihistamines should be avoided in *porphyria*, but chlorpheniramine and cyclizine have been used (see section 9.8.2). **Interactions:** Appendix 1 (antihistamines). **Pregnancy** and **breast-feeding:** Appendixes 4 and 5 (antihistamines).

---

NON-SEDATIVE ANTIHISTAMINES

---

DRIVING. Although drowsiness is rare, nevertheless patients should be advised that it can occur and may affect performance of skilled tasks (e.g. driving); excess alcohol should be avoided.

## ACRIVASTINE

*Indications:* symptomatic relief of allergy such as hay fever, urticaria

*Cautions:* see notes above; pending specific studies avoid in renal impairment

*Side-effects:* see notes above; incidence of sedation and antimuscarinic effects low

*Dose:* 8 mg 3 times daily; CHILD under 12 years, not yet recommended

PoM **Semprex**® (Wellcome)
*Capsules*, acrivastine 8 mg. Net price 84-cap pack = £5.92. Counselling, driving

## ASTEMIZOLE

*Indications:* symptomatic relief of allergy such as hay fever, urticaria

*Cautions:* see notes above; pregnancy (toxicity at high doses in *animal* studies)

*Side-effects:* see notes above; weight gain occurs infrequently; incidence of sedation is low; antimuscarinic effects and psychomotor impairment have not been reported; ventricular arrhythmias have followed excessive dosage

*Dose:* 10 mg daily (must **not** be exceeded); CHILD 6–12 years, 5 mg daily (must **not** be exceeded)

PoM [1]**Hismanal**® (Janssen)
*Tablets*, scored, astemizole 10 mg. Net price 30-tab pack = £5.70. Counselling, driving
*Suspension*, sugar-free, astemizole 5 mg/5 mL. Net price 100 mL = £2.90;　200 mL = £5.80. Counselling, driving
1. Can be sold to the public provided it is licensed and labelled for the treatment of hay fever in adults and children over 12 years; a proprietary brand of astemizole tablets (Pollon-eze®) is on sale to the public

## CETIRIZINE

*Indications:* symptomatic relief of allergy such as hay fever, urticaria

*Cautions:* see notes above; halve dose in renal impairment; incidence of sedation and antimuscarinic effects low

*Side-effects:* see notes above

*Dose:* 10 mg daily *or* 5 mg twice daily; CHILD under 12 years, not yet recommended

PoM **Zirtek**® (A&H)
*Tablets*, f/c, scored, cetirizine hydrochloride 10 mg. Net price 30-tab pack = £8.95. Counselling, driving

## LORATADINE

*Indications:* symptomatic relief of allergy such as hay fever; urticaria

*Cautions; Side-effects:* see notes above; incidence of sedation and antimuscarinic effects low; pregnancy (toxicity at high doses in *animals*)

*Dose:* 10 mg daily; CHILD under 12 years, not yet recommended

PoM **Clarityn**® (Schering-Plough)
*Tablets*, scored, loratadine 10 mg. Net price 30-tab pack = £6.90. Counselling, driving

## TERFENADINE

*Indications:* symptomatic relief of allergy such as hay fever, urticaria
*Cautions:* see notes above; **interactions:** Appendix 1 (antihistamines)
*Side-effects:* see notes above; incidence of sedation is low; antimuscarinic effects and psychomotor impairment have not been reported; possibly associated with hair loss; ventricular arrhythmias (torsade de pointes) have followed excessive dosage
*Dose:* 60 mg twice daily *or* 120 mg in the morning; CHILD 3–6 years 15 mg twice daily; 6–12 years 30 mg twice daily

**Triludan**® (Merrell)
*Tablets*, scored, terfenadine 60 mg. Net price 60-tab pack = £5.80. Counselling, driving
*Forte tablets*, terfenadine 120 mg. Net price 7-tab pack = £2.02; 30-tab pack = £5.80. Counselling, driving
*Suspension*, sugar-free, terfenadine 30 mg/5 mL. Net price 200 mL = £4.24. Counselling, driving
*Note.* A proprietary brand of terfenadine (Seldane®) is on sale to the public

## SEDATIVE ANTIHISTAMINES

DRIVING. Drowsiness may affect performance of skilled tasks (e.g. driving); effects of alcohol enhanced.

## AZATADINE MALEATE

*Indications:* symptomatic relief of allergy such as hay fever, urticaria
*Cautions; Side-effects:* see notes above
*Dose:* 1 mg, increased if necessary to 2 mg, twice daily; CHILD 1–6 years 250 micrograms twice daily, 6–12 years 0.5–1 mg twice daily

**Optimine**® (Schering-Plough)
*Tablets*, scored, azatadine maleate 1 mg. Net price 56-tab pack = £4.48. Label: 2
*Syrup*, azatadine maleate 500 micrograms/5 mL. Diluent syrup, life of diluted syrup 28 days. Net price 120 mL = £1.43. Label: 2

## BROMPHENIRAMINE MALEATE

*Indications:* symptomatic relief of allergy such as hay fever, urticaria
*Cautions; Side-effects:* see notes above
*Dose:* 4–8 mg 3–4 times daily; CHILD up to 3 years 0.4–1 mg/kg daily in 4 divided doses, 3–6 years 2 mg 3–4 times daily, 6–12 years 2–4 mg 3–4 times daily

**Dimotane**® (Wyeth)
*Tablets*, peach, scored, brompheniramine maleate 4 mg. Net price 20 = 70p. Label: 2
*Elixir*, yellow-green, brompheniramine maleate 2 mg/5 mL. Diluent syrup, life of diluted elixir 14 days. Net price 100 mL = 84p. Label: 2

**Dimotane LA**® (Wyeth)
*Tablets*, m/r, peach, s/c, brompheniramine maleate 12 mg. Net price 20 = £1.05. Label: 2, 25
*Dose:* 12–24 mg twice daily; CHILD 6–12 years 12 mg at bedtime, increased if necessary to 12 mg twice daily

## CHLORPHENIRAMINE MALEATE

*Indications:* symptomatic relief of allergy such as hay fever, urticaria; emergency treatment of anaphylactic reactions (section 3.4.3)
*Cautions; Side-effects:* see notes above. Injections may be irritant and cause transitory hypotension or CNS stimulation
*Dose: by mouth*, 4 mg every 4–6 hours, max. 24 mg daily; CHILD 1–2 years 1 mg twice daily, 2–5 years 1 mg every 4–6 hours, max. 6 mg daily, 6–12 years 2 mg every 4–6 hours, max. 12 mg daily
*By subcutaneous or intramuscular injection*, 10–20 mg, repeated if required; max. 40 mg in 24 hours
*By slow intravenous injection* over 1 minute, 10–20 mg diluted in syringe with 5–10 mL blood

**Chlorpheniramine** (Non-proprietary)
*Tablets*, chlorpheniramine maleate 4 mg. Net price 20 = 9p. Label: 2
Available from Cox
**Piriton**® (A&H)
*Tablets*, ivory, chlorpheniramine maleate 4 mg. Net price 20 = 19p. Label: 2
*Syrup*, chlorpheniramine maleate 2 mg/5 mL. Diluent syrup (without preservative), life of diluted syrup 14 days. Net price 150 mL = 29p. Label: 2
PoM *Injection*, chlorpheniramine maleate 10 mg/mL. Net price 1-mL amp = 12p

## CINNARIZINE
See section 4.6

## CLEMASTINE

*Indications:* symptomatic relief of allergy such as hay fever, urticaria
*Cautions; Side-effects:* see notes above
*Dose:* 1 mg twice daily; CHILD 1–3 years 250–500 micrograms twice daily; 3–6 years 500 micrograms twice daily; 6–12 years 0.5–1 mg twice daily; CHILD under 1 year, no longer recommended

**Tavegil**® (Sandoz)
*Tablets*, scored, clemastine 1 mg (as hydrogen fumarate). Net price 50-tab pack = £2.10. Label: 2
*Elixir*, sugar-free, clemastine 500 micrograms (as hydrogen fumarate)/5 mL. Diluent syrup or sorbitol solution 70%, life of diluted elixir 14 days. Net price 150 mL = 98p. Label: 2
*Note.* A proprietary brand of clemastine hydrogen fumarate (Aller-Eze®) is on sale to the public

## CYCLIZINE
See section 4.6

---

## CYPROHEPTADINE HYDROCHLORIDE

*Indications:* symptomatic relief of allergy such as hay fever, urticaria

*Cautions; Side-effects:* see notes above; may cause weight gain

*Dose:* allergy, usual dose 4 mg 3–4 times daily; usual range 4–20 mg daily, max. 32 mg daily; CHILD 2–6 years 2 mg 2–3 times daily, max. 12 mg daily; 7–14 years 4 mg 2–3 times daily, max. 16 mg daily

Migraine, 4 mg with a further 4 mg after 30 minutes if necessary; maintenance, 4 mg every 4–6 hours

Stimulation of appetite—not recommended therefore no dose stated

**Periactin®** (MSD)
*Tablets,* scored, cyproheptadine hydrochloride 4 mg. Net price 20 = 57p. Label: 2
*Syrup,* yellow, cyproheptadine hydrochloride 2 mg/5 mL. Diluent syrup, life of diluted syrup 14 days. Net price 200 mL = £1.27. Label: 2

## DIMENHYDRINATE

See section 4.6

## DIMETHINDENE MALEATE

*Indications:* symptomatic relief of allergy such as hay fever, urticaria

*Cautions; Side-effects:* see notes above

**Fenostil Retard®** (Zyma)
*Tablets,* m/r, greyish-white, dimethindene maleate 2.5 mg. Net price 20 = 57p. Label: 2, 25
*Dose:* 2.5 mg twice daily

## DIPHENHYDRAMINE HYDROCHLORIDE

*Indications:* symptomatic relief of allergy such as hay fever

*Cautions; Side-effects:* see notes above

**Preparations**
Ingredient of compound cough preparations (section 3.9.2)

## DIPHENYLPYRALINE HYDROCHLORIDE

*Indications:* symptomatic relief of allergy such as hay fever, urticaria

*Cautions; Side-effects:* see notes above

**Histryl®** (SK&F)
*Spansule®* (= capsules m/r), pink/clear, enclosing pink and white pellets, diphenylpyraline hydrochloride 5 mg. Net price 30-cap pack = £1.79. Label: 2, 25
*Dose:* 5–10 mg twice daily
*Paediatric Spansule®* (= capsules m/r), pink/clear, enclosing pink and white pellets, diphenylpyraline hydrochloride 2.5 mg. Net price 30-cap pack = £1.36. Label: 1, 25
*Dose:* CHILD over 7 years 2.5 mg twice daily

## HYDROXYZINE HYDROCHLORIDE

See section 4.1.2

## KETOTIFEN

See section 3.3

## MEBHYDROLIN

*Indications:* symptomatic relief of allergy such as hay fever, urticaria

*Cautions:* see notes above

*Side-effects:* see notes above; also very rarely granulocytopenia or agranulocytosis

*Dose:* ADULT and CHILD over 10 years, 50–100 mg 3 times daily

**PoM Fabahistin®** (Bayer)
*Tablets,* orange, s/c, mebhydrolin 50 mg. Net price 20 = 68p. Label: 2

## MEQUITAZINE

*Indications:* symptomatic relief of allergy such as hay fever, urticaria

*Cautions; Side-effects:* see notes above

*Dose:* 5 mg twice daily; CHILD under 12 years, not yet recommended

**PoM Primalan®** (Rhône-Poulenc Rorer)
*Tablets,* mequitazine 5 mg. Net price 56-tab pack = £5.00. Label: 2

## OXATOMIDE

*Indications:* symptomatic relief of allergy such as hay fever, food allergy, urticaria

*Cautions; Side-effects:* see notes above; drowsiness most common; increased appetite with weight gain may occur above 120 mg daily

*Dose:* 30 mg twice daily after food, increased if necessary to 60 mg twice daily; ELDERLY 30 mg twice daily; CHILD 5–14 years 15–30 mg twice daily

**PoM Tinset®** (Janssen)
*Tablets,* scored, oxatomide 30 mg. Net price 25-tab pack = £4.90. Label: 2, 21

## PHENINDAMINE TARTRATE

*Indications:* symptomatic relief of allergy such as hay fever, urticaria

*Cautions; Side-effects:* see notes above; may cause mild CNS stimulation

*Dose:* 25–50 mg 1–3 times daily; CHILD over 10 years 25 mg 1–3 times daily

**Thephorin®** (Sinclair)
*Tablets,* s/c, phenindamine tartrate 25 mg. Net price 50-tab pack = £2.42. Label: 2

## PHENIRAMINE MALEATE

*Indications:* symptomatic relief of allergy such as hay fever, urticaria

*Cautions; Side-effects:* see notes above

**Daneral SA®** (Hoechst)
*Tablets,* m/r, pink, s/c, pheniramine maleate 75 mg. Net price 30-tab pack = £2.61. Label: 2, 25
*Dose:* 75–150 mg at night or 75 mg night and morning

---

## PROMETHAZINE HYDROCHLORIDE

*Indications:* symptomatic relief of allergy such as hay fever, urticaria, emergency treatment of anaphylactic reactions (section 3.4.3)

For use in premedication see section 15.1.4.1; sedation see section 4.1.1

*Cautions; Side-effects:* see notes above; intra-muscular injection may be painful

*Dose: by mouth,* 25 mg at night increased to 50 mg if necessary *or* 10–20 mg 2–3 times daily; CHILD 1–5 years 5–15 mg daily (1–2 years on doctor's advice only), 5–10 years 10–25 mg daily

*By deep intramuscular injection,* 25–50 mg; max. 100 mg; CHILD 5–10 years 6.25–12.5 mg

*By slow intravenous injection* in emergencies, 25–50 mg, max. 100 mg, as a solution containing 2.5 mg/mL in water for injections

**Phenergan**® (Rhône-Poulenc Rorer)
*Tablets,* both blue, f/c, promethazine hydro-chloride 10 mg, net price 56-tab pack = £1.03; 25 mg, 56-tab pack = £1.53. Label: 2

*Elixir,* golden, promethazine hydrochloride 5 mg/5 mL. Net price 100 mL = £1.15. Label: 2

PoM *Injection,* promethazine hydrochloride 25 mg/mL. Net price 1-mL amp = 28p; 2-mL amp = 34p

*Note.* A proprietary brand of promethazine hydro-chloride tablets 20 mg (Sominex®) is on sale to the public for the treatment of occasional insomnia in adults

## PROMETHAZINE THEOCLATE

See section 4.6

## TRIMEPRAZINE TARTRATE

*Indications:* urticaria and pruritus; premedication, see section 15.1.4.1

*Cautions; Side-effects:* see notes above

*Dose:* 10 mg 2–3 times daily, in severe cases up to max. 100 mg daily has been used; ELDERLY 10 mg 1–2 times daily; CHILD over 2 years 2.5–5 mg 3–4 times daily

PoM **Vallergan**® (Rhône-Poulenc Rorer)
*Tablets,* blue, f/c, trimeprazine tartrate 10 mg. Net price 28-tab pack = £1.06. Label: 2

*Syrup,* straw coloured, trimeprazine tartrate 7.5 mg/5 mL. Diluent syrup (without preserv-atives), life of diluted syrup 14 days. Net price 100 mL = £1.20. Label: 2

*Syrup forte,* trimeprazine tartrate 30 mg/5 mL. Diluent as above. Net price 100 mL = £2.48. Label: 2

*Note.* For use of Forte Syrup see section 15.1.4.2

## TRIPROLIDINE HYDROCHLORIDE

*Indications:* symptomatic relief of allergy such as hay fever, urticaria

*Cautions; Side-effects:* see notes above

*Dose:* see preparation

**Pro-Actidil**® (Wellcome)
*Tablets,* m/r, white/pink/blue, triprolidine hydrochloride 10 mg. Net price 20 = £5.48. Label: 2, 25

*Dose:* 10 mg early evening or 5–6 hours before retiring increased to 20 mg daily if symptoms very severe; CHILD under 12 years not rec-ommended

## 3.4.2  Hyposensitisation

Except for wasp and bee sting allergy the value of specific hyposensitisation is uncertain; administration of allergen extract desensitising vaccines is associated with a significant risk of anaphylaxis, see CSM warn-ing below. Most atopic (allergic) patients are sensitive to a wide range of allergens hence hyposensitisation with an extract of a single allergen is usually more than partially successful.

Diagnostic skin tests are unreliable and can only be used in conjunction with a detailed history of allergen exposure.

**CSM Warning.** The CSM has warned that since 1980, in the UK alone, 11 patients, most of whom were young, have died from anaphylaxis caused by allergen extract desensitising vaccines; patients with asthma appear to be particularly susceptible. The CSM is not aware of such problems when these allergens are used for diagnostic purposes (skin testing). Although some vaccines can prevent anaphylactic reactions (e.g. to bee stings) the effectiveness of the others is con-troversial. The CSM therefore recommends that it is important for doctors to balance carefully the known risks of desensitising vaccines against potential ben-efits before embarking on treatment. *Such treatment should only be carried out where facilities for full cardiorespiratory resuscitation are immediately avail-able, and patients should be kept under medical obser-vation for at least 2 hours after treatment.*

For details of the management of anaphylactic shock, see section 3.4.3.

### ALLERGEN EXTRACT VACCINES

Each set usually contains vials for the admin-istration of graded amounts to patients undergoing hyposensitisation. Maintenance sets containing vials at the highest strength are also available. Manufacturer's literature must be consulted for details of allergens, vial strengths, and adminis-tration

*Indications:* hypersensitivity to one or more com-mon allergens (see notes above)

*Cautions:* see notes above including CSM warning; manufacturers recommend that patients should be warned not to eat a heavy meal before the injection

*Contra-indications:* pregnancy, febrile conditions, acute asthma

*Side-effects:* allergic reactions, especially in small children

*Dose: by subcutaneous injection,* see manufacturer's literature; very sensitive patients may be given an antihistamine tablet one hour before the injection

Pollen allergy (hay fever) preparations

PoM **Spectralgen Single Species**® (Kabi Pharmacia)
Prepared from Timothy grass. Net price treatment set = £59.29

PoM **Spectralgen 4 Grass Mix**® (Kabi Pharmacia)
Prepared from 4 varieties of common grasses. Net price treatment set = £64.99

PoM **Spectralgen 3 Tree Mix**® (Kabi Pharmacia)
Prepared from 3 varieties of common trees. Net price treatment set = £63.06

Wasp and bee venom allergy preparations

PoM **Pharmalgen**® (Kabi Pharmacia)
Bee venom extract (*Apis mellifera*) or wasp venom extract (*Vespula* spp.). Net price treatment set = £45.50 (bee), £55.80 (wasp)

### 3.4.3    Allergic emergencies

*Anaphylactic shock* requires prompt energetic treatment of laryngeal oedema, bronchospasm, and hypotension. It is relatively uncommon and is usually precipitated by blood products, vaccines, insect stings, and certain drugs such as antibiotics, iron injections, anti-inflammatory analgesics, heparin, hyposensitising (allergen) preparations, and neuromuscular blocking drugs. It is more likely to occur after parenteral administration and atopic individuals are particularly susceptible.

First-line treatment includes restoration of blood pressure, laying the patient flat, raising the feet, and administration of **adrenaline**\* injection. This is given intramuscularly in a dose of 0.5–1 mg (0.5–1 mL adrenaline injection 1 in 1000), repeated every 10 minutes, according to blood pressure and pulse, until improvement occurs. Antihistamines, e.g. **chlorpheniramine**, given by slow intravenous injection (section 3.4.1), are a useful adjunctive treatment. This is given after adrenaline injection and continued for 24 to 48 hours to prevent relapse.

Continuing deterioration requires further treatment including intravenous fluids (see section 9.2.2), intravenous aminophylline (section 3.1.3) or a nebulised beta₂-adrenoceptor stimulant (such as salbutamol or terbutaline, section 3.1.1.1), oxygen, assisted respiration, and possibly emergency tracheotomy.

Intravenous **corticosteroids** are of secondary value in anaphylactic shock as their onset of action is delayed for several hours but they should be used to prevent further deterioration in severely affected patients (see section 6.3.4).

Some patients with severe allergy to insect stings are encouraged to carry pre-filled adrenaline syringes for emergency administration during periods of risk; adrenaline inhalations (Medihaler-epi®) are much less effective.

*Angioedema* is dangerous when it affects respiration. If obstruction is present, adrenaline injection should be given as described above; antihistamine injections are also helpful but corticosteroids are of secondary value (see also

\* In patients on non-cardioselective beta-blockers severe anaphylaxis may not respond to adrenaline injection, calling for addition of salbutamol by intravenous injection

above). Tracheal intubation as well as other measures may be necessary.

## ADRENALINE

*Indications:* emergency treatment of acute anaphylaxis; cardiopulmonary resuscitation, section 2.7

*Cautions:* hyperthyroidism, diabetes mellitus, ischaemic heart disease, hypertension, elderly patients; **interactions:** Appendix 1 (sympathomimetics)

*Side-effects:* anxiety, tremor, tachycardia, arrhythmias, dry mouth, cold extremities

*Dose:* acute anaphylaxis, *by intramuscular injection,* see table below:

IMPORTANT. Intravenous route is for cardiac resuscitation **only** (see section 2.7)

| Age | Volume of adrenaline 1 in 1000 |
|---|---|
| Under 1 year | 0.05 mL |
| 1 year | 0.1 mL |
| 2 years | 0.2 mL[1] |
| 3–4 years | 0.3 mL[1] |
| 5 years | 0.4 mL[1] |
| 6–12 years | 0.5 mL[1] |
| Adult | 0.5–1 mL |

Volume of adrenaline injection 1 in 1000 (1 mg/mL) for intramuscular injection in anaphylactic shock

These doses may be repeated every 10 minutes, according to blood pressure and pulse, until improvement occurs (may be repeated several times).

1. Suitable for robust children in these age groups; for underweight children use half these doses.

PoM **Adrenaline Injection, BP,** adrenaline 1 in 1000 (adrenaline 1 mg/mL as acid tartrate). Net price 0.5-mL amp = 31p; 1-mL amp = 32p
Available from Boots, Evans, Martindale
*Note.* For 1 in 10000 strength, see section 2.7

PoM **Min-I-Jet**® **Adrenaline** (IMS)
*Injection*, adrenaline 1 in 1000 (1 mg/mL as hydrochloride). Net price 0.5-mL = £3.46; 1-mL = £2.97 (both disposable syringe)
*Injection*, adrenaline 1 in 10000, see section 2.7

Inhalation

PoM **Medihaler-epi**® (3M)
*Aerosol inhalation*, adrenaline acid tartrate 280 micrograms/metered inhalation. Net price 400-inhalation unit = £2.73
*Dose: by aerosol inhalation*, adjunct to anaphylaxis treatment only, min. of 20 puffs

## 3.5    Respiratory stimulants and surfactants

3.5.1  Respiratory stimulants
3.5.2  Respiratory surfactants

### 3.5.1    Respiratory stimulants

Respiratory stimulants (analeptic drugs) have a limited place in the treatment of ventilatory failure in patients with chronic obstructive airways disease. They are effective only when given by intravenous injection or infusion and have a short duration of action. Their use has largely been replaced by ventilatory support. However, occasionally when the latter is contra-indicated and in patients with hypercapnic respiratory failure who are becoming drowsy or comatose, respiratory stimulants in the short term may arouse patients sufficiently to co-operate and clear their secretions.

Respiratory stimulants may be harmful in respiratory failure since they stimulate non-respiratory as well as respiratory muscles. They should only be given under **expert supervision** in hospital and must be combined with active physiotherapy. There is at present no oral respiratory stimulant available for long-term use in chronic respiratory failure.

**Doxapram** is given by continuous intravenous infusion in a dosage of 2 mg per minute. Frequent arterial blood gas studies and pH measurements are necessary during treatment to ensure the correct dosage.

Nikethamide and ethamivan were formerly used as respiratory stimulants but are no longer recommended; the effective doses were close to those causing toxic effects, especially convulsions. Respiratory stimulants such as ethamivan and nikethamide have no place whatsoever in the management of asphyxia in the newborn.

## DOXAPRAM HYDROCHLORIDE

*Indications:* ventilatory failure (see notes above)
*Cautions:* epilepsy, hepatic impairment; see also notes above; **interactions:** Appendix 1 (doxapram)
*Contra-indications:* severe hypertension, status asthmaticus, coronary artery disease, thyrotoxicosis
*Side-effects:* increase in blood pressure and heart rate, dizziness, perineal warmth
*Dose: by intravenous infusion,* 1.5–4 mg per minute according to patient's response
*By intravenous injection* over at least 30 seconds, 1–1.5 mg/kg repeated if necessary at intervals of 1 hour
Postoperative respiratory depression, see section 15.1.7

PoM **Dopram**® (Wyeth)
*Injection,* doxapram hydrochloride 20 mg/mL. Net price 5-mL amp = £2.14
*Intravenous infusion,* doxapram hydrochloride 2 mg/mL in glucose 5%. Net price 500-mL bottle = £22.34

## NIKETHAMIDE

*Indications:* not recommended, see notes above
*Cautions:* see notes above, severe hypertension
*Contra-indications:* respiratory failure due to neurological disease or drug overdose; status asthmaticus, coronary artery disease, thyrotoxicosis; porphyria (see section 9.8.2)
*Side-effects:* nausea, restlessness, convulsions, dizziness, tremor, vasoconstriction, arrhythmias
*Dose: by slow intravenous injection,* 0.5–1 g but not recommended see notes above

PoM **Nikethamide Injection,** nikethamide 250 mg/mL. Net price 2-mL amp = £1.40 (hosp. only)

## ETHAMIVAN

*Indications; Cautions; Contra-indications; Side-effects:* see under Nikethamide and notes above
*Dose: by intravenous injection,* 100 mg, but not recommended see notes above

PoM **Clairvan**® (Sinclair)
*Injection,* ethamivan 50 mg/mL (5%). Net price 2-mL amp = £3.05

## 3.5.2   Respiratory surfactants

## COLFOSCERIL PALMITATE

*Indications:* newborn babies with birthweight of 700 g or more undergoing mechanical ventilation for respiratory distress syndrome, whose heart rate and arterial oxygenation are continuously monitored
*Cautions:* continuous monitoring required to avoid hyperoxaemia (due to rapid improvement in arterial oxygen concentration)
*Side-effects:* may increase incidence of pulmonary haemorrhage; obstruction of endotracheal tube by mucous secretions
*Dose: by endotracheal tube,* 67.5 mg/kg; if still intubated, may be repeated after 12 hours

▼ PoM **Exosurf Neonatal**® (Wellcome)
*Suspension,* colfosceril palmitate 108 mg for reconstitution with 8 mL water for injections (when reconstituted, contains 67.5 mg/5 mL). Net price per vial = £314.29

# 3.6   Oxygen

Oxygen should be regarded as a drug. It is prescribed for hypoxaemic patients to increase alveolar oxygen tension and decrease the work of breathing necessary to maintain a given arterial oxygen tension. The concentration depends on the condition being treated; an inappropriate concentration may have serious or even lethal effects.

*High concentration oxygen therapy,* with concentrations of up to 60% for short periods, is safe in conditions such as pneumonia, pulmonary thromboembolism, and fibrosing alveolitis. In such conditions low arterial oxygen ($P_aO_2$) is usually associated with low or normal arterial carbon dioxide ($P_aCO_2$), therefore there is little risk of hypoventilation and carbon dioxide retention.

In severe acute asthma, the arterial carbon dioxide ($P_aCO_2$) is usually subnormal but as asthma deteriorates may rise steeply (particularly in children). These patients usually require high concentrations of oxygen and if the arterial carbon dioxide ($P_aCO_2$) remains high despite other treatment intermittent positive pressure ventilation needs to be considered urgently. Where facilities for blood gas measurements are not immediately available, for example while transferring the patient to hospital, 35% to 50% oxygen delivered through a conventional mask is recommended. Exceptionally, asthma is diagnosed in patients with a long history of chronic bronchitis and probable respiratory failure; in these patients a lower concentration (24% to 28%) may be needed to limit oxygen-induced reduction of respiratory drive.

*Low concentration oxygen therapy* (controlled oxygen therapy) is reserved for patients with ventilatory failure due to chronic obstructive airways disease or other causes. The concentration should not exceed 28% and in some patients a concentration above 24% may be excessive. The aim is to provide the patient with just enough oxygen to improve hypoxaemia without worsening pre-existing carbon dioxide retention and respiratory acidosis. Treatment should be initiated in hospital as repeated blood gas measurements are required to estimate the correct concentration.

DOMICILIARY OXYGEN. Oxygen should only be prescribed for patients in the home after careful evaluation in hospital by respiratory experts; it should never be prescribed on a placebo basis.

Patients should be advised of the fire risks when receiving oxygen therapy.

## OXYGEN CYLINDERS

Oxygen is occasionally prescribed for *intermittent* use for episodes of hypoxaemia of short duration, for example asthma. It is important, however, that the patient does not rely on oxygen instead of obtaining medical help or taking more specific treatment.

Alternatively, intermittent oxygen may be prescribed for patients with advanced irreversible respiratory disorders to increase mobility and capacity for exercise and to ease discomfort, for example in chronic obstructive bronchitis, emphysema, widespread fibrosis, and primary or thromboembolic pulmonary hypertension. These patients may be prescribed portable equipment through the hospital service, refillable from cylinders in the home.

Under the NHS oxygen may be supplied by chemist contractors as cylinders. Oxygen flow can be adjusted as the cylinders are equipped with an oxygen flow meter with 'medium' (2 litres/minute) and 'high' (4 litres/minute) settings. The FHSAs have lists of pharmacy contractors who provide domiciliary oxygen services.

Patients are supplied with either constant or variable performance masks. The Intersurgical 010 28% or Ventimask Mk 4 28% are constant performance masks and provide a nearly constant supply of oxygen (28%) over a wide range irrespective of the patient's breathing pattern. The variable performance masks include the Intersurgical 005 Mask and the MC Mask; the concentration of oxygen supplied to the patient varies with the rate of flow of oxygen and also with the patient's breathing pattern.

## OXYGEN CONCENTRATORS

*Long-term* administration of oxygen (at least 15 hours daily) may prolong survival in patients with severe chronic obstructive airways disease with cor pulmonale.

Department of Health guidelines suggest that this treatment should be provided for patients who fulfil the following criteria:

$P_aO_2 < 7.3$ kPa; $P_aCO_2 > 6$ kPa;
$FEV_1 < 1.5$ litre and FVC < 2 litre

The measurements should be stable on two occasions at least three weeks apart after the patient has received appropriate bronchodilator therapy.

Less information is available on long-term oxygen in patients with a similar degree of hypoxaemia and airflow obstruction but no hypercapnia; the Department of Health suggests that these patients should not be denied this form of treatment but the effects of long-term therapy have not yet been assessed completely.

Increased respiratory depression from low concentrations of oxygen is seldom a problem in patients with stable respiratory failure although it may occur during exacerbations; patients and relatives should be warned to call for medical help if drowsiness or confusion occur.

Oxygen concentrators are more economical for patients requiring oxygen for long periods, and in England and Wales are now prescribable on the NHS on a regional tendering basis (see below). A concentrator was formerly only provided for a patient who required oxygen for 15 hours a day but it has been found to be cost-effective to provide one for a patient requiring it for 8 hours a day (or 21 cylinders per month).

## PRESCRIBING ARRANGEMENTS FOR OXYGEN CONCENTRATORS

Prescribe concentrator and accessories (face mask, nasal cannula, and humidifier) on form FP10. Specify amount of oxygen required (hours per day) and flow rate. If required, prescribe back-up oxygen set and cylinder at same time. Inform patient that the supplier will be in contact to make arrangements and that the prescription form is to be given to the person who installs the concentrator.

Inform supplier by telephone (see table below) that a concentrator has been prescribed. The supplier will send written confirmation of the order to the prescriber, the patient, and the FHSA.

Follow the same procedure if a back-up oxygen set and cylinder are required later.

| FHSA regional group | Supplier |
|---|---|
| Eastern | De Vilbiss Health Care Ltd |
| North Western | *to order:* |
| London North | Dial 100 |
| South Western | *and ask for:* |
| Wales | Freephone Oxygen |
| West Midlands | Concentrator |
| | |
| London South | Omnicare Health Group Ltd |
| (includes Kent, | *to order:* |
| Surrey, and Sussex) | Dial 100 |
| | *and ask for:* |
| | Freephone Omnicare Oxygen |
| | |
| Northern | Rimer-Alco Ltd |
| Yorkshire (South and | *to order:* |
| West) and | Dial 0800 373580 |
| Humberside | |

In **Scotland** refer the patient for assessment by a respiratory consultant. If the need for a concentrator is confirmed the consultant will arrange for the provision of a concentrator through the Common Services Agency.

# 3.7 Mucolytics

Mucolytics are often prescribed to facilitate expectoration by reducing sputum viscosity in chronic asthma and bronchitis. Few patients, however, have been shown to derive much benefit from them although they do render sputum less viscid. Steam inhalation with postural drainage, is good expectorant therapy in bronchiectasis and some chronic bronchitics.

## ACETYLCYSTEINE
*Indications:* reduction of sputum viscosity
*Side-effects:* occasional gastro-intestinal irritation, headache, urticaria, tinnitus, and sensitivity
*Dose:* adults and children over 6 years, 200 mg in water 3 times daily, usually for 5–10 days but if necessary may be extended to 6 months or longer; CHILD up to 2 years 200 mg daily, 2–6 years 200 mg twice daily

NHS * PoM **Acetylcysteine Granules,** acetylcysteine 200 mg/sachet. Net price 30 sachets = £5.74. Label: 13
* except for abdominal complications associated with cystic fibrosis and endorsed 'S3B' ('S2B' in Scotland)
*Note.* The brand name NHS Fabrol® (Zyma) is used for acetylcysteine granules

## CARBOCISTEINE
*Indications:* reduction of sputum viscosity
*Side-effects:* occasional gastro-intestinal irritation, rashes
*Dose:* 750 mg 3 times daily initially, then 1.5 g daily in divided doses; CHILD 2–5 years 62.5–125 mg 4 times daily, 6–12 years 250 mg 3 times daily

NHS *PoM **Carbocisteine Capsules,** carbocisteine 375 mg. Net price 30-cap pack = £3.20

NHS *PoM **Carbocisteine Syrup,** carbocisteine 125 mg/5 mL. Diluent syrup, life of diluted syrup 14 days, net price 300 mL = £3.51; 250 mg/5 mL, 300 mL = £4.50
* except, for patients under the age of 18 years, any condition which, through damage or disease, affects the airways and has required a tracheostomy and endorsed 'S3B' ('S2B' in Scotland)
*Note.* The brand name NHS Mucodyne® (Rhône-Poulenc Rorer) is used for carbocisteine preparations; capsules and 250 mg/5 mL strength of syrup contain tartrazine

## METHYLCYSTEINE HYDROCHLORIDE
*Indications:* reduction of sputum viscosity
*Dose:* 100–200 mg 3–4 times daily before meals reduced to 200 mg twice daily after 6 weeks; CHILD over 5 years 100 mg 3 times daily
Prophylaxis, 100–200 mg 2–3 times every other day during winter months

NHS **Visclair®** (Sinclair)
*Tablets,* yellow, s/c, e/c, methylcysteine hydrochloride 100 mg. Net price 20 = £3.43. Label: 5, 22, 25

# 3.8 Aromatic inhalations

Inhalations containing volatile substances such as eucalyptus oil are traditionally used and although the vapour may contain little of the additive it encourages deliberate inspiration of warm moist air which is often comforting in bronchitis; boiling water should not be used owing to the risk of scalding. Inhalations are also used for the relief of nasal obstruction in acute rhinitis or sinusitis.

CHILDREN. The use of strong aromatic decongestants (applied as rubs or to pillows) could be hazardous to infants less than one month of age, since in certain circumstances, apnoea could be induced. Mothers with young infants in whom nasal obstruction with mucus is a problem can readily be taught appropriate techniques of suction aspiration.

**Benzoin Tincture, Compound, BP,** Friars' Balsam, balsamic acids approx. 4.5%. Label: 15
Directions for use: add one teaspoonful to a pint of hot, **not** boiling, water and inhale the vapour

NHS **Menthol and Benzoin Inhalation, BP,** menthol 2 g, benzoin inhalation to 100 mL. Label: 15
Directions for use: add one teaspoonful to a pint of hot, **not** boiling, water and inhale the vapour

**Menthol and Eucalyptus Inhalation, BP 1980,** menthol 2 g, eucalyptus oil 10 mL, light magnesium carbonate 7 g, water to 100 mL
Directions for use: add one teaspoonful to a pint of hot, **not** boiling, water and inhale the vapour

NHS **Karvol®** (Crookes)
*Inhalation capsules,* menthol 35.33 mg, with chlorbutol, pine oils, terpineol, and thymol. Net price 10 = 99p
Directions for use: inhale vapour from contents of 1 capsule expressed into handkerchief or a pint of hot, **not** boiling, water; avoid in infants under 3 months

# 3.9   Antitussives

3.9.1 Cough suppressants
3.9.2 Expectorant, demulcent, and compound cough preparations

## 3.9.1   Cough suppressants

The drawbacks of prescribing cough suppressants are rarely outweighed by the benefits of treatment and only occasionally are they useful, as, for example, if sleep is disturbed by a dry cough. Cough suppressants may cause sputum retention and this may be harmful in patients with chronic bronchitis and bronchiectasis. Though commonly used in acute bronchitis and pneumonia they can be harmful; such conditions are best treated by prompt administration of antibacterial drugs (see section 5.1, Table 1).

Cough suppressants such as codeine, dextromethorphan, and pholcodine are seldom sufficiently potent to be effective and all tend to cause constipation.

CHILDREN. The use of cough suppressants containing codeine or similar opioid analgesics is not generally recommended in children and should be avoided altogether in those under 1 year of age.

## CODEINE PHOSPHATE

*Indications:* dry or painful cough
*Cautions:* asthma; hepatic and renal impairment; history of drug abuse; see also notes above and section 4.7.2; **interactions:** Appendix 1 (opioid analgesics)
*Contra-indications:* liver disease, ventilatory failure
*Side-effects:* constipation, in large doses respiratory depression

PoM[1] **Codeine Linctus, BP,** codeine phosphate 15 mg/5 mL. Net price 100 mL = 35p (diabetic, 63p)
*Dose:* 5–10 mL 3–4 times daily; CHILD 5–12 years, 2.5–5 mL
Available from APS, Evans, Galen (Galcodine®, sugar-free), Kerfoot
*Note.* Addendum 1991 to BP 1988 directs that when Diabetic Codeine Linctus is prescribed, Codeine Linctus formulated with a vehicle appropriate for administration to diabetics, whether or not labelled 'Diabetic Codeine Linctus', shall be dispensed or supplied
1. Can be sold to the public provided the maximum single dose does not exceed 5 mL
**Codeine Linctus, Paediatric, BP,** codeine phosphate 3 mg/5 mL. Net price 100 mL = 18p
*Dose:* CHILD 1–5 years 5 mL 3–4 times daily
Available from Evans, Galen (Galcodine®, sugar-free)
*Note.* Sugar-free versions are available
Paediatric Codeine Linctus may be prepared extemporaneously by diluting Codeine Linctus with a suitable vehicle in accordance with the manufacturer's instructions

## DEXTROMETHORPHAN

*Indications:* dry or painful cough
*Cautions; Contra-indications; Side-effects:* see under Codeine Phosphate; avoid in porphyria (see section 9.8.2)

**Preparations**
Ingredient of compound cough preparations (section 3.9.2)
*Note.* A proprietary brand of dextromethorphan modified-release capsules (NHS Coughcaps®) is on sale to the public

## ISOAMINILE CITRATE

*Indications:* dry or painful cough
*Cautions:* see notes above
*Side-effects:* occasionally constipation, dizziness, nausea
*Dose:* see below

PoM **Isoaminile Linctus,** isoaminile citrate 40 mg/5 mL. Life of diluted linctus 14 days. Net price 150 mL = £1.88
*Dose:* 5 mL 3–5 times daily; CHILD, 2.5–5 mL
The brand name NHS Dimyril® (Fisons) is used for isoaminile linctus

## PHOLCODINE

*Indications:* dry or painful cough
*Cautions; Contra-indications; Side-effects:* see under Codeine Phosphate

**Pholcodine Linctus, BP,** pholcodine 5 mg/5 mL in a suitable flavoured vehicle, containing citric acid monohydrate 1%. Net price 100 mL = 29p
*Dose:* 5–10 mL 3–4 times daily; CHILD 5–12 years 2.5–5 mL
Available from APS, Boehringer Ingelheim (Pavacol-D®, sugar-free), Evans, Galen (Galenphol®, sugar-free), Kerfoot, Medo (NHS Pholcomed D®, sugar-free)
**Pholcodine Linctus, Strong, BP,** pholcodine 10 mg/5 mL in a suitable flavoured vehicle, containing citric acid monohydrate 2%. Net price 100 mL = 48p
*Dose:* 5 mL 3–4 times daily
Available from APS, Evans, Kerfoot, Medo (NHS Pholcomed Diabetic Forte®, sugar-free)
**Galenphol®** (Galen)
*Paediatric linctus,* orange, sugar-free, pholcodine 2 mg/5 mL. Diluent as above. Net price 100 mL = 17p
*Dose:* CHILD 1–5 years 5 mL 3 times daily; 6–12 years 5–10 mL
*Note.* A proprietary brand of pholcodine pastilles (NHS Pholcomed®) is on sale to the public

## TERMINAL CARE

Diamorphine and methadone are available in linctuses to control distressful cough in terminal lung cancer although morphine is now preferred (see Terminal Care, p. 12). In other circumstances they are contra-indicated because they induce sputum retention and ventilatory failure as well as causing opioid dependence.

## DIAMORPHINE HYDROCHLORIDE

*Indications:* cough in terminal disease
*Cautions; Contra-indications; Side-effects:* see notes in section 4.7.2; more potent than morphine
*Dose:* see below

**CD Diamorphine Linctus, BPC 1973,** diamorphine hydrochloride 3 mg, oxymel 1.25 mL, glycerol 1.25 mL, compound tartrazine solution 0.06 mL, syrup to 5 mL. It should be recently prepared. Label: 2
*Dose:* 2.5–10 mL every 4 hours

## METHADONE HYDROCHLORIDE

*Indications:* cough in terminal disease
*Cautions; Contra-indications; Side-effects:* see notes in section 4.7.2; longer-acting than morphine therefore effects may be cumulative
*Dose:* see below

**CD Methadone Linctus,** methadone hydrochloride 2 mg/5 mL in a suitable vehicle with a tolu flavour. Label: 2
*Dose:* 2.5–5 mL every 4–6 hours, reduced to twice daily on prolonged use

## MORPHINE HYDROCHLORIDE

*Indications:* cough in terminal disease (see also p. 12)
*Cautions; Contra-indications; Side-effects:* see notes in section 4.7.2
*Dose:* initially 5 mg every 4 hours

**Preparations**
See section 4.7.2

## 3.9.2 Expectorant, demulcent, and compound cough preparations

Although there is no scientific basis for prescribing any of the preparations listed in this section, it may be that a harmless expectorant such as ammonia and ipecacuanha mixture or a demulcent such as simple linctus has a useful placebo role in minor respiratory disorders. Certainly this is preferable to the indiscriminate prescribing of antibiotics.

**Expectorants** are claimed to promote expulsion of bronchial secretions but there is no evidence that any drug can specifically facilitate expectoration.

The assumption that sub-emetic doses of expectorants, such as ammonium chloride, ipecacuanha, and squill promote expectoration is a myth. However, a simple expectorant mixture may serve a useful placebo function and has the advantage of being inexpensive.

**Demulcent cough preparations** contain soothing substances such as syrup or glycerol and certainly some patients believe that such preparations relieve a dry irritating cough. Preparations such as **simple linctus** have the advantage of being harmless and inexpensive and **paediatric simple linctus** is particularly useful in children.

**Compound cough preparations** have no place in the treatment of respiratory disorders. Many contain an unnecessarily large number of ingredients, often in individually subtherapeutic doses, and often with similar therapeutic properties. Others incorporate ingredients with opposing effects such as expectorants and cough sup-

pressants, and claim dual benefits. All such preparations are to be **deprecated** not only as irrational but also for leading to patients receiving inappropriate drugs; for example, the sedative effect of antihistamines may lead to carbon dioxide retention in patients with chronic bronchitis or emphysema. It is therefore best to prescribe one of the simple cough mixtures recommended above; if any other component is needed it may then be prescribed separately, tailored to the needs of the patient.

CHILDREN. The use of cough suppressants containing codeine or similar opioid analgesics is not generally recommended in children and should be avoided altogether in those under 1 year of age.

**NHS Ammonia and Ipecacuanha Mixture, BP,** ammonium bicarbonate 200 mg, liquorice liquid extract 0.5 mL, ipecacuanha tincture 0.3 mL, concentrated camphor water 0.1 mL, concentrated anise water 0.05 mL, double-strength chloroform water 5 mL, water to 10 mL. It should be recently prepared
*Dose:* 10–20 mL 3–4 times daily

**NHS Ammonium Chloride and Morphine Mixture, BP,** ammonium chloride 300 mg, ammonium bicarbonate 200 mg, chloroform and morphine tincture 0.3 mL, liquorice liquid extract 0.5 mL, water to 10 mL. It should be recently prepared. Contains 500 micrograms of anhydrous morphine in 10 mL
*Dose:* 10–20 mL 3–4 times daily

**NHS Ipecacuanha and Morphine Mixture BP, 1980,** ipecacuanha tincture 0.2 mL, chloroform and morphine tincture 0.4 mL, liquorice liquid extract 1 mL, water to 10 mL. It should be recently prepared. 10 mL contains 700 micrograms of anhydrous morphine
*Dose:* 10 mL 3–4 times daily

**Simple Linctus, BP,** citric acid monohydrate 125 mg, concentrated anise water 0.05 mL, chloroform spirit 0.3 mL, amaranth solution 0.075 mL, syrup to 5 mL. Net price 100 mL = 24p
*Dose:* 5 mL 3–4 times daily

**Simple Linctus, Paediatric, BP,** simple linctus 1.25 mL, syrup to 5 mL. Net price 100 mL = 20p
*Dose:* CHILD, 5–10 mL 3–4 times daily

**NHS Squill Linctus, Opiate, BP,** Gee's Linctus, equal volumes of camphorated opium tincture, squill oxymel, and tolu syrup. It contains 800 micrograms of anhydrous morphine in 5 mL
*Dose:* 5 mL 3–4 times daily

**NHS Tolu Linctus, Compound, Paediatric,** citric acid monohydrate 30 mg/5 mL in a suitable vehicle with a tolu flavour
*Dose:* CHILD, 5–10 mL 3–4 times daily

**NHS Actifed Compound Linctus®** (Wellcome)
*Linctus,* dextromethorphan hydrobromide, pseudoephedrine hydrochloride, triprolidine hydrochloride. Net price 100 mL = £1.23; 200 mL = £1.98. Label: 2

**NHS Actifed Expectorant®** (Wellcome)
*Elixir,* guaiphenesin, pseudoephedrine hydrochloride, triprolidine hydrochloride. Net price 100 mL = £1.23; 200 mL = £1.98. Label: 2

**NHS Benylin Chesty Cough Linctus¹®** (W-L)
*Syrup,* diphenhydramine hydrochloride, menthol. Net price 125 mL = £1.37; 300 mL = £2.69. Label: 2
1. Has replaced Benylin Expectorant

**NHS Benylin Childrens Cough Linctus²®** (W-L)
*Syrup,* diphenhydramine hydrochloride, menthol. Net price 125 mL = £1.25. Label: 1
2. Has replaced Benylin Paediatric

NHS **Benylin with Codeine**® (W-L)
*Syrup*, codeine phosphate, diphenhydramine hydrochloride, menthol, sodium citrate. Net price 300 mL = £3.24. Label: 2

NHS **Benylin Dry Cough Linctus3**® (W-L)
*Syrup*, diphenhydramine hydrochloride, dextromethorphan hydrobromide, menthol. Net price 125 mL = £1.37. Label: 2
3. Has replaced Benylin Fortified

NHS **Benylin Mentholated Linctus**® (W-L)
*Syrup*, diphenhydramine hydrochloride, dextromethorphan hydrobromide, pseudoephedrine hydrochloride, menthol. Net price 125 mL = £1.37. Label: 2

NHS **Copholco**® (Fisons)
*Linctus*, pholcodine, cineole, menthol, terpin hydrate. Net price 100 mL = £1.05

NHS **Davenol**® (Whitehall)
*Linctus*, carbinoxamine maleate, ephedrine hydrochloride, pholcodine. Net price 100 mL = 46p. Label: 2

NHS **Dimotane Expectorant**® (Whitehall)
*Elixir*, brompheniramine maleate, guaiphenesin, pseudoephedrine hydrochloride. Net price 100 mL = £1.31. Label: 2

NHS **Dimotane Co**® (Whitehall)
*Elixir*, brompheniramine maleate, codeine phosphate, pseudoephedrine hydrochloride. Net price 100 mL = £1.31. Label: 2

NHS **Dimotane Co Paediatric**® (Whitehall)
*Elixir*, brompheniramine maleate, codeine phosphate, pseudoephedrine hydrochloride. Net price 100 mL = £1.28. Label: 1

NHS **Expulin**® (Galen)
*Linctus*, chlorpheniramine maleate, pseudoephedrine hydrochloride, pholcodine, menthol. Net price 100 mL = £1.14. Label: 2
*Paediatric linctus*, chlorpheniramine maleate, pholcodine, menthol. Net price 100 mL = £1.10. Label: 1

NHS **Guanor Expectorant**® (RP Drugs)
*Syrup*, ammonium chloride, diphenhydramine hydrochloride, menthol, sodium citrate. Net price 200 mL = £1.25. Label: 2

NHS **Histalix**® (Wallace Mfg)
*Syrup*, ammonium chloride, diphenhydramine hydrochloride, menthol, sodium citrate. Net price 150 mL = £1.14. Label: 2

NHS **Phensedyl**® (Rhône-Poulenc Rorer)
*Linctus*, codeine phosphate, promethazine hydrochloride. Net price 100 mL = £1.43. Label: 2

NHS **Sudafed Expectorant**® (Wellcome)
*Syrup*, guaiphenesin, pseudoephedrine hydrochloride. Net price 100 mL = £1.23

NHS **Sudafed Linctus**® (Wellcome)
*Linctus*, dextromethorphan hydrobromide, pseudoephedrine hydrochloride. Net price 100 mL = £1.23. Label: 2

NHS **Tancolin**® (Ashe)
*Linctus* (paediatric), ascorbic acid, citric acid, dextromethorphan hydrobromide, glycerol, sodium citrate. Net price 100 mL = £1.22

NHS **Tercoda**® (Sinclair)
*Elixir*, codeine phosphate, terpin hydrate. Net price 100 mL = £1.07

NHS **Terpoin**® (Hough)
*Elixir*, codeine phosphate with cineole and menthol. Net price 225 mL = £3.28

NHS **Tixylix**® (Intercare)
*Linctus*, pholcodine (as citrate), promethazine hydrochloride. Net price 100 mL = £1.28. Label: 1 *or* 2

# 3.10 Systemic nasal decongestants

These preparations are of doubtful value but unlike the preparations for local application (see section 12.2.2) they do not give rise to rebound nasal congestion. They contain sympathomimetics, and should therefore be **avoided** in patients with hypertension, hyperthyroidism, coronary heart disease, or diabetes, and in patients taking monoamine-oxidase inhibitors; **interactions:** Appendix 1 (sympathomimetics). Many of the preparations also contain antihistamines which may cause drowsiness and affect ability to drive or operate machinery.

NHS **Actifed**® (Wellcome)
*Tablets*, pseudoephedrine hydrochloride, triprolidine hydrochloride. Net price 12-tab pack = 94p. Label: 2
*Syrup*, pseudoephedrine hydrochloride, triprolidine hydrochloride. Net price 100 mL = £1.11. Label: 2

**Dimotane Plus**® (Wyeth)
*Liquid*, brown, sugar-free, brompheniramine maleate 4 mg, pseudoephedrine hydrochloride 30 mg/5 mL. Net price 100 mL = 81p. Label: 2
*Dose:* 10 mL 3 times daily; CHILD 2–6 years 2.5 mL, 6–12 years 5 mL
*Paediatric liquid*, brown, sugar-free, brompheniramine maleate 2 mg, pseudoephedrine hydrochloride 15 mg/5 mL. Net price 100 mL = 74p. Label: 1
*Dose:* CHILD 2–6 years 5 mL, 6–12 years 10 mL, 3 times daily

PoM **Dimotane® Plus LA** (Wyeth)
*Tablets*, m/r, f/c, brompheniramine maleate 12 mg, pseudoephedrine hydrochloride 120 mg. Net price 14-tab pack = 91p. Label: 2, 25
*Dose:* 1 tablet twice daily

NHS **Dimotapp**® (Whitehall)
*Elixir*, brompheniramine maleate, phenylephrine hydrochloride, phenylpropanolamine hydrochloride. Net price 100 mL = £1.19. Label: 2
*Paediatric elixir*, brompheniramine maleate, phenylephrine hydrochloride, phenylpropanolamine hydrochloride. Net price 100 mL = £1.13. Label: 1

NHS **Dimotapp LA**® (Whitehall)
*Tablets*, brompheniramine maleate, phenylephrine hydrochloride, phenylpropanolamine hydrochloride. Net price 30 = £2.45. Label: 2, 25, counselling, gluten

NHS **Eskornade**® (SK&F)
*Spansule*® (= capsules m/r), diphenylpyraline hydrochloride, phenylpropanolamine hydrochloride. Net price 30-cap pack = £3.02. Label: 2, 25
*Syrup*, diphenylpyraline hydrochloride, phenylpropanolamine hydrochloride. Net price 150 mL = £3.11. Label: 2

NHS **Expurhin**® (Galen)
*Paediatric linctus*, chlorpheniramine maleate, ephedrine hydrochloride, menthol. Net price 100 mL = £1.10. Label: 1

**Galpseud**® (Galen)
*Tablets*, pseudoephedrine hydrochloride 60 mg. Net price 20 = 72p
*Dose:* 1 tablet 3 times daily
*Linctus*, orange, sugar-free, pseudoephedrine hydrochloride 30 mg/5 mL. Net price 100 mL = 57p
*Dose:* 10 mL 3 times daily; CHILD 2–6 years 2.5 mL, 6–12 years 5 mL

---

**Haymine**® (Pharmax)
*Tablets*, m/r, yellow, chlorpheniramine maleate 10 mg, ephedrine hydrochloride 15 mg. Net price 30-tab pack = £2.79. Label: 2, 25
*Dose:* 1 tablet 1–2 times daily
**Sudafed**® (Wellcome)
*Tablets*, red, f/c, pseudoephedrine hydrochloride 60 mg. Net price 20 = £1.17
*Dose:* 1 tablet 3 times daily
*Elixir*, pink, pseudoephedrine hydrochloride 30 mg/5 mL. Net price 100 mL = 94p
*Dose:* 10 mL 3 times daily; CHILD 2–5 years 2.5 mL, 6–12 years 5 mL
**Sudafed Plus**® (Wellcome)
*Tablets*, pseudoephedrine hydrochloride 60 mg, triprolidine hydrochloride 2.5 mg. Net price 100-tab pack = £6.49. Label: 2
*Dose:* 1 tablet 3 times daily
*Syrup*, yellow, pseudoephedrine hydrochloride 30 mg, triprolidine hydrochloride 1.25 mg/5 mL. Net price 100 mL = £1·06. Label: 2
*Dose:* 10 mL 3 times daily; CHILD 2–5 years 2.5 mL 3 times daily, 6–12 years 5 mL 3 times daily

PoM **Sudafed SA**® (Wellcome)
*Capsules*, m/r, red/clear, pseudoephedrine hydrochloride 120 mg. Net price 20 = £1.44. Label: 25
*Dose:* 1 capsule every 12 hours
NHS **Sudafed-Co**® (Wellcome)
*Tablets*, paracetamol, pseudoephedrine hydrochloride. Net price 12-tab pack = 99p
NHS **Triogesic**® (Beecham)
*Tablets*, paracetamol, phenylpropanolamine hydrochloride. Net price 30-tab pack = £1.77
NHS **Triominic**® (Beecham)
*Tablets*, pheniramine maleate, phenylpropanolamine hydrochloride. Net price 30-tab pack = £1.77. Label: 2
NHS **Uniflu with Gregovite C**® (Unigreg)
*Tablets*, composite pack of pairs of tablets: Uniflu *tablets*, caffeine, codeine phosphate, diphenhydramine hydrochloride, paracetamol, phenylephrine hydrochloride; Gregovite C *tablets*, ascorbic acid. Net price 6 of each tablet = £1.38; or 12 of each tablet = £2.30. Label: 2
*Dose:* 1 of each tablet every 6 hours

# 4: Drugs acting on the

# CENTRAL NERVOUS SYSTEM

In this chapter, drug treatments are discussed under the following headings:

## 4.1 Hypnotics and anxiolytics

Most anxiolytics ('sedatives') will induce sleep when given in large doses at night and most hypnotics will sedate when given in divided doses during the day. Prescribing of these drugs is widespread but dependence (either physical or psychological) and tolerance to their effects occurs. This may lead to difficulty in withdrawing the drug after the patient has been taking it regularly for more than a few weeks (see Dependence and Withdrawal, below). Hypnotics and anxiolytics should not therefore be prescribed indiscriminately and should, instead, be reserved for short courses to alleviate acute conditions after causal factors have been established.

Prescribing of more than one anxiolytic or hypnotic at the same time is **not** recommended. It may constitute a hazard and there is no evidence that side-effects are minimised.

**Benzodiazepines** are the most commonly used anxiolytics and hypnotics; they act at benzodiazepine receptors which are associated with gamma-aminobutyric acid (GABA) receptors. Barbiturates (section 4.1.3) are no longer recommended.

Benzodiazepines have fewer side-effects than barbiturates and are much less dangerous in overdosage. They are also less likely to interact with other drugs because, unlike barbiturates, they do not induce liver microsomal enzymes.

A paradoxical increase in hostility and aggression may be reported by patients taking benzodiazepines. The effects range from talkativeness and excitement, to aggressive and antisocial acts. Adjustment of the dose (up or down) usually attenuates the impulses. Increased anxiety and perceptual disorders are other paradoxical effects. Increased hostility and aggression after barbiturates and alcohol usually indicates intoxication.

DEPENDENCE AND WITHDRAWAL. The benzodiazepine withdrawal syndrome may not develop until up to 3 weeks after stopping a long-acting benzodiazepine, but may occur within a few hours in the case of a short-acting one. It is characterised by insomnia, anxiety, loss of appetite and body weight, tremor, perspiration, and perceptual disturbances. These symptoms may be similar to the original complaint and encourage further prescribing; some symptoms may continue for weeks or months after stopping benzodiazepines entirely.

Withdrawal of a benzodiazepine should be gradual as abrupt withdrawal may produce confusion, toxic psychosis, convulsions, or a condition resembling delirium tremens.

DRIVING. Hypnotics and anxiolytics may impair judgement and increase reaction time, and so affect ability to drive or operate machinery; they increase the effects of alcohol. Moreover, the hangover effects of a night dose may impair driving on the following day.

---

BENZODIAZEPINE WITHDRAWAL

A suggested protocol for patients unable to reduce existing benzodiazepine[1]:
1. Transfer patient to equivalent daily dose of diazepam[2] preferably taken at night
2. Reduce diazepam dose in fortnightly steps of 2 or 2.5 mg; if withdrawal symptoms occur, maintain this dose until symptoms improve
3. Reduce dose further, if necessary in smaller fortnightly steps[3]; it is better to reduce too slowly rather than too quickly
4. Stop completely; time needed for withdrawal can vary from about 4 weeks to a year or more
Counselling may help; beta-blockers should **only** be tried if other measures fail; antidepressants should **only** be used if clinical depression present; **avoid** antipsychotics (which may aggravate withdrawal symptoms)

---

1. Existing benzodiazepines can be withdrawn in steps of about $\frac{1}{8}$ (range $\frac{1}{10}-\frac{1}{4}$) of daily dose every fortnight
2. Approximate equivalent doses, diazepam 5 mg
   ≡ chlordiazepoxide 15 mg
   ≡ lorazepam 500 micrograms
   ≡ nitrazepam 5 mg
   ≡ oxazepam 15 mg
   ≡ temazepam 10 mg
   ≡ triazolam 125–250 micrograms
3. Steps may be adjusted according to initial dose and duration of treatment and can range from diazepam 500 micrograms ($\frac{1}{4}$ of a 2-mg tablet) to 2.5 mg

---

## 4.1.1  Hypnotics

Before a hypnotic is prescribed the cause of the insomnia should be established and, where possible, underlying factors should be treated. However, it should be noted that some patients have unrealistic sleep expectations, and others understate their alcohol consumption which is often the cause of the insomnia.

*Transient insomnia* may occur in those who normally sleep well and may be due to extraneous factors such as noise, shift work, and jet lag. If a hypnotic is indicated one that is rapidly eliminated should be chosen, and only one or two doses should be given.

*Short-term insomnia* is usually related to an emotional problem or serious medical illness. It may last for a few weeks, and may recur; a hypnotic can be useful but should not be given for more than three weeks (preferably only one week). Intermittent use is desirable with omission of some doses. A rapidly eliminated drug is generally appropriate.

*Chronic insomnia* is rarely benefited by hypnotics and is more often due to mild dependence caused by injudicious prescribing. Psychiatric disorders such as anxiety, depression, and abuse of drugs and alcohol are common causes. Sleep disturbance is very common in depressive illness and early wakening is often a useful pointer. The underlying psychiatric complaint should be treated, adapting the drug regimen to alleviate insomnia. For example, amitriptyline, prescribed for depression, will also help to promote sleep if it is taken at night. Other causes of insomnia include daytime cat-napping and physical causes such as pain, pruritus, and dyspnoea.

Hypnotics should **not** be prescribed indiscriminately and routine prescribing is undesirable. Ideally, they should be reserved for short courses in the acutely distressed. Tolerance to their effects develops within 3 to 14 days of continuous use and long-term efficacy cannot be assured. A major drawback of long-term use is that withdrawal causes rebound insomnia and precipitates a withdrawal syndrome (section 4.1).

Where prolonged administration is unavoidable hypnotics should be discontinued as soon as feasible and the patient warned that sleep may be disturbed for a few days before normal rhythm is re-established; broken sleep with vivid dreams and increased REM (rapid eye movement) may persist for several weeks. This represents a mild form of dependence even if clinical doses are used.

CHILDREN. The prescribing of hypnotics to children, except for occasional use such as for night terrors and somnambulism (sleep-walking), is not justified.

ELDERLY. Hypnotics should be avoided in the elderly, who are at risk of becoming ataxic and confused and so liable to fall and injure themselves.

## BENZODIAZEPINES

Benzodiazepines used as hypnotics include **nitrazepam**, **flunitrazepam**, and **flurazepam** which have a prolonged action and may give rise to residual effects on the following day; repeated doses tend to be cumulative.

**Loprazolam**, **lormetazepam**, and **temazepam** act for a shorter time and they have little or no hangover effect. Withdrawal phenomena however are more common with the short-acting benzodiazepines.

Benzodiazepine anxiolytics such as **diazepam** given as a single dose at night may also be used as hypnotics.

For general guidelines on benzodiazepine prescribing see section 4.1.2 and for benzodiazepine withdrawal see section 4.1.

## NITRAZEPAM

*Indications:* insomnia (short-term use)

*Cautions:* respiratory disease, muscle weakness, history of drug abuse, marked personality disorder, pregnancy, breast-feeding; reduce dose in elderly and debilitated, and in hepatic and renal impairment; avoid prolonged use (and abrupt withdrawal thereafter); **interactions:** Appendix 1 (benzodiazepines)

DRIVING. Drowsiness may persist the next day and affect performance of skilled tasks (e.g. driving); effects of alcohol enhanced

*Contra-indications:* respiratory depression; acute pulmonary insufficiency; phobic or obsessional states, chronic psychosis; porphyria (see section 9.8.2)

*Side-effects:* drowsiness and lightheadedness the next day; confusion and ataxia (especially in the elderly); dependence. See also under Diazepam (section 4.1.2). Overdosage: see Emergency Treatment of Poisoning, p. 19.

*Dose:* 5–10 mg at bedtime; ELDERLY (or debilitated) 2.5–5 mg

PoM **Nitrazepam** (Non-proprietary)
*Tablets,* nitrazepam 5 mg, net price 20 = 7p. Label: 19
Available from APS, Cox, DDSA (NHS Remnos®), Evans, Kerfoot, Roche (NHS Mogadon®), Unigreg (NHS Unisomnia®)
*Oral suspension,* nitrazepam 2.5 mg/5 mL. Net price 150 mL = £3.74. Label: 19
Available from Norgine (NHS Somnite®)
NHS *Capsules,* nitrazepam 5 mg. Net price 20 = 26p. Label: 19
Available from Roche (NHS Mogadon®)

---

## FLUNITRAZEPAM

*Indications:* insomnia (short-term use)
*Cautions; Contra-indications; Side-effects:* see under Nitrazepam
*Dose:* 0.5–1 mg at bedtime; max. 2 mg; ELDERLY 500 micrograms (max. 1 mg)

NHS PoM **Rohypnol**® (Roche)
*Tablets*, purple, f/c, scored, flunitrazepam 1 mg. Net price 30-tab pack = £3.66. Label: 19

## FLURAZEPAM

*Indications:* insomnia (short-term use)
*Cautions; Contra-indications; Side-effects:* see under Nitrazepam
*Dose:* 15–30 mg at bedtime; ELDERLY 15 mg

NHS PoM **Dalmane**® (Roche)
*Capsules*, flurazepam (as hydrochloride), 15 mg (grey/yellow), net price 30-cap pack = £2.42; 30 mg (black/grey), 30-cap pack = £3.12. Label: 19

## LOPRAZOLAM

*Indications:* insomnia (short-term use)
*Cautions; Contra-indications; Side-effects:* see under Nitrazepam
*Dose:* 1 mg at bedtime, increased to 1.5 or 2 mg if required; ELDERLY 0.5–1 mg

PoM **Loprazolam** (Non-proprietary)
*Tablets*, loprazolam 1 mg (as mesylate). Net price 28-tab pack = £1.68. Label: 19
Available from Roussel (previously known as NHS Dormonoct®)

## LORMETAZEPAM

*Indications:* insomnia (short-term use)
*Cautions; Contra-indications; Side-effects:* see under Nitrazepam; shorter acting
*Dose:* 0.5–1.5 mg at bedtime; ELDERLY 500 micrograms

PoM **Lormetazepam** (Non-proprietary)
*Tablets*, lormetazepam 500 micrograms, net price 20 = 84p; 1 mg, 20 = £1.09. Label: 19
Available from APS, Cox, Wyeth

## TEMAZEPAM

*Indications:* insomnia (short-term use); see also section 15.1.4.1 for peri-operative use
*Cautions; Contra-indications; Side-effects:* see under Nitrazepam; shorter acting
*Dose:* 10–30 mg (severe insomnia, up to 40–60 mg) at bedtime; ELDERLY 5–15 mg

PoM **Temazepam** (Non-proprietary)
*Gel-filled capsules* (soft gelatin), temazepam 10 mg, net price 20 = 48p; 15 mg, 20 = 62p; 20 mg, 20 = 84p; 30 mg, 20 = £1.24. Label: 19
Available from APS, Berk, Cox, CP, Evans, Farmitalia Carlo Erba, Kerfoot, Wyeth; the name NHS Temazepam Gelthix® is used for some gel-filled capsules
*Note.* The Advisory Council on the Misuse of Drugs has warned that the gel-filled capsules may be subject to abuse

*Capsules* (hard gelatin), temazepam 10 mg, net price 20 = 36p; 20 mg, 20 = 58p. Label: 19
*Tablets*, temazepam 10 mg, net price 20 = 48p; 20 mg, 20 = 84p. Label: 19
*Oral solution*, temazepam 10 mg/5 mL, net price 100 mL = £2.65. Label: 19

NHS PoM **Temazepam Planpak** (Farmitalia Carlo Erba)
*Capsules* (soft gelatin), all green, 14 capsules each of temazepam 2 mg, 5 mg, and 10 mg. Net price per pack = £8.57. Label: 19
*Dose:* withdrawal, 1 capsule at bedtime, commencing with highest strength and finishing with lowest

## CHLORAL AND DERIVATIVES

**Chloral hydrate** and chloral derivatives are useful hypnotics for children (but see notes above). There is no convincing evidence that they are particularly useful in the elderly. **Triclofos sodium** causes fewer gastro-intestinal upsets than chloral hydrate.

## CHLORAL HYDRATE

*Indications:* insomnia (short-term use)
*Cautions:* respiratory disease, history of drug abuse, marked personality disorder, pregnancy, breast-feeding; reduce dose in elderly and debilitated; avoid prolonged use (and abrupt withdrawal thereafter); avoid contact with skin and mucous membranes; **interactions:** Appendix 1 (chloral)
DRIVING. Drowsiness may persist the next day and affect performance of skilled tasks (e.g. driving); effects of alcohol enhanced
*Contra-indications:* severe cardiac disease, gastritis, marked hepatic or renal impairment
*Side-effects:* gastric irritation; *occasionally:* rashes, headache, ketonuria, excitement, delirium; dependence and renal damage on prolonged use
*Dose:* insomnia, 0.5–1 g (max. 2 g) with plenty of water at bedtime; CHILD 30–50 mg/kg up to a max. single dose of 1 g

PoM **Chloral Mixture** (BP)
(Chloral Oral Solution)
*Mixture*, chloral hydrate 10% in a suitable vehicle. Extemporaneous preparations should be recently prepared according to the following formula: chloral hydrate 1 g, syrup 2 mL, water to 10 mL. Net price 100 mL = 15p. Label: 19, 27
*Dose:* 5–20 mL; CHILD 1–5 years 2.5–5 mL, 6–12 years 5–10 mL, taken well diluted with water at bedtime

PoM **Chloral Elixir, Paediatric** (BP)
(Chloral Oral Solution, Paediatric)
*Elixir*, chloral hydrate 4% in a suitable vehicle with a blackcurrant flavour. Extemporaneous preparations should be recently prepared according to the following formula: chloral hydrate 200 mg, water 0.1 mL, blackcurrant syrup 1 mL, syrup to 5 mL. Net price 100 mL = 32p. Label: 1, 27
*Dose:* up to 1 year 5 mL, well diluted with water

---

PoM **Noctec**® (Squibb)

*Capsules*, red, chloral hydrate 500 mg. Net price 50-cap pack = £1.90. Label: 19, 27

*Dose*: 1–2 capsules with plenty of water at bedtime (max. 4 capsules); CHILD not recommended

PoM **Welldorm**® (S&N Pharm.)

*Tablets*, blue-purple, f/c, chloral betaine 707 mg (≡chloral hydrate 414 mg). Net price 30-tab pack = £2.54. Label: 19, 27

*Dose*: 1–2 tablets with water or milk at bedtime, max. 5 tablets (2 g chloral hydrate) daily

*Elixir*, red, chloral hydrate 143 mg/5 mL. Net price 150-mL pack = £2.68. Label: 19, 27

*Dose*: 15–45 mL (0.4–1.3 g chloral hydrate) with water or milk, at bedtime, max. 70 mL (2 g chloral hydrate) daily; CHILD 1–1.75 mL/kg (30–50 mg/kg chloral hydrate), max. 35 mL (1 g chloral hydrate) daily

*Note*. Previous formulations of Welldorm® Tablets and Elixir contained dichloralphenazone

## TRICLOFOS SODIUM

*Indications:* insomnia (short-term use)

*Cautions; Contra-indications; Side-effects:* see under Chloral Hydrate; less gastric irritation

*Dose:* see under preparation below

PoM **Triclofos** (Non-proprietary)

*Elixir*, triclofos sodium 500 mg/5 mL. Net price 100 mL = £6.10. Label: 19

*Dose*: 10–20 mL (1–2 g triclofos sodium) at bedtime; CHILD up to 1 year 1–2.5 mL (100–250 mg triclofos sodium), 1–5 years 2.5–5 mL (250–500 mg triclofos sodium), 6–12 years 5–10 mL (0.5–1 g triclofos sodium)

## OTHER HYPNOTICS

**Chlormethiazole** may be a useful hypnotic for elderly patients because of its freedom from hangover but, as with all hypnotics, routine administration is undesirable and dependence occurs occasionally. It is used in the treatment of acute withdrawal symptoms in alcohol dependence but to minimise the risk of dependence administration should be limited to 9 days under inpatient supervision.

**Promethazine** is popular for use in children (but see notes above).

**Zopiclone** is a newly introduced hypnotic; although not a benzodiazepine it acts on the same receptors as benzodiazepines. As with other hypnotics it should not be used for long-term treatment.

**Alcohol** is a poor hypnotic as its diuretic action interferes with sleep during the latter part of the night. With chronic use, alcohol disturbs sleep patterns and causes insomnia; **interactions:** Appendix 1 (alcohol).

## CHLORMETHIAZOLE

*Indications:* see under Dose

*Cautions:* cardiac and respiratory disease, history of drug abuse, marked personality disorder, pregnancy, breast-feeding; reduce dose in elderly and debilitated, and in hepatic and renal impairment; avoid prolonged use (and abrupt withdrawal thereafter); during intravenous infusion the sleep induced may quickly lapse into deep unconsciousness and patients must be observed constantly; resuscitation facilities must be available; see also section 4.8.2; **interactions:** Appendix 1 (chlormethiazole)

DRIVING. Drowsiness may persist the next day and affect performance of skilled tasks (e.g. driving); effects of alcohol enhanced

*Contra-indications:* acute pulmonary insufficiency; alcohol-dependent patients who continue to drink

*Side-effects:* sneezing, conjunctival irritation, headache, gastro-intestinal disturbances; rarely, paradoxical excitement, confusion, dependence. Localised thrombophlebitis on intravenous infusion, and at rapid infusion rates cardiovascular and respiratory depression

*Dose: by mouth*, severe insomnia in the elderly (short-term use), 1–2 capsules at bedtime

Restlessness and agitation in the elderly, 1 capsule 3 times daily

Alcohol withdrawal, initially 2–4 capsules, if necessary repeated after some hours;

day 1 (first 24 hours), 9–12 capsules in 3–4 divided doses;

day 2, 6–8 capsules in 3–4 divided doses;

day 3, 4–6 capsules in 3–4 divided doses; then gradually reduced over days 4–6; total treatment for not more than 9 days

*Note*. For an equivalent therapeutic effect 1 capsule ≡ 5 mL elixir

*By intravenous infusion*, acute alcohol withdrawal, 40–100 mL (320–800 mg) initially as 0.8% solution over 5–10 minutes, then continued if necessary at a reduced rate adjusted according to the patient's condition

*Note*. Special care on prolonged intravenous administration since accumulation may occur; also, contains no electrolytes

PoM **Heminevrin**® (Astra)

*Capsules*, grey-brown, chlormethiazole base 192 mg in an oily basis. Net price 60 = £4.45. Label: 19

*Syrup*, sugar-free, chlormethiazole edisylate 250 mg/5 mL. Net price 300-mL pack = £3.72. Label: 19

*Intravenous infusion 0.8%*, chlormethiazole edisylate 8 mg/mL. Net price 500-mL = £5.25

## PROMETHAZINE HYDROCHLORIDE

*Indications:* insomnia (short-term use); other indications, see sections 3.4.1, 4.6, 15.1.4.1

*Cautions; Side-effects:* see section 3.4.1

*Dose: by mouth*, 25 mg at bedtime increased to 50 mg if necessary; CHILD 1–5 years 15–20 mg (1–2 years on doctors advice only), 5–10 years 20–25 mg, at bedtime

**Preparations:** see section 3.4.1

## ZOPICLONE

*Indications:* insomnia (short-term use)

*Cautions:* hepatic impairment; pregnancy and breast-feeding; elderly; history of drug abuse, psychiatric illness; avoid prolonged use (and abrupt withdrawal thereafter); **interactions:** Appendix 1 (zopiclone)

DRIVING. Drowsiness may persist the next day and affect performance of skilled tasks (e.g. driving); effects of alcohol enhanced

*Side-effects:* bitter or metallic taste; gastro-intestinal disturbances including nausea and vomiting; irritability, confusion, depressed mood; drowsiness, dizziness, lightheadedness, and incoordination on the next day; dependence; rarely urticaria and rashes; hallucinations, amnesia, and behavioural disturbances (including aggression) reported

*Dose:* 7.5 mg at bedtime increased to 15 mg in severe insomnia; ELDERLY initially 3.75 mg at bedtime

▼ PoM **Zimovane**® (Rhône-Poulenc Rorer)
*Tablets,* f/c, scored, zopiclone 7.5 mg. Net price 28-tab pack = £27.44. Label: 19

### 4.1.2   Anxiolytics

**Benzodiazepine** anxiolytics can be effective in alleviating definite anxiety states and they are widely prescribed. Although there has been a tendency to prescribe these drugs to almost anyone with stress-related symptoms, unhappiness, or minor physical disease, their use in many situations is unjustified. In particular, they should not be used to treat depression, phobic or obsessional states, or chronic psychosis. In bereavement, psychological adjustment may be inhibited by benzodiazepines. In children anxiolytic treatment should be used only to relieve acute anxiety (and related insomnia) caused by fear e.g. before surgery.

Anxiolytic treatment should be limited to the lowest possible dose for the shortest possible time (see CSM advice, section 4.1). Dependence is particularly likely in patients with a history of alcohol or drug abuse and in patients with marked personality disorders.

Anxiolytics, particularly the benzodiazepines, have been termed 'minor tranquillisers'. This term is misleading because not only do they differ markedly from the antipsychotic drugs ('major tranquillisers') but their use is by no means minor. Antipsychotics, in low doses, are also sometimes used in severe anxiety for their sedative action but long-term use should be avoided in view of a possible risk of tardive dyskinesia (section 4.2.1).

### BENZODIAZEPINES

**Benzodiazepines** are indicated for the short-term relief of severe anxiety but long-term use should be avoided (see notes above). Diazepam, alprazolam, bromazepam, chlordiazepoxide, clo-bazam, clorazepate, and medazepam have a sustained action. Shorter-acting compounds such as **lorazepam** and **oxazepam** may be preferred in patients with hepatic impairment but they carry a greater risk of withdrawal symptoms.

Diazepam or lorazepam are very occasionally administered intravenously for the control of panic attacks. This route is the most rapid but the procedure is not without risk (section 4.8.2) and should be used only when alternative measures have failed. The intramuscular route has no advantage over the oral route.

For guidelines on benzodiazepine withdrawal, see section 4.1.

## DIAZEPAM

*Indications:* short-term use in anxiety or insomnia, adjunct in acute alcohol withdrawal; epilepsy (section 4.8); muscle spasm see section 10.2.2; peri-operative use see section 15.1.4.1

*Cautions:* respiratory disease, muscle weakness, history of drug abuse, marked personality disorder, pregnancy, breast-feeding; reduce dose in elderly and debilitated, and in hepatic and renal impairment; avoid prolonged use (and abrupt withdrawal thereafter); special precautions for intravenous injection (section 4.8.2); **interactions:** Appendix 1 (benzodiazepines)

DRIVING. Drowsiness may affect performance of skilled tasks (e.g. driving); effects of alcohol enhanced

*Contra-indications:* respiratory depression; acute pulmonary insufficiency; phobic or obsessional states, chronic psychosis; porphyria (but see section 9.8.2)

*Side-effects:* drowsiness and lightheadedness the next day; confusion and ataxia (especially in the elderly); amnesia may occur; dependence; *occasionally:* headache, vertigo, hypotension, salivation changes, gastro-intestinal disturbances, rashes, visual disturbances, changes in libido, urinary retention; blood disorders and jaundice reported; on intravenous injection, pain, thrombophlebitis, and rarely apnoea or hypotension; overdosage: see Emergency Treatment of Poisoning, p. 19.

*Dose: by mouth,* anxiety, 2 mg 3 times daily increased if necessary to 15–30 mg daily in divided doses; ELDERLY (or debilitated) half adult dose

Insomnia associated with anxiety, 5–15 mg at bedtime

CHILD night terrors and somnambulism, 1–5 mg at bedtime

*By intramuscular injection or slow intravenous injection* (at a rate of not more than 5 mg/minute), for severe anxiety, control of acute panic attacks, and acute alcohol withdrawal, 10 mg, repeated if necessary after 4 hours

Note. Only use intramuscular route when oral and intravenous routes not possible

*By intravenous infusion*—section 4.8.2

*By rectum* as rectal solution, for acute anxiety and agitation, adults and children over 3 years 10 mg (elderly 5 mg), repeated after 5 minutes if necessary; CHILD 1–3 years, 5 mg

PoM **Diazepam** (Non-proprietary)
*Tablets*, diazepam 2 and 5 mg, net price (both), 20 = 2p; 10 mg, 20 = 5p. Label: 2 *or* 19
Available from APS, Berk (NHS Atensine®), Cox, DDSA (NHS Tensium®), Evans, Kerfoot, Rima (NHS Rimapam®), Roche (NHS Valium®)
*Oral solution*, diazepam 2 mg/5 mL, net price 100 mL = £1.54. Label: 2 *or* 19
Available from Cox, Lagap, Roche (NHS Valium®)
NHS *Strong oral solution*, diazepam 5 mg/5 mL, net price 100-mL pack = £3.30. Label: 2 *or* 19
Available from Lagap
*Injection* (solution), diazepam 5 mg/mL. Do not dilute (except for intravenous infusion). Net price 2-mL amp = 25p
Available from CP, Roche (Valium®)
*Injection* (emulsion), diazepam 5 mg/mL. For intravenous injection or infusion. Net price 2-mL amp = 69p
Available from Dumex (Diazemuls®)
*Rectal tubes* (= rectal solution), diazepam 2 mg/mL, net price 5 × 2.5-mL (5 mg) tubes = £5.25; 4 mg/mL, 5 × 2.5-mL (10 mg) tubes = £6.70
Available from CP (Stesolid®)
*Suppositories*, diazepam 10 mg, net price 5 = £1.08. Label: 2 *or* 19
Available from Sinclair

## ALPRAZOLAM

*Indications:* anxiety (short-term use)
*Cautions; Contra-indications; Side-effects:* see under Diazepam
*Dose:* 250–500 micrograms 3 times daily (elderly or debilitated 250 micrograms 2–3 times daily), increased if necessary to a total of 3 mg daily

NHS PoM **Xanax**® (Upjohn)
*Tablets*, both scored, alprazolam 250 micrograms, net price 60-tab pack = £2.75; 500 micrograms (pink), 60-tab pack = £5.27. Label: 2

## BROMAZEPAM

*Indications:* anxiety (short-term use)
*Cautions; Contra-indications; Side-effects:* see under Diazepam
*Dose:* 3–18 mg daily in divided doses; ELDERLY (or debilitated) half adult dose; max. (in exceptional circumstances in hospitalised patients) 60 mg daily in divided doses

NHS PoM **Lexotan**® (Roche)
*Tablets*, both scored, bromazepam 1.5 mg (lilac), net price 60-tab pack = £4.90; 3 mg (pink), 60-tab pack = £6.22. Label: 2

## CHLORDIAZEPOXIDE

*Indications:* anxiety (short-term use), adjunct in acute alcohol withdrawal
*Cautions; Contra-indications; Side-effects:* see under Diazepam
*Dose:* anxiety, 10 mg 3 times daily increased if necessary to 60–100 mg daily in divided doses; ELDERLY (or debilitated) half adult dose
Note. The doses stated above refer equally to chlordiazepoxide and to its hydrochloride

PoM **Chlordiazepoxide Capsules,** chlordiazepoxide hydrochloride 5 mg, net price 20 = 28p; 10 mg, 20 = 35p. Label: 2
Available from APS, Cox, DDSA (NHS Tropium®), Kerfoot, Roche (NHS Librium®)
PoM **Chlordiazepoxide Hydrochloride Tablets,** chlordiazepoxide hydrochloride 5 mg, net price 20 = 20p; 10 mg, 20 = 22p; 25 mg, 20 = 44p. Label: 2
PoM **Chlordiazepoxide Tablets,** chlordiazepoxide 5 mg, net price 20 = 28p; 10 mg, 20 = 35p; 25 mg, 20 = 78p. Label: 2
Available from Roche (NHS Librium®)

## CLOBAZAM

*Indications:* anxiety (short-term use); adjunct in epilepsy
*Cautions; Contra-indications; Side-effects:* see under Diazepam
*Dose:* anxiety, 20–30 mg daily in divided doses or as a single dose at bedtime, increased in severe anxiety (in hospital patients) to a max. of 60 mg daily in divided doses; ELDERLY (or debilitated) 10–20 mg daily
Epilepsy, 20–30 mg daily; max. 60 mg daily; CHILD over 3 years, not more than half adult dose

NHS [1]PoM **Clobazam** (Non-proprietary)
*Capsules,* clobazam 10 mg. Net price 30-cap pack = £2.60. Label: 2 *or* 19
1. except for epilepsy and endorsed 'S3B' ('S2B'in Scotland)
Note. The brand name NHS Frisium® (Hoechst) is used for clobazam capsules

## CLORAZEPATE DIPOTASSIUM

*Indications:* anxiety (short-term use)
*Cautions; Contra-indications; Side-effects:* see under Diazepam
*Dose:* 7.5–22.5 mg daily in 2–3 divided doses *or* a single dose of 15 mg at bedtime; ELDERLY (or debilitated) half adult dose

NHS PoM **Tranxene**® (Boehringer Ingelheim)
*Capsules,* clorazepate dipotassium 7.5 mg (maroon/grey), net price 20-cap pack = £1.97; 15 mg (pink/grey), 20-cap pack = £2.08. Label: 2 *or* 19

## LORAZEPAM

*Indications:* short-term use in anxiety or insomnia; status epilepticus (section 4.8.2); peri-operative (section 15.1.4.1)
*Cautions; Contra-indications; Side-effects:* see under Diazepam; short acting
*Dose: by mouth*, anxiety, 1–4 mg daily in divided doses; ELDERLY (or debilitated) half adult dose
Insomnia associated with anxiety, 1–2 mg at bedtime

*By intramuscular or slow intravenous injection*, for the control of acute panic attacks, 25–30 micrograms/kg every 6 hours if necessary
Note. Only use intramuscular route when oral and intravenous routes not possible

---

Cautionary label wordings, see inside back cover

PoM **Lorazepam** (Non-proprietary)
*Tablets,* lorazepam 1 mg, net price 20 = 23p; 2.5 mg, 20 = 37p. Label: 2 *or* 19
Available from APS, Cox, Evans, Kerfoot, Wyeth (NHS Ativan®)
*Injection,* lorazepam 4 mg/mL. Net price 1-mL amp = 40p.
For intramuscular injection it should be diluted with an equal volume of water for injections or physiological saline
Available from Wyeth (Ativan®)

## MEDAZEPAM

*Indications:* anxiety (short-term use)
*Cautions; Contra-indications; Side-effects:* see under Diazepam
*Dose:* anxiety, 15–30 mg daily in divided doses, increased in severe anxiety to max. 40 mg daily in divided doses; ELDERLY (or debilitated) half adult dose

NHS PoM **Nobrium®** (Roche)
*Capsules,* medazepam 5 mg (orange/yellow), net price 20 = 62p; 10 mg (orange/black), 20 = 94p. Label: 2

## OXAZEPAM

*Indications:* anxiety (short-term use)
*Cautions; Contra-indications; Side-effects:* see under Diazepam; short acting
*Dose:* anxiety, 15–30 mg (elderly or debilitated 10–20 mg) 3–4 times daily
Insomnia associated with anxiety, 15–25 mg (max. 50 mg) at bedtime

PoM **Oxazepam** (Non-proprietary)
*Tablets,* oxazepam 10 mg, net price 20 = 24p; 15 mg, 20 = 27p; 30 mg, 20 = 33p. Label: 2
Available from APS, Berk, Cox, Kerfoot, Wyeth

## OTHER DRUGS FOR ANXIETY

**Buspirone** is a new drug for the treatment of anxiety; it is thought to act at specific serotonin ($5HT_{1A}$) receptors. Response to treatment may take up to 2 weeks. It does not alleviate the symptoms of benzodiazepine withdrawal. Therefore a patient taking a benzodiazepine still needs to have the benzodiazepine withdrawn gradually; it is advisable to do this before starting buspirone. The dependence and abuse liability of buspirone has not yet been established.

**Meprobamate** is **less effective** than the benzodiazepines, more hazardous in overdosage, and can also induce dependence.

**Beta-blockers** (e.g. propranolol, oxprenolol) (see section 2.4) do not affect psychological symptoms, such as worry, tension, and fear, but they do reduce autonomic symptoms, such as palpitations, sweating, and tremor; they do not reduce non-autonomic symptoms, such as muscle tension. Beta-blockers are therefore indicated for patients with predominantly somatic symptoms; this, in turn, may prevent the onset of worry and fear. Patients with predominantly psychological symptoms may obtain no benefit.

## BUSPIRONE HYDROCHLORIDE

*Indications:* anxiety (short-term use)
*Cautions:* does not alleviate benzodiazepine withdrawal (see notes above); history of hepatic or renal impairment; **interactions:** Appendix 1 (buspirone)
DRIVING. May affect performance of skilled tasks (e.g. driving); effects of alcohol may be enhanced
*Contra-indications:* epilepsy, severe hepatic or renal impairment, pregnancy and breast-feeding
*Side-effects:* nausea, dizziness, headache, nervousness, lightheadedness, excitement; rarely tachycardia, palpitations, chest pain, drowsiness, confusion, dry mouth, fatigue, and sweating
*Dose:* initially 5 mg 2–3 times daily, increased as necessary every 2–3 days; usual range 15–30 mg daily in divided doses; max. 45 mg daily (30 mg in elderly)

PoM **Buspar®** (Bristol-Myers)
*Tablets,* buspirone hydrochloride 5 mg, net price 126-tab pack = £40.32; 10 mg, 100-tab pack = £48.00. Counselling, driving

## CHLORMEZANONE

*Indications:* short-term use in anxiety or insomnia; muscle spasm (but see section 10.2.2)
*Cautions:* respiratory disease, muscle weakness, history of drug abuse, marked personality disorder, pregnancy, breast-feeding; reduce dose in elderly and debilitated, and in hepatic and renal impairment; avoid prolonged use (and abrupt withdrawal thereafter); **interactions:** Appendix 1 (chlormezanone)
DRIVING. Drowsiness may persist the next day and affect performance of skilled tasks (e.g. driving); effects of alcohol enhanced
*Contra-indications:* acute pulmonary insufficiency; respiratory depression; porphyria (see section 9.8.2)
*Side-effects:* drowsiness and lethargy, dizziness, nausea, headache, dry mouth, rashes, dependence; cholestatic jaundice reported
*Dose:* 200 mg 3–4 times daily *or* 400 mg at bedtime; elderly patients half adult dose

PoM **Trancopal®** (Sanofi Winthrop)
*Tablets,* yellow, chlormezanone 200 mg. Net price 60 = £5.73. Label: 2 *or* 19

## HYDROXYZINE HYDROCHLORIDE

*Indications:* anxiety (short-term use), pruritus
*Cautions; Side-effects:* see under Antihistamines (section 3.4.1)
*Dose:* anxiety (adults only) 50–100 mg 4 times daily
Pruritus, initially 25 mg at night increased if necessary to 25 mg 3–4 times daily; CHILD 6 months–6 years initially 5–15 mg daily increased if necessary to 50 mg daily in divided doses; over 6 years initially 15–25 mg daily increased if necessary to 50–100 mg daily in divided doses

PoM **Atarax**® (Pfizer)

*Tablets*, both s/c, hydroxyzine hydrochloride 10 mg (orange), net price 84-tab pack = £1.52; 25 mg (green), 28-tab pack = £1.02. Label: 2

*Syrup*, hydroxyzine hydrochloride 10 mg/5 mL. Net price 150-mL pack = 85p. Label: 2

PoM **Ucerax**® (UCB Pharma)

*Tablets*, f/c, scored, hydroxyzine hydrochloride 25 mg, net price 25-tab pack = £1.77. Label: 2

*Syrup*, hydroxyzine hydrochloride 10 mg/5 mL. Net price 200-mL pack = £1.96. Label: 2

---

## MEPROBAMATE

*Indications:* short-term use in anxiety, but see notes above

*Cautions:* respiratory disease, muscle weakness, epilepsy (may induce seizures), history of drug abuse, marked personality disorder, pregnancy; elderly and debilitated; hepatic and renal impairment; avoid prolonged use, abrupt withdrawal may precipitate convulsions; **interactions:** Appendix 1 (meprobamate)

DRIVING. Drowsiness may affect performance of skilled tasks (e.g. driving); effects of alcohol enhanced

*Contra-indications:* acute pulmonary insufficiency; respiratory depression; porphyria (see section 9.8.2); breast-feeding

*Side-effects:* see under Diazepam, but the incidence is greater and drowsiness is the most common side-effect. Also gastro-intestinal disturbances, hypotension, paraesthesia, weakness, CNS effects which include headache, paradoxical excitement, disturbances of vision; rarely agranulocytosis and rashes

*Dose:* 400 mg 3–4 times daily; elderly patients half adult dose or less

CD **Equanil**® (Wyeth)

*Tablets*, meprobamate 200 mg, net price 20 = 15p; 400 mg (scored), 20 = 22p. Label: 2

---

## 4.1.3  Barbiturates

The intermediate-acting **barbiturates** only have a place in the treatment of severe intractable insomnia in patients already taking barbiturates; they should be avoided in the elderly. The long-acting barbiturates, phenobarbitone and methylphenobarbitone, are of value in epilepsy (section 4.8.1) but their use as sedatives is unjustified. The very short-acting barbiturates, methohexitone and thiopentone, are used in anaesthesia (see section 15.1.1).

---

## BARBITURATES

*Indications:* severe intractable insomnia in patients already taking barbiturates

*Cautions:* avoid use where possible; dependence and tolerance readily occur; abrupt withdrawal may precipitate a serious withdrawal syndrome (rebound insomnia, anxiety, tremor, dizziness, nausea, convulsions, delirium, and death); repeated doses are cumulative and may lead to excessive sedation; caution in respiratory disease, renal disease, hepatic impairment; **interactions:** Appendix 1 (barbiturates and primidone)

DRIVING. Drowsiness may persist the next day and affect performance of skilled tasks (e.g. driving); effects of alcohol enhanced

*Contra-indications:* insomnia caused by pain; porphyria (see section 9.8.2), pregnancy, breast-feeding; avoid in children, young adults, elderly and debilitated patients, also patients with a history of drug or alcohol abuse

*Side-effects:* hangover with drowsiness, dizziness, ataxia, respiratory depression, hypersensitivity reactions, headache, particularly in elderly; paradoxical excitement and confusion occasionally precede sleep; overdosage: see Emergency Treatment of Poisoning, p. 19

*Dose:* see under preparations below

CD **Amytal**® (Lilly)

*Tablets*, amylobarbitone 50 mg, net price 20 = 28p; 100 mg, 20 = 56p. Label: 19

*Dose:* 100–200 mg at bedtime

CD **Sodium Amytal**® (Lilly)

*Capsules*, both blue, amylobarbitone sodium 60 mg, net price 20 = 46p; 200 mg, 20 = 91p. Label: 19

*Dose:* 60–200 mg at bedtime

*Injection*, powder for reconstitution, amylobarbitone sodium. 500-mg vial

*Dose:* status epilepticus, by deep intramuscular injection (max. 5 mL at any one site) or by slow intravenous injection (max. 50 mg/minute), 0.25–1 g; max. single dose, intramuscular 500 mg, intravenous 1 g

CD **Soneryl**® (Rhône-Poulenc Rorer)

*Tablets*, pink, scored, butobarbitone 100 mg. Net price 56-tab pack = 73p. Label: 19

*Dose:* 100–200 mg at bedtime

Quinalbarbitone

*Note.* Quinalbarbitone has been transferred from schedule 3 to schedule 2 of the Misuse of Drugs Regulations 1985; receipt and supply must therefore be recorded in the CD register.

CD **Seconal Sodium**® (Lilly)

*Capsules*, both orange, quinalbarbitone sodium 50 mg, net price 20 = 85p; 100 mg, 20 = £1.29. Label: 19

*Dose:* 50–100 mg at bedtime

CD **Tuinal**® (Lilly)

*Capsules*, orange/blue, a mixture of amylobarbitone sodium 50 mg, quinalbarbitone sodium 50 mg. Net price 20 = 54p. Label: 19

*Dose:* 1–2 capsules at bedtime

*Note.* Only one strength available therefore prescriptions need only specify 'Tuinal capsules'

---

## 4.2  Drugs used in psychoses and related disorders

4.2.1 Antipsychotic drugs
4.2.2 Antipsychotic depot injections
4.2.3 Antimanic drugs

## 4.2.1  Antipsychotic drugs

Antipsychotic drugs are also known as 'neuroleptics' and (misleadingly) as 'major tranquillisers'. Antipsychotic drugs generally tranquillise without impairing consciousness and without causing paradoxical excitement but they should not be regarded merely as tranquillisers. For conditions such as schizophrenia the tranquillising effect is of secondary importance.

In the short term they are used to quieten disturbed patients whatever the underlying psychopathology, which may be brain damage, mania, toxic delirium, agitated depression, or acute behavioural disturbance.

They are used to alleviate severe anxiety but this too should be a short-term measure. Some antipsychotic drugs (e.g. chlorpromazine, thioridazine, flupenthixol) also have an antidepressant effect while others may exacerbate depression (e.g. fluphenazine, pimozide, pipothiazine).

SCHIZOPHRENIA. Antipsychotic drugs relieve florid psychotic symptoms such as thought disorder, hallucinations, and delusions, and prevent relapse. Although they are usually less effective in apathetic withdrawn patients, they sometimes appear to have an activating influence. For example, chlorpromazine may restore an acutely ill schizophrenic to normal activity and social behaviour who was previously withdrawn or even mute and akinetic. Patients with acute schizophrenia generally respond better than those with chronic symptoms.

Long-term treatment of a patient with a definite diagnosis of schizophrenia may be necessary even after the first episode of illness in order to prevent the manifest illness from becoming chronic. Withdrawal of drug treatment requires careful surveillance because the patient who appears well on medication may suffer a disastrous relapse if treatment is withdrawn inappropriately. In addition the need for continuation of treatment may not become immediately evident because relapse is often delayed for several weeks after cessation of treatment.

Antipsychotic drugs are considered to act by interfering with dopaminergic transmission in the brain by blocking dopamine receptors and may give rise to the extrapyramidal effects described below, and also to hyperprolactinaemia. Antipsychotic drugs also affect cholinergic, alpha-adrenergic, histaminergic, and serotonergic receptors.

SIDE-EFFECTS. Extrapyramidal symptoms are the most troublesome. They are caused most frequently by the piperazine phenothiazines (fluphenazine, perphenazine, prochlorperazine, and trifluoperazine), the butyrophenones (benperidol, droperidol, haloperidol, and trifluperidol), and the depot preparations. They are easy to recognise but cannot be accurately predicted because they depend partly on the dose and partly on the type of drug, and on patient susceptibility. They consist of parkinsonian symptoms (including tremor) which may occur gradually, dystonia (abnormal face and body movements) which may appear after only a few doses, akathisia (restlessness) which may resemble an exacerbation of the condition being treated, and tardive dyskinesia (which usually takes longer to develop).

Parkinsonian symptoms remit if the drug is withdrawn and may be suppressed by the administration of **antimuscarinic** drugs (section 4.9.2). Routine administration of such drugs is **not** justified as not all patients are affected and because tardive dyskinesia may be unmasked or worsened by them. Furthermore, these drugs are sometimes abused for their mood-altering effects. Tardive dyskinesia is of particular concern because it may be irreversible on withdrawing therapy and treatment may be ineffective. It occurs fairly frequently in patients (especially the elderly) on long-term therapy and with high dosage, and the treatment of such patients must be carefully and regularly reviewed. Tardive dyskinesia may also occur occasionally after short-term treatment with low dosage.

Hypotension and interference with temperature regulation are dose-related side-effects and are liable to cause dangerous falls and hypothermia in the elderly; very serious consideration should be given before prescribing these drugs for patients over 70 years of age.

Neuroleptic malignant syndrome (hyperthermia, fluctuating level of consciousness, muscular rigidity and autonomic dysfunction with pallor, tachycardia, labile blood pressure, sweating, and urinary incontinence) is a rare but potentially fatal side-effect of some drugs. Drugs for which it has been reported in the UK include haloperidol, chlorpromazine, and flupenthixol decanoate. Discontinuation of drug therapy is essential as there is no proven effective treatment but bromocriptine and dantrolene have been used. The syndrome, which usually lasts for 5–10 days after drug discontinuation, may be unduly prolonged if depot preparations have been used.

Overdosage: see Emergency Treatment of Poisoning, p. 20.

CLASSIFICATION OF ANTIPSYCHOTICS. The **phenothiazine** derivatives can be divided into 3 main groups.

*Group 1:* chlorpromazine, methotrimeprazine, and promazine, generally characterised by pronounced sedative effects and moderate antimuscarinic and extrapyramidal side-effects.

*Group 2:* pericyazine, pipothiazine, and thioridazine, generally characterised by moderate sedative effects, marked antimuscarinic effects, but fewer extrapyramidal side-effects than groups 1 or 3.

*Group 3:* fluphenazine, perphenazine, prochlorperazine, and trifluoperazine, generally characterised by fewer sedative effects, fewer antimuscarinic effects, but more pronounced extrapyramidal side-effects than groups 1 and 2.

Drugs of other chemical groups tend to resemble the phenothiazines of *group 3*. They include the **butyrophenones** (benperidol, droperidol, haloperidol, and trifluperidol); **diphenylbutylpiperidines** (fluspirilene and pimozide); **thioxanthenes** (flupenthixol and zuclopenthixol); **oxypertine**; and **loxapine. Clozapine** differs in that it is sedative with fewer extrapyramidal effects.

---

DOSAGE. In some patients it is necessary to raise the dose of an antipsychotic drug above that which is normally recommended. This should be done with caution and under specialist supervision.

*Once-daily dose.* After an initial period of stabilisation, in most patients, the long half-life of antipsychotic drugs allows the total daily dose to be given as a single dose.

---

CHOICE. As indicated above, the various drugs differ somewhat in predominant actions and side-effects. Selection is influenced by the degree of sedation required and the patient's susceptibility to extrapyramidal side-effects. However, the differences between antipsychotic drugs are less important than the great variability in patient response; moreover, tolerance to these secondary effects usually develops.

Prescribing of more than one antipsychotic at the same time is **not** recommended; it may constitute a hazard and there is no significant evidence that side-effects are minimised.

**Chlorpromazine** is widely used. It has a marked sedating effect and is particularly useful for treating violent patients without causing stupor. Agitated states in the elderly can be controlled without confusion, a dose of 25 mg usually being adequate.

**Flupenthixol** and **pimozide** (see CSM advice p.145) are less sedating than chlorpromazine.

**Sulpiride** is structurally distinct from other antipsychotic drugs. In high doses it controls florid positive symptoms, but in lower doses it has an alerting effect on apathetic withdrawn schizophrenics. **Remoxipride** is a new antipsychotic drug said to have a low level of extrapyramidal and sedative side-effects.

**Fluphenazine, haloperidol**, and **trifluoperazine** are also of value but their use is limited by the high incidence of extrapyramidal symptoms. Haloperidol may be preferred for the rapid control of hyperactive psychotic states.

**Thioridazine** is popular for treating the elderly as there is a reduced incidence of extrapyramidal symptoms.

**Promazine** is not sufficiently active by mouth to be used as an antipsychotic drug

**Clozapine** is indicated only for the treatment of schizophrenia in patients unresponsive to, or intolerant of, conventional antipsychotic drugs. As it can cause agranulocytosis, its use is restricted to patients registered with the Clozaril Patient Monitoring Service (see under Clozapine, below).

**Loxapine** causes relatively little sedation; in overdosage it has a high potential for serious neurological and cardiac toxicity.

OTHER USES. Nausea and vomiting (section 4.6), choreas, motor tics (section 4.9.3), and intractable hiccup (see under Chlorpromazine Hydrochloride and under Haloperidol). **Benperidol** is used in deviant antisocial sexual behaviour but its value is not established.

WITHDRAWAL. Withdrawal of antipsychotic drugs after long-term therapy should always be gradual and closely monitored to avoid the risk of acute withdrawal syndromes or rapid relapse.

DOSAGE. In some patients it is necessary to raise the dose of an antipsychotic drug above that which is normally recommended. This should be done with caution and under specialist supervision.
*Once-daily dose.* After an initial period of stabilisation, in most patients, the long half-life of antipsychotic drugs allows the total daily dose to be given as a single dose.

## CHLORPROMAZINE HYDROCHLORIDE
WARNING. Owing to the risk of contact sensitisation, pharmacists, nurses, and other health workers should avoid direct contact with chlorpromazine; tablets should not be crushed and solutions should be handled with care

*Indications:* see under Dose; antiemetic (in terminal illness), section 4.6; peri-operative use, see section 15.1.4.1

*Cautions:* cardiovascular and cerebrovascular disease, respiratory disease, phaeochromocytoma, parkinsonism, epilepsy, acute infections, pregnancy, breast-feeding, renal and hepatic impairment (avoid if severe), history of jaundice, leucopenia (blood counts if unexplained infections); hypothyroidism, myasthenia gravis, prostatic hypertrophy, closed-angle glaucoma; caution in elderly particularly in very hot or very cold weather. On prolonged use examinations for eye defects and abnormal skin pigmentation are required. Avoid abrupt withdrawal. Patients should remain supine for 30 minutes after intramuscular injection; **interactions:** Appendix 1 (phenothiazines and other antipsychotics)
DRIVING. Drowsiness may affect performance of skilled tasks (e.g. driving); effects of alcohol enhanced

*Contra-indications:* coma caused by CNS depressants; bone-marrow depression; avoid in phaeochromocytoma

*Side-effects:* extrapyramidal symptoms (reversed by dose reduction or antimuscarinic drugs) and, on prolonged administration, occasionally tardive dyskinesia; hypothermia (occasionally pyrexia), drowsiness, apathy, pallor, nightmares, insomnia, depression, and, more rarely, agitation, EEG changes, convulsions. Antimuscarinic symptoms such as dry mouth, nasal congestion, constipation, difficulty with micturition, and blurred vision; cardiovascular symptoms such as hypotension, tachycardia, and arrhythmias; ECG changes; endocrine effects such as menstrual disturbances, galactorrhoea, gynaecomastia, impotence, and weight gain; sensitivity reactions such as agranulocytosis, leucopenia, leucocytosis, and haemolytic anaemia, photosensitisation (more common with chlorpromazine than with other antipsychotics), contact sensitisation and rashes, jaundice and alterations in liver function; neuroleptic malignant syndrome; lupus erythematosus-like syndrome reported. With prolonged high dosage, corneal and lens opacities and purplish pigmentation of the skin, cornea, conjunctiva, and retina. Intramuscular injection may be painful, cause hypotension and tachycardia (see Cautions), and give rise to nodule formation. Overdosage: see Emergency Treatment of Poisoning, p. 20

*Dose: by mouth*,

Schizophrenia and other psychoses, mania, short-term adjunctive management of severe anxiety, psychomotor agitation, excitement, and violent or dangerously impulsive behaviour initially 25 mg 3 times daily (*or* 75 mg at night), adjusted according to response, to usual maintenance dose of 75–300 mg daily (but up to 1 g daily may be required in psychoses); CHILD 1–5 years 500 micrograms/kg every 4–6 hours (max. 40 mg daily); 6–12 years third to half adult dose (max. 75 mg daily)

ELDERLY (or debilitated) third to half adult dose Intractable hiccup, 25–50 mg 3–4 times daily

*By deep intramuscular injection*, (for relief of acute symptoms), 25–50 mg every 6–8 hours; CHILD, as dose by mouth

*By rectum* in suppositories, chlorpromazine 100 mg every 6–8 hours

Note. For equivalent therapeutic effect 100 mg chlorpromazine base given *rectally* as a suppository = 20–25 mg chlorpromazine hydrochloride *by intramuscular injection* = 40–50 mg of chlorpromazine base or hydrochloride *by mouth*

PoM **Chlorpromazine** (Non-proprietary)

*Tablets*, coated, chlorpromazine hydrochloride 10 mg, net price 20 = 12p; 25 mg, 20 = 8p; 50 mg, 20 = 28p; 100 mg, 20 = 53p. Label: 2
Available from APS, DDSA (Chloractil®)

*Elixir*, chlorpromazine hydrochloride 25 mg/5 mL. Net price 100 mL = 26p. Label: 2

*Injection*, chlorpromazine hydrochloride 25 mg/mL, net price 1-mL amp = 21p; 2-mL amp = 27p

*Suppositories*, chlorpromazine 100 mg. Net price 10 = £1.91. Label: 2
Available from Penn (special order)

PoM **Largactil**® (Rhône-Poulenc Rorer)

*Tablets*, all off-white, f/c, chlorpromazine hydrochloride 10 mg. Net price 56-tab pack = 33p; 25 mg, 56-tab pack = 50p; 50 mg, 56-tab pack = £1.16; 100 mg, 56-tab pack = £2.16. Label: 2

*Syrup*, brown, chlorpromazine hydrochloride 25 mg/5 mL. Diluent syrup (without preservative), life of diluted syrup 14 days. Net price 100-mL pack = 59p. Label: 2

*Suspension forte*, orange, sugar-free, chlorpromazine hydrochloride 100 mg (as embonate)/5 mL. Diluent syrup (without preservative), life of diluted suspension 7 days. Net price 100-mL pack = £1.19. Label: 2

*Injection*, chlorpromazine hydrochloride 25 mg/mL. Net price 2-mL amp = 28p

## BENPERIDOL

*Indications:* control of deviant antisocial sexual behaviour (but see notes above)

*Cautions; Contra-indications; Side-effects:* see under Haloperidol; avoid in children

*Dose:* 0.25–1.5 mg daily in divided doses, adjusted according to the response; ELDERLY (or debilitated) initially half adult dose

PoM **Anquil**® (Janssen)

*Tablets*, benperidol 250 micrograms. Net price 20 = £5.36. Label: 2

## CLOZAPINE

*Indications:* schizophrenia in patients unresponsive to, or intolerant of, conventional antipsychotic drugs

*Cautions:* see under Chlorpromazine Hydrochloride; leucocyte and differential blood counts must be normal before treatment and must be monitored weekly for first 18 weeks then fortnightly; avoid drugs which depress leucopoiesis; withdraw treatment if leucocyte count falls below 3000/mm³ or absolute neutrophil count falls below 1500/mm³; patients should report any infections; avoid in children; **interactions**: Appendix 1 (clozapine)

*Contra-indications:* history of drug-induced neutropenia/agranulocytosis; bone marrow disorders; alcoholic and toxic psychoses; drug intoxication; coma or severe CNS depression; pregnancy and breast-feeding

*Side-effects:* see under Chlorpromazine Hydrochloride but more sedating and high incidence of antimuscarinic symptoms; extrapyramidal symptoms may occur less frequently; neutropenia and potentially fatal agranulocytosis, headache and dizziness, hypersalivation, urinary incontinence, myocarditis, and delirium also reported

*Dose:* initially 25–50 mg daily (elderly 25 mg), increased as necessary by 25–50 mg daily (elderly 25 mg) over 7–14 days to 300 mg daily in divided doses (larger dose at night; up to 200 mg daily may be given as a single dose at bedtime); usual antipsychotic dose 200–450 mg daily (max. 900 mg daily), and subsequently adjusted to usual maintenance of 150–300 mg daily

▼ PoM **Clozaril**® (Sandoz)

*Tablets*, both yellow, scored, clozapine 25 mg, net price 84-tab pack = £38.50; 100 mg, 84-tab pack = £154.00 (hosp. only, patient, prescriber, and supplying pharmacist must be registered with the Sandoz Clozaril Patient Monitoring Service). Label: 2, 10 patient information leaflet

## DROPERIDOL

*Indications:* see under Dose; peri-operative use, see section 15.1.4.1

*Cautions; Contra-indications; Side-effects:* see under Haloperidol

*Dose: by mouth*, tranquillisation and emergency control in mania, 5–20 mg repeated every 4–8 hours if necessary (elderly, initially half adult dose); CHILD, 0.5–1 mg daily

*By intramuscular injection*, up to 10 mg repeated every 4–6 hours if necessary (elderly, initially half adult dose); CHILD, 0.5–1 mg daily

*By intravenous injection*, 5–15 mg repeated every 4–6 hours if necessary (elderly, initially half adult dose)

Cancer chemotherapy-induced nausea and vomiting, *by intramuscular or intravenous injection*, 1–10 mg 30 minutes before starting therapy, followed by *continuous intravenous infusion* of 1–3 mg/hour *or* 1–5 mg *by intramuscular or intravenous injection* every 1–6 hours as necessary; CHILD *by intramuscular or intravenous injection*, 20–75 micrograms/kg

PoM **Droleptan**® (Janssen)
*Tablets*, yellow, scored, droperidol 10 mg. Net price 50-tab pack = £12.62. Label: 2
*Oral liquid*, sugar-free, droperidol 1 mg/mL. Net price 100-mL pack (with graduated cap) = £4.59; 500-mL pack = £21.79. Label: 2
*Injection*, droperidol 5 mg/mL. Net price 2-mL amp = 92p

## FLUPENTHIXOL

*Indications:* schizophrenia and other psychoses, particularly with apathy and withdrawal but not mania or psychomotor hyperactivity; depression, section 4.3.4
*Cautions; Contra-indications; Side-effects:* see under Chlorpromazine Hydrochloride but less sedating; extrapyramidal symptoms more frequent (25% of patients); avoid in children, senile confusional states, excitable and overactive patients, and in porphyria (see section 9.8.2)
*Dose:* initially 3–9 mg twice daily adjusted according to the response; max. 18 mg daily

PoM **Depixol**® (Lundbeck)
*Tablets*, yellow, s/c, flupenthixol 3 mg (as dihydrochloride). Net price 20 = £2.59. Label: 2
*Depot injection* (flupenthixol decanoate): section 4.2.2
PoM **Fluanxol**® (depression), see section 4.3.4

## FLUPHENAZINE HYDROCHLORIDE

*Indications:* see under Dose
*Cautions; Contra-indications; Side-effects:* see under Chlorpromazine Hydrochloride, but less sedating and fewer antimuscarinic or hypotensive symptoms; extrapyramidal symptoms, particularly dystonic reactions and akathisia, are more frequent; avoid in depression; avoid in children
*Dose:* schizophrenia and other psychoses, mania, initially 2.5–10 mg daily in 2–3 divided doses, adjusted according to response to 20 mg daily; doses above 20 mg daily (10 mg in elderly) only with special caution
Short-term adjunctive management of severe anxiety, psychomotor agitation, excitement, and violent or dangerously impulsive behaviour, initially 1 mg twice daily, increased as necessary to 2 mg twice daily

PoM **Moditen**® (Squibb)
*Tablets*, all s/c, fluphenazine hydrochloride 1 mg (pink), net price 20 = £1.09; 2.5 mg (yellow), 20 = £1.36; 5 mg, 20 = £1.82. Label: 2
*Depot injections* (fluphenazine decanoate): section 4.2.2

## HALOPERIDOL

*Indications:* see under Dose; motor tics, section 4.9.3
*Cautions; Contra-indications; Side-effects:* see under Chlorpromazine Hydrochloride but less sedating, and fewer antimuscarinic or hypotensive symptoms; pigmentation and photosensitivity reactions rare. Extrapyramidal symptoms, particularly dystonic reactions and akathisia are more frequent especially in thyrotoxic patients. Rarely weight loss. Avoid in basal ganglia disease
*Dose: by mouth*
Schizophrenia and other psychoses, mania, short-term adjunctive management of psychomotor agitation, excitement, and violent or dangerously impulsive behaviour, initially 1.5–20 mg daily in divided doses, gradually increased to 100 mg (and occasionally 200 mg) daily in severely disturbed patients; ELDERLY (or debilitated) initially half adult dose; CHILD initially 25–50 micrograms/kg daily to a max. of 10 mg; adolescents up to 30 mg daily (exceptionally 60 mg)
Short-term adjunctive management of severe anxiety, adults 500 micrograms twice daily
Intractable hiccup, 1.5 mg 3 times daily adjusted according to response
*By intramuscular injection*, 2–10 mg (increasing to 30 mg for emergency control) then 5 mg up to every hour if necessary (intervals of 4–8 hours may be satisfactory)
Nausea and vomiting, 1–2 mg

PoM **Haloperidol** (Non-proprietary)
*Tablets*, haloperidol 1.5 mg, net price 20 = 24p; 5 mg, 20 = 52p; 10 mg, 20 = £1.36; 20 mg, 20 = £2.48. Label: 2
PoM **Dozic**® (RP Drugs)
*Oral liquid*, sugar-free, haloperidol 1 mg/mL, net price 100-mL pack (with pipette) = £5.00; 2 mg/mL, 100-mL pack (with pipette) = £5.10. Label: 2
PoM **Haldol**® (Janssen)
*Tablets*, both scored, haloperidol 5 mg (blue), net price 20 = £1.69; 10 mg (yellow), 20 = £3.30. Label: 2
*Oral liquid*, sugar-free, haloperidol 2 mg/mL. Net price 100-mL pack (with pipette) = £5.21. Label: 2
*Oral liquid concentrate*, sugar-free, haloperidol 10 mg/mL. Net price 100-mL pack = £22.84. Label: 2
Diluent purified water, freshly boiled and cooled, life of diluted concentrate 14 days. Alternatively, purified water, freshly boiled and cooled, containing 0.05% of methyl hydroxybenzoate and 0.005% of propyl hydroxybenzoate, life of diluted concentrate 2 months.

*Injection*, haloperidol 5 mg/mL. Net price 1-mL amp = 33p; 2-mL amp = 63p
*Depot injection* (haloperidol decanoate): section 4.2.2

PoM **Serenace**® (Searle)
*Capsules*, green, haloperidol 500 micrograms. Net price 20 = 67p. Label: 2
*Tablets*, all scored, haloperidol 1.5 mg, net price 20 = £1.19;  5 mg (pink), 20 = £3.36;  10 mg (pale pink), 20 = £6.02;  20 mg (dark pink), 20 = £10.85. Label: 2
*Oral liquid*, sugar-free, haloperidol 2 mg/mL. Net price 100-mL pack = £8.99. Label: 2
Diluent syrup or purified water, freshly boiled and cooled, or syrup for dilutions containing 1% or less of the elixir, life of diluted elixir 2 months.
*Injection*, haloperidol 5 mg/mL, net price 1-mL amp = 59p; 10 mg/mL, 2-mL amp = £2.03

## LOXAPINE

*Indications:* acute and chronic psychoses
*Cautions; Contra-indications:* see under Chlorpromazine Hydrochloride
*Side-effects:* see under Chlorpromazine Hydrochloride; nausea and vomiting, weight gain or loss, dyspnoea, ptosis, hyperpyrexia, flushing and headache, paraesthesia, and polydipsia also reported; no endocrine effects yet reported; avoid in porphyria (see section 9.8.2)
*Dose:* initially 20–50 mg daily in 2 divided doses, increased as necessary over 7–10 days to 60–100 mg daily (max. 250 mg) in 2–4 divided doses, then adjusted to usual maintenance dose of 20–100 mg daily

▼ PoM **Loxapac**® (Novex)
*Capsules*, loxapine (as succinate) 10 mg (yellow/green), net price 100 = £9.52;  25 mg (light green/dark green), 100 = £19.05;  50 mg (blue/dark green), 100 = £34.27. Label: 2

## METHOTRIMEPRAZINE

*Indications:* see under Dose
*Cautions; Contra-indications; Side-effects:* see under Chlorpromazine Hydrochloride but more sedating; risk of postural hypotension particularly in patients over 50 years
*Dose: by mouth*, schizophrenia, initially 25–50 mg daily in divided doses increased as necessary; bedpatients initially 100–200 mg daily in 3 divided doses, increased if necessary to 1 g daily
Adjunctive treatment in terminal care (including management of pain and associated restlessness, distress, or vomiting), 12.5–50 mg every 4–8 hours
*By intramuscular injection or by intravenous injection* (after dilution with an equal volume of sodium chloride 0.9% injection), adjunct in terminal care, 12.5–25 mg (severe agitation up to 50 mg) every 6–8 hours if necessary
*By continuous subcutaneous infusion*, adjunct in terminal care (via syringe driver), 25–200 mg daily (over 24-hour period), diluted in a suitable volume of sodium chloride 0.9% injection

PoM **Nozinan**® (Rhône-Poulenc Rorer)
*Tablets*[1], scored, methotrimeprazine maleate 25 mg. Net price 20 = £2.11. Label: 2
*Injection*, methotrimeprazine hydrochloride 25 mg/mL. Net price 1-mL amp = £1.23
1. Formerly named Veractil®

## OXYPERTINE

*Indications:* see under Dose
*Cautions; Contra-indications; Side-effects:* see under Chlorpromazine Hydrochloride, but extrapyramidal symptoms may occur less frequently. With low doses agitation and hyperactivity occur and with high doses sedation. Occasionally photophobia may occur
*Dose:* schizophrenia and other psychoses, mania, short-term adjunctive management of psychomotor agitation, excitement, and violent or dangerously impulsive behaviour, initially 80–120 mg daily in divided doses adjusted according to the response; max. 300 mg daily
Short-term adjunctive management of severe anxiety, initially 10 mg 3–4 times daily preferably after food; max. 60 mg daily

PoM **Integrin**® (Sanofi Winthrop)
*Capsules*, oxypertine 10 mg. Net price 20 = £1.93. Label: 2
*Tablets*, scored, oxypertine 40 mg. Net price 20 = £6.04. Label: 2

## PERICYAZINE

*Indications:* see under Dose
*Cautions; Contra-indications; Side-effects:* see under Chlorpromazine Hydrochloride, but more sedating; hypotension commonly occurs when treatment initiated
*Dose:* schizophrenia and other psychoses, initially 75 mg daily in divided doses increased at weekly intervals by steps of 25 mg according to response; usual max. 300 mg daily (elderly initially 15–30 mg daily).
Short-term adjunctive management of severe anxiety, psychomotor agitation, and violent or dangerously impulsive behaviour, initially 15–30 mg (elderly 5–10 mg) daily divided into 2 doses, taking the larger dose at bedtime, adjusted according to response
CHILD (severe mental or behavioural disorders only), initially, 500 micrograms daily for 10-kg child, increased by 1 mg for each additional 5 kg to max. total daily dose of 10 mg; dose may be gradually increased according to response but maintenance should not exceed twice initial dose

PoM **Neulactil**® (Rhône-Poulenc Rorer)
*Tablets*, all yellow, scored, pericyazine 2.5 mg, net price 84-tab pack = £1.87;  10 mg, 84-tab pack = £5.04;  25 mg,  50-tab  pack = £8.29. Label: 2
*Syrup forte*, brown, pericyazine 10 mg/5 mL. Diluent syrup, life of diluted syrup 14 days. Net price 100-mL pack = £2.45. Label: 2

## PERPHENAZINE

*Indications:* see under Dose; anti-emetic, section 4.6

*Cautions; Contra-indications; Side-effects:* see under Chlorpromazine Hydrochloride, but less sedating; extrapyramidal symptoms, especially dystonia, more frequent, particularly at high dosage; avoid in children under 14 years; not indicated for agitation and restlessness in the elderly

*Dose:* schizophrenia and other psychoses, mania, short-term adjunctive management of severe anxiety, psychomotor agitation, excitement, and violent or dangerously impulsive behaviour, initially 4 mg 3 times daily adjusted according to the response; max. 24 mg daily; elderly quarter to half adult dose (but see Cautions)

PoM **Fentazin**® (A&H)
*Tablets*, both s/c, perphenazine 2 mg, net price 20 = 52p; 4 mg, 20 = 62p. Label: 2

## PIMOZIDE

*Indications:* see under Dose

*Cautions; Contra-indications; Side-effects:* see under Chlorpromazine Hydrochloride, but less sedating; avoid in children; contra-indicated in breast-feeding; serious arrhythmias reported (contra-indicated if history of arrhythmias or pre-existing congenital QT prolongation); following reports of sudden unexplained death, the CSM recommends ECG before treatment in all patients, periodic ECGs at doses over 16 mg daily and review of need for pimozide if repolarisation changes or arrhythmias develop (close supervision and preferably dose reduction advised); concurrent cardioactive or antipsychotic drugs, or electrolyte disturbances (notably hypokalaemia) may predispose to cardiotoxicity

*Dose:* schizophrenia, initially 10 mg daily in acute conditions, adjusted according to response in increments of 2–4 mg at intervals of not less than 1 week; max. 20 mg daily; prevention of relapse, initially 2 mg daily (range 2–20 mg daily)
Monosymptomatic hypochondriacal psychosis, paranoid psychoses, initially 4 mg daily, adjusted according to response in increments of 2–4 mg at intervals of not less than 1 week; max. 16 mg daily
Mania, hypomania, short-term adjunctive management of excitement and psychomotor agitation, initially 10 mg daily adjusted according to response in increments of 2–4 mg at intervals of not less than 1 week; max. 20 mg daily
ELDERLY half usual starting dose

PoM **Orap**® (Janssen)
*Tablets*, all scored, pimozide 2 mg, net price 20 = £3.25; 4 mg (green), 20 = £6.29; 10 mg, 20 = £12.06. Label: 2

## PROCHLORPERAZINE

*Indications:* see under Dose; anti-emetic, section 4.6

*Cautions; Contra-indications; Side-effects:* see under Chlorpromazine Hydrochloride, but less sedating; extrapyramidal symptoms, particularly dystonic reactions, more frequent; avoid in children (but see section 4.6 for use as anti-emetic)

*Dose: by mouth*, schizophrenia and other psychoses, mania, prochlorperazine maleate or mesylate, 12.5 mg twice daily for 7 days adjusted to 75–100 mg daily according to response
Short-term adjunctive management of severe anxiety, 15–20 mg daily in divided doses; max. 40 mg daily
*By deep intramuscular injection*, psychoses, mania, prochlorperazine mesylate 12.5–25 mg 2–3 times daily
*By rectum* in suppositories, psychoses, mania, the equivalent of prochlorperazine maleate 25 mg 2–3 times daily

**Preparations:**
Section 4.6

## PROMAZINE HYDROCHLORIDE

*Indications:* see under Dose

*Cautions; Contra-indications; Side-effects:* see under Chlorpromazine Hydrochloride

*Dose: by mouth*, short term adjunctive management of psychomotor agitation, 100–200 mg 4 times daily
Agitation and restlessness in elderly, 25–50 mg 4 times daily
*By intramuscular injection*, short-term adjunctive management of psychomotor agitation, 50 mg (25 mg in elderly or debilitated), repeated if necessary after 6–8 hours

PoM **Promazine** (Non-proprietary)
*Tablets*, coated, promazine hydrochloride 25 mg, 50 mg, and 100 mg. Label: 2
Available from Biorex
PoM **Sparine**® (Wyeth)
*Suspension*, yellow, promazine hydrochloride 50 mg (as embonate)/5 mL. Diluent syrup, life of diluted suspension 14 days. Net price 150-mL pack = £1.29. Label: 2.
*Note.* Not recommended for children
*Injection*, promazine hydrochloride 50 mg/mL. Net price 1-mL amp = 26p

## REMOXIPRIDE HYDROCHLORIDE

*Indications:* schizophrenia and other psychoses (except due to depressive illness)

*Cautions; Contra-indications:* see under Chlorpromazine Hydrochloride; avoid in children; **interactions:** Appendix 1 (remoxipride)

*Side-effects:* see under Chlorpromazine Hydrochloride but less sedating and extrapyramidal symptoms may occur less frequently; insomnia, concentration difficulties, anxiety, aggression, nausea, headache, and hypersalivation also reported

*Dose:* initially 300 mg daily (elderly 150 mg daily), adjusted according to response; usual range 150–450 mg daily (max. 600 mg daily); usual maintenance 150–300 mg daily

▼ PoM **Roxiam**® (Astra)
*Capsules*, both blue, m/r, remoxipride hydrochloride 150 mg, net price 28-cap pack = £12.80; 300 mg, 28-cap pack = £21.56. Label: 3, 25

## SULPIRIDE
*Indications:* schizophrenia
*Cautions; Contra-indications; Side-effects:* see under Chlorpromazine Hydrochloride, but less sedating; structurally distinct from chlorpromazine hence not associated with jaundice or skin reactions; avoid in porphyria (see section 9.8.2) and breast-feeding; reduce dose (preferably avoid) in renal impairment
*Dose:* 200–400 mg twice daily; max. 800 mg daily in patients with predominantly negative symptoms, and 2.4 g daily in patients with mainly positive symptoms; ELDERLY, initially 100–200 mg

PoM **Dolmatil**® (Squibb)
*Tablets*, scored, sulpiride 200 mg. Net price 20 = £4.20. Label: 2
PoM **Sulpitil**® (Tillotts)
*Tablets*, scored, sulpiride 200 mg. Net price 28-tab pack = £5.75; 112-tab pack = £23.00. Label: 2

## THIORIDAZINE
*Indications:* see under Dose
*Cautions; Contra-indications; Side-effects:* see under Chlorpromazine Hydrochloride, but less sedating and extrapyramidal symptoms and hypothermia rarely occur; more likely to induce hypotension. Pigmentary retinopathy (with reduced visual acuity, brownish colouring of vision, and impaired night vision) occurs rarely with high doses. Sexual dysfunction, particularly retrograde ejaculation, may occur; avoid in porphyria (see section 9.8.2)
*Dose:* schizophrenia and other psychoses, mania, 150–600 mg daily (initially in divided doses); max. 800 mg daily (hospital patients only) for up to 4 weeks
Short-term adjunctive management of psychomotor agitation, excitement, violent or dangerously impulsive behaviour, 75–200 mg daily
Short-term adjunctive management of severe anxiety, and agitation and restlessness in the elderly, 30–100 mg daily
CHILD (severe mental or behavioural problems only) under 5 years 1 mg/kg daily, 5–12 years 75–150 mg daily (in severe cases, up to 300 mg daily)

PoM **Thioridazine** (Non-proprietary)
*Tablets*, coated, thioridazine hydrochloride 25 mg, net price 20 = 32p; 50 mg, 20 = 61p; 100 mg, 20 = £1.16. Label: 2

PoM **Melleril**® (Sandoz)
*Tablets*, all f/c, thioridazine hydrochloride 10 mg, net price 20 = 23p; 25 mg, 20 = 32p; 50 mg, 20 = 61p; 100 mg, 20 = £1.16. Label: 2
*Suspension 25 mg/5 mL*, thioridazine 25 mg/5 mL. Net price 100 mL = 58p. Label: 2
*Suspension 100 mg/5 mL*, thioridazine 100 mg/5 mL. Net price 100 mL = £2.13. Label: 2
*Note.* These suspensions should not be diluted but the two preparations may be mixed with each other to provide intermediate doses
*Syrup*, orange, thioridazine 25 mg (as hydrochloride)/5 mL. Net price 100-mL pack = 78p. Label: 2

## TRIFLUOPERAZINE
*Indications:* see under Dose; anti-emetic, section 4.6
*Cautions; Contra-indications; Side-effects:* see under Chlorpromazine Hydrochloride but less sedating, and hypotension, hypothermia, and antimuscarinic side-effects occur less frequently; extrapyramidal symptoms, particularly dystonic reactions and akathisia, are more frequent (particularly when the daily dose exceeds 6 mg); caution in children
*Dose: by mouth*
Schizophrenia and other psychoses, short-term adjunctive management of psychomotor agitation, excitement, and violent or dangerously impulsive behaviour, initially 5 mg twice daily, *or* 10 mg daily in modified-release form, increased by 5 mg after 1 week, then at intervals of 3 days, according to the response; CHILD up to 12 years, initially up to 5 mg daily in divided doses, adjusted according to response, age, and body-weight
Short-term adjunctive management of severe anxiety, 2–4 mg daily in divided doses *or* 2–4 mg daily in modified-release form, increased if necessary to 6 mg daily; CHILD 3–5 years up to 1 mg daily, 6–12 years up to 4 mg daily, in divided doses
*By deep intramuscular injection* 1–3 mg daily in divided doses to a max. of 6 mg daily; CHILD 50 micrograms/kg daily in divided doses

PoM **Trifluoperazine** (Non-proprietary)
*Tablets*, coated, trifluoperazine (as hydrochloride) 1 mg, net price 20 = 30p; 5 mg; 20 = 39p. Label: 2
PoM **Stelazine**® (SK&F)
*Tablets*, both blue, s/c, trifluoperazine (as hydrochloride) 1 mg, net price 20 = 42p; 5 mg, 20 = 60p. Label: 2
*Spansule*® (= capsules m/r), all clear/yellow, enclosing dark blue, light blue, and white pellets, trifluoperazine (as hydrochloride) 2 mg, net price 60-cap pack = £2.71; 10 mg, 30-cap pack = £1.77; 15 mg, 30-cap pack = £2.66. Label: 2, 25
*Syrup*, yellow, sugar-free, trifluoperazine 1 mg (as hydrochloride)/5 mL. Diluent sorbitol solution (70%), life of diluted syrup 28 days. Net price 200-mL pack = £1.65. Label: 2

*Liquid concentrate,* yellow, sugar-free, trifluoperazine 10 mg (as hydrochloride)/mL for dilution before use. Diluent sorbitol solution (70%) or water containing benzoic acid 0.1%, life of diluted liquid 12 weeks. Net price 100 mL = £3.71 (hosp. only)
*Injection,* trifluoperazine 1 mg (as hydrochloride)/mL. Net price 1-mL amp = 47p

## TRIFLUPERIDOL

*Indications:* schizophrenia and other psychoses, particularly those with manic features
*Cautions; Contra-indications; Side-effects:* see under Haloperidol
*Dose:* initially 500 micrograms daily, adjusted by 500 micrograms every 3–4 days according to response; max. 6–8 mg daily; CHILD 5–12 years initially 250 micrograms daily, adjusted according to response; max. 2 mg daily; usual maintenance 1 mg daily

PoM **Triperidol**® (Lagap)
*Tablets,* both scored, trifluperidol 500 micrograms, net price 20 = £2.59; 1 mg, 20 = £2.69. Label: 2

## ZUCLOPENTHIXOL ACETATE

*Indications:* short-term management of acute psychosis, mania, or exacerbations of chronic psychosis
*Cautions; Contra-indications; Side-effects:* see under Chlorpromazine Hydrochloride; avoid in porphyria (see section 9.8.2); treatment duration should not exceed 2 weeks
*Dose: by deep intramuscular injection,* 50–150 mg (elderly 50–100 mg), if necessary repeated after 2–3 days (1 additional dose may be needed 1–2 days after the first injection); max. cumulative dose 400 mg per course and max. 4 injections; if maintenance treatment necessary change to an oral antipsychotic 2–3 days after last injection, *or* to a longer acting antipsychotic depot injection given concomitantly with last injection of zuclopenthixol acetate

PoM **Clopixol Acuphase**® (Lundbeck)
*Injection* (oily), zuclopenthixol acetate 50 mg/mL. Net price 1-mL amp = £4.50; 2-mL amp = £9.01

## ZUCLOPENTHIXOL DIHYDROCHLORIDE

*Indications:* schizophrenia and other psychoses, particularly when associated with agitated, aggressive, or hostile behaviour
*Cautions; Contra-indications; Side-effects:* see under Chlorpromazine Hydrochloride; should not be used in apathetic or withdrawn states; avoid in children and in porphyria (see section 9.8.2)
*Dose:* initially 20–30 mg daily in divided doses, increasing to a max. of 150 mg daily if necessary; usual maintenance dose 20–50 mg daily

PoM **Clopixol**® (Lundbeck)
*Tablets,* all f/c, zuclopenthixol (as dihydrochloride) 2 mg (pink), net price 20 = 61p; 10 mg (light brown), 20 = £1.50; 25 mg (brown), 20 = £3.00. Label: 2
*Depot injection* (zuclopenthixol decanoate): section 4.2.2

## 4.2.2  Antipsychotic depot injections

For maintenance therapy, long-acting depot injections of antipsychotic drugs are used because they are more convenient than oral preparations and ensure better patient compliance. However, they may give rise to a higher incidence of extrapyramidal reactions than oral preparations.

ADMINISTRATION.  Depot antipsychotics are administered by deep intramuscular injection at intervals of 1 to 4 weeks. Patients should first be given a small test-dose as undesirable side-effects are prolonged. In general not more than 2–3 mL of oily injection should be administered at any one site.

Individual responses to neuroleptic drugs are very variable and to achieve optimum effect, dosage and dosage interval must be titrated according to the patient's response.

Equivalent doses of depot antipsychotics

| Antipsychotic | Dose (mg) | Interval |
|---|---|---|
| Flupenthixol decanoate | 40 | 2 weeks |
| Fluphenazine decanoate | 25 | 2 weeks |
| Fluphenazine enanthate | 25 | 2 weeks |
| Haloperidol (as decanoate) | 100 | 4 weeks |
| Pipothiazine palmitate | 50 | 4 weeks |
| Zuclopenthixol decanoate | 200 | 2 weeks |

These equivalences are intended **only** as an approximate guide; patients should be carefully monitored after **any** change in medication

CHOICE.  There is no clear-cut division in the use of these drugs, but **zuclopenthixol** may be suitable for the treatment of agitated or aggressive patients whereas **flupenthixol** can cause over-excitement in such patients. **Fluspirilene** has a shorter duration of action than the other depot injections. The incidence of extrapyramidal reactions is similar for all these drugs.

CAUTIONS.  Treatment requires careful monitoring for optimum effect; extrapyramidal symptoms occur frequently. When transferring from oral to depot therapy, dosage by mouth should be gradually phased out. Caution in arteriosclerosis.

CONTRA-INDICATIONS.  Do not use in children, confusional states, coma caused by CNS depressants, parkinsonism, intolerance to antipsychotics.

SIDE-EFFECTS. Pain may occur at injection site and occasionally erythema, swelling, and nodules. For side-effects of specific antipsychotics see under the relevant monograph.

## FLUPENTHIXOL DECANOATE

*Indications:* maintenance in schizophrenia and other psychoses

*Cautions; Contra-indications; Side-effects:* see under Chlorpromazine Hydrochloride (section 4.2.1) and notes above, but it may have a mood elevating effect; extrapyramidal symptoms usually appear 1–3 days after administration and continue for about 5 days but may be delayed; an alternative antipsychotic may be necessary if symptoms such as aggression or agitation appear; avoid in porphyria (see section 9.8.2)

*Dose: by deep intramuscular injection* into the gluteal muscle, test dose 20 mg, then after 5–10 days 20–40 mg repeated at intervals of 2–4 weeks, adjusted according to response; max. 400 mg weekly; usual maintenance dose 50 mg every 4 weeks to 300 mg every 2 weeks
ELDERLY initially quarter to half adult dose

PoM **Depixol**® (Lundbeck)
*Injection* (oily), flupenthixol decanoate 20 mg/mL. Net price 1-mL amp = £1.55; 1-mL syringe = £1.70; 2-mL amp = £2.60; 2-mL syringe = £2.75; 10-mL vial = £14.74
PoM **Depixol Conc.**® (Lundbeck)
*Injection* (oily), flupenthixol decanoate 100 mg/mL. Net price 0.5-mL amp = £3.49; 1-mL amp = £6.40; 5-mL vial = £28.27

## FLUPHENAZINE DECANOATE

*Indications:* maintenance in schizophrenia and other psychoses

*Cautions; Contra-indications; Side-effects:* see under Chlorpromazine Hydrochloride (section 4.2.1) and notes above. Extrapyramidal symptoms usually appear a few hours after the dose has been administered and continue for about 2 days but may be delayed. Contra-indicated in severely depressed states

*Dose: by deep intramuscular injection* into the gluteal muscle, test dose 12.5 mg (6.25 mg in elderly), then after 4–7 days 12.5–100 mg repeated at intervals of 14–35 days, adjusted according to response

PoM **Modecate**® (Squibb)
*Injection* (oily), fluphenazine decanoate 25 mg/mL. Net price 0.5-mL amp = £1.45; 1-mL amp = £2.52; 1-mL syringe = £2.79; 2-mL amp = £4.97; 2-mL syringe = £5.05; 10-mL vial = £24.05
PoM **Modecate Concentrate**® (Squibb)
*Injection* (oily), fluphenazine decanoate 100 mg/mL. Net price 0.5-mL amp = £5.00; 1-mL amp = £9.77

## FLUPHENAZINE ENANTHATE

*Indications; Cautions; Contra-indications; Side-effects:* see under Fluphenazine Decanoate but it has less prolonged effect and higher incidence of extrapyramidal symptoms

*Dose: by deep intramuscular injection* into the gluteal muscle, test dose 12.5 mg (6.25 mg in elderly patients), then after 4–7 days 12.5–100 mg repeated at intervals of 10–21 days, adjusted according to the response

PoM **Moditen Enanthate**® (Squibb)
Product discontinued

## FLUSPIRILENE

*Indications:* maintenance in schizophrenia

*Cautions; Contra-indications; Side-effects:* see under Chlorpromazine Hydrochloride (section 4.2.1) and notes above, but less sedating. Extrapyramidal symptoms usually appear 6–12 hours after the dose and continue for about 48 hours but may be delayed. Common side-effects are restlessness and sweating. With prolonged use, tissue damage (subcutaneous nodules) may occur at injection site

*Dose: by deep intramuscular injection,* 2 mg, increased by 2 mg at weekly intervals, according to response; usual maintenance dose 2–8 mg weekly; max. 20 mg weekly
ELDERLY initially quarter to half adult dose

PoM **Redeptin**® (SK&F)
*Injection* (aqueous suspension), fluspirilene 2 mg/mL. Net price 1-mL amp = 90p; 3-mL amp = £1.59; 6-mL vial = £2.76

## HALOPERIDOL DECANOATE

*Indications:* maintenance in schizophrenia and other psychoses

*Cautions; Contra-indications; Side-effects:* see under Haloperidol (section 4.2.1) and notes above

*Dose: by deep intramuscular injection* into the gluteal muscle, haloperidol (as decanoate) initially 50 mg every 4 weeks, if necessary increasing after 2 weeks by 50-mg increments to 300 mg every 4 weeks; higher doses may be needed in some patients; elderly, initially 12.5–25 mg every 4 weeks

PoM **Haldol Decanoate**® (Janssen)
*Injection* (oily), haloperidol (as decanoate) 50 mg/mL, net price 1-mL amp = £4.66; 100 mg/mL, 1-mL amp = £5.91

## PIPOTHIAZINE PALMITATE

*Indications:* maintenance in schizophrenia and other psychoses

*Cautions; Contra-indications; Side-effects:* see under Chlorpromazine Hydrochloride (section 4.2.1) and notes above

*Dose: by deep intramuscular injection* into the gluteal muscle, test dose 25 mg, then a further 25–50 mg after 4–7 days, then adjusted according to response at intervals of 4 weeks; usual maintenance range 50–100 mg (max. 200 mg) every 4 weeks
ELDERLY initially 5–10 mg

PoM **Piportil Depot**® (Rhône-Poulenc Rorer)
*Injection* (oily), pipothiazine palmitate 50 mg/mL. Net price 1-mL amp = £6.28; 2-mL amp = £10.27

## ZUCLOPENTHIXOL DECANOATE
*Indications:* maintenance in schizophrenia and other psychoses, particularly with aggression and agitation
*Cautions; Contra-indications; Side-effects:* see under Chlorpromazine Hydrochloride (section 4.2.1) and notes above, but less sedating; avoid in porphyria (see section 9.8.2)
*Dose: by deep intramuscular injection* into the gluteal muscle, test dose 100 mg, then after 7–28 days 100–200 mg or more, followed by 200–400 mg repeated at intervals of 2–4 weeks, adjusted according to the response; max. 600 mg weekly

PoM **Clopixol**® (Lundbeck)
*Injection* (oily), zuclopenthixol decanoate 200 mg/mL. Net price 1-mL amp = £3.01; 10-mL vial = £28.63
PoM **Clopixol Conc.**® (Lundbeck)
*Injection* (oily), zuclopenthixol decanoate 500 mg/mL. Net price 1-mL amp with needle = £7.25

## 4.2.3 Antimanic drugs
Drugs are used in mania both to control acute attacks and also to prevent their recurrence.

### ANTIPSYCHOTIC DRUGS

In an acute attack of mania, treatment with an antipsychotic drug (section 4.2.1) is usually required because it may take a few days for lithium to exert its antimanic effect. Lithium may be given concurrently with the antipsychotic drug, and treatment with the antipsychotic gradually tailed off as lithium becomes effective. Alternatively, lithium therapy may be commenced once the patient's mood has been stabilised with the antipsychotic. Haloperidol may be preferred for rapid control of acute mania. However, high doses of haloperidol, fluphenazine, or flupenthixol may be hazardous when used with lithium; irreversible toxic encephalopathy has been reported.

### LITHIUM

Lithium salts are used in the *prophylaxis and treatment of mania*, in the *prophylaxis of manic-depressive illness* (bipolar illness or bipolar depression) and in the *prophylaxis of recurrent depression* (unipolar illness or unipolar depression). Lithium is unsuitable for children.

The decision to give prophylactic lithium usually requires specialist advice, and must be based on careful consideration of the likelihood of recurrence in the individual patient, and the benefit weighed against the risks. In long-term use, therapeutic concentrations have been thought to cause histological and functional changes in the kidney. The significance of such changes is not clear but is of sufficient concern to discourage long-term use of lithium unless it is definitely indicated. Patients should therefore be maintained on lithium after 3–5 years only if, on assessment, benefit persists.

PLASMA CONCENTRATIONS. Lithium salts have a narrow therapeutic/toxic ratio and should therefore not be prescribed unless facilities for monitoring plasma concentrations are available. There seem few if any reasons for preferring one or other of the salts of lithium available. Doses are adjusted to achieve plasma concentrations of 0.4 to 1.0 mmol $Li^+$/litre (lower end of the range for maintenance therapy and elderly patients) on samples taken 12 hours after the preceding dose. It is important to determine the optimum range for each individual patient.

Overdosage, usually with plasma concentrations over 1.5 mmol $Li^+$/litre, may be fatal and toxic effects include tremor, ataxia, dysarthria, nystagmus, renal impairment, and convulsions. If these potentially hazardous signs occur, treatment should be stopped, plasma-lithium concentrations redetermined, and steps taken to reverse lithium toxicity. In mild cases withdrawal of lithium and administration of generous amounts of sodium and fluid will reverse the toxicity. Plasma concentrations in excess of 2.0 mmol $Li^+$/litre require emergency treatment as indicated under Emergency Treatment of Poisoning, p. 19. When toxic concentrations are reached there may be a delay of 1 or 2 days before maximum toxicity occurs.

INTERACTIONS. Lithium toxicity is made worse by sodium depletion, therefore concurrent use of diuretics (particularly thiazides) is hazardous and should be avoided. For other **interactions** with lithium, see Appendix 1 (lithium).

> LITHIUM CARDS. A lithium treatment card available from pharmacies tells patients how to take lithium preparations, what to do if a dose is missed, and what side-effects to expect. It also explains why regular blood tests are important and warns that some medicines and illnesses can change lithium plasma concentrations.
> The cards are available from the Royal Pharmaceutical Society of Great Britain.

## LITHIUM CARBONATE
*Indications:* treatment and prophylaxis of mania, manic-depressive illness, and recurrent depression (see also notes above); aggressive or self-mutilating behaviour

*Cautions:* measure plasma concentrations regularly (every 3 months on stabilised regimens); monitor thyroid function; maintain adequate sodium and fluid intake; avoid in renal impairment, cardiac disease, and conditions with sodium imbalance such as Addison's disease (dose adjustment may be necessary in diarrhoea, vomiting and heavy sweating), also avoid during intercurrent infection; caution in pregnancy, breast-feeding, elderly patients (reduce dose), diuretic treatment, myasthenia gravis; surgery (see section 15.1); **interactions:** Appendix 1 (lithium)

*Side-effects:* gastro-intestinal disturbances, fine tremor, polyuria and polydipsia; also weight gain and oedema (may respond to dose reduction). Signs of lithium intoxication are blurred vision, increasing gastro-intestinal disturbances (anorexia, vomiting, diarrhoea), muscle weakness, increasing CNS disturbances (mild drowsiness and sluggishness increasing to giddiness with ataxia, coarse tremor, lack of co-ordination, dysarthria), and require withdrawal of treatment. With severe overdosage (plasma concentrations above 2 mmol/litre) hyperreflexia and hyperextension of limbs, convulsions, toxic psychoses, syncope, oliguria, circulatory failure, coma, and occasionally, death. Goitre, raised antidiuretic hormone concentration, hypothyroidism, hypokalaemia, ECG changes, exacerbation of psoriasis, and kidney changes may also occur. See also Poisoning, p. 19

*Dose:* see under preparations below, adjusted to achieve a plasma concentration of 0.4–1.0 mmol Li$^+$/litre 12 hours after the preceding dose on the fourth or seventh day of treatment, then every week until dosage has remained constant for 4 weeks and every 3 months thereafter; doses are initially divided throughout the day, but once daily administration is preferred when plasma concentrations stabilised

COUNSELLING. Patients should maintain an adequate fluid intake and should avoid dietary changes which might reduce or increase sodium intake; lithium treatment cards are available from pharmacies (see above)

*Note.* **Different preparations vary widely in bioavailability**; a change in the preparation used requires the same precautions as initiation of treatment.

PoM **Camcolit**® (Norgine)
*Camcolit 250*® *tablets*, f/c, scored, lithium carbonate 250 mg (6.8 mmol Li$^+$). Net price 20 = 59p. Label: 10 lithium card, counselling, see above
*Camcolit 400*® *tablets*, m/r, f/c, scored, lithium carbonate 400 mg (10.8 mmol Li$^+$). Net price 20 = 79p. Label: 10 lithium card, 25, counselling, see above
*Dose* (plasma monitoring, see above):
Treatment, initially 1.5–2 g daily (elderly, 0.5–1 g daily)
Prophylaxis, initially 0.5–1.2 g daily (elderly, 0.5–1 g daily)
Camcolit 250® should be given in divided doses, whereas Camcolit 400® may be given in single or divided doses

PoM **Liskonum**® (SK&F)
*Tablets*, m/r, f/c, scored, lithium carbonate 450 mg (12.2 mmol Li$^+$). Net price 60-tab pack = £2.82. Label: 10 lithium card, 25, counselling, see above
*Dose* (plasma monitoring, see above):
Treatment, initially 450–675 mg twice daily (elderly, initially 225 mg twice daily)
Prophylaxis, initially 450 mg twice daily (elderly, 225 mg twice daily)

PoM **Phasal**® (Lagap)
*Tablets*, m/r, lithium carbonate 300 mg (8.1 mmol Li$^+$). Net price 60-tab pack = £3.82. Label: 10 lithium card, 25, counselling, see above
*Dose* (plasma monitoring, see above):
Treatment, initially 600 mg twice daily (elderly, 0.5–1 g daily in divided doses)
Prophylaxis, initially 600 mg daily

PoM **Priadel**® (Delandale)
*Tablets*, both m/r, scored, lithium carbonate 200 mg (5.4 mmol Li$^+$), net price 20 = 42p; 400 mg (10.8 mmol Li$^+$), 20 = 62p. Label: 10 lithium card, 25, counselling, see above
*Dose* (plasma monitoring, see above):
Treatment and prophylaxis, initially 0.4–1.2 g daily as a single dose or in 2 divided doses (elderly or patients less than 50 kg, 400 mg daily)
*Liquid*, see under Lithium Citrate, below

## LITHIUM CITRATE

*Indications; Cautions; Side-effects:* see under Lithium Carbonate and notes above
*Dose:* see under preparations below, adjusted to achieve plasma concentrations of 0.4–1.0 mmol Li$^+$/litre as described under Lithium Carbonate

PoM **Litarex**® (CP)
*Tablets*, m/r, lithium citrate 564 mg (6 mmol Li$^+$). Net price 20 = 72p. Label: 10 lithium card, 25, counselling, see under Lithium Carbonate
*Dose* (plasma monitoring, see above):
Treatment and prophylaxis, initially 564 mg twice daily

PoM **Priadel**® (Delandale)
*Liquid*, yellow, sugar-free, lithium citrate 520 mg/5 mL (5.4 mmol Li$^+$/5 mL). Net price 150-mL pack = £6.75. Label: 10 lithium card, counselling, see under Lithium Carbonate
*Dose* (plasma monitoring, see above):
Treatment and prophylaxis, initially 1.04–3.12 g daily in 2 divided doses (elderly or patients less than 50 kg, 520 mg twice daily)

## CARBAMAZEPINE

Carbamazepine may be used for the prophylaxis of manic-depressive illness in patients unresponsive to lithium; it seems to be particularly effective in patients with rapid cycling manic-depressive illness (4 or more affective episodes per year).

---

**CARBAMAZEPINE**

*Indications:* prophylaxis of manic-depressive illness unresponsive to lithium; for use in epilepsy see section 4.8.1

*Cautions; Contra-indications; Side-effects:* see section 4.8.1

*Dose:* initially 400 mg daily in divided doses increased until symptoms controlled; usual range 400–600 mg daily; max. 1.6 g daily

**Preparations**
    Section 4.8.1

# 4.3  Antidepressant drugs

**4.3.1** Tricyclic and related antidepressant drugs

**4.3.2** Monoamine-oxidase inhibitors (MAOIs)

**4.3.3** Compound antidepressant preparations

**4.3.4** Other antidepressant drugs

Tricyclic and related antidepressants (antidepressives) are the drugs of choice in the treatment of depressive illness, unless it is so severe that electroconvulsive therapy is immediately indicated. They are preferred to MAOIs because they are more effective antidepressants and do not show the dangerous interactions with some foods and drugs that are characteristic of the MAOIs. **Lithium** (section 4.2.3) has a mood-regulating action and is used in the treatment and prophylaxis of mania, manic depressive illness, and recurrent depression.

Prescribing more than one antidepressant of the tricyclic type at the same time is **not** recommended. It may constitute a hazard and there is no evidence that side-effects are minimised.

Mixtures of antidepressants with tranquillisers are in section 4.3.3; they are **not** recommended.

Other drugs used to treat depression are in section 4.3.4.

It should be noted that although anxiety is often present in depressive illness and may be the presenting symptom, the use of antipsychotics or anxiolytics may mask the true diagnosis. They should therefore be used with caution though they are useful adjuncts in agitated depression.

## 4.3.1  Tricyclic and related antidepressant drugs

The term 'tricyclic' is misleading as there are now 1-, 2-, and 4-ring structured drugs with broadly similar properties.

These drugs are most effective for treating moderate to severe *endogenous depression* associated with psychomotor and physiological changes such as loss of appetite and sleep disturbances; improvement in sleep is usually the first benefit of therapy. Since there may be an interval of 2 to 4 weeks before the antidepressant action takes place electroconvulsive treatment may be

required in severe depression when delay is hazardous or intolerable.

Tricyclic antidepressants are also effective in the management of *panic disorder*.

*Oral and facial pain* may respond to a tricyclic antidepressant, particularly if associated with depression.

Some tricyclic antidepressants are used for the treatment of *nocturnal enuresis* in children, see section 7.4.2.

DOSAGE. About 10 to 20% of patients fail to respond to tricyclic and related antidepressant drugs and inadequate plasma concentrations may account for some of these failures. It is important to achieve plasma concentrations which are sufficiently high for effective treatment but not high enough to cause toxic effects. Low doses should be used for initial treatment in the **elderly** (see under Side-effects, below).

In most patients the long half-life of tricyclic antidepressant drugs allows **once-daily** administration, usually at night; the use of modified-release preparations is therefore unnecessary.

MANAGEMENT. The patient's condition must be checked frequently, especially in the early weeks of treatment, to detect any suicidal tendencies. Limited quantities of antidepressant drugs should be prescribed at any one time as they are dangerous in overdosage. Some of the newer drugs, for example mianserin and trazodone, seem less dangerous in overdose than the older tricyclics.

Treatment should be continued for 2 to 4 weeks before suppression of symptoms can be expected and thereafter should be maintained at the optimum level for at least another month before any attempt is made at dose reduction. Treatment should not be withdrawn prematurely, otherwise symptoms are likely to recur. The natural history of depressive illness suggests that remission usually occurs after 3 months to a year or more and some patients appear to benefit from maintenance therapy with about half the therapeutic dosage for several months to prevent relapse. In recurrent depression, prophylactic maintenance therapy may need to be continued for several years.

In patients who do not respond to antidepressants, the diagnosis, dosage, compliance, and possible continuation of psychosocial or physical aggravating causes should all be carefully reviewed; other drug treatment may be successful. The patient may respond to low-dose **flupenthixol** (Fluanxol®, section 4.3.4) or to MAOIs (section 4.3.2), but see **Interactions**, below.

WITHDRAWAL. Gastro-intestinal symptoms of nausea, vomiting, and anorexia, accompanied by headache, giddiness, 'chills', and insomnia, and sometimes by hypomania, panic-anxiety, and extreme motor restlessness may occur if an antidepressant (particularly an MAOI) is stopped suddenly after regular administration for 8 weeks or more. Reduction in dosage should preferably be carried out gradually over a period of about 4 weeks.

CHOICE. Antidepressant drugs can be roughly divided into those with additional sedative properties, for example **amitriptyline**, and those with less, for example **imipramine**. Agitated and anxious patients tend to respond best to the sedative compounds whereas withdrawn and apathetic patients will often obtain most benefit from less sedating compounds.

Antidepressants with **sedative** properties include amitriptyline, dothiepin, doxepin, maprotiline, mianserin, trazodone, and trimipramine.

**Less sedative** antidepressants include amoxapine, butriptyline, clomipramine, desipramine, imipramine, iprindole, lofepramine, nortriptyline, and viloxazine. Protriptyline has a **stimulant** action.

**Amitriptyline** may be given in divided doses or the entire daily dose may be given at night to promote sleep and avoid daytime drowsiness. **Imipramine** can also be given once daily but as it has a much less sedative action there is less need.

Imipramine and amitriptyline are well established and relatively safe and effective, but nevertheless have more marked antimuscarinic or cardiac side-effects than some of the newer compounds (**doxepin, lofepramine, mianserin, trazodone**, and **viloxazine**); this may be important in individual patients.

**Amoxapine** is related to the antipsychotic loxapine and its side-effects include tardive dyskinesia; overdosage has been associated with seizures.

SIDE-EFFECTS. Arrhythmias and heart block occasionally follow the use of tricyclic antidepressants, particularly amitriptyline, and may be a factor in the sudden death of patients with cardiac disease. Although the use of the older tricyclic antidepressants has been associated with reports of convulsions and of hepatic and haematological reactions, the frequency of these side-effects appears to be much higher, and deaths have been reported, with the newer non-tricyclic antidepressants. In particular, mianserin has been associated with haematological and hepatic reactions and maprotiline has been associated with convulsions. Patients being treated with these drugs therefore require careful supervision. In the case of **mianserin** a full **blood count** is recommended every 4 weeks during the first 3 months of treatment; subsequent clinical monitoring should continue and treatment should be stopped and a full blood count obtained if fever, sore throat, stomatitis, or other signs of infection develop.

Other side-effects of tricyclic and related antidepressants include drowsiness, dry mouth, blurred vision, constipation, and urinary retention (all attributed to antimuscarinic activity), and sweating. The patient should be encouraged to persist with treatment as some tolerance to these side-effects seems to develop. They are further reduced if low doses are given initially and then gradually increased.

This gradual introduction of treatment is particularly important in the elderly, who, because of the hypotensive effects of these drugs, are prone to attacks of dizziness or even syncope. The tricyclic and related antidepressants should be prescribed with caution in epilepsy as they lower the convulsive threshold.

Neuroleptic malignant syndrome (section 4.2.1) may, very rarely, arise in the course of antidepressant treatment.

Overdosage: see Emergency Treatment of Poisoning, p. 19.

INTERACTIONS. MAOIs should preferably not be started until at least a week after tricyclics and related antidepressants have been stopped; tricyclics and related antidepressants should not be given for 2 weeks after stopping MAOI treatment. For other tricyclic **interactions**, see Appendix 1 (antidepressants, tricyclic).

## TRICYCLIC ANTIDEPRESSANTS

### AMITRIPTYLINE HYDROCHLORIDE

*Indications:* depressive illness, particularly where sedation is required; nocturnal enuresis in children (see section 7.4.2)

*Cautions:* cardiac disease (particularly with arrhythmias, see contra-indications below), epilepsy, pregnancy and breast-feeding, elderly, hepatic impairment, thyroid disease, psychoses (may aggravate mania), closed-angle glaucoma, urinary retention, concurrent electroconvulsive therapy. Avoid abrupt cessation of therapy. Also caution in anaesthesia (increased risk of arrhythmias). See section 7.4.2 for nocturnal enuresis; **interactions:** Appendix 1 (antidepressants, tricyclic)
DRIVING. Drowsiness may affect performance of skilled tasks (e.g. driving); effects of alcohol enhanced

*Contra-indications:* recent myocardial infarction, heart block, mania; porphyria (see section 9.8.2)

*Side-effects:* dry mouth, sedation, blurred vision, constipation, nausea, difficulty with micturition (due to antimuscarinic action). Other common side-effects are cardiovascular (arrhythmias, postural hypotension, tachycardia, syncope, particularly with high doses), sweating, tremor, rashes, behavioural disturbances (particularly children), hypomania, confusion (particularly elderly), interference with sexual function, blood sugar changes; increased appetite and weight gain (occasionally weight loss). Less common, black tongue, paralytic ileus, convulsions, agranulocytosis, leucopenia, eosinophilia, purpura, thrombocytopenia, and jaundice; overdosage: see Emergency Treatment of Poisoning, p. 19

*Dose: by mouth,* initially 50–75 mg (elderly and adolescents 25–50 mg) daily in divided doses *or* as a single dose at bedtime increased gradually as necessary to max. 150–200 mg; usual maintenance 50–100 mg daily

Nocturnal enuresis, CHILD 7–10 years 10–20 mg, 11–16 years 25–50 mg at night; max. period of treatment (including gradual withdrawal) 3 months

*By intramuscular or intravenous injection*, 10–20 mg 4 times daily

PoM **Amitriptyline** (Non-proprietary)
*Tablets*, coated, amitriptyline hydrochloride 10 mg, net price 20 = 22p; 25 mg, 20 = 8p; 50 mg, 20 = 48p. Label: 2
Available from APS, Berk (Domical®), Cox, DDSA (Elavil®), Evans, Kerfoot

PoM **Lentizol**® (P-D)
*Capsules*, m/r, both enclosing white pellets, amitriptyline hydrochloride 25 mg (pink), net price 100-cap pack = £4.61; 50 mg (pink/red), 100-cap pack = £8.56. Label: 2, 25

PoM **Tryptizol**® (Morson)
*Tablets*, all f/c, amitriptyline hydrochloride 10 mg (blue), net price 20 = 22p; 25 mg (yellow), 20 = 46p; 50 mg (brown), 20 = 95p. Label: 2
*Capsules*, m/r, orange, amitriptyline hydrochloride 75 mg. Net price 20 = £1.78. Label: 2, 25
*Mixture*, pink, sugar-free, amitriptyline 10 mg (as embonate)/5 mL. Diluent syrup, life of diluted mixture 14 days. Net price 200-mL pack = £1.87. Label: 2
*Injection*, amitriptyline hydrochloride 10 mg/mL. Net price 10-mL vial = 47p

## AMOXAPINE

*Indications:* depressive illness
*Cautions; Contra-indications; Side-effects:* see under Amitriptyline Hydrochloride; tardive dyskinesia reported; menstrual irregularities, breast enlargement, and galactorrhoea reported in women
*Dose:* initially 100–150 mg daily in divided doses *or* as a single dose at bedtime increased as necessary to max. 300 mg daily; usual maintenance 150–250 mg daily
ELDERLY initially 25 mg twice daily increased as necessary after 5–7 days to max. 50 mg 3 times daily

PoM **Asendis**® (Novex)
*Tablets*, amoxapine 25 mg, net price 20 = £2.18; 50 mg (orange, scored), 20 = £3.63; 100 mg (blue, scored), 20 = £6.05; 150 mg (scored), 20 = £9.02. Label: 2

## BUTRIPTYLINE

*Indications:* depressive illness
*Cautions; Contra-indications; Side-effects:* see under Amitriptyline Hydrochloride, but less sedating
*Dose:* 25 mg 3 times daily, increased gradually as necessary to max. 150 mg; usual maintenance dose 25 mg 3 times daily

PoM **Evadyne**® (Wyeth)
*Tablets*, both f/c, butriptyline (as hydrochloride) 25 mg (orange), net price 20 = 77p; 50 mg (pink), 20 = £1.35. Label: 2

## CLOMIPRAMINE HYDROCHLORIDE

*Indications:* depressive illness, adjunctive treatment of phobic and obsessional states; cataplexy associated with narcolepsy

*Cautions; Contra-indications; Side-effects:* see under Amitriptyline Hydrochloride. Postural hypotension may occur on intravenous infusion
*Dose: by mouth*, initially 10 mg daily, increased gradually as necessary to 30–150 mg (elderly 75 mg) in divided doses *or* as a single dose at bedtime; max. 250 mg daily; usual maintenance 30–50 mg daily (severe cases 50–100 mg daily)
Phobic and obsessional states, initially 25 mg daily (elderly 10 mg daily) increased over 2 weeks to 100–150 mg daily
*By intramuscular injection*, initially 25–50 mg daily, increased by 25 mg daily to 100–150 mg daily
*By intravenous infusion*, initially to assess tolerance, 25–50 mg, then usually about 100 mg daily for 7–10 days

PoM **Clomipramine** (Non-proprietary)
*Capsules*, clomipramine hydrochloride 10 mg, net price 84 = £2.73; 25 mg, 84 = £5.42; 50 mg, 56 = £6.86. Label: 2
Available from Generics, Hillcross

PoM **Anafranil**® (Geigy)
*Capsules*, clomipramine hydrochloride 10 mg (yellow/caramel), net price 84-cap pack = £2.76; 25 mg (orange/caramel), 84-cap pack = £5.43; 50 mg (blue/caramel), 56-cap pack = £6.89. Label: 2
*Syrup*, clomipramine hydrochloride 25 mg/5 mL. Net price 150-mL pack = £6.18. Label: 2
*Injection*, clomipramine hydrochloride 12.5 mg/mL. Net price 2-mL amp = 40p

PoM **Anafranil SR**® (Geigy)
*Tablets*, m/r, pink, f/c, clomipramine hydrochloride 75 mg. Net price 28-tab pack = £6.86. Label: 2, 25

## DESIPRAMINE HYDROCHLORIDE

*Indications:* depressive illness
*Cautions; Contra-indications; Side-effects:* see under Amitriptyline Hydrochloride, but less sedating
*Dose:* 75 mg daily in divided doses *or* as a single dose at bedtime, increased as necessary to a max. of 200 mg
ELDERLY initially 25 mg daily

PoM **Pertofran**® (Ciba)
*Tablets*, pink, s/c, desipramine hydrochloride 25 mg. Net price 20 = 71p. Label: 2

## DOTHIEPIN HYDROCHLORIDE

*Indications:* depressive illness, particularly where sedation is required
*Cautions; Contra-indications; Side-effects:* see under Amitriptyline Hydrochloride
*Dose:* initially 75 mg (elderly 50–75 mg) daily in divided doses *or* as a single dose at bedtime, increased gradually as necessary to 150 mg daily (elderly 75 mg may be sufficient); up to 225 mg daily in hospital patients

PoM **Dothiepin** (Non-proprietary)
*Capsules*, dothiepin hydrochloride 25 mg, net price 20 = 95p. Label: 2
Available from APS, Generics, Hillcross, Norton

---

*Tablets*, dothiepin hydrochloride 75 mg, net price 28-tab pack = £3.80. Label: 2
Available from APS, Generics, Hillcross, Norton

PoM **Prothiaden**® (Boots)
*Capsules*, red/brown, dothiepin hydrochloride 25 mg. Net price 20 = £1.00. Label: 2
*Tablets*, red, s/c, dothiepin hydrochloride 75 mg. Net price 28 = £4.00. Label: 2

## DOXEPIN

*Indications:* depressive illness, particularly where sedation is required
*Cautions; Contra-indications; Side-effects:* see under Amitriptyline Hydrochloride; avoid in breast-feeding (see Appendix 5)
*Dose:* initially 75 mg (elderly 10– 50 mg) daily in 3 divided doses, increased gradually to max. 300 mg daily in divided doses; range 30–300 mg daily; up to 100 mg may be given as a single dose at bedtime

PoM **Sinequan**® (Pfizer)
*Capsules*, doxepin (as hydrochloride) 10 mg (orange), net price 56-cap pack = £1.10; 25 mg (orange/blue), 28-cap pack = 79p; 50 mg (blue), 28-cap pack = £1.30; 75 mg (yellow/blue), 28-cap pack = £2.06. Label: 2

## IMIPRAMINE HYDROCHLORIDE

*Indications:* depressive illness; nocturnal enuresis in children (see section 7.4.2)
*Cautions; Contra-indications; Side-effects:* see under Amitriptyline Hydrochloride, but less sedating
*Dose:* initially up to 75 mg daily in divided doses increased gradually to 150–200 mg (up to 300 mg in hospital patients); up to 150 mg may be given as a single dose at bedtime; usual maintenance 50–100 mg daily; ELDERLY initially 10 mg daily, increased gradually to 30–50 mg daily
Nocturnal enuresis, CHILD 7 years 25 mg, 8–11 years 25–50 mg, over 11 years 50–75 mg at bedtime; max. period of treatment (including gradual withdrawal) 3 months

PoM **Imipramine** (Non-proprietary)
*Tablets*, coated, imipramine hydrochloride 10 mg, net price 20 = 15p; 25 mg, 20 = 14p. Label: 2
PoM **Tofranil**® (Geigy)
*Tablets*, both red-brown, s/c, imipramine hydrochloride 10 mg, net price 84-tab pack = £1.39; 25 mg, 84-tab pack = £2.65. Label: 2
*Syrup*, imipramine hydrochloride 25 mg/5 mL. Net price 150-mL pack = £2.70. Label: 2

## LOFEPRAMINE

*Indications:* depressive illness
*Cautions; Contra-indications; Side-effects:* see under Amitriptyline Hydrochloride, but less sedating; hepatic disorders reported; contra-indicated in hepatic and severe renal impairment
*Dose:* 140–210 mg daily in divided doses

PoM **Gamanil**® (Merck)
*Tablets*, f/c, brown-violet, lofepramine 70 mg (as hydrochloride). Net price 56-tab pack = £9.97. Label: 2

## NORTRIPTYLINE

*Indications:* depressive illness; nocturnal enuresis in children (see section 7.4.2)
*Cautions; Contra-indications; Side-effects:* see under Amitriptyline Hydrochloride but less sedating
*Dose:* initially 20–40 mg (elderly 30 mg) daily in single *or* divided doses, increased gradually as necessary to max. 100 mg daily; usual maintenance dose 30–75 mg daily
Nocturnal enuresis, CHILD 7 years 10 mg, 8–11 years 10–20 mg, over 11 years 25–35 mg, at night; max period of treatment (including gradual withdrawal) 3 months

PoM **Allegron**® (Dista)
*Tablets*, nortriptyline (as hydrochloride) 10 mg, net price 20 = 67p; 25 mg (orange, scored), 20 = £1.36. Label: 2
PoM **Aventyl**® (Lilly)
*Capsules*, both yellow/white, nortriptyline (as hydrochloride) 10 mg, net price 20 = 67p; 25 mg, 20 = £1.36. Label: 2

## PROTRIPTYLINE HYDROCHLORIDE

*Indications:* depressive illness, particularly with apathy and withdrawal
*Cautions; Contra-indications; Side-effects:* see under Amitriptyline Hydrochloride but less sedating; anxiety, agitation, tachycardia, and hypotension more common; rashes associated with photosensitisation (avoid direct sunlight); daily dose above 20 mg in elderly (increased risk of cardiovascular side-effects)
*Dose:* initially 10 mg 3–4 times daily (elderly 5 mg 3 times daily initially) if insomnia, last dose not after 4 p.m.; usual range 15–60 mg daily

PoM **Concordin**® (MSD)
*Tablets*, both f/c, protriptyline hydrochloride 5 mg (pink), net price 20 = 37p; 10 mg, 20 = 54p. Label: 2, 11

## TRIMIPRAMINE

*Indications:* depressive illness, particularly where sedation is required
*Cautions; Contra-indications; Side-effects:* see under Amitriptyline Hydrochloride
*Dose:* 50–75 mg daily as a single dose 2 hours before bedtime *or* as 25 mg midday and 50 mg evening, increased as necessary to max. of 300 mg daily; usual maintenance dose 75–150 mg daily
ELDERLY 10–25 mg 3 times daily initially, half adult maintenance dose may be sufficient

PoM **Surmontil**® (Rhône-Poulenc Rorer)
*Capsules*, green/white, trimipramine 50 mg (as maleate). Net price 28-tab pack = £4.63. Label: 2
*Tablets*, trimipramine (as maleate) 10 mg, net price 50 = £2.48; 25 mg, 50 = £4.12. Label: 2

---

## RELATED ANTIDEPRESSANTS

## IPRINDOLE
*Indications:* depressive illness
*Cautions; Contra-indications; Side-effects:* see under Amitriptyline Hydrochloride, but less sedating. Caution in liver disease; jaundice, although rare, may develop, usually in the first 21 days
*Dose:* initially 15–30 mg 3 times daily, increased gradually to max. 60 mg 3 times daily; usual maintenance 30 mg 3 times daily

PoM **Prondol**® (Wyeth)
*Tablets*, yellow, iprindole (as hydrochloride) 15 mg, net price 20 = 42p. Label: 2

## MAPROTILINE HYDROCHLORIDE
*Indications:* depressive illness, particularly where sedation is required
*Cautions; Contra-indications; Side-effects:* see under Amitriptyline Hydrochloride, antimuscarinic effects may occur less frequently but rashes common and increased risk of convulsions at higher dosage; contra-indicated if history of epilepsy
*Dose:* initially 25–75 mg (elderly 30 mg) daily in 3 divided doses *or* as a single dose at bedtime, increased gradually as necessary to max. 150 mg daily

PoM **Ludiomil**® (Ciba)
*Tablets*, all f/c, maprotiline hydrochloride 10 mg (pale orange), net price 20 = 60p; 25 mg (greyish-red), 20 = £1.10; 50 mg (light orange), 20 = £2.15; 75 mg (brownish-orange), 28-tab pack = £4.40. Label: 2
*Additives: include gluten*

## MIANSERIN HYDROCHLORIDE
*Indications:* depressive illness, particularly where sedation is required
*Cautions; Contra-indications; Side-effects:* see under Amitriptyline Hydrochloride; leucopenia, agranulocytosis and aplastic anaemia (particularly in the elderly); jaundice; arthritis, arthralgia; influenza-like syndrome may occur; **blood counts needed, p. 152** Fewer and milder antimuscarinic and cardiovascular effects; **interactions:** Appendix 1 (mianserin)
*Dose:* initially 30–40 mg (elderly 30 mg) daily in divided doses *or* as a single dose at bedtime, increased gradually as necessary; usual dose range 30–90 mg

PoM **Mianserin** (Non-proprietary)
*Tablets*, mianserin hydrochloride 10 mg, net price 20 = £1.36; 20 mg, 20 = £2.74; 30 mg, 20 = £4.00. Label: 2, 25
PoM **Bolvidon**® (Organon)
*Tablets*, all f/c, mianserin hydrochloride 10 mg, net price 20 = £1.16; 20 mg, 20 = £2.33; 30 mg, 20 = £3.49. Label: 2, 25
PoM **Norval**® (Bencard)
*Tablets*, all orange, f/c, mianserin hydrochloride 10 mg, net price 84-tab pack = £5.50; 20 mg, 28-tab pack = £3.66; 30 mg, 28-tab pack = £5.50. Label: 2, 25

## TRAZODONE HYDROCHLORIDE
*Indications:* depressive illness, particularly where sedation is required
*Cautions; Contra-indications; Side-effects:* see under Amitriptyline Hydrochloride but fewer antimuscarinic and cardiovascular effects; rarely priapism; **interactions:** Appendix 1 (trazodone)
*Dose:* initially 150 mg (elderly 100 mg) daily in divided doses after food *or* as a single dose at bedtime; may be increased to 300 mg daily; hospital patients up to max. 600 mg daily in divided doses

PoM **Molipaxin**® (Roussel)
*Capsules*, trazodone hydrochloride 50 mg (violet/green), net price 84-cap pack = £17.30; 100 mg (violet/fawn), 56-cap pack = £20.38. Label: 2, 21
*Tablets*, pink, f/c, trazodone hydrochloride 150 mg. Net price 28-tab pack = £11.62. Label: 2, 21
*Liquid*, sugar-free, trazodone hydrochloride 50 mg/5 mL. Net price 150-mL pack = £7.74. Label: 2, 21
*CR tablets*, m/r, blue, f/c, trazodone hydrochloride 150 mg. Net price 28-tab pack = £11.62. Label: 2, 21, 25
*Dose:* initially 1 tablet daily (elderly, dose form not appropriate for initial dose titration), increased if necessary to 2 tablets daily (up to 4 tablets daily in hospital patients)

## VILOXAZINE HYDROCHLORIDE
*Indications:* depressive illness
*Cautions; Contra-indications; Side-effects:* see under Amitriptyline Hydrochloride, but less sedating and antimuscarinic and cardiovascular side-effects are fewer and milder; nausea and headache may occur; **interactions:** Appendix 1 (viloxazine)
*Dose:* 300 mg daily (preferably as 200 mg in the morning and 100 mg at midday), increased gradually as necessary; max. 400 mg daily; last dose not later than 6 p.m.
ELDERLY 100 mg daily initially, half adult maintenance dose may be sufficient

PoM **Vivalan**® (ICI)
*Tablets*, f/c, viloxazine 50 mg (as hydrochloride). Net price 20 = £1.27. Label: 2

---

## 4.3.2  Monoamine-oxidase inhibitors (MAOIs)

Monoamine-oxidase inhibitors are used much less frequently than tricyclic and related antidepressants because of the dangers of dietary and drug interactions and the fact that it is easier to prescribe MAOIs when tricyclic antidepressants have been unsuccessful than vice versa. **Tranylcypromine**, is the most **hazardous** of the MAOIs because of its stimulant action. The drugs of choice are **phenelzine** or **isocarboxazid** which are less stimulant and therefore safer.

Phobic patients and depressed patients with atypical, hypochondriacal, or hysterical features are said to respond best to MAOIs. However, MAOIs should be tried in any patients who are refractory to treatment with other antidepressants as there is occasionally a dramatic response. Response to treatment may be delayed for 3 weeks or more and may take an additional 1 or 2 weeks to become maximal.

WITHDRAWAL. See section 4.3.1

INTERACTIONS. MAOIs inhibit monoamine oxidase, thereby causing an accumulation of amine neurotransmitters. The metabolism of some amine drugs such as indirect-acting sympathomimetics is also inhibited and their pressor action may be potentiated; the pressor effect of tyramine (in some foods) may also be dangerously potentiated.

Sympathomimetics are present in many proprietary cough mixtures and decongestant nasal drops. See Appendix 1 (MAOIs) and Treatment Card. These interactions may cause a dangerous rise in blood pressure. An early warning symptom may be a throbbing headache. The danger of interaction persists for up to 14 days after treatment with MAOIs is discontinued. Treatment cards which list the necessary precautions are distributed by the Royal Pharmaceutical Society and given to patients at pharmacies etc.

Other antidepressants should **not** be given to patients for 14 days after treatment with MAOIs has been discontinued. Some psychiatrists use selected tricyclics in conjunction with MAOIs but this is hazardous, indeed potentially lethal, except in experienced hands and there is no evidence that the combination is more effective than when either constituent is used alone. The combination of tranylcypromine with clomipramine is particularly **dangerous**.

MAOIs should preferably not be started until at least a week after tricyclics and related antidepressants have been stopped; they should not be started until 2 weeks after a serotonin uptake inhibitor antidepressant (5 weeks in the case of fluoxetine).

For other interactions with monoamine-oxidase inhibitors including those with opioid analgesics (notably pethidine), see Appendix 1 (MAOIs).

**Other MAOIs.** Discontinue first MAOI for at least a week before starting another.

---

**TREATMENT CARD**

*Carry this card with you at all times. Show it to any doctor who may treat you other than the doctor who prescribed this medicine, and to your dentist if you require dental treatment.*

**INSTRUCTIONS TO PATIENTS**
**Please read carefully**
While taking this medicine and for 14 days after your treatment finishes you must observe the following simple instructions:–

1  Do not eat CHEESE, PICKLED HERRING OR BROAD BEAN PODS.

2  Do not eat or drink BOVRIL, OXO, MARMITE or ANY SIMILAR MEAT OR YEAST EXTRACT.

3  Eat only FRESH foods and avoid food that you suspect could be stale or 'going off'. This is especially important with meat, fish, poultry or offal. Avoid game.

4  Do not take any other MEDICINES (including tablets, capsules, nose drops, inhalations or suppositories) whether purchased by you or previously prescribed by your doctor, without first consulting your doctor or your pharmacist.

   NB *Treatment for coughs and colds, pain relievers, tonics and laxatives are medicines.*

5  Avoid alcoholic drinks and de-alcoholised (low alcohol) drinks.

**Keep a careful note of any food or drink that disagrees with you, avoid it and tell your doctor.**

**Report any unusual or severe symptoms to your doctor and follow any other advice given by him.**

| M.A.O.I. | Prepared by The Pharmaceutical Society and the British Medical |

Association on behalf of the Health Departments of the United Kingdom.

Printed in the UK for HMSO 8217411/150M/9.89/4529
Revised Sep. 1989

---

## PHENELZINE

*Indications:* depressive illness

*Cautions:* diabetes mellitus, cardiovascular disease, epilepsy, blood disorders, concurrent electroconvulsive therapy; avoid abrupt discontinuation of treatment; severe hypertensive reactions to certain drugs and foods (see Treatment Card); avoid in elderly and agitated patients; pregnancy and breast-feeding; **interactions:** Appendix 1 (MAOIs)

DRIVING. Drowsiness may affect performance of skilled tasks (e.g. driving)

*Contra-indications:* hepatic impairment (see Appendix 2), cerebrovascular disease, phaeochromocytoma, porphyria (see section 9.8.2), children

*Side-effects:* adverse effects commonly associated with phenelzine and other MAOIs include postural hypotension and dizziness; other common side-effects include drowsiness, headache, weakness and fatigue, dryness of mouth, constipation and other gastro-intestinal disturbances, and oedema; agitation and tremors, nervousness, blurred vision, difficulty in micturition, sweating, convulsions, rashes, leucopenia, sexual disturbances, and weight gain with inappropriate appetite may also occur; psychotic episodes with hypomanic behaviour, confusion, and hallucinations, may be induced

---

in susceptible persons; jaundice has been reported and, on rare occasions, fatal progressive hepatocellular necrosis; peripheral neuropathy may be due to pyridoxine deficiency
*Dose:* 15 mg 3 times daily, increased if necessary to 4 times daily after 2 weeks (hospital patients, max. 30 mg 3 times daily), then reduced gradually to lowest possible maintenance dose (15 mg on alternate days may be adequate)

PoM **Nardil**® (P-D)
*Tablets,* orange, f/c, phenelzine 15 mg (as sulphate). Net price 20 = £1.33. Label: 3, 10 MAOI card

## ISOCARBOXAZID

*Indications:* depressive illness
*Cautions; Contra-indications; Side-effects:* see under Phenelzine
*Dose:* initially up to 30 mg daily in single or divided doses increased after 4 weeks if necessary to max. 60 mg daily for up to 6 weeks under close supervision only; then reduced to usual maintenance dose 10–20 mg daily (but up to 40 mg daily may be required)

PoM **Marplan**® (Roche)
*Tablets,* pink, scored, isocarboxazid 10 mg. Net price 50 = 98p. Label: 3, 10 MAOI card

## TRANYLCYPROMINE

*Indications:* depressive illness
*Cautions; Contra-indications:* see under Phenelzine; also contra-indicated in hyperthyroidism
*Side-effects:* see under Phenelzine; insomnia if given in evening; hypertensive crises with throbbing headache requiring discontinuation of treatment occur more frequently than with other MAOIs; liver damage occurs less frequently than with phenelzine
*Dose:* initially 10 mg twice daily not later than 3 p.m., increasing the second daily dose to 20 mg after 1 week if necessary; doses above 30 mg daily under close supervision only; usual maintenance dose 10 mg daily

PoM **Parnate**® (SK&F)
*Tablets,* red, s/c, tranylcypromine 10 mg (as sulphate). Net price 20 = 91p. Label: 3, 10 MAOI card

## 4.3.3 Compound antidepressant preparations

The use of preparations listed below is **not** recommended because the dosage of the individual components should be adjusted separately. Whereas antidepressants are given continuously over several months, anxiolytics are prescribed on a short-term basis.

NHS PoM **Limbitrol**® (Roche)
*'5' Capsules,* pink/green, amitriptyline 12.5 mg (as hydrochloride), chlordiazepoxide 5 mg. Net price 20 = £1.15. Label: 2

*'10' Capsules,* pink/dark green, amitriptyline 25 mg (as hydrochloride), chlordiazepoxide 10 mg. Net price 20 = £1.67. Label: 2
PoM **Motipress**® (Squibb)
*Tablets,* yellow, s/c, fluphenazine hydrochloride 1.5 mg, nortriptyline 30 mg (as hydrochloride). Net price 28-tab pack = £2.90. Label: 2
PoM **Motival**® (Squibb)
*Tablets,* pink, s/c, fluphenazine hydrochloride 500 micrograms, nortriptyline 10 mg (as hydrochloride). Net price 20 = 70p. Label: 2
PoM **Parstelin**® (SK&F)
*Tablets,* green, s/c, tranylcypromine 10 mg (as sulphate), trifluoperazine 1 mg (as hydrochloride). Net price 20 = 93p. Label: 3, 10 MAOI card
*Caution:* contains MAOI
PoM **Triptafen**® (A&H)
*Tablets,* pink, s/c, amitriptyline hydrochloride 25 mg, perphenazine 2 mg. Net price 20 = 54p. Label: 2
PoM **Triptafen-M**® (A&H)
*Tablets,* pink, s/c, amitriptyline hydrochloride 10 mg, perphenazine 2 mg. Net price 20 = 48p. Label: 2

## 4.3.4 Other antidepressant drugs

### FLUPENTHIXOL

The thioxanthene **flupenthixol** (Fluanxol®) has antidepressant properties, and low doses (1 to 3 mg daily) are given by mouth for this purpose. Its advantages over the tricyclic and related antidepressants are that, with the low doses employed, side-effects are fewer, and that overdosage is less toxic.

### FLUPENTHIXOL

*Indications:* depressive illness (short-term use). For use in psychoses, see section 4.2.1
*Cautions:* cardiovascular disease (including cardiac disorders and cerebral arteriosclerosis), senile confusional states, parkinsonism, renal and hepatic disease; avoid in excitable and overactive patients; avoid in porphyria (see section 9.8.2); **interactions:** Appendix 1 (phenothiazines and other antipsychotics)
DRIVING. Drowsiness may affect performance of skilled tasks (e.g. driving); effects of alcohol enhanced
*Side-effects:* restlessness, insomnia; hypomania reported; rarely dizziness, tremor, visual disturbances, headache, hyperprolactinaemia, extrapyramidal symptoms
*Dose:* initially 1 mg (elderly 500 micrograms) in the morning, increased after 1 week to 2 mg (elderly 1 mg) if necessary. Max. 3 mg (elderly 2 mg) daily, doses above 2 mg (elderly 1 mg) being divided in 2 portions, second dose not after 4 p.m. Discontinue if no response after 1 week at maximum dosage
COUNSELLING. Although drowsiness may occur, can also have an alerting effect so should not be taken in the evening

PoM **Depixol**® (psychoses), see section 4.2.1
PoM **Fluanxol**® (Lundbeck)
*Tablets,* both red, s/c, flupenthixol (as dihydrochloride) 500 micrograms, net price 20 = £1.18; 1 mg, 60-tab pack = £7.16. Label: 2, counselling, administration

## TRYPTOPHAN

**Tryptophan** appeared to benefit some patients when given alone or as adjunctive therapy but tryptophan products have been withdrawn following evidence of an association with the eosino-philia-myalgia syndrome; they remain available on a named-patient basis for patients for whom no alternative treatment is suitable.

## SEROTONIN UPTAKE INHIBITORS

**Fluvoxamine, fluoxetine, paroxetine,** and **sertraline** selectively inhibit the re-uptake of serotonin (5-hydroxytryptamine, 5-HT); they appear to be effective antidepressants. They are less sedative than the tricyclics, with few antimuscarinic effects and with low cardiotoxicity. They do not cause weight gain. Gastro-intestinal side-effects (diarrhoea, nausea and vomiting) are dose-related; headache, restlessness and anxiety may also occur.

INTERACTIONS. MAOIs should preferably not be started until at least 2 weeks after a serotonin uptake inhibitor antidepressant has been stopped (5 weeks after stopping in the case of fluoxetine). Serotonin uptake inhibitor antidepressants should preferably not be started until at least 2 weeks after an MAOI has been stopped.
Other interactions, see Appendix 1.

## FLUOXETINE HYDROCHLORIDE
*Indications:* see under Dose
*Cautions:* hepatic impairment, renal impairment (avoid if severe), epilepsy (avoid if poorly controlled), diabetes mellitus, pregnancy; long half-life (delayed response to dose change or cessation); rare reports of prolonged seizures with electroconvulsive therapy; **interactions:** Appendix 1 (antidepressants, serotonin uptake inhibitor)
DRIVING. May impair performance of skilled tasks (e.g. driving)
*Contra-indications:* breast-feeding
*Side-effects:* rash (discontinue treatment, may be associated with vasculitis, anaphylaxis, and pulmonary inflammation or fibrosis), nausea, vomiting, diarrhoea, anorexia with weight loss, headache, nervousness, insomnia, anxiety, tremor, dry mouth, dizziness, hypomania, drowsiness, convulsions, fever, sexual dysfunction, sweating; other side-effects reported are vaginal bleeding on withdrawal, hyper-prolactinaemia, thrombocytopenia, altered platelet function and abnormal bleeding, confusion; rarely hyponatraemia
*Dose:* depressive illness, 20 mg daily
Bulimia nervosa, 60 mg daily

▼ PoM **Prozac**® (Dista)
*Capsules,* green/off-white, fluoxetine hydrochloride 20 mg. Net price 30-cap pack = £32.05. Counselling, driving

## FLUVOXAMINE MALEATE
*Indications:* depressive illness
*Cautions:* renal and hepatic impairment; pregnancy and breast-feeding; **interactions:** Appendix 1 (antidepressants, serotonin uptake inhibitor)
DRIVING. May impair performance of skilled tasks (e.g. driving); effects of alcohol enhanced
*Contra-indications:* history of epilepsy
*Side-effects:* nausea and vomiting, diarrhoea, drowsiness, dizziness, agitation, anxiety, headache, tremor; bradycardia; convulsions; rarely increase in liver enzymes with symptoms (discontinue)
*Dose:* 100–200 mg daily (up to 100 mg as single dose in evening); max. 300 mg daily

PoM **Faverin**® (Duphar)
*Tablets,* both yellow, e/c, fluvoxamine maleate 50 mg, net price 60-tab pack = £25.00; 100 mg, 30-tab pack = £25.00. Label: 5, 25, counselling, driving

## PAROXETINE
*Indications:* depressive illness
*Cautions:* cardiac disease, epilepsy, hepatic or renal impairment, pregnancy, breast-feeding, history of mania; avoid abrupt withdrawal; **interactions:** Appendix 1 (antidepressants, serotonin uptake inhibitor)
DRIVING. May affect performance of skilled tasks (e.g. driving)
*Side-effects:* nausea, drowsiness, sweating, tremor, asthenia, dry mouth, insomnia, sexual dysfunction
*Dose:* usually 20 mg each morning, if necessary increased gradually in increments of 10 mg to max. 50 mg daily (elderly, 40 mg daily)

▼ PoM **Seroxat**® (SmithKline Beecham)
*Tablets,* both f/c, scored, paroxetine 20 mg (as hydrochloride), net price 30-tab pack = £33.90; 30 mg (blue), 30-tab pack = £50.85. Label: 21, 25, counselling, driving

## SERTRALINE
*Indications:* depressive illness
*Cautions:* epilepsy (avoid if unstable); avoid in hepatic and renal impairment, and in electroconvulsive therapy; pregnancy and breast-feeding; **interactions:** Appendix 1 (antidepressants, serotonin uptake inhibitor)
DRIVING. May affect performance of skilled tasks (e.g. driving)
*Side-effects:* dry mouth, nausea, diarrhoea, delayed ejaculation, tremor, increased sweating, dyspepsia; rarely, increase in serum transaminases (discontinue)
*Dose:* initially 50 mg daily, increased if necessary by increments of 50 mg over several weeks to max. 200 mg daily, then reduced to usual maintenance of 50–100 mg daily; doses of 150 mg or greater should not be used for more than 8 weeks

▼ PoM **Lustral**® (Invicta)
*Tablets*, sertraline (as hydrochloride) 50 mg, net price 28-tab pack = £26.51; 100 mg, 28-tab pack = £39.77. Label: 21, counselling, driving

## 4.4 Central nervous stimulants

Central nervous system stimulants have very few indications and in particular, should **not** be used to treat depression, obesity, senility, debility, or for relief of fatigue.

**Caffeine** is a weak stimulant present in tea and coffee. It is included in many analgesic preparations (section 4.7.1.1) but does not contribute to their analgesic or anti-inflammatory effect. Over-indulgence may lead to a state of anxiety.

The **amphetamines** have a limited field of usefulness and their use should be **discouraged** as they may cause dependence and psychotic states. Patients with narcolepsy may derive benefit from treatment with amphetamines.

Amphetamines have been advocated for the management of hyperactive children; beneficial effects have been described. However, they must be used very selectively as they retard growth and the effect of long-term therapy has not been evaluated.

Amphetamines have **no place** in the management of **depression** or **obesity**.

**Pemoline** is a weak central nervous system stimulant that has been advocated for the management of hyperactive children. The same general reservations apply as for amphetamines and treatment should be carried out only under specialist supervision.

### DEXAMPHETAMINE SULPHATE

*Indications:* narcolepsy, adjunct in the management of hyperkinesia in children (under specialist supervision)

*Cautions:* mild hypertension (contra-indicated if moderate or severe); monitor growth in children; avoid abrupt withdrawal; **interactions:** Appendix 1 (sympathomimetics)

*Contra-indications:* cardiovascular disease or moderate to severe hypertension (caution if mild), hyperexcitable states, hyperthyroidism, history of drug abuse, glaucoma, extrapyramidal disorders, pregnancy and breast-feeding, porphyria (see section 9.8.2)
DRIVING. May affect performance of skilled tasks (e.g. driving); effects of alcohol unpredictable

*Side-effects:* insomnia, restlessness, irritability, nervousness, night terrors, euphoria, tremor, dizziness, headache; dependence, tolerance, sometimes psychosis; anorexia, gastro-intestinal symptoms, growth retardation in children; dry mouth, sweating, tachycardia, palpitations, increased blood pressure; rarely cardiomyopathy reported with chronic use; overdosage: see Emergency Treatment of Poisoning, p. 20

*Dose:* narcolepsy, 10 mg (elderly, 5 mg) daily in divided doses increased by 10 mg (elderly, 5 mg) daily at intervals of 1 week to a max. of 60 mg daily

Hyperkinesia, CHILD over 6 years 5–10 mg in the morning, increased if necessary by 5 mg at intervals of 1 week to usual max. 20 mg daily (older children have received max. 40 mg daily)

**CD Dexedrine**® (Evans)
*Tablets*, scored, dexamphetamine sulphate 5 mg. Net price 20 = 15p. Counselling, driving

## PEMOLINE

*Indications:* adjunct in the management of hyperkinesia in children (under specialist supervision)

*Cautions; Contra-indications; Side-effects:* see under Dexamphetamine Sulphate; chorea, tics, mania, depression, neutropenia, and liver enzyme abnormalities also reported

*Dose:* CHILD over 6 years, initially 20 mg every morning increased by increments of 20 mg at intervals of 1 week to 60 mg every morning, followed, if no improvement, by gradual increase to max. 120 mg every morning

PoM **Volital**® (LAB)
*Tablets*, scored, pemoline 20 mg. Net price 25-tab pack = £1.10

## STIMULANT WITH VITAMINS

**Prolintane** is contained in a preparation with vitamins; it is **not** recommended and is specifically **contra-indicated** in epilepsy and hyperthyroidism.

NHS PoM **Villescon**® (Boehringer Ingelheim)
*Liquid*, red, prolintane hydrochloride 2.5 mg/5 mL with vitamins B group and C. Net price 150-mL pack = 85p
*Dose:* 10 mL twice daily before 4 p.m. for 1–2 weeks but see notes above.

## COCAINE

**Cocaine** is a drug of addiction which causes central nervous stimulation. Its clinical use is mainly as a topical local anaesthetic (see sections 11.7 and 15.2). It has been included in analgesic elixirs for the relief of pain in terminal care but this use is obsolete.

## 4.5 Appetite suppressants

4.5.1 Bulk-forming drugs
4.5.2 Centrally acting appetite suppressants

The development of obesity appears to be multifactorial. Aggravating factors may be depression or other psychosocial problems or drug treatment.

The main treatment of the obese patient is an appropriate diet, carefully explained to the patient, with support and encouragement from the doctor. Attendance at groups (for example 'weight-watchers') helps some individuals. Drugs can play only a limited role and should never be used as the sole element of treatment; their effects tend to be disappointing.

The use of diuretics is **not** appropriate for weight reduction.

## 4.5.1   Bulk-forming drugs

The most commonly used bulk-forming drug is **methylcellulose**. It is claimed to reduce intake by producing feelings of satiety but there is little evidence to support this claim.

### METHYLCELLULOSE

*Indications:* obesity; other indications, see section 1.6.1

*Cautions:* maintain adequate fluid intake

*Contra-indications:* gastro-intestinal obstruction

*Side-effects:* flatulence, abdominal distension, intestinal obstruction

*Dose:* see under preparations below

COUNSELLING. Preparations that swell in contact with liquid should always be carefully swallowed with water and should not be taken immediately before going to bed

**Celevac®** (Boehringer Ingelheim)

*Tablets*, pink, methylcellulose '450' 500 mg. Net price 112-tab pack = 93p. Counselling, see above and dose

*Dose:* 3 tablets, chewed or crushed, with a tumblerful of liquid half an hour before food or when hungry

**Nilstim®** (De Witt)

*Tablets*, green, cellulose (microcrystalline) 220 mg, methylcellulose '2500' 400 mg. Net price 20 = 25p. Counselling, see above and dose

*Dose:* 2 tablets, chewed or crushed, with a tumblerful of liquid 15 minutes before the 2 main meals or when hungry

### STERCULIA

*Indications; Cautions; Contra-indications; Side-effects:* see under Methylcellulose

*Dose:* see under preparation below

**Prefil®** (Norgine)

*Granules*, brown, coated, sterculia 55%. Net price 200 g = £2.27. Label: 22, 27, counselling, administration

*Dose:* two 5-mL spoonfuls followed by a tumblerful of liquid ½–1 hour before food, reduced in patients accustomed to a low-residue diet

## 4.5.2   Centrally acting appetite suppressants

Centrally acting appetite suppressants are of no real value in the treatment of obesity since they do not improve the long-term outlook. They are sympathomimetics and most have a pronounced stimulant effect on the central nervous system.

Use of the amphetamine-like drugs **diethylpropion**, **mazindol**, and **phentermine** is **not** justified as any possible benefits are outweighed by the risks involved; abuse, particularly of diethylpropion, is an increasing problem.

Although **fenfluramine** is also related to amphetamine, in standard doses it has a sedative rather than a stimulant effect. Nevertheless, abuse has occurred and abrupt withdrawal may induce depression. It should preferably be avoided but may be considered for short-term adjunctive treatment in selected patients with severe obesity, given close support and supervision. It should **not** be given to patients with a past history of epilepsy, drug abuse or psychiatric illness and is **not recommended** for periods of treatment beyond 3 months. It should **not** be used for cosmetic reasons in mild to moderate obesity.

**Dexfenfluramine** is the dextro isomer of fenfluramine.

**Thyroid** hormones have no place in the treatment of obesity except in hypothyroid patients.

CHILDREN. These drugs should be avoided in children because of the possibility of growth suppression.

### DEXFENFLURAMINE HYDROCHLORIDE

*Indications:* see notes above

*Cautions; Contra-indications; Side-effects:* see under Fenfluramine Hydrochloride; so far, no reports of schizophrenia-like reactions

*Dose:* 15 mg morning and evening, at mealtimes; max. period of treatment should not exceed 3 months

▼ PoM **Adifax®** (Servier)

*Capsules*, dexfenfluramine hydrochloride 15 mg, net price 60-cap pack = £8.29. Label: 2

### DIETHYLPROPION HYDROCHLORIDE

*Indications:* see notes above

*Cautions:* severe hepatic or renal impairment; cardiovascular disease (avoid if severe), avoid in peptic ulceration, prostatic hypertrophy, depression; **interactions:** Appendix 1 (sympathomimetics)

DRIVING. May impair performance of skilled tasks (e.g. driving); effects of alcohol unpredictable

*Contra-indications:* glaucoma, hyperthyroidism, epilepsy, unstable personality, severe hypertension, history of drug abuse, porphyria (see section 9.8.2); pregnancy (congenital malformations reported) and breast-feeding; avoid in children and elderly

*Side-effects:* dry mouth, headache, rashes, dependence; less common, insomnia, increased nervousness, depression, psychosis, hallucinations, tachycardia, hypertension, constipation; rarely, gynaecomastia

**CD Apisate®** (Wyeth)

*Tablets*, m/r, yellow, diethylpropion hydrochloride 75 mg, thiamine hydrochloride 5 mg, pyridoxine hydrochloride 2 mg, riboflavine 4 mg, nicotinamide 30 mg. Net price 20 = 52p. Label: 25, counselling, driving

*Dose:* 1 tablet mid-morning; to reduce risk of dependence max. continuous period of treatment should not exceed 4–8 weeks (followed by similar period without treatment)

**CD Tenuate Dospan®** (Merrell)

*Tablets*, m/r, scored, diethylpropion hydrochloride 75 mg. Net price 30-tab pack = 96p. Label: 25, counselling, driving

*Dose:* 1 tablet mid-morning; to reduce risk of dependence max. continuous period of treatment should not exceed 8 weeks (followed by similar period without treatment)

*Note.* Brand name prescriptions for Tenuate Dospan must also specify the word 'tablets' (i.e. 'Tenuate Dospan Tablets').

## FENFLURAMINE HYDROCHLORIDE

*Indications:* see notes above

*Cautions:* dependence reported, depression on sudden withdrawal; elderly; **interactions:** Appendix 1 (sympathomimetics)

DRIVING. Drowsiness may affect performance of skilled tasks (e.g. driving); effects of alcohol enhanced

*Contra-indications:* history of depressive illness, drug or alcohol abuse; personality disorders; epilepsy; pregnancy and breast-feeding; porphyria (see section 9.8.2); avoid in children

*Side-effects:* diarrhoea and other gastro-intestinal disturbances; drowsiness, dizziness, and lethargy; also dry mouth, headache, nervousness, irritability, sleep disturbances, depression, visual disorders, hypotension, urinary frequency, impotence and loss of libido; rarely rashes, blood disorders, pulmonary hypertension, schizophrenia-like reactions; neurotoxicity reported in *animal* studies

*Dose:* see below

PoM **Ponderax**® (Servier)

*Pacaps*® (= capsules m/r), clear/blue, enclosing white pellets, fenfluramine hydrochloride 60 mg. Net price 60-cap pack = £7.26. Label: 2, 25

*Dose:* 1 capsule daily; max. period of treatment should not exceed 3 months (see also notes above)

## MAZINDOL

*Indications:* see notes above

*Cautions; Contra-indications; Side-effects:* see under Diethylpropion Hydrochloride

*Dose:* 2 mg after breakfast; to reduce the risk of dependence max. continuous period of treatment should not exceed 4–8 weeks (followed by similar period without treatment)

CD **Teronac** ® (Sandoz)

*Tablets*, scored, mazindol 2 mg. Net price 30-tab pack = £3.02. Counselling, driving

## PHENTERMINE

*Indications:* see notes above

*Cautions; Contra-indications; Side-effects:* see under Diethylpropion Hydrochloride

*Dose:* 15–30 mg before breakfast; to reduce the risk of dependence max. continuous period of treatment should not exceed 4–8 weeks (followed by similar period without treatment)

CD **Duromine** ® (3M)

*Capsules*, both m/r, phentermine (as resin complex) 15 mg (green/grey), net price · 30-cap pack = £1.24; 30 mg (maroon/grey), 30-cap pack = £1.63. Label: 25, counselling, driving

CD **Ionamin** ® (Lipha)

*Capsules*, both m/r, phentermine (as resin complex) 15 mg (grey/yellow), net price 20 = 99p; 30 mg (yellow), 20 = £1.26. Label: 25, counselling, driving

# 4.6 Drugs used in nausea and vertigo

Anti-emetics should be prescribed only when the cause of vomiting is known, particularly in children, otherwise the symptomatic relief that they produce may delay diagnosis. Anti-emetics are unnecessary and sometimes harmful when the cause can be treated, e.g. as in diabetic keto-acidosis, or in excessive digoxin or antiepileptic dosage.

If antinauseant drug treatment is indicated the choice of drug depends on the aetiology of vomiting.

## VESTIBULAR DISORDERS

Anti-emetics may be required in motion sickness, Ménière's disease, positional vertigo, labyrinthitis, and operative manipulation of the otovestibular apparatus. **Hyoscine** and the **antihistamines**, which act on the vomiting centre, are the drugs of choice. If possible they should be administered prophylactically at least 30 minutes before the emetic stimulus. Patients should be **warned** that these compounds may cause drowsiness, impair driving performance, and enhance the effects of alcohol and central nervous depressants.

MOTION SICKNESS. The most effective drug for the prevention of motion sickness is **hyoscine**. Adverse effects (drowsiness, blurred vision, dry mouth, urinary retention) are more frequent than with the antihistamines but are not generally prominent at the doses employed.

Antihistamines such as cinnarizine, cyclizine, dimenhydrinate, and promethazine are slightly less effective but generally better tolerated. There is no evidence that one antihistamine is superior to another but their duration of action and incidence of adverse effects (drowsiness and antimuscarinic effects) differ. If a sedative effect is desired **promethazine** and **dimenhydrinate** are useful, but generally a less sedating antihistamine like **cyclizine** or **cinnarizine** is preferred. To prevent motion sickness the first dose is usually taken half an hour (2 hours for cinnarizine) before the start of the journey. **Metoclopramide** and the **phenothiazines** (except promethazine), which act selectively on the chemoreceptor trigger zone, are ineffective in motion sickness.

OTHER LABYRINTHINE DISORDERS. Vertigo and nausea associated with Ménière's disease and middle-ear surgery disorders may be difficult to treat. **Hyoscine, antihistamines**, and **phenothiazines** (such as prochlorperazine and thiethylperazine) are effective in the prophylaxis and treatment of such conditions. **Betahistine** and **cinnarizine** have been promoted as specific treatment for Ménière's disease. In the acute attack **cyclizine, prochlorperazine**, or **thiethylperazine** may be given rectally or by intramuscular injection.

Treatment of vertigo in its chronic forms is seldom fully effective but antihistamines (such as dimenhydrinate) or phenothiazines (such as prochlorperazine) may help.

For advice to avoid the inappropriate prescribing of drugs (notably phenothiazines) for dizziness in the elderly, see Prescribing for the Elderly, p. 14.

## VOMITING OF PREGNANCY

Nausea in the first trimester of pregnancy does **not** require drug therapy. On rare occasions if vomiting is severe, an antihistamine or a phenothiazine (promethazine or thiethylperazine) may be required. If symptoms have not settled in 24 to 48 hours then a specialist opinion should be sought.

## SYMPTOMATIC RELIEF OF NAUSEA FROM UNDERLYING DISEASE

The **phenothiazines** are dopamine antagonists and act centrally by blocking the chemoreceptor trigger zone. In low doses they are the drugs of choice for the prophylaxis and treatment of nausea and vomiting associated with uraemia, diffuse neoplastic disease, radiation sickness, and the emesis caused by drugs such as opioid analgesics, general anaesthetics, and cytotoxic drugs. Rectal or parenteral administration is required if the vomiting has already started. **Prochlorperazine, perphenazine, trifluoperazine**, and **thiethylperazine** are less sedating than chlorpromazine but severe dystonic reactions sometimes occur, especially in children.

**Metoclopramide** is an effective anti-emetic with a spectrum of activity closely resembling that of the phenothiazines but it has a peripheral action on the gut in addition to its central effect and therefore may be superior to the phenothiazines in the emesis associated with gastroduodenal, hepatic, and biliary disease. The high-dose preparation is of value in the prevention of nausea and vomiting associated with cytotoxic drug therapy. Acute dystonic reactions may occur, particularly with children and young women, but they are less frequent than with phenothiazines.

**Domperidone** is used for the relief of nausea and vomiting, especially when associated with cytotoxic drug therapy. It has the advantage over metoclopramide and the phenothiazines of being less likely to cause central effects such as sedation and dystonic reactions because it does not readily cross the blood-brain barrier. It may be given for the treatment of levodopa- and bromocriptine-induced vomiting in parkinsonism (section 4.9.1). Domperidone acts at the chemoreceptor trigger zone and so is unlikely to be effective in motion sickness and other vestibular disorders.

Antihistamines are active in most of these conditions, but are not usually drugs of choice.

**Nabilone** is a synthetic cannabinoid with anti-emetic properties, reported to be superior to prochlorperazine. It is beneficial in the relief of nausea and vomiting associated with cytotoxic drug therapy. Side-effects occur in most patients given standard doses.

**Ondansetron**, a specific ($5HT_3$) serotonin antagonist, may have a valuable role in the management of nausea and vomiting in patients receiving cytotoxics who are unable to tolerate, or whose nausea and vomiting is not controlled by, less expensive drugs.

**Granisetron** is another specific ($5HT_3$) serotonin antagonist.

## BETAHISTINE HYDROCHLORIDE

*Indications:* vertigo, tinnitus, and hearing loss in Ménière's disease
*Cautions:* asthma; **interactions:** Appendix 1 (betahistine)
*Contra-indications:* phaeochromocytoma
*Side-effects:* nausea; rarely headache, rashes
*Dose:* initially 16 mg 3 times daily, preferably with food; maintenance 24–48 mg daily

PoM **Serc**® (Duphar)
*Tablets*, scored, betahistine hydrochloride 8 mg, net price 20 = £2.15; 16 mg (Serc®-16), 84-tab pack = £18.03. Label: 21

## CHLORPROMAZINE HYDROCHLORIDE

*Indications:* nausea and vomiting of terminal illness (where other drugs have failed or are not available); other indications, see sections 4.2.1, 15.1.4.2
*Cautions; Contra-indications; Side-effects:* see section 4.2.1
*Dose:* *by mouth*, 10–25 mg every 4–6 hours
*By deep intramuscular injection* 25 mg initially then 25–50 mg every 3–4 hours until vomiting stops
*By rectum* in suppositories, chlorpromazine 100 mg every 6–8 hours

**Preparations**
Section 4.2.1

## CINNARIZINE

*Indications:* vestibular disorders, such as vertigo, tinnitus, nausea, and vomiting in Ménière's disease; motion sickness; vascular disease, see section 2.6.3
*Cautions; Side-effects:* see under Cyclizine; also allergic skin reactions and fatigue; caution in hypotension (high doses); rarely, extrapyramidal symptoms in elderly on prolonged therapy; avoid in porphyria (see section 9.8.2)
*Dose:* vestibular disorders, 30 mg 3 times daily; CHILD 5–12 years half adult dose
Motion sickness, 30 mg 2 hours before travel then 15 mg every 8 hours during journey if necessary; CHILD 5–12 years half adult dose

**Stugeron**® (Janssen)
*Tablets*, scored, cinnarizine 15 mg. Net price 20 = 98p. Label: 2
*Note.* A proprietary brand of cinnarizine 15 mg tablets (Marzine RF®) is on sale to the public for travel sickness
**Stugeron Forte**®: see section 2.6.3

## CYCLIZINE

*Indications:* nausea, vomiting, vertigo, motion sickness, labyrinthine disorders

*Cautions; Side-effects:* drowsiness, occasional dry mouth and blurred vision; see also section 3.4.1 (Disadvantages of Antihistamines); cyclizine may aggravate severe heart failure and counteract the haemodynamic benefits of opioids; **interactions:** Appendix 1 (antihistamines)

DRIVING. Drowsiness may affect performance of skilled tasks (e.g. driving); effects of alcohol enhanced

*Dose: by mouth,* cyclizine hydrochloride 50 mg up to 3 times daily; CHILD 6–12 years 25 mg

*By intramuscular or intravenous injection,* cyclizine lactate 50 mg 3 times daily

**Valoid**® (Wellcome)

*Tablets,* scored, cyclizine hydrochloride 50 mg. Net price 20 = 99p. Label: 2

PoM *Injection,* cyclizine lactate 50 mg/mL. Net price 1-mL amp = 57p

## DIMENHYDRINATE

*Indications:* nausea, vomiting, vertigo, motion sickness, labyrinthine disorders

*Cautions; Side-effects:* see under Cyclizine; avoid in porphyria (see section 9.8.2)

*Dose:* 50–100 mg 2–3 times daily; CHILD 1–6 years 12.5–25 mg, 7–12 years 25–50 mg

Motion sickness, first dose 30 minutes before journey

**Dramamine**® (Searle)

*Tablets,* scored, dimenhydrinate 50 mg. Net price 20 = 93p. Label: 2

## DOMPERIDONE

*Indications:* see under Dose

*Cautions:* renal impairment; pregnancy and breast-feeding; not recommended for chronic administration; **interactions:** Appendix 1 (domperidone)

*Side-effects:* raised prolactin concentrations (possible galactorrhoea and gynaecomastia); acute dystonic reactions reported

*Dose: by mouth,* acute nausea and vomiting, (including nausea and vomiting induced by levodopa and bromocriptine), 10–20 mg every 4–8 hours, max. period of treatment 3 months; CHILD, nausea and vomiting following cytotoxic therapy or radiotherapy only, 200–400 micrograms/kg every 4–8 hours

*By rectum in suppositories,* 30–60 mg every 4–8 hours; CHILD, 2–12 years 30–120 mg daily according to body-weight (approximately 4 mg/kg)

PoM **Motilium**® (Sanofi Winthrop)

*Tablets,* f/c, domperidone 10 mg (as maleate). Net price 30-tab pack = £2.52; 100-tab pack = £8.42

*Suspension,* sugar-free, domperidone 5 mg/5 mL. Net price 200-mL pack = £1.85

*Suppositories,* domperidone 30 mg. Net price 10 = £2.72

## GRANISETRON

*Indications:* nausea and vomiting induced by cytotoxic chemotherapy or radiotherapy

*Cautions:* pregnancy and breast-feeding

*Side-effects:* constipation, headache; transient increases in liver enzymes

*Dose: by intravenous infusion* over 5 minutes, prevention, 3 mg (up to 2 additional 3-mg infusions may be given within 24 hours); treatment, as for prevention (the two additional infusions must not be given less than 10 minutes apart); max. 9 mg in 24 hours; CHILD not yet recommended

▼ PoM **Kytril**® (SmithKline Beecham)

*Infusion,* granisetron (as hydrochloride) 1 mg/mL, for dilution and use as infusion, net price 3-mL amp = £36.00

## HYOSCINE HYDROBROMIDE
(Scopolamine hydrobromide)

*Indications:* motion sickness; premedication, see section 15.1.3

*Cautions:* elderly, urinary retention, cardiovascular disease, gastro-intestinal obstruction, hepatic or renal impairment; pregnancy and breast-feeding; **interactions:** Appendix 1 (antimuscarinics)

DRIVING. Drowsiness may affect performance of skilled tasks (e.g. driving): effects of alcohol enhanced

*Contra-indications:* closed-angle glaucoma

*Side-effects:* drowsiness, dry mouth, dizziness, blurred vision, difficulty with micturition

*Dose:* motion sickness, *by mouth,* 300 micrograms 30 minutes before start of journey followed by 300 micrograms every 6 hours if required; max. 3 doses in 24 hours; CHILD 4–10 years 75–150 micrograms, over 10 years 150–300 micrograms

PoM **Hyoscine** (Non-proprietary)

*Tablets,* hyoscine hydrobromide 300 micrograms, net price 20 = 23p; 600 micrograms, 20 = 41p. Label: 2

*Note.* Proprietary brands of hyoscine tablets (Joyrides®, Kwells®) are on sale to the public for motion sickness

PoM **Scopoderm TTS**® (Ciba)

*Dressing,* self-adhesive, pink, releasing hyoscine approx. 500 micrograms/72 hours when in contact with skin. Net price 2 = £2.84. Label: 2, counselling, see below

*Administration:* motion sickness prevention, apply 1 dressing to hairless area of skin behind ear 5–6 hours before journey; replace if necessary after 72 hours, siting replacement dressing behind other ear

COUNSELLING. Explain accompanying instructions to patient and in particular emphasise advice to wash hands after handling and to wash application site after removing, and to use one at a time

## METOCLOPRAMIDE HYDROCHLORIDE

*Indications:* adults, nausea and vomiting, particularly in gastro-intestinal disorders and treatment with cytotoxics or radiotherapy; gastro-intestinal—section 1.2; migraine—section 4.7.4.1

PATIENTS UNDER 20 YEARS. Use restricted to severe intractable vomiting of known cause, vomiting of radiotherapy and cytotoxics, aid to gastro-intestinal intubation, pre-medication

*Cautions:* hepatic and renal impairment; elderly, young adults, and children (measure dose accurately, preferably with a pipette); may mask underlying disorders such as cerebral irritation; avoid for 3–4 days following gastro-intestinal surgery, may cause acute hypertensive response in phaeochromocytoma; pregnancy and breast-feeding; avoid in porphyria (see section 9.8.2); **interactions:** Appendix 1 (metoclopramide)

*Side-effects:* extrapyramidal effects (especially in children/young adults), hyperprolactinaemia, occasionally tardive dyskinesia on prolonged administration; also reported, drowsiness, restlessness, diarrhoea

*Dose: by mouth, or by intramuscular injection or by intravenous injection* over 1–2 minutes, 10 mg (5 mg in young adults 15–19 years under 60 kg) 3 times daily; CHILD up to 1 year (up to 10 kg) 1 mg twice daily, 1–3 years (10–14 kg) 1 mg 2–3 times daily, 3–5 years (15–19 kg) 2 mg 2–3 times daily, 5–9 years (20–29 kg) 2.5 mg 3 times daily, 9–14 years (30 kg and over) 5 mg 3 times daily

Note. Daily dose of metoclopramide should not normally exceed 500 micrograms/kg, particularly for children and young adults (restricted use, see above)

For radiological examinations, as a single dose 5–10 minutes before examination, 10–20 mg (10 mg in young adults 15–19 years); CHILD under 3 years 1 mg, 3–5 years 2 mg, 5–9 years 2.5 mg, 9–14 years 5 mg

*By continuous intravenous infusion* (preferred method), initially (before starting chemotherapy), 2–4 mg/kg over 15–30 minutes, then 3–5 mg/kg over 8–12 hours; max. in 24 hours, 10 mg/kg

*By intermittent intravenous infusion,* initially (before starting chemotherapy), up to 2 mg/kg over at least 15 minutes then up to 2 mg/kg over at least 15 minutes every 2 hours; max. in 24 hours, 10 mg/kg

PoM **Metoclopramide** (Non-proprietary)

*Tablets*, metoclopramide hydrochloride 10 mg, net price 20 = 45p

Available from APS, Ashbourne (Gastroflux®), Berk (Primperan®), Cox, Evans, Kerfoot, Lagap (Parmid®), Nicholas (Metramid®)

*Oral solution*, metoclopramide hydrochloride 5 mg/5 mL, net price 100-mL pack = £1.05

Available from Berk (Primperan®, sugar-free), Lagap (Parmid®)

*Injection*, metoclopramide hydrochloride 5 mg/mL, net price 2-mL amp = 24p

Available from Berk (Primperan®)

PoM **Maxolon**® (Beecham)

*Tablets*, scored, metoclopramide hydrochloride 10 mg. Net price 21-tab pack = £2.20, 84-tab pack = £8.53

*Syrup*, sugar-free, metoclopramide hydrochloride 5 mg/5 mL. Net price 200-mL pack = £3.48

*Paediatric liquid*, sugar-free, metoclopramide hydrochloride 1 mg/mL. Net price 15-mL pack with pipette = £1.37. Counselling, use of pipette

*Injection*, metoclopramide hydrochloride 5 mg/mL. Net price 2-mL amp = 24p

PoM **Maxolon High Dose**® (Beecham)

*Injection*, metoclopramide hydrochloride 5 mg/mL. Net price 20-mL amp = £2.43.

For dilution and use as an intravenous infusion in nausea and vomiting associated with cytotoxic chemotherapy only

Modified-release preparations

*Note.* All unsuitable for patients under 20 years

PoM **Gastrobid Continus**® (Napp)

*Tablets*, m/r, metoclopramide hydrochloride 15 mg. Net price 56-tab pack = £8.06. Label: 25

*Dose:* patients over 20 years, 1 tablet twice daily

PoM **Gastromax**® (Farmitalia Carlo Erba)

*Capsules*, m/r, orange/yellow, enclosing white to light beige pellets, metoclopramide hydrochloride 30 mg. Net price 28-cap pack = £11.85. Label: 22, 25

*Dose:* patients over 20 years, 1 capsule daily

PoM **Maxolon SR**® (Beecham)

*Capsules*, m/r, clear, enclosing white granules, metoclopramide hydrochloride 15 mg. Net price 56-cap pack = £9.78. Label: 25

*Dose:* patients over 20 years, 1 capsule twice daily

## NABILONE

*Indications:* nausea and vomiting caused by cytotoxic chemotherapy, unresponsive to conventional anti-emetics

*Cautions:* severe hepatic impairment; history of psychiatric disorder; elderly; hypertension; heart disease; **interactions:** Appendix 1 (nabilone)

DRIVING. Drowsiness may affect performance of skilled tasks (e.g. driving); effects of alcohol enhanced

*Side-effects:* drowsiness, vertigo, euphoria, dry mouth, ataxia, visual disturbance, concentration difficulties, sleep disturbance, dysphoria, hypotension, headache and nausea; also confusion, disorientation, hallucinations, psychosis, depression, decreased coordination, tremors, tachycardia, decreased appetite, and abdominal pain

*Dose:* patients over 18 years, initially 1 mg twice daily, increased if necessary to 2 mg twice daily, throughout each cycle of cytotoxic therapy and, if necessary, for 48 hours after the last dose of each cycle; max. 6 mg daily given in 3 divided doses. The first dose should be taken the night before initiation of cytotoxic treatment and the second dose 1–3 hours before the first dose of cytotoxic drug

PoM **Cesamet**® (Lilly)

*Capsules*, blue/white, nabilone 1 mg. Net price 20 = £31.76 (hosp. only). Label: 2

## ONDANSETRON

*Indications:* nausea and vomiting induced by cytotoxic chemotherapy or by radiotherapy

*Cautions:* pregnancy and breast-feeding; moderate or severe hepatic impairment (max. 8 mg daily)

*Side-effects:* constipation; headache, sensation of warmth or flushing in head and over stomach; occasional alterations in liver enzymes; hypersensitivity reactions reported

*Dose:* moderately emetogenic chemotherapy or radiotherapy, *by mouth*, 8 mg 1–2 hours before treatment *or*, *by slow intravenous injection*, 8 mg immediately before treatment, *then* 8 mg *by mouth* every 12 hours for up to 5 days

Severely emetogenic chemotherapy, *by slow intravenous injection*, 8 mg immediately before treatment, followed by 8 mg at intervals of 2–4 hours for 2 further doses (*or* followed by 1 mg/hour *by continuous intravenous infusion* for up to 24 hours) *then* 8 mg *by mouth* every 12 hours for up to 5 days

*alternatively*, *by intravenous infusion* over 15 minutes, 32 mg immediately before treatment *then* 8 mg *by mouth* every 12 hours for up to 5 days

*Note.* Efficacy may be enhanced by addition of a single dose of dexamethasone sodium phosphate 20 mg by intravenous injection

CHILD, *by slow intravenous injection or by intravenous infusion* over 15 minutes, 5 mg/m$^2$ immediately before chemotherapy then, 4 mg *by mouth* every 12 hours for up to 5 days

▼ PoM **Zofran**® (Glaxo)

*Tablets*, both yellow, f/c, ondansetron (as hydrochloride) 4 mg, net price 30-tab pack = £187.50; 8 mg, 10-tab pack = £90.00

*Injection*, ondansetron (as hydrochloride) 2 mg/mL, net price 2-mL amp = £10.50; 4-mL amp = £15.00

## PERPHENAZINE

*Indications:* severe nausea, vomiting (see notes above); other indications, section 4.2.1

*Cautions; Contra-indications; Side-effects:* see section 4.2.1; extrapyramidal symptoms may occur, particularly in young adults, elderly, and debilitated; avoid in children under 14 years

*Dose:* 4 mg 3 times daily, adjusted according to response; max. 24 mg daily (chemotherapy-induced); ELDERLY quarter to half adult dose

**Preparations:** section 4.2.1

## PROCHLORPERAZINE

*Indications:* severe nausea, vomiting, vertigo, labyrinthine disorders (see notes above); other indications, section 4.2.1

*Cautions; Contra-indications:* see under Chlorpromazine Hydrochloride (section 4.2.1). Oral route only for children (avoid if less than 10 kg); elderly (see notes above)

*Side-effects:* see under Chlorpromazine Hydrochloride; extrapyramidal symptoms may occur, particularly in children, elderly, and debilitated

*Dose:* by *mouth*, nausea and vomiting, prochlorperazine maleate or mesylate, acute attack, 20 mg initially then 10 mg after 2 hours; prevention 5–10 mg 2–3 times daily; CHILD (over 10 kg only) 250 micrograms/kg 2–3 times daily Labyrinthine disorders, 5 mg 3 times daily, gradually increased if necessary to 30 mg daily in divided doses, then reduced after several weeks to 5–10 mg daily

*By deep intramuscular injection*, nausea and vomiting, 12.5 mg when required followed if necessary after 6 hours by an oral dose, as above; CHILD not recommended

*By rectum* in suppositories, nausea and vomiting, 25 mg followed if necessary after 6 hours by oral dose, as above; *or* due to migraine, 5 mg 3 times daily; CHILD not recommended

PoM **Prochlorperazine** (Non-proprietary)

*Tablets*, prochlorperazine maleate 5 mg, net price 20 = 71p. Label: 2

PoM **Stemetil**® (Rhône-Poulenc Rorer)

*Tablets*, prochlorperazine maleate 5 mg (off-white), net price 84-tab pack = £2.95; 25 mg (scored), 56-tab pack = £5.19. Label: 2

*Syrup*, straw-coloured, prochlorperazine mesylate 5 mg/5 mL. Net price 100-mL pack = £1.66. Label: 2

*Eff sachets*, granules, effervescent, sugar-free, prochlorperazine mesylate 5 mg/sachet. Net price 21-sachet pack = £3.09. Label: 2, 13

*Injection*, prochlorperazine mesylate 12.5 mg/mL. Net price 1-mL amp = 32p; 2-mL amp = 41p

*Suppositories*, prochlorperazine maleate (as prochlorperazine), 5 mg, net price 10 = £4.16; 25 mg, 10 = £5.47. Label: 2

PoM **Vertigon**® (SK&F)

*Spansule*® (= capsules m/r), both clear/purple, enclosing yellowish-green and white pellets, prochlorperazine (as maleate), 10 mg, net price 60-cap pack = £2.24; 15 mg, 60-cap pack = £2.74. Label: 2, 25

*Dose:* initially 10–15 mg once or twice daily (elderly 10 mg daily). Maintenance 10–15 mg daily

Buccal preparation

PoM **Buccastem**® (R&C)

*Tablets (buccal)*, pale yellow, prochlorperazine maleate 3 mg. Net price 4 × 15-tab pack = £6.90. Label: 2, counselling, administration, see under Dose below

*Dose:* 1–2 tablets twice daily; tablets are placed high between upper lip and gum and left to dissolve

## PROMETHAZINE HYDROCHLORIDE

*Indications:* nausea, vomiting, vertigo, labyrinthine disorders, motion sickness; other indications, see sections 3.4.1, 4.1.1, 15.1.4.1

*Cautions; Side-effects:* see under Cyclizine but more sedating; intramuscular injection may be painful; avoid in porphyria (see section 9.8.2)

*Dose: by mouth,* 25–50 mg daily in single or divided doses; max. 75 mg

CHILD, motion sickness prevention, 1–5 years, 5 mg at night and following morning (1–2 years on doctors advice only); 5–10 years, 10 mg at night and following morning

*By deep intramuscular injection,* 25–50 mg when necessary; CHILD 5–10 years 6.25–12.5 mg

*By slow intravenous injection,* see section 3.4.1

**Preparations:** see section 3.4.1

## PROMETHAZINE THEOCLATE

*Indications:* nausea, vertigo, labyrinthine disorders, motion sickness (acts longer than the hydrochloride)

*Cautions; Side-effects:* see under Promethazine Hydrochloride

*Dose:* 25–75 mg, max. 100 mg, daily; CHILD 5–10 years, 12.5–37.5 mg daily

Motion sickness prevention, 25 mg at bedtime on night before travelling *or* 25 mg 1–2 hours before travelling; CHILD 5–10 years, half adult dose

For severe vomiting in pregnancy, 25 mg at bedtime, increased if necessary to a max. of 100 mg daily (but see also Vomiting of Pregnancy in notes above)

**Avomine®** (Rhône-Poulenc Rorer)
*Tablets,* scored, promethazine theoclate 25 mg. Net price 10-tab pack = 88p; 28-tab pack = 93p. Label: 2

## THIETHYLPERAZINE

*Indications:* severe nausea, vomiting, vertigo, labyrinthine disorders

*Cautions; Contra-indications; Side-effects:* see under Chlorpromazine Hydrochloride (section 4.2.1); young adults, elderly, and debilitated particularly susceptible to extrapyramidal effects; avoid in children under 15 years

*Dose: by mouth,* thiethylperazine maleate 10 mg 2–3 times daily

*By intramuscular injection,* thiethylperazine [base] 6.5 mg

*By rectum* in suppositories, thiethylperazine [base] 6.5 mg night and morning

*Note:* Thiethylperazine 6.5 mg ≡ thiethylperazine maleate 10.86 mg ≡ thiethylperazine maleate 10.28 mg

PoM **Torecan®** (Sandoz)
*Tablets,* s/c, thiethylperazine *maleate* 10 mg. Net price 50 = £1.42. Label: 2
*Injection,* thiethylperazine 6.5 mg (as *malate*)/mL. Net price 1-mL amp = 18p
*Suppositories,* thicthylperazine 6.5 mg (as *maleate*). Net price 5 = 91p. Label: 2

## TRIFLUOPERAZINE

*Indications:* severe nausea and vomiting (see notes above); other indications, section 4.2.1

*Cautions; Contra-indications; Side-effects:* see section 4.2.1; extrapyramidal symptoms may occur, particularly in children, elderly, and debilitated

*Dose: by mouth,* 2–4 mg daily in divided doses *or* as a single dose of a modified-release preparation; max. 6 mg daily; CHILD 3–5 years up to 1 mg daily, 6–12 years up to 4 mg daily

*By deep intramuscular injection,* 1–3 mg daily in divided doses, max. 6 mg daily

**Preparations:** section 4.2.1

# 4.7    Analgesics

Terminal Care, see p. 12.

## 4.7.1   Non-opioid analgesics

The non-opioid drugs, aspirin and paracetamol, are particularly suitable for pain in musculoskeletal conditions, whereas the opioid analgesics are more suitable for severe pain of visceral origin.

**Aspirin** is the analgesic of choice for headache, transient musculoskeletal pain, and dysmenorrhoea. It also has anti-inflammatory properties which may be useful, and is an antipyretic. Aspirin tablets or dispersible aspirin tablets are adequate for most purposes as they act rapidly.

Gastric irritation may be a problem; it is minimised by taking the dose after food. Numerous formulations are available which improve gastric tolerance, e.g. the buffered aspirin preparations such as aloxiprin (Palaprin Forte®) and enteric-coated aspirin. Some of these preparations have a slow onset of action and are therefore unsuitable for single-dose analgesic use though their prolonged action may be useful for night pain.

**Paracetamol** is similar in efficacy to aspirin, but has no demonstrable anti-inflammatory activity; it is less irritant to the stomach. Overdosage with paracetamol is particularly dangerous as it may cause hepatic damage which is sometimes not apparent for 4 to 6 days. **Benorylate** is an aspirin–paracetamol ester.

**Nefopam** may have a place in the relief of persistent pain unresponsive to other non-opioid analgesics. It causes little or no respiratory depression, but sympathomimetic and antimuscarinic side-effects may be troublesome.

**Anti-inflammatory analgesics** (see section 10.1.1) are particularly useful for the treatment of patients with chronic disease accompanied by pain and inflammation. Some of them are also used in the short-term treatment of mild to moderate pain including transient musculoskeletal pain. They are also suitable for the relief of pain in *dysmenorrhoea* and to treat pain caused by *secondary bone tumours,* many of which produce lysis of bone and release prostaglandins (see Prescribing in Terminal Care, p. 12).

**CSM advice.**
The CSM has considered available evidence on possible links between Reye's syndrome and aspirin use by feverish children, and recommends that aspirin should no longer be given to children aged under 12 years, unless specifically indicated, e.g. for juvenile rheumatoid arthritis. It is therefore important to advise families that aspirin is not, on the evidence now available, a suitable medicine for children with minor illnesses. Paracetamol (see below) is an effective alternative treatment for fever in children.

## ASPIRIN

*Indications:* mild to moderate pain, pyrexia (see notes above); see also section 10.1.1; antiplatelet, see section 2.9

*Cautions:* asthma, allergic disease, impaired renal or hepatic function (avoid if severe), dehydration, pregnancy; G6PD-deficiency (see section 9.1.5); **interactions:** Appendix 1 (aspirin)

*Contra-indications:* children under 12 years and in breast-feeding (Reye's syndrome, see notes above); gastro-intestinal ulceration, haemophilia; not for treatment of gout

*Side-effects:* generally mild and infrequent but high incidence of gastro-intestinal irritation with slight asymptomatic blood loss, increased bleeding time, bronchospasm and skin reactions in hypersensitive patients. Prolonged administration, see section 10.1.1. Overdosage: see Emergency Treatment of Poisoning, p. 17

*Dose:* 300–900 mg every 4–6 hours when necessary; max. 4 g daily

**Aspirin** (Non-proprietary)
*Tablets*, aspirin 300 mg. Net price 20 = 9p. Label: 21, 32
Available from APS, Evans, Kerfoot
*Dispersible tablets*, aspirin 300 mg, net price 20 = 9p; 75 mg, see section 2.9. Label: 13, 21, 32
Available from APS, Cox, Evans, Kerfoot
*Note.* Addendum 1989 to BP 1988 directs that when soluble aspirin tablets are prescribed, dispersible aspirin tablets shall be dispensed.

**NHS Laboprin DL®** (LAB)
*Powder*, lysine acetylsalicylate 900 mg (≡ aspirin 500 mg), glycine 100 mg/sachet. Net price 10-sachet pack = £2.39. Label: 13, 21, 33

**Palaprin Forte®** (Nicholas)
*Tablets*, orange, scored, aloxiprin[1] 600 mg ≡ aspirin 500 mg. To be taken dispersed in water, chewed, sucked, or swallowed whole. Net price 20 = 50p. Label: 21, 33
*Dose:* ½–2 tablets up to 4 times daily; max. 8 daily
1. Aloxiprin is a polymeric condensation product of aluminium oxide and aspirin

Preparations for intestinal release
**Caprin®** (Sinclair)
*Tablets*, e/c, pink, aspirin 324 mg. Net price 20 = 69p. Label: 5, 25, 32
**Nu-Seals® Aspirin** (Lilly)
*Tablets*, e/c, red, aspirin 300 mg, net price 100-tab pack = £5.27. Label: 5, 25, 32

## PARACETAMOL

*Indications:* mild to moderate pain, pyrexia
*Cautions:* hepatic and renal impairment, alcohol dependence; **interactions:** Appendix 1 (paracetamol)
*Side-effects:* side-effects rare, but rashes, blood disorders, and acute pancreatitis reported; **important:** liver damage (and less frequently renal damage) following overdosage, see Emergency Treatment of Poisoning, p. 18
*Dose:* 0.5–1 g every 4–6 hours to a max. of 4 g daily; CHILD 2 months 60 mg for post-immunisation pyrexia; otherwise under 3 months (on doctor's advice only), 10 mg/kg (5 mg/kg if jaundiced); 3 months–1 year 60–120 mg, 1–5 years 120–250 mg, 6–12 years 250–500 mg; these doses may be repeated every 4–6 hours when necessary (max. of 4 doses in 24 hours)
For full Joint Committee on Vaccination and Immunisation recommendation on post-immunisation pyrexia, see p. 434
Rectal route, see below

**Paracetamol** (Non-proprietary)
*Tablets*, paracetamol 500 mg. Net price 20 = 8p. Label: 29, 30
Available from APS, Cox, Evans, Kerfoot, Sterling Health (NHS Panadol®)
*Soluble Tablets* (= Dispersible tablets), paracetamol 500 mg. Net price 60 = £1.44. Label: 13, 29, 30
Available from Sanofi Winthrop (NHS Panadol Soluble®)
*Paediatric Soluble Tablets* (= Paediatric dispersible tablets), paracetamol 120 mg. Net price 24-tab pack = 62p. Label: 13, 30
Available from R&C (NHS Disprol® Junior)
*Paediatric Oral Solution* (= Paediatric Elixir), paracetamol 120 mg/5 mL. Net price 100 mL = 50p. Label: 30
*Note.* Sugar-free versions are available and can be ordered by specifying 'sugar-free' on the prescription.
Available from Berk, Evans, RP Drugs (Paldesic®), Wallace Mfg (NHS Salzone®)
*Oral Suspension 120 mg/5 mL* (= Paediatric Mixture), paracetamol 120 mg/5 mL. Net price 100 mL = 43p. Label: 30
*Note.* BP directs that when Paediatric Paracetamol Oral Suspension or Paediatric Paracetamol Mixture is prescribed Paracetamol Oral Suspension 120 mg/5 mL should be dispensed; sugar-free versions are available and can be ordered by specifying 'sugar-free' on the prescription
Available from Cupal (Cupanol® Under 6, sugar-free), R&C (Disprol®, sugar-free), Sterling Health (Panadol®, sugar-free), Wellcome (Calpol®, Calpol® sugar-free)
*Oral Suspension 250 mg/5 mL* (= Mixture), paracetamol 250 mg/5 mL. Net price 100 mL = £1.28. Label: 30
Available from Cupal (NHS Cupanol® Over 6, sugar-free), Wellcome (NHS Calpol® Six Plus)
*Suppositories*, paracetamol 125 mg. Net price 10 = £10.50. Label: 30
*Dose:* by rectum, CHILD 1–5 years 125–250 mg (1–2 suppositories) up to 4 times daily
Available from Astra (Alvedon®)

NHS **Pameton**® (Sanofi Winthrop)
*Tablets*, paracetamol 500 mg, DL-methionine 250 mg. Net price 60 tab = £2.77. Label: 29, 30
*Dose:* 2 tablets when required up to 4 times daily; CHILD 6–12 years ½–1 tablet when required; not more often than every 4 hours and max. of 4 doses in 24 hours

## BENORYLATE
(Aspirin-paracetamol ester; 2 g benorylate is equivalent to approximately 1.15 g aspirin and 970 mg paracetamol)
*Indications:* mild to moderate pain; pyrexia; see also section 10.1.1
*Cautions; Contra-indications; Side-effects:* see under Aspirin and under Paracetamol
Note. Preparations containing aspirin are contra-indicated in children under 12 years of age owing to an association with Reye's syndrome, see notes above
*Dose:* 2 g twice daily, preferably after food

**Preparations:** see section 10.1.1

## DICLOFENAC SODIUM
See section 10.1.1

## DIFLUNISAL
*Indications:* mild to moderate pain; see also section 10.1.1
*Cautions; Contra-indications; Side-effects:* see section 10.1.1
*Dose:* 250–500 mg twice daily after food

**Preparations:** section 10.1.1

## FENOPROFEN
*Indications:* mild to moderate pain, pyrexia; see also section 10.1.1
*Cautions; Contra-indications; Side-effects:* See section 10.1.1
*Dose:* 200–600 mg 3–4 times daily, after food; max. 3 g daily

PoM **Progesic**® (Lilly)
*Tablets*, yellow, fenoprofen 200 mg (as calcium salt). Net price 20 = £2.20. Label: 21
PoM **Fenopron**®: see section 10.1.1

## IBUPROFEN
*Indications:* mild to moderate pain; see also section 10.1.1
*Cautions; Contra-indications; Side-effects:* see section 10.1.1
*Dose:* 1.2–1.8 g daily in divided doses, preferably after food, increased if necessary to a max. of 2.4 g daily; CHILD, fever and pain, see below
▼ PoM **Junifen**® (Boots)
*Suspension*, ibuprofen 100 mg/5 mL, net price 150-mL pack = £2.67. Label: 21
*Dose:* fever and pain in children, under 1 year not recommended, 1–12 years 20 mg/kg daily in divided doses *or* 1–2 years 2.5 mL 3–4 times daily, 3–7 years 5 mL, 8–12 years 10 mL

**Other preparations:** see section 10.1.1

## KETOPROFEN
See section 10.1.1

## KETOROLAC
See section 15.1.4.2

## MEFENAMIC ACID
*Indications:* mild to moderate pain, pyrexia in children; menorrhagia; see also section 10.1.1
*Cautions; Contra-indications; Side-effects:* see section 10.1.1; exclude pathological conditions before treating menorrhagia
*Dose:* 500 mg 3 times daily after food; CHILD over 6 months 25 mg/kg daily in divided doses for max. 7 days, except in juvenile arthritis (Still's disease)

**Preparations:** see section 10.1.1

## NAPROXEN SODIUM
*Indications:* mild to moderate pain; rheumatic disease, see Naproxen, section 10.1.1
*Cautions; Contra-indications; Side-effects:* see section 10.1.1
*Dose:* 550 mg twice daily when necessary, preferably after food
Note. 275 mg naproxen sodium ≡ 250 mg naproxen but the sodium salt has a more rapid action.

PoM **Synflex**® (Syntex)
*Tablets*, orange, naproxen sodium 275 mg. Net price 20 = £2.90. Label: 21

## NEFOPAM HYDROCHLORIDE
*Indications:* moderate pain
*Cautions:* hepatic or renal disease, elderly, urinary retention; **interactions:** Appendix 1 (nefopam)
*Contra-indications:* convulsive disorders; not indicated for myocardial infarction
*Side-effects:* nausea, nervousness, urinary retention, dry mouth, lightheadedness; less frequently vomiting, blurred vision, drowsiness, sweating, insomnia, tachycardia, headache; confusion and hallucinations also reported; may colour urine (pink)
*Dose: by mouth*, initially 60 mg (elderly, 30 mg) 3 times daily, adjusted according to response; usual range 30–90 mg 3 times daily
*By intramuscular injection*, 20 mg every 6 hours
Note. Nefopam hydrochloride 20 mg by injection ≡ 60 mg by mouth

PoM **Acupan**® (3M)
*Tablets*, f/c, nefopam hydrochloride 30 mg. Net price 90-tab pack = £11.73. Label: 2, 14
*Injection*, nefopam hydrochloride 20 mg/mL. Net price 1-mL amp = 74p

---

## 4.7.1.1 COMPOUND ANALGESIC PREPARATIONS

Compound analgesic preparations of, for example, aspirin, paracetamol, and codeine are **not** recommended. Single-ingredient preparations should be prescribed in preference because compound preparations rarely have any advantage and complicate the treatment of overdosage. The dangers of co-proxamol (dextropropoxyphene-paracetamol) overdosage call for rapid treatment as described in Emergency Treatment of Poisoning, p. 18.

It is even more desirable to **avoid** mixtures of analgesics with antihistamines or muscle relaxants; the individual components should be prescribed separately so that the dose of each can be adjusted as appropriate.

**Caffeine** is a weak stimulant that is often included, in small doses, in analgesic preparations. It does not contribute to the analgesic or anti-inflammatory effect of the preparation and may possibly aggravate the gastric irritation caused by aspirin. Moreover, in excessive dosage or on withdrawal caffeine may itself induce headache.

> Patients should be warned when compound analgesics contain paracetamol so that they can avoid other paracetamol-containing preparations.

### Co-codamol
**Co-codamol** (Non-proprietary)
*Tablets*, co-codamol 8/500 (codeine phosphate 8 mg, paracetamol 500 mg). Net price 20 = 28p. Label: 29, 30
*Dose:* 1–2 tablets every 4–6 hours; max. 8 tablets daily; CHILD 6–12 years ½–1 tablet
Available from APS, Cox, Evans, Galen (NHS Parake®), Kerfoot, Sterling Health (NHS Panadeine®)
*Effervescent* or *dispersible tablets*, co-codamol 8/500 (paracetamol 500 mg, codeine phosphate 8 mg). Net price 20 = 59p. Label: 13, 29, 30
*Dose:* 1–2 tablets in water every 4–6 hours, max. 8 tablets daily; CHILD 6–12 years ½–1 tablet, max. 4 tablets daily
Available from Fisons (NHS Paracodol®), Sterwin
*Note.* The Drug Tariff allows tablets of co-codamol labelled 'dispersible' to be dispensed against an order for 'effervescent' and *vice versa*
*Capsules*, co-codamol 8/500 (paracetamol 500 mg, codeine phosphate 8 mg). Net price 30 = £1.68. Label: 29, 30
*Dose:* 1–2 capsules every 4 hours; max. 8 capsules daily
Available from Fisons (NHS Paracodol®)
When co-codamol tablets, dispersible (or effervescent) tablets, or capsules are prescribed and no strength is stated tablets, dispersible (or effervescent) tablets, or capsules, respectively, containing codeine phosphate 8 mg and paracetamol 500 mg should be dispensed.

### Co-codaprin
**Co-codaprin** (Non-proprietary)
*Tablets*, co-codaprin 8/400 (codeine phosphate 8 mg, aspirin 400 mg). Net price 20 = 34p. Label: 21, 32
*Dose:* 1–2 tablets every 4–6 hours when necessary; max. 8 tablets daily
Available from Cox

*Dispersible tablets*, co-codaprin 8/400 (codeine phosphate 8 mg, aspirin 400 mg). Net price 20 = 31p. Label: 13, 21, 32
*Dose:* 1–2 tablets in water every 4–6 hours; max. 8 tablets daily
Available from Cox
When co-codaprin tablets or dispersible tablets are prescribed and no strength is stated tablets, or dispersible tablets, respectively, containing codeine phosphate 8 mg and aspirin 400 mg should be dispensed.

### Co-dydramol
**PoM Co-dydramol** (Non-proprietary)
*Tablets*, scored, co-dydramol 10/500 (dihydrocodeine tartrate 10 mg, paracetamol 500 mg). Net price 20 = 33p. Label: 21, 29, 30
*Dose:* 1–2 tablets every 4–6 hours; max. 8 tablets daily
Available from APS, Cox, Evans, Galen (NHS Galake®), Kerfoot, Napp (NHS Paramol®), Sterwin
When co-dydramol tablets are prescribed and no strength is stated tablets containing dihydrocodeine tartrate 10 mg and paracetamol 500 mg should be dispensed.

### Co-proxamol
**PoM Co-proxamol** (Non-proprietary)
*Tablets*, co-proxamol 32.5/325 (dextropropoxyphene hydrochloride 32.5 mg, paracetamol 325 mg). Net price 20 = 28p. Label: 2, 10 patient information leaflet (if available), 29, 30
*Dose:* 2 tablets 3–4 times daily; max. 8 tablets daily
Available from APS, Cox (NHS Cosalgesic®), Dista (NHS Distalgesic®), Evans, Kerfoot, Sterwin
When co-proxamol tablets are prescribed and no strength is stated tablets containing dextropropoxyphene hydrochloride 32.5 mg and paracetamol 325 mg should be dispensed.

### Other compound analgesic preparations
**NHS Antoin®** (Cox)
*Dispersible tablets*, scored, aspirin 400 mg, codeine phosphate 5 mg, caffeine citrate 15 mg. Net price 50 = £1.33. Label: 13, 21
*Dose:* 1–2 tablets in water 3–4 times daily; max. 10 tablets daily
**NHS Cafadol®** (Typharm)
*Tablets*, yellow, scored, paracetamol 500 mg, caffeine 30 mg. Net price 20 = 60p. Label: 29, 30
*Dose:* 1–2 tablets every 4 hours; max. 8 tablets daily; CHILD not recommended in view of caffeine content
**NHS Calpol® Extra** (Wellcome)
*Tablets*, pink, paracetamol 500 mg, codeine phosphate 5 mg, caffeine 10 mg. Net price 12-tab pack = 65p. Label: 29, 30
*Dose:* 2 tablets up to 4 times daily
**NHS CD Equagesic®** (Wyeth)
*Tablets*, pink/white/yellow, ethoheptazine citrate 75 mg, meprobamate 150 mg, aspirin 250 mg. Net price 20 = 66p. Label: 2, 21, 32
*Dose:* muscle pain, 1–2 tablets 3–4 times daily
**NHS Hypon®** (Wellcome)
*Tablets*, yellow, aspirin 325 mg, caffeine 10 mg, codeine phosphate 5 mg. Net price 20 = 54p. Label: 21, 32
*Dose:* 1–2 tablets every 4 hours; max. 12 tablets daily
**NHS PoM Lobak®** (Sanofi Winthrop)
*Tablets*, scored, chlormezanone 100 mg, paracetamol 450 mg. Net price 50 = £7.67. Label: 2, 29, 30
*Dose:* muscle pain, 1–2 tablets 3 times daily; max. 8 tablets daily
**NHS Medised®** (Panpharma)
*Suspension*, paracetamol 120 mg, promethazine hydrochloride 2.5 mg/5 mL. Net price 140-mL pack = £1.23. Label: 1, 30
*Note.* Dose excluded because combination not recommended

NHS **Propain**® (Panpharma)

*Tablets*, yellow, scored, codeine phosphate 10 mg, diphenhydramine hydrochloride 5 mg, paracetamol 400 mg, caffeine 50 mg. Net price 12-tab pack = 85p. Label: 2, 29, 30

*Dose:* 1–2 tablets every 4 hours; max. 8 tablets daily

NHS PoM **Robaxisal Forte**® (Wyeth)

*Tablets*, pink/white, scored, methocarbamol 400 mg, aspirin 325 mg. Net price 20 = £1.90. Label: 2, 21, 32

*Dose:* muscle pain, 2 tablets 4 times daily

NHS **Solpadeine**® (Sterling Health)

*Effervescent tablets*, paracetamol 500 mg, codeine phosphate 8 mg, caffeine 30 mg. Contains 18.5 mmol Na⁺/ tablet; avoid in renal impairment. Net price 24-tab pack = £1.61. Label: 13, 29, 30

*Dose:* 2 tablets in water 3–4 times daily; CHILD not recommended in view of caffeine content

*Capsules*, ingredients as for Effervescent Tablets. Net price 24-cap pack = £1.52. Label: 29, 30

*Dose:* 2 capsules up to 4 times daily

NHS **Syndol**® (Merrell)

*Tablets*, yellow, scored, paracetamol 450 mg, codeine phosphate 10 mg, doxylamine succinate 5 mg, caffeine 30 mg. Net price 20 = £1.36. Label: 2, 29, 30

*Dose:* 1–2 tablets every 4–6 hours; max. 8 tablets daily

NHS **Veganin**® (W-L)

*Tablets*, scored, aspirin 250 mg, paracetamol 250 mg, codeine phosphate 6.8 mg. Net price 20 = 86p. Label: 21, 29, 31

*Dose:* 1–2 tablets every 4 hours; max. 8 tablets daily

---

## HIGHER OPIOID CONTENT

The following preparations have a higher opioid analgesic content than most compound analgesic preparations. For cautions and side-effects, see section 4.7.2.

PoM **Aspav**® (Roussel)

*Dispersible tablets*, aspirin 500 mg, papaveretum 10 mg. Net price 20 = £1.35. Label: 2, 13, 21, 32

*Dose:* 1–2 tablets in water every 4–6 hours if necessary; max. 8 tablets daily. Contra-indicated in women of child-bearing potential (see Appendix 4)

NHS PoM **Doloxene Compound**® (Lilly)

*Capsules*, grey/red, dextropropoxyphene napsylate 100 mg, aspirin 375 mg, caffeine 30 mg. Net price 20 = £1.34. Label: 2, 21, 32

*Dose:* 1 capsule 3–4 times daily; max. 4 capsules daily

NHS CD **Fortagesic**® (Sanofi Winthrop)

*Tablets*, pentazocine 15 mg (as hydrochloride), paracetamol 500 mg. Net price 20 = £1.40. Label: 2, 21, 29, 30

*Dose:* 2 tablets up to 4 times daily; CHILD 7–12 years 1 tablet every 4 hours, max. 4 tablets daily

PoM **Solpadol**® (Sanofi Winthrop)

*Effervescent tablets*, paracetamol 500 mg, codeine phosphate 30 mg. Contains 18.6 mmol Na⁺/tablet; avoid in renal impairment. Net price 60-tab pack = £5.83. Label: 2, 13, 29, 30

*Dose:* 2 tablets in water every 4 hours; max. 8 daily

PoM **Tylex**® (Cilag)

*Capsules*, paracetamol 500 mg, codeine phosphate 30 mg. Net price 100 = £8.60. Label: 2, 29, 30

*Dose:* 1–2 capsules every 4 hours; max. 8 capsules daily

Paediatric

NHS PoM **Formulix**® (Cilag)

Product discontinued

---

## 4.7.2   Opioid analgesics

Opioid analgesics are used to relieve moderate to severe pain particularly of visceral origin. Repeated administration may cause dependence and tolerance, but this is no deterrent in the control of pain in terminal illness, for guidelines see Prescribing in Terminal Care, p. 12.

SIDE-EFFECTS. Opioid analgesics share many side-effects though qualitative and quantitative differences exist. The most common include nausea, vomiting, constipation, and drowsiness. Larger doses produce respiratory depression and hypotension. Overdosage, see Emergency Treatment of Poisoning, p. 18.

INTERACTIONS. See Appendix 1 (opioid analgesics) (**important**: special hazard with *pethidine and possibly other opioids* and MAOIs).

DRIVING. Drowsiness may affect performance of skilled tasks (e.g. driving); effects of alcohol enhanced.

CHOICE. **Morphine** remains the most valuable opioid analgesic for severe pain although it frequently causes nausea and vomiting. It is the standard against which other opioid analgesics are compared. In addition to relief of pain, morphine also confers a state of euphoria and mental detachment.

Morphine is the opioid of choice for the oral treatment of *severe pain in terminal care*. It is given regularly every 4 hours as an oral solution, or every 12 hours as modified-release tablets. For guidelines on dosage adjustment in terminal care, see p. 12.

**Buprenorphine** has both opioid agonist and antagonist properties and may precipitate withdrawal symptoms, including pain, in patients dependent on other opioids. It has abuse potential and may itself cause dependence. It has a much longer duration of action than morphine and sublingually is an effective analgesic for 8 to 12 hours. Vomiting may be a problem. Unlike most opioid analgesics its effects are only partially reversed by naloxone.

**Codeine** is effective for the relief of mild to moderate pain but is too constipating for long-term use.

**Dextromoramide** is less sedating than morphine and has a short duration of action.

**Dipipanone** used alone is less sedating than morphine but the only preparation available contains an anti-emetic and is therefore not suitable for regular regimens in terminal care (see p. 12).

**Dextropropoxyphene** given alone is a very mild analgesic somewhat less potent than codeine. Combinations of dextropropoxyphene with paracetamol (co-proxamol) or aspirin have little more analgesic effect than paracetamol or aspirin alone. An important disadvantage of co-proxamol

---

is that overdosage (which may be combined with alcohol) is complicated by respiratory depression and acute heart failure due to the dextropropoxyphene and by hepatotoxicity due to the paracetamol. Rapid treatment is essential (see Emergency Treatment of Poisoning, p. 18).

**Diamorphine** (heroin) is a powerful opioid analgesic. It may cause less nausea and hypotension than morphine. In *terminal care* the greater solubility of diamorphine allows effective doses to be injected in smaller volumes and this is important in the emaciated patient.

**Dihydrocodeine** is similar in potency to codeine. It is suitable for use in ambulant patients with moderate pain but may cause dizziness and constipation.

**Meptazinol** is claimed to have a low incidence of respiratory depression. It has a reported length of action of 2 to 7 hours with onset within 15 minutes, but there is an incidence of nausea and vomiting.

**Methadone** is less sedating than morphine and acts for longer periods. In prolonged use, methadone should not be administered more often than twice daily to avoid the risk of accumulation and opioid overdosage.

**Nalbuphine** has a similar efficacy to that of morphine for pain relief, but may have fewer side-effects and less abuse potential. Nausea and vomiting occur less than with other opioids but respiratory depression is similar to that with morphine.

**Oxycodone** is used as the pectinate in suppositories (special order, Boots) for the control of *pain in terminal care.*

**Pentazocine** has both agonist and antagonist properties and precipitates withdrawal symptoms, including pain in patients dependent on other opioids. By injection it is more potent than dihydrocodeine or codeine, but hallucinations and thought disturbances may occur. It is not recommended and, in particular, should be avoided after myocardial infarction as it may increase pulmonary and aortic blood pressure as well as cardiac work.

**Pethidine** produces a prompt but short-lasting analgesia and even in high doses it is a less potent analgesic than morphine. It is not suitable for the relief of pain in terminal care. It is used for analgesia in labour, and in the neonate is associated with less respiratory depression than other opioid analgesics (probably because its action is weaker). See also section 15.1.4.3 (perioperative use).

**Phenazocine** is effective in severe pain and has less tendency to increase biliary pressure than other opioid analgesics. It can be administered sublingually if nausea and vomiting are a problem.

ADDICTS. Although caution is necessary addicts (and ex-addicts) may be treated with analgesics in the same way as other people when there is a real clinical need. Doctors are reminded that they do not require a special licence to prescribe opioid analgesics for addicts for relief of pain due to organic disease or injury.

## MORPHINE SALTS

*Indications:* see notes above; acute pulmonary oedema; see also section 15.1.4.3

*Cautions:* hypotension, hypothyroidism, asthma, and decreased respiratory reserve; pregnancy and breast-feeding; may precipitate coma in hepatic impairment (but many such patients tolerate morphine well); reduce dose in renal impairment, elderly and debilitated; dependence (severe withdrawal symptoms if withdrawn abruptly); use of cough suppressants containing opioid analgesics not generally recommended in children and should be avoided altogether in those under 1 year; **interactions:** Appendix 1 (opioid analgesics)

*Contra-indications:* avoid in raised intracranial pressure or head injury (in addition to interfering with respiration, affect pupillary responses vital for neurological assessment)

*Side-effects:* nausea and vomiting (particularly in initial stages), constipation, and drowsiness; larger doses produce respiratory depression and hypotension; other side-effects include difficulty with micturition, ureteric or biliary spasm, dry mouth, sweating, facial flushing, vertigo, bradycardia, palpitations, postural hypotension, hypothermia, hallucinations, mood changes, dependence, miosis, urticaria and pruritus; overdosage: see p. 18

*Dose:* acute pain, *by subcutaneous or intramuscular injection*, 10 mg every 4 hours if necessary (15 mg for heavier well-muscled patients); CHILD up to 1 month 150 micrograms/kg, 1–12 months 200 micrograms/kg, 1–5 years 2.5–5 mg, 6–12 years 5–10 mg

*By slow intravenous injection*, quarter to half corresponding intramuscular dose

Myocardial infarction, *by slow intravenous injection* (2 mg/minute), 10 mg followed by a further 5–10 mg if necessary; elderly or frail patients, reduce dose by half

Acute pulmonary oedema, *by slow intravenous injection* (2 mg/minute) 5–10 mg

Chronic pain, *by mouth or by subcutaneous or intramuscular injection*, 5–20 mg regularly every 4 hours; dose may be increased according to needs; oral dose should be approximately double corresponding intramuscular dose and triple to quadruple corresponding intramuscular *diamorphine* dose (see also Prescribing in Terminal Care, p. 12); *by rectum*, as suppositories, 15–30 mg regularly every 4 hours

Note. The doses stated above refer equally to morphine hydrochloride, sulphate, and tartrate; for dose of **modified-release** tablets, see p. 172.

### PoM or **CD Morphine Oral Solutions**

Oral solutions of morphine can be prescribed by writing the formula:

Morphine hydrochloride 5 mg
Chloroform water to 5 mL

Note. The proportion of morphine hydrochloride may be altered when specified by the prescriber; if above 13 mg per 5 mL the solution becomes **CD**. For sample prescription see Controlled Drugs and Drug Dependence, p. 7. It is usual to adjust the strength so that the dose volume is 5 or 10 mL.

**Oramorph®** (Boehringer Ingelheim)

PoM *Oral solution*, morphine sulphate 10 mg/ 5 mL. Net price 100-mL pack = £2.31; 250-mL pack = £5.10; 500-mL pack = £9.24. Label: 2

**CD** *Concentrated oral solution*, sugar-free, morphine sulphate 100 mg/5 mL. Net price 30-mL pack = £6.16; 120-mL pack = £23.00 (both with calibrated dropper). Label: 2

**CD Sevredol®** (Napp)

*Tablets*, both f/c, scored, morphine sulphate 10 mg (blue), net price 56-tab pack = £6.47; 20 mg (pink), 56-tab pack = £12.94. Label: 2

Modified-release tablets

**CD MST Continus®** (Napp)

*Tablets*, all m/r, f/c, morphine sulphate 10 mg (brown), net price 60-tab pack = £7.70; 30 mg (purple), 60-tab pack = £18.49; 60 mg (orange), 60-tab pack = £36.06; 100 mg (grey), 60-tab pack = £57.10; 200 mg (green), 60-tab pack = £114.20. Label: 2, 25

*Dose:* severe pain uncontrolled by weaker opioids, 30 mg every 12 hours, increased to 60 mg every 12 hours when required, then further increments of 25–50% if necessary. For lower initial doses in patients who have not received other opioids, see Terminal Care, p. 12 CHILD severe, intractable pain in cancer, initially 200–800 micrograms/kg every 12 hours, then further increments of 30–50% if necessary

*Note.* Brand name prescriptions for MST Continus must also specify 'tablets' (i.e. 'MST Continus Tablets').

**CD SRM-Rhotard®** (Farmitalia Carlo Erba)

*Tablets*, all m/r, f/c, morphine sulphate 10 mg (buff), net price 60-tab pack = £6.93; 30 mg (violet), 60-tab pack = £16.41; 60 mg (orange), 60-tab pack = £32.45; 100 mg (grey), 60-tab pack = £51.39. Label: 2, 25

*Dose:* severe pain uncontrolled by weaker opioids, 30 mg every 12 hours, increased to 60 mg every 12 hours when required, then further increments of 25–50% if necessary. For lower initial doses in patients who have not received other opioids, see Terminal Care, p. 12 CHILD not yet recommended

*Note.* Brand name prescriptions for SRM-Rhotard must also specify 'tablets' (i.e. 'SRM-Rhotard Tablets')

Injections

**CD Morphine Sulphate Injection,** morphine sulphate 10, 15, and 30 mg/mL, net price 1- and 2-mL amp (all) = 51–86p

**CD Min-I-Jet® Morphine Sulphate** (IMS)

*Injection*, morphine sulphate 10 mg/mL, net price 2-mL disposable syringe = £5.50

Injection with anti-emetic

**CD Cyclimorph®** (Wellcome)

*Cyclimorph-10® Injection*, morphine tartrate 10 mg, cyclizine tartrate 50 mg/mL. Net price 1-mL amp = £1.16

*Dose:* by subcutaneous, intramuscular, or intravenous injection, 1 mL, repeated not more often than every 4 hours, with not more than 3 doses in any 24-hour period; CHILD 1–5 years 0.25–0.5 mL as a single dose, 6–12 years 0.5–1 mL as a single dose

*Cyclimorph-15® Injection*, morphine tartrate 15 mg, cyclizine tartrate 50 mg/mL. Net price 1-mL amp = £1.21

*Dose:* by subcutaneous, intramuscular, or intravenous injection, 1 mL, repeated not more often than every 4 hours, with not more than 3 doses in any 24-hour period

Suppositories

**CD Morphine Suppositories,** morphine hydrochloride or sulphate 15 mg, net price 12 = £3.52; 30 mg, 12 = £5.51. Label: 2.

*Note.* Both the strength of the suppositories and the morphine salt contained in them must be specified by the prescriber

Mixed opium alkaloids

Mixed opium alkaloids do not have any advantage over morphine alone; alcoholic solutions are liable to evaporation and are **not** recommended.

**CD Nepenthe** (Evans)

*Oral solution* (= elixir), brown, anhydrous morphine 8.4 mg/mL (500 micrograms from opium tincture, 7.9 mg from morphine). Diluent syrup, life of diluted elixir 4 weeks. Net price 100-mL pack = £22.45. Label: 2

*Dose:* 1–2 mL, repeated not more often than every 4 hours when necessary; CHILD 6–12 years 0.5–1 mL, as a single dose

*Note.* This product must always be diluted when being dispensed.

CAUTION. *Nepenthe Oral Solution may become concentrated through evaporation of the solvent. It should be stored in a cool place in the original airtight container. If evaporation occurs during storage the solution should not be used because of risk of overdosage.*

---

# ALFENTANIL

See section 15.1.4.3

# BUPRENORPHINE

*Indications:* moderate to severe pain; peri-operative analgesia, see section 15.1.4.3

*Cautions; Contra-indications; Side-effects:* see under Morphine Salts, but side-effects less marked; can give rise to mild withdrawal symptoms in patients dependent on opioids; effects only partially reversed by naloxone; **interactions:** Appendix 1 (opioid analgesics)

*Dose:* by *sublingual administration*, initially 200–400 micrograms every 8 hours, increasing if necessary to 200–400 micrograms every 6–8 hours; CHILD over 6 months, 16–25 kg, 100 micrograms; 25–37.5 kg, 100–200 micrograms; 37.5–50 kg, 200–300 micrograms

By *intramuscular or slow intravenous injection*, 300–600 micrograms every 6–8 hours; CHILD over 6 months 3–6 micrograms/kg every 6–8 hours; max. 9 micrograms/kg

**CD Temgesic®** (R&C)

*Tablets* (sublingual), buprenorphine (as hydrochloride), 200 micrograms, net price 50 = £6.00; 400 micrograms, 50 = £12.00. Label: 2, 26

*Injection*, buprenorphine 300 micrograms (as hydrochloride)/mL. Net price 1-mL amp = 55p

---

## CODEINE PHOSPHATE

*Indications:* mild to moderate pain

*Cautions; Contra-indications; Side-effects:* see under Morphine Salts but side-effects less marked; use of cough suppressants containing codeine or similar opioid analgesics not generally recommended in children and should be avoided altogether in those under 1 year; **interactions:** Appendix 1 (opioid analgesics)

*Dose: by mouth,* 30–60 mg every 4 hours when necessary, to a max. of 240 mg daily; CHILD 1–12 years, 3 mg/kg daily in divided doses

*By intramuscular injection,* 30–60 mg every 4 hours when necessary

**Codeine Phosphate** (Non-proprietary)
PoM *Tablets,* codeine phosphate 15 mg, net price 20 = 38p; 30 mg, 20 = 39p; 60 mg, 20 = £1.24. Label: 2
*Note.* As for schedule 2 controlled drugs, travellers needing to take codeine phosphate preparations abroad may require a doctor's letter explaining why they are necessary.
PoM *Syrup,* codeine phosphate 25 mg/5 mL. Net price 100 mL = 75p. Label: 2
CD *Injection,* codeine phosphate 60 mg/mL. Net price 1-mL amp = £1.35
**Codeine Linctuses**
See section 3.9.1

Compound preparations, section 4.7.1.1

---

## DEXTROMORAMIDE

*Indications:* severe pain

*Cautions; Contra-indications; Side-effects:* see under Morphine Salts, but less sedating than morphine; only short duration of action (2–3 hours); avoid in obstetric analgesia (increased risk of neonatal depression); **interactions:** Appendix 1 (opioid analgesics)

*Dose: by mouth,* 5 mg increasing to 20 mg, when required
*By subcutaneous or intramuscular injection,* 5 mg increasing to 15 mg, when required
*By rectum* in suppositories, 10 mg when required

CD **Palfium**® (Boehringer Mannheim)
*Tablets,* both scored, dextromoramide (as tartrate) 5 mg, net price 60-tab pack = £4.78; 10 mg (peach), 60-tab pack = £9.45. Label: 2
*Injection,* dextromoramide (as tartrate) 5 mg/mL, net price 1-mL amp = 20p; 10 mg/mL, 1-mL amp = 24p
*Suppositories,* dextromoramide 10 mg (as tartrate). Net price 10 = £2.35. Label: 2

---

## DEXTROPROPOXYPHENE HYDROCHLORIDE

*Indications:* mild to moderate pain

*Cautions; Contra-indications; Side effects:* see under Morphine Salts but side-effects less marked; occasional hepatotoxicity; avoid in porphyria (see section 9.8.2); compound preparations special hazard in overdose, see notes above; convulsions reported in overdose

*Dose:* 65 mg every 6–8 hours when necessary
*Note.* 65 mg dextropropoxyphene hydrochloride = 100 mg dextropropoxyphene napsylate

PoM **Dextropropoxyphene Capsules,** the equivalent of dextropropoxyphene hydrochloride 65 mg (as napsylate). Net price 20 = £1.19. Label: 2
*Note.* The brand name NHS Doloxene®(Lilly) is used for dextropropoxyphene capsules, net price 20 = £1.19

Compound preparations, section 4.7.1.1

---

## DIAMORPHINE HYDROCHLORIDE

*Indications:* see notes above; acute pulmonary oedema

*Cautions; Contra-indications; Side-effects:* see under Morphine Salts; **interactions:** Appendix 1 (opioid analgesics)

*Dose:* acute pain, *by subcutaneous or intramuscular injection,* 5 mg repeated every 4 hours if necessary (up to 10 mg for heavier well-muscled patients)
*By slow intravenous injection,* quarter to half corresponding intramuscular dose
Myocardial infarction, *by slow intravenous injection* (1 mg/minute), 5 mg followed by a further 2.5–5 mg if necessary; elderly or frail patients, reduce dose by half
Acute pulmonary oedema, *by slow intravenous injection* (1 mg/minute) 2.5–5 mg
Chronic pain, *by mouth or by subcutaneous or intramuscular injection,* 5–10 mg regularly every 4 hours; dose may be increased according to needs; intramuscular dose should be approximately half corresponding oral dose, and quarter to third corresponding oral *morphine* dose; see also Prescribing in Terminal Care, p. 12

CD **Diamorphine** (Non-proprietary)
*Tablets,* diamorphine hydrochloride 10 mg. Net price 20 = 91p. Label: 2
*Injection,* powder for reconstitution, diamorphine hydrochloride. Net price 5-mg amp = £1.16, 10-mg amp = £1.34, 30-mg amp = £1.60, 100-mg amp = £4.42, 500-mg amp = £20.68
CD **Diamorphine Linctus**
See section 3.9.1

---

## DIHYDROCODEINE TARTRATE

*Indications:* moderate to severe pain

*Cautions; Contra-indications; Side-effects:* see under Morphine Salts

*Dose: by mouth,* 30 mg every 4–6 hours when necessary, preferably after food; CHILD over 4 years 0.5–1 mg/kg every 4–6 hours
*By deep subcutaneous or intramuscular injection,* up to 50 mg every 4–6 hours

**Dihydrocodeine** (Non-proprietary)
PoM *Tablets,* dihydrocodeine tartrate 30 mg. Net price 20 = 62p. Label: 2, 21
PoM *Elixir,* dihydrocodeine tartrate 10 mg/5 mL. Net price 150 mL = £1.28. Label: 2, 21

---

**CD** *Injection*, dihydrocodeine tartrate 50 mg/mL. Net price 1-mL amp = 30p
Available from Napp (NHS DF 118®)

PoM **DHC Continus®** (Napp)
*Tablets*, m/r, dihydrocodeine tartrate 60 mg (scored), net price 56-tab pack = £6.75; 90 mg, 56-tab pack = £10.63; 120 mg, 56-tab pack = £14.18. Label: 2, 25
*Dose:* chronic severe pain, 60–120 mg every 12 hours

Compound preparations, section 4.7.1.1

## DIPHENOXYLATE
See Co-phenotrope, section 1.4.2

## DIPIPANONE HYDROCHLORIDE
*Indications:* moderate to severe pain
*Cautions; Contra-indications; Side-effects:* see under Morphine Salts; **interactions:** Appendix 1 (opioid analgesics)

**CD Diconal®** (Wellcome)
*Tablets*, pink, scored, dipipanone hydrochloride 10 mg, cyclizine hydrochloride 30 mg. Net price 50 = £6.90. Label: 2
*Dose:* 1 tablet gradually increased to 3 tablets every 6 hours
CAUTION. **Not recommended** in terminal care, see p. 12

## FENTANYL
See section 15.1.4.3

## MEPTAZINOL
*Indications:* moderate to severe pain, including postoperative and obstetric pain and renal colic; peri-operative analgesia, see section 15.1.4.3
*Cautions; Contra-indications; Side-effects:* see under Morphine Salts
*Dose: by mouth*, 200 mg every 3–6 hours as required
*By intramuscular injection*, 75–100 mg every 2–4 hours if necessary; obstetric analgesia, 100–150 mg according to patient's weight (2 mg/kg)
*By slow intravenous injection*, 50–100 mg every 2–4 hours if necessary

PoM **Meptid®** (Wyeth)
*Tablets*, orange, f/c, meptazinol 200 mg. Net price 20 = £1.80. Label: 2
*Injection*, meptazinol 100 mg (as hydrochloride)/mL. Net price 1-mL amp = 79p

## METHADONE HYDROCHLORIDE
*Indications:* severe pain, see notes above; adjunct in treatment of opioid dependence, section 4.10
*Cautions; Contra-indications; Side-effects:* see under Morphine Salts, but less sedating than morphine; **interactions:** Appendix 1 (opioid analgesics)
*Dose: by mouth or by subcutaneous or intramuscular injection*, 5–10 mg every 6–8 hours, adjusted according to response

**CD Methadone Linctus,** see section 3.9.1
**CD Methadone Mixture 1 mg/mL,** section 4.10
**CD Physeptone®** (Wellcome)
*Tablets*, scored, methadone hydrochloride 5 mg. Net price 50 = £2.83. Label: 2
*Injection*, methadone hydrochloride 10 mg/mL. Net price 1-mL amp = 78p

## NALBUPHINE HYDROCHLORIDE
*Indications:* moderate to severe pain; peri-operative analgesia, see section 15.1.4.3
*Cautions; Contra-indications; Side-effects:* see under Morphine Salts; **interactions:** Appendix 1 (opioid analgesics)
*Dose: by subcutaneous, intramuscular, or intravenous injection*, 10–20 mg for 70-kg patient every 3–6 hours, adjusted as required; CHILD 300 micrograms/kg repeated once or twice as necessary
Myocardial infarction, *by slow intravenous injection*, 10–20 mg repeated after 30 minutes if necessary

PoM **Nubain®** (Du Pont)
*Injection*, nalbuphine hydrochloride 10 mg/mL. Net price 1-mL amp = 75p; 2-mL amp = £1.16

## PAPAVERETUM
See section 15.1.4.3

## PENTAZOCINE
*Indications:* moderate to severe pain, but see notes above
*Cautions; Contra-indications; Side-effects:* see under Morphine Salts; occasional hallucinations; avoid in patients dependent on opioids and in arterial or pulmonary hypertension and heart failure; avoid in porphyria (see section 9.8.2)
*Dose: by mouth*, pentazocine hydrochloride 50 mg every 3–4 hours preferably after food (range 25–100 mg); CHILD 6–12 years 25 mg
*By subcutaneous, intramuscular, or intravenous injection*, moderate pain, pentazocine 30 mg, severe pain 45–60 mg every 3–4 hours when necessary; CHILD over 1 year, *by subcutaneous or intramuscular injection*, up to 1 mg/kg, *by intravenous injection* up to 500 micrograms/kg
*By rectum* in suppositories, pentazocine 50 mg up to 4 times daily

**CD Pentazocine** (Non-proprietary)
*Capsules*, pentazocine hydrochloride 50 mg. Net price 20 = £3.48. Label: 2, 21
*Tablets*, pentazocine hydrochloride 25 mg. Net price 20 = £1.65. Label: 2, 21
*Injection*, pentazocine 30 mg (as lactate)/mL. Net price 1-mL amp = 80p; 2-mL amp = £1.34
*Suppositories*, pentazocine 50 mg (as lactate). Net price 20 = £9.60. Label: 2
*Note.* The brand name NHS Fortral® (Sanofi Winthrop) is used for all the above preparations of pentazocine

## PETHIDINE HYDROCHLORIDE
*Indications:* moderate to severe pain, obstetric analgesia; peri-operative analgesia, see section 15.1.4.3

*Cautions; Contra-indications; Side-effects:* see under Morphine Salts, but less constipating than morphine; avoid in severe renal impairment; convulsions reported in overdosage; **interactions:** Appendix 1 (opioid analgesics)

*Dose: by mouth*, 50–150 mg every 4 hours; CHILD 0.5–2 mg/kg

*By subcutaneous or intramuscular injection*, 25–100 mg, repeated after 4 hours; CHILD, *by intramuscular injection*, 0.5–2 mg/kg

*By slow intravenous injection*, 25–50 mg, repeated after 4 hours

Obstetric analgesia, *by subcutaneous or intramuscular injection*, 50–100 mg, repeated 1–3 hours later if necessary; max. 400 mg in 24 hours

**CD Pethidine** (Roche)
*Tablets*, pethidine hydrochloride 50 mg, net price 20 = 39p. Label: 2
*Injection*, pethidine hydrochloride 50 mg/mL. Net price 1-mL amp = 11p; 2-mL amp = 14p. 10 mg/mL see section 15.1.4.3

**CD Pamergan P100®** (Martindale)
*Injection*, pethidine hydrochloride 50 mg, promethazine hydrochloride 25 mg/mL. Net price 2-mL amp = 45p
*Dose:* by intramuscular injection, for obstetric analgesia, 1–2 mL every 4 hours if necessary; severe pain, 1–2 mL every 4–6 hours if necessary; premedication, see section 15.1.4.3
*Note.* Although usually given intramuscularly, may be given intravenously after dilution to at least 10 mL with water for injections

## PHENAZOCINE HYDROBROMIDE

*Indications:* severe pain

*Cautions; Contra-indications; Side-effects:* see under Mophine Salts, but less sedating than morphine; **interactions:** Appendix 1 (opioid analgesics)

*Dose: by mouth or sublingually*, 5 mg every 4–6 hours when necessary; single doses may be increased to 20 mg

**CD Narphen®** (Napp)
*Tablets*, scored, phenazocine hydrobromide 5 mg. Net price 100-tab pack = £20.33. Label: 2

## PHENOPERIDINE

See section 15.1.4.3

## 4.7.3  Trigeminal neuralgia

**Carbamazepine** (section 4.8.1), taken during the acute stages of trigeminal neuralgia, reduces the frequency and severity of attacks if given continuously. It has no effect on other forms of headache. A dose of 100 mg once or twice a day should be given initially and the dose slowly increased until the best response is obtained; most patients require 200 mg 3–4 times daily but a few may require an increased total daily dosage of up to 1.6 g. Plasma concentrations should be monitored when high doses are given. Occasionally extreme dizziness is encountered which is a further reason

for starting treatment with a small dose and increasing it slowly.

Some cases of trigeminal neuralgia respond to **phenytoin** (section 4.8.1) given alone or in conjunction with carbamazepine. A combination of phenytoin and carbamazepine is only required in very refractory cases or in those unable to tolerate high doses of carbamazepine.

## 4.7.4  Antimigraine drugs

### 4.7.4.1  TREATMENT OF THE ACUTE MIGRAINE ATTACK

Most migraine headaches respond to analgesics such as **aspirin** or **paracetamol** (section 4.7.1) but as peristalsis is often reduced during migraine attacks the medication may not be sufficiently well absorbed to be effective; dispersible or effervescent preparations should therefore preferably be used.

**Ergotamine** is used in patients who do not respond to analgesics. It relieves migraine headache by constricting cranial arteries but visual and other prodromal symptoms are not affected and vomiting may be made worse. This can be relieved by the addition of an **anti-emetic** (see below).

The value of ergotamine is limited by difficulties in absorption and by its side-effects, particularly nausea, vomiting, abdominal pain, and muscular cramps. In some patients repeated administration may cause habituation. Rarely headache may be provoked, either by chronic overdosage or by rapid withdrawal of the drug. Doses of 6 to 8 mg per attack and 10 to 12 mg per week should **not** be exceeded. Ergotamine treatment should **not** be repeated at intervals of less than 4 days and it should **never** be prescribed prophylactically[1]; it should not be given in hemiplegic migraine.

There are various ergotamine preparations designed to improve absorption and best results are obtained when the dose is given early in an attack. An aerosol form (Medihaler-Ergotamine®) is acceptable to some patients. Sublingual ergotamine (Lingraine®) probably has no advantage over oral treatment.

**Dihydroergotamine** is of doubtful value.

**Sumatriptan** is a new 5-HT$_1$ agonist currently only available by injection. It appears to be of considerable value in the treatment of an acute attack but experience is relatively limited.

Anti-emetics (section 4.6), such as **metoclopramide** by mouth or, if vomiting is likely, by intramuscular injection, or the phenothiazine and antihistamine anti-emetics, relieve the nausea associated with migraine attacks. Prochlorperazine may be given rectally if vomiting is a problem. Metoclopramide has the added advantage of promoting gastric emptying and normal peristalsis. A single dose should be given at the onset of symptoms. Oral analgesic preparations containing metoclopramide are available.

1. In the management of cluster headache, a low dose of ergotamine is occasionally given on a daily basis for 1–2 weeks; ergotamine is not licensed for this purpose.

## ANALGESICS

Section 4.7.1

## ANALGESICS WITH ANTI-EMETICS

**Migraleve**® (Charwell)

*Tablets*, all f/c, *pink tablets*, buclizine hydrochloride 6.25 mg, paracetamol 500 mg, codeine phosphate 8 mg; *yellow tablets*, paracetamol 500 mg, codeine phosphate 8 mg. Net price 48-tab Duopack (32 pink + 16 yellow) = £4.68; 48 pink = £5.10; 48 yellow = £4.31. Label: 2, 17, 30

*Dose:* 2 pink tablets at onset of attack, or if it is imminent, then 2 yellow tablets every 4 hours if necessary; max. in 24 hours 2 pink and 6 yellow; CHILD 10–14 years, half adult dose

PoM **Migravess**® (Bayer)

*Tablets*, effervescent, scored, metoclopramide hydrochloride 5 mg, aspirin 325 mg. Net price 30-tab pack = £3.60. Label: 13, 17

*Forte tablets*, effervescent, scored, metoclopramide hydrochloride 5 mg, aspirin 450 mg. Net price 30-tab pack = £4.94. Label: 13, 17

*Dose:* tablets or Forte tablets, 2 dissolved in water at onset of attack then every 4 hours when necessary; max. 6 tablets in 24 hours; CHILD 12–15 years, half adult dose

PoM **Paramax**® (Bencard)

*Tablets*, scored, paracetamol 500 mg, metoclopramide hydrochloride 5 mg. Net price 42-tab pack = £3.63. Label: 17, 30

*Sachets*, effervescent powder, sugar-free, the contents of 1 sachet = 1 tablet; to be dissolved in ¼ tumblerful of liquid before administration. Net price 42-sachet pack = £4.79. Label: 13, 17, 30

*Dose:* (tablets or sachets): 2 at onset of attack then every 4 hours when necessary to max. of 6 in 24 hours (young adult 15–19 years, over 60 kg, max. of 5 in 24 hours); ADOLESCENT and YOUNG ADULT 12–19 years, 30–59 kg, 1 at onset of attack then 1 every 4 hours when necessary to max. of 3 in 24 hours

## ERGOTAMINE TARTRATE

*Indications:* acute attacks of migraine and migraine variants unresponsive to analgesics

*Cautions:* withdraw treatment immediately if numbness or tingling of extremities develops; should not be used for migraine prophylaxis; **interactions:** Appendix 1 (ergotamine)

*Contra-indications:* peripheral vascular disease, coronary heart disease, obliterative vascular disease and Raynaud's syndrome, hepatic or renal impairment, sepsis, severe or inadequately controlled hypertension, hyperthyroidism, pregnancy and breast-feeding, porphyria (see section 9.8.2)

*Side-effects:* headache, nausea, vomiting, and abdominal pain; repeated high dosage may cause ergotism with gangrene and confusion; pleural and peritoneal fibrosis may occur with excessive use

*Dose:* see under preparations below

PoM **Cafergot**® (Sandoz)

*Tablets*, ergotamine tartrate 1 mg, caffeine 100 mg. Net price 20 = 91p. Label: 18, counselling, dosage

*Dose:* 1–2 tablets at onset; max. 4 tablets in 24 hours; not to be repeated at intervals of less than 4 days; max. 10 tablets weekly

*Suppositories*, ergotamine tartrate 2 mg, caffeine 100 mg. Net price 30 = £4.99. Label: 18, counselling, dosage

*Dose:* 1 suppository at onset; max. 2 in 24 hours; not to be repeated at intervals of less than 4 days; max. 5 suppositories weekly

PoM **Lingraine**® (Sanofi Winthrop)

*Tablets* (for sublingual use), green, ergotamine tartrate 2 mg. Net price 12 = £6.93. Label: 18, 26, counselling, dosage

*Dose:* 1 tablet at onset repeated after 30 minutes if necessary; max. 3 in 24 hours and 6 weekly

PoM **Medihaler-Ergotamine**® (3M)

*Aerosol inhalation* (oral), ergotamine tartrate 360 micrograms/metered inhalation. Net price 75-dose unit = £3.44. Label: 18, counselling, dosage

*Dose:* 360 micrograms (1 puff) repeated if necessary after 5 minutes; max. 6 inhalations in 24 hours and 15 inhalations weekly

PoM **Migril**® (Wellcome)

*Tablets*, scored, ergotamine tartrate 2 mg, cyclizine hydrochloride 50 mg, caffeine hydrate 100 mg. Net price 20 = £10.61. Label: 2, 18, counselling, dosage

*Dose:* 1 tablet at onset, followed after 30 minutes by ½–1 tablet, repeated every 30 minutes if necessary; max. 4 tablets per attack and 6 tablets weekly

## DIHYDROERGOTAMINE MESYLATE

*Indications:* migraine attack unresponsive to analgesics

*Cautions; Contra-indications; Side-effects:* see under Ergotamine Tartrate, as well as numbness and tingling of extremities, precordial pain reported; also contra-indicated in shock; avoid intra-arterial injection

*Dose: by subcutaneous or intramuscular injection,* 1 mg repeated once after 30–60 minutes if necessary; max. 3 mg daily and 6 mg weekly

PoM **Dihydergot**® (Sandoz)

*Injection*, dihydroergotamine mesylate 1 mg/mL. Net price 1-mL amp = 21p

## ISOMETHEPTENE MUCATE

*Indications:* migraine attack

*Cautions:* cardiovascular disease; **interactions:** Appendix 1 (sympathomimetics)

*Contra-indications:* glaucoma; porphyria (see section 9.8.2)

*Side-effects:* dizziness, circulatory disturbances

*Dose:* see under preparation below

**Midrid**® (Shire)

*Capsules*, red, isometheptene mucate 65 mg, paracetamol 325 mg. Net price 20 = £2.72. Label: 17, 30

*Dose:* migraine, 2 capsules at onset of attack, followed by 1 capsule every hour if necessary; max. 5 capsules in 12 hours

---

## SUMATRIPTAN

*Indications:* acute treatment of migraine attacks (with or without aura) and cluster headache

*Cautions:* not for prophylaxis; conditions which predispose to ischaemic heart disease; hepatic or renal impairment; pregnancy and breast-feeding; **interactions:** Appendix 1 (sumatriptan)

DRIVING. Drowsiness may affect performance of skilled tasks (e.g. driving)

*Contra-indications:* ischaemic heart disease; previous myocardial infarction or Prinzmetal's angina; uncontrolled hypertension; not for hemiplegic migraine

*Side-effects:* transient pain at injection site; sensations of tingling, heat, heaviness, pressure, or tightness in any part of body; flushing, dizziness, feeling of weakness; fatigue, drowsiness, altered liver function tests, transient increase in blood pressure reported; nausea and vomiting

*Dose: by subcutaneous injection* using auto-injector, 6 mg as soon as possible after onset, repeated once after at least 1 hour if symptoms persist; max. 12 mg in 24 hours;

ELDERLY over 65 years and CHILD not yet recommended

IMPORTANT. **Not** for intravenous injection which may cause coronary vasospasm and angina.

▼ PoM **Imigran**® (Glaxo)

*Injection*, sumatriptan (as succinate) 12 mg/mL (= 6 mg/0.5-mL syringe), net price, treatment pack (2 × 0.5-mL pre-filled syringes and auto-injector) = £41.14; refill pack (2 × 0.5-mL pre-filled syringes) = £39.14. Label: 3, 10 patient information leaflet

### 4.7.4.2 PROPHYLAXIS OF MIGRAINE

Where migraine attacks are frequent, search should be made for provocative factors such as stress or diet (chocolate, cheese, alcohol, etc.). Benzodiazepines should be avoided because of the risk of dependence. In patients with more than one attack a month, one of three main prophylactic agents may be tried: pizotifen, beta-blockers, or tricyclic antidepressants (even when the patient is not obviously depressed). Long-term treatment with any of these prophylactic drugs is undesirable; the need for continuing therapy should be reviewed at intervals of about 6 months. Oral contraceptives may precipitate or worsen migraine; patients reporting a sharp increase in frequency of migraine or focal features should be recommended alternative contraceptive measures.

**Pizotifen** is an antihistamine and serotonin antagonist structurally related to the tricyclic antidepressants. It affords good prophylaxis but may cause weight gain. To avoid undue drowsiness treatment may be started at 500 micrograms at night and gradually increased to 3 mg; it is rarely necessary to exceed this dose.

The **beta-blockers** propranolol, metoprolol, nadolol, and timolol (see section 2.4) are all effective. Propranolol is the most commonly used in

an initial dose of 40 mg 2 to 3 times daily by mouth. Beta-blockers may also be given as a single daily dose of a long-acting preparation. The value of beta-blockers is limited by their contra-indications (see section 2.4) and by interaction with ergotamine (see Appendix 1, beta-blockers).

**Tricyclic antidepressants** (section 4.3.1) may usefully be prescribed in a dose, for example, of amitriptyline 10 mg at night, increasing to a maintenance dose of 50 to 75 mg at night.

There is some evidence that the **calcium-channel blockers** (see section 2.6.2), e.g. verapamil and nifedipine may be useful in migraine prophylaxis.

**Cyproheptadine** (see section 3.4.1), an antihistamine with serotonin-antagonist and calcium channel-blocking properties, may also be tried in refractory cases.

**Clonidine** (Dixarit®) is probably little better than placebo and may aggravate depression or produce insomnia. **Methysergide** has dangerous side-effects (retroperitoneal fibrosis and fibrosis of the heart valves and pleura); **important:** it should only be administered under hospital supervision.

### CLONIDINE HYDROCHLORIDE

*Indications:* prevention of recurrent migraine (but see notes above), vascular headache, menopausal flushing; hypertension, see section 2.5.2

*Cautions:* depressive illness, concurrent antihypertensive therapy; avoid in porphyria (see section 9.8.2); **interactions:** Appendix 1 (clonidine)

*Side-effects:* dry mouth, sedation, dizziness, nausea, nocturnal restlessness; occasionally rashes

*Dose:* 50 micrograms twice daily, increased after 2 weeks to 75 micrograms twice daily if necessary

PoM **Dixarit**® (Boehringer Ingelheim)

*Tablets*, blue, s/c, clonidine hydrochloride 25 micrograms. Net price 112-tab pack = £6.13

PoM **Catapres**® (hypertension), see section 2.5.2

### METHYSERGIDE

*Indications:* prevention of severe recurrent migraine and cluster headache in patients who are refractory to other treatment and whose lives are seriously disrupted (**important:** hospital supervision only, see notes above)

*Cautions:* history of peptic ulceration; avoid abrupt withdrawal of treatment; after 6 months withdraw for reassessment for at least 1 month (see also notes above)

*Contra-indications:* renal, hepatic, pulmonary, and cardiovascular disease, severe hypertension, collagen disease, cellulitis, urinary tract disorders, cachectic or septic conditions, pregnancy, breast-feeding

*Side-effects:* nausea, vomiting, heartburn, abdominal discomfort, drowsiness, and dizziness occur frequently in initial treatment; psychic reactions, insomnia, oedema, weight gain, rashes, loss of scalp hair, cramps, arterial spasm, paraesthesias of extremities, arterial hypotension, and tachycardia also occur. Retroperitoneal and other abnormal fibrotic

reactions may occur on prolonged administration, requiring immediate withdrawal of
treatment
*Dose:* 1 mg at bedtime, gradually increased to 1–
2 mg 2–3 times daily with food (see notes above)
Carcinoid syndrome, usual range, 12–20 mg
daily (hospital supervision)

PoM **Deseril**® (Sandoz)
*Tablets*, s/c, methysergide 1 mg (as maleate). Net price
50 = £4.58. Label: 2, 21

## PIZOTIFEN

*Indications:* prevention of vascular headache
including classical migraine, common migraine,
and cluster headache
*Cautions:* urinary retention; closed-angle glaucoma, renal impairment; pregnancy and breast-
feeding; **interactions:** Appendix 1 (pizotifen)
DRIVING. Drowsiness may affect performance of skilled
tasks (e.g. driving); effects of alcohol enhanced
*Side-effects:* antimuscarinic effects, drowsiness,
increased appetite and weight gain; occasionally nausea, dizziness
*Dose:* 1.5 mg at night *or* 500 micrograms 3 times
daily (but see also notes above), adjusted
according to response within the usual range
0.5–3 mg daily; max. single dose 3 mg, max.
daily dose 6 mg; CHILD up to 1.5 mg daily; max.
single dose at night 1 mg

PoM **Sanomigran**® (Sandoz)
*Tablets*, both ivory-yellow, s/c, pizotifen (as
hydrogen malate), 500 micrograms, net price
20 = £1.60; 1.5 mg, 28-tab pack = £7.98.
Label: 2
*Elixir*, sugar-free, pizotifen 250 micrograms (as
hydrogen malate)/5 mL. Net price 300-mL
pack = £4.23. Label: 2

# 4.8   Antiepileptics

**4.8.1** Control of epilepsy
**4.8.2** Drugs used in status epilepticus
**4.8.3** Febrile convulsions

## 4.8.1   Control of epilepsy

The object of treatment is to prevent the occurrence of seizures by maintaining an effective
plasma concentration of the drug. Careful adjustment of doses is necessary, starting with low doses
and increasing gradually until seizures are controlled or there are overdose effects.
    The frequency of administration is determined
by the plasma half-life, and should be kept as low
as possible to encourage better patient
compliance. Most antiepileptics, when used in
average dosage, may be given twice daily. Phenobarbitone and sometimes phenytoin, which have
long half-lives, may often be given as a daily dose
at bedtime. However, with large doses, some
antiepileptics may need to be administered 3 times
daily to avoid adverse effects associated with high

peak plasma concentrations. Young children
metabolise antiepileptics more rapidly than adults
and therefore require more frequent doses and a
higher amount per kilogram body-weight.

COMBINATION THERAPY. Therapy with several
drugs concurrently should be avoided. Patients
are best controlled with one antiepileptic. Combinations of drugs have been used on the grounds
that their therapeutic effects were additive while
their individual toxicity was reduced but there is
no evidence for this. In fact, toxicity may be
enhanced with combination therapy. A second
drug should only be added to the regimen if seizures continue despite high plasma concentrations
or toxic effects. The use of more than two antiepileptics is rarely justified.

INTERACTIONS. Another disadvantage of multiple
therapy is that drug interactions occur between
the various antiepileptics (see Appendix 1, antiepileptics) and other drugs. Because of liver
enzyme induction, phenobarbitone, phenytoin,
primidone, and carbamazepine may increase each
other's metabolism and reduce plasma concentrations. The reduction of carbamazepine
concentration by concurrent phenytoin administration is a most important example. Moreover,
it is illogical to combine primidone and phenobarbitone as the former is largely metabolised to
phenobarbitone in the liver, which is responsible
for most, if not all, of its antiepileptic action.

WITHDRAWAL. Abrupt withdrawal of antiepileptics, particularly the barbiturates and benzodiazepines, should be avoided, as this may
precipitate severe rebound seizures. Reduction in
dosage should be carried out in stages and, in the
case of the barbiturates, the withdrawal process
may take months. The changeover from one antiepileptic drug regimen to another should be made
cautiously, withdrawing the first drug only when
the new regimen has been largely established.
    The decision to withdraw all antiepileptics from
a seizure-free patient, and its timing, is often
difficult and may depend on individual patient
factors. Even in patients who have been seizure-
free for several years, there is a significant risk of
seizure recurrence on drug withdrawal.

DRIVING. Patients suffering from epilepsy may
drive a motor vehicle (but not a heavy goods or
public service vehicle) provided that they have
had a seizure-free period of two years or, if subject
to attacks only while asleep, have established a
three-year period of asleep attacks without awake
attacks. Patients affected by drowsiness should
not drive or operate machinery.

PREGNANCY AND BREAST-FEEDING. During pregnancy, plasma concentrations of antiepileptics
should be frequently monitored as they may fall,
particularly in the later stages. There is an
increased risk of teratogenicity associated with
the use of anticonvulsant drugs but, generally,
prescribing in pregnancy should follow the same

principles as that in non-pregnant patients. **Important** see also under Prescribing in Pregnancy (Appendix 4).

Breast-feeding is acceptable with all antiepileptic drugs, taken in normal doses, with the possible exception of the barbiturates see Prescribing during Breast-feeding (Appendix 5).

## TONIC-CLONIC (GRAND MAL) AND PARTIAL (FOCAL) SEIZURES

The drugs of choice for *tonic-clonic seizures* occurring as part of a syndrome of *primary generalised epilepsy* are carbamazepine, phenytoin, and sodium valproate. Phenobarbitone and primidone are also effective but may be more sedating.

*Partial epilepsy* is more difficult to control. Carbamazepine and phenytoin are the drugs of choice for secondary generalised tonic-clonic seizures and for partial seizures themselves; controlled trials with sodium valproate suggest similar efficacy but more evidence is awaited. Phenobarbitone and primidone are also effective but, once again, are likely to be more sedating. Second-line drugs for both tonic-clonic and partial seizures include clonazepam, clobazam, and acetazolamide.

**Phenytoin** is effective in tonic-clonic and partial seizures. It has a narrow therapeutic index and the relationship between dose and plasma concentration is non-linear; small dosage increases in some patients may produce large rises in plasma concentrations with acute toxic side-effects. Monitoring of plasma concentration greatly assists dosage adjustment. A few missed doses or a small change in drug absorption may result in a marked change in plasma concentration.

Phenytoin may cause coarse facies, acne, hirsutism, and gingival hyperplasia and so may be particularly undesirable in adolescent patients.

**Carbamazepine** is a drug of choice for simple and complex partial seizures and for tonic-clonic seizures regardless of whether they are primary or secondary to a focal discharge. It has a wider therapeutic index than phenytoin and the relationship between dose and plasma concentration is linear, but monitoring of plasma concentrations may be helpful in determining optimum dosage. It has generally fewer side-effects than phenytoin or the barbiturates, but reversible blurring of vision, dizziness, and unsteadiness are dose-related, and may be dose-limiting. These side-effects may be reduced by altering the timing of medication. It is essential to initiate carbamazepine therapy at a low dose and build this up over one or two weeks.

**Phenobarbitone** is an effective drug but may be sedative in adults and cause behavioural disturbances and hyperkinesia in children. Rebound seizures may be a problem on withdrawal. Monitoring plasma concentrations is less useful than with other drugs because tolerance occurs. **Methylphenobarbitone** is largely converted to phenobarbitone in the liver and has no advantages. **Primidone** is largely converted to pheno-

barbitone in the body and this is probably responsible for its antiepileptic action. A small starting dose (125 mg) is essential, and the drug should be introduced over several weeks.

**Sodium valproate** is effective in controlling tonic-clonic seizures, particularly in primary generalised epilepsy. Plasma concentrations are not a useful index of efficacy, therefore routine monitoring is unhelpful. The drug has widespread metabolic effects, and may have dose-related side-effects. There has been recent concern over severe hepatic or pancreatic toxicity, although these effects are rare.

**Vigabatrin** is a new antiepileptic for use in chronic epilepsy not satisfactorily controlled by other antiepileptics. It is useful in tonic-clonic and partial seizures but has prominent behavioural side-effects in some patients.

**Clonazepam** is occasionally used in tonic-clonic or partial seizures, but its sedative side-effects may be prominent. **Clobazam** may be used as adjunctive therapy in the treatment of epilepsy (section 4.1.2), but the effectiveness of these and other **benzodiazepines** may wane considerably after weeks or months of continuous therapy.

## ABSENCE SEIZURES (PETIT MAL)

**Ethosuximide** and **sodium valproate** are the drugs of choice in simple absence seizures. Sodium valproate is also highly effective in treating the tonic-clonic seizures which may co-exist with absence seizures in primary generalised epilepsy. Monitoring plasma-ethosuximide concentrations is helpful in determining optimum dosage.

## MYOCLONIC SEIZURES (MYOCLONIC JERKS)

Myoclonic seizures occur in a variety of syndromes, and response to treatment varies considerably. **Sodium valproate** is the drug of choice and **clonazepam**, **ethosuximide**, and other antiepileptic drugs may be used.

## ATYPICAL ABSENCE, ATONIC, AND TONIC SEIZURES

These seizure types are usually seen in childhood, in specific epileptic syndromes, or associated with cerebral damage or mental retardation. They may respond poorly to the traditional drugs. **Phenytoin**, **sodium valproate**, **clonazepam**, **ethosuximide**, and **phenobarbitone** may be tried. Other second-line antiepileptic drugs are occasionally helpful, including acetazolamide and corticosteroids.

## ACETAZOLAMIDE

*Indications:* see notes above
*Cautions; Side-effects:* see section 11.6
*Dose:* 0.25–1 g daily in divided doses; CHILD 125–750 mg daily

**Preparations**
See section 11.6

## CARBAMAZEPINE

*Indications:* all forms of epilepsy except absence seizures; trigeminal neuralgia (section 4.7.3); prophylaxis in manic-depressive illness (section 4.2.3)

*Cautions:* see notes above; hepatic impairment; pregnancy (**important** see notes above and Appendix 4 (neural tube screening)) and breast-feeding (see notes above); avoid sudden withdrawal; **interactions:** Appendix 1 (carbamazepine)

*Contra-indications:* atrioventricular conduction abnormalities (unless paced); porphyria (see section 9.8.2); patients on MAOIs or within 2 weeks of MAOI therapy (theoretical grounds only)

*Side-effects:* gastro-intestinal disturbances, dizziness, drowsiness, headache, ataxia, confusion and agitation (elderly), visual disturbances (especially double vision and often associated with peak plasma concentrations); constipation, anorexia; generalised erythematous rash may occur in about 3% of patients; leucopenia and other blood disorders have occurred rarely; cholestatic jaundice, acute renal failure, Stevens-Johnson syndrome, toxic epidermal necrolysis, alopecia, thromboembolism, fever, proteinuria, lymph node enlargement, cardiac conduction disturbances, and hepatitis reported; hyponatraemia and oedema also reported (with higher doses)

*Dose:* epilepsy, initially, 100–200 mg 1–2 times daily, increased slowly to usual dose of 0.8–1.2 g daily in divided doses; in some cases 1.6 g daily may be needed; CHILD daily in divided doses, up to 1 year 100–200 mg, 1–5 years 200–400 mg, 5–10 years 400–600 mg, 10–15 years 0.6–1 g

Note. Plasma concentration for optimum response 4–12 mg/litre (20–50 micromol/litre)

PoM **Carbamazepine** (Non-proprietary)
*Tablets,* carbamazepine 100 mg, net price 20 = 53p; 200 mg, 20 = £1.04; 400 mg, 20 = £2.21. Label: 3

PoM **Tegretol**® (Geigy)
*Tablets,* all scored, carbamazepine 100 mg, net price 20 = 62p; 200 mg, 20 = £1.15; 400 mg, 56-tab pack = £6.56. Label: 3

*Chewtabs,* orange, carbamazepine 100 mg, net price 20 = £1.05; 200 mg, 20 = £1.96. Label: 3, 21, 24

*Liquid,* sugar-free, carbamazepine 100 mg/5 mL. Diluent tragacanth mucilage for 1 + 1 dilution, life of diluted liquid 14 days. Net price 300-mL pack = £5.72. Label: 3

PoM **Tegretol**® **Retard** (Geigy)
*Tablets,* modified-release, both scored, carbamazepine 200 mg (beige-orange), net price 20 = £1.50; 400 mg (brown-orange), 20 = £2.94. Label: 3, 25

*Dose:* epilepsy (ADULT and CHILD over 5 years), as above; trigeminal neuralgia, as section 4.7.3; total daily dose given in 2 divided doses

## CLOBAZAM

Section 4.1.2

## CLONAZEPAM

*Indications:* all forms of epilepsy; myoclonus; status epilepticus, section 4.8.2

*Cautions:* see notes above; respiratory disease; hepatic and renal impairment; elderly and debilitated; pregnancy and breast-feeding (see notes above); avoid sudden withdrawal; **interactions:** Appendix 1 (clonazepam)

DRIVING. Drowsiness may affect the performance of skilled tasks (e.g. driving); effects of alcohol enhanced

*Contra-indications:* respiratory depression; acute pulmonary insufficiency; porphyria (see section 9.8.2)

*Side-effects:* drowsiness, fatigue, dizziness, muscle hypotonia, coordination disturbances; hypersalivation in infants, paradoxical aggression, irritability and mental changes; rarely, blood disorders, abnormal liver-function tests; overdosage: see p. 19

*Dose:* 1 mg (elderly, 500 micrograms), initially at night for 4 nights, increased over 2–4 weeks to a usual maintenance dose of 4–8 mg daily in divided doses; CHILD up to 1 year 250 micrograms increased as above to 0.5–1 mg, 1–5 years 250 micrograms increased to 1–3 mg, 5–12 years 500 micrograms increased to 3–6 mg

PoM **Rivotril**® (Roche)
*Tablets,* both scored, clonazepam 500 micrograms (beige), net price 20 = 88p; 2 mg, 20 = £1.84. Label: 2

## ETHOSUXIMIDE

*Indications:* absence seizures

*Cautions:* see notes above; hepatic and renal impairment; pregnancy and breast-feeding (see notes above); avoid sudden withdrawal; avoid in porphyria (see section 9.8.2); **interactions:** Appendix 1 (ethosuximide)

*Side-effects:* gastro-intestinal disturbances, drowsiness, dizziness, ataxia, dyskinesia, hiccup, photophobia, headache, depression, and mild euphoria. Psychotic states, rashes, liver changes, and haematological disorders such as leucopenia and agranulocytosis occur rarely; systemic lupus erythematosus reported

*Dose:* initially, 500 mg daily, increased by 250 mg at intervals of 4–7 days to usual dose of 1–1.5 g daily; occasionally up to 2 g daily may be needed; CHILD up to 6 years 250 mg daily, over 6 years 500 mg, increased gradually to a max. of 1 g daily

Note. Plasma concentration for optimum response 40–100 mg/litre (300–700 micromol/litre)

PoM **Emeside**® (LAB)
*Capsules,* orange, ethosuximide 250 mg. Net price 112-cap pack = £9.64

*Syrup,* black currant or orange, ethosuximide 250 mg/5 mL. Net price 200 mL = £5.22

PoM **Zarontin**® (P-D)
*Capsules,* orange, ethosuximide 250 mg. Net price 50 = £3.82

*Syrup,* red, ethosuximide 250 mg/5 mL. Diluent syrup, life of diluted syrup 14 days. Net price 250-mL pack = £4.67

## LAMOTRIGINE
New preparation, see p. xii

## METHYLPHENOBARBITONE
*Indications; Cautions; Side-effects:* see under
Phenobarbitone
*Dose:* 100–600 mg daily

**CD Prominal**® (Sanofi Winthrop)
*Tablets,* methylphenobarbitone 30 mg, net price
20 = 72p; 60 mg, 20 = 96p; 200 mg, 20 = £2.05.
Label: 2

## PHENOBARBITONE
*Indications:* all forms of epilepsy except absence
seizures; status epilepticus, section 4.8.2
*Cautions:* elderly, debilitated, children, impaired
renal or hepatic function, respiratory depression (avoid if severe), pregnancy and breast-
feeding (see notes above); avoid sudden withdrawal; see also notes above; avoid in porphyria
(see section 9.8.2); **interactions:** Appendix 1
(barbiturates and primidone)
*Side-effects:* drowsiness, lethargy, mental
depression, ataxia and allergic skin reactions;
paradoxical excitement, restlessness and confusion in the elderly and hyperkinesia in
children; megaloblastic anaemia (may be
treated with folic acid); overdosage: see p. 19
*Dose: by mouth,* 60–180 mg at night; CHILD 5–
8 mg/kg daily (febrile convulsions, see 4.8.3)
*By intramuscular or intravenous injection,* 50–
200 mg, repeated after 6 hours if necessary;
max. 600 mg daily; dilute injection 1 in 10 with
water for injections before intravenous
administration
*Note.* For therapeutic purposes phenobarbitone and
phenobarbitone sodium may be considered equivalent
in effect. Plasma concentration for optimum response
15–40 mg/litre (60–180 micromol/litre)

**CD ¹Phenobarbitone Tablets,** phenobarbitone
15 mg, net price 20 = 6p; 30 mg, 20 = 7p; 60 mg,
20 = 10p; 100 mg, 20 = 18p. Label: 2
**CD ¹Phenobarbitone Sodium Tablets,** phenobarbitone sodium 30 mg, net price 20 = 13p;
60 mg, 20 = 29p. Label: 2
**CD ¹Phenobarbitone Elixir,** phenobarbitone 15 mg/
5 mL in a suitable flavoured vehicle, containing alcohol
38%. Net price 100 mL = 54p. Label: 2
*Note.* Some hospitals supply alcohol-free formulations
**CD ¹Phenobarbitone Injection,** phenobarbitone
sodium 200 mg/mL in propylene glycol 90% and
water for injections 10%. Net price 1-mL amp =
63p
*Note.* Must be diluted before intravenous administration
(see under Dose)
Available from Rhône-Poulenc Rorer (**CD** ¹Gardenal
Sodium®). Martindale; other strengths also available
from Martindale.
1. See p. 7 for prescribing requirements for phenobarbitone

## PHENYTOIN
*Indications:* all forms of epilepsy except absence
seizures; trigeminal neuralgia (see also section
4.7.3)

*Cautions:* hepatic impairment (reduce dose),
pregnancy and breast-feeding (see notes
above); change-over from other drugs should
be made cautiously; avoid sudden withdrawal;
avoid in porphyria (see section 9.8.2); see also
notes above; **interactions:** Appendix 1 (phenytoin)
*Side-effects:* nausea, vomiting, mental confusion,
dizziness, headache, tremor, transient nervousness, insomnia occur commonly; rarely
dyskinesias, peripheral neuropathy; ataxia,
slurred speech, nystagmus and blurred vision
are signs of overdosage; rashes (discontinue,
if mild re-introduce cautiously but discontinue
immediately if recurrence), coarse facies, acne
and hirsutism, fever and hepatitis; lupus erythematosus, erythema multiforme (Stevens–
Johnson syndrome), toxic epidermal necrolysis,
polyarteritis nodosa; lymphadenopathy; gingival hypertrophy and tenderness; rarely haematological effects, including megaloblastic
anaemia (may be treated with folic acid), leucopenia, thrombocytopenia, agranulocytosis,
and aplastic anaemia; plasma calcium may be
lowered (rickets and osteomalacia)
*Dose: by mouth,* initially 3–4 mg/kg daily *or* 150–
300 mg daily (as a single dose *or* in two divided
doses) increased gradually as necessary (plasma
monitoring, see notes above); usual dose 300–
400 mg daily; max. 600 mg daily; CHILD 5–8 mg/
kg daily (in 1 or 2 doses)
*By intravenous injection*—section 4.8.2
*Note.* Plasma concentration for optimum response 10–
20 mg/litre (40–80 micromol/litre)
COUNSELLING. Take preferably with or after food

PoM **Phenytoin** (Non-proprietary)
*Tablets,* coated, phenytoin sodium 50 mg, net
price 20 = 14p; 100 mg, 20 = 14p. Label: 27,
counselling, administration
PoM **Epanutin**® (P-D)
*Capsules,* phenytoin sodium 25 mg (white/
purple), net price 20 = 39p; 50 mg (white/
pink), 20 = 40p; 100 mg (white/orange), 20 =
43p. Label: 27, counselling, administration
*Infatabs*® (= tablets, chewable), yellow, scored,
phenytoin 50 mg. Net price 20 = £1.10.
Label: 24
*Suspension,* red, phenytoin 30 mg/5 mL. Diluent
syrup, life of diluted suspension 14 days. Net
price 100 mL = 71p. Counselling, administration
*Note.* For an equivalent therapeutic effect, phenytoin
90 mg as phenytoin suspension 90 mg in 15 mL ≡
phenytoin sodium 100 mg as tablets or capsules. The
MCA now advises that there are no clinically relevant
differences in bioavailability between available phenytoin sodium tablets and capsules

## PRIMIDONE
*Indications:* all forms of epilepsy except absence
seizures; essential tremor (section 4.9.3)
*Cautions; Side-effects:* see under Phenobarbitone. Drowsiness, ataxia, nausea, visual disturbances, and rashes, particularly at first,

usually reversible on continued administration; **interactions:** Appendix 1 (barbiturates and primidone)

*Dose:* epilepsy, initially, 125 mg daily at bedtime, increased by 125 mg every 3 days to 500 mg daily in 2 divided doses then increased by 250 mg every 3 days to a max. of 1.5 g daily in divided doses; CHILD 20–30 mg/kg daily in 2 divided doses

Note. Monitor plasma concentrations of derived phenobarbitone. Optimum range as for phenobarbitone.

PoM **Mysoline**® (ICI)
*Tablets*, scored, primidone 250 mg.  Net price 20 = 36p. Label: 2
*Oral suspension*, primidone 250 mg/5 mL.  Net price 250-mL pack = £1.04.  Label: 2
Diluent propyl hydroxybenzoate 0.015%, methyl hydroxybenzoate 0.15%, carmellose sodium '50' 1%, sucrose 20%, in freshly boiled and cooled purified water.

## SODIUM VALPROATE
*Indications:* all forms of epilepsy
*Cautions:* in patients most at risk (e.g. children and those with history of liver disease) monitor liver function in first 6 months; pregnancy (**important** see notes above and Appendix 4 (neural tube screening)); breast-feeding; monitor platelet function before major surgery; may give false-positive urine tests for ketones in diabetes mellitus; avoid sudden withdrawal; see also notes above; **interactions:** Appendix 1 (valproate)
*Contra-indications:* active liver disease; porphyria (but see section 9.8.2)
*Side-effects:* gastric irritation, nausea, ataxia and tremor; hyperammonaemia, increased appetite and weight gain; transient hair loss (regrowth may be curly), oedema, thrombocytopenia, and inhibition of platelet aggregation; impaired hepatic function leading rarely to fatal hepatic failure (see Cautions—withdraw treatment immediately if vomiting, anorexia, jaundice, drowsiness, or loss of seizure control occurs); amenorrhoea, rashes; rarely pancreatitis (measure plasma amylase in acute abdominal pain), leucopenia, red cell hypoplasia
*Dose: by mouth,* initially, 600 mg daily in divided doses, preferably after food, increasing by 200 mg/day at 3-day intervals to a max. of 2.5 g daily in divided doses, usual maintenance 1–2 g daily (20–30 mg/kg daily); CHILD up to 20 kg (about 4 years), initially 20 mg/kg daily in divided doses, may be increased gradually providing plasma concentrations monitored to 40 mg/kg daily; over 20 kg, initially 400 mg daily in divided doses increased gradually to 20–30 mg/kg daily; max. 35 mg/kg daily
*By intravenous injection* (over 3–5 minutes) or *by intravenous infusion,* continuation of valproate treatment when oral therapy not possible, same as current dose by oral route
Initiation of valproate therapy (when oral valproate not possible), *by intravenous injection* (over 3–5 minutes), 400–800 mg (up to 10 mg/

kg) followed by *intravenous infusion* up to max. 2.5 g daily
CHILD, usually 20–30 mg/kg daily

PoM **Sodium Valproate** (Non-proprietary)
*Tablets*, e/c, sodium valproate 200 mg, net price 20 = £1.31. Label: 5, 25
Available from Hillcross
PoM **Epilim**® (Sanofi Winthrop)
*Tablets* (crushable), scored, sodium valproate 100 mg.  Net price 20 = 80p
*Tablets*, both e/c, lilac, sodium valproate 200 mg, net price 20 = £1.32;  500 mg,  20 = £3.29.  Label: 5, 25
*Liquid*, red, sugar-free, sodium valproate 200 mg/5 mL.  Net price 300-mL pack = £6.04
*Syrup*, red, sodium valproate 200 mg/5 mL.  Diluent syrup (without preservative), life of diluted syrup 14 days.  Net price 300-mL pack = £6.04
PoM **Epilim**® **Intravenous** (Sanofi Winthrop)
*Injection*, powder for reconstitution, sodium valproate.  Net price 400-mg vial (with 4-mL amp water for injections) = £9.00

## VIGABATRIN
*Indications:* epilepsy not satisfactorily controlled by other antiepileptics
*Cautions:* renal impairment; closely monitor neurological function; avoid sudden withdrawal; history of psychosis or behavioural problems; **interactions:** Appendix 1 (vigabatrin)
*Contra-indications:* pregnancy (high doses teratogenic in *animals*) and breast-feeding
*Side-effects:* drowsiness, fatigue, dizziness, nervousness, irritability, depression, headache; less commonly confusion, aggression, psychosis, memory disturbance, visual disturbance (e.g. diplopia); weight gain and gastro-intestinal disturbances reported; excitation and agitation in children
*Dose:* with current antiepileptic therapy, initially 2 g daily in single or 2 divided doses then increased or decreased according to response in steps of 0.5–1 g; usual max. 4 g daily; CHILD 3–9 years initially 1 g daily

▼ PoM **Sabril**® (Merrell)
*Tablets*, scored, vigabatrin 500 mg, net price 100-tab pack = £46.00.  Label: 3

## 4.8.2  Drugs used in status epilepticus
Major status epilepticus should be treated first with intravenous **diazepam** or **clonazepam** but they should be used with caution because of the risk of respiratory depression; in situations where facilities for resuscitation are not immediately available, *small doses* of diazepam can be given intravenously or the drug can be administered as a rectal solution (Stesolid®). Absorption from suppositories is too slow for treatment of status epilepticus. Intramuscular injection is unsatisfactory as the drugs are too slowly absorbed. When diazepam is given intravenously there may be a high risk of venous thrombophlebitis which is minimised by using an emulsion (Diazemuls®).

---

If status epilepticus continues or returns, **chlormethiazole** may be given by intravenous infusion. Chlormethiazole has a short half-life, and the rate of infusion can be titrated against the patient's clinical condition. It does, however, cause respiratory depression. Alternatively **phenytoin sodium** may be given by slow intravenous injection, with ECG monitoring at a rate of not more than 50 mg/minute (in adults) to a maximum of 1 g followed by the maintenance dosage. Intramuscular use of phenytoin is not recommended (absorption is slow and erratic) and intravenous infusion is not recommended (precipitates).

**Paraldehyde** also remains a valuable drug. It is usually given by deep intramuscular injection; when given intramuscularly it causes little respiratory depression and is therefore useful where facilities for resuscitation are poor. Paraldehyde may also be given rectally. In some specialist centres with intensive care facilities, it has also been given intravenously (**must** be very well diluted, see next page).

**Phenobarbitone sodium** (section 4.8.1) is occasionally used but it is less satisfactory for urgent treatment because of its slow metabolism. **Lorazepam** is rarely used for status epilepticus.

# DIAZEPAM
*Indications:* status epilepticus; convulsions due to poisoning (see Emergency Treatment of Poisoning); other indications, see sections 4.1.2, 10.2.2, 15.1.4.1
*Cautions; Contra-indications; Side-effects:* see section 4.1.2; hypotension and apnoea may occur; when given intravenously facilities for reversing respiratory depression with mechanical ventilation must be at hand (but see also notes above)
*Dose: by intravenous injection,* 10–20 mg at a rate of 0.5 mL (2.5 mg) per 30 seconds, repeated if necessary after 30–60 minutes; may be followed by *intravenous infusion* to max. 3 mg/kg over 24 hours; CHILD 200–300 micrograms/kg
*By rectum* as rectal solution, ADULT and CHILD over 3 years 10 mg; CHILD 1–3 years and ELDERLY 5 mg; repeat after 5 minutes if necessary

PoM **Diazepam** (Non-proprietary)
*Injection* (solution), diazepam 5 mg/mL. See Appendix 6. Net price 2-mL amp = 25p
Available from CP
PoM **Diazemuls**® (Dumex)
*Injection* (emulsion), diazepam 5 mg/mL (0.5%). See Appendix 6. Net price 2-mL amp = 69p
PoM **Stesolid**® (CP)
*Rectal tubes* (= rectal solution), diazepam 2 mg/mL. Net price 5 × 2.5-mL (5 mg) tubes = £5.25; 4 mg/mL, 5 × 2.5-mL (10 mg) tubes = £6.70
PoM **Valium**® (Roche)
*Injection* (solution), diazepam 5 mg/mL. See Appendix 6. Net price 2-mL amp = 30p

Oral preparations, section 4.1.2

# CLONAZEPAM
*Indications:* status epilepticus; other forms of epilepsy, and myoclonus, section 4.8.1
*Cautions; Contra-indications; Side-effects:* see section 4.8.1. Hypotension and apnoea may occur and resuscitation facilities must be available
*Dose: by intravenous injection* (over 30 seconds) *or by intravenous infusion,* 1 mg, repeated if necessary; CHILD all ages, 500 micrograms

PoM **Rivotril**® (Roche)
*Injection,* clonazepam 1 mg/mL in solvent, for dilution with 1 mL water for injections immediately before injection or as described in Appendix 6. Net price 1-mL amp (with 1 mL water for injections) = 71p

Oral preparations, section 4.8.1

# CHLORMETHIAZOLE EDISYLATE
*Indications:* status epilepticus; other indications, see sections 4.1.1, 15.1.4.1
*Cautions:* obstructive pulmonary disease; during continuous infusion the sleep induced may quickly lapse into deep unconsciousness and patients must be observed constantly; resuscitation facilities must be available; **special care** on prolonged administration (see under dose); see also section 4.1.1
*Contra-indications:* acute pulmonary insufficiency
*Side-effects:* tingling in the nose, sneezing, conjunctival irritation, headache, slight hypotension, respiratory depression, local thrombophlebitis at site of continuous infusion and at rapid infusion rates cardiovascular and respiratory depression; see also section 4.1.1
*Dose: by intravenous infusion,* as a 0.8% solution, initially, 40–100 mL (320–800 mg) over 5–10 minutes then continued if necessary at a reduced rate adjusted according to the patient's condition (see notes above)
*Note.* Special care on prolonged administration since accumulation may occur; also, contains no electrolytes

PoM **Heminevrin**® (Astra)
*Intravenous infusion 0.8%,* chlormethiazole edisylate 8 mg/mL. Net price 500-mL bottle = £5.25

Oral preparations, section 4.1.1

# LORAZEPAM
*Indications:* status epilepticus; other indications, section 4.1.2
*Cautions; Contra-indications; Side-effects:* see section 4.1.2; hypotension and apnoea may occur and resuscitation facilities must be available
*Dose: by intravenous injection,* 4 mg; CHILD 2 mg

**Preparations**
    Section 4.1.2

## PARALDEHYDE

*Indications:* status epilepticus

*Cautions:* bronchopulmonary disease, hepatic impairment; avoid intramuscular injection near sciatic nerve (causes severe causalgia); intravenous route, specialist centres only with intensive care facilities (see notes above)

*Side-effects:* rashes; pain and sterile abscess after intramuscular injection; rectal irritation after enema

*Dose: by deep intramuscular injection,* as a single dose, 5–10 mL; usual max. 20 mL daily with not more than 5 mL at any one site; CHILD up to 3 months 0.5 mL, 3–6 months 1 mL, 6–12 months 1.5 mL, 1–2 years 2 mL, 3–5 years 3–4 mL, 6–12 years 5–6 mL

*By intravenous infusion,* up to 4–5 mL diluted to a 4% solution with sodium chloride intravenous infusion 0.9% (specialist centres **only**, see notes above)

*By rectum,* 5–10 mL, administered as a 10% enema in physiological saline; CHILD as for intramuscular dose

*Note.* Do not use paraldehyde if it has a brownish colour or an odour of acetic acid. Avoid contact with rubber and plastics.

---

PoM **Paraldehyde** (Non-proprietary)

*Injection,* sterile paraldehyde. Net price 5-mL amp = £2.89; 10-mL amp = £3.72

---

## PHENYTOIN SODIUM

*Indications:* status epilepticus; seizures in neurosurgery; arrhythmias, see section 2.3.2

*Cautions:* hypotension and heart failure; resuscitation facilities must be available; injection solutions alkaline (irritant to tissues); see also section 4.8.1; **interactions:** Appendix 1 (phenytoin)

*Contra-indications:* sinus bradycardia, sino-atrial block, and second- and third-degree heart block; Stokes-Adams syndrome; porphyria (see section 9.8.2)

*Side-effects:* intravenous injection may cause cardiovascular and CNS depression (particularly if injection too rapid) with arrhythmias, hypotension, and cardiovascular collapse; alterations in respiratory function (including respiratory arrest)

*Dose: by slow intravenous injection* (with blood pressure and ECG monitoring), status epilepticus, 10–15 mg/kg at a rate not exceeding 50 mg per minute, as a loading dose (see also notes above). Maintenance doses of about 100 mg should be given thereafter at intervals of every 6 hours, monitored by measurement of plasma concentrations; rate and dose reduced according to weight

*By intramuscular injection,* not recommended (see notes above)

---

PoM **Epanutin Ready Mixed Parenteral**® (P-D)

*Injection,* phenytoin sodium 50 mg/mL with propylene glycol 40% and alcohol 10% in water for injections. Net price 5-mL amp = £4.07

Oral preparations, section 4.8.1

### 4.8.3   Febrile convulsions

*Brief febrile convulsions* need only simple treatment such as tepid sponging or bathing, or antipyretic medication, e.g. **paracetamol** (section 4.7.1). *Prolonged febrile convulsions* (those lasting 15 minutes or longer), *recurrent convulsions,* or those occurring in a child at known risk must be treated more actively, as there is the possibility of resulting brain damage. **Diazepam** is the drug of choice given either by slow intravenous injection in a dose of 250 micrograms/kg (as Diazemuls®, section 4.8.2) or preferably rectally in solution (Stesolid®, section 4.8.2) in a dose of 500 micrograms/kg, repeated if necessary. The rectal route is preferred as satisfactory absorption is achieved within minutes and administration is much easier. Suppositories are not suitable because absorption is too slow.

Intermittent prophylaxis (i.e. the anticonvulsant administered at the onset of fever) is possible in only a small proportion of children. Again **diazepam** is the treatment of choice, orally or rectally.

The exact role of continuous prophylaxis in children at risk from prolonged or complex febrile convulsions is controversial. It is probably indicated in only a small proportion of children, including those whose first seizure occurred at under 14 months or who have pre-existing neurological abnormalities or who have had previous prolonged or focal convulsions. Thus long-term anticonvulsant prophylaxis is rarely indicated.

---

## 4.9   Drugs used in parkinsonism and related disorders

4.9.1  Dopaminergic drugs used in parkinsonism
4.9.2  Antimuscarinic drugs used in parkinsonism
4.9.3  Drugs used in essential tremor, chorea, tics, and related disorders

In idiopathic Parkinson's disease, progressive degeneration of pigment-containing cells of the substantia nigra leads to deficiency of the neurotransmitter dopamine. This, in turn, results in a neurohumoral imbalance in the basal ganglia, causing the characteristic signs and symptoms of the illness to appear. The pathogenesis of this process is still obscure and current drug therapy aims simply to correct the imbalance. Although this approach fails to prevent the progression of the disease, it greatly improves the quality and expectancy of life of most patients.

The patient should be advised at the outset of the limitations of treatment and possible side-effects. About 10 to 20% of patients are unresponsive to treatment.

ELDERLY. Antiparkinsonian drugs carry a special risk of inducing confusion in the elderly. It is particularly important to initiate treatment with low doses and to use small increments.

---

## 4.9.1 Dopaminergic drugs used in parkinsonism

**Levodopa**, used with a **dopa-decarboxylase inhibitor**, is the treatment of choice for patients disabled by idiopathic Parkinson's disease. It is least valuable in elderly patients and in those with long-standing disease who may not tolerate a dose large enough to overcome their deficit. It is also less valuable in patients with post-encephalitic disease who are particularly susceptible to the side-effects. Parkinsonism caused by generalised degenerative brain disease does not normally respond to levodopa. It should not be used for neuroleptic-induced parkinsonism.

Levodopa, the amino-acid precursor of dopamine, acts mainly by replenishing depleted striatal dopamine. It improves bradykinesia and rigidity more than tremor. It is generally administered in conjunction with an extracerebral dopa-decarboxylase inhibitor which prevents the peripheral degradation of levodopa to dopamine but, unlike levodopa, does not cross the blood-brain barrier. Effective brain concentrations of dopamine can thereby be achieved with lower doses of levodopa. At the same time the reduced peripheral formation of dopamine decreases peripheral side-effects such as nausea and vomiting and cardiovascular effects. There is also less delay in onset of therapeutic effect and a smoother clinical response. A disadvantage is an increased incidence of abnormal involuntary movements.

The extracerebral dopa-decarboxylase inhibitors given with levodopa are benserazide (in **co-beneldopa**) and carbidopa (in **co-careldopa**).

When co-careldopa 10/100 (10 mg of carbidopa for each 100 mg of levodopa) is used the dose of carbidopa may be insufficient to achieve full inhibition of extracerebral dopa-decarboxylase; co-careldopa 25/100 (25 mg of carbidopa for each 100 mg of levodopa) should then be used so that the daily dose of carbidopa is at least 75 mg.

Levodopa therapy should be initiated with low doses and gradually increased, by small increments, at intervals of 2 to 3 days. The final dose is usually a compromise between increased mobility and dose-limiting side-effects. Intervals between doses may be critical and should be chosen to suit the needs of the individual patient. Nausea and vomiting are rarely dose-limiting but doses should be taken after meals. Domperidone (section 4.6) may be useful in controlling vomiting. The most frequent dose-limiting side-effects of levodopa are involuntary movements and psychiatric complications. As the patient ages, the maintenance dose may need to be reduced.

During the first 6 to 18 months of levodopa therapy there may be a slow improvement in the response of the patient which is maintained for 1½ to 2 years; thereafter a slow decline may occur. Particularly troublesome is the 'on-off' effect the incidence of which increases as the treatment progresses. This is characterised by fluctuations in performance with normal performance during the 'on' period and weakness and akinesia lasting for 2 to 4 hours during the 'off' period.

'End-of-dose' deterioration may also occur where the duration of benefit after each dose becomes progressively shorter. Modified-release preparations may help with 'end-of-dose' deterioration or nocturnal immobility and rigidity.

**Selegiline** is a monoamine-oxidase-B inhibitor used in severe parkinsonism in conjunction with levodopa to reduce 'end-of-dose' deterioration. Early treatment with selegiline may also delay the need for levodopa therapy and possibly slow the rate of progression of the disease.

**Bromocriptine** acts by direct stimulation of surviving dopamine receptors. Although effective, it has no advantages over levodopa. It should be reserved for patients for whom levodopa alone is no longer adequate or who despite careful titration cannot tolerate levodopa. Its use is often limited by its side-effects and when used with levodopa, abnormal involuntary movements and confusional states are common.

**Lysuride** is a newly introduced drug for parkinsonism; it is similar to bromocriptine in its action.

**Amantadine** has modest antiparkinsonian effects. It improves mild bradykinetic disabilities as well as tremor and rigidity. Unfortunately only a small proportion of patients derive much benefit from this drug and tolerance to its effects occurs. However it has the advantage of being relatively free from side-effects.

## LEVODOPA

*Indications:* parkinsonism (but not drug-induced extrapyramidal symptoms), see notes above

*Cautions:* pulmonary disease, peptic ulceration, cardiovascular disease, diabetes mellitus, open-angle glaucoma, skin melanoma, psychiatric illness (avoid if severe). In prolonged therapy, psychiatric, hepatic, haematological, renal, and cardiovascular surveillance is advisable. Warn patients who benefit from therapy to resume normal activities gradually; avoid abrupt withdrawal; **interactions:** Appendix 1 (levodopa)

*Contra-indications:* closed-angle glaucoma

*Side-effects:* anorexia, nausea, insomnia, agitation, postural hypotension (rarely labile hypertension), dizziness, tachycardia, arrhythmias, reddish discoloration of urine and other body fluids, rarely hypersensitivity; abnormal involuntary movements and psychiatric symptoms which include hypomania and psychosis may be dose-limiting; occasionally depression, drowsiness, and rarely headache, peripheral neuropathy reported

*Dose:* initially 125–500 mg daily in divided doses after meals, increased according to response (but rarely used alone, see notes above)

PoM **Brocadopa**® (Brocades)
*Capsules*, levodopa 125 mg, net price 20 = 71p; 250 mg, 20 = 85p; 500 mg, 20 = £1.52. Label: 14, 21

PoM **Larodopa**® (Roche)
*Tablets*, scored, levodopa 500 mg. Net price 20 = £1.34. Label: 14, 21

## CO-BENELDOPA

A mixture of benserazide hydrochloride and levodopa in mass proportions corresponding to 1 part of benserazide and 4 parts of levodopa

*Indications; Cautions; Contra-indications; Side-effects:* see under Levodopa and notes above

*Dose:* expressed as levodopa, initially 50–100 mg twice daily, adjusted according to response; usual maintenance dose 400–800 mg daily in divided doses after meals

*Note.* When transferring patients from levodopa, 3 capsules co-beneldopa 25/100 (Madopar 125®) should be substituted for 2 g levodopa; the levodopa should be discontinued 12 hours beforehand

PoM **Madopar**® (Roche)

*Capsules 62.5*, blue/grey, co-beneldopa 12.5/50 (benserazide 12.5 mg (as hydrochloride), levodopa 50 mg). Net price 100-cap pack = £7.76. Label: 14, 21

*Capsules 125*, blue/pink, co-beneldopa 25/100 (benserazide 25 mg (as hydrochloride), levodopa 100 mg). Net price 100-cap pack = £13.51. Label: 14, 21

*Capsules 250*, blue/caramel, co-beneldopa 50/200 (benserazide 50 mg (as hydrochloride), levodopa 200 mg). Net price 100-cap pack = £22.46. Label: 14, 21

*Dispersible tablets 62.5*, scored, co-beneldopa 12.5/50 (benserazide 12.5 mg (as hydrochloride), levodopa 50 mg). Net price 100-tab pack = £8.29. Label: 14, 21, counselling, administration, see below

*Dispersible tablets 125*, scored, co-beneldopa 25/100 (benserazide 25 mg (as hydrochloride) levodopa 100 mg). Net price 100-tab pack = £14.70. Label: 14, 21, counselling, administration, see below

*Note.* The tablets may be dispersed in water or orange squash or swallowed whole

PoM **Madopar**® CR (Roche)

*Capsules 125*, m/r, dark green/light blue, co-beneldopa 25/100 (benserazide 25 mg (as hydrochloride), levodopa 100 mg). Net price 100-cap pack = £17.97. Label: 5, 14, 25

*Dose:* fluctuations in response to conventional levodopa/decarboxylase inhibitor preparations, initially 1 capsule substituted for every 100 mg of levodopa and given at same dosage frequency, subsequently increased every 2–3 days according to response; average increase of 50% needed over previous levodopa dose and titration may take up to 4 weeks; supplementary dose of conventional Madopar® may be needed with first morning dose; if response still poor to total daily dose of Madopar® CR plus Madopar® corresponding to 1.2 g levodopa, consider alternative therapy

## CO-CARELDOPA

A mixture of carbidopa and levodopa; the proportions are expressed in the form $x/y$ where $x$ and $y$ are the strengths in milligrams of carbidopa and levodopa respectively

*Indications; Cautions; Contra-indications; Side-effects:* see under Levodopa and notes above

*Dose:* expressed as levodopa, initially 100–125 mg 3–4 times daily adjusted according to response; usual maintenance dose 0.75–1.5 g daily in divided doses after food. See also under Sinemet-Plus®

*Note.* When transferring patients from levodopa, 3 tablets co-careldopa 25/250 (Sinemet-275®) should be substituted for 4 g levodopa; the levodopa should be discontinued 12 hours beforehand

PoM **Sinemet**® (Du Pont)

*Tablets* (Sinemet-110), blue, scored, co-careldopa 10/100 (carbidopa 10 mg (as monohydrate), levodopa 100 mg). Net price 20 = £1.71. Label: 14, 21

*Tablets* (Sinemet-275), blue, scored, co-careldopa 25/250 (carbidopa 25 mg (as monohydrate), levodopa 250 mg). Net price 20 = £3.57. Label: 14, 21

PoM **Sinemet LS**® (Du Pont)

*Tablets*, yellow, scored, co-careldopa 12.5/50 (carbidopa 12.5 mg (as monohydrate), levodopa 50 mg). Net price 84-tab pack = £6.87. Label: 14, 21

*Note.* 2 tablets Sinemet LS® ≡ 1 tablet Sinemet Plus®

PoM **Sinemet-Plus**® (Du Pont)

*Tablets*, yellow, scored, co-careldopa 25/100 (carbidopa 25 mg (as monohydrate), levodopa 100 mg). Net price 20 = £2.52. Label: 14, 21

*Dose:* initially 1 tablet 3 times daily, adjusted according to response to 8 daily in divided doses; larger doses by gradual substitution of Sinemet® for Sinemet-Plus®

*Note.* The daily dose of carbidopa required to achieve full inhibition of extracerebral dopa-decarboxylase is 75 mg; co-careldopa 25/100 provides an adequate dose of carbidopa when low doses of levodopa are needed

PoM **Sinemet**® CR (Du Pont)

*Tablets*, m/r, peach, co-careldopa 50/200 (carbidopa 50 mg (as monohydrate), levodopa 200 mg). Net price 56-tab pack = £21.84. Label: 14, 25

*Dose:* initial treatment or fluctuations in response to conventional levodopa therapy, 1 tablet twice daily; both dose and interval then adjusted according to response at intervals of not less than 3 days; if transferring from existing levodopa therapy withdraw 8 hours beforehand (12 hours for m/r levodopa preparations); 1 tablet Sinemet® CR twice daily can be substituted for a daily dose of levodopa 300–400 mg in Sinemet® conventional tablets

## AMANTADINE HYDROCHLORIDE

*Indications:* parkinsonism (but not drug-induced extrapyramidal symptoms); antiviral, see section 5.3

*Cautions:* cardiovascular, hepatic, or renal disease (avoid if severe), recurrent eczema, psychosis, elderly, breast-feeding. Avoid abrupt discontinuation of treatment; **interactions:** Appendix 1 (amantadine)

DRIVING. May affect performance of skilled tasks (e.g. driving)

*Contra-indications:* epilepsy, gastric ulceration

*Side-effects:* nervousness, inability to concentrate, insomnia, dizziness, convulsions, hallucinations, gastro-intestinal disturbances, skin discoloration, dry mouth, peripheral oedema; rarely leucopenia

*Dose:* 100 mg daily increased if necessary to 100 mg twice daily (not later than 4 p.m.), usually in conjunction with other treatment; max. 400 mg daily (with close supervision)

PoM **Symmetrel**® (Geigy)

*Capsules*, brownish-red, amantadine hydrochloride 100 mg. Net price 20 = £3.38. Counselling, driving

*Syrup*, amantadine hydrochloride 50 mg/5 mL. Net price 150-mL pack = £3.17. Counselling, driving

## BROMOCRIPTINE

*Indications:* parkinsonism (but not drug-induced extrapyramidal symptoms); endocrine disorders, see section 6.7.1

*Cautions; Side-effects:* see section 6.7.1

HYPOTENSIVE REACTIONS. Hypotensive reactions may be disturbing in some patients during the first few days of treatment and particular care should be exercised when driving or operating machinery; tolerance to bromocriptine reduced by alcohol

*Dose:* first week 1–1.25 mg at night, second week 2–2.5 mg at night, third week 2.5 mg twice daily, then 3 times daily increasing by 2.5 mg every 3–14 days according to response to a usual range of 10–40 mg daily; taken with food

PoM **Bromocriptine** (Non-proprietary)

*Tablets*, bromocriptine (as mesylate), 2.5 mg, net price 20 = £3.43. Label: 21, counselling, hypotensive reactions

PoM **Parlodel**® (Sandoz)

*Tablets*, both scored, bromocriptine (as mesylate), 1 mg, net price 20 = £1.86; 2.5 mg, 20 = £3.59. Label: 21, counselling, hypotensive reactions

*Capsules*, bromocriptine (as mesylate), 5 mg (blue/white), net price 20 = £7.04; 10 mg, 20 = £13.03. Label: 21, counselling, hypotensive reactions

## LYSURIDE MALEATE

*Indications:* Parkinson's disease

*Cautions:* history of pituitary tumour; psychotic disturbance; **interactions:** Appendix 1 (lysuride)

HYPOTENSIVE REACTIONS. Hypotensive reactions may be disturbing in some patients during the first few days of treatment and particular care should be exercised when driving or operating machinery

*Contra-indications:* severe disturbances of peripheral circulation; coronary insufficiency, porphyria (see section 9.8.2)

*Side-effects:* nausea and vomiting; dizziness; headache, lethargy, malaise, drowsiness, psychotic reactions (including hallucinations); occasionally severe hypotension, rashes; rarely abdominal pain and constipation; Raynaud's phenomenon reported

*Dose:* initially 200 micrograms at bedtime with food increased as necessary at weekly intervals to 200 micrograms twice daily (midday and bedtime) then to 200 micrograms 3 times daily (morning, midday, and bedtime); further increases made by adding 200 micrograms each week first to the bedtime dose, then to the midday dose and finally to the morning dose; max. 5 mg daily in 3 divided doses after food

▼ PoM **Revanil**® (Roche)

*Tablets*, scored, lysuride maleate 200 micrograms. Net price 100-tab pack = £24.00. Label: 21, counselling, hypotensive reactions

## PERGOLIDE

*Indications:* adjunct to levodopa in Parkinson's disease

*Cautions:* arrhythmias or underlying cardiac disease, history of confusion or hallucinations, dyskinesia, pregnancy, breast-feeding; increase dose gradually and avoid abrupt withdrawal; avoid in porphyria (see section 9.8.2); **interactions:** Appendix 1 (pergolide)

HYPOTENSIVE REACTIONS. Hypotensive reactions may be disturbing in some patients during the first few days of treatment and particular care should be exercised when driving or operating machinery.

*Side-effects:* hallucinations, confusion, dyskinesia, somnolence, abdominal pain, nausea, dyspepsia, diplopia, rhinitis, dyspnoea, insomnia, constipation or diarrhoea, hypotension, tachycardia and arrhythmias reported

*Dose:* 50 micrograms daily for 2 days, increased gradually by 100–150 micrograms every third day over next 12 days, usually given in 3 divided doses; further increases of 250 micrograms every third day; usual maintenance 3 mg daily (above 5 mg daily not evaluated); during pergolide titration levodopa dose may be reduced cautiously

▼ PoM **Celance**® (Lilly)

*Tablets*, all scored, pergolide (as mesylate) 50 micrograms (ivory), net price 30-tab pack = £10.00; 250 micrograms (green), 20 = £7.56; 1 mg (pink), 20 = £30.00. Counselling, hypotensive reactions

## SELEGILINE

*Indications:* Parkinson's disease or symptomatic parkinsonism (but not drug-induced extrapyramidal symptoms), either used alone (in early disease) or as an adjunct to levodopa therapy

*Cautions:* side-effects of levodopa may be increased, concurrent levodopa dosage may need to be reduced by 20–50%; **interactions:** Appendix 1 (selegiline)

*Side-effects:* hypotension, nausea and vomiting, confusion, agitation

*Dose:* 10 mg in the morning, or 5 mg at breakfast and midday

PoM **Eldepryl**® (Britannia)

*Tablets*, scored, selegiline hydrochloride 5 mg. Net price 20 = £9.30

## 4.9.2 Antimuscarinic drugs used in parkinsonism

Antimuscarinic drugs (less correctly termed 'anticholinergics') are the other main class of drugs used in Parkinson's disease. They are less effective than levodopa in idiopathic Parkinson's disease although they often usefully supplement its action. Patients with mild symptoms, particularly where tremor predominates, may be treated initially with antimuscarinic drugs, levodopa being added or substituted as symptoms progress. They have value in post-encephalitic parkinsonism.

Antimuscarinic drugs exert their antiparkinsonian effect by correcting the relative central cholinergic excess thought to occur in parkinsonism as a result of dopamine deficiency. In most patients their effects are only moderate, reducing tremor and rigidity to some effect but without significant action on bradykinesia. They exert a synergistic effect when used with levodopa and are also useful in reducing sialorrhoea.

The antimuscarinic drugs also reduce the symptoms of drug-induced parkinsonism as seen, for example, with antipsychotic drugs (section 4.2.1) but there is no justification for giving them simultaneously with antipsychotics unless parkinsonian side-effects occur. Tardive dyskinesia is not improved by the antimuscarinic drugs and may be made worse.

No important differences exist between the many synthetic antimuscarinic drugs available but some patients appear to tolerate one better than another. They may be taken before food if dry mouth is troublesome, or after food if gastrointestinal symptoms predominate. Those most commonly used are **orphenadrine** and **benzhexol**; **benztropine** and **procyclidine** are also used. Benztropine is similar to benzhexol but is excreted more slowly; changes in dose therefore need to be carried out very gradually. Both procyclidine and benztropine may be given parenterally and are effective emergency treatment for acute drug-induced dystonic reactions which may be severe.

## BENZHEXOL HYDROCHLORIDE

*Indications:* parkinsonism; drug-induced extrapyramidal symptoms (but not tardive dyskinesia, see notes above)

*Cautions:* urinary retention, closed-angle glaucoma, cardiovascular disease, hepatic or renal impairment; gastro-intestinal obstruction; avoid abrupt discontinuation of treatment; drugs of this type liable to abuse; **interactions:** Appendix 1 (antimuscarinics)
DRIVING. May affect performance of skilled tasks (e.g. driving)

*Side-effects:* dry mouth, gastro-intestinal disturbances, dizziness, blurred vision; less commonly urinary retention, tachycardia, hypersensitivity, nervousness, and with high doses in susceptible patients, mental confusion, excitement, and psychiatric disturbances which may necessitate discontinuation of treatment

*Dose:* 1 mg daily, gradually increased; usual maintenance dose 5–15 mg daily in 3–4 divided doses

PoM **Benzhexol**® (Non-proprietary)
*Tablets*, benzhexol hydrochloride 2 mg, net price 20 = 31p; 5 mg, 20 = 63p. Counselling, before or after food (see notes above), driving

PoM **Artane**® (Lederle)
*Tablets*, both scored, benzhexol hydrochloride 2 mg, net price 20 = 32p; 5 mg, 20 = 65p. Counselling, before or after food (see notes above), driving

PoM **Broflex**® (Bioglan)
*Syrup*, pink, benzhexol hydrochloride 5 mg/5 mL. Net price 200-mL pack = £4.34. Counselling, before or after food (see notes above), driving

## BENZTROPINE MESYLATE

*Indications; Cautions; Side-effects:* see under Benzhexol Hydrochloride, but causes sedation rather than stimulation; avoid in children under 3 years

*Dose: by mouth,* 0.5–1 mg daily usually at bedtime, gradually increased; max. 6 mg daily; usual maintenance dose 1–4 mg daily in single or divided doses

*By intramuscular or intravenous injection,* 1–2 mg, repeated if symptoms reappear

PoM **Cogentin**® (MSD)
*Tablets*, scored, benztropine mesylate 2 mg. Net price 20 = 29p. Label: 2
*Injection*, benztropine mesylate 1 mg/mL. Net price 2-mL amp = 77p

## BIPERIDEN

*Indications; Cautions; Side-effects:* see under Benzhexol Hydrochloride, but may cause drowsiness; injection may cause hypotension

*Dose: by mouth,* biperiden hydrochloride 1 mg twice daily, gradually increased to 2 mg 3 times daily; usual maintenance dose 3–12 mg daily in divided doses

*By intramuscular or slow intravenous injection,* biperiden lactate 2.5–5 mg up to 4 times daily

PoM **Akineton**® (Knoll)
*Tablets*, scored, biperiden hydrochloride 2 mg. Net price 100-tab pack = £4·72. Label: 2
*Injection*, biperiden lactate 5 mg/mL. Net price 1-mL amp = 70p

## METHIXENE HYDROCHLORIDE

*Indications; Cautions; Side-effects:* see under Benzhexol Hydrochloride

*Dose:* 2.5 mg 3 times daily gradually increased; usual maintenance dose 15–60 mg (elderly 15–30 mg) daily in divided doses

PoM **Tremonil**® (Sandoz)
*Tablets*, scored, methixene hydrochloride 5 mg. Net price 50 = £1.71. Label: 2

## ORPHENADRINE HYDROCHLORIDE

*Indications; Cautions; Side-effects:* see under Benzhexol Hydrochloride, but more euphoric; may cause insomnia; avoid in porphyria (see section 9.8.2)

*Dose: by mouth,* 150 mg daily in divided doses, gradually increased; max. 400 mg daily

PoM **Biorphen**® (Bioglan)
*Elixir*, sugar-free, orphenadrine hydrochloride 25 mg/5 mL. Net price 200-mL pack = £5.14. Counselling, driving

PoM **Disipal**® (Brocades)
*Tablets*, yellow, s/c, orphenadrine hydrochloride 50 mg. Net price 20 = 30p. Counselling, driving
*Additives: include* tartrazine

## PROCYCLIDINE HYDROCHLORIDE

**Indications; Cautions; Side-effects:** see under Benzhexol Hydrochloride

**Dose:** *by mouth,* 2.5 mg 3 times daily, gradually increased if necessary; usual max. 30 mg daily (60 mg daily in exceptional circumstances)

Acute dystonia, *by intramuscular injection,* 5–10 mg repeated if necessary after 20 minutes; max. 20 mg daily; *by intravenous injection,* 5 mg (usually effective within 5 minutes); an occasional patient may need 10 mg or more and may require up to half an hour to obtain relief

PoM **Procyclidine** (Non-proprietary)
*Tablets*, procyclidine hydrochloride 5 mg. Net price 20 = £1.02. Counselling, driving

PoM **Arpicolin**® (RP Drugs)
*Syrup*, procyclidine hydrochloride 2.5 mg/5 mL, net price 200-mL pack = £3.10; 5 mg/5 mL, 200-mL pack = £5.50. Counselling, driving

PoM **Kemadrin**® (Wellcome)
*Tablets*, scored, procyclidine hydrochloride 5 mg. Net price 20 = £1.17. Counselling, driving
*Injection*, procyclidine hydrochloride 5 mg/mL. Net price 2-mL amp = £1.49

## 4.9.3  Drugs used in essential tremor, chorea, tics, and related disorders

**Tetrabenazine** is mainly used to control movement disorders in Huntington's chorea and related disorders. It may act by depleting nerve endings of dopamine. It has useful action in only a proportion of patients and its use may be limited by the development of depression.

**Haloperidol** may be useful in improving motor tics and symptoms of Gilles de la Tourette syndrome and related choreas. **Pimozide** (see section 4.2.1 for CSM warning) and more recently **clonidine** (section 4.7.4.2) and **sulpiride** (section 4.2.1), are also used in Gilles de la Tourette syndrome. **Benzhexol** (section 4.9.2) at high dosage may also improve some movement disorders. It is sometimes necessary to build the dose up over many weeks, to 20 to 30 mg daily or higher. **Chlorpromazine** and **haloperidol** are used to relieve intractable hiccup (section 4.2.1).

**Propranolol** or another beta-adrenoceptor blocking drug (see section 2.4) may be useful in treating essential tremor or tremors associated with anxiety or thyrotoxicosis. Propranolol is given in a dosage of 40 mg 2 or 3 times daily, increased if necessary; 80 to 160 mg daily is usually required for maintenance.

**Primidone** in some cases provides relief from benign essential tremor; the dose is increased slowly to reduce side-effects.

## HALOPERIDOL

**Indications:** motor tics, adjunctive treatment in choreas and Gilles de la Tourette syndrome; other indications, section 4.2.1

**Cautions; Contra-indications; Side-effects:** see section 4.2.1

**Dose:** *by mouth,* 0.5–1.5 mg 3 times daily adjusted according to the response; 10 mg daily or more may occasionally be necessary in Gilles de la Tourette syndrome; CHILD, Gilles de la Tourette syndrome up to 10 mg daily

**Preparations**
Section 4.2.1

## PRIMIDONE

**Indications:** essential tremor; epilepsy, see section 4.8.1

**Cautions; Contra-indications; Side-effects:** see section 4.8.1

**Dose:** essential tremor, initially 50 mg daily increased gradually over 2–3 weeks according to response; max. 750 mg daily

**Preparations**
Section 4.8.1

## TETRABENAZINE

**Indications:** movement disorders due to Huntington's chorea, senile chorea, and related neurological conditions

**Cautions:** pregnancy; avoid in breast-feeding; **interactions:** Appendix 1 (tetrabenazine)
DRIVING. May affect performance of skilled tasks (e.g. driving)

**Side-effects:** drowsiness, gastro-intestinal disturbances, depression, extrapyramidal dysfunction, hypotension

**Dose:** initially 12.5 mg twice daily (elderly 12.5 mg daily) gradually increased to 12.5–25 mg 3 times daily; max. 200 mg daily

PoM **Nitoman**® (Roche)
*Tablets*, pale yellow-buff, scored, tetrabenazine 25 mg. Net price 120-tab pack = £5·59. Label: 2

### TORSION DYSTONIAS

## BOTULINUM A TOXIN-HAEMAGGLU-TININ COMPLEX

**Indications:** blepharospasm and hemifacial spasm

**Cautions:** avoid deep or misplaced injection; pregnancy, breast-feeding

**Side-effects:** ptosis, diplopia; exacerbation of eyelid abnormalities, paralysis of mid-facial muscles, reduced blinking leading to keratitis and dry eyes; minor bruising and lid swelling

*Dose: by subcutaneous injection*, initially 120 units per affected eye, divided between 4 sites around affected eye as directed on package insert, repeated approximately every 8 weeks or as necessary (dose may be reduced to 80 or 60 units per eye)

▼ PoM **Dysport**® (Porton)
*Injection*, powder for reconstitution, botulinum A toxin-haemagglutinin complex, net price 500-unit vial = £170.00

# 4.10    Drugs used in substance dependence

This section includes drugs used in alcohol dependence, cigarette smoking, and opioid dependence.

## ALCOHOL DEPENDENCE

**Disulfiram** (Antabuse®) is used as an adjunct to the treatment of alcohol dependence. It gives rise to extremely unpleasant systemic reactions after the ingestion of even small amounts of alcohol because it leads to accumulation of acetaldehyde in the body. Reactions include flushing of the face, throbbing headache, palpitations, tachycardia, nausea, vomiting, and, with large doses of alcohol, arrhythmias, hypotension, and collapse. Even the small amounts of alcohol included in many oral medicines may be sufficient to precipitate a reaction. It may be advisable for patients to carry a card warning of the danger of administration of alcohol.

**Chlormethiazole** (section 4.1.1) and **benzodiazepines** (section 4.1.2) are used to attenuate withdrawal symptoms but themselves have a dependence potential (section 4.1).

## DISULFIRAM

*Indications:* adjunct in the treatment of chronic alcohol dependence (under specialist supervision)
*Cautions:* ensure that alcohol not consumed for at least 12 hours before initiating treatment; see also notes above; variable and occasionally severe reactions on alcohol challenge; hepatic or renal impairment, respiratory disease, diabetes mellitus, epilepsy; **interactions:** Appendix 1 (disulfiram)
ALCOHOL REACTION. Patients should be warned of unpredictable and occasionally severe nature of disulfiram-alcohol interactions. Reactions can occur in 10 minutes and last several hours (may require intensive supportive therapy). Patients should not ingest alcohol at all and should be warned of possible presence of alcohol in liquid medicines
*Contra-indications:* cardiac failure, coronary artery disease, psychosis and drug addiction, pregnancy
*Side-effects:* initially drowsiness and fatigue; nausea, vomiting, halitosis, reduced libido; rarely psychotic reactions (depression, paranoia,

schizophrenia, mania), allergic dermatitis, peripheral neuritis, hepatic cell damage
*Dose:* 800 mg as a single dose on first day, reducing over 5 days to 100–200 mg daily; may be continued for up to 1 year

PoM **Antabuse 200**® (CP)
*Tablets*, scored, disulfiram 200 mg. Net price 50 = £17.50. Label: 2, counselling, alcohol reaction

## CIGARETTE SMOKING

Nicotine chewing gum may be used as an adjunct to counselling; it is not available on the NHS.

NHS **Nicorette**® (Kabi Pharmacia)
*Chewing gum*, sugar-free, nicotine (as resin) 2 mg, net price pack of 30 = £2.61; pack of 105 = £7.04

NHS PoM **Nicorette Plus**® (Kabi Pharmacia)
*Chewing gum*, sugar-free, nicotine (as resin) 4 mg, net price pack of 105 = £10.80.
*Cautions:* angina, coronary artery disease; exacerbation of gastritis or peptic ulcer if swallowed
*Contra-indications:* pregnancy
*Dose:* nicotine replacement, initially one 2-mg piece to be chewed slowly for approx. 30 minutes, when urge to smoke occurs; patients needing more than 15 2-mg pieces daily may need the 4-mg strength; max. 15 pieces of 4-mg strength daily

## OPIOID DEPENDENCE

**Methadone** is an opioid *agonist*. It can be substituted for opioids such as diamorphine, preventing the onset of withdrawal symptoms; it is itself addictive and should only be prescribed for those who are physically dependent on opioids. It is administered in a single daily dose usually as methadone mixture 1 mg/mL. The dose is adjusted according to the degree of dependence with the aim of gradual reduction.

**Naltrexone** is an opioid *antagonist*. It blocks the action of opioids such as diamorphine and precipitates withdrawal symptoms in opioid-dependent subjects. Since the euphoric action of opioid agonists is blocked by naltrexone it is given to former addicts as an aid to relapse prevention. Naltrexone should be initiated in specialist clinics only.

## METHADONE HYDROCHLORIDE

*Indications:* adjunct in treatment of opioid dependence, see notes above; analgesia, section 4.7.2
*Cautions; Contra-indications; Side-effects:* section 4.7.2; overdosage: see Emergency Treatment of Poisoning, p. 18
*Dose:* initially 10–20 mg daily, increased by 10–20 mg daily until no signs of withdrawal or intoxication; usual dose 40–60 mg daily

**CD Methadone Mixture 1 mg/mL**
Net price 500 mL = £6.50. Label: 2
Available from Martindale, Penn (special order)

This preparation is 2½ times the strength of Methadone
Linctus and is intended only for drug dependent per-
sons for whom treatment is normally ordered on form
FP10(HP)(ad) or FP10(MDA), or in Scotland on forms
HBP(A) or GP10
The title includes the strength and prescriptions should be
written accordingly
Syrup preserved with hydroxybenzoate esters may be
incompatible with methadone hydrochloride.

## NALTREXONE HYDROCHLORIDE

*Indications:* adjunct to prevent relapse in detoxified formerly opioid-dependent patients

*Cautions:* hepatic and renal impairment; liver
function tests needed before and during treatment; test for opioid dependence with
naloxone; avoid concomitant use of opioids but
increased dose of opioid analgesic may be
required for pain (monitor for opioid intoxication)

*Contra-indications:* patients currently dependent
on opioids; acute hepatitis or liver failure

*Side-effects:* nausea, vomiting, abdominal pain;
anxiety, nervousness, sleeping difficulty, headache, reduced energy; joint and muscle pain;
less frequently, loss of appetite, diarrhoea, constipation, increased thirst; chest pain; increased
sweating and lachrymation; increased energy,
'feeling down', irritability, dizziness, chills;
delayed ejaculation, decreased potency; rash;
occasionally, liver function abnormalities;
reversible idiopathic thrombocytopenia
reported

*Dose:* 25 mg initially then 50 mg daily; the total
weekly dose may be divided and given on 3
days of the week for improved compliance (e.g.
100 mg on Monday and Wednesday, and 150 mg
on Friday)

PoM **Nalorex**® (Du Pont)
*Tablets,* orange, scored, naltrexone hydrochloride 50 mg. Net price 50-tab pack = £79.49

---

# 5: Drugs used in the treatment of

# INFECTIONS

In this chapter, drug treatment is discussed under the following headings:

    5.1 Antibacterial drugs
    5.2 Antifungal drugs
    5.3 Antiviral drugs
    5.4 Antiprotozoal drugs
    5.5 Anthelmintics

## 5.1   Antibacterial drugs

    5.1.1   Penicillins
    5.1.2   Cephalosporins, cephamycins and other beta-lactam antibiotics
    5.1.3   Tetracyclines
    5.1.4   Aminoglycosides
    5.1.5   Macrolides
    5.1.6   Clindamycin and lincomycin
    5.1.7   Some other antibiotics
    5.1.8   Sulphonamides and trimethoprim
    5.1.9   Antituberculous drugs
    5.1.10  Antileprotic drugs
    5.1.11  Metronidazole and tinidazole
    5.1.12  4-Quinolones
    5.1.13  Urinary-tract infections

CHOICE OF A SUITABLE DRUG. Before selecting an antibiotic the clinician must first consider two factors—the patient and the known or likely causative organism. Factors related to the patient which must be considered include history of allergy, renal and hepatic function, resistance to infection (i.e. whether immunocompromised), ability to tolerate drugs by mouth, severity of illness, ethnic origin, age and, if female, whether pregnant, breast-feeding or taking an oral contraceptive.

The known or likely organism and its antibiotic sensitivity, in association with the above factors, will suggest one or more antibiotics, the final choice depending on the microbiological, pharmacological, and toxicological properties.

An example of a rational approach to the selection of an antibiotic is treatment of a urinary-tract infection in a patient complaining of nausea in early pregnancy. The organism is reported as being resistant to ampicillin but sensitive to nitrofurantoin (can cause nausea), gentamicin (can only be given by injection and best avoided in pregnancy), tetracycline and co-trimoxazole (both contra-indicated in pregnancy), and cephalexin. The safest antibiotics in pregnancy are the penicillins and cephalosporins; therefore, cephalexin would be indicated for this patient.

The principles involved in selection of an antibiotic must allow for a number of variables including changing renal and hepatic function, increasing bacterial resistance, and new information on side-effects. Duration of therapy, dosage, and route of administration depend on site, type and severity of infection.

ANTIBIOTIC POLICIES. Many health authorities now place limits on the antibiotics that may be used in their hospitals, to achieve reasonable economy consistent with adequate cover, and to reduce the development of resistant organisms. An authority may indicate a range of drugs for general use, and permit treatment with other drugs only on the advice of the microbiologist or physician responsible for the control of infectious diseases.

BEFORE STARTING THERAPY. The following precepts should be considered before starting:

**Viral** infections should not be treated with antibiotics.

Samples should be taken for culture and sensitivity testing; 'blind' prescribing of an antibiotic for a patient ill with unexplained pyrexia usually leads to further difficulty in establishing the diagnosis.

An up-to-date knowledge of **prevalent organisms** and their current sensitivity is of great help in choosing an antibiotic before bacteriological confirmation is available.

The **dose** of an antibiotic will vary according to a number of factors including age, weight, renal function, and severity of infection. The prescribing of the so-called 'standard' dose in serious infections may result in failure of treatment or even death of the patient. Most antibiotics are rapidly excreted from the body and should be administered every 6 hours for the treatment of serious infections. Less severe infections as seen in general practice usually respond to administration every 8 hours. Agents with prolonged plasma half-lives such as trimethoprim need only be given every 12 hours. The aminoglycoside antibiotics should not be given more frequently than every 8 hours and the interval between doses must be increased in patients with renal failure.

The **route** of administration of an antibiotic will often depend on the severity of the infection. Life-threatening infections require intravenous therapy. Whenever possible painful intramuscular injections should be avoided in children.

**Duration** of therapy depends on the nature of the infection and the response to treatment. Courses should not be unduly prolonged as they are wasteful and may lead to side-effects. However, in certain infections such as endocarditis and tuberculosis it is necessary to continue treatment for relatively long periods. Conversely a single dose of an antibiotic may cure uncomplicated urinary-tract infections.

Suggested treatment is shown in Table 1. When the pathogen has been isolated treatment may be changed to a more appropriate antibiotic if necessary. If no bacterium is cultured the antibiotic can be continued or stopped on clinical grounds. Infections for which prophylaxis is useful are listed in Table 2.

---

## Table 1. Summary of antibacterial therapy

| Infection | Suggested antibacterial | Comment |
|---|---|---|
| **1: Gastro-intestinal system** | | |
| Gastro-enteritis | Antibiotic not usually indicated | Frequently nonbacterial aetiology |
| *Campylobacter* enteritis | Erythromycin *or* ciprofloxacin | |
| Invasive salmonellosis | Amoxycillin[1] *or* trimethoprim *or* ciprofloxacin | Includes severe infections which may be invasive |
| Shigellosis | Ampicillin *or* trimethoprim *or* ciprofloxacin | Antibiotic not indicated for mild cases. Ciprofloxacin should be used for trimethoprim-resistant strains |
| Typhoid fever | Chloramphenicol *or* ciprofloxacin *or* amoxycillin[1] | Infections from the Indian subcontinent, the Middle-East, and South-East Asia may be chloramphenicol-resistant and ciprofloxacin may be more appropriate |
| Biliary-tract infection | Gentamicin *or* a cephalosporin | |
| Peritonitis | Gentamicin (*or* a cephalosporin) + metronidazole (*or* clindamycin) | |
| Peritoneal dialysis-associated peritonitis | Vancomycin + gentamicin added to dialysis fluid | Discontinue either gentamicin or vancomycin when sensitivity known; treat for 5–10 days |
| **2: Cardiovascular system** | | |
| Endocarditis caused by: | | |
| Penicillin-sensitive streptococci (e.g. viridans streptococci) | Benzylpenicillin (*or* vancomycin if penicillin-allergic) + low-dose gentamicin (i.e. 60–80 mg twice daily) | Treat for 4 weeks; stop gentamicin after 2 weeks if organism fully sensitive to penicillin. Oral amoxycillin[1] may be substituted for benzylpenicillin after 2 weeks |
| Streptococci with reduced sensitivity to penicillin e.g. *Streptococcus faecalis* | Benzylpenicillin (*or* vancomycin if penicillin-allergic) + low-dose gentamicin (i.e. 60–80 mg twice daily) | Treat for at least 4 weeks |
| *Staphylococcus aureus* (and *Staphylococcus epidermidis*) | Flucloxacillin[2] + *either* gentamicin *or* fusidic acid (*or* vancomycin alone if penicillin-allergic) | Treat for at least 4 weeks; stop gentamicin after 2 weeks |
| **3: Respiratory system** | | |
| Haemophilus epiglottitis | Chloramphenicol | Give intravenously |
| Exacerbations of chronic bronchitis | Amoxycillin[1] *or* trimethoprim *or* erythromycin *or* tetracycline | Note that 20% of pneumococci and some *Haemophilus influenzae* strains are tetracycline-resistant |
| Pneumonia: | | |
| Previously healthy chest | Benzylpenicillin *or* amoxycillin[1] | Add flucloxacillin[2] if *Staphylococcus* suspected e.g. in influenza or measles; add erythromycin if *Mycoplasma pneumoniae* or *Legionella* infection is suspected (severe *Legionella* infections may require addition of rifampicin) |
| Previously unhealthy chest | Flucloxacillin[2] + amoxycillin[1] (*or* trimethoprim *or* erythromycin) | Substitute erythromycin (*or* rifampicin and erythromycin, see above) for flucloxacillin if *Legionella* infection is suspected; use erythromycin if *Mycoplasma pneumoniae* infection is suspected |
| Hospital-acquired | An aminoglycoside or a 'third generation' cephalosporin | |
| **4: Central nervous system** | | |
| Meningitis caused by: | | |
| *Meningococcus* | Benzylpenicillin[3] | Give rifampicin for 2 days before hospital discharge |
| *Pneumococcus* | Benzylpenicillin[3] | |
| *Haemophilus influenzae* | Chloramphenicol[3] | For *H. influenzae* type b give rifampicin for 4 days before hospital discharge |
| Listeria | Amoxycillin[1] + gentamicin | |

1. Where amoxycillin is suggested ampicillin or an ester of ampicillin (see section 5.1.1.3) may be used.
2. Where flucloxacillin is suggested cloxacillin may be used.
3. A cephalosporin (e.g. cefotaxime) is an alternative for meningococcal, pneumococcal, or *H. influenzae* meningitis.

## Table 1. Summary of antibacterial therapy (*continued*)

| Infection | Suggested antibacterial | Comment |
|---|---|---|
| **7:   Urinary tract** | | |
| Acute pyelonephritis or prostatitis | Trimethoprim *or* gentamicin *or* cephalosporin *or* ciprofloxacin | Do not give trimethoprim in pregnancy. Treat prostatitis with trimethoprim for 4 weeks |
| 'Lower' UTI | Trimethoprim *or* amoxycillin[1] *or* nitrofurantoin *or* oral cephalosporin | |
| **7:   Genital system** | | |
| Syphilis | Procaine penicillin (*or* tetracycline *or* erythromycin if penicillin-allergic) | Treat for 10–21 days |
| Gonorrhoea | Amoxycillin[1] with probenecid (*or* spectinomycin, *or* ciprofloxacin if penicillin-allergic) | Single-dose treatment in uncomplicated infection; choice depends on locality where infection acquired; contact-tracing advised; remember chlamydia |
| Non-gonococcal urethritis | Tetracycline | Treat for 7–21 days; contact-tracing advised |
| Pelvic inflammatory disease | Metronidazole + doxycycline *or* co-amoxiclav alone | Remember gonorrhoea; co-amoxiclav is not active against chlamydia; severely ill patients may require gentamicin (or a 'second-generation' cephalosporin) + a tetracycline |
| **9:   Blood** | | |
| Septicaemia Initial 'blind' therapy | Aminoglycoside + a penicillin *or* a cephalosporin alone *In immunocompromised*, aminoglycoside + a broad-spectrum penicillin *or* a 'third generation' cephalosporin alone | Choice depends on local resistance patterns and clinical presentation; add metronidazole if anaerobic infection suspected; add flucloxacillin[2] *or* vancomycin if Gram-positive infection suspected |
| **10:   Musculoskeletal system** | | |
| Osteomyelitis and septic arthritis | Clindamycin alone *or* flucloxacillin[2] + fusidic acid. If *Haemophilus influenzae* give amoxycillin[1] *or* cefuroxime | Under 5 years of age may be *H. influenzae*. Treat acute disease for at least 6 weeks and chronic infection for at least 12 weeks |
| **11:   Eye** | | |
| Purulent conjunctivitis | Chloramphenicol *or* gentamicin eye-drops | |
| **12:   Ear, nose, and oropharynx** | | |
| Dental infections | Phenoxymethylpenicillin (*or* amoxycillin[1]) *or* erythromycin *or* metronidazole | Tetracycline for chronic destructive forms of periodontal disease |
| Sinusitis | Amoxycillin[1] *or* doxycycline | |
| Otitis media | Benzylpenicillin Phenoxymethylpenicillin | Initial i/m therapy (if possible) with benzylpenicillin, then oral therapy with phenoxymethylpenicillin |
| | Amoxycillin[1] if under 5 years (*or* erythromycin if penicillin-allergic) | Under 5 years of age may be *Haemophilus influenzae* |
| Otitis externa | Flucloxacillin[2] | |
| Throat infections | Benzylpenicillin Phenoxymethylpenicillin (*or* erythromycin if penicillin-allergic) | Initial i/m therapy (in severe infection) with benzylpenicillin, then oral therapy with phenoxymethylpenicillin; treat beta-haemolytic streptococcal infections for at least 10 days. Most infections are caused by viruses |
| **13:   Skin** | | |
| Impetigo | Topical chlortetracycline *or* oral flucloxacillin[2] or erythromycin if systemic toxicity | |
| Erysipelas | Benzylpenicillin Phenoxymethylpenicillin | Initial i/m therapy (if possible) with benzylpenicillin, then oral therapy with phenoxymethylpenicillin |
| Cellulitis | Phenoxymethylpenicillin + flucloxacillin[2] (*or* erythromycin alone if penicillin-allergic) *or* co-amoxiclav alone | Severe cellulitis may require parenteral benzylpenicillin + flucloxacillin or co-amoxiclav alone |
| Acne | Tetracycline | Treat for at least 3–4 months |

1. Where amoxycillin is suggested ampicillin or an ester of ampicillin (see section 5.1.1.3) may be used.
2. Where flucloxacillin is suggested cloxacillin may be used.

## Table 2. Summary of antibacterial prophylaxis

| Infection | Antibacterial and dose |
|---|---|
| Prevention of recurrence of rheumatic fever | Phenoxymethylpenicillin 250 mg twice daily *or* sulphadimidine 500 mg daily (250 mg for children) |
| Prevention of secondary case of meningococcal meningitis | Rifampicin 600 mg every 12 hours for 2 days; CHILD 10 mg/kg (3 months–1 year, 5 mg/kg) every 12 hours for 2 days *or* sulphadimidine (if strain known to be sensitive) 1 g every 12 hours for 2 days; CHILD 500 mg (3 months–1 year, 250 mg) every 12 hours for 2 days |
| Prevention of secondary case of *Haemophilus influenzae* type b disease | Rifampicin 600 mg once daily for 4 days (optimum regimen for adults); CHILD over 3 months 20 mg/kg once daily for 4 days (max. 600 mg daily) |
| Prevention of secondary case of diphtheria in non-immune patient | Erythromycin 500 mg every 6 hours for 5 days |
| Prevention of endocarditis in patients with heart-valve lesion, septal defect, patent ductus, or prosthetic valve | *Dental procedures under local or no anaesthesia*, patients who have not received a penicillin more than once in the previous month, including those with a prosthetic heart valve (but not those who have had endocarditis), oral amoxycillin 3 g 1 hour before procedure; CHILD under 5 years quarter adult dose; 5–10 years half adult dose<br>patients who are penicillin-allergic or have received a penicillin more than once in the previous month,<br>*either* oral erythromycin 1.5 g (as stearate) 1–2 hours before procedure, then 500 mg 6 hours later; CHILD under 5 years quarter adult dose; 5–10 years half adult dose<br>*or* oral clindamycin 600 mg 1 hour before procedure; CHILD under 10 years 6 mg/kg<br>patients who have had endocarditis, amoxycillin + gentamicin, as under general anaesthesia |
| | *Dental procedures under general anaesthesia*, no special risk, *either* i/m amoxycillin 1 g just before induction, then oral amoxycillin 500 mg 6 hours later; CHILD under 10 years half adult dose<br>*or* oral amoxycillin 3 g 4 hours before induction then oral amoxycillin 3 g as soon as possible after procedure; CHILD under 5 years quarter adult dose; 5–10 years half adult dose<br>*or* oral amoxycillin 3 g + oral probenecid 1 g 4 hours before procedure;<br>*special risk* (patients with a prosthetic heart valve or who have had endocarditis), i/m amoxycillin 1 g + i/m gentamicin 120 mg just before induction, then oral amoxycillin 500 mg 6 hours later; CHILD under 10 years amoxycillin half adult dose, gentamicin 2 mg/kg<br>patients who are penicillin-allergic or who have received a penicillin more than once in the previous month, i/v vancomycin 1 g over at least 100 minutes then i/v gentamicin 120 mg just before induction or 15 minutes before procedure; CHILD under 10 years vancomycin 20 mg/kg, gentamicin 2 mg/kg |
| | *Upper respiratory-tract procedures*, as for dental procedures; post-operative dose may be given parenterally if swallowing is painful |
| | *Genito-urinary procedures*, as for special risk patients undergoing dental procedures under general anaesthesia, see above; if urine infected, prophylaxis should cover infective organism |
| | *Obstetric, gynaecological and gastro-intestinal procedures* (prophylaxis required for patients with prosthetic valves only) as for genito-urinary procedures |
| Prevention of gas-gangrene in high lower-limb amputations or following major trauma | Benzylpenicillin 300–600 mg every 6 hours for 5 days *or* if penicillin-allergic give metronidazole 500 mg every 8 hours |
| Prevention of tuberculosis in susceptible close contacts | Isoniazid 300 mg daily for 6 months; CHILD, isoniazid 5–10 mg/kg daily *or* isoniazid 300 mg daily + rifampicin 600 mg daily (450 mg if less than 50 kg) for 3 months; CHILD isoniazid 5–10 mg/kg daily + rifampicin 10 mg/kg daily |

Prevention of infection in abdominal surgery

| | |
|---|---|
| Operations on stomach or oesophagus for carcinoma, or cholecystectomy in patients with possibly infected bile | Single immediate pre-operative dose of gentamicin *or* a cephalosporin |
| Resections of colon and rectum for carcinoma, and resections in inflammatory bowel disease | Single immediate pre-operative dose of *either* gentamicin + metronidazole *or* cefuroxime + metronidazole |
| Hysterectomy | Metronidazole as suppository *or* single i/v dose |

*Note.* High-dose 3-g amoxycillin regimens are now considered suitable for patients who have received a penicillin not more than once in the previous month

Cautionary label wordings, see inside back cover

Prices are **net**, see p. 1

## 5.1.1  Penicillins

5.1.1.1  Benzylpenicillin and phenoxymethyl-
         penicillin
5.1.1.2  Penicillinase-resistant penicillins
5.1.1.3  Broad-spectrum penicillins
5.1.1.4  Antipseudomonal penicillins
5.1.1.5  Mecillinams

The penicillins are bactericidal and act by interfering with bacterial cell wall synthesis. They diffuse well into body tissues and fluids, but
penetration into the cerebrospinal fluid is poor
except when the meninges are inflamed. They are
excreted in the urine in therapeutic concentrations. Probenecid blocks the renal tubular
excretion of the penicillins, producing higher and
more prolonged plasma concentrations (see section 10.1.4); it is not recommended in children
under 2 years of age.

The most important side-effect of the penicillins
is hypersensitivity, which causes rashes and,
occasionally, anaphylaxis, which can be fatal.
Patients who are allergic to one penicillin will be
allergic to all as the hypersensitivity is related to
the basic penicillin structure. A rare but serious
toxic effect of the penicillins is encephalopathy
due to cerebral irritation. This may result from
excessively high doses but can also develop with
normal doses given to patients with renal failure.
The penicillins should **not** be given by intrathecal
injection as they can cause encephalopathy which
may be fatal.

A second problem relating to high doses of
penicillin, or normal doses given to patients with
renal failure, is the accumulation of electrolyte
since most injectable penicillins contain either
sodium or potassium.

Diarrhoea frequently occurs during oral penicillin therapy. It is most common with ampicillin
and its derivatives, which can also cause pseudomembranous colitis.

---

### 5.1.1.1  BENZYLPENICILLIN AND
PHENOXYMETHYLPENICILLIN

---

**Benzylpenicillin** (Penicillin G), the first of the
penicillins, remains an important and useful antibiotic but is inactivated by bacterial penicillinases
(beta-lactamases). It is the drug of choice for
streptococcal, pneumococcal, gonococcal, and
meningococcal    infections    and    also
for actinomycosis, anthrax, diphtheria, gas-
gangrene, leptospirosis, syphilis, tetanus, yaws,
and treatment of Lyme disease in children. Pneumococci, meningococci, and gonococci which
have decreased sensitivity to penicillin have been
isolated. Benzylpenicillin is inactivated by gastric
acid and absorption from the gut is low; therefore
it is best given by injection. Benzylpenicillin may
cause convulsions after high doses by intravenous
injection or in renal failure.

**Procaine penicillin** is a sparingly soluble salt of
benzylpenicillin. It is used in intramuscular depot

preparations which provide therapeutic tissue
concentrations for up to 24 hours. It is the preferred choice for the treatment of syphilis; neuro-
syphilis requires special consideration.

**Benethamine penicillin** is a benzylpenicillin salt
with very low solubility giving a prolonged action
after intramuscular injection, though producing
low plasma concentrations; it is used, with soluble
and procaine penicillin, in Triplopen® (which is
effective for syphilis).

**Phenoxymethylpenicillin** (Penicillin V) has a
similar antibacterial spectrum to benzylpenicillin,
but is less active. It is gastric acid-stable, so is
suitable for oral administration. It should not be
used for serious infections because absorption
can be unpredictable and plasma concentrations
variable. It is indicated principally for respiratory-
tract infections in children, for streptococcal tonsillitis, and for continuing treatment after one or
more injections of benzylpenicillin when clinical
response has begun. It should not be used
for meningococcal or gonococcal infections.
Phenoxymethylpenicillin is used for prophylaxis
against streptococcal infections following rheumatic fever.

---

## BENZYLPENICILLIN
(Penicillin G)
*Indications:* tonsillitis, otitis media, erysipelas,
   streptococcal endocarditis, meningococcal and
   pneumococcal meningitis, prophylaxis in limb
   amputation
*Cautions:* history of allergy; renal impairment;
   **interactions:** Appendix 1 (penicillins)
*Contra-indications:* penicillin hypersensitivity
*Side-effects:* sensitivity reactions including urticaria, fever, joint pains; angioedema; anaphylactic shock in hypersensitive patients;
   diarrhoea after administration by mouth
*Dose: by intramuscular or by slow intravenous
   injection or by infusion,* 1.2 g daily in 4 divided
   doses, increased if necessary to 2.4 g daily or
   more (see also below); NEONATE,  30 mg/kg
   daily (in 2 divided doses in the first few days of
   life then in 3–4 divided doses); CHILD 1 month–
   12 years, 10–20 mg/kg daily in 4 divided doses
Bacterial endocarditis, *by slow intravenous injection or by infusion,* 7.2 g daily in 4–6 divided
   doses
Meningitis, *by slow intravenous injection or by
   infusion,* 2.4 g every 4–6 hours; CHILD 1 month–
   12 years, 180–300 mg/kg daily in 4–6 divided
   doses
Prophylaxis in limb amputation, section 5.1,
   Table 2
*By intrathecal injection,* **not** recommended, see
   section 5.1.1

PoM **Crystapen**® (Glaxo)
   *Injection,* powder for reconstitution, benzypeni-
   cillin sodium (unbuffered). Net price 600-mg
   vial = 12p
   *Electrolytes:* Na+ 1.68 mmol/600-mg vial

---

## BENETHAMINE PENICILLIN
*Indications:* penicillin-sensitive infections; prophylaxis
*Cautions; Contra-indications; Side-effects:* see under Benzylpenicillin

PoM **Triplopen**® (Glaxo)
*Injection*, powder for reconstitution, benethamine penicillin 475 mg, procaine penicillin 250 mg, benzylpenicillin sodium 300 mg. Net price per vial = 40p
*Electrolytes:* Na+ 1.2 mmol/vial
*Dose:* by deep intramuscular injection, 1 vial every 2–3 days

## BENZATHINE PENICILLIN
*Indications:* penicillin-sensitive infections
*Cautions; Contra-indications; Side-effects:* see under Benzylpenicillin
*Dose:* see below

PoM **Penidural**® (Wyeth)
*Suspension*, pink, benzathine penicillin 229 mg/ 5 mL. Net price 100 mL = £1.49. Label: 9
*Dose:* 10 mL 3–4 times daily; CHILD 5 mL 3–4 times daily
*Paediatric drops*, pink, benzathine penicillin 115 mg/mL. Net price 10 mL = £1.63. Label: 9, counselling, use of pipette
*Dose:* CHILD up to 5 years, 1–2 dropperfuls (approx. 77–154 mg) 3–4 times daily

## PHENOXYMETHYLPENICILLIN
(Penicillin V)
*Indications:* tonsillitis, otitis media, erysipelas, rheumatic fever prophylaxis
*Cautions; Contra-indications; Side-effects:* see under Benzylpenicillin; **interactions:** Appendix 1 (penicillins)
*Dose:* 250–500 mg every 6 hours, at least 30 minutes before food; CHILD, every 6 hours, up to 1 year 62.5 mg, 1–5 years 125 mg, 6–12 years 250 mg

PoM **Phenoxymethylpenicillin** (Non-proprietary)
*Capsules*, phenoxymethylpenicillin (as potassium salt) 250 mg, net price 20 = 38p. Label: 9, 23
*Tablets*, phenoxymethylpenicillin (as potassium salt) 250 mg, net price 20 = 33p. Label: 9, 23
Available from APS (Apsin®), Berk, Cox, Evans, Kerfoot
*Oral solution*, phenoxymethylpenicillin (as potassium salt) for reconstitution with water, 125 mg/5 mL, net price 100 mL = 54p; 250 mg/ 5 mL, 100 mL = 81p. Label: 9, 23
Available from APS (Apsin®), Cox, Evans, Kerfoot
PoM **Distaquaine V-K**® (Dista)
*Tablets*, scored, phenoxymethylpenicillin (as potassium salt) 250 mg, net price 20 = 29p. Label: 9, 23
PoM **Stabillin V-K**® (Boots)
*Tablets*, phenoxymethylpenicillin 250 mg (as potassium salt). Net price 20 = 28p. Label: 9, 23

*Elixir*, phenoxymethylpenicillin (as potassium salt) for reconstitution with water, 62.5 mg/ 5 mL, net price 100 mL = 52p; 125 mg/5 mL, 100 mL = 65p; 250 mg/5 mL 100 mL = £1.04. Label: 9, 23
PoM **V-Cil-K**® (Lilly)
*Capsules*, pink, phenoxymethylpenicillin 250 mg (as potassium salt). Net price 20 = 38p. Label: 9, 23
*Tablets*, phenoxymethylpenicillin (as potassium salt) 250 mg, net price 20 = 29p. Label: 9, 23
*Paediatric syrup*, phenoxymethylpenicillin (as potassium salt) for reconstitution with water, 125 mg/5 mL, net price 100 mL = 44p. Label: 9, 23

## PROCAINE PENICILLIN
*Indications:* penicillin-sensitive infections
*Cautions; Contra-indications; Side-effects:* see under Benzylpenicillin; **not** for intravenous administration
*Dose:* see below

PoM **Bicillin**® (Brocades)
*Injection*, powder for reconstitution, procaine penicillin 1.8 g, benzylpenicillin sodium 360 mg. Net price 6-mL multidose vial = £1.93
*Electrolytes:* Na+ 1 mmol/vial
*Dose:* when reconstituted with 4.6 mL water for injections, 1 mL (procaine penicillin 300 mg, benzylpenicillin sodium 60 mg) every 12–24 hours by intramuscular injection
Early syphilis, by intramuscular injection, 3 mL (4 mL in heavier patients) daily for 10 days
*Note.* Reconstitution with 4.6 mL water for injections produces 6 mL

### 5.1.1.2 PENICILLINASE-RESISTANT PENICILLINS

Most staphylococci are now resistant to benzylpenicillin because they produce penicillinases. **Cloxacillin** and **flucloxacillin**, however, are not inactivated by these enzymes and are thus effective in infections caused by penicillin-resistant staphylococci, which is the sole indication for their use. They are acid-stable and can, therefore, be given by mouth as well as by injection.

Flucloxacillin is better absorbed from the gut than cloxacillin and is, therefore, to be preferred for oral therapy.

**Methicillin** is also effective against penicillin-resistant *Staph. aureus*, but can only be given by injection because it is not acid-stable and is now seldom used.

*Staph. aureus* strains resistant to methicillin and cloxacillin have emerged in some hospitals; some of these organisms are only sensitive to vancomycin (section 5.1.7). Other alternatives include rifampicin, teicoplanin, and ciprofloxacin.

**Temocillin** is a new penicillin with activity against penicillinase-producing Gram-negative bacteria (except *Pseudomonas aeruginosa*); it is not active against Gram-positive bacteria.

---

## CLOXACILLIN

*Indications:* infections due to penicillinase-producing staphylococci

*Cautions; Contra-indications; Side-effects:* see under Benzylpenicillin (section 5.1.1.1)

*Dose: by mouth,* 500 mg every 6 hours, at least 30 minutes before food

*By intramuscular injection,* 250 mg every 4–6 hours

*By slow intravenous injection or by infusion,* 500 mg every 4–6 hours

Doses may be doubled in severe infections

CHILD, any route, under 2 years quarter adult dose; 2–10 years half adult dose

*Note.* Oral liquid preparation no longer marketed

PoM **Cloxacillin** (Non-proprietary)
*Capsules,* cloxacillin (as sodium salt) 250 mg, net price 20 = £3.64; 500 mg, 20 = £7.29. Label: 9, 23

PoM **Orbenin**® (Beecham)
*Capsules,* both orange/black, cloxacillin (as sodium salt) 250 mg, net price 20 = £3.64; 500 mg, 20 = £7.29. Label: 9, 23
*Injection,* powder for reconstitution, cloxacillin (as sodium salt). Net price 250-mg vial = 93p; 500-mg vial = £1.86; also available as 1-g vial
*Electrolytes:* Na$^+$ 0.59 mmol/250-mg vial, 1.18 mmol/500-mg vial

## FLUCLOXACILLIN

*Indications:* infections due to penicillinase-producing staphylococci

*Cautions; Contra-indications; Side-effects:* see under Benzylpenicillin (section 5.1.1.1); hepatitis and cholestatic jaundice reported rarely; avoid in porphyria (see section 9.8.2)

*Dose: by mouth,* 250 mg every 6 hours, at least 30 minutes before food

*By intramuscular injection,* 250 mg every 6 hours

*By slow intravenous injection or by infusion,* 0.25–1 g every 6 hours

Doses may be doubled in severe infections

CHILD, any route, under 2 years quarter adult dose; 2–10 years half adult dose

PoM **Flucloxacillin** (Non-proprietary)
*Capsules,* flucloxacillin (as sodium salt) 250 mg, net price 20 = £2.70; 500 mg, 20 = £5.60. Label: 9, 23
Available from APS, Ashbourne (Fluclomix®), Berk (Ladropen®), Brocades (Stafoxil®), Cox, Evans, Kerfoot

*Oral solution* (= elixir or syrup), flucloxacillin (as sodium salt) for reconstitution with water, 125 mg/5 mL. Net price 100 mL = £3.22. Label: 9, 23
Available from APS, Cox

*Oral suspension* (= mixture), flucloxacillin (as magnesium salt) for reconstitution with water, 125 mg/5 mL, net price 100 mL = £3.32; 250 mg/5 mL, 100 mL = £6.64. Label: 9, 23

PoM **Floxapen**® (Beecham)
*Capsules,* both black/caramel, flucloxacillin (as sodium salt) 250 mg, net price 20-cap pack = £4.62, 28-cap pack = £6.47; 500 mg, 28-cap pack = £12.95. Label: 9, 23

*Syrup,* flucloxacillin 125 mg (as magnesium salt)/5 mL when reconstituted with water. Net price 100 mL = £3.32. Label: 9, 23

*Syrup forte,* flucloxacillin 250 mg (as magnesium salt)/5 mL when reconstituted with water. Net price 100 mL = £6.64. Label: 9, 23

*Injection,* powder for reconstitution, flucloxacillin (as sodium salt). Net price 250-mg vial = 93p; 500-mg vial = £1.86; 1-g vial = £3.71
*Electrolytes:* Na$^+$ 0.57 mmol/250-mg vial, 1.13 mmol/500-mg vial, 2.26 mmol/1-g vial

PoM **Ladropen**® (Berk)
*Injection,* powder for reconstitution, flucloxacillin (as sodium salt). Net price 250-mg vial = 77p; 500-mg vial = £1.76

## METHICILLIN SODIUM

*Indications:* infections due to penicillinase-producing staphylococci

*Cautions; Contra-indications; Side-effects:* see under Benzylpenicillin (section 5.1.1.1)

*Dose: by intramuscular injection or by intravenous injection* over 3–4 minutes *or by intravenous infusion,* 1 g every 4–6 hours; CHILD under 2 years quarter adult dose; 2–10 years half adult dose

PoM **Celbenin**® (Beecham)
*Injection,* powder for reconstitution, methicillin sodium. Net price 1-g vial = £1.88
*Electrolytes:* Na$^+$ 2.44 mmol/g

## TEMOCILLIN

*Indications:* infections due to penicillinase-producing Gram-negative bacteria except pseudomonas.

*Cautions; Contra-indications; Side-effects:* see under Benzylpenicillin (section 5.1.1.1)

*Dose: by intramuscular injection or by intravenous injection* (over 3–4 minutes) *or by intravenous infusion,* 1–2 g every 12 hours

Acute uncomplicated urinary-tract infections, 1 g daily as a single dose or in divided doses

▼ PoM **Temopen**® (Bencard)
*Injection,* powder for reconstitution, temocillin (as sodium salt). Net price 500-mg vial = £7.50; 1-g vial = £15.00
*Electrolytes:* Na$^+$ 5 mmol/g

### 5.1.1.3   BROAD-SPECTRUM PENICILLINS

**Ampicillin** is active against certain Gram-positive and Gram-negative organisms but is inactivated by penicillinases including those produced by *Staphylococcus aureus* and by common Gram-negative bacilli such as *Escherichia coli*. Almost all staphylococci, 40% of *E. coli* strains and up to one-tenth of *Haemophilus influenzae* strains are now resistant. The likelihood of resistance should therefore be considered before using ampicillin for the 'blind' treatment of infections; in particular, it should not be used for hospital patients without checking sensitivity.

Ampicillin is well excreted in the bile and urine. It is principally indicated for the treatment of

---

exacerbations of chronic bronchitis and middle ear infections, both of which are usually due to *Streptococcus pneumoniae* and *H. influenzae*, and for urinary-tract infections (section 5.1.13) and gonorrhoea.

Ampicillin can be given by mouth but less than half the dose is absorbed, and absorption is further decreased by the presence of food in the gut. Higher plasma concentrations are obtained with the ampicillin esters **bacampicillin, pivampicillin** and **talampicillin**; their absorption is little affected by the presence of food, and the incidence of diarrhoea is less than with ampicillin. These antibiotics should be given every 8 hours for moderate or severe infections, especially outside the renal tract.

Maculopapular rashes commonly occur with ampicillin (and amoxycillin) but are not usually related to true penicillin allergy. They almost always occur in patients with glandular fever; broad-spectrum penicillins should not therefore be used for 'blind' treatment of a sore throat. Rashes are also common in patients with chronic lymphatic leukaemia and in patients infected with the human immunodeficiency virus (HIV).

**Amoxycillin** is a derivative of ampicillin which differs by only one hydroxyl group and has a similar antibacterial spectrum. It is, however, better absorbed when given by mouth, producing higher plasma and tissue concentrations; unlike ampicillin, absorption is not affected by the presence of food in the stomach.

**Co-amoxiclav** consists of amoxycillin with the beta-lactamase inhibitor clavulanic acid. Clavulanic acid itself has no significant antibacterial activity but, by inactivating penicillinases, it makes the combination active against penicillinase-producing bacteria that are resistant to amoxycillin. These include most *Staph. aureus*, 40% of *E. coli* strains, and up to 10% of *H. influenzae* strains, as well as many *Bacteroides* and *Klebsiella* spp. **Sulbactam** is another beta-lactamase inhibitor which is available in combination with ampicillin as Dicapen®.

Combinations of ampicillin with flucloxacillin (as co-fluampicil) and ampicillin with cloxacillin (Ampiclox®) are available.

**Mezlocillin** is a ureidopenicillin which is active against certain ampicillin-resistant bacteria. However, like ampicillin, it is inactivated by beta-lactamases. It possesses anti-pseudomonal activity.

## AMOXYCILLIN

**Indications:** see under Ampicillin; also typhoid fever and dental prophylaxis

**Cautions; Contra-indications; Side-effects:** see under Ampicillin

**Dose:** *by mouth*, 250 mg every 8 hours, doubled in severe infections; CHILD up to 10 years, 125 mg every 8 hours, doubled in severe infections

Severe or recurrent purulent respiratory infection, 3 g every 12 hours; CHILD 2–5 years 750 mg every 12 hours, 5–10 years 1.5 g every 12 hours Dental prophylaxis, section 5.1, Table 2

*Short-course oral therapy*
Dental abscess, 3 g repeated after 8 hours
Urinary-tract infections, 3 g repeated after 10–12 hours
Gonorrhoea, single dose of 3 g with probenecid 1 g
Otitis media, CHILD 3–10 years, 750 mg twice daily for 2 days

*By intramuscular injection*, 500 mg every 8 hours; CHILD, 50–100 mg/kg daily in divided doses

*By intravenous injection or infusion.* 500 mg every 8 hours increased to 1 g every 6 hours; CHILD, 50–100 mg/kg daily in divided doses

PoM **Amoxycillin** (Non-proprietary)
*Capsules*, amoxycillin (as trihydrate) 250 mg, net price 20 = £2.80; 500 mg, 20 = £5.60. Label: 9
Available from APS, Ashbourne (Amix®), Berk (Almodan®), BHR (Amrit®), Cox, Eastern (Amoram®), Evans, Galen (Galenamox®), Kerfoot, Lagap, Rima (Rimoxallin®)

*Oral suspension*, amoxycillin (as trihydrate) for reconstitution with water, 125 mg/5 mL, net price 100 mL = £1.75; 250 mg/5 mL, 100 mL = £3.26. Label: 9.
Available from APS, Ashbourne (Amix®), Berk (Almodan®), BHR (Amrit®), Cox, Eastern (Amoram®), Evans, Galen (Galenamox®), Kerfoot, Lagap, Rima (Rimoxallin®)

PoM **Almodan**® (Berk)
*Injection*, powder for reconstitution, amoxycillin (as sodium salt), 250-mg vial, net price = 39p; 500-mg vial = 71p

PoM **Amoxil**® (Bencard)
*Capsules*, both maroon/gold, amoxycillin (as trihydrate), 250 mg, net price 21-cap pack = £3.67; 500 mg, 21-cap pack = £7.35. Label: 9
*Dispersible tablets*, sugar-free, amoxycillin 500 mg (as trihydrate). Net price 21-tab pack = £8.48. Label: 9, 13
*Fiztab* (= chewable tablets), sugar-free, amoxycillin (as trihydrate) 125 mg, net price 20-tab pack = £2.20; 250 mg, 20-tab pack = £4.40; 500 mg, 20-tab pack = £8.80. Label: 9, 10 patient information leaflet
*Note.* Dose form not suitable for children under 3 years
*Syrup SF*, both sugar-free, amoxycillin (as trihydrate) for reconstitution with water, 125 mg/5 mL, net price 100 mL = £2.20; 250 mg/5 mL, 100 mL = £4.40. Label: 9
*Paediatric suspension*, amoxycillin 125 mg (as trihydrate)/1.25 mL when reconstituted with water. Net price 20 mL = £3.30. Label: 9, counselling, use of pipette
*Sachets SF*, powder, sugar-free, amoxycillin 750 mg (as trihydrate)/sachet, net price 4-sachet pack = £2.86; 3 g/sachet, 2-sachet pack = £4.73; 14-sachet pack = £33.11. Label: 9, 13
*Injection*, powder for reconstitution, amoxycillin (as sodium salt). Net price 250-mg vial = 36p; 500-mg vial = 66p; 1-g vial = £1.31
*Electrolytes:* Na+ 3.2 mmol/g

PoM **Flemoxin Solutab®** (Brocades)
*Dispersible tablets*, sugar-free, both scored, amoxycillin (as trihydrate) 375 mg, net price 10-tab pack = £2.62; 750 mg, 10-tab pack = £5.25. Label: 9, 13
*Dose:* 375 mg every 12 hours, doubled in severe infections; CHILD 5–10 years half usual adult dose
Severe or recurrent respiratory-tract infection, see under Dose on p. 199

## AMPICILLIN

*Indications:* urinary-tract infections, otitis media, chronic bronchitis, invasive salmonellosis, gonorrhoea
*Cautions:* history of allergy; renal impairment; erythematous rashes common in glandular fever, chronic lymphatic leukaemia, and HIV infection; **interactions:** Appendix 1 (penicillins)
*Contra-indications:* penicillin hypersensitivity
*Side-effects:* nausea, diarrhoea; rashes (discontinue treatment); rarely, pseudomembranous colitis; see also under Benzylpenicillin (section 5.1.1.1)
*Dose: by mouth*, 0.25–1 g every 6 hours, at least 30 minutes before food
Gonorrhoea, 2 g as a single dose with probenecid 1 g
Urinary-tract infections, 500 mg every 8 hours
*By intramuscular injection or intravenous injection or infusion*, 500 mg every 4–6 hours; higher doses in meningitis
CHILD under 10 years, any route, half adult dose

PoM **Ampicillin** (Non-proprietary)
*Capsules*, ampicillin 250 mg, net price 20 = 67p; 500 mg, 20 = £1.41. Label: 9, 23
Available from APS, Berk (Vidopen®), Brocades (Amfipen®), Cox, Evans, Kerfoot, Lagap, Rima (Rimacillin®)
*Oral suspension*, ampicillin 125 mg/5 mL when reconstituted with water, net price 100 mL = 76p; 250 mg/5 mL, 100 mL = £1.23. Label: 9, 23
Available from APS, Berk, Brocades (Amfipen®), Cox, Evans, Kerfoot, Lagap, Rima (Rimacillin®)
PoM **Penbritin®** (Beecham)
*Capsules*, both black/red, ampicillin (as trihydrate) 250 mg, net price 28-cap pack = £2.05; 500 mg, 28-cap pack = £4.10. Label: 9, 23
*Syrup*, ampicillin 125 mg (as trihydrate)/5 mL when reconstituted with water. Net price 100 mL = £1.09. Label: 9, 23
*Syrup forte*, ampicillin 250 mg (as trihydrate)/5 mL when reconstituted with water. Net price 100 mL = £2.17. Label: 9, 23
*Paediatric suspension*, pink, ampicillin 125 mg (as trihydrate)/1.25 mL. Net price 25 mL = £2.03. Label: 9, 23, counselling, use of pipette
*Injection*, powder for reconstitution, ampicillin (as sodium salt). Net price 250-mg vial = 33p; 500-mg vial = 67p
*Electrolytes:* Na+ 0.73 mmol/250 mg
PoM **Vidopen®** (Berk)
*Injection*, powder for reconstitution, ampicillin (as sodium salt). Net price 250-mg vial = 33p; 500-mg vial = 67p.

With cloxacillin
PoM **Ampiclox®** (Beecham)
*Injection*, ampicillin 250 mg (as sodium salt), cloxacillin 250 mg (as sodium salt). Net price per vial = £1.36
*Electrolytes:* Na+ 1.32 mmol/vial
*Dose:* by intramuscular injection or intravenous injection or infusion, 1–2 vials every 4–6 hours; CHILD up to 2 years quarter adult dose, 2–10 years half adult dose
PoM **Ampiclox Neonatal®** (Beecham)
*Suspension*, sugar-free, ampicillin 60 mg (as trihydrate), cloxacillin 30 mg (as sodium salt)/ 0.6 mL when reconstituted with water. Net price 10 mL = £2.06. Label: 9, counselling, use of pipette
*Dose:* 0.6 mL every 4 hours

## AMPICILLIN WITH SULBACTAM

*Indications:* infections due to beta-lactamase-producing organisms; prophylaxis in abdominal and obstetric procedures
*Cautions; Contra-indications; Side-effects:* see under Ampicillin
*Dose: by intramuscular injection or by intravenous injection* over 3 minutes *or by intravenous infusion*, expressed as ampicillin, 1 g every 6–8 hours, doubled for severe infections (max. 8 g daily); CHILD, expressed as ampicillin, 100 mg/kg in 3–4 divided doses (2 divided doses in neonates)
Surgical prophylaxis, expressed as ampicillin, 1–2 g at induction; may be repeated every 6–8 hours for up to 24 hours

▼ PoM **Dicapen®** (Leo)
*Injection 750 mg*, powder for reconstitution, ampicillin (as sodium salt) 500 mg, sulbactam (as sodium salt) 250 mg. Net price per vial = £1.23
*Electrolytes:* Na+ 2.5 mmol/vial
*Injection 1.5 g*, powder for reconstitution, ampicillin (as sodium salt) 1 g, sulbactam (as sodium salt) 500 mg. Net price per vial = £2.46
*Electrolytes:* Na+ 5 mmol/vial
*Injection 3 g*, powder for reconstitution, ampicillin (as sodium salt) 2 g, sulbactam (as sodium salt) 1 g. Net price per vial = £4.92
*Electrolytes:* Na+ 10 mmol/vial
▼ PoM **Unasyn®** (Pfizer)
*Injection 750 mg*, powder for reconstitution, ampicillin (as sodium salt) 500 mg, sulbactam (as sodium salt) 250 mg. Net price per vial = £1.11
*Electrolytes:* Na+ 2.5 mmol/vial

Sultamicillin (Prodrug of ampicillin–sulbactam)
▼ PoM **Unasyn®** (Pfizer)
*Tablets*, sultamicillin (as tosylate) 375 mg (equivalent to ampicillin 220 mg, sulbactam 147 mg). Net price 14-tab pack = £6.30. Label: 9
*Dose:* ADULT and CHILD over 30 kg, upper respiratory-tract, urinary-tract and other mild infections, 1 tablet twice daily
Lower respiratory-tract, skin and soft tissue infections, sinusitis, and otitis media, 2 tablets twice daily
CHILD under 30 kg, dose form not appropriate

---

## BACAMPICILLIN HYDROCHLORIDE

*Indications; Cautions; Contra-indications; Side-effects:* see under Ampicillin

*Dose:* 400 mg 2–3 times daily, doubled in severe infections; CHILD over 5 years, 200 mg 3 times daily

Uncomplicated gonorrhoea, 1.6 g as a single dose with probenecid 1 g

PoM **Ambaxin**® (Upjohn)
*Tablets*, scored, bacampicillin hydrochloride 400 mg. Net price 20 = £6.34. Label: 9

## CO-AMOXICLAV

A mixture of amoxycillin (as the trihydrate or as the sodium salt) and clavulanic acid (as potassium clavulanate); the proportions are expressed in the form $x/y$ where $x$ and $y$ are the strengths in milligrams of amoxycillin and clavulanic acid respectively

*Indications; Cautions; Contra-indications; Side-effects:* see under Ampicillin and notes above; also caution in severe hepatic impairment; hepatitis, cholestatic jaundice, and erythema multiforme (including Stevens-Johnson syndrome) reported; phlebitis at injection site also reported

*Dose: by mouth*, expressed as amoxycillin, 250 mg every 8 hours, dose doubled in severe infections; CHILD see under preparations below (3 months–6 years Augmentin® Paediatric suspension; 6–12 years Augmentin® Junior suspension)

*By intravenous injection or infusion*, expressed as amoxycillin, 1 g every 8 hours increased to 1 g every 6 hours in more serious infections; INFANTS up to 3 months 25 mg/kg every 8 hours (every 12 hours in the perinatal period and in premature infants); CHILD 3 months–12 years, 25 mg/kg every 8 hours increased to 25 mg/kg every 6 hours in more serious infections

PoM **Augmentin**® (Beecham)
*Tablets*, f/c, co-amoxiclav 250/125 (amoxycillin 250 mg as trihydrate, clavulanic acid 125 mg as potassium salt). Net price 21-tab pack = £7.00; 30-tab pack = £10.13. Label: 9
*Dispersible tablets*, sugar-free, co-amoxiclav 250/125 (amoxycillin 250 mg as trihydrate, clavulanic acid 125 mg as potassium salt). Net price 21-tab pack = £7.86. Label: 9, 13
*Junior suspension*, sugar-free, co-amoxiclav 125/62 (amoxycillin 125 mg as trihydrate, clavulanic acid 62 mg as potassium salt)/5 mL when reconstituted with water. Net price 100 mL = £3.93. Label: 9
*Dose:* CHILD 6–12 years, 5 mL every 8 hours, increased to 10 mL in severe infections

*Paediatric suspension*, sugar-free, co-amoxiclav 125/31 (amoxycillin 125 mg as trihydrate, clavulanic acid 31 mg as potassium salt)/5 mL when reconstituted with water. Diluent not more than an equal volume of water, life of diluted suspension 7 days. Net price 100 mL = £3.12. Label: 9
*Dose:* CHILD 3–9 months, 1.25 mL every 8 hours; 9 months–2 years, 2.5 mL every 8 hours; 2–6 years, 5 mL every 8 hours, increased to 10 mL in severe infections
*Injection 600 mg*, powder for preparing intravenous injections, co-amoxiclav 500/100 (amoxycillin 500 mg as sodium salt, clavulanic acid 100 mg as potassium salt). Net price per vial = £1.35
*Electrolytes:* $Na^+$ 1.6 mmol, $K^+$ 0.5 mmol/600-mg vial
*Injection 1.2 g*, powder for preparing intravenous injections, co-amoxiclav 1000/200 (amoxycillin 1 g as sodium salt, clavulanic acid 200 mg as potassium salt). Net price per vial = £2.70
*Electrolytes:* $Na^+$ 3.1 mmol, $K^+$ 1 mmol/1.2-g vial

## CO-FLUAMPICIL

A mixture of equal parts by mass of flucloxacillin and ampicillin

*Indications:* mixed infections involving penicillinase-producing staphylococci

*Cautions; Contra-indications; Side-effects:* see under Ampicillin and Flucloxacillin

*Dose: by mouth*, co-fluampicil, 250/250 every 6 hours, dose doubled in severe infections; CHILD under 10 years half adult dose, dose doubled in severe infections

*By intramuscular or slow intravenous injection or by intravenous infusion*, co-fluampicil 250/250 every 6 hours, dose doubled in severe infections; CHILD under 2 years quarter adult dose, 2–10 years half adult dose, dose doubled in severe infections

PoM **Co-fluampicil** (Non-proprietary)
*Capsules*, co-fluampicil 250/250 (flucloxacillin 250 mg as sodium salt, ampicillin 250 mg as trihydrate). Net price 20 = £4.00. Label: 9, 23
Available from Generics (Flu-Amp®), Norton
PoM **Magnapen**® (Beecham)
*Capsules*, black/turquoise, co-fluampicil 250/250 (flucloxacillin 250 mg as sodium salt, ampicillin 250 mg as trihydrate). Net price 20-cap pack = £5.08. Label: 9, 23
*Syrup*, co-fluampicil 125/125 (flucloxacillin 125 mg as magnesium salt, ampicillin 125 mg as trihydrate)/5 mL when reconstituted with water. Net price 100 mL = £4.13. Label: 9, 23
*Injection 500 mg*, powder for reconstitution, co-fluampicil 250/250 (flucloxacillin 250 mg as sodium salt, ampicillin 250 mg as sodium salt). Net price per vial = £1.10
*Electrolytes:* $Na^+$ 1.3 mmol/vial
*Injection 1 g*, powder for reconstitution, co-fluampicil 500/500 (flucloxacillin 500 mg as sodium salt, ampicillin 500 mg as sodium salt). Net price per vial = £2.20
*Electrolytes:* $Na^+$ 2.6 mmol/vial

## MEZLOCILLIN

*Indications:* Gram-positive and Gram-negative infections (including enteric bacilli); see also notes above.

*Cautions; Contra-indications; Side-effects:* see under Benzylpenicillin (section 5.1.1.1); **interactions:** Appendix 1 (penicillins)

*Dose: by deep intramuscular injection,* 0.5–2 g every 6–8 hours

*By intravenous injection,* over 2–4 minutes, 2 g every 6–8 hours

Serious infections, *by intravenous infusion,* 5 g every 6–8 hours; NEONATE and PREMATURE INFANT, *by prolonged intravenous infusion,* 75 mg/kg every 12 hours; INFANT and CHILD, *by intravenous injection or infusion,* 75 mg/kg every 8 hours

Gonorrhoea, *by deep intramuscular injection,* 1 g as a single dose

PoM **Baypen**® (Bayer)

*Injection,* powder for reconstitution, mezlocillin (as sodium salt). Net price 500-mg vial = £1.20; 1-g vial = £1.85; 2-g vial = £3.36
*Electrolytes:* Na⁺ 1.85 mmol/g

*Infusion,* powder for reconstitution, mezlocillin (as sodium salt). Net price 5-g vial = £7.64 (also available with 50 mL water for injections, transfer needle, and infusion bag)
*Electrolytes:* Na⁺ 9.27 mmol/5-g vial

## PIVAMPICILLIN

*Indications:* see under Ampicillin

*Cautions; Contra-indications; Side-effects:* see under Ampicillin; hepatic and renal function tests required in long-term use; avoid in porphyria (see section 9.8.2)

*Dose:* 500 mg every 12 hours, doubled in severe infections; CHILD up to 1 year 40–60 mg/kg daily in 2–3 divided doses; 1–5 years 350–525 mg daily; 6–10 years 525–700 mg daily; doses can be doubled in severe infections

PoM **Pondocillin**® (Leo)

*Tablets,* f/c, pivampicillin 500 mg. Net price 20 = £4.22. Label: 5, 9, 21
*Suspension,* sugar-free, pivampicillin 175 mg/5 mL when reconstituted with water. Net price 50 mL = £1.76; 100 mL = £2.84. Label: 5, 9, 21
*Sachets,* granules, off-white, pivampicillin 175 mg/sachet. Net price 10-sachet pack = £1.98. Label: 5, 9, 13, 21

With pivmecillinam

PoM **Miraxid**® (Fisons)

*Tablets,* f/c, pivampicillin 125 mg, pivmecillinam hydrochloride 100 mg. Net price 20 = £2.59. Label: 9, 21, 27, counselling, posture (see below)
*Dose:* 2 tablets twice daily, increased to 3 tablets twice daily for severe infections; CHILD 6–10 years 1 tablet twice daily
COUNSELLING. Swallow whole with plenty of fluid during meals while sitting or standing

*Miraxid*® *450 Tablets,* f/c, pivampicillin 250 mg, pivmecillinam hydrochloride 200 mg. Net price 20 = £5.06. Label: 9, 21, 27, counselling, posture (see below)
*Dose:* 1 tablet twice daily, increased to 2 tablets twice daily for severe infections
COUNSELLING. Swallow whole with plenty of fluid during meals while sitting or standing
*Paediatric suspension,* pivampicillin 62.5 mg, pivmecillinam 46.2 mg/unit-dose sachet. Net price 10-sachet pack = £2.70. Label: 9, 13, 21
*Dose:* under 6 years 1 sachet twice daily increased to 2 sachets twice daily for severe infections, 6–10 years 2 sachets twice daily increased to 3 sachets twice daily for severe infections

PoM **Pondocillin Plus**® (Leo)

*Tablets,* f/c, pivampicillin 250 mg, pivmecillinam hydrochloride 200 mg. Net price 20 = £5.98. Label: 9, 21, 27, counselling, posture (see below)
*Dose:* 1 tablet twice daily, increased to 2 tablets twice daily for severe infections
COUNSELLING. Swallow whole with plenty of fluid during meals while sitting or standing

## TALAMPICILLIN HYDROCHLORIDE

*Indications:* see under Ampicillin

*Cautions; Contra-indications; Side-effects:* see under Ampicillin; avoid in severe hepatic or renal impairment

*Dose:* 250–500 mg every 8 hours

PoM **Talpen**® (Beecham)

*Tablets,* f/c, talampicillin hydrochloride 250 mg. Net price 20 = £2.99. Label: 9
*Syrup,* talampicillin hydrochloride 125 mg (as napsylate)/5 mL when reconstituted with water. Net price 100 mL = £2.13. Label: 9

5.1.1.4  ANTIPSEUDOMONAL PENICILLINS

The carboxypenicillins, **carbenicillin** and **ticarcillin,** are principally indicated for the treatment of serious infections caused by *Pseudomonas aeruginosa* although they also have activity against certain other Gram-negative bacilli including *Proteus* spp. and *Bacteroides fragilis.* Carbenicillin has been replaced by ticarcillin which is more active against these organisms.

Timentin® (ticarcillin with clavulanic acid, section 5.1.1.3), is active against penicillinase-producing bacteria resistant to ticarcillin.

The ureidopenicillins, **azlocillin** and **piperacillin,** have a broad spectrum and are both more active than ticarcillin against *Ps. aeruginosa.*

For pseudomonas septicaemias (especially in neutropenia or endocarditis) these antipseudomonal penicillins should be given with an aminoglycoside (e.g. gentamicin or netilmicin, section 5.1.4) as there is a synergistic effect. Penicillins and aminoglycosides must not, however, be mixed in the same syringe or infusion.

Owing to the sodium content of many of these antibiotics, high doses may lead to hypernatraemia.

---

## AZLOCILLIN

*Indications:* infections due to *Pseudomonas aeruginosa*, see notes above
*Cautions; Contra-indications; Side-effects:* see under Benzylpenicillin (section 5.1.1.1); **interactions:** Appendix 1 (penicillins)
*Dose: by intravenous injection,* 2 g every 8 hours
Serious infections, *by intravenous infusion,* 5 g every 8 hours; PREMATURE INFANT 50 mg/kg every 12 hours; NEONATE 100 mg/kg every 12 hours; INFANT 7 days–1 year 100 mg/kg every 8 hours; CHILD 1–14 years 75 mg/kg every 8 hours

PoM **Securopen**® (Bayer)
*Injection,* powder for reconstitution, azlocillin (as sodium salt). Net price 500-mg vial = £1.62; 1-g vial = £3.21; 2-g vial = £5.02
*Electrolytes:* Na+ 1.08 mmol/500-mg vial, 2.17 mmol/1-g vial, 4.33 mmol/2-g vial
*Infusion,* powder for reconstitution, azlocillin (as sodium salt). Net price 5-g vial = £11·80 (also available with 50 mL water for injections, transfer needle, and infusion bag)
*Electrolytes:* Na+ 10.84 mmol/5-g vial

---

## CARBENICILLIN

*Indications:* infections due to *Pseudomonas aeruginosa* and *Proteus* spp., see notes above
*Cautions; Contra-indications:* see under Benzylpenicillin (section 5.1.1.1)
*Side-effects:* see under Benzylpenicillin (section 5.1.1.1); also hypokalaemia, alteration in platelet function
*Dose: by slow intravenous injection or rapid infusion,* severe systemic infections, 5 g every 4–6 hours; CHILD 250–400 mg/kg daily in divided doses
*By intramuscular injection,* urinary-tract infections, 2 g every 6 hours; CHILD 50–100 mg/kg daily in divided doses

PoM **Pyopen**® (Beecham)
*Injection,* powder for reconstitution, carbenicillin (as sodium salt). Net price 1-g vial = £1.54; 5-g vial = £7.50
*Electrolytes:* Na+ 5.4 mmol/1-g vial, 27.1 mmol/5-g vial

---

## PIPERACILLIN

*Indications:* infections due to *Pseudomonas aeruginosa*, see notes above
*Cautions; Contra-indications; Side-effects:* see under Benzylpenicillin (section 5.1.1.1)
*Dose: by intramuscular or by slow intravenous injection or by intravenous infusion,* 100–150 mg/kg daily (in divided doses), increased to 200–300 mg/kg daily in severe infections, and to at least 16 g daily in life-threatening infections; single doses over 2 g intravenous route only

PoM **Pipril**® (Lederle)
*Injection,* powder for reconstitution, piperacillin (as sodium salt). Net price 1-g vial = £3.07; 2-g vial = £6.08; 4-g vial = £12.01
*Infusion,* powder for reconstitution, piperacillin 4 g (as sodium salt), with 50-mL bottle water for injections and transfer needle. Net price complete unit = £12.80
*Electrolytes:* Na+ 1.94 mmol/g

---

## TICARCILLIN

*Indications:* infections due to *Pseudomonas* and *Proteus* spp, see notes above.
*Cautions; Contra-indications; Side-effects:* see under Benzylpenicillin (section 5.1.1.1)
*Dose: by slow intravenous injection* over 3–4 minutes *or by intravenous infusion,* 15–20 g daily in divided doses; CHILD 200–300 mg/kg daily in divided doses
Urinary-tract infections, *by intramuscular or slow intravenous injection,* 3–4 g daily in divided doses; CHILD 50–100 mg/kg daily in divided doses

PoM **Ticar**® (Beecham)
*Injection,* powder for reconstitution, ticarcillin (as sodium salt). Net price 1-g vial = £1.68; 5-g vial = £6.84
*Infusion,* powder for reconstitution, ticarcillin 5 g (as sodium salt) in infusion bottle, with transfer needle and diluent. Net price complete unit = £8.03
*Electrolytes:* Na+ 5.3 mmol/1-g vial, 26.7 mmol/5-g vial

With clavulanic acid
PoM **Timentin**® (Beecham)
*Injection 1.6 g,* powder for reconstitution, ticarcillin 1.5 g (as sodium salt), clavulanic acid 100 mg (as potassium salt). Net price per vial = £3.04
*Injection 3.2 g,* powder for reconstitution, ticarcillin 3 g (as sodium salt), clavulanic acid 200 mg (as potassium salt). Net price per vial = £6.08
*Electrolytes:* Na+ 16 mmol, K+ 1 mmol/3.2-g vial
*Dose: by intravenous infusion,* 3.2 g every 6–8 hours increased to every 4 hours in more severe infections; CHILD 80 mg/kg every 6–8 hours (every 12 hours in neonates)

---

### 5.1.1.5  MECILLINAMS

**Mecillinam** and **pivmecillinam** have significant activity against many Gram-negative bacteria including salmonellae, but excluding *Ps. aeruginosa.* Pivmecillinam is given by mouth and subsequently hydrolysed to mecillinam, which is the active drug and must itself be given by injection.

---

## MECILLINAM

*Indications:* severe infections due to Gram-negative enteric bacteria
*Cautions; Contra-indications; Side-effects:* see under Benzylpenicillin (section 5.1.1.1); liver and renal function tests on long-term use

---

|

*Dose:* by intramuscular or by slow intravenous injection or by intravenous infusion, 5–15 mg/kg every 6–8 hours

PoM **Selexidin®** (Leo)
*Injection*, powder for reconstitution, mecillinam. Net price 400-mg vial = £1.22

## PIVMECILLINAM
*Indications:* see under Dose below
*Cautions; Contra-indications; Side-effects:* see under Benzylpenicillin (section 5.1.1.1); also liver and renal function tests required in long-term use
*Dose:* acute uncomplicated cystitis, 400 mg initially, then 200 mg every 8 hours for 3 days (10-tab pack)
Chronic or recurrent bacteriuria, 400 mg every 6–8 hours
Salmonellosis, 1.2–2.4 g daily for 14 days (14–28 days for carriers)
COUNSELLING. Tablets should be swallowed whole with plenty of fluid during meals while sitting or standing

PoM **Selexid®** (Leo)
*Tablets*, f/c, pivmecillinam hydrochloride 200 mg. Net price 20 = £4.48. Label: 9, 21, 27, counselling, posture (see Dose above)
*Suspension*, granules, pivmecillinam 100 mg/single-dose sachet. Net price 20 sachets = £4.03. Label: 9, 13, 21

With pivampicillin
See under Pivampicillin (section 5.1.1.3)

## 5.1.2 Cephalosporins, cephamycins, and other beta-lactam antibiotics
Antibiotics discussed in this section include the **cephalosporins**, such as cefotaxime, ceftazidime, cefuroxime, cephalexin and cephradine, the **cephamycin**, cefoxitin, the **monobactam**, aztreonam, and the **carbapenem** imipenem (a thienamycin derivative).

## CEPHALOSPORINS AND CEPHAMYCINS

The cephalosporins are broad-spectrum antibiotics but in spite of the number of cephalosporins currently available there are few absolute indications for their use. All have a similar antibacterial spectrum although individual agents have differing activity against certain organisms. The pharmacology of the cephalosporins is similar to that of the penicillins, excretion being principally renal and blocked by probenecid.

The principal side-effect of the cephalosporins is hypersensitivity and about 10% of penicillin-sensitive patients will also be allergic to the cephalosporins. Haemorrhage due to interference with blood clotting factors has been associated with several cephalosporins.

One of the first cephalosporins was **cephalothin** which is less active and less stable than the newer cephalosporins. It has been replaced by the newer cephalosporins, **cephradine, cephazolin**.

**Cefuroxime** and **cephamandole** are 'second generation' cephalosporins and are less susceptible than the other cephalosporins to inactivation by penicillinases. They are, therefore, active against certain bacteria which are resistant to the other drugs and have greater activity against *H. influenzae* and *Neisseria gonorrhoeae*.

**Cefotaxime, ceftazidime**, and **ceftizoxime** are 'third generation' cephalosporins with greater activity than the 'second generation' cephalosporins against certain Gram-negative bacteria. However, they are less active than cefuroxime and cephamandole against Gram-positive bacteria, most notably *Staphylococcus aureus*. Their broad antibacterial spectrum may encourage superinfection with resistant bacteria or fungi.

**Cefsulodin** and **ceftazidime** have good activity against pseudomonas. Ceftazidime is also active against other Gram-negative bacteria. Cefsulodin has a very much narrower spectrum and should be used only for pseudomonal infections.

**Cefoxitin**, a cephamycin antibiotic, is active against bowel flora including *Bacteroides fragilis* and because of this it has been recommended for abdominal sepsis such as peritonitis.

ORALLY ACTIVE CEPHALOSPORINS. The orally active 'first generation' cephalosporins, **cephalexin, cephradine**, and **cefadroxil** and the 'second generation' cephalosporin, **cefaclor** have a similar antimicrobial spectrum. They are useful for urinary-tract infections which do not respond to other drugs or which occur in pregnancy. Cefaclor has good activity against *Haemophilus influenzae*, but is associated with protracted skin reactions especially in children. Cefadroxil has a longer duration of action than the other cephalosporins but poor activity against *H. influenzae*. **Cefuroxime axetil**, an ester of the 'second generation' cephalosporin cefuroxime, has the same antibacterial spectrum as the parent compound; gastro-intestinal side-effects are quite common.

**Cefixime**, a 'third generation' cephalosporin, has a longer duration of action than the other cephalosporins that are active by mouth. It is presently only indicated for acute infections.

## CEFACLOR
*Indications:* infections due to sensitive Gram-positive and Gram-negative bacteria, but see notes above
*Cautions:* penicillin sensitivity; renal impairment; pregnancy and breast-feeding; false positive urinary glucose (if tested for reducing substances) and false positive Coombs' test; **interactions:** Appendix 1 (cephalosporins)
*Contra-indications:* cephalosporin hypersensitivity; porphyria (see section 9.8.2)

*Side-effects:* diarrhoea and rarely pseudo-membranous colitis (CSM has warned both more likely with higher doses), nausea and vomiting; allergic reactions including rashes, pruritus, urticaria, serum sickness-like reactions with rashes, fever and arthralgia, and anaphylaxis; erythema multiforme, toxic epidermal necrolysis reported; eosinophilia and rarely thrombocytopenia or neutropenia; disturbances in liver enzymes, transient hepatitis and cholestatic jaundice; other side-effects reported include reversible interstitial nephritis, hyperactivity, nervousness, sleep disturbances, confusion, hypertonia, and dizziness.

*Dose:* 250 mg every 8 hours, doubled for severe infections; max. 4 g daily; CHILD over 1 month, 20 mg/kg daily in 3 divided doses, doubled for severe infections, max. 1 g daily; *or* 1 month–1 year, 62.5 mg every 8 hours; 1–5 years, 125 mg; over 5 years, 250 mg; doses doubled for severe infections

PoM **Distaclor**® (Dista)
*Capsules,* cefaclor 250 mg (violet/white), net price 21-cap pack = £10.83; 500 mg (violet/grey), 20 = £18.92. Label: 9
*Suspension,* both pink, cefaclor for reconstitution with water, 125 mg/5 mL, net price 100 mL = £5.01; 250 mg/5 mL, 100 mL = £9.35. Label: 9

## CEFADROXIL

*Indications:* see under Cefaclor; see also notes above
*Cautions; Contra-indications; Side-effects:* see under Cefaclor
*Dose:* patients over 40 kg, 0.5–1 g twice daily; skin, soft tissue, and simple urinary-tract infections, 1 g daily; CHILD under 1 year, 25 mg/kg daily in divided doses; 1–6 years, 250 mg twice daily; over 6 years, 500 mg twice daily

PoM **Baxan**® (Bristol-Myers)
*Capsules,* cefadroxil 500 mg (as monohydrate). Net price 20 = £6.63. Label: 9
*Suspension,* cefadroxil (as monohydrate) for reconstitution with water, 125 mg/5 mL, net price 60 mL = £1.75; 250 mg/5 mL, 60 mL = £3.48; 500 mg/5 mL, 60 mL = £5.21. Label: 9

## CEFIXIME

*Indications:* see under Cefaclor and notes above
*Cautions; Contra-indications; Side-effects:* see under Cefaclor
*Dose:* 200–400 mg daily as a single dose or in 2 divided doses; CHILD 8 mg/kg daily as a single dose or in 2 divided doses *or* 6 months–1 year 75 mg; 1–4 years 100 mg; 5–10 years 200 mg; 11–12 years 300 mg

▼ PoM **Suprax**® (Lederle)
*Tablets,* f/c, scored, cefixime 200 mg. Net price 20 = £27.39. Label: 9

*Paediatric oral suspension,* cefixime 100 mg/5 mL when reconstituted with water. Net price 37.5 mL (with double-ended spoon for measuring 3.75 mL or 5 mL since dilution not recommended) = £6.53; 75 mL = £11.72. Label: 9

## CEFOTAXIME

*Indications:* see under Cefaclor; surgical prophylaxis; see also notes above
*Cautions; Contra-indications; Side-effects:* see under Cefaclor
*Dose: by intramuscular or intravenous injection,* moderate to serious infection, 1 g every 8 hours; life-threatening infection, 2 g every 8 hours; exceptionally, for life-threatening infections due to organisms less sensitive to cefotaxime, up to 12 g daily
Urinary-tract and mild to moderate infections, 1 g every 12 hours
Gonorrhoea 1 g as a single dose
In severe renal impairment, doses to be halved after initial dose of 1 g. NEONATE, 50 mg/kg daily in 2–4 divided doses; in severe infections 150–200 mg/kg daily. CHILD, 100–150 mg/kg daily in 2–4 divided doses; in severe infections, up to 200 mg/kg daily
*By intravenous infusion,* 1–2 g over 20–60 minutes

PoM **Claforan**® (Roussel)
*Injection,* powder for reconstitution, cefotaxime (as sodium salt). Net price 500-mg vial = £2.48; 1-g vial = £4.95; 2-g vial = £9.90
*Electrolytes:* Na+ 2.09 mmol/g

## CEFOXITIN

*Indications:* see under Cefaclor; surgical prophylaxis; more active against Gram-negative bacteria
*Cautions; Contra-indications; Side-effects:* see under Cefaclor
*Dose: by intramuscular or by slow intravenous injection or by infusion,* 1–2 g every 6–8 hours, increased in severe infections; max. 12 g daily; CHILD up to 1 week 20–40 mg/kg every 12 hours; 1–4 weeks 20–40 mg/kg every 8 hours; over 1 month 20–40 mg/kg every 6–8 hours

PoM **Mefoxin**® (MSD)
*Injection,* powder for reconstitution, cefoxitin (as sodium salt). Net price 1-g vial = £4.92; 2-g vial = £9.84
*Electrolytes:* Na+ 2.3 mmol/g

## CEFSULODIN SODIUM

*Indications:* infections due to sensitive strains of *Ps. aeruginosa*; surgical prophylaxis
*Cautions; Contra-indications; Side-effects:* see under Cefaclor
*Dose: by intramuscular injection, or by slow intravenous injection, or by intravenous infusion,* 1–4 g daily in 2–4 divided doses increased in severe infections to 6 g daily or more; CHILD 20–50 mg/kg daily

PoM **Monaspor**® (Ciba)
*Injection*, powder for reconstitution, cefsulodin sodium. Net price 500-mg vial = £5.65; 1-g vial = £11.30
*Electrolytes:* Na⁺ 1.8 mmol/g

## CEFTAZIDIME

*Indications:* see under Cefaclor; see also notes above
*Cautions; Contra-indications; Side-effects:* see under Cefaclor
*Dose: by intramuscular injection or intravenous injection or infusion*, 1 g every 8 hours *or* 2 g every 12 hours; 2 g every 8–12 hours in severe infections; single doses over 1 g intravenous route only; elderly usual max. 3 g daily; CHILD, up to 2 months 25–60 mg/kg daily in 2 divided doses, over 2 months 30–100 mg/kg daily in 2–3 divided doses; up to 150 mg/kg daily if immunocompromised or meningitis; intravenous route recommended for children
Urinary-tract and less serious infections, 0.5–1 g every 12 hours
Pseudomonal lung infection in cystic fibrosis, ADULT with normal renal function 100–150 mg/kg daily in 3 divided doses; CHILD up to 150 mg/kg daily; intravenous route recommended for children

PoM **Fortum**® (Glaxo)
*Injection*, powder for reconstitution, ceftazidime (as pentahydrate), with sodium carbonate. Net price 250-mg vial = £2.48; 500-mg vial = £4.95; 1-g vial = £9.90; 2-g vial (for injection and for infusion) = £19.80
*Electrolytes:* Na⁺ 2.3 mmol/g

## CEFTIZOXIME

*Indications:* see under Cefaclor; see also notes above
*Cautions; Contra-indications; Side-effects:* see under Cefaclor
*Dose: by deep intramuscular or slow intravenous injection or by intravenous infusion*, 1–2 g every 8–12 hours increased in severe infections up to 8 g daily, in 3 divided doses; CHILD over 3 months 30–60 mg/kg daily in 2–4 divided doses, increased to 100–150 mg/kg daily for severe infections
Gonorrhoea, *by intramuscular injection*, 1 g as a single dose
Urinary-tract infections, *by deep intramuscular or slow intravenous injection or by infusion*, 0.5–1 g every 12 hours

PoM **Cefizox**® (Wellcome)
*Injection*, powder for reconstitution, ceftizoxime (as sodium salt). Net price 500-mg vial = £2.76; 1-g vial = £5.50; 2-g vial = £11.00
*Electrolytes:* Na⁺ 2.6 mmol/g

## CEFUROXIME

*Indications:* see under Cefaclor; surgical prophylaxis; more active against *H. influenzae* and *N. gonorrhoeae*

*Cautions; Contra-indications; Side-effects:* see under Cefaclor
*Dose: by mouth* (as cefuroxime axetil), 250 mg twice daily in most infections including mild to moderate lower respiratory-tract infections (e.g. bronchitis); doubled for more severe lower respiratory-tract infections or if pneumonia suspected
Urinary-tract infection, 125 mg twice daily, doubled in pyelonephritis
Gonorrhoea, 1 g as a single dose
CHILD over 3 months, 125 mg twice daily, if necessary doubled in child over 2 years with otitis media
*By intramuscular injection or intravenous injection or infusion*, 750 mg every 6–8 hours; 1.5 g every 6–8 hours in severe infections; single doses over 750 mg intravenous route only
CHILD usual dose 60 mg/kg daily (range 30–100 mg/kg daily) in 3–4 divided doses (2–3 divided doses in neonates)
Gonorrhoea, 1.5 g as a single dose by intramuscular injection (divided between 2 sites)
Surgical prophylaxis, 1.5 g by intravenous injection at induction; may be supplemented with 750 mg intramuscularly 8 and 16 hours later (abdominal, pelvic, and orthopaedic operations) *or* followed by 750 mg intramuscularly every 8 hours for further 24–48 hours (cardiac, pulmonary, oesophageal, and vascular operations)
Meningitis, 3 g intravenously every 8 hours; CHILD, 200–240 mg/kg daily (in 3–4 divided doses) reduced to 100 mg/kg daily after 3 days or on clinical improvement; NEONATE, 100 mg/kg daily reduced to 50 mg/kg daily

PoM **Zinacef**® (Glaxo)
*Injection*, powder for reconstitution, cefuroxime (as sodium salt). Net price 250-mg vial = 88p; 750-mg vial = £2.64; 1.5-g vial (for injection and for infusion) = £5.29
*Electrolytes:* Na⁺ 1.8 mmol/750-mg vial

PoM **Zinnat**® (Glaxo)
*Tablets*, both f/c, cefuroxime 125 mg (as cefuroxime axetil), net price 14-tab pack = £6.30; 250 mg, 14-tab pack = £12.60. Label: 9, 21, 25
*Suspension*, cefuroxime (as cefuroxime axetil) 125 mg/5 mL when reconstituted with water. Net price 70 mL = £7.20. Label: 9, 21
*Sachets*, cefuroxime (as cefuroxime axetil) 125 mg/sachet, net price 14-sachet pack = £7.20. Label: 9, 13 21

## CEPHALEXIN

*Indications:* see under Cefaclor
*Cautions; Contra-indications; Side-effects:* see under Cefaclor
*Dose:* 250 mg every 6 hours *or* 500 mg every 8–12 hours increased to 1–1.5 g every 6–8 hours for severe infections; CHILD, 25 mg/kg daily in divided doses, doubled for severe infections, max. 100 mg/kg daily; *or* under 1 year, 125 mg every 12 hours; 1–5 years, 125 mg every 8 hours; 6–12 years, 250 mg every 8 hours

---

PoM **Cephalexin** (Non-proprietary)
*Capsules*, cephalexin 250 mg, net price 20 = £2.44; 500 mg, 20 = £4.80. Label: 9
*Tablets*, cephalexin 250 mg, net price 20 = £2.44; 500 mg, 20 = £4.80. Label: 9
*Oral suspension*, cephalexin for reconstitution with water, 125 mg/5 mL, net price 100 mL = £1.27; 250 mg/5 mL, 100 mL = £2.55. Label: 9

PoM **Ceporex®** (Glaxo)
*Capsules*, both caramel/grey, cephalexin 250 mg, net price 20 = £3.00, 28-cap pack = £4.47; 500 mg, 20 = £5.88, 28-cap pack = £8.72. Label: 9
*Tablets*, all pink, f/c, cephalexin 250 mg, net price 20 = £3.00, 28-tab pack = £4.47; 500 mg, 20 = £5.88, 28-tab pack = £8.72; 1 g (scored), 14-tab pack = £8.72. Label: 9
*Paediatric drops*, orange, cephalexin 125 mg/1.25 mL when reconstituted with water. Net price 10 mL = £1.52. Label: 9, counselling, use of pipette
*Suspension*, both yellow, cephalexin 125 mg/5 mL, net price 100 mL = £1.59; 250 mg/5 mL, 100 mL = £3.19. Do not dilute. Label: 9
*Syrup*, all orange, cephalexin for reconstitution with water, 125 mg/5 mL, net price 100 mL = £1.59; 250 mg/5 mL, 100 mL = £3.19; 500 mg/5 mL, 100 mL = £6.19. Label: 9

PoM **Keflex®** (Lilly)
*Capsules*, cephalexin 250 mg (green/white), net price 28-cap pack = £3.57; 500 mg (pale green/dark green), 28-cap pack = £6.97. Label: 9
*Tablets*, both peach, cephalexin 250 mg, net price 28-tab pack = £3.57; 500 mg (scored), 28-tab pack = £6.97. Label: 9
*Suspension*, cephalexin for reconstitution with water, 125 mg/5 mL (pink), net price 100 mL = £1.27; 250 mg/5 mL (orange), 100 mL = £2.55. Label: 9

## CEPHAMANDOLE

*Indications:* see under Cefaclor; surgical prophylaxis
*Cautions; Contra-indications; Side-effects:* see under Cefaclor
*Dose: by deep intramuscular injection or intravenous injection or infusion*, 0.5–2 g every 4–8 hours; CHILD, 50–100 mg/kg daily in divided doses

PoM **Kefadol®** (Dista)
*Injection*, powder for reconstitution, cephamandole (as nafate) with sodium carbonate. Net price 1-g vial = £3.91
*Electrolytes:* Na⁺ 1.19 mmol/1-g vial

## CEPHAZOLIN

*Indications:* see under Cefaclor; surgical prophylaxis
*Cautions; Contra-indications; Side-effects:* see under Cefaclor

*Dose: by intramuscular injection or intravenous injection or infusion*, 0.5–1 g every 6–12 hours; CHILD, 25–50 mg/kg daily (in divided doses), increased to 100 mg/kg daily in severe infections

PoM **Kefzol®** (Lilly)
*Injection*, powder for reconstitution, cephazolin (as sodium salt). Net price 500-mg vial = £2.45; 1-g vial = £4.63
*Electrolytes:* Na⁺ 2.1 mmol/g

## CEPHRADINE

*Indications:* see under Cefaclor; surgical prophylaxis
*Cautions; Contra-indications; Side-effects:* see under Cefaclor
*Dose: by mouth*, 250–500 mg every 6 hours *or* 0.5–1 g every 12 hours; CHILD, 25–50 mg/kg daily in divided doses
*By intramuscular injection or intravenous injection or infusion*, 0.5–1 g every 6 hours, increased to 8 g daily in severe infections; CHILD 50–100 mg/kg daily in 4 divided doses

PoM **Velosef®** (Squibb)
*Capsules*, cephradine 250 mg (orange/blue), net price 20-cap pack = £3.55; 500 mg, 20-cap pack = £7.00. Label: 9
*Syrup*, cephradine 250 mg/5 mL when reconstituted with water. Diluent syrup, life of diluted syrup 7 days. Net price 100 mL = £4.22. Label: 9
*Injection*, powder for reconstitution, cephradine. Net price 500-mg vial = 99p; 1-g vial = £1.95

## OTHER BETA-LACTAM ANTIBIOTICS

**Aztreonam** is a monocyclic beta-lactam ('monobactam') antibiotic with an antibacterial spectrum limited to Gram-negative aerobic bacteria including *Pseudomonas aeruginosa*, *Neisseria meningitidis*, and *Haemophilus influenzae*; it should not be used alone for 'blind' treatment since it is not active against Gram-positive organisms. Aztreonam is also effective against *Neisseria gonorrhoeae* (but not against concurrent chlamydial infection). Side-effects are similar to those of the other beta-lactams although aztreonam may be less likely to cause hypersensitivity in penicillin-sensitive patients.

**Imipenem**, a carbapenem, is the first thienamycin beta-lactam antibiotic; it has a broad spectrum of activity which includes many aerobic and anaerobic Gram-positive and Gram-negative bacteria. Imipenem is partially inactivated in the kidney by enzymatic activity and is therefore administered in combination with **cilastatin**, a specific enzyme inhibitor, which blocks its renal metabolism. Side-effects are similar to those of other beta-lactam antibiotics; neurotoxicity has been observed at very high dosage or in renal failure.

## AZTREONAM

*Indications:* Gram-negative infections including *Pseudomonas aeruginosa*, *Haemophilus influenzae*, and *Neisseria meningitidis*

*Cautions:* hypersensitivity to beta-lactam antibiotics; hepatic impairment; reduce dose in renal impairment; **interactions:** Appendix 1 (aztreonam)

*Contra-indications:* aztreonam hypersensitivity; pregnancy and breast-feeding

*Side-effects:* nausea, vomiting, diarrhoea, abdominal cramps; mouth ulcers, altered taste; jaundice and hepatitis; blood disorders (including thrombocytopenia and neutropenia); urticaria and rashes

*Dose: by intramuscular injection or intravenous injection or infusion:* 1 g every 8 hours *or* 2 g every 12 hours; 2 g every 6–8 hours for severe infections (including systemic *Pseudomonas aeruginosa* and lung infections in cystic fibrosis); single doses over 1 g intravenous route only

CHILD over 1 week, *by intravenous injection or infusion,* 30 mg/kg every 6–8 hours increased in severe infections for child of 2 years or older to 50 mg/kg every 6–8 hours; max. 8 g daily

Urinary-tract infections, 0.5–1 g every 8–12 hours

Gonorrhoea/cystitis, *by intramuscular injection,* 1 g as a single dose

PoM **Azactam**® (Squibb)

*Injection,* powder for reconstitution, aztreonam. Net price 500-mg vial = £4.48; 1-g vial = £8.95; 2-g vial and 2-g bottle (for preparing infusion) (both) = £17.90

## IMIPENEM WITH CILASTATIN

*Indications:* aerobic and anaerobic Gram-positive and Gram-negative infections

*Cautions:* hypersensitivity to penicillins, cephalosporins and other beta-lactam antibiotics; renal impairment; CNS disorders (e.g. epilepsy); pregnancy

*Contra-indications:* hypersensitivity to imipenem or cilastatin; breast-feeding

*Side-effects:* nausea, vomiting, diarrhoea (pseudomembranous colitis reported), taste disturbances; blood disorders, positive Coombs test; allergic reactions (with rash, pruritus, urticaria, fever, anaphylactic reactions, rarely toxic epidermal necrolysis); myoclonic activity, convulsions, confusion and mental disturbances reported; slight increases in liver enzymes and bilirubin reported; increases in serum creatinine and blood urea; local reactions: erythema, pain and induration, and thrombophlebitis

*Dose: by deep intramuscular injection,* mild to moderate infections, in terms of imipenem, 500–750 mg every 12 hours; gonococcal urethritis or cervicitis, 500 mg as a single dose

*By intravenous infusion,* in terms of imipenem, 1–2 g daily in 3–4 divided doses; less sensitive

organisms, up to 50 mg/kg daily (to max. 4 g daily); CHILD 3 months and older, 60 mg/kg (up to max. of 2 g) daily in 4 divided doses

PoM **Primaxin**® (MSD)

*Intramuscular injection,* powder for reconstitution, imipenem (as monohydrate) 500 mg with cilastatin (as sodium salt) 500 mg. Net price 15-mL vial = £15.00
*Electrolytes:* Na+ 1.47 mmol/vial

*Intravenous infusion,* powder for reconstitution, imipenem (as monohydrate) 250 mg with cilastatin (as sodium salt) 250 mg. Net price 60-mL vial = £9.00
*Electrolytes:* Na+ 0.86 mmol/vial

*Intravenous infusion,* powder for reconstitution, imipenem (as monohydrate) 500 mg with cilastatin (as sodium salt) 500 mg. Net price 120-mL vial = £15.00
*Electrolytes:* Na+ 1.72 mmol/vial

### 5.1.3  Tetracyclines

The tetracyclines are broad-spectrum antibiotics whose value has decreased owing to increasing bacterial resistance. They remain, however, the treatment of choice for infections caused by chlamydia (trachoma, psittacosis, salpingitis, urethritis, and lymphogranuloma venereum), rickettsia (including Q-fever), mycoplasma (respiratory and genital infections), brucellosis (doxycycline with rifampicin), and the spirochaete, *Borrelia burgdorferi* (Lyme disease). They are also used in acne, in destructive (refractory) periodontal disease, in exacerbations of chronic bronchitis (because of their activity against *Haemophilus influenzae*), and for leptospirosis in penicillin hypersensitivity (as an alternative to erythromycin).

Microbiologically, there is little to choose between the various tetracyclines, the only exception being **minocycline** which has a broader spectrum, is active against *Neisseria meningitidis* and has been used for meningococcal prophylaxis; however it may cause dizziness and vertigo.

The tetracyclines are deposited in growing bone and teeth (being bound to calcium) causing staining and occasionally dental hypoplasia, and should **not** be given to children under 12 years or to pregnant women. With the exception of **doxycycline** and **minocycline** the tetracyclines may exacerbate renal failure and should **not** be given to patients with kidney disease. Absorption of tetracyclines is decreased by milk (except doxycycline and minocycline), antacids, and calcium, iron, and magnesium salts.

## TETRACYCLINE

*Indications:* exacerbations of chronic bronchitis; brucellosis (see also notes above), chlamydia, mycoplasma, and rickettsia; pleural effusions due to malignancy or cirrhosis; acne vulgaris (see section 13.6)

*Cautions:* breast-feeding; hepatic impairment (avoid intravenous administration); renal

impairment (avoid if severe); rarely causes photosensitivity; **interactions:** Appendix 1 (tetracyclines)
*Contra-indications:* severe renal impairment, pregnancy (see also Appendix 4), children under 12 years of age, systemic lupus erythematosus
*Side-effects:* nausea, vomiting, diarrhoea; erythema (discontinue treatment); headache and visual disturbances may indicate benign intracranial hypertension; pseudomembranous colitis reported
*Dose: by mouth,* 250 mg every 6 hours, increased in severe infections to 500 mg every 6–8 hours
Acne, see section 13.6
Early syphilis, 500 mg every 6 hours for 15 days
Non-gonococcal urethritis, 500 mg every 6 hours for 7–21 days
*By intramuscular injection,* 100 mg every 8–12 hours, or every 4–6 hours in severe infections
*By intravenous infusion,* 500 mg every 12 hours; max. 2 g daily
Pleural effusions, see under Achromycin® intravenous infusion
COUNSELLING. Tablets or capsules should be swallowed whole with plenty of fluid while sitting or standing

PoM **Tetracycline Tablets,** coated, tetracycline hydrochloride 250 mg. Net price 20 = 30p. Label: 7, 9, 23, counselling, posture, see above
PoM **Achromycin®** (Lederle)
*Capsules,* orange, tetracycline hydrochloride 250 mg. Net price 20 = 95p. Label: 7, 9, 23, counselling, posture, see above
*Tablets,* orange, f/c, tetracycline hydrochloride 250 mg. Net price 20 = 67p. Label: 7, 9, 23, counselling, posture, see above
*Intramuscular injection,* powder for reconstitution, tetracycline hydrochloride 100 mg, procaine hydrochloride 40 mg. Net price per vial = £1.09
*Intravenous infusion,* powder for reconstitution, tetracycline hydrochloride. Net price 250-mg vial = £1.27; 500-mg vial = £2.03
*Dose:* infections, see above
Recurrent pleural effusions, by intrapleural instillation, 500 mg in 30–50 mL sodium chloride intravenous infusion 0.9%
PoM **Panmycin®** (Upjohn)
*Capsules,* grey/yellow, tetracycline hydrochloride 250 mg. Net price 20 = 80p. Label: 7, 9, 23, counselling, posture, see above
PoM **Sustamycin®** (Boehringer Mannheim)
*Capsules,* m/r, light blue/dark blue, tetracycline hydrochloride 250 mg. Net price 20 = £2.12. Label: 7, 9, 23, 25
*Dose:* 2 capsules initially, then 1 every 12 hours
PoM **Tetrabid-Organon®** (Organon)
*Capsules,* m/r, purple/yellow, tetracycline hydrochloride 250 mg. Net price 20 = £1.73. Label: 7, 9, 23, 25
*Dose:* 2 capsules initially, then 1 every 12 hours; acne, 1 daily

PoM **Tetrachel®** (Berk)
*Capsules,* orange, tetracycline hydrochloride 250 mg. Net price 20 = 29p. Label: 7, 9, 23, counselling, posture, see above
*Tablets,* orange, f/c, tetracycline hydrochloride 250 mg. Net price 20 = 27p. Label: 7, 9, 23, counselling, posture, see above

Compound preparations
PoM **Deteclo®** (Lederle)
*Tablets,* blue, f/c, tetracycline hydrochloride 115.4 mg, chlortetracycline hydrochloride 115.4 mg, demeclocycline hydrochloride 69.2 mg. Net price 20 = £2.54. Label: 7, 9, 11, 23, counselling, posture, see above
*Dose:* 1 tablet every 12 hours; 3–4 tablets daily in more severe infections
PoM **Mysteclin®** (Squibb)
*Tablets,* orange, s/c, tetracycline hydrochloride 250 mg, nystatin 250 000 units. Net price 20 = £1.34. Label: 7, 9, 23, counselling, posture, see above

## CHLORTETRACYCLINE HYDROCHLORIDE
*Indications; Cautions; Contra-indications; Side-effects:* see under Tetracycline
*Dose:* 250–500 mg every 6 hours

PoM **Aureomycin®** (Lederle)
*Capsules,* yellow, chlortetracycline hydrochloride 250 mg. Net price 20 = £2.36. Label: 7, 9, 23

## DEMECLOCYCLINE HYDROCHLORIDE
*Indications:* see under Tetracycline; also inappropriate secretion of antidiuretic hormone, section 6.5.2
*Cautions; Contra-indications; Side-effects:* see under Tetracycline, but photosensitivity is more common
*Dose:* 150 mg every 6 hours *or* 300 mg every 12 hours

PoM **Ledermycin®** (Lederle)
*Capsules,* red, demeclocycline hydrochloride 150 mg. Net price 20 = £4.24. Label: 7, 9, 11, 23

## DOXYCYCLINE
*Indications:* see under Tetracycline; brucellosis (with rifampicin); also chronic prostatitis and sinusitis
*Cautions; Contra-indications; Side-effects:* see under Tetracycline, but may be used in renal impairment; avoid in porphyria (see section 9.8.2)
*Dose:* 200 mg on first day, then 100 mg daily; severe infections (including chronic urinary-tract infections), 200 mg daily
Acne, 50 mg daily for 6–12 weeks or longer
COUNSELLING. Capsules should be swallowed whole with plenty of fluid during meals while sitting or standing

PoM **Doxycycline** (Non-proprietary)
*Capsules*, doxycycline 100 mg (as hydrochloride). Net price 20 = £9.80. Label: 6, 9, 27, counselling, posture, see above

PoM **Nordox**® (Panpharma)
*Capsules*, green, doxycycline 100 mg (as hydrochloride). Net price 10-cap pack = £4.66. Label: 6, 9, 27, counselling, posture, see above

PoM **Vibramycin**® (Invicta)
*Capsules*, doxycycline (as hydrochloride) 50 mg (green/ivory), net price 28-cap pack = £7.74; 100 mg (green), 8-cap pack = £4.18. Label: 6, 9, 27, counselling, posture, see above

PoM **Vibramycin-D**® (Invicta)
*Dispersible tablets*, off-white, doxycycline 100 mg. Net price 8-tab pack = £4.91. Label: 6, 9, 13

## LYMECYCLINE
*Indications; Cautions; Contra-indications; Side-effects:* see under Tetracycline
*Dose:* 408 mg every 12 hours

PoM **Tetralysal 300**® (Farmitalia Carlo Erba)
*Capsules*, lymecycline 408 mg (≡ tetracycline 300 mg). Net price 20 = £3.03. Label: 6, 9

## MINOCYCLINE
*Indications:* see under Tetracycline; also meningococcal carrier state
*Cautions; Contra-indications:* see under Tetracycline, but may be used in renal impairment
*Side-effects:* see under Tetracycline; also dizziness and vertigo (more common in women); severe exfoliative rashes and liver damage reported
*Dose:* 100 mg twice daily
Acne, 50 mg twice daily for minimum course of 6 weeks (*caution:* higher doses associated with hyperpigmentation of acne lesions)

PoM **Minocin**® (Lederle)
*Tablets*, both f/c, minocycline (as hydrochloride) 50 mg (beige), net price 84-tab pack = £27.68; 100 mg (orange), 20-tab pack = £13.17. Label: 6, 9

## OXYTETRACYCLINE
*Indications; Cautions; Contra-indications; Side-effects:* see under Tetracycline; avoid in porphyria (see section 9.8.2)
*Dose:* 250–500 mg every 6 hours

PoM **Oxytetracycline** (Non-proprietary)
*Tablets*, coated, oxytetracycline dihydrate 250 mg, net price 20 = 24p. Label: 7, 9, 23
Available from APS, Ashbourne (Oxytetramix®), Berk (Berkmycen®, contain tartrazine), Cox, DDSA (Oxymycin®), Evans, Kerfoot

PoM **Imperacin**® (ICI)
*Tablets*, yellow, f/c, oxytetracycline dihydrate 250 mg. Net price 20 = 49p. Label: 7, 9, 23
*Additives:* include tartrazine

PoM **Terramycin**® (Pfizer)
*Capsules*, yellow, oxytetracycline 250 mg (as hydrochloride). Net price 28-cap pack = 96p. Label: 7, 9, 23

*Tablets*, yellow, s/c, oxytetracycline 250 mg (as dihydrate). Net price 28-tab pack = 96p. Label: 7, 9, 23

## 5.1.4   Aminoglycosides
These include amikacin, gentamicin, kanamycin, neomycin, netilmicin, streptomycin, and tobramycin. All are bactericidal and active against some Gram-positive and many Gram-negative organisms. Amikacin, gentamicin, and tobramycin are also active against *Pseudomonas aeruginosa*; streptomycin is active against *Mycobacterium tuberculosis* and is now almost entirely reserved for tuberculosis (section 5.1.9).

The aminoglycosides are not absorbed from the gut (although there is a risk of absorption in inflammatory bowel disease and liver failure) and must therefore be given by injection for systemic infections.

Excretion is principally via the kidney and accumulation occurs in renal impairment.

Most side-effects of this group of antibiotics are dose-related therefore care must be taken with dosage and whenever possible treatment should not exceed 7 days. The important side-effects are ototoxicity, and to a lesser degree nephrotoxicity; they occur most commonly in the elderly and in patients with renal failure.

If there is impairment of renal function (or high pre-dose plasma concentrations) the interval between doses must be increased; if the renal impairment is severe the dose itself should be reduced as well.

Aminoglycosides may impair neuromuscular transmission and should not be given to patients with myasthenia gravis; large doses given during surgery have been responsible for a transient myasthenic syndrome in patients with normal neuromuscular function.

Aminoglycosides should not be given with potentially ototoxic diuretics (e.g. frusemide and ethacrynic acid); if concurrent use is unavoidable administration of the aminoglycoside and of the diuretic should be separated by as long a period as practicable.

---

PLASMA CONCENTRATIONS. Plasma concentration monitoring avoids both excessive and subtherapeutic concentrations, thus preventing toxicity and, at the same time, ensuring efficacy.

If possible plasma concentrations of aminoglycosides should be measured in all patients and **must** be determined in infants *or* if high doses are being given, *or* if there is renal impairment, *or* if treatment lasts longer than 7 days.

*Note.* Plasma concentrations should be measured approximately one hour after intravenous or intramuscular injection, and also just before the next dose.

---

**Gentamicin** is the most important of the aminoglycosides and is widely used for the treatment of serious infections. It is the aminoglycoside of choice in the UK. It has a broad spectrum but is inactive against anaerobes and has poor activity against haemolytic streptococci and pneumococci. When used for the 'blind' therapy of undiagnosed

---

serious infections it is usually given in conjunction with a penicillin and/or metronidazole.

The daily dose is up to 5 mg/kg given in divided doses every 8 hours (if renal function is normal); whenever possible treatment should not exceed 7 days. Higher doses are occasionally indicated for serious infections, especially in the neonate or the compromised host. A lower dose of 80 mg twice daily (60 mg for lighter or elderly patients) in association with benzylpenicillin is sufficient for endocarditis due to oral streptococci (often termed *Streptococcus viridans*) and gut streptococci.

**Amikacin** is a derivative of kanamycin and has one important advantage over gentamicin in that it is stable to 8 of the 9 classified aminoglycoside-inactivating enzymes whereas gentamicin is inactivated by 5. It is principally indicated for the treatment of serious infections caused by Gram-negative bacilli resistant to gentamicin.

**Kanamycin** has been superseded by other aminoglycosides.

**Netilmicin** has similar activity to gentamicin, but may cause less ototoxicity in those needing treatment for longer than 10 days. Netilmicin is active against a number of gentamicin-resistant Gram-negative bacilli but is less active against *Ps. aeruginosa* than gentamicin or tobramycin.

**Tobramycin** is similar to gentamicin. It is slightly more active against *Ps. aeruginosa* but shows less activity against certain other Gram-negative bacteria.

**Neomycin** is too toxic for parenteral administration and can only be used for infections of the skin or mucous membranes or to reduce the bacterial population of the colon prior to bowel surgery or in hepatic failure. Oral administration may lead to malabsorption. Small amounts of neomycin may be absorbed from the gut in patients with hepatic failure and, as these patients may also be uraemic, cumulation may occur with resultant ototoxicity.

PREGNANCY. Where possible, the aminoglycosides should be avoided in pregnancy as they cross the placenta and can cause fetal eighth nerve damage.

## GENTAMICIN

*Indications:* septicaemia and neonatal sepsis; meningitis and other CNS infections; biliary tract infection, acute pyelonephritis or prostatitis, endocarditis caused by *Strep. viridans* or *strep. faecalis* (with a penicillin)

*Cautions:* renal impairment, infants and elderly (adjust dose and monitor renal, auditory and vestibular function together with plasma gentamicin concentrations); avoid prolonged use; **interactions:** Appendix 1 (aminoglycosides)

*Contra-indications:* pregnancy, myasthenia gravis

*Side-effects:* vestibular damage, reversible nephrotoxicity; rarely, hypomagnesaemia on prolonged therapy, pseudomembranous colitis; see also notes above

*Dose: by intramuscular or by slow intravenous injection* over at least 3 minutes *or by intra-venous infusion*, 2–5 mg/kg daily (in divided doses every 8 hours). In renal impairment the interval between successive doses should be increased to 12 hours when the creatinine clearance is 30–70 mL/minute, 24 hours for 10–30 mL/minute, 48 hours for 5–10 mL/minute, and after twice-weekly dialysis for less than 5 mL/minute

CHILD up to 2 weeks, 3 mg/kg every 12 hours; 2 weeks–12 years, 2 mg/kg every 8 hours

*By intrathecal injection*, 1 mg daily (increased if necessary to 5 mg daily), with 2–4 mg/kg daily *by intramuscular injection* (in divided doses every 8 hours)

Endocarditis prophylaxis, section 5.1, table 2

*Note.* One-hour ('peak') concentration should not exceed 10 mg/litre; pre-dose ('trough') concentration should be less than 2 mg/litre

PoM **Cidomycin**® (Roussel)
*Injection*, gentamicin 40 mg (as sulphate)/mL. Net price 2-mL amp or vial = £1.59
*Paediatric injection*, gentamicin 10 mg (as sulphate)/mL. Net price 2-mL vial = 67p
*Intrathecal injection*, gentamicin 5 mg (as sulphate)/mL. Net price 1-mL amp = 79p

PoM **Genticin**® (Nicholas)
*Injection*, gentamicin 40 mg (as sulphate)/mL. Net price 2-mL amp or vial = £1.58

PoM **Isotonic Gentamicin Injection** (Baxter)
*Intravenous infusion*, gentamicin 800 micrograms (as sulphate)/mL in sodium chloride intravenous infusion 0.9%. Net price 100-mL (80-mg) Viaflex® bag = £1.50
*Electrolytes:* Na⁺ 15.4 mmol/100-mL bag

## AMIKACIN

*Indications:* serious Gram-negative infections resistant to gentamicin

*Cautions; Contra-indications; Side-effects:* see under Gentamicin

*Dose: by intramuscular or by slow intravenous injection or by infusion*, 15 mg/kg daily in 2 divided doses

*Note.* One-hour ('peak') concentration should not exceed 30 mg/litre; pre-dose ('trough') concentration should be less than 10 mg/litre

PoM **Amikin**® (Bristol-Myers)
*Injection*, amikacin 250 mg (as sulphate)/mL. Net price 2-mL vial = £10.14
*Paediatric injection*, amikacin 50 mg (as sulphate)/mL. Net price 2-mL vial = £2.36

## KANAMYCIN

*Indications:* superseded by other aminoglycosides (see notes above)

*Cautions; Contra-indications; Side-effects:* see under Gentamicin

*Dose: by intramuscular injection*, 250 mg every 6 hours *or* 500 mg every 12 hours

*By intravenous infusion*, 15–30 mg/kg daily in divided doses every 8–12 hours

*Note.* One-hour ('peak') concentration should not exceed 30 mg/litre; pre-dose ('trough') concentration should be less than 10 mg/litre

PoM **Kannasyn**® (Sanofi Winthrop)
*Powder* (for preparing injections), kanamycin (as acid sulphate). Net price 1-g vial = £22.16

## NEOMYCIN SULPHATE

*Indications:* bowel sterilisation prior to surgery, see also notes above
*Cautions; Contra-indications; Side-effects:* see under Gentamicin but too toxic for systemic use, see notes above; avoid in renal impairment
*Dose: by mouth,* bowel sterilisation, 1 g every 4 hours

PoM **Neomycin Elixir,** neomycin sulphate 100 mg/5 mL. Net price 100 mL = 66p
PoM **Mycifradin**® (Upjohn)
*Tablets,* neomycin sulphate 500 mg. Net price 20 = £3.60
PoM **Nivemycin**® (Boots)
*Tablets,* neomycin sulphate 500 mg. Net price 20 = £2.06
*Elixir,* neomycin sulphate 100 mg/5 mL. Net price 100 mL = 66p

## NETILMICIN

*Indications:* serious Gram-negative infections resistant to gentamicin
*Cautions; Contra-indications; Side-effects:* see under Gentamicin
*Dose: by intramuscular injection or by intravenous injection over 3–5 minutes or by intravenous infusion,* 4–6 mg/kg daily, as a single daily dose or in divided doses every 8 or 12 hours; in severe infections, up to 7.5 mg/kg daily in divided doses every 8 hours (reduced as soon as clinically indicated, usually within 48 hours) NEONATE up to 1 week, 3 mg/kg every 12 hours; INFANT over 1 week, 2.5–3 mg/kg every 8 hours; CHILD 2–2.5 mg/kg every 8 hours
Urinary-tract infection, 150 mg as a single daily dose for 5 days
Gonorrhoea, 300 mg as a single dose
*Note.* For divided daily dose regimens, one-hour ('peak') concentration should not exceed 12 mg/litre; pre-dose ('trough') concentration should be less than 2 mg/litre

PoM **Netillin**® (Schering-Plough)
*Injection,* netilmicin (as sulphate) 10 mg/mL, net price 1.5-mL (15-mg) amp = £1.49; 50 mg/mL, 1-mL (50-mg) amp = £2.21; 100 mg/mL, 1-mL (100-mg) amp = £2.88; 1.5-mL (150-mg) amp = £4.11, 2-mL (200-mg) amp = £5.33

## TOBRAMYCIN

*Indications:* see under Gentamicin and notes above
*Cautions; Contra-indications; Side-effects:* see under Gentamicin
*Dose: by intramuscular injection or by slow intravenous injection or by intravenous infusion,* 3 mg/kg daily in divided doses every 8 hours; in severe infections up to 5 mg/kg daily in divided doses every 6–8 hours (reduced to 3 mg/kg as soon as clinically indicated); NEONATE 2 mg/kg every 12 hours; CHILD over 1 week 2–2.5 mg/kg every 8 hours

Urinary-tract infection, *by intramuscular injection,* 2–3 mg/kg daily as a single dose
*Note.* One-hour ('peak') concentration should not exceed 10 mg/litre; pre-dose ('trough') concentration should be less than 2 mg/litre

PoM **Nebcin**® (Lilly)
*Injection,* tobramycin (as sulphate) 10 mg/mL, net price 2-mL (20-mg) vial = £1.08; 40 mg/mL, 1-mL (40-mg) vial = £1.46, 2-mL (80-mg) vial = £2.63

## 5.1.5   Macrolides

**Erythromycin** has an antibacterial spectrum that is similar but not identical to that of penicillin; it is thus an alternative to penicillin in penicillin-allergic patients.

Indications for erythromycin include respiratory infections in children, whooping-cough, legionnaires' disease, and campylobacter enteritis. It has activity against gut anaerobes and has been used with neomycin for prophylaxis before bowel surgery. It is active against many penicillin-resistant staphylococci but some are now also resistant to erythromycin. Erythromycin is also active against chlamydia and mycoplasmas.

Erythromycin causes nausea in some patients; in mild to moderate infections this can be avoided by giving a lower dose (250 mg 4 times daily) but if a more serious infection, such as Legionella pneumonia, is suspected higher doses are needed.

**Azithromycin** is a new macrolide with similar activity to erythromycin against Gram-positive bacteria but enhanced activity against some Gram-negative organisms. Plasma concentrations are very low but tissue concentrations are much higher. Once daily dosage is recommended.

**Clarithromycin** is an erythromycin derivative with greater activity than the parent compound. Tissue concentrations are higher than with erythromycin.

## ERYTHROMYCIN

*Indications:* alternative to penicillin in hypersensitive patients; sinusitis, diphtheria and whooping cough prophylaxis; legionnaires' disease; chronic prostatitis; acne vulgaris (see section 13.6)
*Cautions:* hepatic and renal impairment; pregnancy and breast-feeding; **interactions:** Appendix 1 (erythromycin)
*Contra-indications:* porphyria (see section 9.8.2); estolate contra-indicated in liver disease
*Side-effects:* nausea, vomiting, abdominal discomfort, diarrhoea after large doses; reversible hearing loss also reported after large doses; if given for more than 14 days may occasionally cause cholestatic jaundice
*Dose: by mouth,* ADULT and CHILD over 8 years, 250–500 mg every 6 hours *or* 0.5–1 g every 12 hours (see notes above); up to 4 g daily in severe infections; CHILD up to 2 years 125 mg every 6 hours, 2–8 years 250 mg every 6 hours, doses doubled for severe infections

Endocarditis prophylaxis, section 5.1, Table 2

Acne, see section 13.6

Early syphilis, 500 mg 4 times daily for 14 days

*By intravenous infusion*, ADULT and CHILD severe infections, 50 mg/kg daily by continuous infusion *or* in divided doses every 6 hours; mild infections (oral treatment not possible), 25 mg/kg daily

PoM **Erythromycin** (Non-proprietary)

*Tablets*, e/c, erythromycin 250 mg, net price 20 = 86p; 500 mg, 20 = £2.06. Label: 5, 9, 25

*Note.* Erythromycin Tablets are not recommended for the dental prophylaxis of bacterial endocarditis; a Working Party of the British Society for Antimicrobial Chemotherapy has recommended that Erythromycin Stearate Tablets should be specified

*Mixture*, erythromycin (as ethyl succinate) 125 mg/5 mL, net price 100 mL = £1.47; 250 mg/5 mL, 100 mL = £2.17; 500 mg/5 mL, 100 mL = £3.59. Label: 9

PoM **Erythromycin Stearate** (Non-proprietary)

*Tablets*, erythromycin 250 and 500 mg (both as stearate). Label: 9

PoM **Arpimycin**® (RP Drugs)

*Mixture*, all pink, erythromycin (as ethyl succinate) for reconstitution with water, 125 mg/5 mL, net price 100 mL = £1.36; 250 mg/5 mL, 100 mL = £2.03; 500 mg/5 mL, 100 mL = £3.85. Label: 9

PoM **Erycen**® (Berk)

*Tablets*, both orange, e/c, f/c, erythromycin 250 mg, net price 20 = 97p; 500 mg, 20 = £2.41. Label: 5, 9, 25

PoM **Erymax**® (P-D)

*Capsules*, opaque orange/clear orange, enclosing orange and white e/c pellets, erythromycin 250 mg. Net price 28-cap pack = £5.66. Label: 5, 9, 25

*Dose:* 1 every 6 hours *or* 2 every 12 hours; acne, 1 twice daily then 1 daily after 1 month

PoM **Erythrocin**® (Abbott)

*Tablets*, both f/c, erythromycin (as stearate), 250 mg, net price 20 = £2.13; 500 mg, 20 = £4.48. Label: 9

*Intravenous infusion*, powder for reconstitution, erythromycin (as lactobionate). Net price 1-g vial = £8.63

PoM **Erythromid**® (Abbott)

*Tablets*, orange, e/c, f/c, erythromycin 250 mg. Net price 20 = 86p. Label: 5, 9, 25

PoM **Erythromid DS**® (Abbott)

*Tablets*, e/c, f/c, erythromycin 500 mg. Net price 20 = £1.94. Label: 5, 9, 25

PoM **Erythroped**® (Abbott)

*Suspension PI*, erythromycin 125 mg (as ethyl succinate)/5 mL when reconstituted with water. Net price 140 mL = £2.07. Label: 9

*Granules PI*, erythromycin (as ethyl succinate) 125 mg/sachet. Net price 28-sachet pack = £2.91. Label: 9, 13

*Suspension*, erythromycin 250 mg (as ethyl succinate)/5 mL when reconstituted with water. Net price 140 mL = £3.86. Label: 9

*Granules*, erythromycin (as ethyl succinate) 250 mg/sachet. Net price 28-sachet pack = £4.83. Label: 9, 13

*Sugar-free granules*, erythromycin 250 mg (as ethyl succinate)/sachet. Net price 28-sachet pack = £9.02. Label: 9, 13

*Suspension forte*, erythromycin 500 mg (as ethyl succinate)/5 mL when reconstituted with water. Net price 140 mL = £6.85. Label: 9

*Granules forte*, erythromycin (as ethyl succinate) 500 mg/sachet. Net price 28-sachet pack = £7.82. Label: 9, 13

PoM **Erythroped A**® (Abbott)

*Tablets*, yellow, f/c, erythromycin 500 mg (as ethyl succinate). Net price 28-tab pack = £6.47. Label: 9

*Granules*, erythromycin 1 g (as ethyl succinate)/sachet. Net price 14-sachet pack = £7.50. Label: 9, 13

PoM **Ilosone**® (Dista)

*Capsules*, ivory/red, erythromycin 250 mg (as estolate). Net price 20 = £4.15. Label: 9

*Tablets*, pink, erythromycin 500 mg (as estolate). Net price 12-tab pack = £4.96. Label: 9

*Suspension*, orange, erythromycin 125 mg (as estolate)/5 mL. Net price 100 mL = £2.51. Label: 9

*Suspension forte*, orange, erythromycin 250 mg (as estolate)/5 mL. Net price 100 mL = £4.89. Label: 9

## AZITHROMYCIN

*Indications:* respiratory-tract infections; otitis media; skin and soft-tissue infections; uncomplicated genital chlamydial infections

*Cautions; Side-effects:* see under Erythromycin; caution in renal impairment; mild neutropenia reported; pregnancy and breast-feeding; **interactions:** Appendix 1 (azithromycin)

*Contra-indications:* hepatic impairment

*Dose:* 500 mg once daily for 3 days *or* 500 mg once daily on first day then 250 mg daily for 4 days; CHILD 10 mg/kg on first day then 5 mg/kg once daily for 4 days; *or* 15–25 kg, 200 mg on first day then 100 mg once daily for 4 days; 26–35 kg, 300 mg on first day then 150 mg once daily; 36–45 kg, 400 mg on first day then 200 mg once daily

Genital chlamydial infections, 1 g as a single dose

▼ PoM **Zithromax**® (Richborough)

*Capsules*, azithromycin (as dihydrate) 250 mg. Net price 4-cap pack = £9.99, 6-cap pack = £14.99. Label: 9, 23

*Oral suspension*, azithromycin (as dihydrate) 200 mg/5 mL when reconstituted with water. Net price 15-mL pack = £7.05, 22.5-mL pack = £10.35, 30-mL pack = £13.80. Label: 9, 23

## CLARITHROMYCIN

*Indications:* respiratory-tract infections; mild to moderate skin and soft tissue infections

*Cautions; Side-effects:* see under Erythromycin; reduce dose in renal impairment; headache reported rarely

*Dose:* 250 mg every 12 hours for 7 days, increased in severe infections to 500 mg every 12 hours for up to 14 days; CHILD under 12 years not yet recommended

▼ PoM **Klaricid**® (Abbott)
*Tablets*, yellow, f/c, clarithromycin 250 mg. Net price 14-tab pack = £10.36. Label: 9

## 5.1.6   Clindamycin and lincomycin

These antibiotics have only a limited use because of their serious side-effects. Their most serious toxic effect is pseudomembranous colitis (see section 1.5) which may be fatal and is most common in middle-aged and elderly women, especially following operation. Although it can occur with most antibiotics it is more frequently seen with clindamycin. Patients should therefore discontinue treatment immediately if diarrhoea develops.

**Clindamycin**, which is more active and better absorbed from the gut, has generally replaced **lincomycin**. Both are active against Gram-positive cocci, including penicillin-resistant staphylococci and also against many anaerobes, especially *Bacteroides fragilis*. They are well concentrated in bone and excreted in bile and urine.

**Clindamycin** is recommended for staphylococcal joint and bone infections such as osteomyelitis, and intra-abdominal sepsis.

### CLINDAMYCIN

*Indications:* staphylococcal bone and joint infections, peritonitis; endocarditis prophylaxis, section 5.1, Table 2
*Cautions:* discontinue immediately if diarrhoea or colitis develops; impaired hepatic or renal function; **interactions:** Appendix 1 (clindamycin)
*Contra-indications:* diarrhoeal states
*Side-effects:* diarrhoea (discontinue treatment), nausea, vomiting, pseudomembranous colitis
*Dose: by mouth,* 150–300 mg every 6 hours; up to 450 mg every 6 hours in severe infections; CHILD, 3–6 mg/kg every 6 hours
Endocarditis prophylaxis, section 5.1, Table 2
COUNSELLING. Patients should discontinue immediately and contact doctor if diarrhoea develops; capsules should be swallowed with a glass of water.
*By intramuscular injection or by slow intravenous infusion,* 0.6–2.7 g daily in 2–4 divided doses; CHILD, 15–40 mg/kg daily in 3–4 divided doses

PoM **Dalacin C**® (Upjohn)
*Capsules*, clindamycin (as hydrochloride) 75 mg (lavender), net price 20 = £4.92; 150 mg, (lavender/maroon), 20 = £9.07. Label: 9, 27, counselling, see above (diarrhoea)
*Paediatric suspension*, pink, clindamycin 75 mg (as palmitate hydrochloride)/5 mL when reconstituted with purified water (freshly boiled and cooled). Net price 100 mL = £6.62. Label: 9, 27, counselling, see above (diarrhoea)
*Injection*, clindamycin 150 mg (as phosphate)/mL. Net price 2-mL amp = £5.17; 4-mL amp = £10.29

### LINCOMYCIN

*Indications:* see under Clindamycin, also notes above
*Cautions; Contra-indications; Side-effects:* see under Clindamycin; **interactions:** Appendix 1 (lincomycin)
*Dose: by mouth,* 500 mg every 6–8 hours
COUNSELLING. Patients should discontinue immediately and contact doctor if diarrhoea develops
*By deep intramuscular injection,* 600 mg every 12–24 hours
*By intravenous infusion,* 600 mg every 8–12 hours

PoM **Lincocin**® (Upjohn)
*Capsules*, blue, lincomycin 500 mg (as hydrochloride). Net price 12-cap pack = £7.21. Label: 9, 23, counselling, see above (diarrhoea)
*Injection*, lincomycin 300 mg (as hydrochloride)/mL. Net price 2-mL amp = £2.64

## 5.1.7   Some other antibiotics

Antibacterials discussed in this section include chloramphenicol, fusidic acid, spectinomycin, glycopeptide antibiotics (vancomycin and teicoplanin), and the polymyxins (colistin and polymyxin B).

**Chloramphenicol** is a potent, potentially toxic, broad-spectrum antibiotic which should be reserved for the treatment of life-threatening infections, particularly those caused by *Haemophilus influenzae*, and also for typhoid fever.

Its toxicity renders it unsuitable for systemic use except in the circumstances indicated above.

Eye-drops of chloramphenicol (see section 11.3.1) are useful for bacterial conjunctivitis.

### CHLORAMPHENICOL

*Indications:* see notes above
*Cautions:* avoid repeated courses and prolonged treatment; reduce doses in hepatic or renal impairment; blood counts required before and periodically during treatment; may cause 'grey syndrome' in neonates (monitor plasma concentrations); **interactions:** Appendix 1 (chloramphenicol)
*Contra-indications:* pregnancy (see also Appendix 4), breast-feeding, porphyria (see section 9.8.2)
*Side-effects:* blood disorders including irreversible aplastic anaemia (aplastic anaemia attributed to chloramphenicol has terminated in leukaemia), peripheral neuritis, optic neuritis, erythema multiforme, nausea, vomiting, diarrhoea; nocturnal haemoglobinuria reported)
*Dose: by mouth or by intravenous injection or infusion,* 50 mg/kg daily in 4 divided doses (exceptionally, can be doubled for severe infections such as septicaemia and meningitis, providing high doses reduced as soon as clinically

indicated); CHILD, haemophilus epiglottitis and pyogenic meningitis, 50–100 mg/kg daily in divided doses (high dosages decreased as soon as clinically indicated); INFANTS under 2 weeks 25 mg/kg daily (in 4 divided doses), 2 weeks–1 year 50 mg/kg daily (in 4 divided doses)

*Note.* Plasma concentration monitoring required in neonates and preferred in those under 4 years of age; recommended peak plasma concentration 15–25 mg/ litre; pre-dose ('trough') concentration should not exceed 15 mg/litre

### PoM **Chloromycetin®** (P-D)
*Capsules,* white/grey, chloramphenicol 250 mg. Net price 20 = £1.64

*Suspension,* chloramphenicol 125 mg (as palmitate)/5 mL. Net price 100 mL = £3.85

*Injection,* powder for reconstitution, chloramphenicol (as sodium succinate). Net price 300 mg vial = £5.16; 1.2-g vial = £5.03

*Electrolytes:* Na⁺ 0.94 mmol/300-mg vial, 3.75 mmol/1.2-g vial

### PoM **Kemicetine®** (Farmitalia Carlo Erba)
*Injection,* powder for reconstitution, chloramphenicol (as sodium succinate). Net price 1-g vial = 79p

*Electrolytes:* Na⁺ 3.14 mmol/g

---

**Fusidic acid** and its salts are narrow-spectrum antibiotics. The only indication for their use is in infections caused by penicillin-resistant staphylococci, especially osteomyelitis, as they are well concentrated in bone; a second antistaphylococcal antibiotic is usually required to prevent emergence of resistance.

## SODIUM FUSIDATE
*Indications:* see notes above
*Cautions:* liver-function tests required
*Side-effects:* nausea, vomiting, rashes, reversible jaundice, especially after high dosage or rapid infusion (withdraw therapy if persistent)
*Dose:* see under Preparations, below

### PoM **Fucidin®** (Leo)
*Tablets,* f/c, sodium fusidate 250 mg. Net price 20 = £13.89. Label: 9

*Dose:* 500 mg every 8 hours, doubled for severe infections

*Suspension,* orange, fusidic acid 250 mg (≡ sodium fusidate 175 mg)/5 mL. Do not dilute. Net price 50 mL = £7.77. Label: 9, 21

*Dose:* as fusidic acid, ADULT 750 mg every 8 hours; CHILD up to 1 year 50 mg/kg daily (in 3 divided doses), 1–5 years 250 mg every 8 hours, 5–12 years 500 mg every 8 hours

*Note.* Fusidic acid is incompletely absorbed and doses recommended for suspension are proportionately higher than those for sodium fusidate tablets

*Intravenous infusion,* powder for reconstitution, diethanolamine fusidate 580 mg (≡ sodium fusidate 500 mg), with buffer. Net price per vial (with diluent) = £4.65

*Electrolytes:* Na⁺ 14 mmol/vial when reconstituted with buffer

*Dose:* as diethanolamine fusidate, by intravenous infusion, ADULT over 50 kg, 580 mg 3 times daily; ADULT under 50 kg and CHILD, 6–7 mg/kg 3 times daily

---

**Spectinomycin** is active against Gram-negative organisms, including *N. gonorrhoeae.* Its only indication is the treatment of gonorrhoea caused by penicillin-resistant organisms or in a penicillin-allergic patient.

## SPECTINOMYCIN
*Indications:* see notes above
*Cautions:* pregnancy and breast-feeding; **interactions:** Appendix 1 (spectinomycin)
*Side-effects:* nausea, dizziness, urticaria, fever
*Dose: by deep intramuscular injection,* 2 g; up to 4 g in difficult-to-treat cases and in geographical areas of resistance; CHILD over 2 years, if no alternative treatment, 40 mg/kg

### PoM **Trobicin®** (Upjohn)
*Injection,* powder for reconstitution, spectinomycin (as hydrochloride). Net price 2-g vial (with diluent) = £8.16

---

## VANCOMYCIN AND TEICOPLANIN

---

The glycopeptide antibiotics vancomycin and teicoplanin have bactericidal activity against aerobic and anaerobic Gram-positive bacteria.

**Vancomycin** is the drug of choice for antibiotic-associated pseudomembranous colitis, for which it is given by mouth; a dose of 125 mg every 6 hours for 7 to 10 days is considered to be adequate; it is not absorbed by mouth. It has a limited use by the intravenous route in the prophylaxis and treatment of endocarditis and other serious infections caused by Gram-positive cocci including multi-resistant staphylococci. It has a relatively long duration of action and can therefore be given every 12 hours; plasma concentrations should be monitored (especially in patients with renal impairment in whom the dose may need marked reduction). It is ototoxic and nephrotoxic.

**Teicoplanin** is very similar to vancomycin but has a significantly longer duration of action allowing once daily administration. Unlike vancomycin, teicoplanin can be given by intramuscular as well as by intravenous injection.

## VANCOMYCIN
*Indications:* see notes above
*Cautions:* extravasation at injection site may cause necrosis and thrombophlebitis, blood counts and hearing, liver, and kidney function tests required; reduce dose in elderly; **interactions:** Appendix 1 (vancomycin)
*Contra-indications:* if possible avoid parenteral administration in patients with renal impairment or a history of deafness

---

*Side-effects:* after parenteral administration nausea, chills, fever, urticaria, rashes, 'red man' syndrome (on rapid intravenous injection), eosinophilia, tinnitus (discontinue use), renal impairment

*Dose: by mouth*, 125 mg every 6 hours for 7–10 days, see notes above; CHILD, half adult dose

*By intravenous infusion*, 500 mg over at least 60 minutes every 6 hours *or* 1 g over at least 100 minutes every 12 hours; NEONATE up to 1 week, 15 mg/kg initially then 10 mg/kg every 12 hours; INFANT 1–4 weeks, 15 mg/kg initially then 10 mg/kg every 8 hours; CHILD over 1 month, 10 mg/kg every 6 hours

Note. Plasma concentration monitoring required

Endocarditis prophylaxis, section 5.1, table 2

### PoM **Vancocin**® (Lilly)

*Matrigel capsules*, vancomycin (as hydrochloride) 125 mg (blue/peach), net price 20-cap pack = £63.08; 250 mg (blue/grey), 20-cap pack = £126.16

*Injection*, powder for reconstitution, vancomycin (as hydrochloride). Net price 500-mg vial = £13.36

## TEICOPLANIN

*Indications:* potentially serious Gram-positive infections including endocarditis, dialysis-associated peritonitis, and serious infections due to *Staphylococcus aureus*

*Cautions:* blood counts and liver and kidney function tests required; reduce dose in renal impairment (and monitor renal and auditory function on prolonged administration or if other nephrotoxic drugs given); reduce dose in elderly

*Side-effects:* nausea, vomiting, diarrhoea; rash, fever, bronchospasm, anaphylactic reactions; dizziness, headache; blood disorders including eosinophilia, leucopenia, and thrombocytopenia; disturbances in liver enzymes, transient increase of serum creatinine; tinnitus, mild hearing loss, and vestibular disorders also reported; local reactions include erythema, pain, and thrombophlebitis

*Dose: by intravenous injection or infusion*, 400 mg initially, subsequently 200 mg daily; severe infections, 400 mg every 12 hours for 3 doses initially, subsequently 400 mg daily; the subsequent doses can alternatively be given by intramuscular injection

CHILD *by intravenous injection or infusion*, initially 6 mg/kg every 12 hours for 3 doses, subsequently 3 mg/kg daily (severe infections, 6 mg/kg daily)

### ▼ PoM **Targocid**® (Merrell)

*Injection*, powder for reconstitution, teicoplanin, net price 200-mg vial (with diluent) = £26.72; 400-mg vial (with diluent) = £53.44

*Electrolytes:* Na⁺ <0.5 mmol/200- and 400-mg vial

## POLYMYXINS

The polymyxin antibiotics, colistin and polymyxin B, are active against Gram-negative organisms, including *Pseudomonas aeruginosa*. They are **not** absorbed by mouth and thus need to be given by injection to obtain a systemic effect; however, they are toxic and have few, if any, indications for systemic use.

Colistin is used in bowel sterilisation regimens in neutropenic patients; it is **not** recommended for gastro-intestinal infections.

Both colistin and polymyxin B are included in some preparations for topical application. For reference to use as a bladder irrigation see section 7.4.4.

## COLISTIN

*Indications:* see notes above

*Cautions:* reduce dose in renal impairment; **interactions:** Appendix 1 (polymyxins)

*Contra-indications:* myasthenia gravis; porphyria (see section 9.8.2)

*Side-effects:*    perioral    and    peripheral paraesthesia, vertigo, muscle weakness, apnoea, nephrotoxicity

*Dose: by mouth*, bowel sterilisation, 1.5–3 million units every 8 hours

*By intramuscular injection or intravenous injection or infusion*, 2 million units every 8 hours (but see notes above)

### PoM **Colomycin**® (Pharmax)

*Tablets*, scored, colistin sulphate 1.5 million units. Net price 50 = £63.60

*Syrup*, pink, colistin sulphate 250 000 units/5 mL when reconstituted with water. Net price 80 mL = £3.79

*Injection*, powder for reconstitution, colistin sulphomethate sodium. Net price 500 000-unit vial = £1.25; 1 million-unit vial = £1.83

*Electrolytes*, (before reconstitution) Na⁺ < 0.5 mmol/ 500 000- and 1 million-unit vial

## POLYMYXIN B SULPHATE

*Indications; Cautions; Contra-indications; Side-effects:* see under Colistin

*Dose: by slow intravenous infusion*, 15 000–25 000 units/kg daily in divided doses

### PoM **Aerosporin**® (Wellcome)

*Injection*, powder for reconstitution, polymyxin B sulphate. Net price 500 000-unit vial = £13.81

### PoM **Polybactrin**® (Wellcome)

*Soluble GU*, powder for reconstitution, polymyxin B sulphate 75 000 units, neomycin sulphate 20 000 units, bacitracin 1000 units. For bladder irrigation. Net price per vial = £6.62

## 5.1.8    Sulphonamides and trimethoprim

The importance of the sulphonamides as chemotherapeutic agents has decreased as a result of increasing bacterial resistance and their replacement by antibiotics which are generally more active and less toxic.

The principal indication for sulphonamides used alone is urinary-tract infections caused by sensitive organisms.

Sulphamethoxazole and trimethoprim have been used in combination (as co-trimoxazole) because of their synergistic activity. Increasing bacterial resistance to sulphonamides and the high incidence of sulphonamide-related side-effects have however diminished the value of co-trimoxazole.

Indications for **co-trimoxazole** include urinary-tract infections, prostatitis, exacerbations of chronic bronchitis, and invasive salmonella infections, but trimethoprim alone is now preferred. High doses of co-trimoxazole are used for *Pneumocystis carinii* infections. Co-trimoxazole is no longer recommended for gonorrhoea.

**Trimethoprim** can be used alone for the treatment of urinary- and respiratory-tract infections and for prostatitis and invasive salmonella infections. Side-effects are less than with co-trimoxazole especially in older patients.

Side-effects of the sulphonamides include rashes, which are common, the Stevens-Johnson syndrome (erythema multiforme), renal failure (especially with the less soluble preparations), and blood dyscrasias, notably marrow depression and agranulocytosis.

Side-effects of co-trimoxazole are similar to those of the sulphonamides but a particular watch should be kept for haematological effects and special care should be taken in patients who may be folate deficient such as the elderly and chronic sick. There have been recent reports of deaths in patients over the age of 65 years being treated with co-trimoxazole and almost certainly associated with the sulphonamide component. For this reason co-trimoxazole should be used with care in the elderly and preferably only if there is no acceptable alternative. The effect on the fetus is unknown and the drugs should not be used in pregnancy.

The **longer-acting sulphonamide**, sulfametopyrazine which is highly bound to plasma proteins, has the advantage of requiring less frequent administration, but toxic effects due to accumulation are more likely to occur.

For *topical preparations* of sulphonamides used in the treatment of burns see section 13.10.1.1.

## CO-TRIMOXAZOLE

A mixture of trimethoprim and sulphamethoxazole in the proportions of 1 part to 5 parts

*Indications:* invasive salmonellosis, typhoid fever, bone and joint infections due to *Haemophilus influenzae*, urinary-tract infections, sinusitis, exacerbations of chronic bronchitis, gonorrhoea in penicillin-allergic patients

*Cautions:* blood counts in prolonged treatment, maintain adequate fluid intake, renal impairment, breast-feeding; photosensitivity; elderly patients (**important:** see notes above); **interactions:** Appendix 1 (co-trimoxazole)

*Contra-indications:* pregnancy, infants under 6 weeks (risk of kernicterus), renal or hepatic failure, jaundice, blood disorders; porphyria (see section 9.8.2)

*Side-effects:* nausea, vomiting, glossitis, rashes, erythema multiforme (includes Stevens-Johnson syndrome), epidermal necrolysis, eosinophilia, agranulocytosis, granulocytopenia, purpura, leucopenia; megaloblastic anaemia due to trimethoprim

*Dose: by mouth,* 960 mg every 12 hours, increased to 1.44 g in severe infections; 480 mg every 12 hours if treated for more than 14 days; CHILD, every 12 hours, 6 weeks to 5 months, 120 mg; 6 months to 5 years, 240 mg; 6–12 years, 480 mg

Prophylaxis of recurrent urinary-tract infection, 480 mg at night; CHILD 6–12 mg/kg at night

Gonorrhoea, 1.92 g every 12 hours for 2 days, or 2.4 g followed by a further dose of 2.4 g after 8 hours but see notes above

High-dose therapy for *Pneumocystis carinii* infections, 120 mg/kg daily in divided doses for 14 days

*By intramuscular injection or intravenous infusion,* 960 mg every 12 hours

Note. 480 mg of co-trimoxazole consists of sulphamethoxazole 400 mg and trimethoprim 80 mg

PoM **Co-trimoxazole** (Non-proprietary)

*Tablets,* co-trimoxazole 480 mg; net price 20 = 97p; 960 mg, 20 = £3.17. Label: 9

Available from APS, Ashbourne (Comixco®), Cox (480 mg), CP, DDSA (Fectrim®, Fectrim® Forte), Evans (480 mg), Kerfoot (960 mg), Lagap (Laratrim® 960 mg), Norton (Comox®)

*Dispersible tablets,* co-trimoxazole 480 mg. Net price 20 = £1.44. Label: 9, 13

Available from APS, Kerfoot, Norton (Comox®)

*Paediatric oral suspension,* co-trimoxazole 240 mg/5 mL. Net price 100 mL = £2.09. Label: 9

Available from APS, Ashbourne (Comixco®), CP, Evans, Kerfoot, Lagap (Laratrim®), Norton (Comox®), RP Drugs (Chemotrim®)

*Oral suspension,* co-trimoxazole 480 mg/5 mL. Net price 100 mL = £3·00. Label: 9

Available from APS, CP, Evans, Kerfoot, Lagap (Laratrim®)

PoM **Bactrim®** (Roche)

*Drapsules®*(= tablets), orange, f/c, co-trimoxazole 480 mg. Net price 20 = £2.26. Label: 9

*Tablets* (dispersible), yellow, scored, co-trimoxazole 480 mg. Net price 20 = £2.49. Label: 9, 13

*Double-strength tablets,* scored, co-trimoxazole 960 mg. Net price 20 = £3.54. Label: 9

*Paediatric tablets,* co-trimoxazole 120 mg. Net price 20 = 64p. Label: 9

*Adult suspension,* yellow, co-trimoxazole 480 mg/5 mL. Net price 100 mL = £3.00. Label: 9

*Paediatric syrup,* sugar-free, yellow, co-trimoxazole 240 mg/5 mL. Net price 100 mL = £2.09. Label: 9

PoM **Septrin**® (Wellcome)
*Tablets*, co-trimoxazole 480 mg. Net price 20 = £3.03. Label: 9
*Dispersible tablets*, orange, sugar-free, co-trimoxazole 480 mg. Net price 20 = £3.22. Label: 9, 13
*Forte tablets*, scored, co-trimoxazole 960 mg. Net price 20 = £5.05. Label: 9
*Paediatric dispersible tablets*, orange, sugar-free, co-trimoxazole 120 mg. Net price 20 = £1.01. Label: 9, 13
*Adult suspension*, co-trimoxazole 480 mg/5 mL. Net price 100 mL = £4.74. Label: 9
*Paediatric suspension*, sugar-free, co-trimoxazole 240 mg/5 mL. Diluent syrup or sorbitol solution 70%, life of diluted suspension 14 days. Net price 100 mL = £2.63. Label: 9
*Intramuscular injection*, co-trimoxazole 320 mg/mL. Net price 3-mL amp = £2.71
*Intravenous infusion*, co-trimoxazole 96 mg/mL. To be diluted before use. Net price 5-mL amp = £1.59

## SULFAMETOPYRAZINE

*Indications:* urinary-tract infections, chronic bronchitis
*Cautions; Contra-indications; Side-effects:* see under Co-trimoxazole
*Dose:* 2 g once weekly

PoM **Kelfizine W**® (Farmitalia Carlo Erba)
*Tablets*, sulfametopyrazine 2 g. Tablets to be taken in water. Net price 1 = £1.25. Label: 9, 13

## SULPHADIAZINE

*Indications:* meningococcal meningitis
*Cautions; Contra-indications; Side-effects:* see under Co-trimoxazole; avoid in severe renal impairment
*Dose: by deep intramuscular injection or intravenous infusion*, 2 g initially then 1 g every 6 hours for 2 days, followed by oral treatment for a further 5 days

PoM **Sulphadiazine** (Non-proprietary)
*Tablets*, sulphadiazine 500 mg. Net price 20 = £1.34. Label: 9, 27
*Injection*, sulphadiazine 250 mg (as sodium salt)/mL. Net price 4-mL amp = 94p

## SULPHADIMIDINE

*Indications:* urinary-tract infections; meningococcal meningitis
*Cautions; Contra-indications; Side-effects:* see under Co-trimoxazole
*Dose: by mouth*, 2 g initially, then 0.5–1 g every 6–8 hours
Meningitis prophylaxis, see section 5.1, table 2

PoM **Sulphadimidine** (Non-proprietary)
*Tablets*, sulphadimidine 500 mg. Net price 20 = £1.22. Label: 9, 27

## TRIMETHOPRIM

*Indications:* urinary-tract infections, acute and chronic bronchitis
*Cautions:* renal impairment, breast-feeding, predisposition to folate deficiency, blood counts required on long-term therapy; **interactions:** Appendix 1 (trimethoprim)
*Contra-indications:* severe renal impairment, pregnancy, neonates; porphyria (see section 9.8.2)
*Side-effects:* gastro-intestinal disturbances including nausea and vomiting, pruritus, rashes, depression of haemopoiesis
*Dose: by mouth*, acute infections, 200 mg every 12 hours; urinary-tract infections, 300 mg daily *or* 200 mg twice daily; CHILD, twice daily, 2–5 months 25 mg, 6 months–5 years 50 mg, 6–12 years 100 mg
Chronic infections and prophylaxis, 100 mg at night; CHILD 1–2 mg/kg at night
*By slow intravenous injection or infusion*, 150–250 mg every 12 hours; CHILD under 12 years, 6–9 mg/kg daily in 2–3 divided doses

PoM **Trimethoprim** (Non-proprietary)
*Tablets*, trimethoprim 100 mg, net price 20 = 62p; 200 mg, 20 = 91p. Label: 9
PoM **Ipral**® (Squibb)
*Tablets*, trimethoprim 100 mg, net price 20 = 80p; 200 mg, 20 = £1.71. Label: 9
PoM **Monotrim**® (Duphar)
*Tablets*, both scored, trimethoprim 100 mg, net price 20 = 80p; 200 mg, 20 = £1.71. Label: 9
*Suspension*, sugar-free, trimethoprim 50 mg/5 mL. Diluents sorbitol solution or water, life of diluted suspension 14 days. Net price 100 mL = £1.77.
*Injection*, trimethoprim 20 mg (as lactate)/mL. Net price 5-mL amp = 68p
PoM **Syraprim**® (Wellcome)
*Tablets*, scored, trimethoprim 300 mg, net price 20 = £13.04. Label: 9
*Injection*, trimethoprim 20 mg (as lactate)/mL. Net price 5-mL amp = £1.86
PoM **Trimogal**® (Lagap)
*Tablets*, trimethoprim 100 mg, net price 20 = 61p; 200 mg, 20 = 91p. Label: 9
PoM **Trimopan**® (Berk)
*Tablets*, both scored, trimethoprim 100 mg, net price 20 = 97p; 200 mg, 20 = £1.75. Label: 9
*Suspension*, sugar-free, trimethoprim 50 mg/5 mL. Net price 100 mL = £1.37. Label: 9

## 5.1.9   Antituberculous drugs

Tuberculosis is treated in two phases—an *initial phase* using at least three drugs and a *continuation phase* using two drugs. Treatment requires specialised knowledge, particularly where the disease involves resistant organisms or non-respiratory organs.

The regimens given below are recommended by the Joint Tuberculosis Committee of the British Thoracic Society for the treatment of tuberculosis in the UK; variations occur in other countries.

INITIAL PHASE. The concurrent use of at least three drugs during the initial phase is designed to reduce the population of viable bacteria as rapidly as possible and to prevent the emergence of drug-resistant bacteria. Treatment of choice for the initial phase is the daily use of isoniazid, rifampicin, and pyrazinamide; ethambutol is added if drug resistance is thought likely. Streptomycin is now rarely used in the UK but it may be added if the organism is resistant to isoniazid. The initial phase drugs should be continued for 2 months.

CONTINUATION PHASE. After the initial phase, treatment is continued for a further 4 months with isoniazid and rifampicin; longer treatment may be necessary for bone and joint infections, for meningitis, or for resistant organisms.

*Recommended dosage for standard unsupervised 6-month regimen*

| Isoniazid (for 6 months) | ADULT 300 mg daily; CHILD 10 mg/kg (max. 300 mg) daily |
| Rifampicin (for 6 months) | ADULT under 50 kg 450 mg daily, 50 kg and over 600 mg daily; CHILD 10 mg/kg daily |
| Pyrazinamide (for first 2 months only) | ADULT under 50 kg 1.5 g, 50 kg and over 2 g daily; CHILD 35 mg/kg daily |

*Note.* Ethambutol and streptomycin are included in treatment regimens if resistance is suspected; see notes below for doses

PREGNANCY AND BREAST-FEEDING. The standard regimen (above) may be used during pregnancy and breast-feeding; pyridoxine supplements are advisable. Streptomycin should not be given in pregnancy

CHILDREN. As for adults, children are given isoniazid, rifampicin, and pyrazinamide for the first 2 months followed by isoniazid and rifampicin during the next 4 months. If pyrazinamide is omitted from the initial phase, then treatment with isoniazid and rifampicin should be given for 9 months. Ethambutol should be **avoided** in young children because of the difficulty in testing eyesight and in obtaining reports of visual symptoms (see below).

NON-COMPLIANT PATIENTS. Treatment needs to be fully supervised in patients who cannot be relied upon to comply with the treatment regimen. These patients are given isoniazid, rifampicin, and pyrazinamide 3 times a week under supervision for the first 2 months followed by isoniazid and rifampicin three times a week for a further 4 months.

*Recommended dosage for intermittent supervised treatment*

| Isoniazid (for 6 months) | ADULT and CHILD 15 mg/kg 3 times a week |
| Rifampicin (for 6 months) | ADULT 600–900 mg 3 times a week; CHILD 15 mg/kg 3 times a week |
| Pyrazinamide (for first 2 months only) | ADULT under 50 kg 2 g 3 times a week, 50 kg and over 2.5 g; CHILD 50 mg/kg 3 times a week |
| | *or* |
| | ADULT under 50 kg 3 g twice a week, 50 kg and over 3.5 g; CHILD 75 mg/kg twice a week |

*Note.* Ethambutol and streptomycin are included in treatment regimens if resistance is suspected; see notes below for doses

> Major causes of treatment failure are incorrect prescribing by the physician and inadequate compliance by the patient. Avoid both excessive and inadequate dosage.

**Isoniazid** is cheap and highly effective. Like rifampicin it should always be included in any antituberculous regimen unless there is a specific contra-indication. Its only common side-effect is peripheral neuropathy which is more likely to occur where there are pre-existing risk factors such as diabetes and alcoholism and in chronic renal failure and malnutrition. In these circumstances pyridoxine 10 mg daily should be given prophylactically from the start of treatment. Other side-effects such as hepatitis and psychosis are rare.

**Rifampicin** is a key component of any antituberculous regimen. Like isoniazid it should always be included unless there is a specific contra-indication.

During the first two months of rifampicin administration transient disturbance of liver function with elevated serum transaminases is common but generally does not require interruption of treatment. Occasionally more serious liver toxicity requires a change of treatment particularly in those with pre-existing liver disease.

On intermittent treatment six toxicity syndromes have been recognised—influenzal, abdominal, and respiratory symptoms, shock, renal failure, and thrombocytopenic purpura—and can occur in 20 to 30% of patients.

Rifampicin induces hepatic enzymes which accelerate the metabolism of several drugs including oestrogens, corticosteroids, phenytoin, sulphonylureas, and anticoagulants. The effectiveness of oral contraceptives is reduced and alternative family planning advice should be offered.

**Pyrazinamide** is a bactericidal drug only active against intracellular dividing forms of *Mycobacterium tuberculosis*; it exerts its main effect only in the first two or three months. It is particularly useful in tuberculous meningitis because of good meningeal penetration. It is not active against *M. bovis*.

**Ethambutol** is included in a treatment regimen if resistance is suspected; it can be omitted if the risk of resistance is low. For unsupervised treatment ethambutol is given in a dose of 25 mg/kg daily in the initial phase followed by 15 mg/kg daily in the continuation phase (*or* 15 mg/kg daily throughout); in fully supervised intermittent treatment ethambutol is given in a dose of 30 mg/kg 3 times a week *or* 45 mg/kg twice a week.

Side-effects of ethambutol are largely confined to visual disturbances in the form of loss of acuity, colour blindness, and restriction of visual fields. These toxic effects are more common where excessive dosage is used or the patient's renal function is impaired, in which case the drug should be **avoided**. The earliest features of ocular toxicity are subjective and patients should be advised to discontinue therapy immediately if they develop deterioration in vision and promptly seek further advice. Early discontinuation of the drug is almost always followed by recovery of eyesight. Patients who cannot understand warnings about visual side-effects should, if possible, be given an alternative drug. In particular, ethambutol should be **avoided** in children until they are at least 6 years old and capable of reporting symptomatic visual changes accurately.

Ophthalmic examination should be performed prior to treatment and at intervals during treatment.

**Streptomycin** is now rarely used in the UK except for resistant organisms. It is given intramuscularly in a standard dose of 1 g daily, reduced to 500–750 mg in patients under 50 kg or those over 40 years of age. For fully supervised intermittent treatment streptomycin is given in a dose of 1 g 3 times a week, reduced to 750 mg 3 times a week in patients under 50 kg. Children are given streptomycin in a dose of 15–20 mg/kg daily or for fully supervised intermittent treatment, 15–20 mg/kg 3 times a week. Plasma drug concentrations should be measured, particularly in patients with impaired renal function in whom streptomycin must be used with great care. Side-effects increase after a cumulative dose of 100 g, which should only be exceeded in exceptional circumstances.

Second-line drugs available for infections caused by resistant organisms, or when first-line drugs cause unacceptable side-effects, include capreomycin, cycloserine, and prothionamide (no longer on UK market).

## CAPREOMYCIN

*Indications:* in combination with other drugs, tuberculosis resistant to first-line drugs
*Cautions:* renal, hepatic, or auditory impairment; monitor renal, hepatic, auditory, and vestibular function and electrolytes; pregnancy (teratogenic in *animals*) and breast-feeding; **interactions:** Appendix 1 (capreomycin)
*Side-effects:* hypersensitivity reactions including urticaria and rashes; leucocytosis or leucopenia, rarely thrombocytopenia; changes in liver function tests; nephrotoxicity, electrolyte disturbances; hearing loss with tinnitus and vertigo; neuromuscular block after large doses, pain and induration at injection site
*Dose: by deep intramuscular injection*, 1 g daily (not more than 20 mg/kg) for 2–4 months, then 1 g 2–3 times each week

PoM **Capastat**® (Dista)
*Injection*, powder for reconstitution, capreomycin sulphate 1 million units (≡ capreomycin approx. 1 g). Net price per vial = £2.28

## CYCLOSERINE

*Indications:* in combination with other drugs, tuberculosis resistant to first-line drugs
*Cautions:* reduce dose in renal impairment; monitor haematological, renal, and hepatic function; pregnancy and breast-feeding; **interactions:** Appendix 1 (cycloserine)
*Contra-indications:* epilepsy, depression, severe anxiety, psychotic states, alcohol dependence, porphyria (see section 9.8.2)
*Side-effects:* mainly neurological, including headache, dizziness, vertigo, drowsiness, tremor, convulsions; psychosis, depression; rashes; megaloblastic anaemia; changes in liver function tests
*Dose:* usually 250 mg every 12 hours; max. 1 g daily
Note. Blood concentration monitoring required especially in renal impairment or if dose exceeds 500 mg daily or if signs of toxicity; blood concentration should not exceed 30 mg/litre

PoM **Cycloserine** (Lilly)
*Capsules*, red/grey cycloserine 250 mg, net price 20 = £11.35. Label: 2, 8

## ETHAMBUTOL HYDROCHLORIDE

*Indications:* tuberculosis, in combination with other drugs
*Cautions:* warn patients to report visual changes—see notes above
*Contra-indications:* renal impairment; young children (see notes), elderly patients, optic neuritis, poor vision
*Side-effects:* optic neuritis, red/green colour blindness, peripheral neuritis
*Dose:* ADULT and CHILD over 6 years, see notes above

PoM **Myambutol**® (Lederle)
*Tablets*, ethambutol hydrochloride 100 mg (yellow), net price 20 = £1.45; 400 mg (grey), 20 = £5.23. Label: 8
PoM **Mynah**® (Lederle)
*Mynah 200 tablets*, ethambutol hydrochloride 200 mg, isoniazid 100 mg. Net price 84-tab pack = £13.27. Label: 8, 23
*Mynah 250 tablets*, yellow, ethambutol hydrochloride 250 mg, isoniazid 100 mg. Net price 84-tab pack = £16.45. Label: 8, 23
*Mynah 300 tablets*, orange, ethambutol hydrochloride 300 mg, isoniazid 100 mg. Net price 84-tab pack = £19.66. Label: 8, 23

## ISONIAZID

*Indications:* tuberculosis, in combination with other drugs; prophylaxis—section 5.1, Table 2

*Cautions:* impaired liver and kidney function, epilepsy, history of psychosis, alcoholism, breast-feeding; **interactions:** Appendix 1 (isoniazid)

*Contra-indications:* drug-induced liver disease, porphyria (see section 9.8.2)

*Side-effects:* nausea, vomiting, hypersensitivity reactions including rashes, peripheral neuritis with high doses (pyridoxine prophylaxis, see notes above), convulsions, psychotic episodes, agranulocytosis; hepatitis (especially over age of 35); systemic lupus erythematosus-like syndrome reported

*Dose: by mouth or by intramuscular or intravenous injection*, see notes above

PoM **Isoniazid Tablets,** isoniazid 50 mg, net price 20 = 28p; 100 mg, 20 = 32p. Label: 8, 22

PoM **Isoniazid Elixir** (BPC)
*Elixir*, isoniazid 50 mg, citric acid monohydrate 12.5 mg, sodium citrate 60 mg, concentrated anise water 0.05 mL, compound tartrazine solution 0.05 mL, glycerol 1 mL, double-strength chloroform water 2 mL, water to 5 mL. Label: 8, 22
Isoniazid oral solution (isoniazid 50 mg/5 mL) available from Penn, RP Drugs (both special order)

▼ PoM **Rimifon®** (Roche)
*Injection*, isoniazid 25 mg/mL. Net price 2-mL amp = 9p.

## PYRAZINAMIDE

*Indications:* tuberculosis in combination with other drugs

*Cautions:* impaired renal function, diabetes, gout; **interactions:** Appendix 1 (pyrazinamide)

*Contra-indications:* liver damage, porphyria (see section 9.8.2)

*Side-effects:* hepatotoxicity including fever, anorexia, hepatomegaly, jaundice, liver failure; nausea, vomiting, arthralgia, sideroblastic anaemia, urticaria

*Dose:* see notes above

PoM **Zinamide®** (MSD)
*Tablets*, scored, pyrazinamide 500 mg. Net price 20 = £1.44. Label: 8

## RIFAMPICIN

*Indications:* see under Dose

*Cautions:* reduce dose in hepatic impairment (see Appendix 2; liver function tests and blood counts in hepatic disorders and on prolonged therapy); pregnancy (see Appendix 4); advise patients on oral contraceptives to use additional means; discolours soft contact lenses; see also notes above; **interactions:** Appendix 1 (rifampicin)
*Note.* If treatment interrupted re-introduce with low dosage; discontinue permanently if serious side-effects develop

*Contra-indications:* jaundice, porphyria (see section 9.8.2)

*Side-effects:* gastro-intestinal symptoms including anorexia, nausea, vomiting, diarrhoea (pseudomembranous colitis reported); those occurring mainly on intermittent therapy include influenzal syndrome (with chills, fever, dizziness, bone pain), respiratory symptoms (including shortness of breath), collapse and shock, haemolytic anaemia, acute renal failure, and thrombocytopenic purpura; alterations of liver function, jaundice; flushing, urticaria, and rashes; other side-effects reported include oedema, muscular weakness and myopathy, leucopenia, eosinophilia, menstrual disturbances; urine, saliva, and other body secretions coloured orange-red

*Dose:* brucellosis, legionnaires' disease and serious staphylococcal infections, in combination with other drugs, *by mouth or by intravenous infusion*, 0.6–1.2 g daily in 2–4 divided doses

Tuberculosis, in combination with other drugs, see notes above

Leprosy, section 5.1.10

Prophylaxis of meningococcal meningitis and *Haemophilus influenzae* (type b) infection, section 5.1, Table 2

PoM **Rifampicin** (Non-proprietary)
*Capsules*, rifampicin 150 mg, net price 20 = £3.44; 300 mg, 20 = £6.88. Label: 8, 14, 22, counselling, see lenses above
Available from Generics

PoM **Rifadin®** (Merrell)
*Capsules*, rifampicin 150 mg (blue/red), net price 20 = £3.82; 300 mg (red), 20 = £7.64. Label: 8, 14, 22, counselling, see lenses above
*Syrup*, red, rifampicin 100 mg/5 mL. Do not dilute. Net price 120 mL = £3.71. Label: 8, 14, 22, counselling, see lenses above
*Intravenous infusion*, powder for reconstitution, rifampicin. Net price 600-mg vial (with solvent) = £8.00
*Electrolytes:* Na+ <0.5 mmol/vial

PoM **Rimactane®** (Ciba)
*Capsules*, rifampicin 150 mg (red), net price 20 = £3.44; 300 mg (red/brown), 20 = £6.88. Label: 8, 14, 22, counselling, see lenses above
*Syrup*, red, rifampicin 100 mg/5 mL. Do not dilute. Net price 100 mL = £2.78. Label: 8, 14, 22, counselling, see lenses above
*Intravenous infusion*, powder for reconstitution, rifampicin. Net price 300-mg vial (with diluent) = £7.28
*Electrolytes:* Na+ < 0.5 mmol/vial
*Note.* Owing to risk of contact sensitisation care must be taken to avoid contact during preparation and infusion

**Combined preparations**
PoM **Rifater®** (Merrell)
*Tablets*, pink-beige, s/c, rifampicin 120 mg, isoniazid 50 mg, pyrazinamide 300 mg. Net price 20 = £4.40. Label: 8, 14, 22, counselling, see lenses above
*Dose:* initial treatment of pulmonary tuberculosis, patients up to 40 kg 3 tablets daily preferably before breakfast, 40–49 kg 4 tablets daily, 50–64 kg 5 tablets daily, 65 kg or more, 6 tablets daily; not suitable for use in children

---

PoM **Rifinah 150**® (Merrell)
*Tablets*, pink, rifampicin 150 mg, isoniazid
100 mg. Net price 84-tab pack = £16.59. Label:
8, 14, 22, counselling, see lenses above
*Dose:* ADULT under 50 kg, 3 tablets daily, preferably before breakfast

PoM **Rifinah 300**® (Merrell)
*Tablets*, orange, rifampicin 300 mg, isoniazid
150 mg. Net price 56-tab pack = £21.93. Label:
8, 14, 22, counselling, see lenses above
*Dose:* ADULT 50 kg and over, 2 tablets daily,
preferably before breakfast

PoM **Rimactazid 150**® (Ciba)
*Tablets*, pink, s/c, rifampicin 150 mg, isoniazid
100 mg. Net price 84-tab pack = £14.93. Label:
8, 14, 22, counselling, see lenses above
*Additives: include gluten*
*Dose:* ADULT under 50 kg, 3 tablets daily, preferably before breakfast

PoM **Rimactazid 300**® (Ciba)
*Tablets*, orange, s/c, rifampicin 300 mg, isoniazid
150 mg. Net price 56-tab pack = £19.74. Label:
8, 14, 22, counselling, see lenses above
*Additives: include gluten*
*Dose:* ADULT 50 kg and over, 2 tablets daily,
preferably before breakfast

---

## STREPTOMYCIN
*Indications:* tuberculosis, in combination with
other drugs
*Cautions; Contra-indications; Side-effects:* see
under Aminoglycosides, section 5.1.4; also hypersensitivity reactions, paraesthesia of mouth
*Dose: by deep intramuscular injection*, see notes
above

PoM **Streptomycin Sulphate** (Evans)
*Injection*, powder for reconstitution, streptomycin (as sulphate). Net price 1-g vial = £5.62

## 5.1.10   Antileprotic drugs
Advice from a member of the Panel of Leprosy
Opinion is essential for the treatment of leprosy
(Hansen's disease). Details of the Panel can be
obtained from the Department of Health tele-
phone 071-972 3272.

For over twenty years the mainstay of leprosy
treatment was dapsone monotherapy but resistance to dapsone became an increasing concern.
The World Health Organization has made recommendations to overcome this problem of dapsone resistance and to prevent the emergence
of resistance to other antileprotic drugs. These
recommendations are based on the same principles as for the chemotherapy of tuberculosis.
Drugs recommended are **dapsone**, **rifampicin**, and
**clofazimine**; ethionamide or prothionamide
(which are not marketed in the UK) are no longer
recommended unless absolutely necessary.

A three-drug regimen is recommended for *multibacillary leprosy* (lepromatous, borderline-lep-
romatous, and borderline leprosy) and a two-drug
regimen for those suffering from *paucibacillary
leprosy* (borderline-tuberculoid, tuberculoid, and
indeterminate). These regimens, which are widely

applicable throughout the world (with minor local
variations), are as follows:

*Multibacillary leprosy (3-drug regimen)*
| | | |
|---|---|---|
| Rifampicin | 600 mg | once-monthly, supervised (450 mg for those weighing less than 35 kg) |
| Dapsone | 100 mg daily, self-administered | |
| Clofazimine | 300 mg once-monthly, supervised, *and* 50 mg daily, self-administered | |

*Note.* Substitution of clofazimine with ethionamide or
prothionamide is no longer recommended unless absolutely necessary; administration (in a dose of 250–375 mg
daily) should be under medical supervision, with periodic
checks for hepatotoxicity

Treatment should be given for at least 2 years and
be continued, wherever possible, up to smear
negativity. It should be continued unchanged during both type I (reversal) or type II (erythema
nodosum leprosum) reactions which, if severe,
should receive their own specific treatment (e.g.
prednisolone or increased clofazimine dosage).

*Paucibacillary leprosy (2-drug regimen)*
| | | |
|---|---|---|
| Rifampicin | 600 mg | once-monthly, supervised (450 mg for those weighing less than 35 kg) |
| Dapsone | 100 mg daily, self-administered | |

Treatment should be given for 6 months. If treatment is interrupted the regimen should be recommenced where it was left off to complete the full
course.

Neither the multibacillary nor the
paucibacillary antileprosy regimen is sufficient to
treat tuberculosis, therefore patients who also
have tuberculosis should be given appropriate
antituberculous drugs in addition to the antileprosy regimen.

## DAPSONE
*Indications:* leprosy, dermatitis herpetiformis
*Cautions:* cardiac or pulmonary disease; anaemia
(treat severe anaemia before starting); G6PD-
deficiency (including breast-feeding of affected
children, see section 9.1.5); pregnancy; avoid
in porphyria (see section 9.8.2); **interactions:**
Appendix 1 (dapsone)
*Side-effects:* (dose-related and uncommon at
doses used for leprosy), neuropathy, allergic
dermatitis, anorexia, nausea, vomiting, headache, insomnia, tachycardia, anaemia, hepatitis, agranulocytosis
*Dose:* leprosy, 1–2 mg/kg daily, see notes above
Dermatitis herpetiformis, see specialist literature

PoM **Dapsone Tablets**, dapsone 50 mg, net price
20 = 50p; 100 mg, 20 = 67p. Label: 8

## CLOFAZIMINE
*Indications:* leprosy
*Cautions:* hepatic and renal impairment—func-
tion tests required

---

*Side-effects:* nausea, giddiness, headache, and diarrhoea with high doses, skin and urine coloured (red), lesions discoloured (blue-black)
*Dose:* leprosy, see notes above
Lepromatous lepra reactions, dosage increased to 300 mg daily for max. of 3 months

PoM **Lamprene**® (Geigy)
*Capsules*, brown, clofazimine 100 mg. Net price 20 = £1.65. Label: 8, 14, 21

## RIFAMPICIN
Section 5.1.9

## 5.1.11   Metronidazole and tinidazole

**Metronidazole** is an antimicrobial drug with high activity against anaerobic bacteria and protozoa; indications include trichomonal vaginitis (section 5.4.3), bacterial vaginosis (notably *Gardnerella vaginalis* infections), and *Entamoeba histolytica* and *Giardia lamblia* infections (section 5.4.2). It is also used for surgical and gynaecological sepsis in which its activity against colonic anaerobes, especially *Bacteroides fragilis*, is important. Metronidazole is also effective in the treatment of pseudomembranous colitis (in a dose of 400 mg by mouth three times daily).

**Tinidazole** is similar to metronidazole but has a longer duration of action.

## METRONIDAZOLE
*Indications:* anaerobic infections, see under Dose below; protozoal infections, section 5.4.2
*Cautions:* disulfiram-like reaction with alcohol, hepatic impairment; pregnancy and breast-feeding (manufacturer advises avoidance of high-dose regimens); **interactions:** Appendix 1 (metronidazole)
*Side-effects:* nausea, vomiting, unpleasant taste, and gastro-intestinal disturbances; rashes, urticaria and angioedema; rarely drowsiness, headache, dizziness, ataxia, and darkening of urine; on prolonged or intensive therapy peripheral neuropathy, transient epileptiform seizures, and leucopenia
*Dose:* anaerobic infections (usually treated for 7 days), *by mouth*, 800 mg initially then 400 mg every 8 hours; *by rectum*, 1 g every 8 hours for 3 days, then 1 g every 12 hours; *by intravenous infusion*, 500 mg every 8 hours; CHILD, any route, 7.5 mg/kg every 8 hours
Leg ulcers and pressure sores, *by mouth*, 400 mg every 8 hours for 7 days
Bacterial vaginosis, *by mouth*, 400 mg twice daily for 7 days *or* 2 g as a single dose
Acute ulcerative gingivitis, *by mouth*, 200 mg every 8 hours for 3 days; CHILD 1–3 years 50 mg every 8 hours for 3 days; 3–7 years 100 mg every 12 hours; 7–10 years 100 mg every 8 hours
Acute dental infections, *by mouth*, 200 mg every 8 hours for 3–7 days

Surgical prophylaxis, *by mouth*, 400 mg every 8 hours during 24 hours before surgery; CHILD 7.5 mg/kg every 8 hours, then until oral administration can be resumed *either by rectum*, 1 g every 8 hours; CHILD 125–250 mg every 8 hours *or by intravenous infusion*, 500 mg shortly before surgery then every 8 hours; CHILD 7.5 mg/kg every 8 hours

PoM **Metronidazole** (Non-proprietary)
*Tablets*, metronidazole 200 mg, net price 20 = 58p; 400 mg, 20 = £1.45. Label: 4, 9, 21, 25, 27
Available from APS, Cox, DDSA (Vaginyl®), Evans, Kerfoot, Lagap (Metrolyl®), Lederle (Zadstat®)
PoM **Elyzol**® (CP)
*Suppositories*, metronidazole 500 mg, net price 10 = £4.50; 1 g, 10 = £7.00. Label: 4
PoM **Flagyl**® (Rhône-Poulenc Rorer)
*Tablets*, both f/c, ivory, metronidazole 200 mg, net price 21-tab pack = £2.19; 400 mg, 14-tab pack = £3.11. Label: 4, 9, 21, 25, 27
*Intravenous infusion*, metronidazole 5 mg/mL. Net price 20-mL amp = £2.06; 100-mL bottle = £4.34; 100-mL Viaflex® bag = £4.78
*Electrolytes:* Na+ 13.6 mmol/100-mL bottle or bag
*Suppositories*, metronidazole 500 mg, net price 10 = £6.77; 1 g, 10 = £10.28. Label: 4, 9
PoM **Flagyl S**® (Rhône-Poulenc Rorer)
*Suspension*, metronidazole 200 mg (as benzoate)/5 mL. Net price 100 mL = £4.53. Label: 4, 9, 23
PoM **Metrotop**®: see section 13.10.1.2
PoM **Metrolyl**® (Lagap)
*Intravenous infusion*, metronidazole 5 mg/mL. Net price 100-mL Steriflex® bag = £4.05
*Electrolytes:* Na+ 14.53 mmol/100-mL bag
*Suppositories*, metronidazole 500 mg, net price 10 = £4.25; 1 g, 10 = £6.80. Label: 4, 9
PoM **Zadstat**® (Lederle)
*Suppositories*, metronidazole 500 mg, net price 10 = £4.25; 1 g, 10 = £6.80. Label: 4, 9

With antifungal
PoM **Flagyl Compak**® (Rhône-Poulenc Rorer)
*Treatment pack*, tablets, off-white, f/c, metronidazole 400 mg, with pessaries, yellow, nystatin 100 000 units. Net price 14 tablets and 14 pessaries (with applicator) = £4.24
*Dose:* for mixed trichomonal and candidal infections, 1 tablet twice daily for 7 days and 1 pessary inserted twice daily for 7 days *or* 1 pessary at night for 14 nights

## TINIDAZOLE
*Indications:* anaerobic infections, see under Dose below; protozoal infections, section 5.4.2
*Cautions; Side-effects:* see under Metronidazole; pregnancy (manufacturer advises avoidance in first trimester)
*Dose:* anaerobic infections *by mouth*, 2 g initially, followed by 1 g daily *or* 500 mg twice daily, usually for 5–6 days
Bacterial vaginosis and acute ulcerative gingivitis, a single 2-g dose
Abdominal surgery prophylaxis, a single 2-g dose approximately 12 hours before surgery

PoM **Fasigyn**® (Pfizer)
*Tablets*, f/c, tinidazole 500 mg. Net price 20-tab
pack = £11.50. Label: 4, 9, 21, 25

## 5.1.12   4-Quinolones

Antibacterials discussed in this section include
acrosoxacin, ciprofloxacin, enoxacin, ofloxacin,
temafloxacin, and the urinary antiseptics cinoxacin, nalidixic acid, and norfloxacin.

**Acrosoxacin** is used only in the treatment of
gonorrhoea in patients allergic to penicillins or
who have strains resistant to penicillins and other
antibiotics.

**Nalidixic acid** and **cinoxacin** are effective in
uncomplicated urinary-tract infections; **norfloxacin** has also been introduced for the treatment
of urinary-tract infections.

**Ciprofloxacin** is active against both Gram-positive and Gram-negative bacteria. It is particularly
active against Gram-negative bacteria, including
salmonella, shigella, campylobacter, neisseria,
and pseudomonas. Ciprofloxacin only has moderate activity against Gram-positive bacteria such
as *Streptococcus pneumoniae* and *Strep. faecalis*;
it is not the drug of first choice for pneumococcal
pneumonia. It is active against chlamydia and
some mycobacteria. Most anaerobic organisms
are not susceptible. Uses for ciprofloxacin include
infections of the respiratory and urinary tracts,
and of the gastro-intestinal system, and
gonorrhoea and septicaemia caused by sensitive
organisms. Whenever possible, ciprofloxacin
should be reserved for the treatment of infections
caused by organisms resistant to standard drugs.

**Enoxacin** is used for urinary-tract infections,
skin and soft-tissue infections, gonorrhoea, and
shigellosis.

**Ofloxacin** is used for urinary-tract infections,
lower respiratory-tract infections, gonorrhoea,
and non-gonococcal urethritis and cervicitis.

**Temafloxacin** is another new 4-quinolone which
is indicated for the treatment of lower respiratory-
tract infections, urinary-tract infections,
gonorrhoea, and skin infection.

CAUTIONS. 4-Quinolones should be used with caution in patients with epilepsy or a history of
epilepsy, in hepatic or renal impairment, in pregnancy, during breast-feeding, and in children or
adolescents (arthropathy has developed in weight-
bearing joints in young *animals*); **interactions:**
Appendix 1 (4-quinolones).
**CSM warning (convulsions).**
The CSM has warned that 4-quinolones may
induce convulsions in patients with or without a
history of convulsions; taking NSAIDs at the same
time may also induce them.

SIDE-EFFECTS. Common side-effects of the 4-qui-
nolones include nausea, vomiting, abdominal
pain, diarrhoea (rarely pseudomembranous
colitis), headache, dizziness, sleep disorders,
rash, pruritus, anaphylaxis, photosensitivity,
increase in blood urea and creatinine, transient
disturbances in liver enzymes and bilirubin,

arthralgia and myalgia, blood disorders (including
eosinophilia, leucopenia, thrombocytopenia, and
altered prothrombin concentration). Less frequent side-effects include anorexia, restlessness,
hallucinations, confusion, and disturbances in
vision, taste and smell.

## CIPROFLOXACIN

*Indications:* Gram-negative and Gram-positive
infections, see notes above
*Cautions; Side-effects:* see notes above; avoid
excessive alkalinity of urine and ensure
adequate fluid intake (risk of crystalluria); not
recommended in children or growing adolescents; G6PD deficiency (see section 9.1.5);
anaphylaxis reported, particularly in AIDS
patients, also reported dyspepsia, tremor, convulsions, jaundice and hepatitis with necrosis,
renal failure, nephritis, vasculitis, Stevens-
Johnson syndrome and tachycardia
DRIVING. May impair performance of skilled tasks (e.g.
driving); effects of alcohol enhanced
*Dose: by mouth*, respiratory-tract infections,
250–750 mg twice daily
Urinary-tract infections, 250–500 mg twice
daily
Gonorrhoea, 250 mg as a single dose
Most other infections, 500–750 mg twice daily
*By intravenous infusion* (over 30–60 minutes),
200 mg twice daily
Urinary-tract infections, 100 mg twice daily
Gonorrhoea, 100 mg as a single dose
CHILD not recommended (see above) but where
benefit outweighs risk, *by mouth*, 7.5–15 mg/
kg daily in 2 divided doses *or by intravenous
infusion*, 5–10 mg/kg daily in 2 divided doses

PoM **Ciproxin**® (Baypharm)
*Tablets*, f/c, scored, ciprofloxacin (as hydrochloride) 250 mg. Net price 20 = £15.00. Label:
5, 9, 25, counselling, driving
*Intravenous infusion*, ciprofloxacin 2 mg (as
lactate)/mL. Net price 50-mL bottle = £12.00;
100-mL bottle = £24.00
*Electrolytes:* Na+ 15.4 mmol/100-mL bottle

## ACROSOXACIN

(Rosoxacin)
*Indications:* gonorrhoea
*Cautions; Side-effects:* see notes above; avoid
frequent repeat doses in patients under 18 years
DRIVING. May impair performance of skilled tasks (e.g,
driving)
*Dose:* 300 mg as a single dose on an empty
stomach

PoM **Eradacin**® (Sanofi Winthrop)
*Capsules*, red/yellow, acrosoxacin 150 mg. Net
price 20-cap pack = £29.04. Label: 2, 23

## CINOXACIN

*Indications:* urinary-tract infections
*Cautions; Side-effects:* see notes above; avoid in
severe renal impairment; also reported, peripheral and oral oedema, tinnitus, perineal
burning

*Dose:* 500 mg every 12 hours; prophylaxis, 500 mg at night

PoM **Cinobac®** (Lilly)
*Capsules,* green/orange, cinoxacin 500 mg. Net price 14-cap pack = £6.88. Label: 9

## ENOXACIN

*Indications:* urinary-tract and skin infections, gonorrhoea, shigellosis
*Cautions; Side-effects:* see notes above; also reported, dyspepsia, dry mouth and throat, stomatitis, palpitation and tachycardia, oedema, fatigue, tremor, convulsions, tinnitus
*Dose:* urinary-tract infections, 200 mg twice daily for 3 days; complicated infections, 400 mg (elderly 200 mg) twice daily for 7–14 days
Skin infections, 400 mg (elderly 200 mg) twice daily for 7–14 days
Chancroid, 400 mg (elderly 200 mg) every 12 hours for 3 doses
Gonorrhoea, 400 mg as a single dose
Shigellosis, 400 mg (elderly 200 mg) twice daily for 5 days

PoM **Comprecin®** (P-D)
*Tablets,* f/c, blue, enoxacin 200 mg. Net price 6-tab pack = £2.50. Label: 9

## NALIDIXIC ACID

*Indications:* urinary-tract infections
*Cautions; Side-effects:* see notes above; avoid in porphyria (see section 9.8.2) and if history of convulsive disorders, avoid strong sunlight, false positive urinary glucose (if tested for reducing substances); caution in G6PD deficiency (see section 9.1.5); also reported toxic psychosis and convulsions, weakness, increased intracranial pressure, paraesthesia, cranial nerve palsy, cholestasis, metabolic acidosis
*Dose:* 1 g every 6 hours for 7 days, reduced in chronic infections to 500 mg every 6 hours; CHILD over 3 months max. 50 mg/kg daily in divided doses; reduced in prolonged therapy to 30 mg/kg daily

PoM **Nalidixic Acid** (Non-proprietary)
*Tablets,* nalidixic acid 500 mg. Net price 56-tab pack = £10.34. Label: 9, 11
PoM **Mictral®** (Sanofi Winthrop)
*Granules,* effervescent, nalidixic acid 660 mg, sodium citrate (as sodium citrate and citric acid) 4.1 g/sachet (Na⁺ 41 mmol/sachet). Net price 9-sachet pack = £5.11. Label: 9, 11, 13
*Dose:* 1 sachet in water 3 times daily for 3 days
PoM **Negram®** (Sanofi Winthrop)
*Tablets,* beige, nalidixic acid 500 mg. Net price 56-tab pack = £11.96. Label: 9, 11
*Suspension,* pink, sugar-free, nalidixic acid 300 mg/5 mL. Diluent syrup, life of diluted suspension 14 days. Net price 150 mL = £11.98. Label: 9, 11

PoM **Uriben®** (RP Drugs)
*Suspension,* pink, nalidixic acid 300 mg/5 mL. Diluent syrup, life of diluted suspension 14 days. Net price 200 mL = £15.00; 500 mL = £30.00. Label: 9, 11

## NORFLOXACIN

*Indications:* see under Dose
*Cautions; Side-effects:* see notes above; avoid in prepubital children and growing adolescents; also reported, anorexia, depression, anxiety, tinnitus, toxic epidermal necrolysis, Stevens-Johnson syndrome
*Dose:* urinary-tract infections, 400 mg twice daily for 7–10 days (for 3 days in uncomplicated lower urinary-tract infections)
Chronic relapsing urinary-tract infections, 400 mg twice daily for 12 weeks; may be reduced to 400 mg once daily if adequate suppression within first 4 weeks

▼ PoM **Utinor®** (MSD)
*Tablets,* norfloxacin 400 mg. Net price 6-tab pack = £2.88, 14-tab pack = £6.72. Label: 5, 9

## OFLOXACIN

*Indications:* see under Dose
*Cautions; Side-effects:* see notes above; caution in history of psychiatric illness; avoid strong sunlight; avoid in epilepsy or history of epilepsy and in children and adolescents; also reported, loss of appetite, anxiety, unsteady gait and tremor, paraesthesia, neuropathy, psychotic reactions (discontinue treatment); tachycardia, anaemia and agranulocytosis
DRIVING. May affect performance of skilled tasks (e.g. driving)
*Dose:* urinary-tract infections, 200–400 mg daily preferably in the morning, increased if necessary in upper urinary-tract infections to 400 mg twice daily
Lower respiratory-tract infections, 400 mg daily preferably in the morning, increased if necessary to 400 mg twice daily
Uncomplicated gonorrhoea, 400 mg as a single dose
Non-gonococcal urethritis and cervicitis, 400 mg daily in single or divided doses

▼ PoM **Tarivid®** (Hoechst, Roussel)
*Tablets,* scored, yellow-white, ofloxacin 200 mg, net price 10-tab pack = £7.38, 20-tab pack = £14.75. Label: 5, 9, counselling, driving

## TEMAFLOXACIN

*Indications:* see under Dose
*Cautions; Side-effects:* see notes above; also reported, constipation, dyspepsia, flatulence, asthenia

*Dose:* lower respiratory-tract infections, 300–600 mg twice daily for 7–14 days
Pneumonia, 600 mg twice daily for 7–14 days
Urinary-tract infections, 400 mg once daily for 3 days; complicated infections, 400 mg twice daily for 10 days (28 days in prostatitis)
Gonococcal urethritis and cervicitis, 400 mg as a single dose
Non-gonococcal urethritis and cervicitis, 400 mg twice daily for 7 days
Skin infections, 600 mg twice daily for 7–10 days (28 days for serious or complicated infections)

▼ PoM **Teflox**® (Abbott)
*Tablets*, f/c, temafloxacin, 300 mg, net price 14-tab pack = £17.70; also 400 mg, 20-tab pack. Label: 5, 9

## 5.1.13   Urinary-tract infections

Urinary-tract infection is more common in women than in men; when it occurs in men there is frequently an underlying abnormality of the renal tract. Recurrent episodes of infection are an indication for radiological investigation especially in children in whom untreated pyelonephritis may lead to permanent kidney damage.

*Escherichia coli* is the most common cause of urinary-tract infection. Less common causes include Proteus and Klebsiella spp. *Pseudomonas aeruginosa* infections are almost invariably associated with functional or anatomical abnormalities of the renal tract. *Staphylococcus epidermidis* and *Enterococcus faecalis* infection may complicate catheterisation or instrumentation. Whenever possible a specimen of urine should be collected for culture and sensitivity testing before starting antibiotic therapy.

*Uncomplicated lower urinary-tract infections* often respond to ampicillin, nalidixic acid, nitrofurantoin, or trimethoprim given for 5–7 days; those caused by fully sensitive bacteria respond to two 3-g doses of amoxycillin (section 5.1.1.3). Bacterial resistance, however, especially to ampicillin (to which approximately 40% of *E. coli* are now resistant), has increased the importance of urine culture prior to therapy. Alternatives for resistant organisms include co-amoxiclav (amoxycillin with clavulanic acid), an oral cephalosporin, and ciprofloxacin. Hexamine should **not** be used as it is only bacteriostatic, requires acid urine, and frequently causes side-effects.

Long-term low dose therapy may be required in selected patients to prevent *recurrence of infection*; indications include frequent relapses and significant kidney damage. Trimethoprim and nitrofurantoin have been recommended for long-term therapy.

*Acute pyelonephritis* can be associated with septicaemia and is best treated initially by injection of a broad-spectrum antibiotic such as cefuroxime or gentamicin especially if the patient is vomiting or severely ill.

*Prostatitis* can be difficult to cure and requires treatment for several weeks with an antibiotic which penetrates prostatic tissue such as trimethoprim, erythromycin, or ciprofloxacin.

Where infection is localised and associated with an indwelling *catheter* a bladder instillation is often effective (see section 7.4.4).

Patients with *heart-valve lesions* undergoing instrumentation of the urinary tract should be given a parenteral antibiotic to prevent bacteraemia and endocarditis (section 5.1, Table 2).

Urinary-tract infection in *pregnancy* may be asymptomatic and requires prompt treatment to prevent progression to acute pyelonephritis. Penicillins and cephalosporins can be given in pregnancy but trimethoprim, sulphonamides, 4-quinolones, and tetracyclines should be avoided.

In *renal failure* antibiotics normally excreted by the kidney accumulate with resultant toxicity unless the dose is reduced. This applies especially to the aminoglycosides which should be used with great caution; tetracyclines, hexamine, and nitrofurantoin should be avoided altogether.

## NITROFURANTOIN

*Indications:* urinary-tract infections
*Cautions:* monitor lung and liver function on long-term therapy, especially in the elderly; susceptibility to peripheral neuropathy; false positive urinary glucose (if tested for reducing substances); urine may be coloured yellow or brown; **interactions:** Appendix 1 (nitrofurantoin)
*Contra-indications:* impaired renal function, infants less than 1 month old, G6PD deficiency (including late pregnancy, and breast-feeding of affected infants, see section 9.1.5), porphyria (see section 9.8.2)
*Side-effects:* anorexia, nausea, vomiting, and diarrhoea; acute and chronic pulmonary reactions; peripheral neuropathy; also reported, angioedema, urticaria, rash and pruritus; rarely, cholestatic jaundice, hepatitis, exfoliative dermatitis, erythema multiforme, pancreatitis, arthralgia, blood disorders (including agranulocytosis, thrombocytopenia, and aplastic anaemia), and transient alopecia
*Dose:* 50–100 mg every 6 hours with food; CHILD 3 mg/kg daily in 4 divided doses
Prophylaxis (but see Cautions), 50–100 mg at night; CHILD 1 mg/kg at night

PoM **Nitrofurantoin** (Non-proprietary)
*Tablets,* nitrofurantoin 50 mg, net price 20 = 75p. Label: 9, 14, 21
PoM **Furadantin**® (Norwich Eaton)
*Tablets*, all yellow, scored, nitrofurantoin 50 mg, net price 20 = £1.96; 100 mg, 20 = £3.29. Label: 9, 14, 21
*Suspension,* yellow, sugar-free, nitrofurantoin 25 mg/5 mL. Do not dilute. Net price 300 mL = £4.50. Label: 9, 14, 21

PoM **Macrodantin**® (Norwich Eaton)
*Capsules*, nitrofurantoin 50 mg (yellow/white), net price 28-cap pack = £3.05; 100 mg (yellow), 20 = £3.49. Label: 9, 14, 21

## HEXAMINE HIPPURATE
(Methenamine hippurate)
*Indications:* prophylaxis and long-term treatment of recurrent urinary-tract infections
*Cautions:* pregnancy; **interactions:** Appendix 1 (hexamine)
*Contra-indications:* severe renal impairment, dehydration, metabolic acidosis
*Side-effects:* gastro-intestinal disturbances, bladder irritation, rash
*Dose:* 1 g every 12 hours (may be increased in patients with catheters to 1 g every 8 hours); CHILD 6–12 years 500 mg every 12 hours

**Hiprex**® (3M)
*Tablets*, scored, hexamine hippurate 1 g. Net price 60-tab pack = £5.75. Label: 9

## 5.2 Antifungal drugs

Fungal infections are frequently associated with a defect in host resistance which should, if possible, be corrected otherwise drug therapy may fail. Similarly, treatment of dermatophyte infection may be unsuccessful until the animal source has been removed or controlled.

For local treatment of fungal infections see also sections 7.2.2 (genital), 7.4.4 (bladder), 11.3.2 (eye), 12.1.1 (ear), 12.3.3 (oropharynx), and 13.10.2 (skin).

POLYENE ANTIFUNGALS. The polyene antifungals include amphotericin and nystatin.

**Amphotericin** is not absorbed from the gut and is the only polyene antibiotic which can be given parenterally. It is used for the treatment of systemic fungal infections and is active against most fungi and yeasts. It is highly protein bound and penetrates poorly into body fluids and tissues. When given parenterally amphotericin is toxic and side-effects are common.

A formulation of amphotericin encapsulated in liposomes has just become available and is apparently significantly less toxic than the parent compound. It is therefore being recommended for systemic mycoses when amphotericin alone is contra-indicated because of toxicity, especially nephrotoxicity.

**Nystatin** is not absorbed when given by mouth and is too toxic for parenteral use. It is active against a number of yeasts and fungi but is principally used for *Candida albicans* infections of skin and mucous membranes. It is also used in the treatment of intestinal candidiasis.

IMIDAZOLE ANTIFUNGALS. The imidazole antifungals include clotrimazole, econazole, isoconazole, ketoconazole, miconazole, sulconazole, and tioconazole; they are active against a wide range of fungi and yeasts. Their main indications are vaginal candidiasis and der-

matophyte infections. Clotrimazole, econazole, isoconazole, sulconazole, and tioconazole are used for local treatment.

**Miconazole** is used for local treatment and can be given by mouth for oral and intestinal infection; it can also be given parenterally for systemic infections including aspergillosis, candidiasis, and cryptococcosis but the injection contains polyethoxylated castor oil which may give rise to hypersensitivity reactions.

**Ketoconazole** is significantly better absorbed after oral administration than the other imidazoles, but has been associated with fatal hepatotoxicity. The CSM has advised that prescribers should weigh the potential benefits of ketoconazole treatment against the liver damage risk and should carefully monitor patients both clinically and biochemically. It should **not** be given for superficial fungal infections.

TRIAZOLE ANTIFUNGALS. The triazole antifungals include fluconazole and itraconazole which are absorbed by mouth.

**Fluconazole** is an oral triazole antifungal indicated for local and systemic candidiasis and cryptococcal infections.

**Itraconazole** is indicated for oropharyngeal and vulvovaginal candidiasis, pityriasis versicolor, and tinea corporis and pedis; it is metabolised in the liver and should not be given to patients with a history of liver disease.

OTHER ANTIFUNGALS. **Flucytosine** is a synthetic antifungal drug which is only active against yeasts and has been used for the treatment of systemic candidiasis, cryptococcosis, and torulopsosis. It is well absorbed from the gut and distributed widely in the body. Side-effects are uncommon but bone-marrow depression can occur and weekly blood counts are necessary during prolonged therapy. Synergy has been demonstrated with amphotericin. Resistance to flucytosine is not uncommon and can develop during therapy; sensitivity testing is, therefore, essential before and during treatment.

**Griseofulvin** is selectively concentrated in keratin and is the drug of choice for widespread or intractable dermatophyte infections. It is well absorbed from the gut but is inactive when applied topically. It is more effective in skin than in nail infections and treatment must be continued for several weeks or even months. Side-effects are uncommon.

**Terbinafine**, an allylamine antifungal, has recently been introduced for ringworm infections where oral treatment is considered appropriate; it is ineffective against pityriasis versicolor.

## AMPHOTERICIN
*Indications:* See under Dose
*Cautions:* when given parenterally, toxicity common (close supervision necessary); hepatic and renal-function tests, blood counts, and plasma

electrolyte monitoring required; other nephrotoxic drugs, corticosteroids (avoid except to control reactions), antineoplastics; frequent change of injection site (irritant); **interactions:** Appendix 1 (amphotericin)

*Side-effects:* when given parenterally, anorexia, nausea and vomiting, diarrhoea, epigastric pain; febrile reactions, headache, muscle and joint pain; anaemia; disturbances in renal function (including hypokalaemia and hypomagnesaemia) and renal toxicity; also cardiovascular toxicity (including arrhythmias), blood disorders, neurological disorders (including hearing loss, diplopia, convulsions, peripheral neuropathy), abnormal liver function (discontinue treatment), rash, anaphylactoid reactions

*Dose: by mouth,* intestinal candidiasis, 100–200 mg every 6 hours

*By slow intravenous infusion,* systemic fungal infections, 250 micrograms/kg daily, gradually increased if tolerated to 1 mg/kg daily; max. (severe infection) 1.5 mg/kg daily or on alternate days

*Note.* Prolonged treatment usually necessary; if interrupted for longer than 7 days recommence at 250 micrograms/kg daily and increase gradually

PoM **Fungilin**® (Squibb)
*Tablets,* yellow, scored, amphotericin 100 mg. Net price 56-tab pack = £8.32. Label: 9
*Lozenges*—see section 12.3.2
*Suspension,* yellow, sugar-free, amphotericin 100 mg/mL. Net price 12 mL = £2.31. Label: 9, counselling, use of pipette

PoM **Fungizone**® (Squibb)
*Intravenous infusion,* powder for reconstitution, amphotericin (as sodium deoxycholate complex). Net price 50-mg vial = £3.70
*Electrolytes:* Na⁺ <0.5 mmol/vial

Liposomal amphotericin
▼ PoM **AmBisome**® (Vestar)
*Intravenous infusion,* powder for reconstitution, amphotericin 50 mg encapsulated in liposomes. Net price 50-mg vial = £140.00
*Electrolytes:* Na⁺ < 0.5 mmol/vial
*Dose:* systemic mycoses where toxicity (particularly nephrotoxicity) precludes use of conventional amphotericin, by intravenous infusion, initially 1 mg/kg daily as a single dose increased gradually if necessary to 3 mg/kg daily as a single dose

## FLUCONAZOLE

*Indications:* see under Dose
*Cautions:* renal impairment; pregnancy (toxicity at high doses in *animal* studies) and breast-feeding; children (use only if imperative and if no alternative treatment; not recommended under 1 year); raised liver enzymes **interactions:** Appendix 1 (fluconazole)
*Side-effects:* nausea, abdominal discomfort, diarrhoea, and flatulence; occasionally abnormalities of liver enzymes; rarely rash (discontinue treatment)

*Dose:* acute or recurrent vaginal candidiasis, *by mouth,* a single dose of 150 mg
Mucosal candidiasis (except vaginal), *by mouth,* 50 mg daily (100 mg daily in unusually difficult infections) given for 7–14 days in oropharyngeal candidiasis (max. 14 days except in severely immunocompromised patients); for 14 days in atrophic oral candidiasis associated with dentures; for 14–30 days in other mucosal infections (e.g. oesophagitis, candiduria)
Systemic candidiasis and cryptococcal infections (including meningitis), *by mouth or intravenous infusion,* 400 mg initially then 200 mg daily, increased if necessary to 400 mg daily; treatment continued according to response (at least 6–8 weeks for cryptococcal meningitis)
Prevention of relapse of cryptococcal meningitis in AIDS patients after completion of primary therapy, at least 100 mg daily
Prevention of fungal infections in immunocompromised patients following cytotoxic chemotherapy or radiotherapy, 50 mg daily; 100 mg daily if risk of severe recurrent infections
CHILD over 1 year (see Cautions), *by mouth or by intravenous infusion,* superficial candidal infections, 1–2 mg/kg daily; systemic candidiasis and cryptococcal infections, 3–6 mg/kg daily

PoM **Diflucan**® (Pfizer)
*Capsules,* fluconazole 50 mg (blue/white), net price 7-cap pack = £16.61; 150 mg (blue), single-capsule pack = £7.12; 200 mg (purple/white), 7-cap pack = £66.42. Label: 50 and 200 mg, 9
*Oral suspension,* fluconazole for reconstitution with water, 50 mg/5 ml, net price 35 mL = £16.61; 200 mg/5 ml, 35 mL = £66.42. Label: 9
*Intravenous infusion,* fluconazole 2 mg/mL in sodium chloride intravenous infusion 0.9%, net price 25-mL bottle = £7.32; 100-mL bottle = £29.28
*Electrolytes:* Na⁺ 15 mmol/100-mL bottle

## FLUCYTOSINE

*Indications:* systemic yeast infections
*Cautions:* hepatic impairment, renal impairment (reduce dose and monitor plasma concentrations), blood disorders, liver-function tests and blood counts required; pregnancy, breast-feeding
*Side-effects:* nausea, vomiting, diarrhoea, rashes, thrombocytopenia, leucopenia
*Dose: by mouth or intravenous infusion,* 200 mg/kg daily in 4 divided doses; extremely sensitive organisms, 100–150 mg/kg daily may be sufficient
*Note.* Plasma concentration for optimum response 25–50 mg/litre (200–400 micromol/litre)

PoM **Alcobon**® (Roche)
*Tablets,* scored, flucytosine 500 mg. Net price 20 = £9.43 (hosp. only)

---

*Intravenous infusion*, flucytosine 10 mg/mL. Net price 250-mL infusion bottle and giving set = £16.56 (hosp. only)
*Electrolytes:* Na+ 34.44 mmol/250-mL bottle

## GRISEOFULVIN

*Indications:* dermatophyte infections of the skin, scalp, hair and nails, where topical therapy has failed or is inappropriate
*Cautions:* rarely aggravation or precipitation of systemic lupus erythematosus; **interactions:** Appendix 1 (griseofulvin)
DRIVING. May impair performance of skilled tasks (e.g. driving); effects of alcohol enhanced
*Contra-indications:* liver failure, porphyria (see section 9.8.2); pregnancy
*Side-effects:* headache, nausea, vomiting, rashes, photosensitivity
*Dose:* 0.5–1 g daily, in divided doses or as a single dose; CHILD, 10 mg/kg daily in divided doses or as a single dose

PoM **Fulcin**® (ICI)
*Tablets*, griseofulvin 125 mg (scored), net price 20 = 63p; 500 mg (f/c), 20 = £2.35. Label: 9, 21, counselling, driving
*Oral suspension*, brown, griseofulvin 125 mg/5 mL. Net price 100 mL = £1.13. Label: 9, 21, counselling, driving
PoM **Grisovin**® (Glaxo)
*Tablets*, both f/c, griseofulvin 125 mg, net price 20 = 47p; 500 mg, 20 = £1.75. Label: 9, 21, counselling, driving

## ITRACONAZOLE

*Indications:* oropharyngeal and vulvovaginal candidiasis; pityriasis versicolor and other dermatophyte infections
*Cautions:* avoid if history of liver disease; pregnancy (toxicity in *animal* studies) and breast-feeding; **interactions:** Appendix 1 (itraconazole)
*Side-effects:* nausea, abdominal pain, dyspepsia, headache
*Dose:* oropharyngeal candidiasis, 100 mg daily (200 mg daily in AIDS or neutropenia) for 15 days
Vulvovaginal candidiasis, 200 mg twice daily for 1 day
Pityriasis versicolor, 200 mg daily for 7 days
Tinea corporis and tinea cruris, 100 mg daily for 15 days
Tinea pedis and tinea manuum, 100 mg daily for 30 days
Max. period of treatment, 30 days
CHILD not yet recommended

PoM **Sporanox**® (Janssen)
*Capsules*, blue/pink, enclosing coated beads, itraconazole 100 mg. Net price 4-cap pack = £5.99; 15-cap pack = £22.46. Label: 5, 9, 21, 25

## KETOCONAZOLE

*Indications:* systemic mycoses, serious chronic resistant mucocutaneous candidiasis, serious resistant gastro-intestinal mycoses, chronic resistant vaginal candidiasis, resistant dermatophyte infections of skin or finger nails (not toe nails); prophylaxis of mycoses in immunosuppressed patients
*Cautions:* **important:** monitor liver function clinically and biochemically—for treatment lasting longer than 14 days perform liver function tests before starting, 14 days after starting, then at monthly intervals (for details see data sheet); pregnancy (teratogenicity in *animal* studies); avoid in porphyria (see section 9.8.2); **interactions:** Appendix 1 (ketoconazole)
*Contra-indications:* hepatic impairment
*Side-effects:* nausea, vomiting, abdominal pain; headache; rashes, urticaria, pruritus; rarely thrombocytopenia, gynaecomastia; fatal liver damage—for CSM advice see notes above, risk of developing hepatitis greater if given for longer than 14 days
*Dose:* 200 mg once daily with food, usually for 14 days; if response inadequate after 14 days continue until at least 1 week after symptoms have cleared and cultures become negative; max. 400 mg daily
CHILD, 3 mg/kg daily
Chronic resistant vaginal candidiasis, 400 mg daily with food for 5 days

PoM **Nizoral**® (Janssen)
*Tablets*, scored, ketoconazole 200 mg. Net price 30-tab pack = £15.69. Label: 5, 9, 21
*Suspension*, pink, ketoconazole 100 mg/5 mL. Net price 100 mL with pipette = £7.16. Label: 5, 9, 21, counselling, use of pipette

## MICONAZOLE

*Indications:* see under Dose
*Cautions:* change infusion site to avoid phlebitis; pregnancy; avoid in porphyria (see section 9.8.2); **interactions:** Appendix 1 (miconazole)
*Side-effects:* nausea and vomiting, pruritus, rashes
*Dose: by mouth* as tablets, oral and intestinal fungal infections, 250 mg every 6 hours for 10 days or up to 2 days after symptoms clear; as oral gel, see under Daktarin® oral gel
*By intravenous infusion*, systemic fungal infections, initially, 600 mg every 8 hours; CHILD, max. 15 mg/kg every 8 hours up to 40 mg/kg/day

**Daktarin**® (Janssen)
PoM *Tablets*, scored, miconazole 250 mg. Net price 20 = £14.89. Label: 9, 21
*Note.* Can be sucked for oral treatment
PoM [1]*Oral gel*, sugar-free, miconazole 25 mg/mL. Net price 80 g = £5.00. Label: 9, counselling advised, hold in mouth, after food
*Dose:* oral and intestinal fungal infections, 5–10 mL in the mouth after food 4 times daily; retain near lesions before swallowing; CHILD under 2 years, 2.5 mL twice daily, 2–6 years, 5 mL twice daily, over 6 years, 5 mL 4 times daily
Localised lesions, smear affected area with clean finger; a 15-g tube (net price £1.70) also available
1. 15-g tube can be sold to public

PoM *Intravenous solution*, miconazole 10 mg/mL. For dilution and use as an infusion. Net price 20-mL amp = £1.47 (hosp. only)
*Note.* Contains polyethoxylated castor oil which has been associated with anaphylaxis

## NYSTATIN

*Indications:* candidiasis
*Side-effects:* nausea, vomiting, diarrhoea at high doses
*Dose: by mouth*, intestinal candidiasis 500 000 units every 6 hours, doubled in severe infections; CHILD 100 000 units 4 times daily
For use as a mouthwash in oral candidiasis, see section 12.3.2

PoM **Nystatin** (Non-proprietary)
*Oral suspension*, nystatin 100000 units/mL. Net price 30 mL with pipette = £2.50. Label: 9, counselling, use of pipette
PoM **Nystan**® (Squibb)
*Tablets*, brown, s/c, nystatin 500 000 units. Net price 56-tab pack = £4.70. Label: 9
*Pastilles*—see section 12.3.2
*Suspension*, yellow, nystatin 100000 units/mL. Net price 30 mL with pipette = £2.50. Label: 9, counselling, use of pipette
*Suspension*, gluten-, lactose-, and sugar-free, nystatin 100000 units/mL when reconstituted with water. Net price 24 mL with pipette = £1.67. Label: 9, counselling, use of pipette
PoM **Nystatin-Dome**® (Lagap)
*Suspension*, yellow, nystatin 100000 units/mL. Net price 30 mL with 1-mL spoon = £2.86. Label: 9, counselling, use of 1-mL spoon

## TERBINAFINE

*Indications:* tinea pedis, cruris, and corporis where oral therapy appropriate
*Cautions:* hepatic and renal impairment; pregnancy, breast-feeding
*Side-effects:* abdominal discomfort, loss of appetite, nausea, diarrhoea; rash, urticaria
*Dose:* 250 mg daily usually for 2–6 weeks in tinea pedis, 2–4 weeks in tinea cruris, 4 weeks in tinea corporis; CHILD not yet recommended

▼ PoM **Lamisil**® (Sandoz)
*Tablets*, off-white, scored, terbinafine 250 mg (as hydrochloride), net price 14-tab pack = £23.75, 28-tab pack = £45.80. Label: 9

# 5.3   Antiviral drugs

The specific therapy of virus infections is generally unsatisfactory and treatment is, therefore, primarily symptomatic. Fortunately, the majority of infections resolve spontaneously.

## HERPES SIMPLEX AND VARICELLA–ZOSTER

**Acyclovir** is active against herpes viruses but does not eradicate them. It is effective only if started at the onset of infection. Uses of acyclovir include the systemic treatment of varicella–zoster and the systemic and topical treatment of herpes simplex infections of the skin and mucous membranes (including initial and recurrent genital herpes); it is also used topically in the eye. It can be life-saving in herpes simplex and varicella–zoster infections in the immunocompromised, and is also used in the immunocompromised for prevention of recurrence and prophylaxis. See also section 11.3.3 (eye) and section 13.10.3 (skin, including herpes labialis).

**Idoxuridine** is also only effective if started at the onset of infection; it is too toxic for systemic use. It has been used topically in the treatment of herpes simplex lesions of the skin and external genitalia with variable results; it has also been used topically in the treatment of zoster, but evidence of its value is dubious. See also section 11.3.3 (eye) and section 13.10.3 (skin, including herpes labialis).

**Inosine pranobex** has been used by mouth for herpes simplex infections; its effectiveness has not been established. **Amantadine** has also been used by mouth but, again, its effectiveness has not been established; it has also been used for the prophylaxis of influenza A infections.

## ACYCLOVIR

*Indications:* herpes simplex and varicella–zoster
*Cautions:* maintain adequate hydration; reduce dose in renal impairment; pregnancy; **interactions:** Appendix 1 (acyclovir)
*Side-effects:* rashes; gastro-intestinal disturbances; rises in bilirubin and liver-related enzymes, increases in blood urea and creatinine, decreases in haematological indices, headache, neurological reactions, fatigue
*Dose: by mouth*,
Herpes simplex, treatment, 200 mg (400 mg in the immunocompromised) 5 times daily, usually for 5 days; CHILD under 2 years, half adult dose, over 2 years, adult dose
Herpes simplex, prevention of recurrence, 200 mg 4 times daily *or* 400 mg twice daily possibly reduced to 200 mg 2 or 3 times daily and interrupted every 6–12 months
Herpes simplex, prophylaxis in the immunocompromised, 200–400 mg 4 times daily; CHILD under 2 years, half adult dose, over 2 years, adult dose
Herpes zoster, 800 mg 5 times daily for 7 days
*By slow intravenous infusion*, herpes simplex or zoster 5 mg/kg over 1 hour, repeated every 8 hours; doubled in zoster in the immunocompromised, and in simplex encephalitis; CHILD 3 months–12 years, 250 mg/m$^2$ doubled in the immunocompromised and in simplex encephalitis
*By topical application*, herpes simplex (*cream or eye ointment* as appropriate) every 4 hours (5 times daily), see sections 13.10.3 and 11.3.3
*Note.* Cream should not be used on mucous membranes

PoM **Zovirax**® (Wellcome)
*Tablets*, acyclovir 200 mg (blue), net price 25-tab pack = £28.89; 400 mg (pink), 56-tab pack = £105.95; 800 mg (blue, scored), 35-tab pack = £113.00. Label: 9
*Suspension*, off-white, sugar-free, acyclovir 200 mg/5 mL. Diluent syrup or sorbitol solution for 1 + 1 dilution, life of diluted mixture 28 days. Net price 125 mL = £28.89. Label: 9
*Intravenous infusion*, powder for reconstitution, acyclovir (as sodium salt). Net price 250-mg vial = £10.80; 500-mg vial = £19.44
*Electrolytes:* Na$^+$ 1.1 mmol/250-mg vial
*Cream*, see section 13.10.3
*Eye ointment*, see section 11.3.3

---

## AMANTADINE HYDROCHLORIDE
*Indications:* see under Dose; parkinsonism, see section 4.9.1
*Cautions; Contra-indications; Side-effects:* see section 4.9.1
*Dose:* herpes zoster, 100 mg twice daily for 14 days, if necessary extended for a further 14 days for post-herpetic neuralgia
Influenza A$_2$, treatment, 100 mg twice daily for 5–7 days; prophylaxis 100 mg twice daily for as long as required (usually 7–10 days); CHILD 10–15 years, 100 mg daily

**Preparations**
See section 4.9.1

---

## IDOXURIDINE
See sections 11.3.3 (eye) and 13.10.3 (skin including herpes labialis)

---

## INOSINE PRANOBEX
*Indications:* see under Dose
*Cautions:* avoid in renal impairment; history of gout or hyperuricaemia
*Side-effects:* reversible increases in serum and urinary uric acid
*Dose:* mucocutaneous herpes simplex, 1 g 4 times daily for 7–14 days
Adjunctive treatment of genital warts, 1 g 3 times daily for 14–28 days

PoM **Imunovir**® (Leo)
*Tablets*, inosine pranobex 500 mg. Net price 100 = £37.24. Label: 9

---

## HUMAN IMMUNODEFICIENCY VIRUS

---

**Zidovudine** inhibits the human immunodeficiency virus (HIV) but does not eradicate it from the body; it is not therefore a cure for AIDS but may delay progression of the disease. It is now also being recommended for asymptomatic HIV antibody positive individuals.

Zidovudine is toxic and expensive and should only be prescribed by those experienced in its use.

## ZIDOVUDINE
(Azidothymidine, AZT)
*Indications:* management of advanced human immunodeficiency virus (HIV) disease such as acquired immunodeficiency syndrome (AIDS) or AIDS-related complex; early symptomatic or asymptomatic HIV infection with markers indicating risk of disease progression
*Cautions:* haematological toxicity (blood tests at least every 2 weeks for first 3 months then at least once a month, early disease with good bone marrow reserves may require less frequent tests e.g. every 1–3 months); adjust dose according to data sheet if anaemia or myelosuppression; renal and hepatic impairment; elderly; pregnancy; avoid in breast-feeding; *interactions:* Appendix 1 (zidovudine)
*Contra-indications:* abnormally low neutrophil counts or haemoglobin values (see data sheet)
*Side-effects:* anaemia (often requiring transfusion), neutropenia, and leucopenia (all more frequent with high dose and advanced disease); also include, nausea and vomiting, anorexia, abdominal pain, headache, rash, fever, myalgia, paraesthesia, insomnia, malaise, and asthenia
*Dose: by mouth*, symptomatic disease, 200 mg every 4 hours (total 1.2 g daily) for 70-kg patient; for advanced disease with poorer tolerance dose may be reduced to maintenance of 100 mg every 4 hours (total 600 mg daily); daily dosage can be given in 4–5 divided doses
Asymptomatic disease, initially 500 mg daily increased if disease progresses to 1.5 g daily
CHILD initially 180 mg/m$^2$ every 6 hours
*By intravenous infusion*, patients temporarily unable to take oral zidovudine, 2.5 mg/kg every 4 hours; not to be given for more than 2 weeks

PoM **Retrovir**® (Wellcome)
*Capsules*, white/blue band, zidovudine 100 mg, net price 100 = £108.18; 250 mg (blue/white), 40-cap pack = £108.18
*Syrup*, zidovudine 50 mg/5 mL. Net price 200-mL pack with 10-mL oral syringe = £21.64. Counselling, use of oral syringe
▼*Injection*, zidovudine 20 mg/mL. For dilution and use as an intravenous infusion. Net price 10 mL vial = £10.86

---

## CYTOMEGALOVIRUS (CMV)

---

**Ganciclovir** is related to acyclovir but with enhanced activity against cytomegalovirus; it is much more toxic than acyclovir and indicated only for life- or sight-threatening *cytomegalovirus infections in immunocompromised* patients. It can cause leucopenia and thrombocytopenia and is also a potential carcinogen. It should therefore only be prescribed when the potential benefit outweighs the risks of adverse reactions. Ganciclovir causes profound myelosuppression when given with zidovudine; the two should not normally be given together particularly during initial ganciclovir therapy.

**Foscarnet** is also active against cytomegalovirus and is indicated for cytomegalovirus retinitis in patients with AIDS in whom ganciclovir is contra-indicated or is inappropriate. It is not recommended for the treatment of CMV infections other than retinitis or for use in non-AIDS patients. Foscarnet is a toxic drug which can cause impairment of renal function in up to 50% of patients.

## GANCICLOVIR

*Indications:* life-threatening or sight-threatening cytomegalovirus infections in immunocompromised patients only (consult data sheet)

*Cautions:* haematological toxicity (blood counts required every 1–2 days for first 14 days—see data sheet); renal impairment; concomitant administration of drugs that inhibit replication of rapidly dividing cells (e.g. pentamidine, co-trimoxazole); history of exposure to irradiation or to drugs toxic to bone marrow (avoid concomitant zidovudine during induction); increased risk of seizures with imipenem; potential carcinogen; ensure adequate hydration after administration; vesicant—infuse only into veins with adequate blood flow; **not** for neonatal or congenital cytomegalovirus; **interactions:** Appendix 1 (ganciclovir)

*Contra-indications:* pregnancy (includes effective contraception during treatment and barrier contraception for men for 90 days after treatment); breast-feeding (until 72 hours after last dose); hypersensitivity to ganciclovir or acyclovir; abnormally low neutrophil counts (see data sheet)

*Side-effects:* most frequent, neutropenia and thrombocytopenia; anaemia and eosinophilia; fever, rash, abnormal liver function tests; raised blood urea nitrogen or serum creatinine; also sepsis, facial oedema, sore throat, epistaxis, malaise; other side-effects reported have included all body systems, including cardio-vascular, CNS and special senses, gastro-intestinal, metabolic, musculoskeletal, respiratory, dermatological, urogenital (see data sheet); local reactions at injection site

*Dose: by intravenous infusion* over 1 hour, initially 5 mg/kg every 12 hours for 14–21 days; maintenance (for patients at risk of relapse of retinitis) 6 mg/kg daily on 5 days per week *or* 5 mg/kg daily every day
In renal impairment, consult data sheet for dosage reduction

PoM **Cymevene**® (Syntex)
*Intravenous infusion*, powder for reconstitution, ganciclovir (as sodium salt). Net price 500-mg vial = £29.48
*Electrolytes:* Na+ 2.0 mmol/500-mg vial
CAUTION IN HANDLING. Wear polythene gloves and safety glasses when reconstituting; if solution contacts skin or mucosa immediately wash with soap and water

## FOSCARNET SODIUM

*Indications:* cytomegalovirus retinitis in patients with AIDS in whom ganciclovir is inappropriate

*Cautions:* renal impairment (avoid if severe), hypocalcaemia, monitor serum creatinine and serum calcium concentrations every second day; ensure adequate hydration

*Contra-indications:* pregnancy, breast-feeding

*Side-effects:* nausea, vomiting, headache, fatigue, rash; impairment of renal function including acute renal failure, symptomatic hypocalcaemia; decreased haemoglobin concentration; rarely hypoglycaemia, convulsions; thrombophlebitis if given undiluted by peripheral vein

*Dose: by intravenous infusion*, 20 mg/kg over 30 minutes then 21–200 mg/kg daily according to renal function for 2–3 weeks

▼ PoM **Foscavir**® (Astra)
*Intravenous infusion*, foscarnet sodium hexahydrate 24 mg/mL. Net price 500-mL bottle = £53.58

---

RESPIRATORY SYNCYTIAL VIRUS

**Tribavirin** inhibits a wide range of DNA and RNA viruses. It is given by inhalation for the treatment of severe bronchiolitis caused by the respiratory syncytial virus in infants, especially when they have other serious diseases.

## TRIBAVIRIN
(Ribavirin)

*Indications:* severe respiratory syncytial virus bronchiolitis in infants and children

*Cautions:* maintain standard supportive respiratory and fluid management therapy; monitor equipment for precipitation

*Contra-indications:* pregnancy

*Side-effects:* reticulocytosis; also worsening respiration, bacterial pneumonia, and pneumothorax reported

*Dose: by aerosol inhalation or nebulisation* (via small particle aerosol generator) of solution containing 20 mg/mL for 12–18 hours for at least 3 days; max. 7 days

PoM **Virazid**® (Britannia)
*Inhalation*, tribavirin 6 g for reconstitution with 300 mL water for injections. Net price 3 × 6-g vials = £585.00

---

# 5.4 Antiprotozoal drugs

5.4.1 Antimalarials
5.4.2 Amoebicides
5.4.3 Trichomonacides
5.4.4 Antigiardial drugs
5.4.5 Leishmaniacides
5.4.6 Trypanocides
5.4.7 Drugs for toxoplasmosis
5.4.8 Drugs for pneumocystis pneumonia

Advice on specific problems available from:

| | |
|---|---|
| Birmingham | 021-772 4311 |
| Glasgow | 041-946 7120 (travel prophylaxis) |
| | 041-946 7120 Extn 277 (treatment) |
| Liverpool | 051-708 9393 |
| London | 071-387 4411 (treatment) |
| | 071-388 9600 (travel prophylaxis) |
| | 071-636 8636 (travel prophylaxis) |
| | 071-636 7921 (recorded advice) |
| Oxford | (0865) 225570 |

## 5.4.1 Antimalarials

Recommendations on the prophylaxis and treatment of malaria reflect guidelines agreed by UK malaria specialists.

The centres listed above should be consulted for advice on special problems.

## TREATMENT OF MALARIA

If the infective species is **not known** or if the infection is **mixed** initial treatment should be with quinine, mefloquine, or halofantrine as for *falciparum malaria* (next column).

1. For chloroquine-sensitive strains of falciparum malaria chloroquine is effective *by mouth* in the dosage schedule outlined under benign malarias but it should **not** be used unless there is an **unambiguous exposure history** in one of the few remaining areas of chloroquine sensitivity.

   In the patient with a *chloroquine-sensitive infection* is seriously ill, chloroquine is given by *continuous intravenous infusion*. The dosage (for adults and children) is chloroquine 10 mg/kg (of base) infused over 8 hours, followed by three 8-hour infusions of 5 mg/kg (of base) each. *Oral therapy* is started as soon as possible to complete the course; the total cumulative dose for the course should be 25 mg/kg of base.

2. Valid for quinine hydrochloride, dihydrochloride, and sulphate; not valid for quinine bisulphate which contains a correspondingly smaller amount of quinine.

3. If quinine is not available quinidine may be given by intravenous infusion in a loading dose of 15 mg/kg (of base) infused over 4 hours followed by 7.5 mg/kg (of base) infused over 4 hours every 8 hours but cardiotoxicity is more likely (ECG monitoring).

4. In intensive care units the loading dose can alternatively be given as quinine salt[2] 7 mg/kg infused over 30 minutes followed immediately by 10 mg/kg salt over 4 hours then (after 8 hours) maintenance dose as described.

5. **Important:** the loading dose of 20 mg/kg should **not** be used if the patient has received quinine (or quinidine) or mefloquine or possibly chloroquine during the previous 24 hours

6. Maintenance dose should be reduced to 5–7 mg/kg of salt if parenteral treatment is required for more than 48 hours.

## FALCIPARUM MALARIA (TREATMENT)

Falciparum malaria (malignant malaria) is caused by *Plasmodium falciparum*. In most parts of the world *P. falciparum* is now resistant to chloroquine which should not therefore be given for treatment[1].

**Quinine, mefloquine,** or **halofantrine** can be given *by mouth* if the patient can swallow tablets and there are no serious manifestations (e.g. impaired consciousness); quinine should be given *by intravenous infusion* (see below) if the patient is seriously ill or unable to take tablets.

The adult dosage regimen for **quinine** *by mouth* is:

600 mg (of quinine salt[2]) every 8 hours for 7 days *and* (if quinine resistance known or suspected) *either followed by* **Fansidar®** 3 tablets as a single dose

*or* (if Fansidar®-resistant) *given with* **tetracycline** 250 mg every 6 hours for 7 days.

Alternatively **mefloquine** or **halofantrine** may be given instead of quinine.

The adult dosage regimen for **mefloquine** *by mouth* is:

20 mg/kg (of mefloquine base) as a single dose (up to maximum 1.5 g) *or preferably* as 2 divided doses 6–8 hours apart.

The adult dosage regimen for **halofantrine** *by mouth* is:

1.5 g of halofantrine hydrochloride divided into three doses of 500 mg given at intervals of 6 hours; this course should be repeated after an interval of 1 week.

It is not necessary to give Fansidar® or tetracycline after mefloquine or halofantrine treatment.

If the patient is seriously ill, **quinine**[3] should be given *by intravenous infusion.* The adult dosage regimen for quinine *by infusion* is:

loading dose[4] of 20 mg/kg[5] (up to maximum 1.4 g) of quinine salt[2] infused over 4 hours *then after 8–12 hours* maintenance dose of 10 mg/kg[6] (up to maximum 700 mg) of quinine salt[2] infused over 4 hours every 8–12 hours (until patient can swallow tablets to complete the 7-day course) *either followed by* Fansidar® *or given with* tetracycline as above.

CHILDREN.
*Oral.* Quinine is well tolerated by children although the salts are bitter. The dosage regimen for quinine *by mouth* for children is:

10 mg/kg (of quinine salt[2]) every 8 hours for 7 days *then* (if quinine resistance known or suspected)
Fansidar® as a single dose: up to 4 years ½ tablet, 5–6 years 1 tablet, 7–9 years 1½ tablets, 10–14 years 2 tablets.

Alternatively mefloquine or halofantrine may be given instead of quinine; it is not necessary to give Fansidar® after mefloquine or halofantrine

treatment. The dosage regimen for mefloquine *by mouth* for children is calculated on a mg/kg basis as for adults (see above). The dosage regimen for halofantrine *by mouth* for children over 37 kg is the same as for adults (see above); there is no suitable dose form for children under 37 kg.
*Parenteral.* The dosage regimen for quinine *by intravenous infusion* for children is calculated on a mg/kg basis as for adults (see above).

---

## BENIGN MALARIAS (TREATMENT)

Benign malaria is usually caused by *Plasmodium vivax* and less commonly by *P. ovale* and *P. malariae*. **Chloroquine** is the drug of choice for the treatment of benign malarias.

The adult dosage regimen for **chloroquine** *by mouth* is:
initial dose of 600 mg (of base) *then*
a single dose of 300 mg after 6 to 8 hours *then*
a single dose of 300 mg daily for 2 days
(approximate total cumulative dose of 25 mg/kg of base)
Chloroquine alone is adequate for *P. malariae* infections but in the case of *P. vivax* and *P. ovale*, a *radical cure* (to destroy parasites in the liver and thus prevent relapses) is required. This is achieved with **primaquine**[1] in an adult dosage of 15 mg daily for 14 to 21 days given after the chloroquine; a 21-day course is recommended for Chesson-type strains of *P. vivax* from south-east Asia and western Pacific.

CHILDREN. The dosage regimen of chloroquine for benign malaria in children is:
initial dose of 10 mg/kg (of base) *then*
a single dose of 5 mg/kg after 6–8 hours *then*
a single dose of 5 mg/kg daily for 2 days
For a *radical cure* children are then given primaquine[1] in a dose of 250 micrograms/kg daily.

---

1. Before starting primaquine the blood should be tested for glucose-6-phosphate dehydrogenase (G6PD) activity as the drug can cause haemolysis in patients who are deficient in the enzyme. If the patient is G6PD deficient primaquine, in a dose for adults of 30 mg once a week (children 500–750 micrograms/kg once a week) for 8 weeks, has been found useful and without undue harmful effects.

---

Advice on specific problems available from:
Birmingham    021-772 4311
Glasgow        041-946 7120 (travel prophylaxis)
               041-946 7120 Extn 277 (treatment)
Liverpool      051-708 9393
London         071-387 4411 (treatment)
               071-388 9600 (travel prophylaxis)
               071-636 8636 (travel prophylaxis)
               071-636 7921 (recorded advice)
Oxford         (0865) 225570

---

## PROPHYLAXIS AGAINST MALARIA

The recommendations on prophylaxis reflect guidelines agreed by UK malaria specialists; the advice is aimed at residents of the UK who travel to endemic areas for short stays. The choice of drug takes account of:
risk of exposure to malaria;
extent of drug resistance;
efficacy of the recommended drugs;
side-effects of the drugs;
patient-related criteria (e.g. age, pregnancy, renal or hepatic impairment).

NETS AND REPELLENTS. The most important point to remember is that **prophylaxis is relative and not absolute**, and that breakthrough can occur with any of the drugs recommended anywhere in the world. Personal protection against being bitten, e.g. use of mosquito nets, repellents etc. is **very important**.

LENGTH OF PROPHYLAXIS. Prophylaxis should be started one week before travel into an endemic area (or if not possible at earliest opportunity up to 1 or 2 days before travel); it should be continued for at least 4 weeks after leaving (except for mefloquine).

CHILDREN. The following prophylactic doses are based on guidelines agreed by UK malaria experts and may differ from advice in data sheets. If in doubt telephone centres listed in the box in the previous column.

| Age | Weight (kg) | Fraction of adult dose | | |
|---|---|---|---|---|
| | | Chloroquine Proguanil | | Maloprim® |
| 0–5 weeks | | $\frac{1}{8}$ | | — |
| 6 weeks–11 months | | $\frac{1}{4}$ | | — |
| 1–5 years | 10–19 | $\frac{1}{2}$ | | $\frac{1}{4}$ |
| 6–11 years | 20–39 | $\frac{3}{4}$ | | $\frac{1}{2}$ |
| 12 years | 40 | adult dose | | adult dose |

*Note.* Weight is a better guide than age for children over 6 months old. Specialist advice should be obtained for use of Maloprim® in children under 1 year of age.
Prophylaxis is required in **breast-fed infants**; although antimalarials are excreted in milk, the amounts are too variable to give reliable protection.

PREGNANCY. Chloroquine and proguanil may be given in usual doses in areas where *P. falciparum* strains are sensitive; in the case of proguanil folate supplements should be given. Maloprim® is contra-indicated in the first trimester; folate supplements should be given if Maloprim® is prescribed in the second and third trimester. The centres listed in the box in the previous column should be consulted for advice on prophylaxis in resistant areas.

---

SPECIFIC RECOMMENDATIONS. Specific recommendations by geographical regions are given below.

**North Africa and the Middle East**
(risk: generally low; transmission confined to rural areas and may be seasonal)

> chloroquine 300 mg (as base) once weekly

*or*

> proguanil hydrochloride 200 mg once daily

Above recommendations apply to some areas of Turkey (south coast and border with Syria) and also to Mauritius. No chemoprophylaxis needed for Algeria, Libya, Morocco, Tunisia, or tourist areas of Egypt; *both* chloroquine *and* proguanil needed for Afghanistan, Iran, and Oman.

**Sub-Saharan Africa** (includes East, Central and West Africa, north-east corner of South Africa (including Kruger National Park) and also Madagascar) (risk: very high)

> *both*
> chloroquine 300 mg (as base) once weekly
> *and*
> proguanil hydrochloride 200 mg once daily

Mefloquine alone is an option for short-term travellers (max. 3 weeks abroad) to Cameroon, Kenya, Malawi, Tanzania, Uganda, Zaire, and Zambia; see Mefloquine p. 236 for details of regimen.

**South Asia** (Bangladesh, Bhutan, India, Nepal, Pakistan, and Sri Lanka) (risk: variable)

> *both*
> chloroquine 300 mg (as base) once weekly
> *and*
> proguanil hydrochloride 200 mg once daily

**South-East Asia**
(risk: varies from very low to substantial)

> *both*
> chloroquine 300 mg (as base) once weekly
> *and*
> proguanil hydrochloride 200 mg once daily

Mefloquine alone is an option for short-term travellers (max. 3 weeks abroad); see Mefloquine p. 236 for details of regimen.

No chemoprophylaxis needed for tourist areas and cities of Brunei, China, Hong Kong, peninsular west Malaysia, Philippines, Sarawak, Singapore, and Thailand (all very low risk).

**Oceania** (Papua New Guinea, Solomon Islands, Vanuatu) (risk: very high)

> *both*
> Maloprim® 1 tablet once weekly
> *and*
> chloroquine 300 mg (as base) once weekly

Mefloquine alone is an option for short-term travellers (max. 3 weeks abroad); see Mefloquine (p. 236) for details of regimen.

**Latin America**
(risk: variable to high)

*Variable risk areas:*

> chloroquine 300 mg (as base) once weekly

*or*

> proguanil hydrochloride 200 mg once daily

Used for variable risk areas which include Argentina (a few areas), Belize, rural Costa Rica, Dominican Republic, El Salvador, Guatemala, Haiti, Honduras, rural Mexico, Nicaragua, rural Paraguay, and Peru (below 1500 m)

*Variable to high risk areas:*

> *both*
> chloroquine 300 mg (as base) once weekly
> *and*
> proguanil hydrochloride 200 mg once daily

Used for variable to high risk areas which include Bolivia (below 2500 m), rural Brazil, Colombia, Equador, French Guiana, Guyana, Panama, Suriname, and rural Venezuela.

Mefloquine alone is an option for short-term travellers (max. 3 weeks abroad) to the Amazonas region of Brazil; see Mefloquine (p. 236) for details of regimen.

> TREATMENT COURSES. Adults travelling to areas of chloroquine-resistance who are unlikely to have easy access to medical care should carry a treatment course. Self-medication should be **avoided** if medical help is accessible; prophylaxis should be continued during and after the attack. In view of the continuing emergence of resistant strains and of the different regimens required for different areas expert advice should be sought on the best treatment course for an individual patient.

## CHLOROQUINE

*Indications:* chemoprophylaxis and treatment of malaria; rheumatoid arthritis and lupus erythematosus—see section 10.1.3

*Cautions:* hepatic and renal impairment, pregnancy (but for malaria benefit outweighs risk, see Appendix 4, Antimalarials), may exacerbate psoriasis, neurological disorders (especially history of epilepsy), severe gastrointestinal disorders, G6PD deficiency (see section 9.1.5); elderly; regular ophthalmic examinations if prophylaxis treatment given for more than 3 years; avoid concurrent therapy with hepatotoxic drugs—other **interactions**: Appendix 1 (chloroquine)

*Side-effects:* gastro-intestinal disturbances, headache, visual disturbances, irreversible retinal damage, corneal opacities, depigmentation or loss of hair, skin reactions; rarely blood disorders (thrombocytopenia, agranulocytosis, and aplastic anaemia)

*Dose:* see notes above

PoM\* **Avloclor**® (ICI)
*Tablets*, scored, chloroquine phosphate 250 mg (≡chloroquine base 155 mg). Net price 20-tab pack = 70p. Label: 5
\* Can be sold to the public provided it is licensed and labelled for the prophylaxis of malaria

**Nivaquine**® (Rhône-Poulenc Rorer)
PoM\* *Tablets*, f/c, yellow, chloroquine sulphate 200 mg (≡chloroquine base 150 mg). Net price 28-tab pack = £1.04. Label: 5
\* Can be sold to the public provided it is licensed and labelled for the prophylaxis of malaria

PoM\* *Syrup*, golden, chloroquine sulphate 68 mg/5 mL (≡chloroquine base 50 mg/5 mL). Net price 60 mL = £1.31. Label: 5
\* Can be sold to the public provided it is licensed and labelled for the prophylaxis of malaria

PoM *Injection*, chloroquine sulphate 54.5 mg/mL (≡chloroquine base 40 mg/mL). Net price 5-mL amp = 52p

## HALOFANTRINE HYDROCHLORIDE

*Indications:* treatment of uncomplicated chloroquine-resistant falciparum malaria, see notes above

*Cautions:* pregnancy; discontinue breast-feeding during treatment; not indicated for cerebral or complicated malaria

*Side-effects:* diarrhoea, abdominal pain, nausea, vomiting; transient elevation of serum transaminases; pruritus also reported

*Dose:* see notes above

▼ PoM **Halfan**® (SK&F)
*Tablets*, scored, halofantrine hydrochloride 250 mg. Net price 12-tab pack = £13.96

## MEFLOQUINE

*Indications:* chemoprophylaxis and treatment of chloroquine-resistant falciparum malaria, see notes above

*Cautions:* exclude pregnancy before starting chemoprophylaxis (**important teratogenic risk**) avoid for chemoprophylaxis in severe hepatic and in renal impairment; avoid frequent or prolonged administration (accumulation occurs due to long half-life); not recommended in young children (under 15 kg); **interactions**: Appendix 1 (mefloquine)
COUNSELLING. May affect performance of skilled tasks

*Contra-indications:* chemoprophylaxis in pregnancy (teratogenic in *animals*, **avoid** pregnancy **during** and for **3 months after**), breast-feeding, and history of psychiatric disturbances or convulsions

*Side-effects:* nausea, vomiting, diarrhoea, abdominal pain, anorexia; dizziness and loss of balance; rarely bradycardia, headache, neuropsychiatric disturbances (discontinue treatment), weakness, rash, pruritus, and disturbances in liver function tests

*Dose:* short-term chemoprophylaxis (max. 3 weeks in endemic area), 250 mg each week for 6 weeks starting 1 week before departure; CHILD 15–19 kg (2–5 years) quarter adult dose, 20–30 kg (6–8 years) half adult dose, 31–45 kg (9–11 years) three-quarters adult dose
Longer chemoprophylaxis (more than 3 weeks in endemic area), not recommended by UK experts
Treatment, see notes above

▼ PoM **Lariam**® (Roche)
*Tablets*, scored, mefloquine 250 mg (as hydrochloride). Net price 6-tab pack = £10.90. Label: 21, 25, 27

## PRIMAQUINE

*Indications:* eradication of *Plasmodium vivax* and *P. ovale* malaria

*Cautions:* G6PD deficiency (see notes above); systemic diseases associated with granulocytopenia (e.g. rheumatoid arthritis, lupus erythematosus); pregnancy and breast-feeding; **interactions**: Appendix 1 (primaquine)

*Side-effects:* nausea, vomiting, abdominal pain; less commonly methaemoglobinaemia, haemolytic anaemia especially in G6PD deficiency

*Dose:* see notes above

**Primaquine** (ICI)
*Tablets*, brown, s/c, primaquine 7.5 mg (as phosphate). Net price 20 = 12p

## PROGUANIL HYDROCHLORIDE

*Indications:* chemoprophylaxis of malaria

*Cautions:* severe renal impairment; pregnancy (folate supplements needed); **interactions**: Appendix 1 (proguanil)

*Side-effects:* mild gastric intolerance; occasionally mouth ulcers and stomatitis; skin reaction and hair loss reported

*Dose:* see notes above

**Paludrine®** (ICI)
*Tablets,* scored, proguanil hydrochloride 100 mg. Net price 20 = 64p. Label: 21

## PYRIMETHAMINE

*Indications:* malaria (but used only in combination with dapsone or sulphadoxine); toxoplasmosis (section 5.4.7)
*Cautions:* hepatic or renal impairment, folate supplements in pregnancy, blood counts required with prolonged treatment; **interactions:** Appendix 1 (pyrimethamine)
*Side-effects:* depression of haematopoiesis with high doses, rashes, insomnia

**Daraprim®** (Wellcome)
*Tablets,* scored, pyrimethamine 25 mg. Net price 30-tab pack = £2.22
*Dose:* not recommended alone

With sulfadoxine
ADDITIONAL CAUTIONS: Severe adverse reactions on long-term use therefore not for prophylaxis; pregnancy (see also Appendix 4) and breast-feeding (see also Appendix 5); **interactions:** Appendix 1
PoM **Fansidar®** (Roche)
*Tablets,* scored, pyrimethamine 25 mg, sulfadoxine 500 mg. Net price 10-tab pack = £2.52
*Dose:* treatment, see notes above
Chemoprophylaxis, not recommended by UK experts.

With dapsone
ADDITIONAL CAUTIONS: G6PD deficiency (see section 9.1.5); pregnancy (see also Appendix 4) and breast-feeding (see also Appendix 5); **interactions:** Appendix 1
PoM **Maloprim®** (Wellcome)
*Tablets,* scored, pyrimethamine 12.5 mg, dapsone 100 mg. Net price 30-tab pack = £2.76
*Dose:* limited use, see Chemoprophylaxis

## QUININE

*Indications:* falciparum malaria; nocturnal leg cramps, see section 10.2.2
*Cautions:* atrial fibrillation, conduction defects, heart block, pregnancy; G6PD deficiency (see section 9.1.5); **interactions:** Appendix 1 (quinine)
*Contra-indications:* haemoglobinuria, optic neuritis
*Side-effects:* cinchonism, including tinnitus, headache, nausea, abdominal pain, rashes, visual disturbances (including temporary blindness), confusion; hypersensitivity reactions including angioedema, blood disorders (including thrombocytopenia and intravascular coagulation), and acute renal failure; hypoglycaemia (especially after parenteral administration)
*Dose:* see notes above
*Note.* Quinine (anhydrous base) 100 mg ≡ quinine bisulphate 169 mg ≡ quinine dihydrochloride 122 mg ≡ quinine hydrochloride 122 mg ≡ quinine sulphate 121 mg. Quinine bisulphate 300-mg tablets are available but provide smaller amounts of quinine than the dihydrochloride, hydrochloride, or sulphate

PoM **Quinine Dihydrochloride Tablets,** quinine dihydrochloride 300 mg. Net price 20 = £2.34
PoM **Quinine Hydrochloride Tablets,** quinine hydrochloride 300 mg. Net price 20 = £1.84
PoM **Quinine Sulphate Tablets,** coated, quinine sulphate 125 mg, net price 20 = 50p; 200 mg, 20 = 74p; 300 mg, 20 = 72p
PoM **Quinine Dihydrochloride Injection,** quinine dihydrochloride 300 mg/mL. For dilution and use as an infusion. 1- and 2-mL amps
Injection available from Martindale and Penn (both special order) or from specialist centres (see p. 223)
*Note.* Intravenous injection of quinine is so hazardous that it has been superseded by infusion

## 5.4.2 Amoebicides

**Metronidazole** is the drug of choice for *acute invasive amoebic dysentery* for it is very effective against vegetative amoebae in ulcers at a dosage of 800 mg three times daily for 5 days; it is also effective against amoebae which have migrated to the liver. It is given either for 10 days, or for 5 days followed by a 10-day course of diloxanide furoate. **Tinidazole** is also effective.
**Diloxanide furoate** is the drug of choice in *chronic intestinal amoebiasis* in which only cysts and not vegetative forms of *Entamoeba histolytica* are present in the faeces; metronidazole and tinidazole are relatively ineffective. Diloxanide furoate is relatively free from toxic effects in therapeutic doses and the usual course is of 10 days, given alone for chronic infections or following 5 days of metronidazole in acute dysenteric infections.
For *amoebic abscesses* of the liver **metronidazole** is effective in doses of 400 mg 3 times daily for 5–10 days; the course may be repeated after 2 weeks if necessary. Aspiration of the abscess is indicated where it is suspected that it may rupture or where there is no improvement after 72 hours of metronidazole; the aspiration may need to be repeated. Aspiration aids penetration of metronidazole and, for abscesses with more than 100 mL of pus, if carried out in conjunction with drug therapy, may reduce the period of disability.
If metronidazole or tinidazole are not available emetine may be used but its side-effects are much more marked. Diloxanide is not effective against hepatic amoebiasis, but a 10-day course should be given at the completion of metronidazole or tinidazole treatment to destroy any amoebae in the gut.

## DILOXANIDE FUROATE

*Indications:* chronic amoebiasis—see notes
*Side-effects:* flatulence, vomiting, urticaria, pruritus
*Dose:* 500 mg every 8 hours for 10 days; CHILD 20 mg/kg daily in 3 divided doses.
See also notes above

PoM **Furamide**® (Boots)
*Tablets*, scored, diloxanide furoate 500 mg.
Label: 9
Available only on direct order from Boots

PoM **Entamizole**® (Boots)
*Tablets*, off-white, diloxanide furoate 250 mg, metronidazole 200 mg. Label: 4, 9, 21, 25
Available only on direct order from Boots
*Dose:* amoebiasis, 2 tablets 3 times daily for 5 days;
CHILD 5–12 years ½–1 tablet, according to age, for 5 days
Treatment may be extended to 10 days in refractory cases; not suitable for prolonged (e.g. prophylactic) use

## METRONIDAZOLE

*Indications:* see under Dose below; anaerobic infections, section 5.1.11
*Cautions; Side-effects:* section 5.1.11
*Dose: by mouth*, invasive intestinal amoebiasis,
800 mg every 8 hours for 5 days; CHILD 1–3 years 200 mg every 8 hours; 3–7 years 200 mg every 6 hours; 7–10 years 400 mg every 8 hours
Extra-intestinal amoebiasis (including liver abscess) and symptomless amoebic cyst passers, 400–800 mg every 8 hours for 5–10 days; CHILD 1–3 years 100–200 mg every 8 hours; 3–7 years 100–200 mg every 6 hours; 7–10 years 200–400 mg every 8 hours
Urogenital trichomoniasis, 200 mg every 8 hours for 7 days *or* 400 mg every 12 hours for 7 days, *or* 800 mg in the morning and 1.2 g at night for 2 days, *or* 2 g as a single dose; CHILD 1–3 years 50 mg every 8 hours for 7 days; 3–7 years 100 mg every 12 hours; 7–10 years 100 mg every 8 hours
Giardiasis, 2 g daily for 3 days; CHILD 1–3 years 500 mg daily; 3–7 years 600–800 mg daily; 7–10 years 1 g daily

**Preparations**
Section 5.1.11

## TINIDAZOLE

*Indications:* see under Dose below; anaerobic infections, section 5.1.11
*Cautions; Side-effects:* section 5.1.11
*Dose:* intestinal amoebiasis, 2 g daily for 2–3 days; CHILD 50–60 mg/kg daily for 3 days
Amoebic involvement of liver, 1.5–2 g daily for 3–5 days; CHILD 50–60 mg/kg daily for 5 days
Urogenital trichomoniasis and giardiasis, single 2-g dose (repeated once if necessary); CHILD single dose of 50–75 mg/kg

**Preparations**
Section 5.1.11

## 5.4.3   Trichomonacides

**Metronidazole** (section 5.4.2) is the treatment of choice for *Trichomonas vaginalis* infection.

If metronidazole is ineffective, **nimorazole** may be tried; it is usually given as a single 2-g dose, with food. A further 2-g dose may be given if there is no clinical improvement.

Alcohol should be avoided during treatment with both metronidazole and nimorazole.

## NIMORAZOLE

*Indications:* trichomoniasis; acute ulcerative gingivitis, see section 12.3.2
*Contra-indications:* active CNS disease, severe renal failure
*Side-effects:* nausea, vomiting, rashes, vertigo, drowsiness, ataxia (discontinue treatment), intolerance to alcohol
*Dose:* see notes above

**Naxogin 500**® (Farmitalia Carlo Erba)
*Tablets*, scored, nimorazole 500 mg. Net price 8-tab pack = £1.74. Label: 4, 21

## 5.4.4   Antigiardial drugs

**Metronidazole** (section 5.4.2) is the treatment of choice for *Giardia lamblia* infections, given by mouth in a dosage of 2 g daily for 3 days or 400 mg every 8 hours for 5 days.

Alternative treatments are **tinidazole** (section 5.4.2) 2 g as a single dose or **mepacrine hydrochloride** 100 mg every 8 hours for 5–7 days.

## MEPACRINE HYDROCHLORIDE

*Indications:* giardiasis
*Cautions:* hepatic impairment, elderly, history of psychosis; avoid in psoriasis; **interactions:** Appendix 1 (mepacrine)
*Side-effects:* gastro-intestinal disturbances; dizziness, headache; with large doses nausea, vomiting and occasionally transient acute toxic psychosis and CNS stimulation; on prolonged treatment yellow discoloration of skin and urine, chronic dermatoses (including severe exfoliative dermatitis), hepatitis, aplastic anaemia; also reported blue/black discoloration of palate and nails and corneal deposits with visual disturbances
*Dose:* 100 mg every 8 hours for 5–7 days; CHILD 2 mg/kg every 8 hours

**Mepacrine Hydrochloride**
*Tablets*, mepacrine hydrochloride 100 mg. Net price 20 = 28p. Label: 4, 9, 14, 21
Available from Boots (special order)

## 5.4.5   Leishmaniacides

Cutaneous leishmaniasis frequently heals spontaneously without specific treatment. If the skin lesions are extensive or unsightly, treatment is indicated, as it is in visceral leishmaniasis (kala-azar).

**Sodium stibogluconate**, an organic pentavalent antimony compound, is the treatment of choice for visceral leishmaniasis. The dose is 20 mg/kg daily (max. 850 mg) for at least 20 days by intramuscular or intravenous injection; the dosage varies with different geographical regions and expert advice should be obtained. Skin lesions are treated for 10 days.

---

**Pentamidine isethionate** (section 5.4.8) has been used in antimony-resistant visceral leishmaniasis, but although the initial response is often good, the relapse rate is high; it is associated with serious side-effects.

---

## SODIUM STIBOGLUCONATE

*Indications:* leishmaniasis

*Cautions:* intravenous injections must be given slowly and stopped if coughing or substernal pain develops; intramuscular injection painful

*Contra-indications:* pneumonia, myocarditis, nephritis, hepatitis

*Side-effects:* anorexia, vomiting, coughing, substernal pain

*Dose:* see notes above

PoM **Pentostam**® (Wellcome)

*Injection,* sodium stibogluconate equivalent to pentavalent antimony 100 mg/mL. Net price 100-mL bottle = £68.01

*Electrolytes:* Na+ 109 mmol/100-mL bottle

---

## 5.4.6 Trypanocides

The prophylaxis and treatment of trypanosomiasis is difficult and differs according to the strain of organism. Expert advice should therefore be obtained.

---

## 5.4.7 Drugs for toxoplasmosis

Most infections caused by *Toxoplasma gondii* are self-limiting, and treatment is not necessary. Exceptions are patients with eye involvement (toxoplasma choroidoretinitis), and those who are immunosuppressed. The treatment of choice is a combination of pyrimethamine and sulphadiazine, given for several weeks. Pyrimethamine is a folate antagonist, and adverse reactions to this combination are relatively common.

If toxoplasmosis is acquired in pregnancy, transplacental infection may lead to severe disease in the fetus. The pyrimethamine and sulphadiazine combination is best avoided in pregnancy but there are encouraging reports with spiramycin (not on UK market).

---

## 5.4.8 Drugs for Pneumocystis pneumonia

Pneumonia caused by *Pneumocystis carinii* occurs in immunosuppressed or severely debilitated patients. It is the commonest cause of pneumonia in AIDS. **Co-trimoxazole** (section 5.1.8) in high dosage is the drug of choice for the treatment of pneumocystis pneumonia. **Pentamidine isethionate** is an alternative to co-trimoxazole and is particularly indicated for patients with a history of adverse reactions to, or who have not responded to, co-trimoxazole. Pentamidine isethionate is a

potentially toxic drug that can cause severe hypotension during or immediately after administration; it should only be administered by those experienced in its use. Pentamidine isethionate is given by intravenous infusion but can also be administered by inhalation which reduces side-effects (although systemic absorption may still occur); intermittent prophylactic inhalation may prevent relapse.

---

## PENTAMIDINE ISETHIONATE

*Indications:* see under Dose (should only be given by specialists)

*Cautions:* risk of severe hypotension following administration (establish baseline blood pressure and administer with patient lying down; monitor blood pressure closely during administration, and at regular intervals, until treatment concluded); hepatic and renal impairment; hypertension or hypotension; hyperglycaemia or hypoglycaemia; leucopenia, thrombocytopenia, or anaemia; carry out laboratory monitoring for all functions according to data sheet

*Side-effects:* severe reactions, sometimes fatal, due to hypotension, hypoglycaemia, pancreatitis, and arrhythmias; also leucopenia, thrombocytopenia, acute renal failure, hypocalcaemia; also reported: azotaemia, abnormal liver-function tests, leucopenia, anaemia, hyperkalaemia, nausea and vomiting, dizziness, syncope, flushing, hyperglycaemia, rash, and taste disturbances; bronchoconstriction reported on inhalation; discomfort, pain, induration, abscess formation, and muscle necrosis at injection site

*Dose: Pneumocystis carinii* pneumonia, *by intravenous infusion,* 4 mg/kg daily for at least 14 days (reduced according to data sheet in renal impairment)

*By inhalation of nebulised solution* (using suitable equipment—see data sheet) 600 mg pentamidine isethionate daily for 3 weeks; secondary prevention, 300 mg every 4 weeks *or* 150 mg every 2 weeks

Visceral leishmaniasis (Kala-azar), *by deep intramuscular injection,* 3–4 mg/kg on alternate days to max. total of 10 injections; course may be repeated if necessary

Cutaneous leishmaniasis, *by deep intramuscular injection,* 3–4 mg/kg once or twice weekly until condition resolves (but see also section 5.4.5)

Trypanosomiasis, *by deep intramuscular injection or intravenous infusion,* 4 mg/kg daily or on alternate days to total of 7–10 injections

*Note.* Direct bolus intravenous injection should be avoided whenever possible and **never** given rapidly; intramuscular injections should be deep and preferably given into the buttock

PoM **Pentacarinat**® (Rhône-Poulenc Rorer)

*Injection,* powder for reconstitution, pentamidine isethionate. Net price 300-mg vial = £15.98

*Nebuliser solution,* pentamidine isethionate. Net price 300-mg bottle = £16.87

---

# 5.5   Anthelmintics

5.5.1   Drugs for threadworms
5.5.2   Ascaricides
5.5.3   Taenicides
5.5.4   Drugs for hookworms
5.5.5   Schistosomicides
5.5.6   Filaricides
5.5.7   Drugs for guinea worms
5.5.8   Drugs for strongyloidiasis

Advice on prophylaxis and treatment of helminth infections is available from:

| | |
|---|---|
| Birmingham | 021-772 4311 |
| Glasgow | 041-946 7120 Extn 277 |
| Liverpool | 051-708 9393 |
| London | 071-387 4411 (treatment) |

## 5.5.1   Drugs for threadworms

(pinworms, *Enterobius vermicularis*)

Anthelmintics are relatively ineffective in threadworm infections, and their use should be combined with hygienic measures to break the cycle of auto-infection. All members of the family require treatment.

Adult threadworms do not live for longer than 6 weeks and for development of fresh worms, ova must be swallowed and exposed to the action of digestive juices in the upper intestinal tract. Direct multiplication of worms does not take place in the large bowel. Adult female worms lay ova on the peri-anal skin which causes pruritus; scratching the area then leads to ova being transmitted on fingers to the mouth, often via food eaten with unwashed hands. Washing hands and scrubbing nails before each meal and after each visit to the toilet is essential. A bath taken immediately after rising will remove ova laid during the night.

**Mebendazole** is the drug of choice for patients of all ages over 2 years. It is given as a single dose; as reinfection is very common, a second dose may be given after 2–3 weeks.

**Piperazine** salts are preferably given daily for 7 days; a further 7-day course may be given if necessary after an interval of 1 week. Single-dose preparations are also available.

**Pyrantel** is equally effective. It is given as a single dose; cure-rates are improved if one or two further doses are given at intervals of 2 weeks.

## MEBENDAZOLE

*Indications:* threadworm, roundworm, whipworm, and hookworm infections

*Cautions:* pregnancy (toxicity in *rats*)
*Note.* The package insert in the Vermox® pack includes the statement that it is not suitable for women known to be pregnant or children under 2 years

*Side-effects:* rarely abdominal pain, diarrhoea

*Dose:* threadworms, ADULT and CHILD over 2 years, 100 mg as a single dose; if reinfection occurs second dose may be needed after 2–3 weeks; CHILD under 2 years, not yet recommended

Roundworms—section 5.5.2

¹PoM **Vermox**® (Janssen)
*Tablets*, pink, scored, chewable, mebendazole 100 mg. Net price 6-tab pack = £1.57
*Suspension* mebendazole 100 mg/5 mL. Net price 30 mL = £1.82

1. Can be sold to the public if supplied for the oral treatment of enterobiasis in a container or package containing only a single dose of not more than 100 mg of mebendazole; a proprietary brand (Ovex®) is also on sale to the public.

## PIPERAZINE

*Indications:* threadworm and roundworm infections

*Cautions:* renal impairment (avoid if severe), liver disease, neurological disease; epilepsy, pregnancy (see also Appendix 4 (packs on sale to the general public carry a warning to avoid in epilepsy and pregnancy); **interactions:** Appendix 1 (piperazine)

*Side-effects:* nausea, vomiting, colic, diarrhoea, allergic reactions including urticaria, bronchospasm, and rare reports of Stevens-Johnson syndrome and angioedema; rarely dizziness, muscular incoordination ('worm wobble'); drowsiness, confusion and clonic contractions in patients with neurological or renal abnormalities

*Dose:* threadworms, as piperazine hydrate, 2 g once daily for 7 days; CHILD under 2 years 50–75 mg/kg once daily for 7 days, 2–4 years 750 mg once daily for 7 days, 5–12 years 1.5 g once daily for 7 days; repeat course after 1 week if necessary

Roundworms—section 5.5.2

*Note.* 100 mg piperazine hydrate ≡ 125 mg piperazine citrate ≡ 104 mg piperazine phosphate

**Antepar**® (Wellcome)
*Tablets*, yellow, scored, piperazine hydrate 500 mg (as phosphate). Net price 28-tab pack = £2.86. Label: 24
*Elixir*—product discontinued.

**Pripsen**® (R&C)
*Oral powder*, cream, piperazine phosphate 4 g and sennosides 15.3 mg/sachet. Net price two-dose sachet pack = £1.31. Label: 13
*Dose:* threadworms, stirred into a small glass of milk or water and drunk immediately, ADULT and CHILD over 6 years, 1 sachet, repeat after 14 days; INFANT 3 months–1 year, one-third sachet (2.5 mL powder); CHILD 1–6 years, two-thirds sachet (5 mL powder), repeat after 14 days

Roundworms, first dose as for threadworms; repeat at monthly intervals for up to 3 months if reinfection risk

## 5.5.2   Ascaricides

(common roundworm infections)

**Levamisole** (not on UK market) is very effective against ascaris and is generally considered to be the drug of choice. It is very well tolerated; mild nausea or vomiting has been reported in about

---

1% of treated patients; it is given as a single dose of 120–150 mg in adults.

**Mebendazole** (section 5.5.1) is also active against *Ascaris lumbricoides*; the usual dose is 100 mg twice daily for 3 days. **Pyrantel** is also an effective broad-spectrum anthelmintic and a single dose of 10 mg/kg (max. 1 g) is usually sufficient to eradicate ascaris; it may occasionally produce mild nausea but experience shows it to be a very safe drug. **Piperazine** may also be given in a single dose equivalent to 4 g of piperazine hydrate.

## PYRANTEL

*Indications:* roundworm, threadworm, and hookworm infections

*Cautions:* liver disease; **interactions:** Appendix 1 (pyrantel)

*Side-effects:* see notes above

*Dose:* ADULT and CHILD over 6 months, *Ascaris lumbricoides* alone, a single dose of 5 mg/kg; mixed infections involving *Ascaris lumbricoides*, single dose of 10 mg/kg

Hookworm—section 5.5.4

Threadworm—section 5.5.1

PoM **Combantrin**® (Pfizer)

*Tablets*, orange, pyrantel 125 mg (as embonate). Net price 6-tab pack = 64p.

## 5.5.3 Taenicides
(tapeworms)

**Niclosamide** is the most widely used drug for tapeworm infections and side-effects are limited to occasional gastro-intestinal upset, light-headedness, and pruritus. Fears of developing cysticercosis in *Taenia solium* infections have proved unfounded. All the same, it is wise to anticipate this possibility by using an anti-emetic on wakening.

**Praziquantel** (not on UK market) is as effective as niclosamide and is given as a single dose of 10–20 mg/kg after a light breakfast.

## NICLOSAMIDE

*Indications:* tapeworm infections—see notes above and Dose

*Side-effects:* gastro-intestinal discomfort

*Dose:* *Taenia solium*, 2 g as a single dose after a light breakfast, followed by a purgative after 2 hours; CHILD up to 2 years, 500 mg, 2–6 years, 1 g

*T. saginata* and *Diphyllobothrium latum*, as for *T. solium* but half the dose may be taken after breakfast and the remainder one hour later followed by a purgative after a further 2 hours

*Hymenolepis nana*, 2 g on first day, then 1 g daily for next 6 days; CHILD up to 2 years, quarter adult dose; 2–6 years, half adult dose

COUNSELLING. To be chewed thoroughly and washed down with water or taken crushed in water

**Yomesan**® (Bayer)

*Tablets*, yellow, chewable, niclosamide 500 mg. Net price 4-tab pack = £1.41. Label: 4, 24, 27, counselling, administration

## 5.5.4 Drugs for hookworms
(ancylostomiasis, necatoriasis)

Hookworms live in the upper small intestine and draw blood from the point of their attachment to their host. An iron-deficiency anaemia may thereby be produced and, if present, effective treatment of the infection requires not only expulsion of the worms but treatment of the anaemia.

**Bephenium** is still widely used and its side-effects are limited to occasional nausea and vomiting. A single dose of 2.5 g is given and repeated after 1–2 days. It is unpleasant to take and activity against *Necator americanus* is unreliable. **Pyrantel** (section 5.5.2) is very effective against hookworms and, like bephenium, has side-effects limited to occasional nausea and vomiting. The usual dose is 10 mg/kg (max. 1 g) given as a single dose.

**Mebendazole** (section 5.5.1) has a useful broad-spectrum activity, and is effective against hookworms; the usual dose is 100 mg twice daily for 3 days.

## BEPHENIUM

*Indications:* roundworm and hookworm infections

*Side-effects:* nausea, vomiting, diarrhoea, headache, vertigo

*Dose:* see notes above

**Alcopar**® (Wellcome)

*Granules*, yellow/green, bephenium 2.5 g (as hydroxynaphthoate)/sachet. Net price per sachet = 84p. Label: 13

## 5.5.5 Schistosomicides
(bilharziasis)

Adult *Schistosoma haematobium* worms live in the genito-urinary veins and adult *S. mansoni* in those of the colon and mesentery. *S. japonicum* is more widely distributed in veins of the alimentary tract and portal system.

**Praziquantel** (Biltricide®, not on UK market) is effective against all human schistosomes. The dose is 40 mg/kg as a single oral dose (60 mg/kg in 3 divided doses on one day for *S. japonicum* infections). No serious toxic effects have been reported. Of all the available schistosomicides, it has the most attractive combination of effectiveness, broad-spectrum activity, and low toxicity.

**Oxamniquine** (Vansil®, *Pfizer*) is effective against *S. mansoni* infections only. It is a quinoline compound given by mouth; the dosage ranges from 15 mg/kg as a single dose to a total of 60 mg/kg over 2 to 3 days according to the geographical region. It can occasionally cause convulsions.

**Metriphonate** (Bilarcil®, not on UK market) is an organophosphorus compound which is only effective against *S. haematobium* infections. It is given by mouth in 3 doses of 7.5 mg/kg at intervals of 2 weeks. As it reduces plasma-cholinesterase concentrations it should be used with caution in patients likely to be frequently exposed to organophosphorus insecticides.

Hycanthone, lucanthone, niridazole, and stibocaptate have now been superseded.

## 5.5.6  Filaricides

**Diethylcarbamazine** is effective against microfilariae and adults of *Loa loa*, *Wuchereria bancrofti*, and *Brugia Malayi*. To minimise reactions treatment is commenced with a dose of 1 mg/kg and increased gradually over 3 days to 6 mg/kg daily in divided doses; this dosage is maintained for 21 days and usually gives a radical cure for these infections. Close medical supervision is necessary particularly in the early phase of treatment.

In heavy infections there may be a febrile reaction, and in heavy *Loa loa* infection there is a small risk of encephalopathy. In such cases treatment must be given under careful in-patient supervision and stopped at the first sign of cerebral involvement (and specialist advice sought).

Diethylcarbamazine can cause such serious reactions in onchocerciasis, that it should no longer be used for this infection. Suramin has also been used for onchocerciasis but is now obsolete because of its toxicity.

**Ivermectin** (Mectizan®, *MSD*, not on UK market) is very effective in *onchocerciasis* and it is now the drug of choice. A single dose of 150 micrograms/kg by mouth produces a prolonged reduction in microfilarial levels. Retreatment at intervals of 6 to 12 months depending on symptoms must be given until the adult worms die out. Reactions are usually slight and most commonly take the form of temporary aggravation of itching and rash.

## DIETHYLCARBAMAZINE CITRATE
*Indications:* filariasis
*Cautions; Side-effects:* see notes above
*Dose:* see notes above

**Banocide®** (Wellcome)
Product discontinued.

## 5.5.7  Drugs for guinea worms
(dracontiasis)

Guinea worms, *Dracunculus medinensis*, may be killed and their removal from the tissues facilitated by a course of **niridazole** (Ambilhar®, not on UK market). Use of niridazole does not obviate the concomitant need for sterile dressing of the ulcer caused by a guinea worm and for its extraction, wherever possible, under sterile conditions. In India, mebendazole has been reported as effective at a dosage of 200 mg twice daily for 7 days. **Metronidazole** has also been reported to be effective in a dose of 400 mg three times daily for 5 days.

## 5.5.8  Drugs for strongyloidiasis

Adult *Strongyloides stercoralis* live in the gut and produce larvae which penetrate the gut wall and invade the tissues, setting up a cycle of autoinfection. **Thiabendazole** is the drug of choice, at a dosage of 25 mg/kg every 12 hours for 3 days. **Albendazole** (SmithKline Beecham, not on UK market) is an alternative with fewer side-effects; it is given in a dose of 400 mg daily for 3 days, repeated after 3 weeks if necessary.

## THIABENDAZOLE
*Indications:* strongyloidiasis, cutaneous and visceral larva migrans, dracontiasis, symptoms of trichinosis; secondary treatment for threadworm when mixed with above infestations; adjunct in hookworm, whipworm, or roundworm
*Cautions:* hepatic or renal impairment, discontinue if hypersensitivity reactions occur; **interactions:** Appendix 1 (thiabendazole)
DRIVING. May impair performance of skilled tasks (e.g. driving)
*Contra-indications:* pregnancy (teratogenesis in *animal* studies)
*Side-effects:* anorexia, nausea, vomiting, dizziness, diarrhoea, headache, pruritus, drowsiness; hypersensitivity reactions including fever, chills, angioedema, rashes, erythema multiforme; rarely tinnitus, collapse, parenchymal liver damage
*Dose:* see notes above

PoM **Mintezol®** (MSD)
*Tablets*, orange, chewable, thiabendazole 500 mg. Net price 6-tab pack = 52p. Label: 3, 21, 24

---

# 6: Drugs used in the treatment of disorders of the
# ENDOCRINE SYSTEM

In this chapter, drug treatment is discussed under the following headings:

**6.1** Drugs used in diabetes
**6.2** Thyroid and antithyroid drugs
**6.3** Corticosteroids
**6.4** Sex hormones
**6.5** Hypothalamic and pituitary hormones
**6.6** Drugs affecting bone metabolism
**6.7** Other endocrine drugs

## 6.1 Drugs used in diabetes

**6.1.1** Insulin
**6.1.2** Oral antidiabetic drugs
**6.1.3** Diabetic ketoacidosis
**6.1.4** Treatment of hypoglycaemia
**6.1.5** Treatment of diabetic neuropathy
**6.1.6** Diagnostic and monitoring agents for diabetes mellitus

### 6.1.1 Insulin

**6.1.1.1** Short-acting insulin
**6.1.1.2** Intermediate- and long-acting insulins
**6.1.1.3** Hypodermic equipment

Insulin plays a key role in the body's regulation of carbohydrate, fat, and protein metabolism. Diabetes mellitus is due to a deficiency in insulin synthesis and secretion. Patients are generally described as insulin-dependent diabetics (type 1) or non-insulin-dependent diabetics (type 2), although many of the latter need insulin to maintain satisfactory control.

Insulin is a polypeptide hormone of complex structure. It is extracted mainly from pork pancreas and purified by crystallisation; it can also be made biosynthetically by recombinant DNA technology using *Escherichia coli* or semisynthetically by enzymatic modification of porcine material (see under Human Insulins, below). All insulin preparations are to a greater or lesser extent immunogenic in man but immunological resistance to insulin action is uncommon.

Insulin is inactivated by gastro-intestinal enzymes, and must therefore be given by injection; the subcutaneous route is ideal for most circumstances. It is usually injected into the upper arms, thighs, buttocks, or abdomen; there may be increased absorption from a limb site if the limb is used in strenuous exercise. Insulin is usually administered using a syringe and needle but portable injection devices (e.g. NovoPen®, Penject®) which hold soluble insulin in cartridge form and meter the required dose are rapidly growing in popularity; they permit greater freedom even though injections may be needed 3 or 4 times daily.

Insulin can also be given by continuous subcutaneous infusion using soluble insulin in an infusion pump. This technique now has an established though limited place in the treatment of diabetes, and provides for continuous basal insulin infusion with preprandial boosts. Its chief benefit is the considerable improvement in quality of life enjoyed by some patients, and, at times, the elimination of troublesome hypoglycaemia. It is unsuitable for emotionally or psychiatrically disturbed patients, and thus does not provide a general solution for 'brittle' diabetics. There are many disadvantages to this technique. Patients using it must be well-motivated, reliable, and able to monitor their own blood glucose, and must have access to expert advice both day and night.

When treating diabetic ketoacidosis (section 6.1.3), insulin should be given by intravenous or intramuscular injection, since absorption from subcutaneous depots may be slow and erratic.

Minor allergic reactions at the sites of injections during the first few weeks of treatment are uncommon, usually transient and require no treatment. Fat hypertrophy sometimes develops at sites of insulin injection and can to some extent be avoided by rotation of injection sites.

CHOICE OF TREATMENT. About 25% of diabetics require insulin treatment; apart from those presenting in ketoacidosis, insulin is needed by most of those with a rapid onset of symptoms, weight loss, weakness, and sometimes vomiting, often associated with ketonuria. The majority of those who are obese can be managed by restriction of carbohydrate or energy intake alone or with the subsequent administration of oral hypoglycaemic drugs. Most children require insulin from the outset.

MANAGEMENT OF DIABETIC PATIENTS. The aim of treatment is to achieve the best possible control of plasma glucose without making the patient obsessional, and avoiding disabling hypoglycaemia; close co-operation is needed between the patient and the medical team. Mixtures of available insulin preparations may be required and these combinations have to be worked out for the individual patient. Insulin requirements may be affected by variations in lifestyle, infection, and corticosteroids, and sometimes by a very small amount when the oral contraceptive pill is taken. In pregnancy insulin requirements should be assessed frequently by an experienced diabetic physician.

The energy and carbohydrate intake must be adequate to allow normal growth and development but obesity must be avoided. The carbohydrate intake must be regulated in those patients on insulin and should be distributed throughout the day. Fine control of plasma glucose can be achieved by moving portions of carbohydrate from one meal to another without altering the total intake.

Insulin doses are determined on an individual basis, by gradually increasing the dose but avoiding troublesome hypoglycaemic reactions.

There are 3 main types of insulin preparations:

1. those of **short** duration which have a relatively rapid onset of action, namely soluble forms of insulin;

2. those with an **intermediate** action, e.g. Isophane Insulin Injection and Insulin Zinc Suspension; and

3. those whose action is slower in onset and lasts for **long** periods, e.g. Human Ultratard®.

The *duration of action* of different insulin preparations varies considerably from one patient to another, and needs to be assessed for every individual; those indicated below are only approximations. The type of insulin used and its dose and frequency of administration depend on the particular needs of the patient. Most patients are best started on insulins of intermediate action twice daily and a short-acting insulin can later be added to cover any hyperglycaemia which may follow breakfast or evening meal.

Some recommended insulin regimens

| Insulin | Regimen |
| --- | --- |
| 1. Short-acting insulin mixed with Intermediate-acting insulin | twice daily (before meals) |
| 2. Short-acting insulin mixed with Intermediate-acting insulin | before breakfast |
| Short-acting insulin | before evening meal |
| Intermediate-acting insulin | bedtime |
| 3. Short-acting insulin | three times daily (before breakfast, midday and evening meal) |
| Intermediate-acting insulin | bedtime |
| 4. Short-acting insulin mixed with Intermediate-acting insulin | before breakfast (sufficient in some cases) |

HUMAN INSULINS. There are differences in the amino-acid sequence in animal and human insulins; most available insulins are either porcine in origin or of human sequence prepared by modification of porcine material (emp) or biosynthetically (crb, prb, or pyr). Preparations of human sequence insulin should theoretically be less immunogenic, but in trials no real advantage has been shown.

HYPOGLYCAEMIA. This is a potential hazard when the type of insulin is changed, especially when converting from beef to human insulin. The conversion from beef to human sequence insulin should always be undertaken with specialist advice; it is usual to reduce the total dose by about 10%, with careful monitoring for the first few days. When changing from porcine to human sequence insulin, a dose change is not usually needed, but careful monitoring is advised. Loss of warning of hypoglycaemia is a common problem among insulin-treated diabetics and can be a serious hazard, especially for drivers. The cause is not known, but very tight control of diabetes appears to lower the blood glucose concentration needed to trigger hypoglycaemic symptoms. Beta-blockers can also blunt hypoglycaemic awareness (and can delay recovery).

Some patients have reported loss of warning of hypoglycaemia after transfer to human insulin. Patients should be warned of this possibility and if they believe that human insulin is responsible for their loss of warning it is reasonable to transfer them back to porcine insulin. When prescribing insulin great care should be taken to specify whether a human or an animal preparation is required. Indications for changing from animal to human preparations must be very carefully considered in the light of these reported problems.

DRIVING. Car drivers need to be particularly careful to avoid hypoglycaemia (see above) and should be warned of the problems. They should normally check their blood glucose concentration before driving and, on long journeys, at intervals of approximately two hours. If hypoglycaemia occurs a car driver should switch off the ignition until recovery is complete, which may take up to 15 minutes or longer. Driving is not permitted when hypoglycaemic awareness has been lost.

UNITS. The word 'unit' should **not** be abbreviated.

### 6.1.1.1   SHORT-ACTING INSULIN

**Soluble Insulin** is a short-acting form of insulin. For maintenance regimens it is usual to inject it 15 to 30 minutes before meals.

Soluble insulin is the only appropriate form of insulin for use in diabetic emergencies and at the time of surgical operations. It has the great advantage that it can be given intravenously and intramuscularly, as well as subcutaneously.

When injected subcutaneously, soluble insulin has a rapid onset of action (after 30 to 60 minutes), a peak action between 2 and 4 hours, and a duration of action of up to 8 hours. Human sequence preparations tend to have a more rapid onset and a shorter overall duration.

When injected intravenously, soluble insulin has a very short half-life of only about 5 minutes and its effect disappears within 30 minutes.

## SOLUBLE INSULIN
(Insulin Injection; Neutral Insulin)
A sterile solution of insulin (i.e. bovine or porcine) or of human insulin; pH 6.6–8.0

*Indications:* diabetes mellitus; diabetic keto-acidosis (section 6.1.3)

*Cautions:* see notes above; reduce dose in renal impairment; **interactions:** Appendix 1 (anti-diabetics)

*Side-effects:* see notes above; local reactions and fat hypertrophy at injection site; overdose causes hypoglycaemia

*Dose: by subcutaneous, intramuscular, or intravenous injection or intravenous infusion, according to patient's requirements*

Highly purified animal

**Hypurin Neutral®** (CP)

*Injection*, soluble insulin (bovine, highly purified) 100 units/mL. Net price 10-mL vial = £8.95

**Velosulin®** (Novo Nordisk Wellcome)

*Injection*, soluble insulin (porcine, highly purified) 100 units/mL. Net price 10-mL vial = £7.85

**Velosulin Cartridge®** (Novo Nordisk Wellcome)

*Injection* (subcutaneous infusion only), soluble insulin (porcine, highly purified) 100 units/mL. Net price 5.7-mL cartridge vial (for use only in Nordisk Wellcome Infuser®) = £5.14

Human sequence

**Human Actrapid®** (Novo Nordisk)

*Injection*, soluble insulin (human, pyr) 100 units/mL. Net price 10-mL vial = £8.45

**Human Actrapid Penfill®** (Novo Nordisk)

*Injection*, soluble insulin (human, pyr) 100 units/mL. Net price 5 × 1.5-mL cartridge (for NHS NovoPen® devices) = £7.69

**Human Velosulin®** (Novo Nordisk Wellcome)

*Injection*, soluble insulin (human, emp) 100 units/mL. Net price 10-mL vial = £8.45

**Humulin S®** (Lilly)

*Injection*, soluble insulin (human, prb) 100 units/mL. Net price 10-mL vial = £9.25, cartridge (for NHS B-D pen®), 5 × 1.5-mL = £8.01

**Pur-In® Neutral** (CP)

*Injection*, soluble insulin (human, emp) 100 units/mL. Net price 10-mL vial = £8.45, 5 × 3-mL cartridge (for NHS Pur-In Pen® device) = £15.38

Mixed preparations, see Biphasic Insulin and Biphasic Isophane Insulin (section 6.1.1.2)

### 6.1.1.2 INTERMEDIATE- AND LONG-ACTING INSULINS

When given by subcutaneous injection intermediate- and long-acting insulins have an onset of action of approximately 1–2 hours, a maximal effect at 4–12 hours, and a duration of 16–35 hours. Some are given twice daily in conjunction with short-acting (soluble) insulin, and others are given once daily, particularly in elderly patients. They can be mixed with soluble insulin in the syringe, essentially retaining the properties of the two components, although there may be some blunting of the initial effect of the soluble insulin component (especially on mixing with protamine zinc insulin, see below).

**Isophane Insulin** is a suspension of insulin with protamine which is of particular value for initiation of twice-daily insulin regimens. Patients usually mix isophane with soluble insulin but ready-mixed preparations may be appropriate (**Biphasic Isophane Insulin**).

**Biphasic Insulin** is another ready-mixed insulin suitable for twice-daily injection.

**Insulin Zinc Suspension (Amorphous)** has an intermediate duration of action and **Insulin Zinc Suspension (Crystalline)** a more prolonged duration of action. These preparations may be used independently or in **Insulin Zinc Suspension** (30% amorphous, 70% crystalline).

**Protamine Zinc Insulin** is usually given once-daily in conjunction with short-acting (soluble) insulin. It has the drawback of binding with the soluble insulin when mixed in the same syringe, and is now rarely used.

### INSULIN ZINC SUSPENSION
(Insulin Zinc Suspension (Mixed); I.Z.S.)

A sterile neutral suspension of bovine and/or porcine insulin or of human insulin in the form of a complex obtained by the addition of a suitable zinc salt; consists of rhombohedral crystals (10–40 microns) and of particles of no uniform shape (not exceeding 2 microns)

*Indications:* diabetes mellitus (long acting)

*Cautions; Side-effects:* see under Soluble Insulin (section 6.1.1.1)

*Dose: by subcutaneous injection*, according to patient's requirements

Highly purified animal

**Hypurin Lente®** (CP)

*Injection*, insulin zinc suspension (bovine, highly purified) 100 units/mL. Net price 10-mL vial = £8.95

**Lentard MC®** (Novo Nordisk)

*Injection*, insulin zinc suspension (bovine and porcine, highly purified) 100 units/mL. Net price 10-mL vial = £6.89

Human sequence

**Human Monotard®** (Novo Nordisk)

*Injection*, insulin zinc suspension (human, pyr) 100 units/mL. Net price 10-mL vial = £8.45

**Humulin Lente®** (Lilly)

*Injection*, insulin zinc suspension (human, prb) 100 units/mL. Net price 10-mL vial = £9.25

### INSULIN ZINC SUSPENSION (AMORPHOUS)
(Amorph. I.Z.S.)

A sterile neutral suspension of bovine or porcine insulin in the form of a complex obtained by the addition of a suitable zinc salt; consists of particles of no uniform shape (not exceeding 2 microns)

*Indications:* diabetes mellitus (intermediate acting)

*Cautions; Side-effects:* see under Soluble Insulin (section 6.1.1.1)

*Dose: by subcutaneous injection*, according to patient's requirements

**Semitard MC®** (Novo Nordisk)

*Injection*, insulin zinc suspension (amorphous) (porcine, highly purified) 100 units/mL. Net price 10-mL vial = £7.49

Cautionary label wordings, see inside back cover

Prices are **net**, see p. 1

## INSULIN ZINC SUSPENSION (CRYSTALLINE)

(Cryst. I.Z.S.)

A sterile neutral suspension of bovine insulin or of human insulin in the form of a complex obtained by the addition of a suitable zinc salt; consists of rhombohedral crystals (10–40 microns)

*Indications:* diabetes mellitus (duration of action, see below)

*Cautions; Side-effects:* see under Soluble Insulin (section 6.1.1.1)

*Dose: by subcutaneous injection*, according to patient's requirements

Human sequence

**Human Ultratard**® (Novo Nordisk) (long acting)

*Injection*, insulin zinc suspension (human, pyr) 100 units/mL. Net price 10-mL vial = £8.45

**Humulin Zn**® (Lilly) (intermediate acting)

*Injection*, insulin zinc suspension, crystalline (human, prb) 100 units/mL. Net price 10-mL vial = £9.25

## ISOPHANE INSULIN

(Isophane Insulin Injection; Isophane Protamine Insulin Injection; Isophane Insulin (NPH))

A sterile suspension of bovine or porcine insulin or of human insulin in the form of a complex obtained by the addition of protamine sulphate or another suitable protamine

*Indications:* diabetes mellitus (intermediate acting)

*Cautions; Side-effects:* see under Soluble Insulin (section 6.1.1.1); protamine may cause allergic reactions

*Dose: by subcutaneous injection*, according to patient's requirements

Highly purified animal

**Hypurin Isophane**® (CP)

*Injection*, isophane insulin (bovine, highly purified) 100 units/mL. Net price 10-mL vial = £8.95

**Insulatard**® (Novo Nordisk Wellcome)

*Injection*, isophane insulin (porcine, highly purified) 100 units/mL. Net price 10-mL vial = £7.85

Human sequence

**Human Insulatard**® (Novo Nordisk Wellcome)

*Injection*, isophane insulin (human, emp) 100 units/mL. Net price 10-mL vial = £8.45

**Human Protaphane**® (Novo Nordisk)

*Injection*, isophane insulin (human, pyr) 100 units/mL. Net price 10-mL vial = £8.45

**Human Protaphane Penfill**® (Novo Nordisk)

*Injection*, isophane insulin (human, pyr) 100 units/mL. Net price 5 × 1.5-mL cartridge (for NHS Novopen® devices) = £8.10

**Humulin I**® (Lilly)

*Injection*, isophane insulin (human, prb) 100 units/mL. Net price 10-mL vial = £9.25, cartridge (for NHS B-D pen®), 5 × 1.5 mL = £8.01

**Pur-In**® **Isophane** (CP)

*Injection*, isophane insulin (human, emp) 100 units/mL. Net price 10-mL vial = £8.45, 5 × 3-mL cartridge (for NHS Pur-In Pen® device) = £16.20

Mixed preparations, see Biphasic Isophane Insulin (below)

## PROTAMINE ZINC INSULIN

(Protamine Zinc Insulin Injection)

A sterile suspension of insulin in the form of a complex obtained by the addition of a suitable protamine and zinc chloride; this preparation was included in BP 1980 but is not included in BP 1988

*Indications:* diabetes mellitus (long acting)

*Cautions; Side-effects:* see under Soluble Insulin (section 6.1.1.1); protamine may cause allergic reactions; see also notes above

*Dose: by subcutaneous injection*, according to patient's requirements

**Hypurin Protamine Zinc**® (CP)

*Injection*, protamine zinc insulin (bovine, highly purified) 100 units/mL. Net price 10-mL vial = £9.60

BIPHASIC INSULINS

## BIPHASIC INSULIN

(Biphasic Insulin Injection)

A sterile suspension of crystals containing bovine insulin in a solution of porcine insulin

*Indications:* diabetes mellitus (intermediate acting)

*Cautions; Side-effects:* see under Soluble Insulin (section 6.1.1.1)

*Dose: by subcutaneous injection*, according to patient's requirements

**Rapitard MC**® (Novo Nordisk)

*Injection*, biphasic insulin (highly purified) 100 units/mL. Net price 10-mL vial = £6.89

## BIPHASIC ISOPHANE INSULIN

(Biphasic Isophane Insulin Injection)

A sterile buffered suspension of porcine insulin complexed with protamine sulphate (or another suitable protamine) in a solution of porcine insulin *or* a sterile buffered suspension of human insulin complexed with protamine sulphate (or another suitable protamine) in a solution of human insulin

*Indications:* diabetes mellitus (intermediate acting)

*Cautions; Side-effects:* see under Soluble Insulin (section 6.1.1.1); protamine may cause allergic reactions

*Dose: by subcutaneous injection*, according to the patient's requirements

Highly purified animal

**Initard 50/50**® (Novo Nordisk Wellcome)
*Injection*, biphasic isophane insulin (porcine, highly purified), 50% soluble, 50% isophane. 100 units/mL. Net price 10-mL vial = £7.85

**Mixtard 30/70**® (Novo Nordisk Wellcome)
*Injection*, biphasic isophane insulin (porcine, highly purified), 30% soluble, 70% isophane, 100 units/mL. Net price 10-mL vial = £7.85

Human sequence

**Human Actraphane 30/70**® (Novo Nordisk)
*Injection*, biphasic isophane insulin (human, pyr), 30% soluble, 70% isophane, 100 units/mL. Net price 10-mL vial = £8.45

**Human Initard 50/50**® (Novo Nordisk Wellcome)
*Injection*, biphasic isophane insulin (human, emp), 50% soluble, 50% isophane, 100 units/mL. Net price 10-mL vial = £8.45

**Human Mixtard 30/70**® (Novo Nordisk Wellcome)
*Injection*, biphasic isophane insulin (human, emp), 30% soluble, 70% isophane, 100 units/mL. Net price 10-mL vial = £8.45

**Humulin M1**® (Lilly)
*Injection*, biphasic isophane insulin (human, prb), 10% soluble, 90% isophane, 100 units/mL. Net price 10-mL vial = £9.25, 5 × 1.5-mL cartridge (for NHS B-D pen®) = £8.01

**Humulin M2**® (Lilly)
*Injection*, biphasic isophane insulin (human, prb), 20% soluble, 80% isophane, 100 units/mL. Net price 10-mL vial = £9.25, 5 × 1.5-mL cartridge (for NHS B-D pen®) = £8.01

**Humulin M3**® (Lilly)
*Injection*, biphasic isophane insulin (human, prb), 30% soluble, 70% isophane, 100 units/mL. Net price 10-mL vial = £9.25, 5 × 1.5-mL cartridge (for NHS B-D pen®) = £8.01

**Humulin M4**® (Lilly)
*Injection*, biphasic isophane insulin (human, prb), 40% soluble, 60% isophane, 100 units/mL. Net price 10-mL vial = £9.25, 5 × 1.5-mL cartridge (for NHS B-D pen®) = £8.01

**PenMix 10/90 Penfill**® (Novo Nordisk)
*Injection*, biphasic isophane insulin (human, pyr), 10% soluble, 90% isophane, 100 units/mL. Net price 5 × 1.5-mL cartridge (for NHS Novopen® devices) = £8.10

**PenMix 20/80 Penfill**® (Novo Nordisk)
*Injection*, biphasic isophane insulin (human, pyr), 20% soluble, 80% isophane, 100 units/mL. Net price 5 × 1.5-mL cartridge (for NHS Novopen® devices) = £8.10

**PenMix 30/70 Penfill**® (Novo Nordisk)
*Injection*, biphasic isophane insulin (human, pyr), 30% soluble, 70% isophane, 100 units/mL. Net price 5 × 1.5-mL cartridge (for NHS Novopen® devices) = £8.10

**PenMix 40/60 Penfill**® (Novo Nordisk)
*Injection*, biphasic isophane insulin (human, pyr), 40% soluble, 60% isophane, 100 units/mL. Net price 5 × 1.5-mL cartridge (for NHS Novopen® devices) = £8.10

**PenMix 50/50 Penfill**® (Novo Nordisk)
*Injection*, biphasic isophane insulin (human, pyr), 50% soluble, 50% isophane, 100 units/mL. Net price 5 × 1.5-mL cartridge (for NHS Novopen® devices) = £8.10

**Pur-In**® **Mix 15/85** (CP)
*Injection*, biphasic isophane insulin (human, emp), 15% soluble, 85% isophane, 100 units/mL. Net price 10-mL vial = £8.45, 5 × 3-mL cartridge (for NHS Pur-In Pen® device) = £16.20

**Pur-In**® **Mix 25/75** (CP)
*Injection*, biphasic isophane insulin (human, emp), 25% soluble, 75% isophane, 100 units/mL. Net price 10-mL vial = £8.45, 5 × 3-mL cartridge (for NHS Pur-In Pen® device) = £16.20

**Pur-In**® **Mix 50/50** (CP)
*Injection*, biphasic isophane insulin (human, emp), 50% soluble, 50% isophane, 100 units/mL. Net price 10-mL vial = £8.45, 5 × 3-mL cartridge (for NHS Pur-In Pen® device) = £16.20

### 6.1.1.3 HYPODERMIC EQUIPMENT

Patients should be advised on the safe disposal of lancets, single-use syringes, and needles. Suitable arrangements for the safe disposal of contaminated waste must be made before these products are prescribed for patients who are carriers of infectious diseases.

Injection devices

NHS **Autopen**® (Owen Mumford)
Injection device, for use with multidose insulin cartridges. Net price = £13.96

NHS **B-D Pen**® (Becton Dickinson)
Injection device, allows adjustment of dosage in multiples of one unit. For use with 1.5-mL insulin cartridges. Net price = £23.86

NHS **NovoPen II**® (Novo Nordisk)
Injection device, for use with Human Actrapid Penfill®

NHS **Penject**® (Hypoguard)
Injection device, for use with Becton Dickinson U100 1-mL syringe

NHS **Pur-In Pen**® (CP)
Injection devices, for use with Pur-In® insulin cartridges; allow adjustment of dosage in multiples of one unit (Pur-In Pen® 1), two units (Pur-In Pen® 2), and four units (Pur-In Pen® 4). All hosp. only

Lancets

Lancets may be used on their own or in an automatic "finger pricking" device such as NHS Autoclix® (BM Diagnostics) or NHS Glucolet® (Bayer Diagnostics). Various devices take different lancets, Monolet® and Unilet G® are compatible with most devices. Available from Bayer Diagnostics (Ames®), Becton Dickinson (B-D Microfine®), Sherwoods (Monolet®, Monolet® Extra), Owen Mumford (Unilet G®, Unilet®)

Needles

**Hypodermic Needle, Sterile single use** (Drug Tariff). For use with re-usable glass syringe, sizes 0.5 mm (25G), 0.45 mm (26G), 0.4 mm (27G). Net price 100-needle pack = £2.20

**Needle Clipping Device** (Drug Tariff). Consisting of a clipper to remove needle from its hub and container from which cut-off needles cannot be retrieved; designed to hold 1200 needles, not suitable for use with lancets. Net price = £1.04

Available from Becton Dickinson (B-D Safe-clip®)

Subcutaneous infusion pumps
NHS **MS36**® (Graseby Medical)
Infusion pump, for use with any brand of U100 soluble insulin. Net price = £782.00

Syringes
**Clickcount**® (Hypoguard). Calibrated glass with Luer taper conical fitting, supplied with dosage chart and strong box for blind patients for whom the Pre-Set syringe is unsuitable. Net price 1 mL = £14.50
**Hypodermic Syringe** (Drug Tariff). Calibrated glass with Luer taper conical fitting, for use with U100 insulin. Net price 0.5 mL and 1 mL = £9.72
Available from Rand Rocket
**Pre-Set U100 Insulin Syringe** (Drug Tariff). Calibrated glass with Luer taper conical fitting, supplied with dosage chart and strong box, for blind patients. Net price 1 mL = £15.81
Available from Rand Rocket
**U100 Insulin Syringe with Needle** (Drug Tariff). Disposable with fixed or separate needle for single use, colour coded orange, sizes 0.5 mm (25G), 0.45 mm (26G), 0.4 mm (27G), 0.36 mm (28G). Net price 0.5 mL and 1 mL (with needle) = 10p
Available from Becton Dickinson (Lo-Dose®, Plasti-pak®), Rand Rocket (Clinipak®)

## 6.1.2   Oral antidiabetic drugs

**6.1.2.1** Sulphonylureas
**6.1.2.2** Biguanides
**6.1.2.3** Guar gum

Oral antidiabetic drugs are used for non-insulin-dependent (type 2) diabetes; they should not be prescribed until patients have been shown not to respond adequately to at least one month's restriction of energy and carbohydrate intake. They should be used to augment the effect of diet, and not to replace it.

### 6.1.2.1   SULPHONYLUREAS

The sulphonylureas act mainly by augmenting insulin secretion and consequently are effective only when some residual pancreatic beta-cell activity is present; during long-term administration they also have an extrapancreatic action. All may lead to hypoglycaemia 4 hours or more after food but this is usually an indication of overdose, and is relatively uncommon.

There are several sulphonylureas but there is no evidence for any difference in their effectiveness. Only **chlorpropamide** has appreciably more side-effects, mainly because of its very prolonged duration of action and the consequent hazard of hypoglycaemia, but also as a result of the common and unpleasant chlorpropamide-alcohol flush phenomenon. Selection of an individual sulphonylurea depends otherwise on the age of the patient and renal function (see below), or more generally just on personal preference.

Elderly patients are particularly prone to the dangers of hypoglycaemia when long-acting sulphonylureas are used; **chlorpropamide**, and also preferably **glibenclamide**, should be avoided in these patients and replaced by others, such as **gliclazide** or **tolbutamide**.

CAUTIONS AND CONTRA-INDICATIONS. These drugs tend to encourage weight gain and should only be prescribed if poor control and symptoms persist despite adequate attempts at dieting. They should not be used during breast-feeding, and caution is needed in the elderly and those with hepatic and renal insufficiency because of the hazard of hypoglycaemia. The short-acting tolbutamide may be used in renal impairment, as may gliquidone and gliclazide which are principally metabolised and inactivated in the liver. Sulphonylureas should be avoided in porphyria (see section 9.8.2).

Insulin therapy should be instituted temporarily during intercurrent illness (such as myocardial infarction, coma, infection, and trauma) and during surgery since control of diabetes with the sulphonylureas is often inadequate in such circumstances. Insulin therapy is also usually substituted during pregnancy. Sulphonylureas are contra-indicated in the presence of ketoacidosis.

SIDE-EFFECTS. These are generally mild and infrequent and include gastro-intestinal disturbances and headache.

Chlorpropamide may cause facial flushing after drinking alcohol; this effect is not normally witnessed with other sulphonylureas. Chlorpropamide may also enhance the effect of antidiuretic hormone and very rarely may cause hyponatraemia.

Sensitivity reactions (usually in first 6–8 weeks of therapy) include transient rashes which rarely progress to erythema multiforme and exfoliative dermatitis, fever, and jaundice; photosensitivity has also rarely been reported with chlorpropamide. Blood disorders are rare too but include thrombocytopenia, agranulocytosis, and aplastic anaemia. All these phenomena are very rare.

## CHLORPROPAMIDE

*Indications:* diabetes mellitus (for use in diabetes insipidus, see section 6.5.2)
*Cautions; Contra-indications; Side-effects:* see notes above; **interactions:** Appendix 1 (antidiabetics)
*Dose:* initially 250 mg daily (elderly patients 100–125 mg but avoid—see notes above), adjusted according to response; max. 500 mg daily; taken with breakfast

PoM **Chlorpropamide** (Non-proprietary)
*Tablets*, chlorpropamide 100 mg, net price 20 = 18p; 250 mg, 20 = 27p. Label: 4
PoM **Diabinese**® (Pfizer)
*Tablets*, scored, chlorpropamide 100 mg, net price 28-tab pack = 56p; 250 mg, 28-tab pack = £1.23. Label: 4

---

## GLIBENCLAMIDE

*Indications:* diabetes mellitus

*Cautions; Contra-indications; Side-effects:* see notes above; **interactions:** Appendix 1 (antidiabetics)

*Dose:* initially 5 mg daily (elderly patients 2.5 mg (but see also notes above)), adjusted according to response; max. 15 mg daily; taken with breakfast

PoM **Glibenclamide** (Non-proprietary)
*Tablets,* glibenclamide 2.5 mg, net price 20 = 63p; 5 mg, 20 = 68p
Available from APS (Libanil®), Ashbourne (Diabetamide®), Berk (Calabren®), Cox, Evans, Generics, Kerfoot, Lagap (Malix®)

PoM **Daonil**® (Hoechst)
*Tablets,* scored, glibenclamide 5 mg. Net price 28-tab pack = £2.70

PoM **Semi-Daonil**® (Hoechst)
*Tablets,* scored, glibenclamide 2.5 mg. Net price 28-tab pack = £1.62

PoM **Euglucon**® (Roussel)
*Tablets,* glibenclamide 2.5 mg, net price 28-tab pack = £1.62; 5 mg (scored), 28-tab pack = £2.70

## GLICLAZIDE

*Indications:* diabetes mellitus

*Cautions; Contra-indications; Side-effects:* see notes above; **interactions:** Appendix 1 (antidiabetics)

*Dose:* initially, 40–80 mg daily, adjusted according to response; up to 160 mg as a single dose, with breakfast; higher doses divided; max. 320 mg daily

PoM **Diamicron**® (Servier)
*Tablets,* scored, gliclazide 80 mg. Net price 60 = £6.48

## GLIPIZIDE

*Indications:* diabetes mellitus

*Cautions; Contra-indications; Side-effects:* see notes above; **interactions:** Appendix 1 (antidiabetics)

*Dose:* initially 2.5–5 mg daily, adjusted according to response; max. 40 mg daily; up to 15 mg may be given as a single dose before breakfast; higher doses divided

PoM **Glibenese**® (Pfizer)
*Tablets,* scored, glipizide 5 mg. Net price 56-tab pack = £3.30

PoM **Minodiab**® (Farmitalia Carlo Erba)
*Tablets,* glipizide 2.5 mg, net price 60 = £3.39; 5 mg (scored), 60 = £4.74

## GLIQUIDONE

*Indications:* diabetes mellitus

*Cautions; Contra-indications; Side-effects:* see notes above; **interactions:** Appendix 1 (antidiabetics)

*Dose:* initially 15 mg daily before breakfast, adjusted to 45–60 mg daily in 2 or 3 divided doses; max. single dose 60 mg, max. daily dose 180 mg

PoM **Glurenorm**® (Sanofi Winthrop)
*Tablets,* scored, gliquidone 30 mg. Net price 100 = £16.35

## TOLAZAMIDE

*Indications:* diabetes mellitus

*Cautions; Contra-indications; Side-effects:* see notes above; **interactions:** Appendix 1 (antidiabetics)

*Dose:* initially 100–250 mg daily with breakfast adjusted according to response; max. 1 g daily; higher doses divided

PoM **Tolanase**® (Upjohn)
*Tablets,* both scored, tolazamide 100 mg, net price 20 = £1.13; 250 mg, 20 = £2.46

## TOLBUTAMIDE

*Indications:* diabetes mellitus

*Cautions; Contra-indications; Side-effects:* see notes above; **interactions:** Appendix 1 (antidiabetics)

*Dose:* 0.5–1.5 g (max. 2 g) daily in divided doses (see notes above)

PoM **Tolbutamide** (Non-proprietary)
*Tablets,* tolbutamide 500 mg. Net price 20 = 29p

PoM **Rastinon**® (Hoechst)
*Tablets,* scored, tolbutamide 500 mg. Net price 20 = 68p

### 6.1.2.2 BIGUANIDES

**Metformin**, the only available biguanide, has a different mode of action from the sulphonylureas, and is not interchangeable with them. It exerts its effect mainly by decreasing gluconeogenesis and by increasing peripheral utilisation of glucose; since it only acts in the presence of endogenous insulin it is only effective in diabetics with some residual functioning pancreatic islet cells. Metformin is used in the treatment of non-insulin-dependent diabetics when strict dieting and sulphonylurea treatment have failed to control diabetes, especially in overweight patients, in whom it may, if necessary, be used first. It can be used alone or with a sulphonylurea. It does not exert a hypoglycaemic action in non-diabetic subjects unless given in overdose. Gastro-intestinal side-effects are initially common, and may persist in some patients, particularly when very high doses such as 3 g daily are given.

Metformin is not free from the hazard of lactic acidosis but this occurs almost exclusively in renal failure patients, in whom it should not be used.

## METFORMIN HYDROCHLORIDE

*Indications:* diabetes mellitus (see notes above)

*Cautions:* see notes above; **interactions:** Appendix 1 (antidiabetics)

*Contra-indications:* hepatic or renal impairment (withdraw if renal impairment suspected), predisposition to lactic acidosis, heart failure, severe infection or trauma, dehydration, alcohol dependence; pregnancy, breast-feeding

*Side-effects:* anorexia, nausea, vomiting, diarrhoea (usually transient), lactic acidosis (withdraw treatment), decreased vitamin-B$_{12}$ absorption

*Dose:* 500 mg every 8 hours *or* 850 mg every 12 hours with or after food; max. 3 g daily in divided doses though most physicians limit this to 2 g daily (see notes above)

PoM **Metformin** (Non-proprietary)
*Tablets*, coated, metformin hydrochloride 500 mg, net price 21-tab pack = 50p, 84-tab pack = £2.02; 850 mg, 20 = 81p. Label: 21
Available from APS, Cox, Evans, Kerfoot, Lagap (Orabet®)

PoM **Glucophage**® (Lipha)
*Tablets*, f/c, metformin hydrochloride 500 mg, net price 84 = £2.11; 850 mg, 56 = £2.34. Label: 21

---

### 6.1.2.3 GUAR GUM

Guar gum, if taken in adequate quantities, results in some reduction of postprandial plasma-glucose concentrations in diabetes mellitus, probably by retarding carbohydrate absorption. It is also used to relieve symptoms of the dumping syndrome.

Flatulence limits its use.

## GUAR GUM

*Indications:* see notes above
*Cautions:* maintain adequate fluid intake; **interactions:** Appendix 1 (guar gum)
COUNSELLING. Preparations that swell in contact with liquid should always be carefully swallowed with water and should not be taken imediately before going to bed.
*Contra-indications:* gastro-intestinal obstruction
*Side-effects:* flatulence, abdominal distension, intestinal obstruction

**Guarem**® (Rybar)
*Granules*, ivory, sugar-free, guar gum 5 g/sachet. Net price 100 sachets = £16.45. Label: 13, counselling, food (see below), administration (see above)
*Dose:* 5 g stirred into 200 mL fluid 3 times daily immediately before main meals (or sprinkled on food and eaten accompanied by 200 mL fluid)

**Guarina**® (Norgine)
*Granules*, dispersible, guar gum 5 g/sachet. Net price 60 sachets = £8.95. Label: 13, counselling, food (see below), administration (see above)
*Dose:* 5 g stirred into 150 mL fluid immediately before main meals up to 3 times daily (or sprinkled on food and eaten accompanied by 150 mL of fluid)

### 6.1.3   Diabetic ketoacidosis

**Soluble insulin,** the only form of insulin that may be given intravenously, is used in the management of diabetic ketoacidotic and hyperosmolar non-ketotic coma. It is preferable to use the type of soluble insulin that the patient has been using previously. It is necessary to achieve and to maintain an adequate plasma-insulin concentration until the metabolic disturbance is brought under control.

Insulin is best given by *intravenous infusion*, using an infusion pump, and diluted to 1 unit/mL (care in mixing, see Appendix 6). Adequate plasma concentrations can usually be maintained with infusion rates of 6 units/hour for adults and 0.1 units/kg/hour for children. Blood glucose is expected to decrease by about 5 mmol/hour; if the response is inadequate the infusion rate can be doubled or quadrupled. When the plasma glucose has fallen to 10 mmol/litre the infusion rate can be reduced to 1 to 2 units/hour for adults (about 0.02 units/kg/hour for children) and continued until the patient is ready to take food by mouth. The insulin infusion should not be stopped before subcutaneous insulin has been started.

No matter how large, a bolus intravenous injection of insulin can only provide an adequate plasma concentration for a short time, therefore if facilities for intravenous infusion are not available the insulin is given by *intramuscular injection*. An initial loading dose of 20 units intramuscularly is followed by 6 units intramuscularly every hour until the plasma glucose concentration has fallen to 10 mmol/litre; intramuscular injections are then given every 2 hours. Although absorption of insulin is usually rapid after intramuscular injection, it may be impaired in the presence of hypotension and poor tissue perfusion; moreover depots of insulin may build up during treatment therefore late hypoglycaemia should be watched for and treated appropriately.

*Intravenous replacement of fluid and electrolytes* with **sodium chloride** intravenous infusion is an essential part of the management of ketoacidosis; **potassium chloride** is included in the infusion as appropriate to prevent the hypokalaemia induced by the insulin. **Sodium bicarbonate** infusion (1.26% or 2.74%) is only used in cases of extreme acidosis and shock since the acid-base disturbance is normally corrected by the insulin. **Glucose** solution (10%) is infused once the blood glucose has decreased below 10 mmol/litre but insulin infusion must continue.

For the role of glucose, see section 9.2.2.

---

### 6.1.4   Treatment of hypoglycaemia

Initially, glucose or 3 or 4 lumps of sugar should be taken with a little water. If necessary, this may be repeated in 10 to 15 minutes.

If hypoglycaemia causes unconsciousness, up to 50 mL of **50% glucose intravenous infusion** should be given intravenously (see section 9.2.2).

**Glucagon** can be given as an alternative to parenteral glucose in hypoglycaemia. It is a polypeptide hormone produced by the alpha cells of the islets of Langerhans. Its action is to increase plasma glucose concentration by mobilising glycogen stored in the liver. It has the advantage that it can be injected by any route (intramuscular, subcutaneous, or intravenous) in a dose of 1 mg (1 unit) in circumstances when an intravenous injection of glucose would be difficult or impossible to administer. It may be issued to close relatives of insulin-treated patients for emergency use in hypoglycaemic attacks. It is often advisable to prescribe on an 'if necessary' basis to all hospitalised insulin-treated patients, so that it may be given rapidly by the nurses during an hypoglycaemic emergency. If not effective in 20 minutes intravenous glucose should be given.

## GLUCAGON

*Indications:* acute hypoglycaemia

*Cautions:* see notes above. Ineffective in chronic hypoglycaemia, starvation, and adrenal insufficiency

*Contra-indications:* insulinoma, phaeochromocytoma, glucagonoma

*Side-effects:* nausea, vomiting, rarely hypersensitivity reactions

*Dose: by subcutaneous, intramuscular, or intravenous injection,* adults and children 0.5–1 unit repeated after 20 minutes if necessary

*Note.* 1 unit of glucagon = 1 mg of glucagon or glucagon hydrochloride

PoM **Glucagon Injection,** powder for reconstitution, glucagon (as hydrochloride, with lactose). Net price 1-unit vial (Lilly) = £5.16; (Novo Nordisk) = £4.62; 10-unit vial (Novo Nordisk) = £27.06 (all with diluent)

CHRONIC HYPOGLYCAEMIA

**Diazoxide,** administered by mouth, is useful in the management of patients with chronic hypoglycaemia from excess endogenous insulin secretion, either from an islet cell tumour or islet cell hyperplasia. It has no place in the management of acute hypoglycaemia.

## DIAZOXIDE

*Indications:* chronic intractable hypoglycaemia (for use in hypertensive crisis see section 2.5.1)

*Cautions:* ischaemic heart disease, pregnancy, labour, impaired renal function; haematological examinations and blood pressure monitoring required during prolonged treatment; growth, bone, and developmental checks in children; **interactions:** Appendix 1 (diazoxide)

*Side-effects:* anorexia, nausea, vomiting, hyperuricaemia, hypotension, oedema, tachycardia, arrhythmias, extrapyramidal effects; hypertrichosis on prolonged treatment

*Dose: by mouth,* adults and children, initially 5 mg/kg daily in 2–3 divided doses

PoM **Eudemine**® (A&H)

*Tablets*—discontinued

*Note.* Diazoxide powder is available on named patient basis for extemporaneous preparation of oral suspension.

## 6.1.5 Treatment of diabetic neuropathy

Optimal diabetic control is beneficial for the management of *painful neuropathy.* Most patients should be treated with insulin, and relief can probably be accelerated by continuous insulin infusion. **Non-opioid analgesics** such as aspirin and paracetamol (see section 4.7.1) are indicated. Relief may also be obtained with the **tricyclic antidepressants,** amitriptyline, imipramine, and nortriptyline (see section 4.3.1) with or without a low dose of a **phenothiazine** (see section 4.2). **Carbamazepine** (see section 4.8.1) or mexiletine may be useful; lignocaine has also been used but needs further evaluation.

In *autonomic neuropathy* diabetic diarrhoea can often be aborted by two or three doses of **tetracycline** 250 mg (see section 5.1.3). Otherwise **codeine phosphate** (see section 1.4.2) is the best drug, but all other antidiarrhoeal preparations can be tried. **Anti-emetics** or **cisapride** may control vomiting in gastroparesis. In the rare cases where they do not, erythromycin (especially when given intravenously) has been shown to be of benefit but further studies are needed.

In *neuropathic postural hypotension* an increased salt intake and the use of the **mineralocorticoid** fludrocortisone 100 to 400 micrograms daily (see section 6.3.1) help by increasing plasma volume but uncomfortable oedema is a common side-effect. Fludrocortisone can also be combined with **flurbiprofen** (see section 10.1.1) and **ephedrine hydrochloride** (see section 3.1.1.2).

*Gustatory sweating* can be treated with **antimuscarinics** (see section 1.2), poldine methylsulphate is the best but propantheline bromide may also be used; side-effects are common. In some patients with *neuropathic oedema,* **ephedrine hydrochloride** 30 to 60 mg three times daily offers impressive relief.

## 6.1.6 Diagnostic and monitoring agents for diabetes mellitus

BLOOD GLUCOSE MONITORING

Blood glucose monitoring gives a direct measure of the glucose concentration at the time of the test and can detect hypoglycaemia as well as hyperglycaemia. It is a method of assessing diabetic control, especially where tight control is essential e.g. in pregnancy. Patients should be properly trained in the use of blood glucose monitoring systems and to take appropriate action on the results obtained. Inadequate understanding of the normal fluctuations in blood glucose may lead to confusion and inappropriate action.

Blood glucose concentration evaluation may be carried out visually (using a colour comparison chart) or by means of a meter. Meters give a more precise reading and are useful for patients with poor eyesight or who are colour blind.

*Note:* In the U.K. blood glucose concentration is expressed in mmol/litre and the British Diabetic Association advises its members that these units should be used for self blood glucose monitoring. In other European countries units of mg/100 mL (or mg/dL) are commonly used.

It is advisable to check that the meter is pre-set in the correct units.

### Test strips

**BM-Test 1–44®** (BM Diagnostics)
*Reagent strips*, for blood glucose monitoring, visual range (1–44 mmol/litre) meter range (0.5–27.7 mmol/litre), suitable for use with Reflolux® S, Hypo-Count® MXR. Net price 50-strip pack = £12.39

**Dextrostix®** (Bayer Diagnostics)
*Reagent strips*, for blood glucose monitoring, visual range (1.4–14 mmol/litre), meter range (0–22.2 mmol/litre), suitable for use with Hypo-Count® MXA, Hypo-Count® IIA. Net price 50-strip pack = £12.36

**ExacTech®** (MediSense)
*Biosensor strips*, for blood glucose monitoring, range (2.2–25mmol/litre), for use with ExacTech® meter only. Net price 50-strip pack = £11.42

**Glucostix®** (Bayer Diagnostics)
*Reagent strips*, for blood glucose monitoring, visual range (1–44 mmol/litre), meter range (2–22 mmol/litre), suitable for use with Glucometer® II with memory, Glucometer® GX. Net price 50-strip pack = £12.36

**Hypoguard® GA** (Hypoguard)
*Reagent strips*, for blood glucose monitoring, visual range (1–22 mmol/litre), meter range (0–22 mmol/litre), suitable for use with Hypo-Count® GA, Hypo-Count® IIA. Net price 50-strip pack = £11.18

### Meters

**NHS ExacTech®** (MediSense)
Meter (Sensor) for blood glucose monitoring for use with ExacTech® test strips. ExacTech Companion = £39.00, ExacTech Companion starter pack = £49.00, ExacTech Pen = £39.00, ExacTech Pen starter pack = £49.00

**NHS Glucometer®** (Bayer Diagnostics)
Meters for blood glucose monitoring for use with Glucostix® test strips. Glucometer II with memory = £49.00, Glucometer GX = £39.00

**NHS Hypo-Count®** (Hypoguard)
Meters for blood glucose monitoring, Hypo-Count GA (for use with Hypoguard GA® test strips) = £55.00

**NHS Reflolux®** (BM Diagnostics)
Meter for blood glucose monitoring for use with BM-Test 1–44® test strips. Reflolux S = £29.00

### URINALYSIS

#### Glucose

Qualitative and semiquantitative tests range from reagent strips specific to glucose in urine to reagent tablets which detect all reducing sugars in urine. They vary in the time taken to perform the test and colour changes. Training of patients in the performance of the test and correct evaluation of results is essential.

**Clinistix®** (Bayer Diagnostics)
*Reagent strips*, for detection of glucose in urine. Net price 50-strip pack = £2.42

**Clinitest®** (Bayer Diagnostics)
*Reagent tablets*, for detection of glucose and other reducing substances in urine. Pocket set (test tube, dropper

and 36 tablets), net price = £2.96, 36-tab pack = £1.49, 6-test tube pack = £1.74, 6-dropper pack = £1.55, NHS test tube rack set (6 tubes and 2 droppers) = £4.38

**Diabur Test 5000®** (BM Diagnostics)
*Reagent strips*, for detection of glucose in urine. Net price 50-strip pack = £2.11

**Diastix®** (Bayer Diagnostics)
*Reagent strips*, for detection of glucose in urine. Net price 50-strip pack = £2.06

#### Ketones

**Acetest®** (Bayer Diagnostics)
*Reagent tablets*, for detection of ketones in urine. Net price 100-tab pack = £2.64

**Ketostix®** (Bayer Diagnostics)
*Reagent strips*, for detection of ketones in urine. Net price 50-strip pack = £2.06

**Ketur Test®** (BM Diagnostics)
*Reagent strips*, for testing ketones in urine. Net price 50-strip pack = £2.02

#### Protein

**Albustix®** (Bayer Diagnostics)
*Reagent strips*, for detection of protein in urine. Net price 50-strip pack = £2.84

**Albym Test®** (BM Diagnostics)
*Reagent strips*, for detection of protein in urine. Net price 50-strip pack = £2.72

### GLUCOSE TOLERANCE TEST

The **glucose** tolerance test is used in the diagnosis of diabetes mellitus. In the UK this generally involves giving 75 g of glucose BP (= dextrose monohydrate) by mouth to the fasting patient, and measuring plasma concentrations at intervals. At an international level, however, confusion has arisen because in different pharmacopoeias the title 'glucose' can mean the anhydrous form or the monohydrate. Sources at the World Health Organisation have therefore suggested that the form of dextrose should be standardised as anhydrous, and that the standard amount should be 75 g. The equivalent value (and titles) in the UK are:

Anhydrous glucose BP (anhydrous dextrose) 75 g = Glucose BP (dextrose monohydrate) 82.5 g

## 6.2   Thyroid and antithyroid drugs

6.2.1 Thyroid hormones
6.2.2 Antithyroid drugs

### 6.2.1   Thyroid hormones

Thyroid hormones are used in hypothyroidism (myxoedema), and also in diffuse non-toxic goitre, Hashimoto's thyroiditis (lymphadenoid goitre), and thyroid carcinoma. Neonatal hypothyroidism requires prompt treatment for normal development.

**Thyroxine sodium** is the treatment of choice for *maintenance* therapy. The initial dose should not exceed 100 micrograms daily, preferably before breakfast, or 25 to 50 micrograms in elderly patients or those with cardiac disease, increased by 25 to 50 micrograms at intervals of at least 4 weeks. The usual maintenance dose to relieve hypothyroidism is 100 to 200 micrograms daily which can be administered as a single dose.

In infants a daily dose of 10 micrograms/kg up to a maximum of 50 micrograms daily should be given; subsequent therapy should reach 100 micrograms daily by 5 years and adult doses by 12 years, guided by clinical response, growth assessment, and measurements of plasma thyroxine and thyroid-stimulating hormone.

**Liothyronine sodium** has a similar action to thyroxine but is more rapidly metabolised; 20 micrograms is equivalent to 100 micrograms of thyroxine. Its effects develop after a few hours and disappear within 24 to 48 hours of discontinuing treatment. It may be used in *severe hypothyroid states* when a rapid response is desired.

Liothyronine by intravenous injection is the treatment of choice in *hypothyroid coma*. Adjunctive therapy includes intravenous fluids, hydrocortisone, and antibiotics; assisted ventilation is often required.

Dried **thyroid** should **not** be used as its effects are unpredictable.

## THYROXINE SODIUM

*Indications:* hypothyroidism
*Cautions:* cardiovascular disorders, prolonged myxoedema, adrenal insufficiency; **interactions:** Appendix 1 (thyroxine)
*Side-effects:* arrhythmias, anginal pain, tachycardia, cramps in skeletal muscles, headache, restlessness, excitability, flushing, sweating, diarrhoea, excessive weight loss
*Dose:* see notes above

PoM **Thyroxine** (Non-proprietary)
*Tablets*, thyroxine sodium 25 micrograms, net price 20 = 7p; 50 micrograms, 20 = 4p; 100 micrograms, 20 = 5p
PoM **Eltroxin®** (Glaxo)
*Tablets*, scored, thyroxine sodium 50 micrograms, net price 20 = 5p; 100 micrograms, 20 = 6p

## LIOTHYRONINE SODIUM

(L-Tri-iodothyronine sodium)
*Indications:* see notes above
*Cautions; Contra-indications; Side-effects:* see under Thyroxine Sodium; has a more rapid effect
*Dose: by mouth,* initially 10–20 micrograms daily in 2–3 divided doses gradually increased to 20 micrograms 3 times daily; eldery patients should receive smaller initial doses, gradually increased; CHILD, adult dose reduced in proportion to body-weight

*By slow intravenous injection,* hypothyroid coma, 5-20 micrograms repeated every 12 hours or more frequently (every 4 hours if necessary); alternatively 50 micrograms initially then 25 micrograms every 8 hours reducing to 25 micrograms twice daily

PoM **Tertroxin®** (Glaxo)
*Tablets*, scored, liothyronine sodium 20 micrograms. Net price 100-tab pack = 90p
PoM **Triiodothyronine** (Glaxo)
*Injection*, powder for reconstitution, liothyronine sodium (with dextran). Net price 20-microgram amp = £3.60

## 6.2.2 Antithyroid drugs

Antithyroid drugs are used to prepare patients for thyroidectomy. They are also used for prolonged periods in the hope of inducing life-long remission. In the UK carbimazole is the most commonly used drug. Propylthiouracil may be used in patients who suffer sensitivity reactions to carbimazole; sensitivity is not necessarily displayed to both drugs. Both drugs act primarily by interfering with the synthesis of thyroid hormones.

---

**CSM warning (neutropenia and agranulocytosis)**
Doctors are reminded of the importance of recognising bone marrow suppression induced by carbimazole and the need to stop treatment promptly.
1. Patient should be asked to report symptoms and signs suggestive of infection, especially sore throat.
2. A white blood cell count should be performed if there is any clinical evidence of infection.
3. Carbimazole should be stopped promptly if there is clinical or laboratory evidence of neutropenia.

---

**Carbimazole** should be given in a daily dose of 30 to 60 mg and maintained at this dose until the patient becomes euthyroid, usually after 4 to 8 weeks; the dose may then be progressively reduced to a maintenance dose of between 5 and 15 mg daily; therapy is usually given for 18 months. Children may be given 15 mg daily, adjusted according to response. Rashes are common, and **propylthiouracil** may then be substituted. Pruritus and rashes can also be treated with antihistamines without discontinuing therapy, however patients should be advised to report any sore throat immediately because of the rare complication of agranulocytosis see CSM warning, above.

Antithyroid drugs may be given *once daily* although divided doses are still commonly used. Over-treatment with the rapid development of hypothyroidism is not uncommon and should be avoided particularly during pregnancy since it can cause fetal goitre.

A combination of carbimazole, 20 to 60 mg daily with thyroxine, 50 to 150 micrograms daily, may be used in a *blocking-replacement regimen*; therapy is again usually given for 18 months. The blocking-replacement regimen is not suitable during pregnancy.

Unless operation or use of radioactive iodine is planned, treatment should be for at least a year.

Before partial thyroidectomy **iodine** may be given for 10 to 14 days in addition to carbimazole or propylthiouracil to assist control and reduce vascularity of the thyroid. Iodine should not be used for long-term treatment since its antithyroid action tends to diminish.

Radioactive sodium iodide ($^{131}$I) solution is used increasingly for the treatment of thyrotoxicosis at all ages, particularly where medical therapy or compliance is a problem, in patients with cardiac disease, and in patients who relapse after thyroidectomy.

**Propranolol** is useful for rapid relief of thyrotoxic symptoms and may be used in conjunction with antithyroid drugs or as an adjunct to radioactive iodine. Beta-blockers are also useful in neonatal thyrotoxicosis and in supra-ventricular arrhythmias due to hyperthyroidism. Propranolol may be used in conjunction with iodine to prepare mildly thyrotoxic patients for surgery but it is still preferable to make the patient euthyroid with carbimazole before surgery. Laboratory tests of thyroid function are not altered by beta-blockers. Most experience in treating thyrotoxicosis has been gained with propranolol but **nadolol** and **sotalol** are also used. For doses and preparations see section 2.4.

*Thyrotoxic crisis* ('thyroid storm') requires emergency treatment with intravenous administration of fluids, propranolol (5 mg) and hydrocortisone (100 mg every 6 hours, as sodium succinate), as well as oral iodine solution and carbimazole or propylthiouracil which may need to be administered by nasogastric tube.

PREGNANCY AND BREAST-FEEDING. Radioactive iodine therapy is contra-indicated during pregnancy. Propylthiouracil and carbimazole can be given. Both drugs cross the placenta and in high doses may cause fetal goitre and hypothyroidism. Rarely, carbimazole has been associated with aplasia cutis of the neonate.

Carbimazole and propylthiouracil transfer to breast milk but this does not preclude breast-feeding as long as neonatal development is closely monitored.

## CARBIMAZOLE

*Indications:* hyperthyroidism
*Cautions:* large goitre; pregnancy, breast-feeding (see notes)
*Side-effects:* nausea, headache, rashes and pruritus, arthralgia; rarely alopecia, agranulocytosis **(see CSM warning above)**, jaundice
*Dose:* see notes above

PoM **Neo-Mercazole 5**® (Nicholas)
*Tablets,* pink, scored, carbimazole 5 mg. Net price 20 = 45p
PoM **Neo-Mercazole 20**® (Nicholas)
*Tablets,* pink, carbimazole 20 mg. Net price 20 = £1.84

## IODINE AND IODIDE

*Indications:* thyrotoxicosis (pre-operative)
*Cautions:* pregnancy, children; not for long-term treatment
*Contra-indications:* breast-feeding
*Side-effects:* hypersensitivity reactions including coryza-like symptoms, headache, lachrymation, conjunctivitis, pain in salivary glands, laryngitis, bronchitis, rashes; on prolonged treatment depression, insomnia, impotence; goitre in infants of mothers taking iodides

**Aqueous Iodine Oral Solution** (Lugol's Solution), iodine 5%, potassium iodide 10% in purified water, freshly boiled and cooled, total iodine 130 mg/mL. Net price 100 mL = £1.35. Label: 27
*Dose:* 0.1–0.3 mL 3 times daily well diluted with milk or water

## PROPYLTHIOURACIL

*Indications:* hyperthyroidism
*Cautions; Side-effects:* see under Carbimazole; also rarely tendency to haemorrhage; reduce dose in renal impairment; systemic lupus erythematosus reported
*Dose:* 300–450 mg daily in divided doses

PoM **Propylthiouracil Tablets,** propylthiouracil 50 mg. Net price 20 = £1.50

# 6.3   Corticosteroids

6.3.1 Replacement therapy
6.3.2 Comparisons of corticosteroids
6.3.3 Disadvantages of corticosteroids
6.3.4 Clinical management

## 6.3.1   Replacement therapy

The adrenal cortex normally secretes hydrocortisone (cortisol) which has glucocorticoid activity and weak mineralocorticoid activity. It also secretes the mineralocorticoid aldosterone.

In deficiency states, physiological replacement is best achieved with a combination of **hydrocortisone**[1] and the mineralocorticoid **fludrocortisone**; hydrocortisone alone does not usually provide sufficient mineralocorticoid activity for complete replacement.

In *Addison's disease* or following adrenalectomy, **hydrocortisone** 20 to 30 mg daily by mouth is usually required. This is given in 2 doses, the larger in the morning and the smaller in the

---

1. Cortisone has generally been superseded by hydrocortisone; management with the more potent synthetic glucocorticoids such as prednisolone (with fludrocortisone) though practicable, offers no advantage. They tend to have less mineralocorticoid activity than hydrocortisone and their greater glucocorticoid activity is only of advantage in the treatment of inflammatory and neoplastic disease.

---

evening, mimicking the normal diurnal rhythm of cortisol secretion. The optimum daily dose is determined on the basis of clinical response. Glucocorticoid therapy is supplemented by fludrocortisone 50 to 300 micrograms daily.

In *acute adrenocortical insufficiency*, **hydrocortisone** is given intravenously (preferably as sodium succinate) in doses of 100 mg every 6 to 8 hours in sodium chloride intravenous infusion 0.9%.

In *hypopituitarism* glucocorticoids should be given as in adrenocortical insufficiency, but since the production of aldosterone is also regulated by the renin-angiotensin system a mineralocorticoid is not usually required. Additional replacement therapy with thyroxine (section 6.2.1) and sex hormones (section 6.4) should be given as indicated by the pattern of hormone deficiency.

Corticosteroid cover for *adrenalectomy*, for *hypophysectomy* or for operations on patients on long-term treatment with corticosteroids is determined logically from the knowledge that in a normal person major stress will not lead to the secretion of more than 300 mg of cortisol in 24 hours; once the stress is over, cortisol production rapidly returns to its usual level of approximately 20 mg per 24 hours. A simple way of mimicking this is to administer hydrocortisone. On the day of operation hydrocortisone 100 mg (usually as the succinate) is given by intramuscular or intravenous injection with the premedication, and repeated every 8 hours. In the absence of complications, the dose can be halved every 24 hours until a normal maintenance dose of 20 to 30 mg per 24 hours is reached on the 5th postoperative day.

## CORTISONE ACETATE
Section 6.3.4

## FLUDROCORTISONE ACETATE

*Indications:* mineralocorticoid replacement in adrenocortical insufficiency
*Cautions; Contra-indications; Side-effects:* section 6.3.3
*Dose:* adrenocortical insufficiency, 50–300 micrograms daily; CHILD 5 micrograms/kg daily

PoM **Florinef**® (Squibb)
*Tablets*, pink, scored, fludrocortisone acetate 100 micrograms. Net price 20 = 96p. Label: 10 steroid card

## HYDROCORTISONE
Section 6.3.4

## 6.3.2 Comparisons of corticosteroids

Betamethasone, dexamethasone, hydrocortisone, prednisolone, and prednisone are used for their anti-inflammatory effect; the following table shows equivalent anti-inflammatory doses.

Equivalent Anti-inflammatory Doses of Glucocorticoids

| Drug | Equivalent anti-inflammatory dose (mg) |
|---|---|
| Betamethasone | 0.75 |
| Cortisone acetate | 25 |
| Dexamethasone | 0.75 |
| Hydrocortisone | 20 |
| Methylprednisolone | 4 |
| Prednisolone | 5 |
| Prednisone | 5 |
| Triamcinolone | 4 |

*Note.* This table takes no account of mineralocorticoid effects (see text below), nor does it take account of variations in duration of action.

In comparing the relative potencies of corticosteroids in terms of their anti-inflammatory (glucocorticoid) effects it should be borne in mind that high anti-inflammatory (glucocorticoid) activity in itself is of no advantage unless it occurs in conjunction with relatively low mineralocorticoid activity so that the mineralocorticoid effect on water and electrolytes is not also increased.

The mineralocorticoid activity of **fludrocortisone** is so high that its anti-inflammatory activity is of no clinical relevance.

The mineralocorticoid effects of **cortisone** and **hydrocortisone** are too high for them to be used on a long-term basis for inflammatory disease suppression since fluid retention would be too great, but they are suitable for adrenal replacement therapy (section 6.3.1); hydrocortisone is preferred because cortisone is only active after conversion in the liver to hydrocortisone. Hydrocortisone is also used by intravenous injection for the emergency management of some conditions (section 6.3.4). The relatively moderate anti-inflammatory potency of hydrocortisone makes it a first-choice topical corticosteroid for the management of inflammatory skin conditions because side-effects (both topical and caused by absorption) are less marked (see section 13.4); cortisone is not active topically.

**Prednisolone** has predominantly glucocorticoid activity and is the corticosteroid most commonly used by mouth for long-term administration. **Prednisone** has a similar level of glucocorticoid activity but is only active after conversion in the liver to prednisolone; it is therefore not recommended.

**Betamethasone** and **dexamethasone** have very high glucocorticoid activity in conjunction with insignificant mineralocorticoid activity. This makes them particularly suitable for high-dose therapy in conditions where water retention would be a disadvantage (see *cerebral oedema*, section 6.3.4).

They also have a long duration of action and this, coupled with their lack of mineralocorticoid action makes them particularly suitable for conditions which require suppression of corticotrophin secretion (see *congenital adrenal hyperplasia*, section 6.3.4). Some esters of betamethasone and of **beclomethasone** exert a considerably more marked topical effect (e.g. on the skin or the lungs) than when given by mouth; use is made of this to obtain topical effects without corresponding systemic activity (e.g. for skin applications and asthma inhalations).

Stimulation of the adrenal cortex by **corticotrophin** or **tetracosactrin** has been used as an alternative to corticosteroids to control certain diseases; there is no close relationship between the dose producing satisfactory clinical improvement and the equivalent dose of oral corticosteroid producing the same degree of improvement.

### 6.3.3 Disadvantages of corticosteroids

Overdosage or prolonged use may exaggerate some of the normal physiological actions of corticosteroids.

**Mineralocorticoid** effects include *hypertension*, *sodium and water retention and potassium loss*. They are most marked with fludrocortisone, but are significant with cortisone, hydrocortisone, corticotrophin, and tetracosactrin. Mineralocorticoid actions are negligible with the high potency glucocorticoids, betamethasone and dexamethasone, and occur only slightly with methylprednisolone, prednisolone, prednisone, and triamcinolone.

**Glucocorticoid** effects include *diabetes* and *osteoporosis* which is a danger, particularly in the elderly, as it may result in osteoporotic fractures for example of the hip or vertebrae; in addition administration of high doses is associated with *avascular necrosis* of the femoral head. *Mental disturbances* may occur; a serious paranoid state or depression with risk of suicide may be induced, particularly in patients with a history of mental disorder. *Euphoria* is frequently observed. *Muscle wasting* (proximal myopathy) may also occur.

Corticosteroid therapy is weakly linked with *peptic ulceration*; the use of soluble or enteric-coated preparations to reduce the risk is speculative only. Modification of tissue reactions may result in spread of *infection*; suppression of clinical signs may allow septicaemia or tuberculosis to reach an advanced stage before being recognised.

High doses of corticosteroids may cause *Cushing's syndrome*, with moon face, striae, and acne; it is usually reversible on withdrawal of treatment, but this must always be gradually tapered to avoid symptoms of acute adrenal insufficiency (see Adrenal Suppression).

In children, administration of corticosteroids may result in *suppression of growth*. Corticosteroids given in high dosage during *pregnancy* may affect adrenal development in the child (but see also Appendix 4).

For details of the adverse effects of topical and of systemic corticosteroid therapy on the *skin*, see sections 13.4 and 13.5.

For details of the adverse effects of topical and of systemic corticosteroid therapy on the *eye*, see section 11.4.

ADRENAL SUPPRESSION. Administration of corticosteroids suppresses the secretion of corticotrophin and may lead to adrenal atrophy; withdrawal of treatment must therefore be gradual to avoid symptoms of *acute adrenal insufficiency*. When long-term treatment is to be discontinued, the dose should be reduced gradually over a period of several weeks or months depending on the dosage and duration of the therapy. Too rapid a reduction of corticosteroid dosage can lead to *acute adrenal insufficiency*, *hypotension*, and *death*. A number of minor withdrawal symptoms may also result such as *rhinitis*, *conjunctivitis*, *loss of weight*, *arthralgia*, and *painful itchy skin nodules*.

Adrenal atrophy can persist for years after stopping prolonged corticosteroid therapy, therefore any illness or surgical emergency may require temporary reintroduction of corticosteroid therapy to compensate for lack of sufficient adrenocortical response. Anaesthetists **must** therefore know whether a patient is taking or has been taking corticosteroids to avoid a precipitous fall in blood pressure during anaesthesia or in the immediate postoperative period. Patients should therefore carry cards giving details of their dosage and possible complications. These 'steroid cards' can be obtained from local Family Practitioner Committees or

DHSS Printing and Stationery Unit,
Room 110, North Fylde Central Office,
Norcross, Blackpool FY5 3TA

In Scotland 'steroid cards' are available from Health Boards.

Pharmacists may obtain 'steroid cards' from the Royal Pharmaceutical Society of Great Britain.

**Interactions**: see Appendix 1 (corticosteroids and corticotrophin).

### 6.3.4 Clinical management

Corticosteroids should not be used unless the benefits justify the hazards; the lowest dose that will produce an acceptable response should be used (see also under Administration, below). Dosage varies widely in different diseases and in different patients.

If the use of a corticosteroid can save or prolong life, as in *exfoliative dermatitis*, *pemphigus*, *acute leukaemia* or *acute transplant rejection*, high doses may need to be given, as the complications of therapy are likely to be less serious than the effects of the disease itself.

When long-term corticosteroid therapy is used in relatively benign chronic diseases such as *rheumatoid arthritis* the danger of treatment may become greater than the disabilities produced by the disease. To minimise side-effects the maintenance dose should be kept as low as possible (see also section 10.1.2.1).

When potentially less harmful measures are ineffective corticosteroids are used topically for the treatment of *inflammatory conditions of the skin* (see section 13.4). Corticosteroids should be avoided or used only under specialist supervision in *psoriasis* (see section 13.5).

Corticosteroids are used both topically (by rectum) and systemically (by mouth or intravenously) in the management of *ulcerative colitis* and *Crohn's disease* (see sections 1.5 and 1.7.2).

Use can be made of the mineralocorticoid activity of fludrocortisone to treat *postural hypotension* in autonomic neuropathy (see section 6.1.5).

Very high doses of corticosteroids have been given by intravenous injection in *septic shock*. However a recent study (using methylprednisolone sodium succinate) did not demonstrate efficacy and, moreover, suggested a higher mortality in some subsets of patients given the high-dose corticosteroid therapy.

Dexamethasone and betamethasone have little if any mineralocorticoid action and their long duration of action makes them particularly suitable for suppressing corticotrophin secretion in *congenital adrenal hyperplasia* where the dose should be tailored to the individual on clinical grounds and by measurement of adrenal androgens and 17-hydroxyprogesterone. In common with all glucocorticoids their suppressive action on the hypothalamic-pituitary-adrenal axis is greatest and most prolonged when they are given at night. In most normal subjects a single dose of 1 mg of dexamethasone at night, depending on weight, is sufficient to inhibit corticotrophin secretion for 24 hours. This is the basis of the 'overnight dexamethasone suppression test' for diagnosing Cushing's syndrome.

Betamethasone and dexamethasone are also appropriate for conditions where water retention would be a disadvantage, as for example in treating traumatic *cerebral oedema* with doses of 12 to 20 mg daily.

In acute hypersensitivity reactions such as *angioedema* of the upper respiratory tract and *anaphylactic shock*, corticosteroids are indicated as an adjunct to emergency treatment with adrenaline (see section 3.4.3). In such cases hydrocortisone (as sodium succinate) by intravenous injection in a dose of 100 to 300 mg may be required.

Corticosteroids are preferably used by inhalation in the management of *asthma* (see section 3.2) but systemic therapy in association with bronchodilators is required for the emergency treatment of severe acute asthma (see section 3.1.1).

Corticosteroids may also be useful in conditions such as *rheumatic fever*, *chronic active hepatitis*, and *sarcoidosis*; they may also lead to remissions of acquired *haemolytic anaemia*, and some cases of the *nephrotic syndrome* (particularly in children) and *thrombocytopenic purpura*.

Corticosteroids can improve the prognosis of serious conditions such as *systemic lupus erythematosus*, *temporal arteritis*, and *polyarteritis nodosa*; the effects of the disease process may be suppressed and symptoms relieved, but the underlying condition is not cured, although it may ultimately burn itself out. It is usual to begin therapy in these conditions at fairly high dose,

such as 40 to 60 mg prednisolone daily, and then to reduce the dose to the lowest commensurate with disease control.

For other reference to the use of corticosteroids see section 11.4 (eye), 12.1.1 (otitis externa), 12.2.1 (allergic rhinitis), and 12.3.1 (aphthous ulcers).

ADMINISTRATION. Whenever possible *local treatment* with creams, intra-articular injections, inhalations, eye-drops, or enemas should be used in preference to *systemic treatment*. The suppressive action of a corticosteroid on cortisol secretion is least when it is given in the morning, therefore in an attempt to reduce pituitary-adrenal suppression a corticosteroid (usually prednisolone) should normally be taken as a single dose in the morning. In an attempt to reduce pituitary-adrenal suppression further, the total dose for two days can sometimes be taken as a single dose on alternate days; alternate-day administration has not been very successful in the management of asthma (see section 3.2) but it can be suitable for rheumatoid arthritis (see section 10.1.2). Pituitary-adrenal suppression can also be reduced by means of intermittent therapy with short courses. In some conditions it may be possible to reduce the dose of corticosteroid by adding a small dose of an immunosuppressive drug (see section 8.2.1).

CHILDREN. In children the indications for corticosteroids are the same as for adults but risks are greater. The implications of starting these drugs are serious, and they should be used only when specifically indicated, in a minimal dosage, and for the shortest possible time. Prolonged or continuous treatment is rarely justified.

## PREDNISOLONE

*Indications:* suppression of inflammatory and allergic disorders; see also notes above

*Cautions; Contra-indications; Side-effects:* section 6.3.3

*Dose: by mouth*, initially, up to 10–20 mg daily (severe disease, up to 60 mg daily), preferably taken in the morning after breakfast; can often be reduced within a few days but may need to be continued for several weeks or months

Maintenance, usual range, 2.5–15 mg daily, but higher doses may be needed; cushingoid side-effects increasingly likely with doses above 7.5 mg daily

See also section 3.2 (asthma), section 8.2.2 (immunosuppression), and section 10.1.2 (rheumatic diseases)

*By intramuscular injection*, prednisolone acetate, 25–100 mg once or twice weekly (for preparation see section 10.1.2.2)

PoM **Prednisolone** (Non-proprietary)

*Tablets,* prednisolone 1 mg, net price 20 = 7p; 5 mg, 20 = 15p. Label: 10 steroid card, 21

PoM **Deltacortril Enteric**® (Pfizer)
*Tablets*, both e/c, prednisolone 2.5 mg (brown),
net price 56-tab pack = 62p; 5 mg (red), 56-tab
pack = £1.18. Label: 5, 10 steroid card, 25

PoM **Deltastab**® (Boots)
*Tablets*, scored, prednisolone 1 mg, net price
20 = 6p; 5 mg, 20 = 14p. Label: 10 steroid card,
21
*Injection*, see section 10.1.2.2

PoM **Precortisyl**® (Roussel)
*Tablets*, prednisolone 1 mg, net price 20 = 7p;
5 mg (scored), 20 = 15p. Label: 10 steroid card,
21

PoM **Precortisyl Forte**® (Roussel)
*Tablets*, scored, prednisolone 25 mg. Net price
20 = £1.56. Label: 10 steroid card, 21

PoM **Prednesol**® (Glaxo)
*Tablets*, pink, scored, soluble, prednisolone 5 mg
(as sodium phosphate). Net price 20 = £1.15.
Label: 10 steroid card, 13, 21

PoM **Sintisone**® (Farmitalia Carlo Erba)
*Tablets*, scored, prednisolone steaglate 6.65 mg
(≡ prednisolone 5 mg). Net price 20 = £1.29.
Label: 10 steroid card, 21

## BETAMETHASONE

*Indications:* suppression of inflammatory and
allergic disorders; congenital adrenal hyperplasia; cerebral oedema; see also notes above

*Cautions; Contra-indications; Side-effects:* section
6.3.3

*Dose: by mouth*, usual range 0.5–5 mg daily. See
also Administration (above)

*By intramuscular injection or slow intravenous
injection or infusion*, 4–20 mg, repeated up to 4
times in 24 hours; CHILD, *by slow intravenous
injection*, up to 1 year 1 mg, 1–5 years 2 mg, 6–
12 years 4 mg

PoM **Betnelan**® (Glaxo)
*Tablets*, scored, betamethasone 500 micrograms.
Net price 20 = 73p. Label: 10 steroid card, 21

PoM **Betnesol**® (Glaxo)
*Tablets*, pink, scored, soluble, betamethasone
500 micrograms (as sodium phosphate). Net
price 20 = 64p. Label: 10 steroid card, 13, 21
*Injection*, betamethasone 4 mg (as sodium
phosphate)/mL. Net price 1-mL amp = 65p.
Label: 10 steroid card

## CORTISONE ACETATE

*Indications:* section 6.3.1

*Cautions; Contra-indications; Side-effects:* section
6.3.3

*Dose: by mouth*, replacement therapy, 25–
37.5 mg daily in divided doses

PoM **Cortisone Acetate** (Non-proprietary)
*Tablets*, cortisone acetate 5 mg, net price 20 =
15p; 25 mg, 20 = 63p. Label: 10 steroid card, 21

PoM **Cortistab**® (Boots)
*Tablets*, both scored, cortisone acetate 5 mg, net price
20 = 15p; 25 mg, 20 = 62p. Label: 10 steroid card, 21

PoM **Cortisyl**® (Roussel)
*Tablets*, scored, cortisone acetate 25 mg. Net price 20 =
£1.19. Label: 10 steroid card, 21

*I am a patient on—*

# STEROID
# TREATMENT

**which must not be
stopped abruptly**

*and in the case of intercurrrent illness
may have to be increased*

*full details are available
from the hospital or general* ➔
*practitioners shown overleaf*

STC1

# INSTRUCTIONS

1   *DO NOT STOP taking the steroid
drug except on medical advice.
Always have a supply in reserve.*

2   *In case of feverish illness, accident, operation (emergency or
otherwise), diarrhoea or vomiting
the steroid treatment MUST be
continued. Your doctor may wish
you to have a LARGER DOSE or
an INJECTION at such times.*

3   *If the tablets cause indigestion
consult your doctor AT ONCE.*

4   *Always carry this card while receiving steroid treatment and show it
to any doctor, dentist, nurse or
midwife or anyone else who is
giving you treatment.*

5   *After your treatment has finished
you must still tell any doctor,
dentist, nurse or midwife or anyone
else who is giving you treatment
that you have had steroid treatment.*

## DEXAMETHASONE

*Indications:* suppression of inflammatory and allergic disorders; shock; diagnosis of Cushing's disease, congenital adrenal hyperplasia; cerebral oedema; see also notes above

*Cautions; Contra-indications; Side-effects:* section 6.3.3; perineal irritation may follow intravenous administration of the phosphate ester

*Dose: by mouth,* usual range 0.5–9 mg daily. See also Administration (above)
See also section 8.1 (chemotherapy emesis)

*By intramuscular injection or slow intravenous injection or infusion* (as dexamethasone phosphate), initially 0.5–20 mg; CHILD 200–500 micrograms/kg daily

Cerebral oedema (as dexamethasone phosphate), *by intravenous injection,* 10 mg initially, then 4 mg *by intramuscular injection* every 6 hours as required for 2–10 days

PoM **Dexamethasone** (Organon)
*Tablets,* dexamethasone 500 micrograms, net price 20 = 64p; 2 mg, 20 = £1.73. Label: 10 steroid card, 21

*Injection,* dexamethasone sodium phosphate 5 mg/mL (≡ dexamethasone 4 mg/mL, dexamethasone phosphate 4.8 mg/mL). Net price 1-mL amp = 83p; 2-mL vial = £1.27. Label: 10 steroid card

PoM **Decadron**® (MSD)
*Tablets,* scored, dexamethasone 500 micrograms. Net price 20 = 91p. Label: 10 steroid card, 21

*Injection,* dexamethasone phosphate 4 mg/mL (≡ dexamethasone 3.33 mg/mL, dexamethasone sodium phosphate 4.17 mg/mL). Net price 2-mL vial = £1.76. Label: 10 steroid card

PoM **Decadron Shock-Pak**® (MSD)
*Injection,* dexamethasone 20 mg/mL (≡ dexamethasone sodium phosphate 25 mg/mL). Net price 5-mL vial = £15.13. Label: 10 steroid card
*Dose:* shock, *by intravenous injection or infusion,* 2–6 mg/kg, repeated if necessary after 2–6 hours (but see section 6.3.2)

## FLUDROCORTISONE

See section 6.3.1

## HYDROCORTISONE

*Indications:* adrenocortical insufficiency (section 6.3.1); suppression of inflammatory and allergic disorders; shock; see also notes above

*Cautions; Contra-indications; Side-effects:* section 6.3.3; perineal irritation may follow intravenous administration of the phosphate ester

*Dose: by mouth,* replacement therapy, 20–30 mg daily in divided doses—see section 6.3.1

*By intramuscular injection or slow intravenous injection or infusion,* 100–500 mg, 3–4 times in 24 hours or as required; CHILD *by slow intravenous injection* up to 1 year 25 mg, 1–5 years 50 mg, 6–12 years 100 mg

Anaphylactic shock—see notes above

Oral preparations
PoM **Hydrocortistab**® (Boots)
*Tablets,* scored, hydrocortisone 20 mg. Net price 20 = 62p. Label: 10 steroid card, 21

PoM **Hydrocortone**® (MSD)
*Tablets,* scored, hydrocortisone 10 mg, net price 20 = 46p; 20 mg, 20 = 71p. Label: 10 steroid card, 21

Parenteral preparations
PoM **Hydrocortisone Sodium Succinate** (Organon)
*Injection,* powder for reconstitution, hydrocortisone (as sodium succinate). Net price 100-mg (amp or vial) = 55p; 500-mg vial = £3.39. Label: 10 steroid card

PoM **Efcortelan Soluble**® (Glaxo)
*Injection,* powder for reconstitution, hydrocortisone (as sodium succinate). Net price 100-mg vial (with 2-mL amp water for injections) = 67p. Label: 10 steroid card

PoM **Efcortesol**® (Glaxo)
*Injection,* hydrocortisone 100 mg (as sodium phosphate)/mL. Net price 1-mL amp = 75p; 5-mL amp = £3.40. Label: 10 steroid card

PoM **Solu-Cortef**® (Upjohn)
*Injection,* powder for reconstitution, hydrocortisone (as sodium succinate). Net price 100-mg vial (with 2-mL amp water for injections) = £1.02; without water for injections = 96p. Label: 10 steroid card

## METHYLPREDNISOLONE

*Indications:* suppression of inflammatory and allergic disorders; cerebral oedema; see also notes above

*Cautions; Contra-indications; Side-effects:* section 6.3.3; rapid intravenous administration of large doses has been associated with cardiovascular collapse

*Dose: by mouth,* usual range 2–40 mg daily. See also Administration (above)

*By intramuscular injection or slow intravenous injection or infusion,* initially 10–500 mg; graft rejection, up to 1 g daily *by intravenous infusion* for up to 3 days

Oral preparations
PoM **Medrone**® (Upjohn)
*Tablets,* scored, methylprednisolone 2 mg (pink), net price 30-tab pack = £2.69; 4 mg, 30-tab pack = £5.16; 16 mg, 14-tab pack = £6.68. Label: 10 steroid card, 21

Parenteral preparations
PoM **Methylprednisolone Sodium Succinate** (Non-proprietary)
*Injection,* powder for reconstitution, methylprednisolone (as sodium succinate) (all with solvent). Net price 125-mg vial = £3.56; 500-mg vial = £10.59; 1-g vial = £19.09
Available from Evans

PoM **Solu-Medrone®** (Upjohn)
*Injection*, powder for reconstitution, methyl-prednisolone (as sodium succinate) (all with solvent). Net price 40-mg vial = £1.32; 125-mg vial = £3.96; 500-mg vial = £11.77; 1-g vial = £21.21; 2-g vial = £40.27. Label: 10 steroid card

*Intramuscular depot*
PoM **Depo-Medrone®** (Upjohn)
*Injection* (aqueous suspension), methylpredni-solone acetate 40 mg/mL. Net price 1-mL vial = £2.59; 2-mL vial = £4.65; 3-mL vial = £6.75. Label: 10 steroid card
*Dose: by deep intramuscular injection*, 40–120 mg, repeated every 2–3 weeks if required

## PREDNISONE
*Indications:* suppression of inflammatory and allergic disorders; see also notes above
*Cautions; Contra-indications; Side-effects:* section 6.3.3. Avoid in liver disease
*Dose:* see Prednisolone

PoM **Prednisone** (Non-proprietary)
*Tablets*, prednisone 5 mg, net price 20 = 15p. Label: 10 steroid card, 21
PoM **Decortisyl®** (Roussel)
*Tablets*, scored, prednisone 5 mg. Net price 20 = 15p. Label: 10 steroid card, 21

## TRIAMCINOLONE
*Indications:* suppression of inflammatory and allergic disorders; see also notes above
*Cautions; Contra-indications; Side-effects:* section 6.3.3. Triamcinolone in high dosage has a greater tendency to cause proximal myopathy and should be avoided in chronic therapy
*Dose: by mouth*, 2–24 mg daily. See also Administration (above)
*By deep intramuscular injection*, into gluteal muscle, 40 mg of acetonide for depot effect, repeated at intervals according to the patient's response; max. single dose 100 mg

PoM **Kenalog®** (Squibb)
*Injection* (aqueous suspension), triamcinolone acetonide 40 mg/mL. Net price 1-mL vial = £1.70; 1-mL syringe = £2.11; 2-mL syringe = £3.66. Label: 10 steroid card
PoM **Ledercort®** (Lederle)
*Tablets*, triamcinolone 2 mg (blue), net price 20 = £1.94; 4 mg, 20 = £3.87. Label: 10 steroid card, 21

# 6.4   Sex hormones

Sex hormones are described under the following section headings:
  6.4.1 Female sex hormones
  6.4.2 Male sex hormones and antagonists
  6.4.3 Anabolic steroids

## 6.4.1   Female sex hormones
  6.4.1.1 Oestrogens and HRT
  6.4.1.2 Progestogens

### 6.4.1.1   OESTROGENS AND HRT

Oestrogens are necessary for the development of female secondary sexual characteristics; they also stimulate myometrial hypertrophy with endometrial hyperplasia.

Oestrogen therapy is given cyclically or continuously for a number of gynaecological conditions. If long-term therapy is required a progestogen should be added cyclically to prevent cystic hyperplasia of the endometrium and possible transformation to cancer. This cyclical addition of a progestogen is not necessary if the patient has had a hysterectomy.

PRIMARY AMENORRHOEA. After assessment by a specialist an oestrogen such as ethinyloestradiol is administered continuously together with cyclical progestogen, or a low-dose combined oral contraceptive is given (see section 7.3.1).

HORMONE REPLACEMENT THERAPY (HRT). Menopausal *vasomotor symptoms* and menopausal *vaginitis* are alleviated by administration of small doses of oestrogen. There is also good evidence that small doses of oestrogen given for several years starting in the perimenopausal period will diminish postmenopausal *osteoporosis* and reduce the incidence of *stroke and myocardial infarction*. There is an increased risk of *endometrial cancer* (countered by cyclical progestogen, see below) and, after some years of use, possibly a slightly increased risk of *breast cancer*.

Hormone replacement therapy (HRT) is indicated for menopausal women whose lives are inconvenienced by *vaginal atrophy* or *vasomotor instability*. Vaginal atrophy may respond to a short course of oestrogen cream given for a few weeks and repeated if necessary. Oral therapy is needed for vasomotor symptoms and should be given for at least a year; in a woman with a uterus cyclical progestogen should be added to reduce the risk of endometrial cancer (see above). Hormone replacement therapy is also indicated for women with *early natural or surgical menopause (before age 45)*, since they are at high risk of osteoporosis; in a woman with a uterus cyclical progestogen should again be added to reduce the risk of endometrial cancer (see above); hormone replacement therapy should be given to the age of at least 50 and possibly for a further 10 years.

Long-term hormone replacement therapy in general is almost certainly favourable in risk benefit terms for menopausal women *without a uterus* because they do not require cyclical progestogen therapy; it should probably be continued for about 10 years. The picture is less clear for menopausal women *with a uterus* because the need for cyclical administration of progestogen may blunt the protective effect of low-dose oestrogen against myocardial infarction and stroke; any effect of the progestogen (favourable or otherwise) on breast cancer is not yet known. Nevertheless, risk factors for osteoporosis should be borne in mind and, if there are several, consideration given to hormone

---

replacement therapy. Risk factors include *recent corticosteroid therapy or any disease predisposing to osteoporosis, thinness, lack of exercise, alcoholism or smoking, and fracture of a hip or forearm before the age of 65; women of Afro-Caribbean origin appear to be less susceptible than those who are white or Asian.*

**Choice.** The choice of oestrogen for hormone replacement therapy is not straightforward and depends on an overall balance of indication, risk, and convenience. Vaginitis in a woman with a uterus can only be treated for a few weeks with an oestrogen, without addition of cyclical progestogen; this constraint includes topical cream (see section 7.2.1) since a significant amount is absorbed through the vaginal mucosa. Ethinyloestradiol is suitable for long-term continuous oral therapy in a woman without a uterus but conjugated oestrogens may be preferred. A woman with a uterus requires a regimen of continuous or cyclical oestrogen with cyclical progestogen for the last 10 to 13 days of the cycle; for this purpose combined oral preparations may be suitable. All oral preparations of oestrogen are subject to first-pass metabolism in the liver and intestine, therefore subcutaneous or transdermal administration reflects more closely endogenous hormone activity. In the case of subcutaneous implants, problems have been encountered with the recurrence of vasomotor symptoms at supraphysiological plasma concentrations; moreover, there is evidence of prolonged endometrial stimulation after discontinuation (calling for continued cyclical progestogen). Transdermal applications are convenient for vasomotor symptoms but oral progestogen is still needed on a cyclical basis if the woman has a uterus; they have not yet been fully assessed for protection against osteoporosis.

Providing calcium intake is adequate calcium supplements do not confer additional benefit on hormone replacement therapy (see section 9.5.1).

SUPPRESSION OF LACTATION. Oestrogens are no longer used to suppress lactation because of their association with thrombo-embolism. **Bromocriptine** (section 6.7.1) is used where necessary.

NEOPLASIA. Stilboestrol is used mainly in neoplastic conditions (see section 8.3.1)

## ETHINYLOESTRADIOL

*Indications:* see notes above

*Cautions:* prolonged exposure to unopposed oestrogens may increase risk of development of endometrial cancer (see notes above); breast-feeding, diabetes, epilepsy, asthma, hypertension, migraine, cardiac or renal disease, history of jaundice, contact lenses (may irritate); may interfere with results of thyroid-function tests and cortisol estimations by increasing concentrations of hormone-binding protein; **interactions:** Appendix 1 (oestrogens)

SURGERY. For a warning on oestrogens and elective surgery, see Combined Oral Contraceptives, section 7.3.1

*Contra-indications:* pregnancy; oestrogen-dependent cancer, history of thrombo-embolism, hepatic impairment, Dubin-Johnson and Rotor syndromes, endometriosis, porphyria (see section 9.8.2), sickle-cell anaemia (but see also Oral Contraceptives), undiagnosed vaginal bleeding, history of herpes gestationis; deterioration of otosclerosis

*Side-effects:* nausea and vomiting, weight gain, breast enlargement and tenderness, withdrawal bleeding, sodium retention with oedema and hypertension (minimal for HRT), changes in liver function, jaundice, thrombosis (but for HRT see notes above), rashes and chloasma, depression, headache, endometrial carcinoma in postmenopausal women

*Dose:* menopausal symptoms 10–20 micrograms daily continuously *or* for 21 days, repeated after 7 days, with progestogen from day 17 to day 26 of cycle if uterus intact

Primary amenorrhoea, 10 micrograms on alternate days increasing to a max. of 50 micrograms daily continuously with a progestogen for the last 5 days of month

Hereditary haemorrhagic telangiectasia, 0.5–1 mg daily (specialist use only)

Oestrogen-only
*Note.* Unsuitable for long-term use alone in women with an intact uterus (who require addition of cyclical progestogen)
PoM **Ethinyloestradiol Tablets,** ethinyloestradiol 10 micrograms, net price 20 = 49p; 20 micrograms, 20 = 60p; 50 micrograms, 20 = 88p; 1 mg, 20 = £1.97

## MESTRANOL

*Indications:* see notes above and under preparations

*Cautions; Contra-indications; Side-effects:* see under Ethinyloestradiol

*Dose:* see below

With progestogen
*Note.* Unsuitable for use as or with an oral contraceptive; not necessary for women who have had a hysterectomy (who can receive oestrogen alone)
PoM **Syntex Menophase®** (Syntex)
*Tablets,* 5 pink, mestranol 12.5 micrograms; 8 orange, mestranol 25 micrograms; 2 yellow, mestranol 50 micrograms; 3 green, mestranol 25 micrograms and norethisterone 1 mg; 6 blue, mestranol 30 micrograms and norethisterone 1.5 mg; 4 lavender, mestranol 20 micrograms and norethisterone 750 micrograms. Net price per pack = £3.33
*Dose:* menopausal symptoms (including osteoporosis prophylaxis), if uterus intact 1 tablet daily, starting with a pink tablet on Sunday, then in sequence (without interruption)

## OESTRADIOL

*Indications:* see notes above and under preparations

*Cautions; Contra-indications; Side-effects:* see under Ethinyloestradiol; transdermal delivery systems may cause erythema and itching

*Dose:* see below

Oestrogen-only

*Note.* Unsuitable for long-term use alone in women with an intact uterus (who require addition of cyclical progestogen)

PoM **Oestradiol Implants** (Organon)

*Implant,* oestradiol 25 mg, net price each = £6.60; 50 mg, each = £13.20; 100 mg, each = £25.30

*Dose: by implantation,* oestrogen replacement, including osteoporosis prophylaxis (with cyclical progestogen on 10–13 days of each cycle if uterus intact, see notes above), 25–100 mg as required (usually every 4–8 months)

PoM **Climaval®** (Sandoz)

*Tablets,* oestradiol valerate 1 mg (grey-blue), net price 28-tab pack = £2.40; 2 mg (blue), 28-tab pack = £2.40

*Dose:* menopausal symptoms (if patient has had a hysterectomy), 1–2 mg daily (for up to 24 months)

PoM **Estraderm TTS®** (Ciba)

*25 Dressing* (TTS 25), self-adhesive, releasing oestradiol approx. 25 micrograms/24 hours when in contact with skin. Net price 8 dressings = £6.75. Label: 10 patient information leaflet, counselling, see below

*50 Dressing* (TTS 50), self-adhesive, releasing oestradiol approx. 50 micrograms/24 hours when in contact with skin. Net price 8 dressings = £7.45. Label: 10 patient information leaflet, counselling, see below

*100 Dressing* (TTS 100), self-adhesive, releasing oestradiol approx. 100 micrograms/24 hours when in contact with skin. Net price 8 dressings = £8.20. Label: 10 patient information leaflet, counselling, see below

*Dose:* menopausal symptoms (but not osteoporosis prophylaxis), 1 patch to be applied twice weekly on continuous basis; give progestogen on 12 days a month (unless patient has had hysterectomy); therapy should be initiated with TTS 50 for first month, subsequently adjusted to lowest effective dose; max. one TTS 100 daily

COUNSELLING. Patch should be removed after 3–4 days and replaced with fresh patch on slightly different site; recommended sites: clean, dry, unbroken areas of skin on trunk below waistline; not to be applied on or near breasts

PoM **Hormonin®** (Shire)

*Tablets,* pink, oestradiol 600 micrograms, oestriol 270 micrograms, oestrone 1.4 mg. Net price 20 = £1.34

*Dose:* menopausal symptoms (including osteoporosis prophylaxis), with progestogen for 12–13 days per cycle if uterus intact, 1–2 tablets daily

*Note.* Hormonin® tablets can be given continuously or cyclically (21 days out of 28)

PoM **Progynova®** (Schering Health Care)

*Tablets,* both s/c, oestradiol valerate 1 mg (beige), net price 21-tab pack = £1.98; 2 mg (blue), 21-tab pack = £1.98

*Dose:* menopausal symptoms (short-term), 1 mg daily for 21 days, interval of at least 7 days before next course; increased to 2 mg daily if required

With progestogen

*Note.* Unsuitable for use as or with an oral contraceptive; not necessary for women who have had a hysterectomy (who can receive oestrogen alone)

PoM **Cyclo-Progynova®** (Schering Health Care)

*1-mg Tablets,* all s/c, 11 beige, oestradiol valerate 1 mg; 10 brown, oestradiol valerate 1 mg and norgestrel 500 micrograms (≡levonorgestrel 250 micrograms). Net price per pack = £3.50

*Dose:* menopausal symptoms (including osteoporosis prophylaxis), if uterus intact, 1 beige tablet daily for 11 days, starting on 5th day of menstruation (or at any time if cycles have ceased or are infrequent), then 1 brown tablet daily for 10 days, followed by a 7-day interval

*2-mg Tablets,* all s/c, 11 white, oestradiol valerate 2 mg; 10 brown, oestradiol valerate 2 mg and norgestrel 500 micrograms (≡levonorgestrel 250 micrograms). Net price per pack = £3.50

*Dose:* see above, but starting with 1 white tablet daily (instead of 1 beige tablet) if symptoms not fully controlled with lower strength

PoM **Estrapak 50®** (Ciba)

*Calendar pack,* 8 self-adhesive dressings, releasing oestradiol approx. 50 micrograms/24 hours when in contact with skin, and 12 tablets, red, norethisterone acetate 1 mg. Net price per pack = £8.45. Label: 10 patient information leaflet, counselling, see below

*Dose:* menopausal symptoms (including osteoporosis prophylaxis) if uterus intact, starting within 5 days of onset of menstruation (or at any time if cycles have ceased or are infrequent), apply 1 dressing twice weekly on continuous basis, and take 1 tablet daily on days 15–26 of each 28-day treatment cycle

COUNSELLING. Patch should be removed after 3–4 days and replaced with fresh patch on slightly different site; recommended sites: clean, dry, unbroken areas of skin on trunk below waistline; not to be applied on or near breasts

PoM **Nuvelle®** (Schering Health Care)

*Tablets,* all s/c, 16 white, oestradiol valerate 2 mg; 12 pink, oestradiol valerate 2 mg and levonorgestrel 75 micrograms. Net price 3 × 28-tab pack = £13.77

*Dose:* climacteric symptoms of menopause, 1 white tablet daily for 16 days, starting on 5th day of menstruation (or any time if cycles have ceased or are infrequent) then 1 pink tablet daily for 12 days; subsequent courses are repeated without interval

---

PoM **Trisequens**® (Novo Nordisk)

*Trisequens*® *tablets*, 12 blue, oestradiol 2 mg, oestriol 1 mg; 10 white, oestradiol 2 mg, oestriol 1 mg, norethisterone acetate 1 mg; 6 red, oestradiol 1 mg, oestriol 500 micrograms. Net price per pack = £3.74

*Dose:* menopausal symptoms (including osteoporosis prophylaxis), if uterus intact, 1 blue tablet daily, starting on 5th day of menstruation (or at any time if cycles have ceased or are infrequent), then 1 tablet daily in sequence (without interruption)

*Trisequens Forte*® *tablets*, 12 yellow, oestradiol 4 mg, oestriol 2 mg; 10 white, oestradiol 4 mg, oestriol 2 mg, norethisterone acetate 1 mg; 6 red, oestradiol 1 mg, oestriol 500 micrograms. Net price per pack = £3.74

*Dose:* menopausal symptoms (but not osteoporosis prophylaxis), see under Trisequens®, starting with 1 yellow tablet daily (instead of 1 blue tablet) if symptoms not fully controlled with lower strength

## OESTRIOL

*Indications:* see notes above and under preparations

*Cautions; Contra-indications; Side-effects:* see under Ethinyloestradiol

*Dose:* see below

PoM **Ovestin**® (Organon)

*Tablets*, oestriol 250 micrograms. Net price 20 = 60p. Label: 25

*Dose:* genito-urinary symptoms associated with oestrogen-deficiency states, 0.5–3 mg daily, as single dose, for up to 1 month, then 0.5–1 mg daily until restoration of epithelial integrity (short-term use)

Infertility associated with poor cervical penetration, 0.25–1 mg daily, as single dose, on days 6–15 of cycle (with regular monitoring)

Ingredient of Hormonin® and (with progestogen) of Trisequens®, see Oestradiol

## OESTROGENS, CONJUGATED

*Indications:* see notes above and under preparations

*Cautions; Contra-indications; Side-effects:* see under Ethinyloestradiol

*Dose:* see below

PoM **Premarin**® (Wyeth)

*Tablets*, all s/c, conjugated oestrogens 625 micrograms (maroon), net price 21-tab pack = £1.13; 1.25 mg (yellow), 21-tab pack = £1.86; 2.5 mg (purple), 20 = £2.09

*Dose:* menopausal symptoms including osteoporosis prophylaxis, (with progestogen for 10–12 days per cycle if uterus intact), 0.625–1.25 mg daily

With progestogen

PoM **Prempak-C**® (Wyeth)

*0.625 Calendar pack*, all s/c, 28 maroon tablets, conjugated oestrogens 625 micrograms; 12 light brown tablets, norgestrel 150 micrograms (≡ levonorgestrel 75 micrograms). Net price per pack = £3.98

*Dose:* menopausal symptoms (including osteoporosis prophylaxis), if uterus intact, 1 maroon tablet daily on continuous basis, starting on 1st day of menstruation (or at any time if cycles have ceased or are infrequent), and 1 brown tablet daily on days 17–28 of each 28-day treatment cycle; subsequent courses are repeated without interval

*1.25 Calendar pack*, all s/c, 28 yellow tablets, conjugated oestrogens 1.25 mg; 12 light brown tablets, norgestrel 150 micrograms (≡ levonorgestrel 75 micrograms). Net price per pack = £3.98

*Dose:* see above, but taking 1 yellow tablet daily on continuous basis (instead of 1 maroon tablet) if symptoms not fully controlled with lower strength

## PIPERAZINE OESTRONE SULPHATE

(Estropipate)

*Indications:* see notes above and under preparations

*Cautions; Contra-indications; Side-effects:* see under Ethinyloestradiol

*Dose:* see below

PoM **Harmogen**® (Abbott)

*Tablets*, peach, scored, piperazine oestrone sulphate 1.5 mg. Net price 20 = £1.58

*Dose:* menopausal symptoms, 1.5–4.5 mg daily in single or divided doses for 21–28 days, repeated after 5–7 days if necessary; if given for longer reduced to lowest dose (and given with progestogen for 12 days per month if uterus intact)

## TIBOLONE

Tibolone combines oestrogenic and progestogenic activity with weak androgenic activity. It has recently been introduced for the treatment of vasomotor symptoms of the menopause. It is given continuously, without cyclical progestogen.

## TIBOLONE

*Indications:* see under Dose

*Cautions:* vaginal bleeding, renal impairment, epilepsy, migraine, diabetes mellitus, hypercholesterolaemia; withdraw if signs of thromboembolic disease, abnormal liver function tests or cholestatic jaundice; induce withdrawal bleeding with a progestogen if transferring from another form of HRT; **interactions:** Appendix 1 (tibolone)

*Contra-indications:* hormone-dependent tumours, history of cardiovascular or cerebrovascular disease (e.g. thrombophlebitis,

---

thrombo-embolism), uninvestigated vaginal bleeding, severe liver disease, pregnancy, breast-feeding

*Side-effects:* weight changes, ankle oedema, dizziness, seborrhoeic dermatitis, vaginal bleeding, headache, gastro-intestinal disturbances, increased facial hair

*Dose:* vasomotor symptoms following natural or surgical menopause, 2.5 mg daily

Note. Unsuitable for use in the premenopause and as or with an oral contraceptive

▼ PoM **Livial**® (Organon)
*Tablets*, tibolone 2.5 mg. Net price 28-tab pack = £13.20

## 6.4.1.2 PROGESTOGENS

Progestogens modify some of the effects of, and act mainly on tissues sensitised by, oestrogens; their effects are inhibited by oestrogen excess. There are two main groups of progestogen, the naturally occurring hormone *progesterone* and its analogues (allyloestrenol, dydrogesterone, hydroxyprogesterone, and medroxyprogesterone) and the *testosterone* analogues e.g. norethisterone. Progesterone and its analogues are less androgenic than the testosterone derivatives and neither progesterone nor dydrogesterone causes virilisation. Other synthetic derivatives are variably metabolised into testosterone and oestrogen; thus side-effects vary with the preparation and the dose.

Progestogens are used in many menstrual disorders, including *severe dysmenorrhoea*, and *menorrhagia*. **Norethisterone** and **dydrogesterone** may be given alone on a cyclical basis during part of the menstrual cycle or in conjunction with an oestrogen. Where contraception is also required in younger women, however, the best choice is a combined oral contraceptive (see section 7.3.1).

Where *endometriosis* requires drug treatment, it may respond to a progestogen, e.g. norethisterone, administered on a continuous basis. Alternatively, danazol (section 6.7.3) may be given.

Progestogens have been widely advocated for the alleviation of *premenstrual symptoms* but no convincing physiological basis for such treatment has been shown.

The progestogens desogestrel, ethynodiol, levonorgestrel, lynoestrenol, and norethisterone are used in combined oral and in progestogen-only *contraceptives* (see sections 7.3.1 and 7.3.2). Levonorgestrel is the active isomer and has twice the potency of racemic norgestrel.

Progestogens are also used in conjunction with oestrogens in *hormone replacement therapy* in menopausal women with an intact uterus (see section 6.4.1.1). See section 8.3.2 for use in *neoplastic disease*.

Progestogens have been used in *habitual abortion* but there is no evidence of benefit. If they are used for this purpose they should be of the true progesterone-derivative type, e.g. **hydroxyprogesterone hexanoate** to avoid any masculinisation of a female fetus.

## PROGESTERONE

*Indications:* see under Dose and notes above
*Cautions:* diabetes, breast-feeding, hypertension; hepatic, cardiac, or renal disease; **interactions:** Appendix 1 (progestogens)
*Contra-indications:* undiagnosed vaginal bleeding, missed or incomplete abortion, past severe arterial disease or current high risk (e.g. family history, together with cholesterol above 6.5 mmol/litre), mammary carcinoma; porphyria (see section 9.8.2)
*Side-effects:* acne, urticaria, oedema, weight gain, gastro-intestinal disturbances, changes in libido, breast discomfort, premenstrual symptoms, irregular menstrual cycles; rarely jaundice. Injection may be painful
*Dose:* by *vagina or rectum*, premenstrual syndrome, 200 mg daily to 400 mg twice daily starting at day 12–14 and continued until onset of menstruation (but not recommended, see notes above); rectally if barrier methods of contraception are used, or if vaginal infection
By *deep intramuscular injection* into buttock, embryo transfer, consult manufacturer's literature

PoM **Cyclogest**® (Hoechst)
*Suppositories*, progesterone 200 mg, net price 15 = £5.40; 400 mg, 15 = £7.83
PoM **Gestone**® (Paines & Byrne)
*Injection*, progesterone 25 mg/mL, 1-mL amp = 34p; 50 mg/mL, 1-mL amp = 44p, 2-mL amp = 58p

## ALLYLOESTRENOL

*Indications:* habitual abortion, but see notes above
*Cautions; Contra-indications; Side-effects:* see under Progesterone and notes above
*Dose:* habitual abortion, 5–10 mg daily for at least 16 weeks (but see notes above)

PoM **Gestanin**® (Organon)
*Tablets*, allyloestrenol 5 mg. Net price 20 = £1.99

## DESOGESTREL

Ingredient of combined oral contraceptives (section 7.3.1)

## DYDROGESTERONE

*Indications:* see under Dose and notes above
*Cautions; Contra-indications; Side-effects:* see under Progesterone and notes above; breakthrough bleeding may occur (increase dose)
*Dose:* endometriosis, 10 mg 2–3 times daily from 5th to 25th day of cycle or continuously
Infertility, irregular cycles, 10 mg twice daily from 11th to 25th day for at least 6 cycles
Habitual abortion, 10 mg twice daily from day 11 to day 25 of cycle until conception, then continuously until 20th week of pregnancy and gradually reduced (but see notes above)
Dysfunctional uterine bleeding, 10 mg twice daily (together with an oestrogen) for 5–7 days to arrest bleeding; 10 mg twice daily (together

---

with an oestrogen) from 11th to 25th day of cycle to prevent bleeding
Dysmenorrhoea, 10 mg twice daily from 5th to 25th day of cycle
Amenorrhoea, 10 mg twice daily from 11th to 25th day of cycle with oestrogen therapy from 1st to 25th day of cycle
Premenstrual syndrome, 10 mg twice daily from 12th to 26th day of cycle increased if necessary (but not recommended, see notes above)
Hormone replacement therapy, with continuous oestrogen therapy, 10 mg twice daily, for the first 12–14 days of each calendar month; with cyclical oestrogen, 10 mg twice daily for the last 12–14 days of each treatment cycle

PoM **Duphaston®** (Duphar)
*Tablets*, scored, dydrogesterone 10 mg. Net price 60-tab pack = £10.05

## ETHYNODIOL DIACETATE
Ingredient of combined and progestogen-only oral contraceptives (sections 7.3.1 and 7.3.2)

## GESTODENE
Ingredient of combined oral contraceptives (section 7.3.1)

## HYDROXYPROGESTERONE HEXANOATE
*Indications:* habitual abortion but see notes above
*Cautions; Contra-indications; Side-effects:* see under Progesterone and notes above
*Dose:* by intramuscular injection, 250–500 mg weekly during first half of pregnancy

PoM **Proluton* Depot®** (Schering Health Care)
*Injection* (oily), hydroxyprogesterone hexanoate 250 mg/mL. Net price 1-mL amp = £2.35; 2-mL amp = £3.69
*formerly Primolut Depot®

## LEVONORGESTREL
Ingredient of combined and progestogen-only oral contraceptives (sections 7.3.1 and 7.3.2)

## MEDROXYPROGESTERONE ACETATE
*Indications:* see under Dose; for use as a contraceptive, see section 7.3.2; for use in malignant disease, see section 8.3.2
*Cautions; Contra-indications; Side-effects:* see under Progesterone and notes above; disturbances of normal menstrual cycle and irregular bleeding may occur; contra-indicated in pregnancy
*Dose:* by mouth, 2.5–10 mg daily for 5–10 days beginning on 16th–21st day of cycle, repeated for 2 cycles in dysfunctional uterine bleeding and 3 cycles in secondary amenorrhoea
Mild to moderate endometriosis, 10 mg 3 times daily for 90 consecutive days, beginning on 1st day of cycle
*By deep intramuscular injection,* endometriosis, 50 mg weekly or 100 mg every 2 weeks

PoM **Depo-Provera® 50mg/mL** (Upjohn)
*Injection* (aqueous suspension), medroxyprogesterone acetate 50 mg/mL. Net price 1-mL vial = £1.55; 3-mL vial = £4.17; 5-mL vial = £6.85
PoM **Provera®** (Upjohn)
*Tablets*, both scored, medroxyprogesterone acetate 5 mg, net price 20-tab pack = £2.58, 100-tab pack = £12.87; 10 mg, 50-tab pack = £12.87

## NORETHISTERONE
*Indications:* see under Dose; for use as a contraceptive see sections 7.3.1 and 7.3.2
*Cautions; Contra-indications; Side-effects:* see under Progesterone but more virilising and greater incidence of liver disturbances and jaundice; avoid in pregnancy; exacerbation of epilepsy and migraine
*Dose:* endometriosis 10 mg daily starting on 5th day of cycle (increased if spotting occurs to 25 mg daily in divided doses to prevent breakthrough bleeding)
Menorrhagia, 5 mg 3 times daily for 10 days to arrest bleeding; to prevent bleeding 5 mg twice daily from 19th to 26th day
Dysmenorrhoea, 5 mg 3 times daily from 5th to 24th day for 3–4 cycles
Premenstrual syndrome, 5 mg 2–3 times daily from 19th to 26th day for several cycles (but not recommended, see notes above)
Postponement of menstruation, 5 mg 3 times daily starting 3 days before anticipated onset

PoM **Menzol®** (Schwarz)
*Tablets*, scored, norethisterone 5 mg. Net price 3 × 24-tab (8-day) 'Planapak' = £7.70; 3 × 60-tab (20-day) 'Planapak' = £19.35
PoM **Primolut N®** (Schering Health Care)
*Tablets*, norethisterone 5 mg. Net price 20 = £1.63
PoM **Utovlan®** (Syntex)
*Tablets*, scored, norethisterone 5 mg. Net price 20 = £1.54

## NORGESTIMATE
Ingredient of combined oral contraceptive (section 7.3.1)

## NORGESTREL
Ingredient of combined and progestogen-only oral contraceptives (section 7.3.1) and of combined preparations for menopausal symptoms (section 6.4.1.1)

## 6.4.2 Male sex hormones and antagonists
Androgens cause masculinisation; they may be used as replacement therapy in castrated adults and in those who are hypogonadal due to either pituitary or testicular disease. In the normal male they depress spermatogenesis and inhibit pituitary gonadotrophin secretion. Androgens also have an anabolic action which led to the development of anabolic steroids (section 6.4.3).

Androgens are useless as a treatment of impotence and impaired spermatogenesis unless there is associated hypogonadism; they should not be given until the hypogonadism has been properly investigated. Treatment should be under expert supervision.

When given to patients with hypopituitarism they can lead to normal sexual development and potency but not to fertility. If fertility is desired, the usual treatment is with gonadotrophins or pulsatile gonadotrophin-releasing hormone (section 6.5.1) which will stimulate spermatogenesis as well as androgen production.

Caution should be used when androgens or chorionic gonadotrophin are used in treating boys with delayed puberty since the fusion of epiphyses is hastened and may result in short stature.

Androgens are still quite useful in occasional women with disseminated cancer of the breast despite their masculinising effects.

Intramuscular depot preparations of **testosterone esters** are preferred for replacement therapy. Testosterone enanthate or propionate or alternatively Sustanon®, which consists of a mixture of testosterone esters and has a longer duration of action, may be used. Satisfactory replacement therapy can sometimes be obtained with 1 mL of Sustanon 250®, given by intramuscular injection once a month, although more frequent dose intervals are often necessary. Implants of testosterone have been superseded for hypogonadism but are still occasionally used. Menopausal women are also sometimes given implants of testosterone (in a dose of 50–100 mg every 4–8 months) as an adjunct to hormone replacement therapy.

Of the orally active preparations, methyltestosterone is no longer on the UK market; like other 17α-alkyl derivatives of testosterone it could sometimes cause dose-related but reversible cholestatic jaundice. **Mesterolone** is not a 17α-alkyl derivative and is less toxic to the liver.

## TESTOSTERONE AND ESTERS

*Indications:* see under preparations
*Cautions:* cardiac, renal, or hepatic impairment (see Appendix 2), ischaemic heart disease, hypertension, epilepsy, migraine, skeletal metastases (risk of hypercalcaemia)
*Contra-indications:* breast cancer in men, prostatic cancer, pregnancy, breast-feeding, nephrosis
*Side-effects:* sodium retention with oedema, increase in weight, hypercalcaemia, increased bone growth, priapism, precocious sexual development and premature closure of epiphyses in pre-pubertal males, prostatism in elderly patients, high doses cause virilism in women, and suppress spermatogenesis in men

PoM **Primoteston Depot**® (Schering Health Care)
*Injection* (oily), testosterone enanthate 250 mg/mL. Net price 1-mL amp = £4.13
*Dose: by intramuscular injection,* hypogonadism, initially 250 mg every 2–3 weeks; maintenance 250 mg every 3–6 weeks
Breast cancer, 250 mg every 2 weeks

PoM **Restandol**® (Organon)
*Capsules*, red-brown, testosterone undecanoate 40 mg in oily solution. Net price 60 = £15.78. Label: 21, 25
*Dose:* androgen deficiency, 120–160 mg daily for 2–3 weeks; maintenance 40–120 mg daily

PoM **Sustanon 100**® (Organon)
*Injection* (oily), testosterone propionate 20 mg, testosterone phenylpropionate 40 mg, and testosterone isocaproate 40 mg/mL. Net price 1-mL amp = £1.11
*Dose: by deep intramuscular injection,* androgen deficiency, 1 mL every 2 weeks

PoM **Sustanon 250**® (Organon)
*Injection* (oily), testosterone propionate 30 mg, testosterone phenylpropionate 60 mg, testosterone isocaproate 60 mg, and testosterone decanoate 100 mg/mL. Net price 1-mL amp = £2.61
*Dose: by deep intramuscular injection,* androgen deficiency, 1 mL usually every 3 weeks

PoM **Virormone**® (Paines & Byrne)
*Injection,* testosterone propionate 50 mg/mL. Net price 2-mL amp = 46p
*Dose: by intramuscular injection,* androgen deficiency, 50 mg 2–3 times weekly
Delayed puberty, 50 mg weekly.
Breast cancer, 100 mg 2–3 times weekly

Testosterone
PoM **Testosterone** (Organon)
*Implant,* testosterone 100 mg, net price = £5.61; 200 mg = £10.45
*Dose: by implantation,* male hypogonadism, 600 mg every 6 months
Menopausal women, see notes above

## MESTEROLONE

*Indications:* see under Dose
*Cautions; Contra-indications; Side-effects:* see under Testosterone Esters; spermatogenesis unimpaired
*Dose:* androgen deficiency, 25 mg 3–4 times daily for several months, reduced to 50–75 mg daily in divided doses for maintenance

PoM **Pro-Viron**® (Schering Health Care)
*Tablets,* scored, mesterolone 25 mg. Net price 50 = £7.91

## ANTI-ANDROGENS

**Cyproterone acetate** is an anti-androgen used in the treatment of severe hypersexuality and sexual deviation in the male; it inhibits spermatogenesis and produces reversible infertility. Abnormal sperm forms are produced. Cyproterone acetate is also used in the treatment of acne and hirsutism in women (see section 13.6) and in prostatic cancer (see section 8.3.4). As hepatic tumours have been produced in *animal* studies, careful consideration should be given to the risk/benefit ratio before treatment.

## CYPROTERONE ACETATE

*Indications:* see notes above; prostate cancer, see section 8.3.4

*Cautions:* impaired ability to drive and operate machinery; ineffective for male hypersexuality in chronic alcoholism (relevance to prostate cancer not known); blood counts and monitor hepatic function, adrenocortical function and blood glucose regularly; diabetes mellitus, adrenocortical insufficiency

*Contra-indications:* (do not apply in prostate cancer) hepatic disease, malignant or wasting disease, severe depression, history of thromboembolic disorders; youths under 18 years (may arrest bone maturation and testicular development)

*Side-effects:* fatigue and lassitude, weight changes, changes in hair pattern, gynaecomastia (rarely leading to galactorrhoea and benign breast nodules); rarely osteoporosis; inhibition of spermatogenesis (see notes above); liver abnormalities reported in *animals*

*Dose:* male hypersexuality, 50 mg twice daily after food

PoM **Androcur**® (Schering Health Care)
*Tablets*, scored, cyproterone acetate 50 mg. Net price 56-tab pack = £32.23. Label: 2, 21

### 6.4.3 Anabolic steroids

All the anabolic steroids have some androgenic activity but they cause less virilisation than androgens in women. Their protein-building property led to the hope that they might be widely useful in medicine but this hope has not been realised. They have, for example, been given for osteoporosis in women and in cases of wasting. Their use as body builders or tonics is quite unjustified; they are abused by some athletes.

Anabolic steroids are also used in the treatment of some *aplastic anaemias* (see section 9.1.3) and to reduce the itching of *chronic biliary obstruction* (see Prescribing in Terminal Care).

## NANDROLONE

*Indications:* osteoporosis in postmenopausal women; aplastic anaemia, see section 9.1.3

*Cautions:* cardiac and renal impairment, hepatic impairment (see Appendix 2), hypertension, diabetes mellitus, epilepsy, migraine; monitor skeletal maturation in young patients; skeletal metastases (risk of hypercalcaemia); **interactions:** Appendix 1 (anabolic steroids)

*Contra-indications:* severe hepatic impairment, prostate cancer, male breast cancer, pregnancy, porphyria (see section 9.8.2)

*Side-effects:* acne, sodium retention with oedema, virilisation with high doses including voice changes (sometimes irreversible), amenorrhoea, inhibition of spermatogenesis, premature epiphyseal closure; abnormal liver function tests reported with high doses; liver tumours reported occasionally on prolonged treatment with anabolic steroids

*Dose:* see below

PoM **Deca-Durabolin**® (Organon)
*Injection* (oily), nandrolone decanoate 25 mg/mL, net price 1-mL amp = £1.75, 1-mL syringe = £1.88; 50 mg/mL, 1-mL amp = £3.37, 1-mL syringe = £3.57
*Dose: by deep intramuscular injection*, 50 mg every 3 weeks

PoM **Deca-Durabolin 100**®, see section 9.1.3

PoM **Durabolin**® (Organon)
*Injection* (oily), nandrolone phenylpropionate 25 mg/mL, net price 1-mL amp = 86p, 1-mL syringe = 91p; 50 mg/mL, 1-mL syringe = £1.70
*Dose: by deep intramuscular injection*, 50 mg weekly

## STANOZOLOL

*Indications:* see under Dose

*Cautions; Contra-indications; Side-effects:* see under Nandrolone. Headache, dyspepsia, euphoria, depression, cramp, and occasionally hair loss, also reported; cholestatic jaundice occasionally reported

*Dose: by mouth*, vascular manifestations of Behcet's disease, 10 mg daily
Hereditary angioedema, 2.5–10 mg daily to control attacks, reduced for maintenance (2.5 mg 3 times weekly may be sufficient); CHILD 1–6 years initially 2.5 mg daily, 6–12 years initially 2.5–5 mg daily, reduced for maintenance

*Note:* In hereditary angioedema restricted to well-established cases who have experienced serious attacks (and not for premenopausal women except in life-threatening situations)

PoM **Stromba**® (Sanofi Winthrop)
*Tablets*, scored, stanozolol 5 mg. Net price 56-tab pack = £24.48

# 6.5 Hypothalamic and pituitary hormones and anti-oestrogens

Hypothalamic and pituitary hormones are described under the following section headings:

6.5.1 Hypothalamic and anterior pituitary hormones and anti-oestrogens

6.5.2 Posterior pituitary hormones and antagonists

Use of preparations in these sections requires detailed prior investigation of the patient and *should be reserved for specialist centres*.

## 6.5.1   Hypothalamic and anterior pituitary hormones and anti-oestrogens

### ANTI-OESTROGENS

The anti-oestrogens **clomiphene**, **cyclofenil**, and **tamoxifen** are used in the treatment of female infertility due to secondary amenorrhoea (e.g. polycystic ovarian disease). They induce gonadotrophin release by occupying oestrogen receptors in the hypothalamus, thereby interfering with feedback mechanisms; chorionic gonadotrophin is sometimes used as an adjunct. Care is taken to avoid hyperstimulation and multiple pregnancies.

### CLOMIPHENE CITRATE

*Indications:* anovulatory infertility—see notes above

*Cautions:* see notes above; polycystic ovary syndrome (cysts may enlarge during treatment), incidence of multiple births increased

*Contra-indications:* hepatic disease, ovarian cysts, endometrial carcinoma, pregnancy, abnormal uterine bleeding

*Side-effects:* visual disturbances (withdraw), ovarian hyperstimulation (withdraw), hot flushes, abdominal discomfort, occasionally nausea, vomiting, depression, insomnia, breast tenderness, weight gain, rashes, dizziness, hair loss

*Dose:* 50 mg daily for 5 days starting on 2nd to 5th day of menstrual cycle or at any time if cycles have ceased; in absence of ovulation second course of 100 mg daily for 5 days may be given; most patients who are going to respond will do so to first course; 3 courses should constitute adequate therapeutic trial; long-term cyclical therapy not recommended

PoM **Clomid**® (Merrell)
*Tablets*, yellow, scored, clomiphene citrate 50 mg. Net price 20 = £6.73

PoM **Serophene**® (Serono)
*Tablets*, scored, clomiphene citrate 50 mg. Net price 20 = £6.73

### CYCLOFENIL

*Indications:* anovulatory infertility—see notes above

*Contra-indications:* see under Clomiphene Citrate

*Side-effects:* hot flushes, abdominal discomfort, nausea; rarely cholestatic jaundice

*Dose:* 200 mg twice daily for 10 days starting on 3rd day of natural or induced bleeding, repeated for at least 3 cycles

PoM **Rehibin**® (Serono)
*Tablets*, scored, cyclofenil 100 mg. Net price 20 = £3.70

### TAMOXIFEN
See section 8.3.4

### ANTERIOR PITUITARY HORMONES

#### CORTICOTROPHINS

**Tetracosactrin** an analogue of corticotrophin (ACTH) is used to test adrenocortical function; corticotrophin itself is no longer commercially available in the UK. Failure of the plasma cortisol concentration to rise after intramuscular administration indicates adrenocortical insufficiency.

Both corticotrophin and tetracosactrin were formerly used as alternatives to corticosteroids in conditions such as Crohn's disease or rheumatoid arthritis; their value was limited by the variable and unpredictable therapeutic response and by the waning of their effect with time.

### TETRACOSACTRIN

*Indications:* see notes above

*Cautions; Contra-indications; Side-effects:* see section 6.3.3 and Corticotrophin; important risk of anaphylaxis (medical supervision; see data sheet)

PoM **Synacthen**® (Ciba)
*Injection*, tetracosactrin 250 micrograms (as acetate)/mL. Net price 1-mL amp = 93p
*Dose:* diagnostic, *by intramuscular or intravenous injection*, 250 micrograms as a single dose

PoM **Synacthen Depot**® (Ciba)
*Injection* (aqueous suspension), tetracosactrin 1 mg (as acetate)/mL, with zinc phosphate complex; also contains benzyl alcohol. Net price 1-mL amp = £1.05; 2-mL vial = £1.92
*Dose: by intramuscular injection,* initially 1 mg daily (or every 12 hours in acute cases); subsequently reduced to 1 mg every 2–3 days, then 1 mg weekly (or 500 micrograms every 2–3 days)

#### GONADOTROPHINS

Follicle-stimulating hormone (FSH) is used in the treatment of infertile women with proven hypopituitarism or who have not responded to clomiphene; it is used in conjunction with luteinising hormone (LH). Follicle-stimulating hormone is contained in **menotrophin** (which also contains luteinising hormone) and **urofollitrophin**; luteinising hormone is contained in **chorionic gonadotrophin**. Treatment requires careful monitoring to avoid the ovarian hyperstimulation syndrome and multiple pregnancy.

The gonadotrophins are also occasionally used in the treatment of oligospermia associated with hypopituitarism. There is no justification for their use in primary gonadal failure.

Chorionic gonadotrophin has also been used in delayed puberty in the male to stimulate endogenous testosterone production, but has little advantage over testosterone (section 6.4.2).

## CHORIONIC GONADOTROPHIN
(Human Chorionic Gonadotrophin; HCG)
A preparation of a glycoprotein fraction secreted by the placenta and obtained from the urine of pregnant women having the action of the pituitary luteinising hormone
*Indications:* see notes above
*Cautions:* see notes above; cardiac or renal impairment, asthma, epilepsy, migraine
*Side-effects:* oedema (particularly in males—reduce dose), headache, tiredness, mood changes, gynaecomastia, local reactions; sexual precocity with high doses; may aggravate ovarian hyperstimulation
*Dose: by intramuscular injection*, according to patient's requirements

PoM **Gonadotraphon LH**® (Paines & Byrne)
*Injection*, powder for reconstitution, chorionic gonadotrophin. Net price 500-unit amp = 98p; 1000-unit amp = £1.25; 5000-unit amp = £3.71 (all with solvent)

PoM **Pregnyl**® (Organon)
*Injection*, powder for reconstitution, chorionic gonadotrophin. Net price 500-unit amp = 69p; 1500-unit amp = £2.07; 5000-unit amp = £3.08 (all with solvent)

PoM **Profasi**® (Serono)
*Injection*, powder for reconstitution, chorionic gonadotrophin. Net price 500-unit amp = 69p; 1000-unit amp = 95p; 2000-unit amp = £1.75; 5000-unit amp = £3.08 (all with solvent)

## MENOTROPHIN
Extract of the urine of postmenopausal women containing primarily follicle-stimulating hormone (with luteinising hormone)
*Indications:* see notes above
*Cautions:* ovarian cysts, adrenal or thyroid disorders, hyperprolactinoma or pituitary tumour
*Side-effects:* ovarian hyperstimulation, multiple pregnancy; local reactions
*Dose: by deep intramuscular injection*, according to patient's response

PoM **Humegon**® (Organon)
*Injection*, powder for reconstitution, menotrophin as follicle-stimulating hormone 75 units, luteinising hormone 75 units. Net price per amp = £8.80; follicle-stimulating hormone 150 units, luteinising hormone 150 units, 1 amp = £16.00 (both with solvent)

PoM **Pergonal**® (Serono)
*Injection*, powder for reconstitution, menotrophin as follicle-stimulating hormone 75 units, luteinising hormone 75 units. Net price per amp (with solvent) = £9.79

## UROFOLLITROPHIN
Extract of the urine of postmenopausal women containing follicle-stimulating hormone
*Indications:* see notes above
*Cautions; Side-effects:* see under Menotrophin
*Dose: by deep intramuscular injection*, according to patient's response

PoM **Metrodin**® (Serono)
*Injection*, powder for reconstitution, urofollitrophin as follicle-stimulating hormone 75 units. Net price per amp (with solvent) = £9.79

GROWTH HORMONE
Growth hormone is used in the treatment of short stature due to growth hormone deficiency (including short stature in Turner syndrome); only the human type is effective as growth hormone is species specific. Growth hormone of human origin (HGH; somatotrophin) has been replaced by a growth hormone of human sequence, **somatropin**, produced using recombinant DNA technology.

## SOMATROPIN
(Biosynthetic Human Growth Hormone)
*Indications:* see notes above
*Cautions:* only patients with open epiphyses; relative deficiencies of other pituitary hormones (notably hypothyroidism); diabetes mellitus (adjustment of antidiabetic therapy may be necessary); avoid in pregnancy (theoretical risk)
*Side-effects:* antibody formation; local reactions (rotate subcutaneous injection sites to prevent lipo-atrophy); in Turner syndrome temporary exacerbation of lymphoedema reported
*Dose:* 0.5–0.7 units/kg (Turner syndrome, 1 unit/kg) weekly divided into 6 or 7 doses for *subcutaneous injection* (alternatively divided into 2 or 3 doses for *intramuscular injection*, but more painful)

▼ PoM **Genotropin**® (Kabi Pharmacia)
*Injection*, powder for reconstitution, somatropin (rbe), net price 4-unit vial (with diluent) = £30.50; 12-unit vial (with diluent) = £91.50
*KabiPen injection*, two-compartment cartridge containing powder for reconstitution, somatropin (rbe) and diluent (for use with NHS Kabi-Pen® device). Net price 16-unit pack = £122.00
*KabiQuick injection*, two-compartment single-dose syringe containing powder for reconstitution, somatropin (rbe) and diluent. Net price 2-unit syringe = £16.00, 3-unit syringe = £24.00, 4-unit syringe = £32.00
*KabiVial injection*, two-compartment cartridge containing powder for reconstitution, somatropin (rbe) and diluent. Net price 4-unit vial = £30.50, 16-unit vial = £122.00

PoM **Humatrope**® (Lilly)
*Injection*, powder for reconstitution, somatropin (rbe) and diluent, net price 4-unit vial = £30.50; 16-unit vial = £122.00

▼ PoM **Norditropin**® (Novo Nordisk)
*Injection*, powder for reconstitution, somatropin (epr), net price 12-unit vial (with diluent) = £91.50
*PenSet 12 injection*, powder for reconstitution, somatropin (epr), net price 12-unit vial (with diluent in cartridge and needle) = £96.08. For use with NHS Nordiject® 12 device

*PenSet 24 injection*, powder for reconstitution, somatropin (epr), net price 24-unit vial (with diluent in cartridge and needle) = £192.15. For use with NHS Nordiject® 24 device

PoM **Saizen**® (Serono)

*Injection*, powder for reconstitution, somatropin (rmc), net price 4-unit vial (with diluent) = £30.50; 10-unit vial (with diluent) = £76.25

---

## HYPOTHALAMIC HORMONES

**Gonadorelin** (gonadotrophin-releasing hormone, LH-RH) when injected intravenously in normal subjects leads to a rapid rise in plasma concentrations of both luteinising hormone (LH) and follicle-stimulating hormone (FSH). It has not proved to be very helpful, however, in distinguishing hypothalamic from pituitary lesions. Gonadorelin is also used for treatment of infertility, particularly in the female. The gonadotrophin-releasing hormone analogues, buserelin and goserelin, are indicated in metastatic prostate cancer (see section 8.3.4); nafarelin is indicated in endometriosis (see section 6.7.2).

Thyrotrophin-releasing hormone (TRH, **protirelin**) may be of value in difficult cases of hyperthyroidism. Failure of plasma thyrotrophin (TSH) concentration to rise after intravenous injection indicates excess circulating thyroid hormones. Impaired or absent responses also occur in some euthyroid patients with single adenoma, multinodular goitre, or endocrine exophthalmos; patients with hypopituitarism show a reduced or delayed rise.

## GONADORELIN

(LH–RH)

*Indications:* see preparations below

*Side-effects:* rarely, nausea, headache, abdominal pain, increased menstrual bleeding; rarely, hypersensitivity reaction on repeated administration of large doses; irritation at injection site

*Dose:* see below

PoM **Fertiral**® (Hoechst)

*Injection*, gonadorelin 500 micrograms/mL. Net price 2-mL amp = £34.30

For amenorrhoea and infertility due to abnormal release of LH–RH (endogenous gonadorelin), *by pulsatile subcutaneous infusion*, initially 10–20 micrograms over 1 minute, repeated every 90 minutes for max. of 6 months; pulsatile intravenous infusion (in association with heparin) may be required

PoM **HRF**® (Wyeth)

*Injection*, powder for reconstitution, gonadorelin. Net price 100-microgram vial = £8.12; 500-microgram vial = £17.73 (both with diluent)

For assessment of pituitary function (adults), *by subcutaneous or intravenous injection*, 100 micrograms

PoM **Relefact LH-RH**® (Hoechst)

*Injection*, gonadorelin 100 micrograms/mL. Net price 1-mL amp = £9.68

For assessment of pituitary function, *by intravenous injection*, 100 micrograms

PoM **Relefact LH-RH/TRH**® (Hoechst)

*Injection*, gonadorelin 100 micrograms, protirelin 200 micrograms/mL. Net price 1-mL amp = £11.18

For assessment of anterior pituitary reserve by intravenous injection, 1 mL

---

## PROTIRELIN

*Indications:* assessment of thyroid function and thyroid stimulating hormone reserve

*Cautions:* severe hypopituitarism, myocardial ischaemia, bronchial asthma and obstructive airways disease, pregnancy

*Side-effects:* after rapid intravenous administration desire to micturate, flushing, dizziness, nausea, strange taste; transient increase in pulse rate and blood pressure; rarely bronchospasm

*Dose: by intravenous injection*, 200 micrograms; CHILD 1 microgram/kg

PoM **TRH** (Roche)

*Injection*, protirelin 100 micrograms/mL. Net price 2-mL amp = £1.50 (hosp. only)

## 6.5.2  Posterior pituitary hormones and antagonists

---

## POSTERIOR PITUITARY HORMONES

DIABETES INSIPIDUS. **Vasopressin** (antidiuretic hormone, ADH) is used in the treatment of *pituitary* ('cranial') *diabetes insipidus* as its analogues **lypressin** or **desmopressin**. Dosage is tailored to produce a slight diuresis every 24 hours to avoid water intoxication. Treatment may be required for a limited period only in diabetes insipidus following trauma or pituitary surgery.

Desmopressin has a longer duration of action than vasopressin or lypressin; unlike vasopressin and lypressin it has no vasoconstrictor effect. It is given intranasally for maintenance therapy, and by injection in the postoperative period or in unconscious patients. Desmopressin is also used in the differential diagnosis of diabetes insipidus. Following a dose of 2 micrograms intramuscularly or 20 micrograms intranasally, restoration of the ability to concentrate urine after water deprivation confirms a diagnosis of cranial diabetes insipidus. Failure to respond occurs in nephrogenic diabetes insipidus.

In *nephrogenic* and *partial pituitary diabetes insipidus* benefit may be gained from the paradoxical antidiuretic effect of thiazides (see section 2.2.1) e.g. chlorthalidone 100 mg twice daily reduced to maintenance dose of 50 mg daily.

Chlorpropamide (section 6.1.2.1) is also useful in partial pituitary diabetes insipidus, and probably acts by sensitising the renal tubules to the action of remaining endogenous vasopressin; it is given in doses of up to 350 mg daily in adults and 200 mg daily in children, care being taken to avoid hypoglycaemia. Carbamazepine (see section 4.8.1) is also sometimes useful (in a dose of 200 mg once or twice daily); its mode of action may be similar to that of chlorpropamide.

---

OTHER USES. Desmopressin injection is also used to boost factor VIII concentrations in mild to moderate haemophilia.

Vasopressin infusion is used to control variceal bleeding in portal hypertension, prior to more definitive treatment and with variable results. Terlipressin, a new derivative of vasopressin, is used similarly.

Oxytocin, another posterior pituitary hormone, is indicated in obstetrics (see section 7.1.1).

## VASOPRESSIN

*Indications:* pituitary diabetes insipidus; bleeding from oesophageal varices
*Cautions:* heart failure, asthma, epilepsy, migraine; adjust fluid intake to avoid hyponatraemia and water intoxication; renal impairment (see also contra-indications)
*Contra-indications:* vascular disease, chronic nephritis (until reasonable blood nitrogen concentrations attained)
*Side-effects:* pallor, nausea, belching, cramp, desire to defaecate, uterine cramps, hypersensitivity reactions, constriction of coronary arteries (may cause anginal attacks and myocardial ischaemia)
*Dose: by subcutaneous or intramuscular injection,* diabetes insipidus, 5–20 units every four hours
*By intravenous infusion,* initial control of variceal bleeding, 20 units over 15 minutes

Synthetic vasopressin
PoM **Pitressin**® (P-D)
*Injection,* argipressin (synthetic vasopressin) 20 units/mL. Net price 1-mL amp = £1.18 (hosp. only)

## DESMOPRESSIN

*Indications:* see under Dose
*Cautions:* see under Vasopressin; less pressor activity, but still need for considerable caution in renal impairment, cardiovascular disease and hypertension (not indicated for nocturnal enuresis or nocturia in these circumstances); also need for considerable caution in cystic fibrosis
*Dose: intranasally,* pituitary diabetes insipidus (diagnosis), adults and children, 20 micrograms
Pituitary diabetes insipidus (treatment), adults and children, 10–20 micrograms once or twice daily (young children, 5 micrograms)
Primary nocturnal enuresis, adults and children over 7 years, 20 micrograms at bedtime, increased to 40 micrograms if necessary (**important:** see also cautions); after 3 months withdraw for reassessment for at least 1 week
Nocturia associated with multiple sclerosis, adults (under 65 years), 10–20 micrograms at bedtime (**important:** see also cautions)

*By intramuscular or intravenous injection,* pituitary diabetes insipidus, 1–4 micrograms daily; CHILD 400 nanograms
Mild to moderate haemophilia and von Willebrand's disease, consult literature

PoM **DDAVP**® (Ferring)
*Intranasal solution,* desmopressin 100 micrograms/mL. Net price 2.5-mL dropper bottle and catheter = £9.50
*Injection,* desmopressin 4 micrograms/mL. Net price 1-mL amp = £1.07
PoM **Desmospray**® (Ferring)
*Nasal spray,* desmopressin 10 micrograms/metered spray. Net price 5-mL unit = £19.92

## LYPRESSIN

*Indications:* pituitary diabetes insipidus
*Cautions; Contra-indications; Side-effects:* see under Vasopressin; less hypersensitivity; also nasal congestion with ulceration of mucosa
*Dose: intranasally,* 2.5–10 units 3–7 times daily

PoM **Syntopressin**® (Sandoz)
*Nasal spray,* lypressin 50 units/mL, 2.5 units/squeeze. Net price 5-mL bottle = £3.49

## TERLIPRESSIN

*Indications:* bleeding from oesophageal varices
*Cautions; Contra-indications; Side-effects:* see under Vasopressin, but effects are milder
*Dose: by intravenous injection,* 2 mg followed by 1 or 2 mg every 4 to 6 hours until bleeding is controlled, for up to 72 hours

PoM **Glypressin**® (Ferring)
*Injection,* terlipressin, powder for reconstitution. Net price 1-mg vial with 5 mL diluent = £19.00 (hosp. only)

### ANTIDIURETIC HORMONE ANTAGONISTS

**Demeclocycline** (see section 5.1.3) may be used in the treatment of hyponatraemia resulting from inappropriate secretion of antidiuretic hormone. It is thought to act by directly blocking the renal tubular effect of antidiuretic hormone. Initially 0.9 to 1.2 g is given daily in divided doses, reduced to 600–900 mg daily for maintenance.

## 6.6 Drugs affecting bone metabolism

See also plicamycin (section 8.1.2), calcium (section 9.5.1.1), phosphorus (section 9.5.2), vitamin D (section 9.6.4), and oestrogens in postmenopausal osteoporosis (section 6.4.1.1).

### 6.6.1 Calcitonin

**Calcitonin** is involved with parathyroid hormone in the regulation of bone turnover and hence in the maintenance of calcium balance and homoeostasis. It is used to lower the plasma-calcium concentration in some patients with hypercalcaemia (notably when associated with malignant disease). In the treatment of severe Paget's disease of bone it is used mainly for relief of pain but it is also effective in relieving some of the neurological complications, for example deafness. The prolonged use of **porcine calcitonin** can lead to the production of neutralising antibodies. **Salcatonin** (synthetic salmon calcitonin) is less immunogenic and thus more suitable for long-term therapy. When changing treatment in Paget's disease, calcitonin (pork) 80 units is equivalent to salcatonin 50 units.

## CALCITONIN (PORK)

*Indications:* Paget's disease of bone; hypercalcaemia

*Cautions:* see notes above; may contain trace of thyroid; skin test if history of allergy; pregnancy and breast-feeding (avoid—inhibits lactation in *animals*)

*Side-effects:* nausea, vomiting, flushing, tingling of hands, unpleasant taste, inflammatory reactions at injection site

*Dose:* hypercalcaemia, *by subcutaneous or intramuscular injection*, initially 4 units/kg daily adjusted according to clinical and biochemical response (higher doses more conveniently given as salcatonin, see below)
Paget's disease of bone, *by subcutaneous or intramuscular injection*, dose range 80 units 3 times weekly to 160 units daily in single or divided doses; in patients with bone pain or nerve compression syndromes, 80–160 units daily for 3–6 months

PoM **Calcitare**® (Rhône-Poulenc Rorer)
*Injection*, powder for reconstitution, porcine calcitonin. Net price 160-unit vial (with gelatin diluent) = £11.36

## SALCATONIN

*Indications:* see under Dose

*Cautions; Side-effects:* see under Calcitonin (pork) and notes above

*Dose:* hypercalcaemia, *by subcutaneous or intramuscular injection*, range from 5–10 units/kg daily *to* 400 units every 6–8 hours adjusted according to clinical and biochemical response (no additional benefit with over 8 units/kg every 6 hours); *by slow intravenous infusion* (Miacalcic® only), 5–10 units/kg over at least 6 hours
Paget's disease of bone, *by subcutaneous or intramuscular injection*, dose range 50 units 3 times weekly to 100 units daily, in single or divided doses; in patients with bone pain or nerve compression syndromes, 50–100 units daily for 3–6 months
Bone pain in neoplastic disease, *by subcutaneous or intramuscular injection*, 200 units every 6 hours *or* 400 units every 12 hours for 48 hours; may be repeated at discretion of physician
Postmenopausal osteoporosis, *by subcutaneous or intramuscular injection*, 100 units daily with dietary calcium and vitamin D supplements (sections 9.5.1.1 and 9.6.4)

PoM **Calsynar**® (Rhône-Poulenc Rorer)
*Injection*, salcatonin 100 units/mL in saline/acetate, net price 1-mL amp = £8.12; 200 units/mL in saline/acetate, 2-mL vial = £29.20
For subcutaneous or intramuscular injection only

PoM **Miacalcic**® (Sandoz)
*Injection*, salcatonin 50 units/mL, net price 1-mL amp = £3.65; 100 units/mL, 1-mL amp = £7.31; 200 units/mL, 2-mL vial = £26.28
For subcutaneous or intramuscular injection and for dilution and use as an intravenous infusion

### 6.6.2    Bisphosphonates

**Disodium etidronate** is used mainly in the treatment of Paget's disease of bone. It is adsorbed onto hydroxyapatite crystals, so slowing both their rate of growth and dissolution, and reduces the increased rate of bone turnover associated with the disease. Disodium etidronate is also highly effective in the treatment of hypercalcaemia of malignancy; more recently **disodium pamidronate** and **sodium clodronate** have been introduced for this purpose as well.

## DISODIUM ETIDRONATE

*Indications:* see under Dose

*Cautions:* enterocolitis; discontinue use if fractures occur; reduce dose in renal impairment (avoid if severe); pregnancy and breast-feeding; **interactions:** Appendix 1 (bisphosphonates)

*Side-effects:* nausea, diarrhoea, increase in bone pain, increased risk of fractures with high doses; transient taste loss reported

*Dose:* Paget's disease of bone, *by mouth*, 5 mg/kg as a single daily dose for up to 6 months; doses above 10 mg/kg daily for up to 3 months may be used with caution but doses above 20 mg/kg daily are not recommended
Hypercalcaemia of malignancy, *by intravenous infusion*, 7.5 mg/kg daily for 3 days; repeat once if necessary after at least 7 days; *by mouth*, on day after last intravenous dose, 20 mg/kg as a single daily dose for 30 days; max. recommended treatment period 90 days

COUNSELLING. Avoid food for at least 2 hours before and after oral treatment, particularly calcium-containing products

PoM **Didronel**® (Norwich Eaton)
*Tablets*, disodium etidronate 200 mg. Net price 60-tab pack = £37.62. Counselling, food and calcium (see above)

PoM **Didronel IV**® (Norwich Eaton)
*Injection*, disodium etidronate 50 mg/mL. Net price 6-mL amp = £16.43

## DISODIUM PAMIDRONATE

*Note.* Disodium pamidronate was formerly called aminohydroxypropylidenediphosphonate disodium (APD)

*Indications:* hypercalcaemia of malignancy

*Cautions:* severe renal impairment; possibility of convulsions due to electrolyte disturbances; transient rise in body temperature; pregnancy and breast-feeding; **interactions:** Appendix 1 (bisphosphonates)

*Dose: by slow intravenous infusion*, according to plasma calcium concentration 15–60 mg in single infusion or in divided doses over 2–4 days; max. 90 mg per treatment course (see Appendix 6)

▼ PoM **Aredia**® (Ciba)
*Intravenous solution*, disodium pamidronate (anhydrous) 3 mg/mL. For dilution and use as infusion. Net price 5-mL amp = £24.16

## SODIUM CLODRONATE

*Indications:* hypercalcaemia of malignancy
*Cautions:* monitor renal and hepatic function and white cell count; **interactions:** Appendix I (bisphosphonates)
*Contra-indications:* pregnancy, breast-feeding, renal impairment; avoid oral administration in severe inflammatory conditions of the gastrointestinal tract
*Side-effects:* nausea, diarrhoea, hypocalcaemia; rarely skin reactions
*Dose: by mouth*, 1.6 g daily in single or 2 divided doses increased if necessary to a max. of 3.2 g daily; max. recommended treatment period 6 months
COUNSELLING. Avoid food for 1-2 hours before and after treatment, particularly calcium-containing products e.g. milk
*By slow intravenous infusion*, 300 mg daily for max. 7–10 days

▼ PoM **Bonefos**® (Boehringer Ingelheim)
*Capsules*, yellow, sodium clodronate 400 mg. Net price 112-cap pack = £194.00. Counselling, food and calcium
*Concentrate* (= intravenous solution), sodium clodronate 60 mg/mL, for dilution and use as infusion. Net price 5-mL amp = £14.80

▼ PoM **Loron**® (Boehringer Mannheim)
*Capsules*, sodium clodronate 400 mg. Net price 120-cap pack = £207.85. Label: 10 patient information leaflet, counselling, food and calcium
*Intravenous solution*, sodium clodronate 30 mg/mL, for dilution and use as infusion. Net price 10-mL amp = £14.80

# 6.7   Other endocrine drugs

This section includes:
**6.7.1** Bromocriptine
**6.7.2** Danazol, gestrinone, and nafarelin
**6.7.3** Metyrapone and trilostane

## 6.7.1   Bromocriptine

Bromocriptine is a stimulant of dopamine receptors in the brain; it also inhibits release of prolactin by the pituitary. Bromocriptine is used for the suppression of lactation when simpler measures fail, for the treatment of galactorrhoea and cyclical benign breast disease, and for the treatment of prolactinomas (when it reduces both plasma prolactin concentration and tumour size). Bromocriptine also inhibits the release of growth hormone and is sometimes used in the treatment of acromegaly, the success rate is much lower than with prolactinomas.

For the use of bromocriptine in parkinsonism, see section 4.9.1.

## BROMOCRIPTINE

*Indications:* see notes above
*Cautions:* monitor for pituitary enlargement, particularly during pregnancy, annual gynaecological assessment (post-menopausal, every 6 months), monitor for peptic ulceration in acromegalic patients; contraceptive advice if appropriate (oral contraceptives may increase prolactin concentrations); at high dosage caution in patients with history of psychotic disorders or with severe cardiovascular disease and monitor for retroperitoneal fibrosis; avoid in porphyria (see section 9.8.2); **interactions:** Appendix 1 (bromocriptine)
HYPOTENSIVE REACTIONS. Hypotensive reactions may be disturbing in some patients during the first few days of treatment and particular care should be exercised when driving or operating machinery; tolerance to bromocriptine reduced by alcohol
*Side-effects:* nausea, vomiting, constipation, headache, dizziness, postural hypotension, drowsiness, reversible pallor of fingers and toes particularly in patients with Raynaud's syndrome; *high doses*, confusion, psychomotor excitation, hallucinations, dyskinesia, dry mouth, leg cramps, pleural effusions (may necessitate withdrawal of treatment), retroperitoneal fibrosis reported (monitoring required)
*Dose:* prevention/suppression of lactation for medical reasons, 2.5 mg on 1st day (prevention) or daily for 2–3 days (suppression); then 2.5 mg twice daily for 14 days
Hypogonadism/galactorrhoea, infertility, initially 1–1.25 mg at bedtime, increased gradually; usual dose 7.5 mg daily in divided doses, increased if necessary to a max. of 30 mg daily. Usual dose in infertility without hyperprolactinaemia, 2.5 mg twice daily
Cyclical benign breast disease and cyclical menstrual disorders (particularly breast pain), 1–1.25 mg at bedtime, increased gradually; usual dose 2.5 mg twice daily
Acromegaly, initially 1–1.25 mg at bedtime, increase gradually to 5 mg every 6 hours
Prolactinoma, initially 1–1.25 mg at bedtime; increased gradually to 5 mg every 6 hours (occasional patients may require up to 30 mg daily)
Doses should be taken with food

PoM **Bromocriptine** (Non-proprietary)
*Tablets*, bromocriptine (as mesylate), 2.5 mg, net price 20 = £5.03. Label: 21, counselling, hypotensive reactions

PoM **Parlodel**® (Sandoz)

*Tablets*, both scored, bromocriptine (as mesylate) 1 mg, net price 20 = £1.86; 2.5 mg, 20 = £3.59. Label: 21, counselling, see above

*Capsules*, bromocriptine (as mesylate) 5 mg (blue/white), net price 20 = £7.04; 10 mg, 20 = £13.03. Label: 21, counselling, hypotensive reactions

## 6.7.2 Danazol, gestrinone and nafarelin

**Danazol** inhibits pituitary gonadotrophins; it combines androgenic activity with antioestrogenic and antiprogestogenic activity. It is used in the treatment of *endometriosis* and has also been used for *menorrhagia* and other *menstrual disorders*, *mammary dysplasia*, and *gynaecomastia* where other measures proved unsatisfactory. It may also be effective in the long-term management of *hereditary angioedema*.

**Gestrinone** has general actions similar to those of danazol and has recently been introduced for the treatment of endometriosis.

**Nafarelin**, a gonadotrophin-releasing hormone analogue, "down-regulates" pituitary gonadotrophin secretion, leading to inhibition of ovarian steroid secretion. It is thus effective in the treatment of endometriosis.

## DANAZOL

*Indications:* see notes above and under Dose

*Cautions:* cardiac, hepatic, or renal impairment (avoid if severe), elderly, polycythaemia, epilepsy, diabetes mellitus, hypertension, migraine, lipoprotein disorder, history of thrombosis; withdraw if virilisation (may be irreversible on continued use); non-hormonal contraceptive methods should be used, if appropriate; **interactions:** Appendix 1 (danazol)

*Contra-indications:* pregnancy, ensure that patients with amenorrhoea are not pregnant; breast-feeding; severe hepatic, renal or cardiac impairment; thrombo-embolic disease; uninvestigated vaginal bleeding; androgen-dependent tumours; porphyria (see section 9.8.2)

*Side-effects:* nausea, dizziness, rashes, backache, nervousness, headache, weight gain; menstrual disturbances, flushing and reduction in breast size; skeletal muscle spasm, hair loss; androgenic effects including acne, oily skin, oedema, hirsutism, voice changes and rarely clitoral hypertrophy (see also Cautions); insulin resistance; leucopenia and thrombocytopenia reported; benign intracranial hypertension and visual disturbances also reported; rarely cholestatic jaundice

*Dose:* usual range 200–800 mg daily in up to 4 divided doses; in women all doses should start during menstruation, preferably on the first day Endometriosis, initially 400 mg daily in up to 4 divided doses, adjusted according to response, usually for 6 months

Menorrhagia, 200 mg daily, usually for 3 months

Severe cyclical mastalgia, 200–300 mg daily usually for 3–6 months

Benign breast cysts 300 mg daily usually for 3–6 months

Gynaecomastia, 400 mg daily in divided doses for 6 months (adolescents 200 mg daily, increased to 400 mg daily if no response after 2 months)

CHILD, precocious puberty, no longer recommended

PoM **Danazol** (Non-proprietary)

*Capsules*, danazol 100 mg, net price 20 = £5.55; 200 mg, 20 = £10.98

Available from Generics

PoM **Danol**® (Sanofi Winthrop)

*Capsules*, danazol 100 mg (grey/white), net price 50-cap pack = £15.40; 200 mg (pink/white), 56-cap pack = £33.83.

## GESTRINONE

*Indications:* endometriosis

*Cautions; Contra-indications; Side-effects:* see under Danazol; **Interactions:** Appendix 1 (gestrinone)

*Dose:* 2.5 mg twice weekly starting on first day of cycle with second dose 3 days later, repeated on same two days preferably at same time each week; duration of treatment usually 6 months
MISSED DOSES. one missed dose — 2.5 mg as soon as possible and maintain original sequence; two or more missed doses — discontinue, re-start on first day of new cycle (following negative pregnancy test)

▼ PoM **Dimetriose**® (Roussel)

*Capsules*, gestrinone 2.5 mg, net price 8-cap pack = £75.00

## NAFARELIN

*Indications:* endometriosis

*Cautions:* ovarian cysts; non-hormonal method of contraception should be used throughout treatment

*Contra-indications:* pregnancy, breast-feeding; undiagnosed vaginal bleeding

*Side-effects:* hot flushes, vaginal dryness, change in libido, headache, emotional lability, myalgia, decreased breast size, irritation of nasal mucosa; rarely sensitivity reactions such as shortness of breath, chest pain, urticaria, rash, pruritus; ovarian cysts (may require withdrawal); decrease in trabecular bone density (repeat courses not recommended)

*Dose:* 200 micrograms twice daily as one spray in one nostril in the morning and one spray in the other nostril in the evening starting between second and fourth day of menstrual cycle, max. duration of treatment 6 months

▼ PoM **Synarel**® (Syntex)

*Nasal spray*, nafarelin 200 micrograms (as acetate)/metered spray. Net price 60-dose unit = £101.35. Label: 10 patient information leaflet

---

### 6.7.3 Metyrapone and trilostane

**Metyrapone** is a competitive inhibitor of 11β-hydroxylation in the adrenal cortex; the resulting inhibition of cortisol production leads to an increase in ACTH production which, in turn, leads to increased synthesis and release of cortisol precursors. It may be used as a test of anterior pituitary function.

Although most types of *Cushing's syndrome* are treated surgically, that which occasionally accompanies carcinoma of the bronchus is not usually amenable to surgery. Metyrapone has been found helpful in controlling the symptoms of the disease; it is also used in other forms of Cushing's syndrome to prepare the patient for surgery. The dosages used are either low, and tailored to cortisol production, or high, in which case corticosteroid replacement therapy is also needed.

**Trilostane** inhibits the synthesis of mineralocorticoids and glucocorticoids by the adrenal cortex, and may be useful in Cushing's syndrome and primary hyperaldosteronism. It appears to be less effective than metyrapone for Cushing's syndrome.

See also aminoglutethimide (section 8.3.4).

### METYRAPONE

*Indications:* see under Dose

*Cautions:* gross hypopituitarism (risk of precipitating acute adrenal failure); many drugs interfere with estimation of steroids

*Contra-indications:* pregnancy, breast-feeding

*Side-effects:* occasional nausea, vomiting, dizziness, headache, hypotension

*Dose:* in the assessment of pituitary function 750 mg every 4 hours for 6 doses; CHILD 15 mg/kg (minimum 250 mg) every 4 hours for 6 doses
Management of Cushing's syndrome, range 0.25–6 g daily, tailored to cortisol production; see also section 6.3.1
Resistant oedema due to increased aldosterone secretion in cirrhosis, nephrosis, and congestive heart failure, 2.5–4.5 g daily in divided doses (with a glucocorticoid)
*Note.* Metyrapone should only be used under specialist advice; corticosteroid replacement therapy needed with high doses

PoM **Metopirone**® (Ciba)
*Capsules*, metyrapone 250 mg. Net price 20 = £4.18. Label: 21

### TRILOSTANE

*Indications:* see notes above

*Cautions:* impaired liver and kidney function, monitor circulating corticosteroids and blood-electrolyte concentrations; non-hormonal contraceptive methods should be used, if appropriate; **interactions:** Appendix 1 (trilostane)

*Contra-indications:* pregnancy

*Side-effects:* rarely flushing, nausea, rhinorrhoea with high doses

*Dose:* 60 mg 4 times daily for at least 3 days, then adjusted according to patient's response; usual dose range 120–480 mg daily in divided doses

PoM **Modrenal**® (Farillon)
*Capsules*, pink/black, trilostane 60 mg. Net price 20 = £7.92

# 7: Drugs used in
# OBSTETRICS, GYNAECOLOGY, and URINARY-TRACT DISORDERS

In this chapter, drugs are discussed under the following headings:

**7.1** Drugs used in obstetrics
**7.2** Treatment of vaginal and vulval conditions
**7.3** Contraceptives
**7.4** Drugs for genito-urinary disorders
**7.5** Appliances for urinary disorders

For hormonal therapy of gynaecological disorders see sections 6.4.1 and 6.5.1.

## 7.1 Drugs used in obstetrics

**7.1.1** Prostaglandins and oxytocics
**7.1.2** Mifepristone
**7.1.3** Myometrial relaxants

> *Note.* Because of the complexity of dosage regimens in obstetrics, in all cases detailed specialist literature should be consulted.

### 7.1.1 Prostaglandins and oxytocics

Prostaglandins and oxytocics are used to induce abortion or induce or augment labour and to minimise blood loss from the placental site. They include oxytocin, ergometrine, and the prostaglandins. All induce uterine contractions with varying degrees of pain according to the strength of contractions induced.

INDUCTION OF ABORTION. **Dinoprostone**, given by the *extra-amniotic* route is the preferred prostaglandin for the induction of late therapeutic abortion. Extra-amniotic **dinoprostone** is also of value as an adjunct in 'priming' the cervix prior to suction termination but is less commonly used nowadays.

**Gemeprost** is a prostaglandin available in the form of pessaries to ripen and soften the cervix before induction of abortion, particularly in primigravida.

INDUCTION AND AUGMENTATION OF LABOUR. **Oxytocin** (Syntocinon®) is administered by slow intravenous infusion, preferably using an infusion pump, to induce or augment labour, often in conjunction with amniotomy. Uterine activity must be monitored carefully and hyperstimulation avoided. Large doses of oxytocin may result in excessive fluid retention.

**Dinoprostone** is available as vaginal tablets and vaginal gels for the induction of labour at term. The intravenous and oral routes are rarely used.

PREVENTION AND TREATMENT OF HAEMORRHAGE. Bleeding due to *incomplete abortion* can be controlled with **ergometrine** and **oxytocin** (Syntometrine®) given intravenously or intramuscularly, the dose being adjusted according to the patient's condition and blood loss. This is commonly used prior to surgical evacuation of the uterus, particularly when surgery is delayed. Oxytocin and ergometrine combined are more effective in early pregnancy than either drug alone.

For the routine management of the *third stage of labour* ergometrine 500 micrograms with oxytocin 5 units (Syntometrine® 1 mL) is given by intramuscular injection with or after delivery of the shoulders. Intravenous injection is recommended for the prevention of postpartum haemorrhage in *high-risk cases*, giving either ergometrine 125–250 micrograms alone *or* oxytocin 5–10 units alone, after delivery of the shoulders (repeated if necessary); alternatively intravenous infusion of oxytocin 10–20 units/ 500 mL can be given after delivery of the shoulders, particularly when the uterus is *atonic*. If these measures are ineffective the use of **carboprost** is considered.

In domiciliary obstetric practice small secondary postpartum haemorrhage may be treated with **ergometrine** by mouth in a dose of 500 micrograms three times daily for 3 days.

## CARBOPROST

*Indications:* postpartum haemorrhage due to uterine atony in patients unresponsive to ergometrine and oxytocin

*Cautions:* history of glaucoma or raised intra-ocular pressure, asthma, hypertension, hypotension, anaemia, jaundice, diabetes, history of epilepsy, uterine scars; excessive dosage may cause uterine rupture

*Contra-indications:* acute pelvic inflammatory disease, cardiac, renal, pulmonary, or hepatic disease

*Side-effects:* nausea, vomiting and diarrhoea, hyperthermia and flushing, bronchospasm; less frequent effects include raised blood pressure, dyspnoea, and pulmonary oedema; chills, headache, diaphoresis, dizziness, and erythema and pain at injection site also reported

*Dose: by deep intramuscular injection*, 250 micrograms repeated if necessary at intervals of 1½ hours (in severe cases the interval may be reduced but should not be less than 15 minutes); total dose should not exceed 12 mg (48 doses)

▼ PoM **Hemabate**® (Upjohn)
*Injection*, carboprost as trometamol salt (tromethamine salt) 250 micrograms/mL, net price 1-mL amp = £16.50 (hosp. only)

---

# DINOPROSTONE

*Indications:* see notes above

*Cautions:* asthma, glaucoma and raised intra-ocular pressure; excessive dosage may cause uterine rupture; continuous administration for more than 2 days not recommended; see also notes above

*Contra-indications:* hypertonic uterine inertia, mechanical obstruction of delivery, placenta praevia, predisposition to uterine rupture, severe toxaemia, untreated pelvic infection, fetal distress, grand multiparas and multiple pregnancy, prior history of difficult or traumatic delivery; avoid extra-amniotic route in cervicitis or vaginitis

*Side-effects:* nausea, vomiting, diarrhoea, flushing, shivering, headache, dizziness, temporary pyrexia and raised white blood cell count, uterine hypertonus, unduly severe uterine contractions; all dose-related and more common after intravenous administration; also local tissue reaction and erythema after intravenous administration

*Dose:* see under Preparations, below

IMPORTANT. Do not confuse dose of **Prostin E2**® vaginal **gel** with that of **Prostin E2**® vaginal **tablets**—not bioequivalent. In addition, do not confuse **Prostin E2**® vaginal gel with **Prepidil**® cervical gel—different site of administration and different indication—see under Preparations, below.

PoM **Prepidil**® (Upjohn)

*Cervical gel*, dinoprostone 200 micrograms/mL in disposable syringe. Net price 2.5-mL syringe (500 micrograms) = £14.12

*Dose:* by cervix, pre-induction cervical softening and dilation, inserted into cervical canal (just below level of internal cervical os), 500 micrograms [single dose gel]

PoM **Prostin E2**® (Upjohn)

*Tablets,* dinoprostone 500 micrograms. Net price 10-tab pack = £14.93 (hosp. only)

*Dose:* by mouth, induction of labour, 500 micrograms, followed by 0.5–1 mg (max. 1.5 mg) at hourly intervals

*Intravenous solution,* for dilution and use as an infusion, dinoprostone 1 mg/mL, net price 0.75-mL amp = £7.43; 10 mg/mL, 0.5-mL amp = £16.05 (both hosp. only; rarely used, see data sheet for dose and indications)

*Extra-amniotic solution,* dinoprostone 10 mg/mL. Net price 0.5-mL amp (with diluent) = £16.05 (hosp. only; less commonly used nowadays, see data sheet for dose and indications)

*Vaginal gel,* dinoprostone 400 micrograms/mL, net price 2.5 mL (1 mg) = £14.52; 800 micrograms/mL, 2.5 mL (2 mg) = £16.00

*Dose:* by vagina, induction of labour, inserted high into posterior fornix (avoid administration into cervical canal), 1 mg (unfavourable primigravida 2 mg), followed after 6 hours by 1–2 mg if required; max. [gel] 3 mg (unfavourable primigravida 4 mg)

*Vaginal tablets,* dinoprostone 3 mg. Net price 8-vaginal tab pack = £65.04

*Dose:* by vagina, induction of labour, inserted high into posterior fornix, 3 mg, followed after 6–8 hours by 3 mg if labour is not established; max. 6 mg [vaginal tablets]

*Note.* Prostin E2 Vaginal Gel and Vaginal Tablets are **not** bioequivalent

# DINOPROST

*Indications:* see notes above

*Cautions; Contra-indications; Side-effects:* see under Dinoprostone and notes above

PoM **Prostin F2 alpha**® (Upjohn)

*Intra-amniotic injection,* dinoprost 5 mg (as trometamol salt)/mL. Net price 4-mL amp = £19.71 (hosp. only; rarely used, see data sheet for dose and indications)

# ERGOMETRINE MALEATE

*Indications:* active management of third stage of labour, postpartum haemorrhage

*Cautions:* toxaemia, cardiac disease, hypertension, sepsis, multiple pregnancy; porphyria (see section 9.8.2)

*Contra-indications:* 1st and 2nd stages of labour, vascular disease, impaired pulmonary, hepatic, and renal function

*Side-effects:* nausea, vomiting, transient hypertension, vasoconstriction

*Dose: by mouth,* 0.5–1 mg (onset about 8 minutes, duration about 1 hour); see also notes above

*By intramuscular injection,* 200–500 micrograms (onset about 5–7 minutes, duration about 45 minutes)

*By intravenous injection* for emergency control of haemorrhage, 100–500 micrograms (onset about 1 minute)

See also notes above

PoM **Ergometrine Tablets,** ergometrine maleate 250 micrograms, net price 20 = £1.50; 500 micrograms, 20 = £1.69

PoM **Ergometrine Injection,** ergometrine maleate 500 micrograms/mL. Net price 1-mL amp = 29p

Combined preparation

PoM **Syntometrine**® (Sandoz)

*Injection,* ergometrine maleate 500 micrograms, oxytocin 5 units/mL. Net price 1-mL amp = 19p

*Dose:* by intramuscular injection, 1 mL; by intravenous injection, 0.5–1 mL

# GEMEPROST

*Indications:* see under Dose

*Cautions:* obstructive airways disease, cardiovascular insufficiency, raised intra-ocular pressure, cervicitis or vaginitis

*Side-effects:* vaginal bleeding and uterine pain; nausea, vomiting, or diarrhoea; headache, muscle weakness, dizziness, flushing, chills, backache, dyspnoea, chest pain, palpitations and mild pyrexia; uterine rupture reported (most commonly in multiparas or if history of uterine surgery)

*Dose: by vagina* in pessaries, softening and dilation of the cervix to facilitate transcervical operative procedures in first trimester, 1 mg 3 hours before surgery

Second trimester abortion, 1 mg every 3 hours for max. of 5 administrations; second course may begin 24 hours after start of treatment
Second trimester intra-uterine death, 1 mg every 3 hours for max. of 5 administrations only; monitor for coagulopathy

PoM **Cervagem**® (Farillon)
*Pessaries*, gemeprost 1 mg. Net price 1 pessary = £20.96

## OXYTOCIN

*Indications:* see under Dose
*Cautions:* hypertension, pressor drugs (may precipitate severe hypertension), multiple pregnancy, high parity, previous Caesarean section
*Contra-indications:* hypertonic uterine action, mechanical obstruction to delivery, failed trial labour, severe toxaemia, predisposition to amniotic fluid embolism, fetal distress, and placenta praevia
*Side-effects:* high doses cause violent uterine contractions leading to rupture and fetal asphyxiation, arrhythmias, maternal hypertension and subarachnoid haemorrhage, water intoxication
*Dose: by slow intravenous infusion*, induction of labour and augmentation of labour in hypotonic uterine inertia, as a solution containing 1 unit per litre, 1–3 milliunits per minute, adjusted according to response
Missed abortion, as a solution containing 10–20 units/500 mL given at a rate of 10–30 drops/minute, increased in strength by 10–20 units/500 mL every hour to a max. strength of 100 units/500 mL
Postpartum haemorrhage, see notes above

PoM **Syntocinon**® (Sandoz)
*Injection*, oxytocin 1 unit/mL, net price 2-mL amp = 18p; 5 units/mL, 1-mL amp = 20p; 10 units/mL, 1-mL amp = 23p, 5-mL amp = 84p

Combined preparation—see Syntometrine

## 7.1.1.1 DUCTUS ARTERIOSUS

MAINTENANCE OF PATENCY
**Alprostadil** (prostaglandin $E_1$) is used to maintain patency of the ductus arteriosus in neonates with congenital heart defects, prior to corrective surgery in centres where intensive care is immediately available.

## ALPROSTADIL

*Indications:* congenital heart defects in neonates prior to corrective surgery
*Cautions:* see notes above; history of haemorrhage, avoid in hyaline membrane disease, monitor arterial pressure
*Side-effects:* apnoea (particularly in infants under 2 kg), flushing, bradycardia, hypotension, tachycardia, cardiac arrest, oedema, diarrhoea, fever, convulsions, disseminated intravascular coagulation, hypokalaemia; cortical proliferation of long bones, weakening of the wall of the ductus arteriosus and pulmonary artery may follow prolonged use

*Dose: by intravenous infusion*, initially 50–100 nanograms/kg/minute, then decreased to lowest effective dose

PoM **Prostin VR**® (Upjohn)
*Intravenous solution*, alprostadil 500 micrograms/mL in alcohol. For dilution and use as an infusion. Net price 1-mL amp = £56.96 (hosp. only)

CLOSURE OF DUCTUS ARTERIOSUS
Prostaglandin $E_1$ has the role of dilating the ductus arteriosus; indomethacin is believed to close it by inhibiting prostaglandin synthesis.

## INDOMETHACIN

*Indications:* patent ductus arteriosus in premature infants (under specialist supervision)
*Cautions:* may mask symptoms of infection; may reduce renal function by 50% or more and precipitate renal insufficiency especially in infants with heart failure, sepsis, or hepatic impairment, or who are receiving nephrotoxic drugs; if urine volume reduced, discontinue until output returns to normal; may induce hyponatraemia; monitor renal function and electrolytes
*Contra-indications:* untreated infection, bleeding, congenital heart disease where patency of ductus arteriosus necessary for satisfactory pulmonary or systemic blood flow; thrombocytopenia, coagulation defects, necrotising enterocolitis, renal impairment
*Side-effects:* include haemorrhagic, renal, gastrointestinal, metabolic, and coagulation disorders; fluid retention, and exacerbation of infection
*Dose: by intravenous injection*, over 5–10 seconds, 3 doses at intervals of 12–24 hours, age less than 48 hours, 200 micrograms/kg then 100 micrograms/kg then 100 micrograms/kg; age 2–7 days, 200 micrograms/kg then 200 micrograms/kg then 200 micrograms/kg; age over 7 days, 200 micrograms/kg then 250 micrograms/kg then 250 micrograms/kg; solution prepared with 1–2 mL sodium chloride 0.9% or water for injections (not glucose and no preservatives)
If ductus arteriosus reopens a second course of 3 injections may be given

PoM **Indocid PDA**® (Morson)
*Injection*, powder for reconstitution, indomethacin (as sodium trihydrate). Net price 3 × 1-mg vials = £22.50 (hosp. only)

## 7.1.2   Mifepristone

## MIFEPRISTONE

*Indications:* medical alternative to surgical termination of intra-uterine pregnancy of up to 63 days gestation (based on first day of last menstrual period and/or ultrasound scan)
*Cautions:* asthma, chronic obstructive airways disease; cardiovascular disease or risk factors; prosthetic heart valves or history of infective endocarditis (prophylaxis recommended, see section 5.1 table 2); not recommended in hepatic or renal impairment; avoid aspirin and NSAIDs for at least 8–12 days after mifepristone administration

*Contra-indications:* pregnancy of 64 days gestation and over, suspected ectopic pregnancy; chronic adrenal failure, long-term corticosteroid therapy, haemorrhagic disorders and anticoagulant therapy; women over 35 years, moderate or heavy smokers (smoking and alcohol must be avoided after taking and for at least 2 days after the gemeprost pessary); porphyria (see section 9.8.2)

*Side-effects:* vaginal bleeding (may be severe), malaise, faintness, nausea, vomiting, rashes; uterine pain after gemeprost (may be severe and require parenteral opioids); uterine and urinary-tract infections reported

*Dose: by mouth,* 600 mg in a single dose in presence of doctor and observed for at least 2 hours after administration; followed 36–48 hours later (unless abortion already complete) by gemeprost 1 mg *by vagina* as pessaries, observed for at least 6 hours after insertion with follow-up visit 8–12 days later (if treatment fails essential that pregnancy be terminated by another method)

Note. Careful monitoring essential for 6 hours after administration of gemeprost pessary (risk of profound hypotension)

▼ PoM **Mifegyne**® (Roussel)

*Tablets,* yellow, mifepristone 200 mg. Net price 3-tab pack = £42.90 (supplied to NHS hospitals and premises approved under Abortion Act 1967). Label: 10 patient information leaflet

## 7.1.3 Myometrial relaxants

Beta$_2$-adrenoceptor stimulants (sympathomimetics) relax uterine muscle and are used in selected cases in an attempt to inhibit *premature labour.*

They should not be used unless a clear benefit is likely. Tachycardia is the commonest side-effect and may be extreme if atropine is also administered.

Drugs used in the treatment of *spasmodic dysmenorrhoea* include aspirin and some other NSAIDs (see section 4.7.1). See section 6.4.1.1 for hormone treatment.

## ISOXSUPRINE HYDROCHLORIDE

*Indications:* uncomplicated premature labour

*Cautions:* may cause hypotension in the newborn; see notes above

*Contra-indications:* recent arterial haemorrhage, heart disease, premature detachment of placenta, severe anaemia, infection

*Side-effects:* hypotension, tachycardia, flushing, nausea, vomiting

*Dose: by intravenous infusion,* initially 200–300 micrograms/minute gradually increased to 500 micrograms/minute until labour is arrested; subsequently *by intramuscular injection,* 10 mg every 3 hours for 24 hours, then every 4–6 hours for 48 hours

PoM **Duvadilan**® (Duphar)

*Injection,* isoxsuprine hydrochloride 5 mg/mL. Net price 2-mL amp = 35p

## RITODRINE HYDROCHLORIDE

*Indications:* uncomplicated premature labour; fetal asphyxia due to hypertonic uterine action

*Cautions:* diabetes mellitus (monitor blood sugar during intravenous treatment), cardiac disorders, thyrotoxicosis, treatment with corticosteroids, anaesthetics, potassium-depleting diuretics (depresses potassium plasma concentrations); monitor blood pressure and pulse; **interactions:** Appendix 1 (sympathomimetics, beta$_2$)

*Contra-indications:* haemorrhage, hypertension, pre-eclampsia, cord compression, infection

*Side-effects:* nausea, vomiting, flushing, sweating, tremor; hypokalaemia, tachycardia and hypotension with high doses

*Dose: by intravenous infusion,* premature labour, initially 50 micrograms/minute, gradually increased to 150–350 micrograms/minute and continued for 12–48 hours after contractions have ceased; or *by intramuscular injection,* 10 mg every 3–8 hours continued for 12–48 hours after contractions have ceased; then *by mouth,* 10 mg 30 minutes before termination of intravenous infusion, repeated every 2 hours for 24 hours, followed by 10–20 mg every 4–6 hours, max. 120 mg daily

Fetal asphyxia due to hypertonic uterine action, *by intravenous infusion,* 50 micrograms/minute increased as necessary to a max. of 350 micrograms/minute, while preparations are made for delivery

PoM **Yutopar**® (Duphar)

*Tablets,* buff, scored, ritodrine hydrochloride 10 mg. Net price 90-tab pack = £19.80

*Injection,* ritodrine hydrochloride 10 mg/mL. Net price 5-mL amp = £2.15

## SALBUTAMOL

*Indications:* uncomplicated premature labour

*Cautions; Contra-indications; Side-effects:* see under Ritodrine Hydrochloride

*Dose: by intravenous infusion,* 10 micrograms/minute gradually increased to max. of 45 micrograms/minute until contractions have ceased, then gradually reduced; or *by intravenous or intramuscular injection,* 100–250 micrograms repeated according to patient's response; subsequently *by mouth* 4 mg every 6–8 hours

**Preparations:** see section 3.1.1.1

## TERBUTALINE SULPHATE

*Indications:* uncomplicated premature labour

*Cautions; Contra-indications; Side-effects:* see under Ritodrine Hydrochloride

*Dose: by intravenous infusion,* 10 micrograms/minute (as a 0.0005% solution) for 1 hour, gradually increased to a max. of 25 micrograms/minute until contractions have ceased, then reduced; subsequently *by subcutaneous injection,* 250 micrograms every 6 hours for 3 days, and *by mouth,* 5 mg every 8 hours until 37th week of pregnancy

**Preparations**
See section 3.1.1.1

# 7.2   Treatment of vaginal and vulval conditions

**7.2.1** Topical hormones
**7.2.2** Anti-infective drugs

Preparations for topical application to the vulva and vagina include pessaries, creams, and medicated tampons.

Symptoms are primarily referable to the vulva, but infections almost invariably involve the vagina which should also be treated. Applications to the vulva alone are likely to give only symptomatic relief without cure.

*Aqueous medicated douches* may disturb normal vaginal acidity and bacterial flora.

*Topical anaesthetic agents* give only symptomatic relief and may cause sensitivity reactions. They are indicated only in cases of pruritus where specific local causes have been excluded.

*Systemic drugs* are required in the treatment of infections such as gonorrhoea and syphilis (see section 5.1).

## 7.2.1   Topical hormones

Application of cream containing an oestrogen may be used on a short-term basis to improve the quality of the vaginal epithelium in menopausal atrophic vaginitis. For further comment see section 6.4.1.1.

Topical oestrogens are also used prior to vaginal surgery in postmenopausal women for prolapse when there is epithelial atrophy.

> Topical oestrogens should be used in the minimum effective amount and treatment discontinued as soon as possible to minimise absorption of the oestrogen.

## OESTROGENS, TOPICAL

*Indications:* see notes above
*Cautions; Contra-indications; Side-effects:* see Ethinyloestradiol (section 6.4.1.1); contra-indicated in pregnancy and lactation; discontinue treatment and examine patients periodically to assess need for further treatment

PoM **Ortho® Dienoestrol** (Cilag)
*Cream*, dienoestrol 0.01%. Net price 78 g with applicator = £2.61
Insert 1–2 applicatorfuls daily for 1–2 weeks, then gradually reduced to 1 applicatorful 1–3 times weekly if necessary; attempts to reduce or discontinue should be made at 3–6 month intervals with re-examination

PoM **Ortho-Gynest®** (Cilag)
*Intravaginal cream*, oestriol 0.01%. Net price 78 g with applicator = £5.40
Insert 1 applicatorful daily, preferably in evening; reduced to 1 applicatorful twice a week; attempts to reduce or discontinue should be made at 3–6 month intervals with re-examination

*Pessaries*, oestriol 500 micrograms. Net price 15 pessaries = £5.29
Insert 1 pessary daily, preferably in the evening, until improvement occurs; maintenance 1 pessary twice a week; attempts to reduce or discontinue should be made at 3–6 month intervals with re-examination

PoM **Ovestin®** (Organon)
*Intravaginal cream*, oestriol 0.1%. Net price 15 g with applicator = £4.74
Insert 1 applicator-dose daily for 2–3 weeks, then reduce to twice a week (discontinue every 2–3 months for 4 weeks to assess need for further treatment); postmenopausal surgery, 1 applicator-dose daily for 2 weeks, resuming 2 weeks after surgery

PoM **Premarin®** (Wyeth)
*Vaginal cream*, conjugated oestrogens 625 micrograms/g. Net price 42.5 g with calibrated applicator = £2.19
Insert 1–2 g daily, starting on 5th day of cycle, for 3 weeks, followed by 1-week interval; if therapy long term, oral progestogen for 10–12 days at end of each cycle essential

PoM **Tampovagan® Stilboestrol and Lactic Acid** (Norgine)
*Pessaries*, stilboestrol 500 micrograms, lactic acid 5%. Net price 10 pessaries = £8.28
Insert 2 pessaries at night for 1–2 weeks then reduce (short-term only, see notes above)

PoM **Vagifem®** (Novo Nordisk)
*Vaginal tablets*, f/c, m/r, oestradiol 25 micrograms in disposable applicators. Net price 15-applicator pack = £14.99
Insert 1 tablet daily for 2 weeks then reduce to 1 tablet twice weekly; discontinue after 3 months to assess need for further treatment

## 7.2.2   Anti-infective drugs

Effective specific treatments are available for the common vaginal infections, therefore the causal organism should be identified before starting treatment.

### FUNGAL INFECTIONS

*Vaginal candidiasis* is treated primarily with antifungal pessaries or cream inserted high into the vagina (including the time of menstruation). *Candidal vulvitis* can be treated locally with cream but is almost invariably associated with vaginal infection which should be treated as well.

**Nystatin** is a well established treatment. One or two pessaries are inserted for 14 to 28 nights; they may be supplemented with cream for vulvitis and to treat other superficial sites of infection.

**Imidazole** drugs (clotrimazole, econazole, isoconazole, and miconazole) appear to be equally effective in shorter courses of 3 to 14 days according to the preparation used; single dose preparations are also available, which is an advantage when compliance is a problem. Vaginal applications may be supplemented with cream for vulvitis and to treat other superficial sites of infection.

Recurrence is common if the full course of treatment is not completed and is also particularly likely if there are predisposing factors such as

---

antibiotic therapy, oral contraceptive use, pregnancy, or diabetes mellitus. Possible reservoirs of infection may also lead to recontamination and should be treated. These include other skin sites such as the digits, nail beds, and umbilicus as well as the gut and the bladder. The partner may also be the source of re-infection and should be treated with cream at the same time.

Oral treatment with fluconazole or itraconazole may be necessary in resistant or recurrent infection (see section 5.2); oral ketoconazole has been associated with fatal hepatotoxicity (see section 5.2 for CSM warning).

## GENITAL ANTIFUNGAL PREPARATIONS

*Indications:* vaginal and vulval candidiasis
*Side-effects:* local irritation, possibly including burning, oedema, erythema
*Administration:* insert pessaries or cream high into the vagina and complete the course regardless of intervening menstruation

**Canesten®** (Baypharm)
*Cream* (topical), clotrimazole 1%. Net price 20 g = £1.82; 50 g = £4.26
Apply to anogenital area 2–3 times daily
PoM *Vaginal cream*, clotrimazole 2%. Net price 35 g (with 5-g applicators) = £5.22
Insert 5 g twice daily for 3 days or once nightly for 6 nights
PoM *Vaginal cream (10% VC®)*, clotrimazole 10%. Net price 5-g applicator pack = £3.43
Insert 5 g at night as a single dose
PoM *Vaginal tablets*, clotrimazole 100 mg, net price 6 tabs with applicator = £2.64; 200 mg, 3 tabs with applicator = £2.58
Insert 200 mg for 3 nights *or* 100 mg for 6 nights
PoM *Vaginal tablets (Canesten 1®)*, clotrimazole 500 mg. Net price 1 with applicator = £2.58
Insert 1 at night as a single dose
PoM *Duopak*, clotrimazole 100-mg vaginal tablets and cream (topical) 1%. Net price 6 tabs and 20 g cream = £4.35

**Ecostatin®** (Squibb)
*Cream* (topical), econazole nitrate 1%. Net price 15 g = £1.49; 30 g = £2.75
Apply to anogenital area twice daily
PoM *Pessaries*, econazole nitrate 150 mg. Net price 3 with applicator = £3.96
Insert 1 pessary for 3 nights
PoM *Pessary (Ecostatin 1®)*, econazole nitrate 150 mg. Net price 1 pessary with applicator = £4.40
Insert 1 pessary at night as a single dose
PoM *Twinpack*, econazole nitrate 150-mg pessaries and cream 1%. Net price 3 pessaries and 15 g cream = £4.98

PoM **Flagyl Compak®**, see section 5.1.11

PoM **Gyno-Daktarin®** (Janssen)
*Intravaginal cream*, miconazole nitrate 2%. Net price 78 g with applicators = £4.95
Insert two 5-g applicatorfuls at night for 7 nights; *topical*, apply to anogenital area twice daily

*Pessaries*, miconazole nitrate 100 mg. Net price 14 = £4.04
Insert 2 pessaries for 7 nights
*Tampons*, coated with miconazole nitrate 100 mg. Net price 10 = £3.83
Insert 1 tampon night and morning for 5 days
*Combipack*, miconazole nitrate 100-mg pessaries and cream (topical) 2%. Net price 14 pessaries and 15 g cream = £5.94
*Ovule* (= vaginal capsule) *(Gyno-Daktarin 1®)*, miconazole nitrate 1.2 g in a fatty basis. Net price 1 ovule (with finger stall) = £3.95
Insert 1 ovule at night as a single dose

PoM **Gyno-Pevaryl®** (Cilag)
*Cream*, econazole nitrate 1%. Net price 15 g = £1.74; 30 g = £3.45
Apply to anogenital area 2–3 times daily for 14 days
*Pessaries*, econazole nitrate 150 mg with applicator. Net price 3 = £3.17
Insert 1 pessary for 3 nights
*Pessary (Gyno-Pevaryl 1®)*, econazole nitrate 150 mg (formulated for single-dose therapy). Net price 1 = £4.40
Insert 1 pessary at night as a single dose
*Combipack*, econazole nitrate 150-mg pessaries, econazole nitrate 1% cream (to be applied to anogenital area). Net price 3 pessaries and 15 g cream = £4.98
*CP pack (Gyno-Pevaryl 1®)*, econazole nitrate 150-mg pessary, econazole nitrate 1% cream (to be applied to anogenital area). Net price 1 pessary and 15 g cream = £5.84

PoM **Nizoral®** (Janssen)
*Cream* (topical), ketoconazole 2%. Net price 30 g = £3.81
Apply to anogenital area once or twice daily

PoM **Nystan®** (Squibb)
*Cream* and *Ointment*, see section 13.10.2
*Gel* (topical), nystatin 100 000 units/g. Net price 30 g = £2.66
Apply to anogenital area 2–4 times daily
*Vaginal cream*, nystatin 100 000 units/4-g application. Net price 60 g with applicator = £3.26
*Pessaries*, yellow, nystatin 100 000 units. Net price 28-pessary pack = £1.96
Insert 1–2 applicatorfuls of cream or 1–2 pessaries at night for at least 14 nights

**Pevaryl®** (Cilag)
*Cream*, econazole nitrate 1%. Net price 30 g = £2.65
Apply to anogenital area 2–3 times daily
*Lotion* and *Dusting powder*, see section 13.10.2

PoM **Travogyn®** (Schering Health Care)
*Cream* (topical), isoconazole nitrate 1%. Net price 20 g = £1.88
Apply to anogenital area twice daily
*Vaginal tablets* (=pessaries), isoconazole nitrate 300 mg. Net price 2 = £3.90
Insert 2 pessaries as a single dose preferably at night

---

## OTHER INFECTIONS

Vaginal preparations intended to restore normal acidity (Aci-Jel®) may prevent recurrence of vaginal infections and permit the re-establishment of the normal vaginal flora.

*Trichomonal infections* commonly involve the lower urinary tract as well as the genital system and need systemic treatment with metronidazole, nimorazole, or tinidazole (see sections 5.4.2 and 5.4.3).

*Bacterial infections* with Gram-negative organisms are particularly common in association with gynaecological operations and trauma. Metronidazole is effective against certain Gram-positive organisms, especially *Bacteroides* spp. and may be used prophylactically in gynaecological surgery.

Antibacterial creams such as Sultrin® are used in the treatment of mixed bacterial infections but are of unproven value; they are ineffective against *Candida* spp. and *Trichomonas vaginalis*.

Acyclovir may be used in the treatment of genital infection due to *herpes simplex virus*, the HSV type 2 being a major cause of genital ulceration. It has a beneficial effect on virus shedding and healing, generally giving relief from pain and other symptoms. See section 5.3 for systemic preparations, and section 13.10.3 for cream.

## PREPARATIONS FOR OTHER VAGINAL INFECTIONS

**Aci-Jel®** (Cilag)

*Vaginal jelly*, acetic acid 0.92% in a buffered (pH 4) basis. Net price 85 g with applicator = £3.37

Non-specific infections, insert 1 applicatorful twice daily to restore vaginal acidity

**Betadine®** (Napp)

*Caution:* avoid in pregnancy (and if planned) and in breast-feeding

*Side-effects:* rarely sensitivity; may interfere with thyroid function

*Vaginal Cleansing Kit*, solution, povidone-iodine 10%. Net price 250 mL with measuring bottle and applicator = £2.78

To be diluted and used once daily, preferably in the morning; may be used with Betadine® pessaries or vaginal gel

*Pessaries*, brown, povidone-iodine 200 mg. Net price 28 pessaries with applicator = £5.11

*Vaginal gel*, brown, povidone-iodine 10%. Net price 80 g with applicator = £2.33

Vaginal infections or pre-operatively, insert 1 moistened pessary night and morning for up to 14 days *or* use morning pessary with 5-g gel at night *or* morning douche with pessary (or 5-g gel) at night

PoM**Gynatren®** (Solco Basle)

Vaccine prepared from inactivated *Lactobacillus acidophilus*. Net price 3 × 0.5-mL amp = £16.00

*Dose:* for recurrent trichomoniasis, by intramuscular injection, 3 doses each of 0.5 mL separated by intervals of 2 weeks

PoM**Sultrin®** (Cilag)

*Indications:* bacterial vaginitis and cervicitis

*Contra-indications:* pregnancy

*Side-effects:* sensitivity

*Cream*, sulphathiazole 3.42%, sulphacetamide 2.86%, sulphabenzamide 3.7%. Net price 78 g with applicator = £3.48

*Vaginal tablets*, sulphathiazole 172.5 mg, sulphacetamide 143.75 mg, sulphabenzamide 184 mg. Net price 20 with applicator = £2.94

Insert 1 pessary or applicatorful of cream twice daily for 10 days, then once daily if necessary

# 7.3    Contraceptives

7.3.1   Combined oral contraceptives
7.3.2   Progestogen-only contraceptives
7.3.3   Spermicidal contraceptives
7.3.4   Contraceptive devices

The criteria by which contraceptive methods should be judged are effectiveness, acceptability, and freedom from side-effects.

**Hormonal contraception** is the most effective method of fertility control, short of sterilisation, but has unwanted major and minor side-effects, especially for certain groups of women.

**Intra-uterine devices** have a high use-effectiveness but may produce undesirable side-effects, especially menorrhagia, or be otherwise unsuitable in a significant proportion of women; their use is generally inadvisable in nulliparous women because of the increased risk of pelvic sepsis and infertility.

**Barrier methods** alone (condoms, diaphragms, and caps) are less effective but can be very reliable for well-motivated couples if used in conjunction with a **spermicide**. Occasionally sensitivity reactions occur.

The health departments of the UK have recently issued a revised edition of the booklet, *Handbook of Contraceptive Practice*, 1990. Copies can be obtained from:

DOH Store, Health Publications Unit,
Central Store, Manchester Road,
Heywood, Lancs OL10 2PZ

## 7.3.1    Combined oral contraceptives

Oral contraceptives containing an oestrogen and a progestogen are the most effective preparations for general use. The oestrogen content ranges from 20 to 50 micrograms and generally a preparation with the lowest oestrogen and progestogen content which gives good cycle control and minimal side-effects in the individual patient is chosen.

DOSAGE. The dosage regimen for *combined oral contraceptives* is usually 1 tablet daily for 21 days, followed by a 7-day interval during which menstrual bleeding occurs. If the first course is started on the 5th day of the cycle ovulation may not be inhibited during that cycle and additional contraceptive precautions should therefore be taken during the first 7 days[1] or when changing from a high to a low oestrogen preparation. Additional contraceptive precautions are unnecessary in the first cycle if the tablets are started on the first day of the cycle as is now usually recommended.

The tablet should be taken at approximately the same time each day. If it is delayed by longer than 12 hours, contraceptive protection may be lost.

MISSED PILL. It is important to bear in mind that the critical time for loss of protection is when a pill is forgotten at the *beginning* or *end* of a cycle. The following advice is now recommended by family planning organisations:

'If you forget a pill, take it as soon as you remember, and the next one at your normal time. If you are 12 or more hours late with any pill (especially the first or last in the packet) the pill may not work. As soon as you remember, continue normal pill taking. However, you will not be protected for the next seven days and must either not have sex or use another method such as the sheath. If these seven days run beyond the end of your packet, start the next packet at once when you have finished the present one, i.e. do not have a gap between packets. This will mean you may not have a period until the end of two packets but this does you no harm. Nor does it matter if you see some bleeding on tablet-taking days. If you are using everyday (ED) pills—miss out the seven inactive pills. If you are not sure which these are, ask your doctor.'

SIDE-EFFECTS. Combined oral contraceptives carry a small risk of thrombo-embolic and cardiovascular complications. This increases with age, obesity, and cigarette smoking, and with predisposing conditions such as diabetes, hypertension, and familial hyperlipidaemia.

Hypertension may develop as the result of therapy but when it is due to contraceptive usage reversion to normotension occurs on cessation of treatment.

Critical factors which limit effectiveness are vomiting and diarrhoea and some antibiotics, for example ampicillin, which interfere with oestrogen absorption. Drugs which induce hepatic enzyme activity (e.g. barbiturates, griseofulvin, phenytoin, rifampicin) also increase the risk of failure.

---

**CSM advice.**
It is important to balance the uncertainties in relation to carcinoma of the breast against the evidence available that combined oral contraceptives protect against ovarian and endometrial carcinoma. Taking into account both the benefits and potential risks of oral contraceptive use, the CSM recommends that there is no need for a change in oral contraceptive prescribing practice on the evidence presently available.

---

CHILDBIRTH. Following childbirth oral contraception can be started at any time after 3 to 4 weeks postpartum (not earlier because of the

increased risk of thrombosis in relation to the combined pill, and of breakthrough bleeding in relation to the progestogen-only pill). If they are started later than 4 weeks postpartum extra contraceptive precautions should be taken for 7 days. Lactation may be affected by combined oral contraceptives as described in Appendix 5.

SURGERY. Oestrogen-containing oral contraceptives should be discontinued (and adequate alternative contraceptive arrangements made) 4 weeks before major elective surgery and all surgery to the legs; they should normally be recommenced at the first menses occurring at least 2 weeks after the procedure. When discontinuation is not possible, e.g. after trauma or if, by oversight, a patient admitted for an elective procedure is still on an oestrogen-containing oral contraceptive, some consideration should be given to subcutaneous heparin prophylaxis. These recommendations do not apply to minor surgery with short duration of anaesthesia, e.g. laparoscopic sterilisation or tooth extraction, or to women taking oestrogen-free hormonal contraceptives.

For hormone replacement therapy the same policy as for oestrogen-containing oral contraceptives may be appropriate, although the evidence of an increased risk is questionable. For reference to supraphysiological concentrations of oestradiol implants see section 6.4.1.

---

## ORAL CONTRACEPTIVES (Combined)

*Indications:* contraception; menstrual symptoms, see section 6.4.1.1

*Cautions:* see notes above; diabetes, hypertension, cardiac or renal disease, migraine, epilepsy, depression, asthma, immobilisation, contact lenses (may irritate), varicose veins; cigarette-smokers, patients over 35 years, obesity, breast-feeding, sickle-cell anaemia (safety not established); **interactions:** Appendix 1 (contraceptives, oral)

*Contra-indications:* pregnancy; thrombosis and history of any thrombo-embolic disease, after evacuation of hydatidiform mole (until return to normal of urine and plasma gonadotrophin values); recurrent jaundice, acute and chronic liver disease, porphyria (see section 9.8.2), Dubin-Johnson and Rotor syndromes, hyperlipidaemia, mammary or endometrial carcinoma, oestrogen-dependent tumours, severe or focal migraine, undiagnosed vaginal bleeding, history of pruritus of pregnancy or herpes gestationis, deterioration of otosclerosis

*Side-effects:* nausea, vomiting, headache, breast tenderness, changes in body weight, thrombosis (more common in blood groups A, B, and AB than O), changes in libido, depression, chloasma, hypertension, impairment of liver function, hepatic tumours, reduced menstrual loss, 'spotting' in early cycles, amenorrhoea; rarely photosensitivity

*Dose:* see notes above

---

1. Formerly 14 days but family planning organisations now consider 7 days to be enough.

---

### Ethinyloestradiol 20 micrograms

Mercilon® has been reported to give much better cycle control than Loestrin 20®. Appropriate for obese patients and for older women (provided oral contraceptive use otherwise suitable).

PoM **Loestrin 20**® (P-D)
*Tablets*, blue-grey, f/c, norethisterone acetate 1 mg, ethinyloestradiol 20 micrograms. Net price 21-tab pack = 86p
PoM **Mercilon**® (Organon)
*Tablets*, desogestrel 150 micrograms, ethinyloestradiol 20 micrograms. Net price 21-tab pack = £2.40

---

### Ethinyloestradiol 30 micrograms

Standard strength from which the initial choice is usually selected. Highly effective if the pill-free interval is not lengthened by dose omissions. Of these, Conova 30®, Eugynon 30®, and Ovran 30® are not good first choices since the others have less of the apparently unfavourable effects on plasma lipids.

PoM **Conova 30**® (Gold Cross)
*Tablets*, f/c, ethynodiol diacetate 2 mg, ethinyloestradiol 30 micrograms. Net price 21-tab pack = 80p
PoM **Eugynon 30**® (Schering Health Care)
*Tablets*, s/c, levonorgestrel 250 micrograms, ethinyloestradiol 30 micrograms. Net price 21-tab pack = 69p
PoM **Femodene**® (Schering Health Care)
*Tablets*, s/c, gestodene 75 micrograms, ethinyloestradiol 30 micrograms. Net price 21-tab pack = £1.90
PoM **Femodene ED**® (Schering Health Care)
As for Femodene and in addition 7 white placebo tablets. Net price 28-tab pack = £1.90
PoM **Loestrin 30**® (P-D)
*Tablets*, green, f/c, norethisterone acetate 1.5 mg, ethinyloestradiol 30 micrograms. Net price 21-tab pack = £1.26
PoM **Marvelon**® (Organon)
*Tablets*, desogestrel 150 micrograms, ethinyloestradiol 30 micrograms. Net price 21-tab pack = £1.48
PoM **Microgynon 30**® (Schering Health Care)
*Tablets*, beige, s/c, levonorgestrel 150 micrograms, ethinyloestradiol 30 micrograms. Net price 21-tab pack = 60p
PoM **Minulet**® (Wyeth)
*Tablets*, s/c, gestodene 75 micrograms, ethinyloestradiol 30 micrograms. Net price 21-tab pack = £1.90
PoM **Ovran 30**® (Wyeth)
*Tablets*, levonorgestrel 250 micrograms, ethinyloestradiol 30 micrograms. Net price 21-tab pack = 57p

PoM **Ovranette**® (Wyeth)
*Tablets*, levonorgestrel 150 micrograms, ethinyloestradiol 30 micrograms. Net price 21-tab pack = 62p

---

### Ethinyloestradiol 35 micrograms

In common with the 30-microgram strength (above), standard strength from which the initial choice is usually selected. Highly effective if the pill-free interval is not lengthened by dose omissions.

PoM **Brevinor**® (Syntex)
*Tablets*, norethisterone 500 micrograms, ethinyloestradiol 35 micrograms. Net price 21-tab pack = 57p
▼ PoM **Cilest**® (Cilag)
*Tablets*, blue, norgestimate 250 micrograms, ethinyloestradiol 35 micrograms. Net price 21-tab pack = £1.90
PoM **Neocon 1/35**® (Ortho)
*Tablets*, peach, norethisterone 1 mg, ethinyloestradiol 35 micrograms. Net price 21-tab pack = 76p
PoM **Norimin**® (Syntex)
*Tablets*, yellow, norethisterone 1 mg, ethinyloestradiol 35 micrograms. Net price 21-tab pack = 65p
PoM **Ovysmen**® (Ortho)
*Tablets*, norethisterone 500 micrograms, ethinyloestradiol 35 micrograms. Net price 21-tab pack = 57p

---

### Ethinyloestradiol 50 micrograms

Increased security but possibility of increased side-effects. Used mainly in circumstances of reduced bioavailability (e.g. during long-term use of enzyme-inducing antiepileptics).

PoM **Ovran**® (Wyeth)
*Tablets*, levonorgestrel 250 micrograms, ethinyloestradiol 50 micrograms. Net price 21-tab pack = 37p

---

### Mestranol 50 micrograms

In common with the ethinyloestradiol 50-microgram strength (above), increased security but possibility of increased side-effects. Used mainly in circumstances of reduced bioavailability (e.g. during long-term use of enzyme-inducing antiepileptics).

PoM **Norinyl-1**® (Syntex)
*Tablets*, norethisterone 1 mg, mestranol 50 micrograms. Net price 21-tab pack = 63p
PoM **Ortho-Novin 1/50**® (Ortho)
*Tablets*, norethisterone 1 mg, mestranol 50 micrograms. Net price 21-tab pack = 78p

---

*Phased formulations*

A little more complex for the user to take, but provide better cycle control (with low metabolic effect) than equivalent fixed-dose levonorgestrel or norethisterone formulations.

PoM **BiNovum**® (Ortho)
*Tablets*, 7 white, norethisterone 500 micrograms, ethinyloestradiol 35 micrograms; 14 peach, norethisterone 1 mg, ethinyloestradiol 35 micrograms. Net price 21-tab pack = 75p
*Dose:* 1 tablet daily for 21 days, starting with a white tablet on 1st day of cycle, and repeated after a 7-day interval

PoM **Logynon**® (Schering Health Care)
*Tablets*, all s/c, 6 light brown, levonorgestrel 50 micrograms, ethinyloestradiol 30 micrograms; 5 white, levonorgestrel 75 micrograms, ethinyloestradiol 40 micrograms; 10 ochre, levonorgestrel 125 micrograms, ethinyloestradiol 30 micrograms. Net price 21-tab pack = 95p
*Dose:* 1 tablet daily for 21 days, starting with tablet marked 1 on 1st day of cycle, and repeated after a 7-day interval

PoM **Logynon ED**® (Schering Health Care)
As for Logynon and in addition 7 white placebo tablets. Net price 28-tab pack = 95p
*Dose:* 1 tablet daily starting in red sector on 1st day of cycle continuing in sequence without interruption

PoM **Synphase**® (Syntex)
*Tablets*, 7 white, norethisterone 500 micrograms, ethinyloestradiol 35 micrograms; 9 yellow, norethisterone 1 mg, ethinyloestradiol 35 micrograms; 5 white, norethisterone 500 micrograms, ethinyloestradiol 35 micrograms. Net price 21-tab pack = £1.11
*Dose:* 1 tablet daily for 21 days, starting with tablet marked 1 on the 5th day of the cycle, and repeated after a 7-day interval

PoM **Tri-Minulet**® (Wyeth)
*Tablets*, s/c, 6 beige, gestodene 50 micrograms, ethinyloestradiol 30 micrograms; 5 dark brown, gestodene 70 micrograms, ethinyloestradiol 40 micrograms; 10 white, gestodene 100 micrograms, ethinyloestradiol 30 micrograms. Net price 21-tab pack = £2.65
*Dose:* 1 tablet daily for 21 days, starting with tablet marked 1 on the 1st day of the cycle, and repeated after a 7-day interval

PoM **Trinordiol**® (Wyeth)
*Tablets*, all s/c, 6 light brown, levonorgestrel 50 micrograms, ethinyloestradiol 30 micrograms; 5 white, levonorgestrel 75 micrograms, ethinyloestradiol 40 micrograms; 10 ochre, levonorgestrel 125 micrograms, ethinyloestradiol 30 micrograms. Net price 21-tab pack = £1.09
*Dose:* 1 tablet daily for 21 days, starting with tablet marked 1 on 1st day of cycle, and repeated after a 7-day interval

PoM **TriNovum**® (Ortho)
*Tablets*, 7 white, norethisterone 500 micrograms, ethinyloestradiol 35 micrograms; 7 light peach, norethisterone 750 micrograms, ethinyloestradiol 35 micrograms; 7 peach, norethisterone 1 mg, ethinyloestradiol 35 micrograms. Net price 21-tab pack = 94p
*Dose:* 1 tablet daily for 21 days, starting with a white tablet on 1st day of cycle, and repeated after a 7-day interval

PoM **TriNovum ED**® (Ortho)
As for TriNovum and in addition 7 green placebo tablets. Net price 28-tab pack = 99p
*Dose:* 1 tablet daily starting in the white sector on 1st day of cycle continuing in sequence without interruption

*Emergency contraception*

Combined oral contraceptives may also be given for occasional emergency use after unprotected intercourse. Two tablets of a preparation containing levonorgestrel 250 micrograms and ethinyloestradiol 50 micrograms ([1]Schering PC4®) are taken within 72 hours, and a further 2 tablets 12 hours later. The patient should be counselled on administration and should always consult her doctor approximately 3 weeks after using this treatment.

PoM **Schering PC4**® (Schering Health Care)
*Tablets*, s/c, levonorgestrel 250 micrograms, ethinyloestradiol 50 micrograms. Net price 4-tab pack = £1.40. For post-coital contraception as an occasional emergency measure; should not be administered if menstrual bleeding overdue or if unprotected intercourse occurred more than 72 hours previously
*Dose:* 2 tablets as soon as possible after coitus (up to 72 hours) then 2 tablets after 12 hours

## 7.3.2 Progestogen-only contraceptives

When oestrogens are contra-indicated, progestogen-only preparations may offer a suitable alternative but the oral preparations have a higher failure rate than combined preparations. They are suitable for older patients who may be at risk from oestrogen, heavy smokers, and those in whom oestrogens cause severe side-effects. Menstrual irregularities (oligomenorrhoea, menorrhagia) are more common but patients tend to revert to a more regular cyclical menstrual pattern on long treatment. Oral preparations are started on the 1st day of the cycle and taken every day at the same time without a break. Additional contraceptive precautions are unnecessary when initiating treatment with progestogen-only contraceptives. When changing from a combined oral contraceptive to a progestogen-only preparation treatment should start on the day following completion of the combined oral contraceptive course so that there is no break in tablet taking.

The tablet should be taken at the same time each day. If it is delayed by longer than 3 hours, contraceptive protection may be lost.

---

1. **Ovran**® (see p. 284) also contains levonorgestrel 250 micrograms and ethinyloestradiol 50 micrograms but is not licensed or packed for post-coital contraception.

MISSED PILL. The following advice is now recommended by family planning organisations:

'If you forget a pill, take it as soon as you remember and carry on with the next pill at the right time. If the pill was more than three hours overdue you are not protected. Continue normal pill-taking but you must also use another method, such as the sheath, for the next 48 hours. If you have vomiting or very severe diarrhoea the pill may not work. Continue to take it, but you may not be protected from the first day of vomiting or diarrhoea. Use another method, such as the sheath, for any intercourse during the stomach upset and for the next 48 hours.'

**Medroxyprogesterone acetate** (Depo-Provera®) is a long-acting progestogen given by intramuscular injection; it is as effective as the combined oral preparations but should never be given without *full counselling backed by the manufacturer's approved leaflet*. It is useful for short-term interim contraception, for example, before vasectomy becomes effective or after rubella vaccination. It may also be used as a long-term contraceptive for women who are unable to use any other method, after counselling on the long and short-term effects. Transient infertility and irregular cycles may occur after discontinuation of treatment. Heavy bleeding has been reported in patients given medroxyprogesterone acetate in the immediate puerperium (the first dose is best delayed until 6 to 7 weeks postpartum). **Norethisterone enanthate** (Noristerat®) is a long-acting progestogen given as an oily injection which provides contraception for 8 weeks.

Progestogen-only preparations can be administered in the early puerperium without adverse effects (except increased bleeding); established lactation is not affected.

## PROGESTOGEN-ONLY CONTRACEPTIVES

*Indications:* contraception

*Cautions:* diabetes, hypertension, heart disease, past ectopic pregnancy (oral preparations only), functional ovarian cysts, malabsorption syndromes; migraine which is severe or focal or has begun for first time on a combined oral contraceptive; active liver disease, recurrent cholestatic jaundice, and history of jaundice in pregnancy; **interactions:** Appendix 1 (contraceptives)

*Contra-indications:* pregnancy, undiagnosed vaginal bleeding, past severe arterial disease or current high risk (e.g. family history, together with cholesterol above 6.5 mmol/litre); liver adenoma; after evacuation of hydatidiform mole (until return to normal of urine and plasma gonadotrophin values); carcinoma of the breast and other sex hormone dependent cancers; porphyria (see section 9.8.2)

*Side-effects:* menstrual irregularities (see also notes above); nausea and vomiting, headache, breast discomfort, depression, skin disorders, weight changes. For other critical factors affecting contraceptive efficacy such as vomiting,

diarrhoea, enzyme induction, and for comment on progestogen-only contraceptives and surgical operations, see under Combined Oral Contraceptives (section 7.3.1)

*Dose: by mouth*, 1 tablet daily at the same time, preferably early in the evening, starting on 1st day of cycle then continuously

Oral preparations

PoM **Femulen**® (Gold Cross)
*Tablets*, ethynodiol diacetate 500 micrograms. Net price 28-tab pack = 94p

PoM **Micronor**® (Ortho)
*Tablets*, norethisterone 350 micrograms. Net price 28-tab pack = 63p

PoM **Microval**® (Wyeth)
*Tablets*, levonorgestrel 30 micrograms. Net price 35-tab pack = £1.00

PoM **Neogest**® (Schering Health Care)
*Tablets*, brown, s/c, norgestrel 75 micrograms (= levonorgestrel 37.5 micrograms). Net price 35-tab pack = 78p

PoM **Norgeston**® (Schering Health Care)
*Tablets*, s/c, levonorgestrel 30 micrograms. Net price 35-tab pack = 78p

PoM **Noriday**® (Syntex)
*Tablets*, norethisterone 350 micrograms. Net price 28-tab pack = 60p

Parenteral preparations

PoM **Depo-Provera**® (Upjohn)
*Injection* (aqueous suspension), medroxyprogesterone acetate 150 mg/mL, net price 1-mL vial = £4.17
*Note*. The 150 mg/mL strength of Depo-Provera is also available in a 3.3-mL vial for use in cancer (see section 8.3.2), and a 50 mg/mL strength is available in 1-, 3-, and 5-mL vials for endometriosis.
*Dose: by deep intramuscular injection*, 150 mg in first 5 days of cycle or first 6 weeks after parturition (delay until 6 weeks after parturition if breast-feeding); for long-term contraception, repeated every 3 months

PoM **Noristerat**® (Schering Health Care)
*Injection* (oily), norethisterone enanthate 200 mg/mL. Net price 1-mL amp = £3.00
*Dose: by deep intramuscular injection into gluteal muscle*, short-term contraception, 200 mg in first 5 days of cycle or immediately after parturition (duration 8 weeks); may be repeated once after 8 weeks (withhold breast-feeding for neonates with severe or persistent jaundice requiring medical treatment)

## 7.3.3  Spermicidal contraceptives

Spermicidal contraceptives are useful additional safeguards but do **not** give adequate protection if used alone; they are suitable for use with barrier methods. They have two components: a spermicide and a vehicle which itself may have some inhibiting effect on sperm migration.

**CSM Advice.** Oil-based vaginal and rectal preparations are likely to damage condoms and contraceptive diaphragms made from latex rubber, and may render them less effective as a barrier method of contraception and as a protection from sexually transmitted diseases (including AIDS).

**C-Film®** (Arun)
*Film*, nonoxinol '9' 67 mg in a water-soluble basis. Net price 10 films = £1.16

**Delfen®** (Ortho)
*Foam*, nonoxinol '9' 12.5%, pressurised aerosol unit in a water-miscible basis. Net price 20 g (with applicator) = £4.65

**Double Check®** (FP)
*Pessaries*, nonoxinol '9' 6% in a water-soluble basis. Net price 10 pessaries = 99p
*Note.* A pack including 10 condoms, called Two's Company®, costs £2.22 (not prescribable on NHS)

**Duracreme®** (LRC)
*Cream*, nonoxinol '9' 2% in a water-soluble basis. Net price 100-g tube = £2.60; applicator = 75p

**Duragel®** (LRC)
*Gel*, nonoxinol '9' 2% in a water-soluble basis. Net price 100-g tube = £2.60; applicator = 75p

**Gynol II®** (Ortho)
*Jelly*, nonoxinol '9' 2% in a water-soluble basis. Net price 81 g = £2.61; applicator = 75p

**Ortho-Creme®** (Ortho)
*Cream*, nonoxinol '9' 2% in a water-miscible basis. Net price 70 g = £2.44; applicator = 75p

**Orthoforms®** (Ortho)
*Pessaries*, nonoxinol '9' 5% in a water-soluble basis. Net price 15 pessaries = £2.40

**Ortho-Gynol®** (Ortho)
*Jelly*, p-di-isobutylphenoxypolyethoxyethanol 1% in a water-soluble basis. Net price 81 g = £2.44; applicator = 75p

**Staycept®** (Syntex)
*Jelly*, octoxinol 1% in a water-soluble basis. Net price 80 g = £1.98
*Pessaries*, nonoxinol '9' 6% in a water-soluble basis. Net price 10 pessaries = £1.43

## 7.3.4 Contraceptive devices

### INTRA-UTERINE DEVICES

The intra-uterine device (IUD) is suitable for older parous women but should be a last-resort contraceptive for young nulliparous women because of the increased risk of pelvic inflammatory disease and infertility. Inert intra-uterine devices are no longer on the UK market but may still be worn by some women.

Smaller devices have now been introduced in order to minimise side-effects; these consist of a plastic carrier wound with copper wire; some also have a central core of silver with the aim of preventing fragmentation of the copper. Family planning organisations now recommend that the replacement time for these devices should be 5 years; any copper intrauterine device licensed currently in the UK, which is fitted in a woman over the age of 40, may remain in the uterus until menopause.

The timing and technique of fitting an intra-uterine device play a critical part in its subsequent performance and call for proper training and experience. Devices should not be fitted during the heavy days of the period; they are best fitted after the end of menstruation and before the calculated time of implantation.

An intra-uterine device should not be removed in mid-cycle unless an additional contraceptive was used for the previous 7 days. If removal is essential (e.g. to treat severe pelvic infection) post-coital contraception should be considered.

If an intra-uterine device fails and the woman wishes to continue to full-term the device should be removed in the first trimester if possible.

## INTRA-UTERINE CONTRACEPTIVE DEVICES

*Indications:* see notes above

*Cautions:* anaemia, heavy menses, history of pelvic inflammatory disease, diabetes, valvular heart disease (antibiotic cover needed), epilepsy, increased risk of expulsion if inserted before uterine involution; gynaecological examination before insertion, 3 months after, and yearly; remove if pregnancy occurs; anticoagulant therapy (avoid if possible); if pregnancy occurs, increased likelihood that it may be tubal

*Contra-indications:* pregnancy, severe anaemia, very heavy menses, history of ectopic pregnancy or tubal surgery, distorted or small uterine cavity, genital malignancy, pelvic inflammatory disease, immunosuppressive therapy, *copper devices:* copper allergy, Wilson's disease, medical diathermy

*Side-effects:* uterine or cervical perforation, displacement, pelvic infection, heavy menses, dysmenorrhoea, allergy; *on insertion:* some pain and bleeding (helped by giving an NSAID, such as ibuprofen half-an-hour before insertion); occasionally, epileptic seizure, vasovagal attack

PoM **Multiload® Cu250** (Organon)
*Intra-uterine device*, copper wire, surface area approx. 250 mm² wound on vertical stem of plastic carrier, 3.6 cm length, with 2 down-curving flexible arms, monofilament thread attached to base of vertical stem; preloaded in inserter. Net price, each = £6.75
For uterine length over 7 cm; replacement every 3 years (but see notes above)

PoM **Multiload® Cu250 Short** (Organon)
*Intra-uterine device*, as above, with vertical stem length 2.5 cm. Net price, each = £6.75
For uterine length 5–7 cm; replacement every 3 years (but see notes above)

PoM **Multiload® Cu375** (Organon)
*Intra-uterine device*, as above, with copper surface area approx. 375 mm². Net price, each = £8.75
For uterine length over 7 cm; replacement every 5 years (see notes above)

PoM **Novagard®** (Kabi Pharmacia)
*Intra-uterine device*, copper wire with silver core, surface area approx. 200 mm² wound on vertical stem of T-shaped plastic carrier, impregnated with barium sulphate for radio-opacity, monofilament thread attached to base of vertical stem; partially preloaded in inserter. Dimensions: transverse arms, vertical stem, both 3.2 cm. Net price, each = £9.90
For uterine length over 5.5 cm; replacement every 5 years (see notes above)

PoM **Nova-T®** (Schering Health Care)
*Intra-uterine device*, copper wire with silver core, surface area approx. 200 mm² wound on vertical stem of T-

shaped plastic carrier, impregnated with barium sulphate for radio-opacity, threads attached to base of vertical stem. Net price, each = £9.90
For uterine length over 6.5 cm; replacement every 5 years (see notes above)

PoM **Ortho Gyne-T®** (Ortho)
*Intra-uterine device*, copper wire, surface area 200 mm², wound on vertical stem of T-shaped plastic carrier, impregnated with barium sulphate for radio-opacity, 2-tail plastic thread attached to base of vertical stem. Net price each = £8.99
For uterine length over 6.5 cm; replacement every 3 years (but see notes above)

PoM **Ortho Gyne-T® 380 Slimline** (Ortho)
*Intra-uterine device*, as above, with copper wire surface area 320 mm² and copper collar surface 30 mm² on distal portion of each arm. Net price = £9.40
For uterine length over 6.5 cm; replacement every 4 years (but see notes above)

## OTHER CONTRACEPTIVE DEVICES

### Contraceptive caps

**Type A contraceptive pessary.** Translucent rubber, sizes 1 to 5 (55–75 mm rising in steps of 5 mm), net price = £5.74
Available from Lamberts (Dumas Vault Cap®)

**Type B contraceptive pessary.** Opaque rubber, sizes 22 to 31 mm (rising in steps of 3 mm), net price = £6.70
Available from Lamberts (Prentif Cavity Rim Cervical Cap®)

**Type C contraceptive pessary.** Translucent rubber, sizes 1 to 3 (45, 48 and 51 mm), net price = £5.74
Available from Lamberts (Vimule Cap®)

### Contraceptive diaphragms

**Type A Diaphragm with flat metal spring.** Transparent rubber with flat metal spring, sizes 55–95 mm (rising in steps of 5 mm), net price = £5.49
Available from Cilag (Ortho-White®), LRC (Durex Flat Spring®)

**Type B Diaphragm with coiled metal rim.** Opaque rubber with coiled metal rim, sizes 55–95 mm (rising in steps of 5 mm), net price = £5.53
Available from Cilag (Ortho®)

NHS **Arcing Spring Diaphragm.** Opaque rubber with arc-ing spring, sizes 60–95 mm (rising in steps of 5 mm)
Available from Cilag (All-Flex®, net price = £6.35), LRC (Durex Arcing Spring®, net price = £6.29)

### Fertility thermometer

**Fertility (Ovulation) Thermometer** (Zeal)
Mercury in glass thermometer, range 35 to 39°C (gradu-ated in 0.1°C). Net price = £1.40
For monitoring ovulation for the rhythm method of con-traception

## 7.4    Drugs for genito-urinary disorders

7.4.1  Drugs for urinary retention
7.4.2  Drugs for urinary frequency, enuresis, and incontinence
7.4.3  Drugs used in urological pain
7.4.4  Bladder instillations and urological sur-gery
7.4.5  Drugs for impotence

For drugs used in the treatment of urinary-tract infections see section 5.1.13.

### 7.4.1    Drugs for urinary retention

*Acute retention* is painful and is treated by cath-eterisation.

*Chronic retention* is painless and often long-standing. Catheterisation is unnecessary unless there is deterioration of renal function. After the cause has initially been established and treated, drugs may be required to increase detrusor muscle tone.

### PARASYMPATHOMIMETICS

Parasympathomimetics produce the effects of par-asympathetic nerve stimulation; they possess the muscarinic rather than the nicotinic effects of acetylcholine and improve voiding efficiency by increasing detrusor muscle contraction. In the absence of obstruction to the bladder outlet they have a limited role in the relief of urinary reten-tion. Generalised parasympathomimetic side-effects such as sweating, bradycardia, and intes-tinal colic may occur, particularly in the elderly.

**Carbachol** and **bethanechol** are choline esters that have been used in postoperative urinary retention. Bethanechol has a more selective action on the bladder than carbachol but the use of both has now been superseded by catheterisation.

**Distigmine** inhibits the breakdown of acetyl-choline. It may help patients with an upper motor neurone neurogenic bladder.

### BETHANECHOL CHLORIDE

*Indications:* urinary retention (but see notes above)
*Contra-indications:* intestinal or urinary obstruction or where increased muscular activity of urinary or gastro-intestinal tract harmful; asthma, bradycardia, hyper-thyroidism, recent myocardial infarction, epilepsy, hypotension, parkinsonism, vagotonia, peptic ulcer-ation, pregnancy; **interactions**: Appendix 1 (chol-inergics)
*Side-effects:* parasympathomimetic effects such as nausea, vomiting, sweating, blurred vision, bradycardia, and intestinal colic
*Dose:* 10–25 mg 3–4 times daily half an hour before food

PoM **Myotonine®** (Glenwood)
*Tablets*, both scored, bethanechol chloride 10 mg, net price 20 = 90p; 25 mg, 20 = £1.15. Label: 22

### CARBACHOL

*Indications:* urinary retention, but see notes above
*Contra-indications; Side-effects:* see under Bethanechol Chloride but side-effects more acute
*Dose: by mouth,* 2 mg 3 times daily half an hour before food
*By subcutaneous injection* (acute symptoms, postop-erative urinary retention) 250 micrograms, repeated twice if necessary at 30-minute intervals
*Note:* Inadvertent intravenous administration of car-bachol is **extremely hazardous** and calls for emergency treatment with atropine.

PoM **Carbachol** (Non-proprietary)
*Tablets*, carbachol 2 mg. Net price 20 = £1.06. Label: 22
*Injection*, carbachol 250 micrograms/mL.

## DISTIGMINE BROMIDE
*Indications:* urinary retention due to upper motor lesions; myasthenia gravis, see section 10.2.1
*Cautions:* asthma, bradycardia, hyperthyroidism, recent myocardial infarction, epilepsy, hypotension, parkinsonism, vagotonia, peptic ulceration, pregnancy; **interactions:** Appendix 1 (cholinergics)
*Contra-indications:* intestinal or urinary obstruction or where increased muscular activity of urinary or gastro-intestinal tract harmful
*Side-effects:* see under Bethanechol Chloride, but action slower therefore side-effects less acute; see also Neostigmine (section 10.2.1)
*Dose: by mouth*, 5 mg daily or on alternate days, half an hour before breakfast
*By intramuscular injection*, 500 micrograms 12 hours after surgery to prevent urinary retention; may be repeated every 24 hours

PoM **Ubretid**® (Rhône-Poulenc Rorer)
*Tablets*, scored, distigmine bromide 5 mg. Net price 20 = £10.80. Label: 22
*Injection*, distigmine bromide 500 micrograms/mL. Net price 1-mL amp = 82p

### ALPHA-BLOCKERS

The selective alpha-blockers **indoramin** and **prazosin** (see section 2.5.4) relax smooth muscle in benign prostatic hyperplasia producing an increase in urinary flow-rate and an improvement in obstructive symptoms. Both have a low incidence of side-effects, although sedation, dizziness, and hypotension may occur; since they are antihypertensives, caution is needed if a patient is receiving antihypertensive treatment (see **Interactions**, Appendix 1, alpha-blockers). Hospital supervision is preferable.

## 7.4.2 Drugs for urinary frequency, enuresis, and incontinence

### URINARY INCONTINENCE

Antimuscarinic drugs such as **oxybutynin** and **flavoxate** are used to treat *urinary frequency*; they increase bladder capacity by diminishing unstable detrusor contractions. All these drugs may cause dry mouth and blurred vision and may precipitate glaucoma. Oxybutynin has a high level of side-effects which limits its use; the dosage needs to be carefully assessed, particularly in the elderly. Flavoxate has less marked side-effects but is also less effective. Propantheline was formerly widely used in urinary incontinence but had a low response rate with a high incidence of side-effects; it is now primarily indicated in adult enuresis. The **tricyclic antidepressants** imipramine, amitriptyline, and nortriptyline (see section 4.3.1) are sometimes effective in the management of the unstable bladder because of their antimuscarinic properties.

## FLAVOXATE HYDROCHLORIDE
*Indications:* urinary frequency and incontinence, dysuria
*Cautions; Contra-indications:* see under Oxybutynin Hydrochloride
*Side-effects:* antimuscarinic side-effects (see Atropine Sulphate, section 1.2); see also notes above
*Dose:* 200 mg 3 times daily

PoM **Urispas**® (Syntex)
*Tablets*, s/c, flavoxate hydrochloride 100 mg. Net price 100 = £4.95

## OXYBUTYNIN HYDROCHLORIDE
*Indications:* urinary frequency and incontinence, neurogenic bladder instability and nocturnal enuresis
*Cautions:* frail elderly; hepatic or renal impairment; hyperthyroidism; cardiac disease where increase in rate undesirable; prostatic hypertrophy; hiatus hernia with reflux oesophagitis; pregnancy and breast-feeding; **interactions:** Appendix 1 (antimuscarinics)
*Contra-indications:* intestinal obstruction or atony, severe ulcerative colitis or toxic megacolon; significant bladder outflow obstruction; glaucoma
*Side-effects:* antimuscarinic side-effects (see under Atropine Sulphate, section 1.2); see also notes above
*Dose:* 5 mg 2–3 times daily increased if necessary to max. 5 mg 4 times daily
ELDERLY 5 mg twice daily
CHILD over 5 years, neurogenic bladder instability, 5 mg twice daily increased if necessary to max. 5 mg 3 times daily; nocturnal enuresis (preferably over 7 years, see notes below), 5 mg 2–3 times daily (last dose before bedtime)

▼ PoM **Ditropan**® (S&N Pharm.)
*Tablets*, both blue, scored, oxybutynin hydrochloride 2.5 mg, net price 84-tab pack = £12.04; 5 mg, 84-tab pack = £24.08. Label: 3

## PROPANTHELINE BROMIDE
*Indications:* adult enuresis, see notes above
*Cautions; Contra-indications:* see under Oxybutynin Hydrochloride
*Side-effects:* antimuscarinic side-effects (see Atropine Sulphate, section 1.2); see also notes above
*Dose:* 15–30 mg 2–3 times daily one hour before meals

**Preparations:**
See section 1.2

### NOCTURNAL ENURESIS

*Nocturnal enuresis* is a normal occurrence in young children but persists in as many as 5% by 10 years of age. In the absence of urinary-tract infection simple measures such as bladder training or the use of an alarm system may be successful.

Drug therapy is not appropriate for children under 7 years of age and should be reserved for when alternative measures have failed. The possible side-effects and potential toxicity of these agents if taken in overdose should be borne in mind when they are prescribed.

The most widely used treatment is with tricyclics such as **amitriptyline**, **imipramine**, and less often **nortriptyline** (see section 4.3.1). They are effective, but behaviour disturbances may occur and relapse is common after withdrawal. Treatment should not normally exceed 3 months unless a full physical examination (including ECG) is given.

**Desmopressin**, an analogue of vasopressin, is also used for nocturnal enuresis (see section 6.5.2).

The sympathomimetic drug **ephedrine** may also be useful.

## AMITRIPTYLINE HYDROCHLORIDE
See section 4.3.1

## DESMOPRESSIN
See section 6.5.2

## EPHEDRINE HYDROCHLORIDE
*Indications:* nocturnal enuresis
*Cautions; Contra-indications; Side-effects:* see under Ephedrine Hydrochloride (section 3.1.1.2)
*Dose:* CHILD 7–8 years 30 mg, 9–12 years 45 mg, 13–15 years 60 mg at bedtime
**Preparations**
See section 3.1.1.2

## IMIPRAMINE HYDROCHLORIDE
See section 4.3.1

## NORTRIPTYLINE HYROCHLORIDE
See section 4.3.1

### 7.4.3   Drugs used in urological pain
The acute pain of *ureteric colic* may be relieved with **pethidine**; **diclofenac** is also effective and compares favourably with pethidine.

**Lignocaine gel** is a useful topical application in *urethral pain* or to relieve the discomfort of catheterisation (see section 15.2).

ALKALINISATION OF URINE

*Alkalinisation* of urine may be undertaken with **sodium bicarbonate**, or alternatively with potassium citrate. The alkalinising action may relieve the discomfort of *cystitis* caused by lower urinary tract infections. Sodium bicarbonate, in particular, is also used as a urinary alkalinising agent in some metabolic and renal disorders (see section 9.2.2).

## POTASSIUM CITRATE
*Indications:* relief of discomfort in mild urinary-tract infections; alkalinisation of urine
*Cautions:* renal impairment, cardiac disease; elderly; **interactions:** Appendix 1 (potassium salts)
*Side-effects:* hyperkalaemia on prolonged high dosage, mild diuresis
*Dose:* see under preparations

**Potassium Citrate Mixture** (BP)
(Potassium Citrate Oral Solution)
*Oral solution*, potassium citrate 30%, citric acid monohydrate 5% in a suitable vehicle with a lemon flavour. Extemporaneous preparations should be recently prepared according to the following formula: potassium citrate 3 g, citric acid monohydrate 500 mg, syrup 2.5 mL, quillaia tincture 0.1 mL, lemon spirit 0.05 mL, double-strength chloroform water 3 mL, water to 10 mL. Contains about 28 mmol K+/10 mL. Label: 27
*Dose:* 10 mL 3 times daily well diluted with water
**Effercitrate®** (Typharm)
*Tablets*, effervescent, the equivalent of potassium citrate 1.5 g (13.9 mmol K+), citric acid 250 mg (1 tablet ≡ 5 mL potassium citrate mixture). Net price 12 = £1.60. Label: 13
*Dose:* ADULT and CHILD over 6 years, 2 tablets dissolved in a tumblerful of water up to 3 times daily; CHILD 1–6 years 1 tablet

## SODIUM BICARBONATE
*Indications:* relief of discomfort in mild urinary-tract infections; alkalinisation of urine
*Cautions; Side-effects:* see section 1.1.2; also caution in elderly
*Dose:* 3 g in water every 2 hours until urinary pH exceeds 7; maintenance of alkaline urine 5-10 g daily

**Sodium Bicarbonate Powder.** Net price 50 g = 5p. Label: 13

ACIDIFICATION OF URINE

*Acidification* of urine has been undertaken with **ascorbic acid** but it is not always reliable.

For pH-modifying solutions for the maintenance of indwelling urinary catheters, see section 7.4.4.

**ASCORBIC ACID**
*Indications:* acidification of urine but see notes above
*Dose: by mouth*, 4 g daily in divided doses

**Preparations**
See section 9.6.3

OTHER PREPARATIONS FOR
URINARY DISORDERS

A terpene mixture (Rowatinex®) is claimed to be of benefit in *urolithiasis* for the expulsion of calculi.

**Rowatinex®** (Monmouth)
*Capsules*, yellow, e/c, anethol 4 mg, borneol 10 mg, camphene 15 mg, cineole 3 mg, fenchone 4 mg, pinene 31 mg. Net price 50 = £7.54. Label: 25
*Dose:* 1 capsule 3–4 times daily

## 7.4.4 Bladder instillations and urological surgery

INFECTED BLADDERS. Various solutions are available as irrigations or washouts.

Initial treatment is with **sterile sodium chloride solution 0.9%** (physiological saline).

Aqueous **chlorhexidine** (see section 13.11.2) is effective against a wide range of common urinary-tract pathogens but not against most *Pseudomonas* spp. Solutions containing 1 in 5000 (0.02%) are used but they may irritate the mucosa and cause burning and haematuria (in which case they should be discontinued); solutions containing 1 in 10000 (0.01%) are usually preferred post-operatively. **Polymyxin B sulphate with neomycin** (Polybactrin®) and **colistin** (both section 5.1.7) are bactericidal to most pathogens and emergence of resistance is slow.

**Noxythiolin** is also bactericidal to most pathogens with slow emergence of resistance, but initial use in the purulent infected bladder is often accompanied by an intense reaction including the passage of large clumps of fibrin. Other indications for noxythiolin include intraperitoneal use during colonic surgery.

Bladder irrigations of **amphotericin** 100 micrograms/mL (see section 5.2) may be of value in mycotic infections.

DISSOLUTION OF BLOOD CLOTS. Clot retention is usually treated by irrigation with sterile **sodium chloride solution 0.9%** but sterile **sodium citrate** solution for bladder irrigation (3%) may also be helpful. **Streptokinase-streptodornase** (Varidase Topical®, see section 13.11.7) is an alternative.

LOCALLY ACTING CYTOTOXIC DRUGS. **Doxorubicin** (see section 8.1.2) is used to treat recurrent superficial bladder tumours, carcinoma-in-situ, and some papillary tumours. An instillation (50 mg in 50 mL of sterile sodium chloride solution 0.9%) is retained in the bladder for one hour and treatment repeated monthly. Although systemic side-effects are few, it may cause frequency, urgency, dysuria, and occasionally reduction in bladder capacity.

**Mitomycin** is used for recurrent bladder tumours. A solution containing 20 to 40 mg in 40 mL of sterile water is instilled weekly for 4 weeks then monthly for at least 11 months.

**Thiotepa** (see section 8.1.1) is used for bladder tumours of low to medium grade malignancy. A solution containing 30–60 mg in 60 mL of sterile water is retained in the bladder for 2 hours. It is given weekly for 4 weeks. The concentration should be reduced in bonemarrow suppression.

INTERSTITIAL CYSTITIS. Dimethyl sulphoxide may be used for symptomatic relief in patients with interstitial cystitis (Hunner's ulcer). 50 mL of a 50% solution (Rimso-50®) is instilled into the bladder, retained for 15 minutes, and voided by the patient. Treatment is repeated at intervals of 2 weeks. Bladder spasm and hypersensitivity reactions may occur and long-term use requires ophthalmic, renal, and hepatic assessment at 6-monthly intervals.

## CHLORHEXIDINE

*Indications:* bladder washouts, see notes above and section 13.11.2

## DIMETHYL SULPHOXIDE

*Indications:* bladder washouts, see notes above

PoM **Rimso-50®** (Britannia)
*Bladder instillation*, sterile, dimethyl sulphoxide 50%, in aqueous solution. Net price 50 mL = £19.80

## NOXYTHIOLIN

*Indications:* see notes above
*Side-effects:* burning sensation on application to bladder (relieved by addition of amethocaine)
*Dose: bladder instillation*, 100 mL of a 2.5% solution instilled 1–2 times daily
*Intraperitoneal use*, 100 mL of a 2.5% solution instilled prior to closure

PoM **Noxyflex S®** (Geistlich)
*Solution*, powder for reconstitution, noxythiolin. Net price 2.5 g in 20 mL vial = £5.32; 2.5 g in 100-mL vial with transfer needle = £6.65

## SODIUM CHLORIDE

*Indications:* bladder washouts, see notes above

Available from Baxter, Kendall

## SODIUM CITRATE

*Indications:* bladder washouts, see notes above

**Sterile Sodium Citrate Solution for Bladder Irrigation,** sodium citrate 3%, dilute hydrochloric acid 0.2%, in purified water, freshly boiled and cooled, and sterilised

## UROLOGICAL SURGERY

Endoscopic surgery within the urinary tract requires an isotonic irrigant as there is a high risk of fluid absorption; if this occurs in excess, hypervolaemia, haemolysis, and renal failure may result. **Glycine irrigation solution 1.5%** is the irrigant of choice for transurethral resection of the prostate gland and bladder tumours; **sterile sodium chloride solution 0.9%** (physiological saline) is used for percutaneous renal surgery.

## GLYCINE

*Indications:* bladder irrigation during urological surgery; see notes above
*Cautions; Side-effects:* see notes above

**Glycine Irrigation Solution** (Non-proprietary)
*Irrigation solution*, glycine 1.5% in water for injections
Available from Baxter, Kendall

## MAINTENANCE OF INDWELLING URINARY CATHETERS

The deposition which occurs in catheterised patients is usually chiefly composed of phosphate and to minimise this the catheter (if latex) should be changed at least as often as every 6 weeks. If the catheter is to be left for longer periods a silicone catheter should be used. If bladder wash-outs are required at frequent intervals this usually indicates that the catheter needs to be changed.

### CATHETER PATENCY SOLUTIONS

**Chlorhexidine 0.02%.** Available from CliniMed (Uro-Tainer Chlorhexidine®, 100-mL sachet = £1.89), Galen (Uriflex C®, 100-mL sachet = £1.56)

**Mandelic acid 1%.** Available from CliniMed (Uro-Tainer Mandelic Acid®, 100-mL sachet = £1.89)

**Sodium chloride 0.9%.** Available from Clini-Med (Uro-Tainer Sodium Chloride®, 100-mL sachet = £1.79, Uro-Tainer M®, with integral drug additive port, 50- and 100-mL sachets = £2.12), Galen (Uriflex S®, 100-mL sachet = £1.47, Uriflex SP® with integral drug additive port, 100-mL sachet = £1.75)

**Solution G**, citric acid 3.23%, magnesium oxide 0.38%, sodium bicarbonate 0.7%, disodium edetate 0.01%. Available from CliniMed (Uro-Tainer Suby G®, 100-mL sachet = £1.89), Galen (Uriflex G®, 100-mL sachet = £1.56)

**Solution R**, citric acid 6%, gluconolactone 0.6%, magnesium carbonate 2.8%, disodium edetate 0.01%. Available from CliniMed (Uro-Tainer Solution R®, 100-mL sachet = £1.89), Galen (Uriflex R®, 100-mL sachet = £1.56)

### 7.4.5   Drugs for impotence

Reasons for failure to produce a satisfactory erection include psychogenic, vascular, neurogenic, and endocrine abnormalities. Intracavernosal injection of vasoactive drugs under careful medical supervision is used for both diagnostic and therapeutic purposes.

The most effective treatment for impotence has been shown to be direct injection of the smooth muscle relaxant **papaverine** into the corpus cavernosum. The usual dose of papaverine by intracavernosal injection is 7.5 mg initially increased according to response to a range of 30–60 mg. Patients with neurological or psychogenic impotence are more sensitive to the effect of papaverine than those with vascular abnormalities. **Phentolamine** (0.25–1.25 mg) can be added if the response is inadequate.

Persistence of the erection for longer than 4 hours is an emergency requiring aspiration of the corpora; if aspiration fails, 1 mg of metaraminol can be diluted to 5 mL with sodium chloride injection 0.9% and given by careful slow injection into the corpora.

Other side-effects include vasovagal attacks and syncope; caution is needed in patients with cardiovascular disease and ischaemic attacks.

Local side-effects include haematoma and burning pain at the site of injection and fibrotic changes in the corpora cavernosa (which may lead to Peyronie-like erectile distortion).

*Note.* Papaverine is available from Boots and Penn (special order)

## 7.5   Appliances for urinary disorders

Urostomy pouches are included here but associated products (e.g. skin protectives and adhesives) are in section 1.8

### UROSTOMY POUCHES

Body's Care range
**Rubber bags** (Body's Care)
  Black butyl, one-piece pouch. Net price 1 day pouch (screwcap outlet) = £23.25; 1 night pouch (screwcap outlet) = £27.12; 1 day or night pouch (both spout outlet) = £24.55; 1 day pouch (tap outlet) = £25.84; 1 night pouch (tap outlet) = £27.12
  White rubber, one-piece pouch. Net price 1 day pouch (screwcap outlet) = £14.89; 1 day pouch (screwcap outlet) = £12.92; 1 day pouch (spout outlet) = £11.62; 1 night pouch (spout outlet) = £11.62

Bullen range
**Lenbul** (Bullen)
  Day bag (= pouch), one-piece pouch. Net price 1 pouch with tap outlet = £12.32; 1 pouch with large opening = £12.78; 1 pouch with metal strip = £13.78
  Night bag (= pouch). Net price 1 pouch with tap outlet = £14.08; 1 pouch with large opening = £14.61
  One-piece flange and bag (= pouch) with tap outlet. Net price 1 (1- or 2-inch) = £25.87
  Baby's bag (= pouch) and flange with tap outlet. Net price 1 (1½-inch or 2-inch, with or without night tube) = £35.96
  Child's rubber cap and bag (= pouch) with non-reflux valve. Net price 1 small, 1 small with metal strip, or 1 large = £24.37; 1 large with metal strip = £26.21
**SR-F** (Bullen)
  Set, comprises 1 waistband, 1 flange standard 3-inch base, 1 closed day pouch with screw outlet, 1 closed night pouch with screw outlet and 30 double-sided acrylic adhesive plasters. Net price 1 set = £53.47
**SR-U** (Bullen)
  Appliance, as SR-F set but pouches have tap outlet. Net price 1 appliance = £58.27
**OPR-F** (Bullen)
  Appliance, comprises 1 waistband, 2 pouches with screw outlet (1- or 2-inch opening), and 30 double-sided acrylic adhesive plasters. Net price 1 appliance = £77.59
**OPR-U** (Bullen)
  Appliance, as OPR-F appliance but pouches have tap outlet. Net price 1 appliance = £77.59
**LOP-F7** (Bullen)
  Appliance, comprises 1 belt, 10 lightweight pouches with one-piece flange and 1-inch opening, and 30 double-sided arylic adhesive plasters. Net price 1 appliance = £37.20
**LOP-U** (Bullen)
  Appliance, as LOP-F7 appliance. Net price 1 appliance = £37.20

Drew range
**Urostomy bags** (Drew)
Urostomy bag (= pouch), one-piece pouch. Net price 50 pouches (D1/2, OSTO 06) = £73.41
**Rubber bags** (Drew)
Rubber bag (= pouch), one-piece pouch. Net price 1 pouch screwcap outlet (OSTO 16) = £12.57; 1 pouch (OSTO 17) tap outlet = £13.19
**Ureterostomy appliance** (Drew)
Ureterostomy appliance .Net price 1 appliance (D1/2, OSTO 05) = £35.57

Coloplast range
**Stoma Urine** (Coloplast)
Maxi, one-piece pouch with zinc oxide adhesive. Net price 30 pouches (13-mm hole) = £63.30
Midi, one-piece pouch with zinc oxide adhesive. Net price 30 pouches (13-mm hole) = £63.30
**URO 2002**® (Coloplast)
Two-piece pouch. Net price 20 small pouches (100 mL, to fit 40 mm base plate) = £46.20; 20 large pouches (375 mL, to fit 40 or 60 mm base plate) = £46.20
Base plate. Net price 5 plates (40 mm, to fit 10–35 mm stoma) or 5 plates (60 mm, to fit 10–55 mm stoma) = £12.20
Night drainage system. Net price 10 pouches (1.65 litre), 1 tube, and 2 connectors = £11.90; hospital pack, 10 pouches (1.65 litre), 5 tubes, and 10 connectors = £17.60

Hollister range
**Classic** (Hollister)
Karaya 5® seal and regular adhesive with gasket for optional belt, one-piece pouch, clear. Net price 20 pouches (23, 30, or 40 cm, *with* 19, 25, 32, 38, 44, or 51 mm gasket), including 1 standard drain tube = £54.03
Regular adhesive with gasket for optional belt, one-piece pouch, clear. Net price 20 pouches (23, 30, or 40 cm pouches *with* 19, 25, 32, 38, 44, or 51 mm gasket), including 1 standard drain tube = £41.10
Regular adhesive only (beltless), one-piece pouch, clear. Net price 20 pouches (23-cm pouch *with* 19, 25, 32, 38, 44, or 51 mm opening size), including 1 standard drain tube = £41.10
**First Choice**® (Hollister)
Urostomy pouch with synthetic skin barrier and Microporous II adhesive. Net price 10 pouches (13–64 mm starter hole, 19, 25, 32, 38, 44, or 51 mm) = £40.00
**Guardian**® (Hollister)
Guardian, two-piece pouch with wide-bore tap and non-reflux valve. Net price 10 pouches (25-cm for max. 25, 38, or 51 mm stomas), including 1 drain tube adapter = £20.00
**Lo-profile**® (Hollister)
Karaya 5® seal and Microporous II adhesive with gasket for optional belt, one-piece pouch, with non-reflux valve, clear. Net price 10 pouches (25-cm pouch *with* 19, 25, 32, 38, 44, or 51 mm gasket), including 1 Lo-profile drain tube = £47.93
Microporous II adhesive only (beltless) one-piece pouch with non-reflux valve. Net price 10 pouches (25-cm pouch *with* 19, 25, 32, 38, 44, or 51 mm opening), including 1 Lo-profile drain tube = £36.40

Leyland range
**Rubber bags** (Leyland)
Black rubber (Birkbeck®), one-piece pouch. Net price 1 day pouch (19 mm hole) = £25.88; 1 night pouch (19 mm hole) = £28.23
Pink rubber, one-piece pouch. Net price 1 day pouch (19 mm hole) = £25.88; 1 night pouch (19 mm hole) = £28.23
White rubber, one-piece pouch. Net price 1 day pouch (19, 25, or 28 mm holes) = £14.06; 1 night pouch (19, 25, or 28 mm holes) = £14.44

White rubber (Glasgow), one-piece pouch. Net price 1 pouch (small or large tap) = £17.17
White rubber transverse, one-piece pouch. net price 1 left or right pouch (small, medium, or large) = £17.17
Latex rubber, one-piece pouch. Net price 1 day pouch (19, 25, or 28 mm holes) = £14.22; 1 night pouch (19, 25, or 28 mm holes) = £15.78

Salts range
**Rubber bags** (Salts)
AR white rubber tap bag (= pouch), one-piece pouch with spout outlet. Net price 1 small or medium pouch (both 25, 32, or 38 mm holes) or 1 large pouch (25, 32, 38, 44, or 51 mm holes) = £13.57
KR AR black rubber tap bag (= pouch), one-piece pouch with spout outlet and non-reflux valve. Net price 1 medium or large pouch (both 19, 25, 32, or 38 mm holes) = £33.28; special size holes also available to order
KR AR MB black rubber tap bag (= pouch), one-piece pouch with tap outlet, bridge, and non-reflux valve. Net price 1 small, medium, or large pouch (both 19, 25, 32, or 38 mm holes) = £37.75; special size holes also available to order
KR WP black rubber tap bag (= pouch), one-piece pouch with spout outlet. Net price 1 medium or large pouch (both 19, 25, 32, or 38 mm holes) = £39.56; special size holes also available to order
KR WP MB black rubber tap bag (= pouch), one-piece pouch with spout outlet. Net price 1 medium or large pouch (both 19, 25, 32, or 38 mm holes) = £45.32; special size holes also available to order
Black rubber tap bag (= pouch) (for use with flange), one-piece pouch with spout outlet. Net price 1 small, medium, or large pouch = £30.56; special size holes also available to order
White rubber tap bag (= pouch) for use with flange, one-piece pouch with spout outlet. Net price 1 small, medium, or large pouch = £8.93
**Light White** (Salts)
Urostomy with Realistic® washer, one-piece pouch, white. Net price 20 large pouches (all 25, 32, or 38 mm holes) = £90.98
Urostomy with Realistic® washer, one-piece pouch, clear. Net price 20 large or small pouches (all 25, 32, or 38 mm holes) = £90.98
Urostomy, one-piece pouch, white. Net price 20 large pouches (25, 32, or 38 mm holes) = £68.36
Urostomy clear, one-piece pouch, clear. Net price 20 large or small pouches (25, 32, or 38 mm holes) = £68.36
Urostomy adhesive, one-piece pouch with adhesive. Net price 20 large pouches (25, 32, or 38 mm holes) = £72.20
Urostomy clear adhesive, one-piece pouch with adhesive, clear. Net price 20 large or small pouches (both 25, 32, or 38 mm holes) = £72.20
**Simplicity 1**® (Salts)
Paediatric Uri-bag, one-piece pouch, 13 mm starter hole. Net price = £34.60

Simcare range
**Carshalton** (Simcare)
Bag (= pouch), one-piece pouch. Net price 10 oval or triangular pouches (both 25, 32, or 38 mm) with acrylic plaster = £16.46
Set, one-piece pouch. Net price 20 oval or triangular pouches with plasters, bodyplate clamp, connector, and belt (both 25, 32, or 38 mm holes) = £56.00
**Chiron Non-disposable** (Simcare)
Butyl rubber bag (= pouch), one-piece pouch with stopcock outlet, black. Net price 1 day bag (22 mm) = £29.46
Latex rubber day bag (= pouch), one-piece pouch with stopcock outlet. Net price 1 day bag (38 mm) = £20.40
Latex rubber night bag (= pouch), one-piece pouch. Net price 1 night bag (38 mm) = £23.14

Cautionary label wordings, see inside back cover

Prices are **net**, see p. 1

Rubber child-size bag (pouch), white, one-piece pouch with stopcock outlet. Net price 1 = £17.12
Rubber day bag (= pouch), one-piece pouch, white with stopcock outlet. Net price 1 (38 mm) = £20.40
Rubber night bag (= pouch), one-piece, white. Net price 1 (38, 44, or 51 mm) = £23.14

**Chiron** (Simcare)
Ileal bladder appliance, set comprises 1 web and elastic belt 25 mm wide, 1 wire pressure frame, 1 St Mark's pattern rubber flange (without diaphragm), 2 rubber day pouches with stopcock outlet, 30 double-sided plasters. Net price = £65.73

**Mitcham** (Simcare)
Maxi, one-piece pouch. Net price 10 pouches with adhesive flange (25, 32, or 38 mm) = £33.54, 10 pouches with nonadhesive flange (25, 32, or 38 mm) = £27.39
Mini, one-piece pouch. Net price 10 pouches with adhesive flange (19, 25, or 32 mm) = £33.54, 10 pouches with nonadhesive flange (25 mm or 32 mm) = £27.39
Standard, one-piece pouch. Net price 10 pouches with adhesive flange (19, 25, 32 or 38 mm) = £33.54, 10 pouches with nonadhesive flange (25, 32, or 38 mm) = £27.39, 1 pouch with nonadhesive flange and foam pads (25, 32, or 38 mm) = £4.78

**Rediflow** (Simcare)
Adhesive set, may be worn with belt. Net price 20 pouches (19, 25, 32, 38, 44, or 51 mm) = £49.29

**Thackraycare range**
**Raymed®** (Thackraycare)
Butyl night bag (= pouch), one-piece pouch. Net price 1 pouch with screwcap outlet = £24.95; 1 pouch with tap outlet = £25.80

## DRAINABLE DRIBBLING APPLIANCES

Re-usable for at least 1 month (with exception of Alexa®)

**Body's Care range**
**Bag** (Body's Care)
Dribbling bag with loops and tapes. Net price 1 = £13.00
**Urinal** (Body's Care)
Drip male urinal with tap. Net price 1 = £34.80; 1 replacement belt = £8.60

**Bullen range**
**Bags** (Bullen)
Net price 10 Dribblet® bags = £20.09; 10 Dribblet® sheath bags = £45.09

**Henleys range**
**Alexa® dribbler bag** (Henleys)
Plain bag, with draw strings.Net price 100 bags = £4.22; 100 bags with non-reflux valve = £16.25

**Leyland range**
**Peoplecare®** (Leyland)
Male drip urinal. Net price 1 = £41.39

**Thackraycare range**
**Aquadry®** (Thackraycare)
Male incontinence pouch. Net price 1 (with short or long tube) = £6.15
Drip type urinal. Net price 1 = £46.25

**Ward range**
**Bags** (Ward)
Male dribbling bad with diaphragm and belt. Net price 1 = £22.71
Plastic dribbling bag. Net price 1 = £11.30

## INCONTINENCE BELTS

Average life 6 months

**Body's Care range**
**Waist belt for kipper bags** (Body's Care)
Net price 1 = £4.55; 1 (with webbing band) = £4.55

**Leyland range**
**Peoplecare®** (Leyland)
Waist and support strap for kipper bag. Net price 1 = £5.56
Rubber belt. Net price 1 = £3.06

**Simcare range**
**Belts** (Simcare)
Rubber belt. Net price 1 = £4.62
Elastic support. Net price 1 (small, medium, or large) = £9.89
Web belt (small, medium, or large) = £9.58

**Ward range**
**Belts** (Ward)
Waist belt for black kipper bag. Net price 1 = £4.16
Rubber belt for PP (pubic pressure) urinal. Net price 1 = £3.60

**Willis range**
**Belts** (Willis)
Waist band 2-inch white web with looped strap to support bag. Net price 1 (38 and 46 inch) = £4.09; 1 (larger than 46 inch) = £4.38

## INCONTINENCE SHEATHS

Unless otherwise indicated the incontinence sheaths (also known as penile sheaths or external catheters) listed below are of the soft, flexible, latex type. Each sheath may be left in place for 1 to 3 days between changes

**Aldington range**
**Dryaid®** (Aldington)
Incontinence sheath. Net price 20 sheaths (with adhesive strip; small, medium, large, or extra-large) = £24.15; 20 sheaths (without adhesive strip; small, medium, large, or extra-large) = £13.98
**Polymed®** (Aldington)
Incontinence sheath. Net price 20 sheaths (with adhesive strip; small, medium, large, or extra-large) = £24.15; 20 sheaths (without adhesive strip; small, medium, large, or extra-large) = £13.98

**Bard range**
**Reliasheath®** (Bard)
Incontinence sheath. Net price 30 sheaths (20, 25, 30, 35, or 40 mm) = £20.90
**Uriplan®** (Bard)
Incontinence sheath. Net price 30 sheaths (without Crix-iline® strip; 20, 25, 30, 35, or 40 mm) = £20.90
Uro sheath® (washable; may be used many times). Net price 1 (25, 35, or 40 mm) = £4.36

**Camp range**
**Posey®** (Camp)
Incontinence sheath. Net price 10 sheaths (incontinence sheath A) = £4.65; 10 sheaths ('Fastflow' incontinence sheath, 25, 30, or 35 mm) = £5.80

**Coloplast range**
**Conveen®** (Coloplast)
Incontinence sheath, with anti-kink design and Uriliner® adhesive strip. Net price 30 sheaths (20, 25, 30, 35, or 40 mm) = £37.50

**Conveen self-sealing Urisheath**® (Coloplast)
Incontinence sheath. Net price 30 sheaths (25, 30, or 35 mm) = £36.90

ConvaTec range
**Accuseal**® (ConvaTec)
Incontinence sheath. Net price 10 sheaths (20, 25, 30, 35, or 40 mm) = £6.99

EMS Medical range
**Sheaths** (EMS Medical)
Incontinence sheath. Net price 100 sheaths (25, 30, or 35 mm) = £42.00; 100 sheaths (with liner; 25, 30, or 35 mm) = £28.30

Fry Surgical range
**Uridom**® (Fry Surgical)
Incontinence sheath, with adhesive strip. Net price 30 sheaths = £26.10

Hospital Management and Supplies range
**Macrodom**® (Hospital Management and Supplies)
Incontinence sheath, including adhesive strip. Net price 30 sheaths (with 2-inch tube) = £18.25; 25 sheaths (with 5-inch tube) = £19.17
**Macrodom Plus**® (Hospital Management and Supplies)
Incontinence sheath, including adhesive strip. Net price 30 sheaths (small, medium, or large) = £23.00

Incare range
**Male incontinence sheath** (Incare)
Incontinence sheath, self adhesive. Net price 15 sheaths (22, 26, 30, or 34 mm) = £20.29

Mediplus range
**Medimates**® (Mediplus)
Incontinence sheath with single-sided adhesive strip. Net price 30 sheaths (straight, 20, 25, 30, 35, or 40 mm; bulb, 25, 30, or 35 mm) = £26.70
Incontinence sheath with double-sided adhesive strip. Net price 30 sheaths (straight, 20, 25, 30, 35, or 40 mm; bulb, 25, 30, or 35 mm) = £28.50

North West Medical range
**Uridrop**® (North West Medical)
Incontinence sheath. Net price 30 sheaths (paediatric = 42 or 55 mm; sizes 1, 2, 3, or 4 = 70, 80, 100, or 107 mm) = £11.20
Incontinence sheath, with Uristrip® adhesive strip. Net price 30 sheaths (paediatric = 42 or 55 mm; sizes 1, 2, 3, or 4 = 70, 80, 100, or 107 mm) = £21.60

Payne range
**Incontiaid**® (Payne)
Incontinence sheath. Net price 10 sheaths, with adhesive strip (sizes 0, 1, 2, 3, or 4) = £11.50; 1 sheath, without adhesive strip (sizes 0, 1, 2, 3, or 4) = 75p; 10 adhesive strips = £3.75

Rüsch range
**Portasheath**® (Rüsch)
Incontinence sheath. Net price 25 sheaths (25, 30, or 35 mm) = £19.50
Secure external catheter kit, with adhesive strip. Net price 10 sheaths (25, 30, or 35 mm) = £8.00

Salts range
**Heritage Cohesive/Sheath**® (Salts)
Incontinence sheath, with adhesive. Net price 30 sheaths (17, 22, 25, 32, or 34 mm) = £28.64
**Male continence sheath** (Salts)
Incontinence sheath. Net price 10 sheaths (17, 22, 25, 32, or 34 mm) = £6.47

Seton range
**Incontinence sheath** (Seton)
Incontinence sheath. Net price 30 sheaths (small, medium, large, or extra-large) = £27.80; 30 sheaths with self-adhesive liner (small, medium, large, or extra-large) = £33.12

Sherwood range
**Texas Catheter**® (Sherwood)
Incontinence sheath, with adhesive strip. Net price 12 sheaths = £8.28
**Uri Drain**® (Sherwood)
Incontinence sheath, with double-sided adhesive strip (25, 30, or 35 mm). Net price 10 = £7.65

Simcare range
**Continence sheath** (Simcare)
Incontinence sheath. Net price 1 sheath (small, medium, large, or extra-large) = £1.19
**Uro Flo**® (Simcare)
Incontinence sheath, straight, including adhesive strip. Net price 30 sheaths (small, medium, or large) = £34.81
**Uro Flo Mk2**® (Simcare)
Incontinence sheath, bulbous, with adhesive strip. Net price 30 sheaths = £34.81
**Male incontinence sheath** (Simcare)
Incontinence sheath. Net price 100 sheaths = £57.67

Simpla range
**Bubble U**® (Simpla)
Incontinence sheath, with adhesive foam strip. Net price 30 sheaths (small, medium, large, or extra-large) = £23.37
Incontinence sheath, with self-adhesive Uriseal® liner. Net price 30 sheaths (small, medium, large, or extra-large) = £33.60

S&N range
**Regard**® (S&N)
Incontinence sheath, with liners. Net price 30 sheaths (small, medium, large, or extra-large) = £30.00

Thackraycare range
**Aquadry**® (Thackraycare)
Incontinence sheath. Net price 10 sheaths (small, medium, large, or extra-large) = £8.78; 10 sheaths with bulbous end (small, medium, or large) = £25.32
**Aquadry Freedom**® (Thackraycare)
Freedom® incontinence sheath, self-adhesive. Net price 30 sheaths (small, medium, or large) = £35.60
Freedom Plus® Incontinence sheath, self-adhesive. Net price 30 sheaths (small, medium, or large) = £35.60

Vygon range
**Peniflow**® (Vygon)
Incontinence sheath. Net price 40 sheaths = £44.38

## FIXING STRIPS AND ADHESIVES

**Aldington**
Dryaid® strip, Polymed® strip. Net price 20 strips (both) = £10.17
**Bio Diagnostics**
Urifix® tape. Net price 5 m = £4.90
**Camp**
Posey® sheath holder. Net price 12 (adult) = £12.00; 12 (paediatric) = £10.20
**ConvaTec**
Urihesive® strips. Net price 15 = £5.50
**Dow Corning**
Adhesive B (Silicone adhesive aerosol). Net price 207 g = £8.97
355 medical adhesive (brush-on silicone adhesive). Net price 1 = £2.72

**EMS Medical**
Urifix® tape. Net price 5 m = £5.30
**North West Medical**
Uristrip® adhesive strip. Net price 30 = £10.40
**Payne**
Incontiaid® sheath holder. Net price 1 = 85p
**Salts**
Heritage® sheath collar pack. Net price 30 = £3.29
NHS Cohesive® strips for use with sheaths. Net price
10 = £4.50
**Thackraycare**
Aquadry® medical adhesive (brush on). Net price 1 =
£3.25 Aquadry® penile liners. Net price 20 = £7.50

---

## LEG BAGS

Most plastic bags suitable for use for 5–7 days; rubber
bags re-usable for 4–6 months

Aldington range
**Leg bags** (Aldington)
Leg bag, plastic. Net price 10 bags (short tube, 350 or
500 mL) = £12.55; 10 bags (long tube, 350 or 500 mL) =
£13.47

Bard range
**Uriplan®** (Bard)
Leg bag, plastic, shaped, with tap outlet and elastic
Velcro straps. Net price 10 bags (350 mL, direct inlet) =
£20.80; 10 bags (350 mL, 12 inch inlet tube) = £20.50; 10
bags (500 mL, direct inlet) = £21.00; 10 bags (500 mL, 4
or 12 inch inlet tube) = £21.09; 10 bags (750 mL, direct
inlet, or 4 or 12 inch inlet tube) = £21.20
**Seton Urisac®** (Bard)
Leg bag, plastic. Net price 10 bags (350 mL, short tube) =
£10.20; 10 bags (350 mL, long tube) = £10.50; 10 bags
(500 mL, short tube) = £11.10; 10 bags (500 mL, long
tube) = £11.40; 10 bags (750 mL, short tube) = £11.70;
10 bags (750 mL, long tube) = £12.20

Body's Care range
**Leg bags** (Body's Care)
Kipper bag, black, white, or clear. Net price 1 bag =
£20.90
Leg drainage bag, plastic, with tap outlet. Net price 10
bags (350 or 500 mL) = £17.90; 10 bags (750 mL) =
£18.70

Coloplast range
**Conveen®** (Coloplast)
Standard leg bag, plastic. Net price, with 1 pair Velcro
straps, 10 bags (500 mL, 10 or 40 cm tube) = £17.40
Contour leg bag, plastic, shaped, sterile with sample
port. Net price, with 1 pair Velcro straps, 10 bags
(600 mL, 5 or 30 cm tube; 800 mL, 45 cm tube) = £21.80

ConvaTec range
**Accuseal®** (ConvaTec)
Leg bag, plastic. Net price 10 bags (350 mL) = £13.26;
10 bags (500 mL) = £15.81; 10 bags (750 mL) = £14.64

EMS Medical range
**Leg drainage bags** (EMS)
Leg bag, plastic. Net price 10 bags = (500 mL, short or
long tube) = £12.85

Incare range
**Urinary leg bag** (Incare)
Leg bag, plastic. Net price 10 bags (540 mL, 37 cm
tube) = £21.10; 10 bags (540 mL, direct inlet) = £20.59

Leyland range
**Kipper bags** (Leyland)
Leg bag. Net price 1 bag (clear/white plastic or all black
plastic or rubber, with strap and buckle) = £23.24; 1
bag (clear/white plastic, without strap and buckle) =
£19.05

Payne range
**Incontiaid®** (Payne)
Leg bag, plastic. Net price 1 bag = £2.10
**Single-chambered Bags** (Payne)
Leg bag, single-chambered. Net price 1 bag (rubber, with
box outlet tap) = £39.20; 1 bag (for night use) = £42.80;
1 bag (for female use) = £31.80; 1 bag (rubber, kipper-
style) = £31.80; 1 bag (rubber, Ross type) = £36.30

Pharma-Plast range
**Careline®** (Bradgate)
Leg bag, plastic, with tap outlet and overnight connection
tube. Net price, with 1 pair Velcro straps, 10 bags
(350 mL, short or long tube) = £18.00; 10 bags (500 mL,
short or long tube) = £18.50; 10 bags (750 mL, short or
long tube) = £19.00

Rüsch range
**Leg bag** (Rüsch)
Leg bag, plastic. Net price (750 mL) = £9.30

Salts range
**Heritage®** (Salts)
Leg bag, plastic. Net price 10 bags (350 mL, short tube) =
£10.20; 10 bags (500 mL, short tube) = £11.81; 10 bags
(500 mL, long tube) = £12.02; 10 bags (500 mL, short
tube) = £13.17; 10 bags (750 mL, long tube) = £13.48;
5 leg bag packs = £8.51

Sherwood range
**Argyle®** (Sherwood)
Leg bag, plastic. Net price (350, 500 or 750 mL, short or
long tube) = £20.50

Simcare range
NHS **Meredith®** (Simcare)
Top outlet bag. Net price 25 bags (2 litres) = £42.89
**PVC drainage bag** (Simcare)
Leg bag, plastic. Net price 1 bag (small or large) = £3.26
**Rubber bags** (Simcare)
Leg bag, rubber, with leg strap. Net price = £30.20
**Uro-Flo®** (Simcare)
Standard leg bag, plastic. Net price (350, 500 or 750 mL,
5 or 30 cm tube) = £12.73
Xtend® leg bag, plastic. Net price (500 mL, 6–20 cm or
22–36 cm tube) = £22.58

Simpla range
**Trident®** (Simpla)
Leg bag, plastic. Net price 10 bags (350 mL, short tube) =
£20.87; 10 bags (500 mL, short or long tube) = £21.09;
10 bags (750 mL, short, long, or adjustable long tube) =
£21.19

S&N range
**Regard®** (S&N)
Leg bag, plastic. Net price 10 bags (350 mL, short tube) =
£20.87; 10 bags (500 mL, short tube or adjustable long
tube) = £21.09; 10 bags (750 mL, adjustable long
tube) = £21.19

Thackraycare range
**Aquadry®** (Thackraycare)
Catheter drainage bag, plastic. Net price 10 bags
(small) = £20.65; 10 bags (large) = £21.20
Leg bag, plastic. Net price 10 bags (350, 500, or 750 mL,
short or long tube) = £19.95

---

Universal range
**Unicorn®** (Universal)

Leg bag, plastic. Net price 10 bags (350 mL, short tube) = £17.60; 10 bags (500 mL, short or long tube) = £17.80; 10 bags (750 mL, short or long tube) = £18.00

Wallace range
**Leg bags** (Wallace)

Leg bag, with valve outlet, natural latex straps, and plastic tube. Net price 10 bags (350 mL, short tube) = £20.22; 10 bags (350 mL, long tube) = £20.78; 10 bags (500 mL, short tube) = £20.65; 10 bags (500 mL, long tube) = £21.18; 10 bags (750 mL, short tube) = £20.96; 10 bags (750 mL, long tube) = £21.08

Leg bag, with twist tap, elastic straps, and plastic tube. Net price 10 bags (750 mL, short tube) = £20.96; 10 bags (750 mL, long tube, 30 cm) = £21.08

Tri-form® leg bag, plastic. Net price 10 bags (500 mL, short tube) = £20.52; 10 bags (500 mL, medium tube) = £20.86; 10 bags (500 mL, long tube) = £21.11

Ward range
**Kipper bag** (Ward)

Leg bag, kipper type, rubber. Net price 1 bag (black, clear, or white) = £18.95

**Leg drainage bag** (Ward)

Leg bag, plastic. Net price 10 bags (350 mL) = £9.15; 10 bags (500 mL) = £9.45; 10 bags (750 mL) = £9.94

**Comfort®** (Ward)

Leg bag, plastic. Net price 10 bags (350 mL) = £9.19; 10 bags (500 mL) = £9.45; 10 bags (750 mL) = £9.94

Willis range
**Leg bags** (Willis)

Rubber bag, for catheter drainage, short neck leg strap. Net price 1 bag = £24.18; 1 bag with web belt and support strap) = £28.29

Rubber bag, female, for catheter drainage, with conical mount. Net price 1 bag = £22.95; 1 bag (with web belt and support strap) = £27.06

Rubber bag, single-chambered, with olive mount. Net price 1 bag = £24.30; 1 bag (with web belt and support strap) = £28.29

---

# NIGHT DRAINAGE BAGS

Suitable for night-time use for collection of urine from indwelling catheters or from incontinence sheaths; bag hangers normally supplied through community nursing service.

Drainage bags have life of 5–7 nights

**Aldington**

2 litre urine drainage bag. Net price 10 bags = £9.64 (C), £10.75 (CV), £11.15 (CVT), £10.21 (DVT)

**Bard**

Uriplan® drainage bag. Net price 10 bags = £9.30

**Body's Care**

2 litre drainage bag with tap outlet. Net price 1 bag = £1.15

**Coloplast**

Conveen® 1.5 litre drainage bag with 90 cm tube. Net price 10 bags = £10.50

**ConvacTec**

Drainage bag. Net price 5 bags (Accuseal®) = £10.50; 5 bags (night) = £6.82

**EMS Medical**

2 litre urine drainage bag. Net price 10 bags = £9.80

**Hospital Management and Supplies**

Macpak® range. Net price 10 bags (Macpak® 1, non-drainable) = £1.47; 5 bags (Macpak® 3, drainable) = £3.81; 10 bags (Macpak® 5, non-drainable) = £1.46

**Pharma-Plast**

Careline® range, 2 litre urine drainage bag with 90 cm inlet tube. Net price 10 bags (Careline® E1, non-drainable) = £1.56; 10 bags (Careline® E2, non-drainable, with non-reflux valve) = £1.65; 5 bags (Careline® E4, with non-reflux valve and tap outlet) = £4.10

**Rand Rocket**

Urine drainage bag (non-drainable, short or long tube). Net price 25 bags = £3.75

**Salts**

2 litre urine drainage bag. Net price 10 bags = £9.67

**Sherwood**

Argyle® 2 litre urinary drainage bag. Net price 10 bags = £9.20

**Simcare**

Uro-flo® night drainage bag. Net price 10 bags (female or male) = £12.41

**Simpla**

Urine drainage bag. Net price 10 bags (S1, non-drainable) = £1.89; 10 bags (S2, non-drainable with non-reflux valve) = £2.01; 10 bags (night, short tube) = £9.39; 10 bags (S4, long tube) = £9.98

**S&N**

Regard® overnight drainage bag. Net price 10 bags = £8.68

**Thackraycare**

Urine drainage bag. Net price 1 bag = £1.15

Aqua® range 2 litre urine drainage bag. Net price 10 bags (Aqua® 2, non-drainable) = £1.90; 10 bags (Aqua® 4) = £8.60

**Wallace**

Community INBEDS night bag. Net price 10 bags = £11.40

**Ward**

2 litre drainage bag with push/pull outlet. Net price 10 bags = £9.94

---

# SUSPENSORY SYSTEMS

Drainage bag with support; bags may be used for 5–7 days

**Bard**

Urisac® Portabag® with belt. Net price 10 bags (plastic) = £10.25; 1 belt = £6.00

**EMS Medical**

Drainage bag with Shepheard Sporran belt. Net price 10 bags (plastic) = £12.85; 1 belt = £6.75

**Rüsch**

Portabag® with Portabelt®. Net price 10 bags (plastic) = £14.30; 1 belt = £8.00

**Wallace**

Holster bag with leg bag holster. Net price 10 bags (400 mL, plastic) = £16.21; 1 holster (24–30, 30–36, or 36–44 inch) = £7.58

---

# TUBING AND ACCESSORIES

**Bard**

General purpose tubing. Net price 96 inch = £1.82

Urinary drainage economy tube. Net price 48 inch = £1.16

Adaptor for Uro sheath® 8 inch. Net price 1 = 92p

Uriplan® leg bag straps (washable). Net price 5 pairs = £10.63

Latex leg bag straps. Net price 10 pairs = £2.18

---

Seton range foam/Velcro leg bag straps. Net price 10 pairs = £4.14

Urisac® tapes. Net price 10 pairs = £4.58

**Body's Care**

Velcro leg straps. Net price 1 pair = £1.40

Leg bag connecting tube. Net price 1 = £1.10; 1 (with mount) = £1.85

**Coloplast**

Velcro bands (washable). Net price 10 pairs = £29.20

**ConvaTec**

Accuseal® leg bag extension tube. Net price 10 tubes = £5.84

Accuseal® catheter adaptor. Net price 10 = £4.78

**EMS Medical**

Velcro leg straps. Net price 10 = £5.00

**Incare**

Leg bag straps. Net price 1 pair (14 inch, calf or 23 inch, thigh) = £2.27

**Leyland**

Connecting tubes, net price 1 tube for kipper bag = £2.31; 1 14 inch connecting tube for drip urinal = £2.30; 1 connecting tube for all urinals with female connector = £3.51

**MMG**

G-Strap. Net price 'adult' or 'short', 5 = £10.00; 'abdomen', 5 = £11.00

**Payne**

Rubber extension tube, 6 inch. Net price = £2.70

Velcro leg strap. Net price 1 = 75p

**Portex**

Tapered adaptor (catheter to leg bag). Net price 1 = £4.90; 1 (stepped) = £6.90

**Salts**

Heritage® leg bag extension tube. Net price 2 tubes = £1.70

**Sherwood**

Argyle® foam and Velcro strap, washable. Net price 10 (75 cm, leg) = £16.20; 5 (150 cm, abdomen) = £15.25

Argyle Suregrip® general purpose tube, internal diameter 7 mm, length 2.7 m. Net price 50 tubes = £34.50

Argyle Penrose® tubing, internal diameter 6, 8, 10, 13, 16, 19, or 25 mm and length 44 cm. Net price 50 = £29.50

**Simcare**

Stopcock for Chiron plastic urinal bags (in place of screwcap). Net price 1 = £3.85

Rubber extension tube (with mounts). Net price = £3.85

Rubber tubing (length, 1.5 m). Net price 1 = £9.00

Plastic connector with tube. Net price 1 = £2.58

Female connector for Mitcham bag. Net price = £1.78

Leg straps. Net price 5 pairs = £11.24

Night bag connector. Net price 1 = £1.09

Spare 'O' rings for pp urinal. Net price 5 = £1.02

Uro-Flo® elastic Velcro leg straps. Net price 5 pairs = £3.66

Paul (Penrose) tubing. Net price 10 (6, 13, 19, or 25 mm) = £11.04; 10 (32, 38, 44, or 51 mm) = £11.04

**Simpla**

Leg bag straps. Net price 20 pairs (foam) = £10.86; 5 pairs (elasticated, washable) = £10.70

**Thackraycare**

Leg bag connecting tube. Net price 10 = £6.55

Aquadry® leg straps. Net price 5 pairs = £8.75

**Wallace**

Leg bag extension tube. Net price 10 (30 cm) = £23.46; 10 (60 cm) = £25.80

Silgrip® leg straps. Net price 5 pairs (elasticated or Side-Fix thigh-fitting) = £10.48; 5 pairs (Side-Fix calf-fitting) = £9.96

# URINAL SYSTEMS

Patients generally have two urinal systems (one to wash and one to wear). Each appliance should last for 6 months

**Bard**

Uriplan Mcguire® urinal and adaptor. Net price (waist sizes 66–81 cm, 81–96 cm, or 96–112 cm) = £48.60

Male day and night urinal. Net price 1 (14 oz) = £38.10; 1 (20 oz) = £33.74

Mobile paraplegic day and night urinal. Net price 1 = £39.67

Uriplan Mcguire® adaptor and tubing. Net price = £6.56

**Bell and Croyden**

Fridjohn male urinal. Net price 1 = £40.61

Male urinal, day and night use. Net price 1 (with long or short bag) = £37.35

**Body's Care**

Male day and night urinal with tap, covered bag, with band and suspensory, and leg strap with air vent. Net price 1 = £43.30

Male night urinal with tap, covered bag, with band and suspensory. Net price 1 = £52.68

Male day and night urinal with tap, long tube, covered bag, with band and suspensory with air vent. Net price 1 = £51.19

Male day and night urinal with tap, double bag, air vent, inflating rim, with band understraps. Net price 1 = £54.21

Male day and night urinal with tap, covered bag, diaphragm top, and air vent. Net price 1 = £46.85

Male day and night urinal with tap, improved pattern, inflating rim, short air vent, with band and understrap. Net price 1 = £51.41; 1 (with extension tube) = £54.27; 1 (with long bag) = £52.15

Male day and night urinal with tap, air vent, diaphragm top, with band and understrap. Net price 1 (with long bag) = £49.87; 1 (with short bag) = £46.21; 1 (with extension tube) = £49.71

Male day and night urinal with tap, air vent, with band and suspensory. Net price 1 (long bag) = £44.41

Male day urinal with tap, to contain penis and scrotum. Net price 1 (short bag, with band and understrap) = £41.87; 1 (with inner sheath and air vent) = £43.51

Male jockey appliance with tap. Net price 1 = £46.32

Spares

Replacement belt. Net price 1 = £9.11

Outer receiver. Net price 1 = £10.60

Inner sheath. Net price 5 = £10.92

Plastic bags. Net price 5 = £11.98

Rubber bag. Net price 1 = £19.45

Ring. Net price 1 = 79p

Stoke Mandeville male urinal with tap (specify sheath size). Net price 1 = £49.18; 1 (with double bag) = £59.04; 1 replacement sheath (specify size) = £4.87

Male pubic pressure urinal with tap (specify sheath size). Net price 1 (with rubber bag) = £52.59; 1 (with 5 plastic bags) = £49.50

Spares

Flange with sheaths. Net price 1 = £24.59

Cone. Net price (curved, small, medium, or large; straight, small, medium, large, or extra-large) = £9.75

Plastic bag. Net price 1 (small or large) = £11.98

Rubber bag. Net price 1 = £19.08

Rubber belt. Net price 1 = £3.50

Progress® long life plastic urinal. Net price 1 (inner sheath or scrotal) = £20.78

Fridjohn urinal. Net price 1 = £62.11

YB wet urinal. Net price 1 = £50.40

Essex appliance. Net price 1 = £42.08

One-piece belt. Net price 1 (rubber or plastic bag cover-let) = £42.20

**Bullen**

Child urinal. Net price 1 (with transverse bag) = £64.58; 1 (with medium-size long bag) = £62.41

Male urinal. Net price 1 (with large-size long bag) = £68.59

**Ellis**

Hallam modular urinal. Net price 1 = £28.75; 1 spare bag = £1.53; 1 spare belt = £3.41

**Leyland**

Thames urinal with bag and connecting tube. Net price 1 (standard or long bag) = £65.08

Severn urinal with bag and connecting tube. Net price 1 (standard bag, long bag, or 5 plastic bags) = £65.08; 5 Severn spare sheaths = £25.51

Mersey urinal with bag and connecting tube. Net price 1 (standard bag, long bag, or 5 plastic bags) = £65.08

Wye urinal. Net price 1 (with separate connecting tube and on/off valve) = £21.03; 1 (with long night extension tube) = £24.51; 1 (with short or long bag) = £35.03

Arizona male urinal. Net price 1 = £65.08

'55' male urinal. Net price 1 = £64.10; 6 spare sheaths = £29.95

Clyde urinal with bag and connecting tube. Net price 1 (standard bag, long bag, or 5 plastic bags) = £65.08

Stoke Mandeville pattern male urinal. Net price 1 (20, 24, 25, 28, 32, 35, 38, 42, 45, 48, 51, 54, 57, 60, or 63 mm sheath) = £65.08; 1 spare sheath = £6.31

Sahara one-piece top pubic pressure urinal with bag. Net price 1 paediatric (with small rubber collection bag or 5 small plastic collection bags) = £62.04; 1 standard or large (with standard or long rubber collection bag or 5 medium plastic collection bags, and connecting tube) = £62.04

Peoplecare® pubic pressure male urinal. Net price 1 paediatric (flange 25 mm and sheath 13, 16, 19, or 22 mm; *or* flange 29 mm and sheath 22 or 25 mm; *or* flange 32 mm and sheath 19, 22, or 25 mm) = £20.15; 1 adult (flange 38 mm and sheath 19, 22, 25, 29, or 32 mm; *or* flange 44 mm and sheath 35, 38, or 41 mm) = £20.15

Spares

Pubic pressure bag. Net price 1 (standard, medium) = £10.40; 1 (standard, large) = £12.89; 1 (curved top, small, medium, or large) = £7.85; 1 (straight top, small, medium, large, or extra-large) = £7.85

Transverse rubber bag with tap. Net price 1 = £21.29

Pubic pressure flange. Net price 1 (double-based) = £20.15; 1 (adult, rubber) = £23.23

Kipper inco set. Net price 1 = £34.87

**LRC**

Dry sheaths. Net price 144 = £14.00

**Payne**

Male incontinence appliance with rubber belt. Net price 1 (with combined rubber flange and understraps) = £53.23; 1 (MK2 with rubber flange and fabric face piece) = £57.24; 1 (with combined rubber flange, understraps, and coned top) = £47.24; (MK9, with rubber flange and fabric facepiece) = £59.65

Lightweight male incontinence appliance. Net price 1 (with fabric face piece and separate long flanged plastic bag with foam pad) = £33.75; 1 (MK5, with fabric facepiece, separate flange, and long flanged plastic bag with rubber belt) = £47.40; 1 (with combined flange and understraps and long flanged plastic bag with rubber belt) = £41.57; 1 (MK10, with fabric facepiece, separate flange, and long flanged plastic bag with rubber belt) = £49.81

Spares

Rubber flange. Net price 1 (with diaphragm, MK5) = £14.40; 1 (with feathered diaphragm, MK1 and MK6) = £23.86; 1 (with feathered diaphragm, MK2) = £15.41; 1 (with feathered diaphragm and large reinforced top, MK3) = £27.07

Material face piece with support belt and loop. Net price 1 = £17.87; 1 (loop and scrotal) = £20.28

Reinforced cone top. Net price 1 (plastic or rubber) = £10.38

Bag. Net price 1 (plastic) = £2.62; 1 (rubber) = £15.68; 1 (plastic, long flange, MK4) = £3.75; 1 (plastic, long flange, MK5, MK6, or MK10) = £3.53

Belt. Net price 1 (elastic) = £7.12; 1 (web) = £4.98; 1 (rubber) = £3.37

Night connector. Net price 1 = £3.15; 1 (drainage) = £3.37

Payne's urine director. Net price 1 = £19.05

Stoke Mandeville condom urinal complete. Net price 1 = £43.92

Spares

Kipper bag. Net price 1 = £24.72

Belt. Net price 1 (38, 46, or 60 inch) = £5.24

Rubber tube and connector. Net price 1 = £1.93; rubber tubing (per metre) = £3.96; nylon connector 1 = £1.12

Dry incontinence sheath. Net price 144 = £12.79

Pubic pressure urinal complete with bag. Net price 1 (rubber or plastic bag) = £53.23

Spares

Pubic pressure flange with sheath (all sizes). Net price 1 = £23.86

Coned top. Net price 1 (straight or curved, small, medium, or large, *or* extra-large) = £10.38

Replacements

Rubber bag with vent tube. Net price 1 = £18.83

Reinforced cone top with vent tube. Net price 1 = £13.64

Latex tubing, 8 or 10 mm bore. Net price per metre = £3.96

Condom set. Net price 1 = £45.80; 1 (with 40 oz bag) = £56.82

Urinal replacement parts

Nylon stud. Net price 1 = £1.05; 1 (with latex tube) = £1.12

Waist belt for single-chambered bag. Net price 1 (38, 46, or 60 inch) = £5.24

**Salts**

Male pubic pressure urinal with rubber bag or 4 plastic bags. Net price 1 = £41.51

Spares

Pubic pressure flange with sheath (all sizes). Net price 1 = £19.92

Cone. Net price 1 (small, medium, or large; straight or curved, extra-large, straight) = £8.87

Pubic pressure flange belt. Net price 1 = £17.50

Bags. Net price 4 (plastic, child or adult) = £9.75; 1 (rubber, child, adult, or transverse) = £9.75

Belt. Net price = £2.97

**Simcare**

Male pubic pressure urinal, child, with integral flange. Net price 1 (rubber bag, straight cone, medium) = £50.93; 1 (plastic bag, curved cone, small or medium) = £49.79

Spares

Pubic pressure flange with integral sheath for child. Net price 1 (all sizes) = £28.03

Cone. Net price 1 (small, medium, or large, straight or curved; extra-large, straight) = £11.86

Pubic pressure flange, double-based. Net price 1 (child, 32 mm; adult, 38 or 44 mm) = £25.07

Chailey male urinal. Net price 1 (child, plastic bag) = £52.41; 1 (adolescent or adult, rubber bag) = £46·99; 1 (adolescent or adult, plastic bag) = £59.52

Spares

Curved top with integral sheath and straps. Net price 1 (various sizes) = £31.36

Belt, rubber. Net price 1 (61 or 91 cm) = £4.62

Bags, rubber (also suitable for pubic pressure and Chiron urinals). Net price 1 (wide neck, adult, or child) = £3.09

Male pubic pressure urinal, adult, with integral flange. Net price 1 (rubber bag, various sizes) = £59.01; 1 (plastic bag, various sizes) = £54.98

Replacement pubic pressure flange. Net price 1 = £28.03

Male pubic pressure urinal, adult, with double-based flange. Net price 1 (rubber bag, various sizes) = £59.01; 1 (plastic bag, various sizes) = £54.98

Replacement sheath. Net price 10 = £1.08

Bag, rubber, for pubic presure urinals. Net price 1 (adult, with vent tube) = £24.46; 1 (adult, double) = £26.19

---

Cautionary label wordings, see inside back cover

Stoke Mandeville urinal. Net price 1 (sheath type) = £53.76; 1 (double rubber bag) = £69.88
Spares
Bag. Net price 1 = £26.19; 1 (with top) = £49.62
Sheath. Net price 1 = £7.33; 10 (for sheath type) = £3.22
Net suspensory. Net price 1 = £15.50
Chiron male rubber urinal with webbing belt. Net price 1 = £48.39
Male one-piece urinal. Net price = £46.07
Surrey model lightweight urinal. Net price = (MKI or MKII) = £43.77
Spares
Bag. Net price 10 = £27.39
Foam pad. Net price 5 (76 mm/32 mm = £5.39
Chiron urinal. Net price 1 (male, plastic, rubber sheaths) = £25.04; 1 (geriatric, film-type sheaths) = £36.36; 1 (rubber sheaths) = £36.36
Spares
Sheath. Net price 1 (rubber) = £4.62; 10 (film type) = 86p
Net suspensory. Net price 1 = £10.87
Male urinal for bed use. Net price 10 = £40.84
Pubic flange, large opening. Net price 1 = £18.77
Transverse rubber bag and stopcock. Net price 1 (child) = £27.65

**Steeper**

Paraplegic male urinal for day and night use with porthole swan-neck top, adjustable elastic belt with linen front 4 buttonholes, and understraps suitable for sitting patients. Net price 1 = £54.36
Male rubber urinal for day use, porthole top, straight neck and inner sheath, adjustable elastic belt with linen front, 4 buttonholes, and understraps. Net price 1 = £40.15; 1 (with swan-neck) = £43.41
Adjustable waistband, elastic, for above urinals. Net price 1 = £6.82
Male urinal, rabbit eared, with inner sheath complete with waistband. Net price 1 = £38.50
Adjustable waistband. Net price 1 = £3.77
Scrotal pouch. Net price 1 = £4.25
Male dribbling bag (rubber), curved with porthole diaphragm and adjustable webbing belt. Net price 1 = £19.61
Pubic pressure urinal with double-based flange, disposable film sheaths, and 4 plastic bags. Net price 1 = £35.86

**Thackraycare**

Aquadry® urinal. Net price 1 (scrotal support, adult or adolescent; pubic pressure, adult or adolescent; rubber understrap, adult or adolescent; paediatric; pubic pressure paediatric with rubber understrap) = £47.90; 1 (long-term) = £46.75
Spares
Bag (except for drip type and long-term). Net price 5 (250 or 325 mL) = £10.85
Flange (range of sizes). Net price 1 = £23.60
Cones. Net price 1 (small, medium, or large, curved or straight) = £9.90
Rubber belt. Net price 1 (adult or child) = £2.75

**Ward**

Jockey male urinal. Net price 1 = £59.44
Varsity male urinal. Net price 1 = £45.88
Male urinal. Net price 1 (day use, covered bag, complete with belt suspensory and thigh strap) = £37.95; 1 (day and night, covered bag, air vent, belt suspensory) = £39.29; 1 (day and night, short bag and belt) = £40.67; 1 (day and night, short covered bag and belt) = £44.07; (day and night, double Chamber bag) = £45.81; 1 (day and night, long bag and belt) = £40.67
Paraplegic male urinal. Net price 1 = £55.57
Stoke Mandeville Pattern. Net price 1 = £53.39; 1 (removable rubber sheath, double chamber rubber bag, thigh strap and belt) = £47.95
Spare sheath. Net price 1 = £4.96

Male pubic pressure urinal. Net price 1 (rubber bag) = £49.75; 1 (plastic bag) = £44.08
Spares
Pubic pressure flange. Net price 1 = £22.82
Pubic pressure cone; Net price 1 = £9.02
Bags. Net price 1 (rubber) = £12.36; 1 (plastic) = £2.48
Male urinal. Net price 1 (day, covered bag complete with belt) = £36.12; 1 (day and night or night, covered bag complete with belt, suspensory, and thigh strap) = £47.73; 1 (day and night, long tube, air vent, rubber bag, complete with belt and thigh strap) = £43.32
Male urinal. Net price 1 (night, covered bag complete with belt, suspensory, and thigh strap) = £47.73
Male dribbling bag and tapes. Net price 1 = £17.63
Male urinal. Net price 1 (day and night, short covered bag or short bag and belt) = £40.67
Male urinal. Net price 1 (sheath and disc type with long rubber belt or sheath and suspensory with short or long covered bag) = £44.33
Male urinal. Net price 1 (conical top with short or long rubber bag) = £25.30
Night urinal. Net price 1 (with long tube) = £21.38
Stoke Mandeville sheath-type urinal, with 30 rubber film sheaths, rubber bag, and thigh strap and belt. Net price 1 = £42.46
St Peters pattern suprapubic bag. Net price 1 = £26.15

**Willis**

Male urinal, day and night, air tube to bag, inner sheath and diaphragm to receiver, web belt and cotton suspensory bag. Net price 1 = £44.68; 1 (bag covered with Coutil®, elastic leg strap) = £46.50; 1 (long narrow Coutil®-covered bag, web belt and cotton suspensory bag) = £46.50
Male urinal, receiver to contain penis and scrotum, web waist band, and tape understraps. Net price 1 (day, night, or small build) = £42.66
Male urinal, long rubber bag with 2 leg straps, loops and straps, flanged receiver, air tube, diaphragm and short conical inner sheath, web band and cotton suspensory bag. Net price 1 (day and night) = £44.14
Male urinal, short rubber bag, detachable bag and night tube, web belt and cotton suspensory bag. Net price 1 (day and night) = £35.57
Spares for above urinals
White web waist band. Net price 1 (29, 36, or 44–48 inch) = £4.00
Suspension bag. Net price 1 (small, medium, or large) = £4.49

## URETHRAL CATHETERS

Urethal catheter sizes are designated by the Charrière (Ch) gauge system; when the size is not stated by the prescriber the Drug Tariff recommends that size 14 or 16 be supplied. For the Foley catheter, if the balloon size is not stated, the 10 mL size should be supplied for adults, 5 mL for paediatric use (balloon sizes are defined as the amount of fluid required to fully inflate the volume of lumen).

**Foley** (indwelling Nelaton catheter with balloon, 2-way), short/medium- or long-term use; male (adult) gauge (Ch) 12–28, female (adult) gauge (Ch) 12–26 both with balloon sizes 10 and 30 mL; paediatric gauge (Ch) 8–10 balloon size 5 mL. Net price male = £1.75, female = £2.25. paediatric = £3.15
Available from Bard, Dow Corning, Rüsch, Sherwood, Simcare, Simpla

**Nelaton** (ordinary cylindrical catheter), male gauge (Ch) 8–24, female gauge (Ch) 8–18, paediatric gauge (Ch) 8–10. Net price male = 31p, female = 28p
Available from Bard, EMS (PVC), Pennine, Portex (PVC), Rüsch, Simcare (PVC).

**Scott** (short curved tubular catheter for women and girls), female gauge (Ch) 8–14. Net price = £1.99
Available from Simcare (polyethylene)

# 8: Drugs used in the treatment of
# MALIGNANT DISEASE and
# for IMMUNOSUPPRESSION

In this chapter, drug treatment is discussed under the following headings:

**8.1** Cytotoxic drugs
**8.2** Drugs affecting the immune response
**8.3** Sex hormones and hormone antagonists in malignant disease

Malignant disease may be treated by surgery, radiotherapy, and/or chemotherapy. Certain tumours are highly sensitive to chemotherapy but many are not, and inappropriate drug administration in these circumstances can only increase morbidity or mortality.

## 8.1 Cytotoxic drugs

**8.1.1** Alkylating drugs
**8.1.2** Cytotoxic antibiotics
**8.1.3** Antimetabolites
**8.1.4** Vinca alkaloids and etoposide
**8.1.5** Other antineoplastic drugs

Great care is needed when prescribing these drugs as damage to normal tissue, which may be irreversible, is an almost invariable consequence of their use. These drugs should rarely, if ever, be used empirically in a patient with cancer, and administration should always be regarded as a clinical trial with clear objectives in mind.

---

**CRM guidelines on cytotoxic drug handling:**

1. Trained personnel should reconstitute cytotoxics;
2. Reconstitution should be carried out in designated areas;
3. Protective clothing (including gloves) should be worn;
4. The eyes should be protected and means of first aid should be specified;
5. Pregnant staff should not handle cytotoxics;
6. Adequate care should be taken in the disposal of waste material, including syringes, containers, and absorbent material.

---

In a minority of cancers, chemotherapy may result in cure, or marked prolongation of survival. Here short-term drug-related toxicity, which may be severe, is acceptable. However, for the majority of patients, modest survival prolongation or palliation of symptoms will be the aim, and an attempt should be made to use relatively non-toxic treatments, or to consider the use of other effective modalities, e.g. radiotherapy.

Cytotoxics may be used either singly, or in combination. In the latter case, the initial letters of the drug names, or proprietary names, identify the regimen used. Drug combinations are frequently more toxic than single drugs but may have the advantage in certain tumours of enhanced

response and increased survival. However for some tumours, single-agent chemotherapy remains the treatment of choice.

---

Most cytotoxic drugs are teratogenic, and all may cause life-threatening toxicity; administration should, where possible, be confined to those experienced in their use.

Because of the complexity of dosage regimens in the treatment of malignant disease, dose statements have been omitted from some of the drug entries in this chapter. *In all cases detailed specialist literature should be consulted.*

Prescriptions should **not** be repeated except on the instructions of a specialist.

---

Cytotoxic drugs fall naturally into a number of classes, each with characteristic antitumour activity, sites of action, and toxicity. A knowledge of sites of metabolism and excretion is important, as impaired drug handling as a result of disease is not uncommon and may result in enhanced toxic effects. A number of side-effects are characteristic of particular agents or groups of drugs, e.g. neurotoxicity of vinca alkaloids, and details will be provided in the appropriate sections. Most toxic effects are, however, common to many of these drugs and will be briefly outlined here.

EXTRAVASATION OF INTRAVENOUS DRUGS. A number of drugs will cause severe local tissue necrosis if leakage into the extravascular compartment occurs. Recommended modes of administration must be adhered to. Infusion of vesicant drugs should be stopped immediately if local pain is experienced. Where doubt exists as to whether significant leakage has occurred, the infusion should be discontinued and the cannula resited in another vein. There are no proven antidotes for extravasation, but general recommendations include elevation of the limb and application of ice packs three or four times daily until pain and swelling settle; if ulceration occurs plastic surgery may be required.

HYPERCALCAEMIA. Hypercalcaemia is a common complication of malignant disease. Treatment of the underlying malignancy may resolve it, but drugs which specifically lower serum calcium are often also required (see section 9.5.1.2).

HYPERURICAEMIA. Hyperuricaemia, which can result in uric acid crystal formation in the urinary tract with associated renal dysfunction is a complication of the treatment of non-Hodgkin's lymphoma and leukemia. Allopurinol (see section 10.1.4) should be started 24 hours before treating such tumours, and should be continued for 7 to 10 days; patients should be adequately hydrated.

---

The dose of mercaptopurine or azathioprine should be reduced if allopurinol needs to be given concomitantly (see Appendix 1).

NAUSEA AND VOMITING. Nausea and vomiting is a source of considerable distress to many patients receiving chemotherapy. It should be anticipated and, where possible, prevented with anti-emetic treatment tailored to the chemotherapy regimen and the response of the patient.

If first-line anti-emetics are ineffective treatment should be escalated as below. Hospital admission may be necessary.

*Group 1: severe emesis unlikely*
Drugs in this group include alkylating drugs by mouth, intravenous fluorouracil, vinca alkaloids, and methotrexate.

Phenothiazines (e.g. prochlorperazine) or domperidone, given by mouth, when necessary, will often suffice. Premedication with these drugs is often useful before intravenous chemotherapy, treatment being continued for up to 24 hours afterwards. Both prochlorperazine and domperidone are also available as suppositories which is useful for patients who develop vomiting despite oral therapy.

*Group 2: moderate emesis*
Drugs in this group include intravenous cyclophosphamide and doxorubicin; premedication is essential for all drugs in this group. Most patients can be treated on an out-patient basis therefore, if possible, the anti-emetics should be given by mouth.

Anti-emetics in group 1 are given when necessary but it is usually preferable to give in addition dexamethasone 10 mg by mouth before and 6 hours after chemotherapy, and/or lorazepam 1 to 2 mg by mouth given similarly. Lorazepam has the advantage of causing drowsiness and amnesia, but patients cannot drive after it. Nabilone is also suitable, but may cause dysphoria. Ondansetron may also have a valuable role.

Patients in group 1 with an unsatisfactory response can be transferred to drugs in this group.

*Group 3: severe emesis*
Drugs in this group include mustine, dacarbazine, and cisplatin. They commonly cause severe emesis, particularly if used in combination.

A simple well-tolerated anti-emetic regimen is dexamethasone 10 mg by mouth with lorazepam 1 to 2 mg by mouth, given before and 6 hours after chemotherapy. Out-patients should be warned not to drive. Dexamethasone and lorazepam can also be given intravenously to inpatients; the dose of lorazepam is titrated according to the patient's level of consciousness (drowsiness should be obtained with 2 to 4 mg). This regimen should be avoided in patients with chronic chest disease and care is necessary in the elderly.

Alternatively, or in addition, high-dose metoclopramide can be given by intravenous infusion but it may cause dystonic reactions in younger patients (see section 4.6).

Ondansetron may be useful for controlling vomiting in the short term.

Patients in group 2 with an unsatisfactory response can be transferred to drugs in this group.

BONE-MARROW SUPPRESSION. All cytotoxic drugs except vincristine and bleomycin cause marrow depression. This commonly occurs 7 to 10 days after administration, but is delayed for certain drugs, such as carmustine, lomustine, and melphalan. Peripheral blood counts must be checked prior to each treatment, and doses should be reduced or therapy delayed if marrow recovery has not occurred. Fever occurring in a neutropenic patient (neutrophil count less than $0.8 \times 10^9$/litre) is an indication for immediate parenteral broad-spectrum antibiotic therapy (see section 5.1, Table 1), once appropriate bacteriological investigations have taken place.

ALOPECIA. Reversible hair loss is a common complication, although it varies in degree between drugs and individual patients. No pharmacological methods of preventing this are available.

REPRODUCTIVE FUNCTION. Most cytotoxic drugs are teratogenic and should not be administered during pregnancy, especially during the first trimester (but for transplant therapy, see below).

Contraceptive advice should be offered where appropriate before cytotoxic therapy begins. Regimens that do not contain an alkylating drug may have less effect on fertility, but those with an alkylating drug will render almost all males permanently sterile early in a treatment course (there is no effect on potency). Pre-treatment counselling and consideration of sperm storage may be appropriate. Females are less severely affected, though the span of reproductive life may be shortened by the onset of a premature menopause. No increase in fetal abnormalities or abortion-rate has been recorded in patients who remain fertile after cytotoxic chemotherapy.

**Transplant therapy.** Female transplanted patients immunosuppressed with azathioprine should not discontinue it on becoming pregnant; although spontaneous abortion may be more common, congenital fetal abnormalities are not increased in successful pregnancies. There is less experience of cyclosporin in pregnancy; although compatible with normal pregnancy, retardation of fetal growth has been reported. Any risk to the offspring of azathioprine-treated men is small.

## 8.1.1   Alkylating drugs

Extensive experience is available with these drugs, which are among the most widely used in cancer chemotherapy. They act by damaging DNA, thus interfering with cell replication. In addition to the side-effects common to many cytotoxic drugs (section 8.1), there are two problems associated with prolonged usage. Firstly, gametogenesis is often severely affected (see above). Secondly, prolonged use of these drugs, par-

---

ticularly when combined with extensive irradiation, is associated with a marked increase in the incidence of acute non-lymphocytic leukaemia.

**Cyclophosphamide** is widely used in the treatment of chronic lymphocytic leukaemia, the lymphomas, and solid tumours. It may be given orally or intravenously and is inactive until metabolised by the liver. A urinary metabolite of cyclophosphamide, acrolein, may cause haemorrhagic cystitis; this is a serious complication and if it occurs cyclophosphamide is not normally used again. An increased fluid intake, for example 3 to 4 litres per day after intravenous injection, will help avoid this complication. When high-dose therapy is used mesna will also help prevent this complication.

**Ifosfamide** is related to cyclophosphamide; like cyclophosphamide it is given with mesna to reduce urothelial toxicity.

**Chlorambucil** is commonly used to treat chronic lymphocytic leukaemia, the indolent non-Hodgkin's lymphomas, Hodgkin's disease, and ovarian cancer. Side-effects, apart from marrow suppression, are uncommon, although rashes may occur.

**Melphalan** is used to treat myeloma and occasionally solid tumours and lymphomas. Marrow toxicity is delayed and it is usually given at intervals of 4–6 weeks.

**Busulphan** is used almost exclusively to treat chronic myeloid leukaemia. Frequent blood counts are necessary as excessive myelosuppression may result in irreversible bone-marrow aplasia. Hyperpigmentation of the skin is a common side-effect and, rarely, progressive pulmonary fibrosis may occur.

**Lomustine** (CCNU) is a lipid-soluble nitrosourea and may be given orally. It is mainly used to treat Hodgkin's disease and certain solid tumours. Marrow toxicity is delayed, and the drug is therefore given at intervals of 4 to 6 weeks. Permanent marrow damage may occur with prolonged use. Nausea and vomiting are common and moderately severe.

**Carmustine** is given intravenously. It has similar activity and toxicities to lomustine and is most commonly given to patients with myeloma, lymphoma, and brain tumours. Cumulative renal damage and delayed pulmonary fibrosis may occur.

**Mustine** is now much less commonly used. It is a very toxic drug which causes severe vomiting. The freshly prepared injection must be given into a fast-running intravenous infusion. Local extravasation causes severe tissue necrosis.

**Estramustine** is a stable combination of an oestrogen and mustine, designed to deliver mustine to the oestrogen receptor site of a tumour, for example prostate cancer. It has both a local cytotoxic effect and (by reducing testosterone concentrations) a hormonal effect.

**Treosulfan** is used to treat ovarian cancer.

**Thiotepa** is usually used as an intracavitary drug for the treatment of malignant effusions or bladder cancer. It is also occasionally used to treat breast cancer, but requires parenteral administration.

**Mitobronitol** is occasionally used to treat chronic myeloid leukaemia; it is available on a named-patient basis only (as *Myelobromol*®, Sinclair).

## BUSULPHAN

*Indications:* chronic myeloid leukaemia

*Cautions; Side-effects:* see section 8.1 and notes above; avoid in porphyria (see section 9.8.2)

*Dose:* induction of remission, 60 micrograms/kg to max. 4 mg daily; maintenance, 0.5–2 mg daily

PoM **Myleran**® (Wellcome)

*Tablets*, busulphan 500 micrograms, net price 25 = £3.21; 2 mg, 25 = £4.84

## CARMUSTINE

*Indications:* see notes above

*Cautions; Side-effects:* see section 8.1 and notes above; irritant to tissues

PoM **BiCNU**® (Bristol-Myers)

*Injection*, powder for reconstitution, carmustine. Net price 100-mg vial (with diluent) = £12.50

## CHLORAMBUCIL

*Indications:* see notes above (for use as an immunosuppressant see section 8.2.1)

*Cautions; Side-effects:* see section 8.1 and notes above; caution in renal impairment; avoid in porphyria (see section 9.8.2)

*Dose:* used alone, usually 100–200 micrograms/kg daily for 4–8 weeks

PoM **Leukeran**® (Wellcome)

*Tablets*, both yellow, chlorambucil 2 mg, net price 25 = £7.77; 5 mg, 25 = £11.85

## CYCLOPHOSPHAMIDE

*Indications:* see notes above

*Cautions; Side-effects:* see section 8.1 and notes above; reduce dose in renal impairment; avoid in porphyria (see section 9.8.2); **interactions:** Appendix 1 (cyclophosphamide)

PoM **Cyclophosphamide** (Farmitalia Carlo Erba)

*Tablets*, pink, s/c, cyclophosphamide (anhydrous) 50 mg. Net price 20 = £1.91. Label: 27

*Injection*, powder for reconstitution, cyclophosphamide. Net price 107-mg vial = 95p; 214-mg vial = £1.35; 535-mg vial = £2.36; 1.07-g vial = £4.12

PoM **Endoxana**® (ASTA Medica)

*Tablets*, s/c, cyclophosphamide 50 mg, net price 100-tab pack = £9.13. Label: 27

*Injection*, powder for reconstitution, cyclophosphamide. Net price 107-mg vial = 79p; 214-mg vial = £1.13; 535-mg vial = £1.97; 1.069-g vial = £3.44

## ESTRAMUSTINE PHOSPHATE

*Indications:* prostate cancer
*Cautions:* see section 8.1
*Contra-indications:* peptic ulceration, severe liver or cardiac disease
*Side-effects:* see section 8.1; also gynaecomastia, altered liver function, cardiovascular disorders (angina and rare reports of myocardial infarction)
*Dose:* 0.14–1.4 g daily in divided doses (usual range 0.56–1.12 g daily)

PoM **Estracyt**® (Kabi Pharmacia)
*Capsules,* estramustine phosphate 140 mg (as disodium salt). Net price 20 = £27.17. Label: 21, counselling, should not be taken with dairy products

## IFOSFAMIDE

*Indications:* see notes above
*Cautions; Side-effects:* see section 8.1 and notes under Cyclophosphamide; reduce dose in renal impairment; **interactions:** Appendix 1 (ifosfamide)

PoM **Mitoxana**® (ASTA Medica)
*Injection,* powder for reconstitution, ifosfamide. Net price 500-mg vial = £6.74; 1-g vial = £11.76; 2-g vial = £21.65 (hosp. only)

## LOMUSTINE

*Indications:* see notes above
*Cautions; Side-effects:* see section 8.1 and notes above
*Dose:* used alone, 120–130 mg/m² body-surface every 6–8 weeks

PoM **CCNU**® (Lundbeck)
*Capsules,* lomustine 10 mg (blue/white), net price 20 = £9.42; 40 mg (blue), 20 = £23.69

## MELPHALAN

*Indications:* myelomatosis; see also notes above
*Cautions; Side-effects:* see section 8.1 and notes above; reduce dose in renal impairment
*Dose: by mouth,* 150–300 micrograms/kg daily for 4–6 days, repeated after 4–8 weeks

PoM **Alkeran**® (Wellcome)
*Tablets,* melphalan 2 mg, net price 25 = £10.66; 5 mg, 25 = £18.86
*Injection,* powder for reconstitution, melphalan. Net price 100-mg vial (with solvent and diluent) = £51.38

## MUSTINE HYDROCHLORIDE

*Indications:* Hodgkin's disease—see notes above
*Cautions; Side-effects:* see section 8.1 and notes above; irritant to tissues (also caution in handling—vesicant and a nasal irritant)

PoM **Mustine Hydrochloride**® (Boots)
*Injection,* powder for reconstitution, mustine hydrochloride. Net price 10-mg vial = £1.48

## THIOTEPA

*Indications:* see notes above and section 7.4.4
*Cautions; Side-effects:* see section 8.1; **interactions:** Appendix 1 (thiotepa)

PoM **Thiotepa** (Lederle)
*Injection,* powder for reconstitution, thiotepa, net price 15-mg vial = £4.85

## TREOSULFAN

*Indications:* see notes above
*Cautions; Side-effects:* see section 8.1
*Dose: by mouth,* courses of 1–2 g daily in 4 divided doses to provide total dose of 21–28 g over initial 8 weeks

PoM **Treosulfan**® (Leo)
*Capsules,* treosulfan 250 mg. Net price 20 = £7.53. Label: 25
*Injection,* powder for reconstitution, treosulfan. Net price 5 g in infusion bottle with transfer needle = £17.19

UROTHELIAL TOXICITY

Urothelial toxicity, commonly manifest by haemorrhagic cystitis, is a problem peculiar to the use of cyclophosphamide or ifosfamide and is caused by a metabolite (acrolein). **Mesna** reacts specifically with this metabolite in the urinary tract, preventing toxicity. Mesna is given simultaneously with cyclophosphamide or ifosfamide, and further doses are given orally or intravenously 4 and 8 hours after treatment.

## MESNA

*Indications:* see notes above
*Side-effects:* above max. therapeutic doses, gastro-intestinal disturbances, fatigue, headache, limb pains, depression, irritability, lack of energy, rash

PoM **Uromitexan**® (ASTA Medica)
*Injection,* mesna 100 mg/mL. Net price 4-mL amp = £1.36; 10-mL amp = £2.95

*Note.* For oral administration contents of ampoule are taken in fruit juice

## 8.1.2   Cytotoxic antibiotics

Drugs within this group are widely used. Many cytotoxic antibiotics act as radiomimetics and simultaneous use of radiotherapy should be avoided as it may result in markedly enhanced normal tissue toxicity.

**Doxorubicin** is one of the most successful and widely used antitumour drugs, and is used to treat the acute leukaemias, lymphomas, and a variety of solid tumours. It is given by fast running infusion, commonly at 21-day intervals. Local extravasation will cause severe tissue necrosis. Common toxic effects include nausea and vomiting, myelosuppression, alopecia, and mucositis. This drug is largely excreted by the biliary tract, and an elevated bilirubin concentration is an indication for reducing the dose. Supraventricular tachycardia related to drug administration is an uncommon complication. Higher cumulative doses are associated with development of a cardiomyopathy. It is customary to limit total cumulative doses to 450–550 mg/m$^2$ body-surface area as symptomatic and potentially fatal heart failure is increasingly common above this level. Patients with pre-existing cardiac disease, the elderly, and those who have received myocardial irradiation should be treated cautiously. Cardiac monitoring, for example by sequential radionuclide ejection fraction measurement, may assist in safely limiting total dosage. Evidence is available to suggest that weekly low dose administration may be associated with less cardiac damage.

**Epirubicin** is structurally related to doxorubicin and clinical trials suggest that it is as effective in the treatment of breast cancer. A maximum cumulative dose of 0.9–1 g/m$^2$ is recommended to help avoid cardiotoxicity.

**Aclarubicin** and **idarubicin** are newly introduced anthracyclines with general properties similar to those of doxorubicin.

**Mitozantrone** is structurally related to doxorubicin and preliminary work suggests that it has equal activity in breast cancer; it is well tolerated apart from myelosuppression and dose-related cardiotoxicity; cardiac examinations are recommended after a cumulative dose of 160 mg/m$^2$ if this complication is to be avoided.

**Bleomycin** is used to treat the lymphomas, certain solid tumours and, by the intracavitary route, malignant effusions. It is unusual in that it causes little marrow suppression. Dermatological toxicity is common; increased pigmentation particularly affecting the flexures and subcutaneous sclerotic plaques may occur. Mucositis is also relatively common and an association with Raynaud's phenomenon is reported. Hypersensitivity reactions manifest by chills and fevers commonly occur a few hours after drug administration and may be prevented by simultaneous administration of a corticosteroid, for example hydrocortisone intravenously. The principal problem associated with the use of bleomycin is progressive pulmonary fibrosis. This is dose related, occurring more commonly at cumulative doses greater than 300 units and in the elderly. Basal lung crepitations or suspicious chest X-ray changes are an indication to stop therapy with this drug. Patients who have received extensive treatment with bleomycin (e.g. cumulative dose more than 100 units) may be at risk of developing respiratory failure if a general anaesthetic is given with high inspired oxygen concentrations. Anaesthetists should be warned of this.

**Dactinomycin** is principally used to treat paediatric cancers. Its side-effects are similar to those of doxorubicin, except that cardiac toxicity is not a problem.

**Plicamycin** (mithramycin) is no longer used as a cytotoxic, but has found a useful (though diminishing) role in low dose in the emergency therapy of hypercalcaemia due to malignant disease (for general management of hypercalcaemia, see section 9.5.1.2).

**Mitomycin** is used to treat upper gastro-intestinal and breast cancers. It causes delayed marrow toxicity and is usually administered at 6-weekly intervals. Prolonged use may result in permanent marrow damage. It is a relatively toxic drug and may cause lung fibrosis and renal damage.

## ACLARUBICIN

*Indications:* acute non-lymphocytic leukaemia in patients who have relapsed or are resistant or refractory to first-line chemotherapy

*Cautions; Side-effects:* see section 8.1 and notes above; caution in hepatic and renal impairment; irritant to tissues

▼ PoM **Aclacin**® (Lundbeck)
*Injection*, powder for reconstitution, aclarubicin 20 mg (as hydrochloride). Net price 20-mg vial = £29.20

## BLEOMYCIN

*Indications:* squamous cell carcinoma; see also notes above

*Cautions; Side-effects:* see section 8.1 and notes above; reduce dose in renal impairment; also caution in handling—irritant to skin

PoM **Bleomycin**® (Lundbeck)
*Injection*, powder for reconstitution, bleomycin (as sulphate). Net price 15-unit amp = £15.97
*Note.* Ampoules previously labelled as containing '15 mg' of bleomycin contained 15 units. The ampoules are now labelled only as units.

## DACTINOMYCIN

(Actinomycin D)
*Indications:* see notes above
*Cautions; Side-effects:* see section 8.1 and notes above; irritant to tissues

PoM **Cosmegen Lyovac**® (MSD)
*Injection*, powder for reconstitution, dactinomycin, net price 500-microgram vial = £1.25

## DOXORUBICIN HYDROCHLORIDE

*Indications:* see notes above and section 7.4.4
*Cautions; Side-effects:* see section 8.1 and notes above; reduce dose in hepatic impairment; also caution in handling—irritant to skin and tissues

PoM **Doxorubicin Rapid Dissolution** (Farmitalia Carlo Erba)
*Injection*, powder for reconstitution, doxorubicin hydrochloride, net price 10-mg vial = £17.66; 50-mg vial = £88.30
*Note.* This preparation has replaced Adriamycin®
PoM **Doxorubicin Solution for Injection** (Farmitalia Carlo Erba)
*Injection*, doxorubicin hydrochloride 2 mg/mL, net price 5-ml vial = £19.43; 25-mL vial = £97.15

## EPIRUBICIN HYDROCHLORIDE

*Indications:* see notes above
*Cautions; Side-effects:* see section 8.1 and notes above; reduce dose in hepatic impairment; irritant to tissues

PoM **Pharmorubicin®  Rapid Dissolution** (Farmitalia Carlo Erba)
*Injection,* powder for reconstitution, epirubicin hydrochloride. Net price 10-mg vial = £17.66; 20-mg vial = £35.32; 50-mg vial = £88.30
PoM **Pharmorubicin®  Solution for Injection** (Farmitalia Carlo Erba)
*Injection,* epirubicin hydrochloride 2 mg/mL, net price 5-mL vial = £19.43; 25-mL vial = £97.15

## IDARUBICIN HYDROCHLORIDE

*Indications:* acute leukaemias—see notes above
*Cautions; Side-effects:* see section 8.1 and notes above; caution in hepatic and renal impairment; also caution in handling—irritant to skin and tissues

▼ PoM **Zavedos®** (Farmitalia Carlo Erba)
*Injection,* powder for reconstitution, idarubicin hydrochloride, net price 5-mg vial = £63.30; 10-mg vial = £126.60

## MITOMYCIN

*Indications:* see notes above
*Cautions; Side-effects:* see section 8.1 and notes above; irritant to tissues

PoM **Mitomycin C Kyowa®** (Martindale)
*Injection,* powder for reconstitution, mitomycin. Net price 2-mg vial = £5.73; 10-mg vial = £18.87; 20-mg vial = £35.98 (hosp. only)

## MITOZANTRONE

*Indications:* see notes above
*Cautions; Side-effects:* see section 8.1 and notes above; intrathecal administration not recommended

PoM **Novantrone®** (Lederle)
*Intravenous infusion,* mitozantrone 2 mg (as hydrochloride)/mL, net price 10-mL vial = £150.43; 12.5-mL vial = £188.05; 15-mL vial = £225.60

## PLICAMYCIN
(Mithramycin)

*Indications:* refractory hypercalcaemia associated with malignancy—see notes above
*Cautions; Side-effects:* see section 8.1 and notes above; caution in hepatic or renal impairment (see Appendixes 2 and 3); irritant to tissues
*Dose: by intravenous infusion,* 25 micrograms/kg daily for 3–4 days, repeated if necessary at intervals of 7 days or longer; maintenance, 25 micrograms/kg 1–3 times each week

PoM **Mithracin®** (Pfizer)
*Injection,* powder for reconstitution, plicamycin, net price 2.5-mg vial = £7.51 (hosp. only)

## 8.1.3   Antimetabolites

Antimetabolites are incorporated into new nuclear material or combine irreversibly with vital cellular enzymes, preventing normal cellular division.

**Methotrexate** inhibits the enzyme dihydrofolate reductase, essential for the synthesis of purines and pyrimidines. It may be given orally, intravenously, intramuscularly, or intrathecally. High-dose methotrexate cannot generally be recommended except in clinical trials.

Methotrexate is used as maintenance therapy for childhood acute lymphoblastic leukaemia. Other uses include choriocarcinoma, non-Hodgkin lymphomas, and a number of solid tumours. Intrathecal methotrexate is used in the CNS prophylaxis of childhood acute lymphoblastic leukaemia, and as a therapy for established meningeal cancer or lymphoma.

Methotrexate causes myelosuppression, mucositis, and rarely pneumonitis. It is **contra-indicated** if significant renal impairment is present, as the kidney is its route of excretion. It should also be **avoided** if a significant pleural effusion or ascites is present as it tends to accumulate at these sites, and its subsequent return to the circulation will be associated with myelosuppression. For similar reasons blood counts should be carefully monitored when intrathecal methotrexate is given.

Oral or parenteral folinic acid (see below) will help prevent, and speed recovery from, methotrexate mucositis or myelosuppression.

**Cytarabine** acts by interfering with pyrimidine synthesis. It may be given subcutaneously, intravenously, or intrathecally. Its predominant use is in the induction of remission and maintenance therapy of acute myeloblastic leukaemia. It is a potent myelosuppressant and requires careful haematological monitoring.

**Fluorouracil** may be given orally but is usually given intravenously. It is used to treat a number of solid tumours, including colon and breast cancer. It may also be used topically for certain malignant skin lesions. Toxicity is unusual, but may include myelosuppression, mucositis, and rarely a cerebellar syndrome.

**Mercaptopurine** is used almost exclusively as maintenance therapy for the acute leukaemias. The dose should be reduced if the patient is receiving concurrent allopurinol as this drug interferes with the metabolism of mercaptopurine.

**Thioguanine** is used orally to induce remission and for maintenance in acute myeloid leukaemia.

**Azathioprine**, a derivative of the antimetabolite mercaptopurine, is commonly used as an immunosuppressant (section 8.2.1).

## CYTARABINE

*Indications:* acute leukaemias
*Cautions; Side-effects:* see section 8.1 and notes above

PoM **Cytarabine** (Non-proprietary)
*Injection*, powder for reconstitution, cytarabine. Net price 100-mg vial = £2.75; 500-mg vial = £14.95; 1-g vial = £25.86
Available from David Bull

PoM **Alexan**® (Pfizer)
*Injection*, cytarabine 20 mg/mL. Net price 2-mL amp = £1.06; 5-mL amp = £2.65

PoM **Alexan**® **100** (Pfizer)
*Injection*, cytarabine 100 mg/mL. Net price 1-mL amp = £2.65; 10-mL amp = £26.46. For intravenous infusion only

PoM **Cytosar**® (Upjohn)
*Injection*, powder for reconstitution, cytarabine. Net price 100-mg vial = £3.17; 500-mg vial = £14.95. For intravenous injection or infusion and subcutaneous injection only

## FLUOROURACIL

*Indications:* see notes above
*Cautions; Side-effects:* see section 8.1; also caution in handling—irritant; **interactions:** Appendix 1 (fluorouracil)
*Dose: by mouth*, maintenance 15 mg/kg weekly; max. in one day 1 g

PoM **Fluorouracil** (Non-proprietary)
*Injection*, fluorouracil 25 mg/mL (as sodium salt). Net price 10-mL vial = £1.42; 20-mL vial = £2.60; 100-mL vial = £12.60

PoM **Fluoro-uracil** (Roche)
*Capsules*, blue/orange, fluorouracil 250 mg. Net price 30-cap pack = £35.38. Label: 21
*Injection*, fluorouracil 25 mg/mL (as sodium salt). Net price 10-mL amp = £1.42
*Note*. The injection solution can also be given by mouth in fruit juice

PoM **Efudix**® (Roche)
*Cream*, fluorouracil 5%. Net price 20 g = £3.75

## MERCAPTOPURINE

*Indications:* acute leukaemias
*Cautions; Side-effects:* see section 8.1 and notes above; reduce dose in renal impairment; avoid in porphyria (see section 9.8.2); **interactions:** Appendix 1 (mercaptopurine)
*Dose:* initially 2.5 mg/kg daily

PoM **Puri-Nethol**® (Wellcome)
*Tablets*, fawn, scored, mercaptopurine 50 mg. Net price 25 = £17.47

## METHOTREXATE

*Indications:* see notes above
*Cautions; Side-effects:* see section 8.1 and notes above; reduce dose in renal impairment; dose-related toxicity in hepatic impairment (avoid in non-malignant conditions, e.g. psoriasis); avoid in porphyria (see section 9.8.2); **interactions:** Appendix 1 (methotrexate)
*Dose: by mouth*, leukaemia in children (maintenance), 15 mg/m$^2$ weekly in combination with other drugs; psoriasis, 10–25 mg weekly

PoM **Methotrexate** (Lederle)
*Tablets*, both yellow, scored, methotrexate 2.5 mg, net price 20 = £2.17.
*Injection*, methotrexate 2.5 mg (as sodium salt)/mL. Net price 2-mL vial = 91p
*Injection*, methotrexate 25 mg (as sodium salt)/mL. Net price 1-mL vial = £1.94; 2-mL vial = £2.69; 4-mL vial = £5.14; 8-mL vial = £10.28; 20-mL vial = £25.71; 40-mL vial = £45.71; 200-mL vial = £205.71
*Injection*, powder for reconstitution, methotrexate (as sodium salt). Net price 500-mg vial = £32.00

PoM **Maxtrex**® (Farmitalia Carlo Erba)
*Tablets*, both yellow, scored, methotrexate 2.5 mg, net price 20 = £2.14; 10 mg, 20 = £9.70

## THIOGUANINE

*Indications:* acute leukaemias
*Cautions; Side-effects:* see section 8.1 and notes above; reduce dose in renal impairment
*Dose:* initially 2–2.5 mg/kg daily

PoM **Lanvis**® (Wellcome)
*Tablets*, yellow, scored, thioguanine 40 mg. Net price 25-tab pack = £42.25

FOLINIC ACID RESCUE

Folinic acid (leucovorin) is used to counteract the folate-antagonist action of methotrexate and thus speed recovery from methotrexate-induced mucositis or myelosuppression. It does not counteract the antibacterial activity of folate antagonists such as trimethoprim.

Folinic acid also interacts with fluorouracil; when the two are used together in metastatic colonic cancer a favourable effect has been demonstrated on response-rate and probably also on survival.

## FOLINIC ACID

*Indications:* see notes above
*Cautions:* avoid simultaneous administration of methotrexate; as for Folic Acid (section 9.1.2) **not** indicated for pernicious anaemia or other megaloblastic anaemias where vitamin B$_{12}$ deficient
*Side-effects:* rarely, pyrexia after parenteral adminstration
*Dose:* as an antidote to methotrexate (started 8–24 hours after the beginning of methotrexate infusion), in general up to 120 mg in divided doses over 12–24 hours *by intramuscular or intravenous injection or infusion*, followed by 12–15 mg *intramuscularly or* 15 mg *by mouth* every 6 hours for the next 48 hours
Suspected methotrexate overdosage, immediate administration of an equal or higher dose of folinic acid

PoM **Calcium Folinate** (Non-proprietary)
*Tablets*, scored, folinic acid (as calcium salt) 15 mg. Net price 10-tab pack = £42.28

PoM **Calcium Leucovorin** (Lederle)
*Tablets*, scored, folinic acid 15 mg (as calcium salt). Net price 10-tab pack = £42.28
*Injection*, folinic acid 3 mg (as calcium salt)/mL. Net price 1-mL amp = £1.09
*Injection*, powder for reconstitution, folinic acid (as calcium salt). Net price 15-mg vial = £4.57; 30-mg vial = £8.57; 350-mg vial (Lederfolin®) = £99.98
PoM **Refolinon®** (Farmitalia Carlo Erba)
*Tablets*, yellow, scored, folinic acid 15 mg (as calcium salt). Net price 30 = £105.00
*Injection*, folinic acid 3 mg (as calcium salt)/mL. Net price 2-mL = £1·60; 10-mL = £6.70

## 8.1.4    Vinca alkaloids and etoposide

These interfere with microtubule assembly, causing metaphase arrest. All have similar activity but vary in the predominant site of toxicity.

The vinca alkaloids are used to treat the acute leukaemias, lymphomas, and some solid tumours (e.g. breast and lung cancer). They commonly cause peripheral and autonomic neuropathy. This side-effect is most obvious with vincristine, and is manifest by peripheral paraesthesia, loss of deep tendon reflexes, and abdominal bloating and constipation. If these symptoms are severe, doses should be reduced. Significant new motor weakness is a **contra-indication** to further use of these drugs. Recovery of the nervous system is generally slow but complete. Intrathecal administration of **all** vinca alkaloids is **contra-indicated** (usually fatal).

**Vincristine** causes virtually no myelosuppression. Its use may be associated with alopecia; hyponatraemia, as a result of inappropriate ADH secretion, has been described.

**Vinblastine** is a more myelosuppressive drug than vincristine, but causes less neurotoxicity.

**Vindesine** is the most recent addition to the vinca alkaloid group. It has a similar range of clinical activity, and side-effects intermediate between those of the above two drugs.

**Etoposide** may be given orally or intravenously, the dose when used orally being double that when given intravenously. There is limited clinical evidence to suggest that administration in divided doses over 3–5 days may be beneficial; courses may not be repeated more frequently than at intervals of 21 days. It has useful activity in small cell carcinoma of the bronchus, the lymphomas, and testicular teratoma. Toxic effects include alopecia, myelosuppression, nausea, and vomiting.

## ETOPOSIDE

*Indications:* see notes above
*Cautions; Contra-indications; Side-effects:* see section 8.1 and notes above; irritant to tissues

PoM **Vepesid®** (Bristol-Myers)
*Capsules*, etoposide 50 mg, net price 20 = £113.95; 100 mg, 10-tab pack = £99.57
*Injection*, etoposide 20 mg/mL. To be diluted. Net price 5-mL vial = £14.58
*Caution:* may dissolve certain types of filter

## VINBLASTINE SULPHATE

*Indications:* see notes above
*Cautions; Contra-indications; Side-effects:* see section 8.1 and notes above; caution in handling—avoid contact with eyes; irritant to tissues
*Note.* IMPORTANT. Intrathecal injection **contra-indicated**

PoM **Vinblastine** (Non-proprietary)
*Injection*, vinblastine sulphate 1 mg/mL. Net price 10-mL vial = £11.00
Available from David Bull
*Injection*, powder for reconstitution, vinblastine sulphate. Net price 10-mg vial (with diluent) = £6.86
Available from David Bull, Lederle
PoM **Velbe®** (Lilly)
*Injection*, powder for reconstitution, vinblastine sulphate. Net price 10-mg amp (with diluent) = £10.29

## VINCRISTINE SULPHATE

*Indications:* see notes above
*Cautions; Contra-indications; Side-effects:* see section 8.1 and notes above; caution in handling—avoid contact with eyes; irritant to tissues
*Note.* IMPORTANT. Intrathecal injection **contra-indicated**

PoM **Vincristine** (Non-proprietary)
*Injection*, vincristine sulphate 1 mg/mL. Net price 1-mL vial = £9.80; 2-mL vial = £19.00; 5-mL vial = £39.60; 1-mL syringe = £10·49; 2-mL syringe = £19.00
Available from David Bull
*Injection*, powder for reconstitution, vincristine sulphate, net price, 1-mg vial = £3.42; 2-mg vial = £6.86; 5-mg vial = £17.14 (all with diluent)
Available from David Bull, Lederle
PoM **Oncovin®** (Lilly)
*Injection*, vincristine sulphate 1 mg/mL, net price 1-mL vial = £10.31; 2-mL vial = £20.40
*Injection*, powder for reconstitution, vincristine sulphate. Net price 1-mg vial = £9.36 (with diluent)

## VINDESINE SULPHATE

*Indications:* see notes above
*Cautions; Contra-indications; Side-effects:* see section 8.1 and notes above; caution in handling—avoid contact with eyes; irritant to tissues
*Note.* IMPORTANT. Intrathecal injection **contra-indicated**

PoM **Eldisine®** (Lilly)
*Injection*, powder for reconstitution, vindesine sulphate, net price 5-mg vial (with diluent) = £51.77 (hosp. only)

## 8.1.5    Other antineoplastic drugs

**Amsacrine** has an action and toxic effects similar to those of doxorubicin (section 8.1.2). It is used as second-line treatment in refractory acute myeloid leukaemia. Side-effects include myelosuppression and mucositis; electrolytes should be monitored as fatal arrhythmias have occurred in association with hypokalaemia.

## AMSACRINE

*Indications:* see notes above
*Cautions; Side-effects:* see section 8.1 and notes above; reduce dose in renal or hepatic impairment; also caution in handling—irritant to skin and tissues

PoM **Amsidine**® (P-D)
*Concentrate for intravenous infusion*, amsacrine 5 mg (as lactate)/mL, when reconstituted by mixing two solutions. Net price 1.5-mL amp with 13.5-mL vial = £32.60 (hosp. only)
*Note.* Use glass apparatus for reconstitution

---

**Carboplatin** is a derivative of cisplatin which has probably equivalent activity in ovarian cancer. It is also active in small cell lung cancer and is under trial in a variety of other malignancies. Carboplatin is better tolerated than cisplatin; nausea and vomiting are reduced in severity and nephrotoxicity, neurotoxicity, and ototoxicity are much less of a problem than with cisplatin. It is, however, more myelosuppressive than cisplatin.

## CARBOPLATIN

*Indications:* see notes above
*Cautions; Side-effects:* see section 8.1 and notes above; reduce dose in renal impairment

PoM **Paraplatin**® (Bristol-Myers)
*Injection*, carboplatin 10 mg/mL. Net price 5-mL vial = £22.86; 15-mL vial = £68.57; 45-mL vial = £205.71

---

**Cisplatin** has an alkylating action. It has useful antitumour activity in certain solid tumours including ovarian cancer and testicular teratoma. It is, however, a toxic drug. Common problems include severe nausea and vomiting, nephrotoxicity (pretreatment hydration mandatory and renal function should be closely monitored), myelotoxicity, ototoxicity (high tone hearing loss and tinnitus), peripheral neuropathy, and hypomagnesaemia. These toxic effects commonly necessitate dose reduction or drug withdrawal. It is preferable that treatment with this drug be supervised by specialists familiar with its use.

## CISPLATIN

*Indications:* see notes above
*Cautions; Side-effects:* see section 8.1 and notes above; reduce dose in renal impairment; **interactions:** Appendix 1 (cisplatin)

PoM **Cisplatin** (Non-proprietary)
*Injection*, cisplatin 1 mg/mL. Net price 10-mL vial = £2.90; 50-mL vial = £14.00; 100-mL vial = £27.00
*Injection*, powder for reconstitution, cisplatin 10-mg vial, net price = £2.50; 50-mg vial = £12.10; 150-mg vial = £68.57; 450-mg vial = £205.71
Various strengths available from David Bull, Farmitalia Carlo Erba, Lederle

---

**Crisantaspase** is the enzyme asparaginase produced by *Erwinia chrysanthemi*. It is used (usually intramuscularly) almost exclusively in acute lymphoblastic leukaemia. Facilities for the management of anaphylaxis should be available. Side-effects also include nausea, vomiting, CNS depression, and liver function and blood lipid changes; careful monitoring is therefore necessary and the urine is tested for glucose to exclude hyperglycaemia.

## CRISANTASPASE

*Indications; Cautions; Side-effects:* see notes above

PoM **Erwinase**® (Porton)
*Injection*, powder for reconstitution, crisantaspase. Net price 20 × 10000-unit vial = £650.00

---

**Dacarbazine** is not commonly used on account of its toxicity. It has been used to treat melanoma and, in combination therapy, the soft tissue sarcomas. It is also a component of a commonly used second-line combination for Hodgkin's disease (ABVD—doxorubicin [Adriamycin®], bleomycin, vinblastine, and dacarbazine). The predominant side-effects are myelosuppression and intense nausea and vomiting.

## DACARBAZINE

*Indications:* see notes above
*Cautions; Side-effects:* see section 8.1; also caution in handling—irritant to skin and tissues

PoM **DTIC-Dome**® (Bayer)
*Injection*, powder for reconstitution, dacarbazine. Net price 100-mg vial = £4.83; 200-mg vial = £7.40

---

**Hydroxyurea** is an orally active drug used mainly in the treatment of chronic myeloid leukaemia. Myelosuppression, nausea, and skin reactions are the most common toxic effects.

## HYDROXYUREA

*Indications:* see notes above
*Cautions; Side-effects:* see section 8.1 and notes above
*Dose:* 20–30 mg/kg daily *or* 80 mg/kg every third day

PoM **Hydrea**® (Squibb)
*Capsules*, pink/green, hydroxyurea 500 mg. Net price 20 = £2.39

---

**Procarbazine** is most often used in Hodgkin's disease, for example in MOPP (mustine, vincristine [Oncovin®], procarbazine, and prednisolone) chemotherapy. It is given orally. Toxic effects include nausea, myelosuppression, and a hypersensitivity rash preventing further use of this drug. It is a mild monoamine-oxidase inhibitor but dietary restriction is not considered necessary. Alcohol ingestion may cause a disulfiram-like reaction.

## PROCARBAZINE
*Indications:* see notes above
*Cautions; Side-effects:* see section 8.1 and notes above; reduce dose in renal impairment; **interactions:** Appendix 1 (procarbazine)
*Dose:* initially 50 mg daily, increased by 50 mg daily to 250–300 mg daily in divided doses; maintenance (on remission) 50–150 mg daily to cumulative total of at least 6 g

PoM **Natulan**® (Roche)
*Capsules,* ivory, procarbazine 50 mg (as hydrochloride). Net price 50-cap pack = £3.44. Label: 4

**Razoxane** has limited activity in the leukaemias, and is little used.

## RAZOXANE
*Indications:* see notes above
*Cautions; Side-effects:* see section 8.1
*Dose:* acute leukaemias, 150–500 mg/m$^2$ daily for 3–5 days

PoM **Razoxin**® (ICI)
*Tablets,* scored, razoxane 125 mg. Net price 30-tab pack = £27.56

# 8.2 Drugs affecting the immune response

8.2.1 Cytotoxic immunosuppressants
8.2.2 Corticosteroids and other immunosuppressants
8.2.3 Immunostimulants
8.2.4 Interferons

## 8.2.1 Cytotoxic immunosuppressants
These drugs are used to suppress rejection in organ transplant recipients and are also used to treat a variety of auto-immune and collagen diseases (see section 10.1.3). They are non-specific in their action and careful monitoring of peripheral blood counts is required, with dose adjustments for marrow toxicity. Patients receiving these drugs will be prone to atypical infections.

**Azathioprine** is widely used for transplant recipients and is also used to treat a number of autoimmune conditions, usually when corticosteroid therapy alone has provided inadequate control. This drug is metabolised to mercaptopurine, and doses should be reduced when concurrent therapy with allopurinol is given. The predominant toxic effect is myelosuppression, although hepatic toxicity is also well recognised.

Cyclophosphamide and chlorambucil (section 8.1.1) are less commonly prescribed as immunosuppressants.

## AZATHIOPRINE
*Indications:* see notes above
*Cautions; Side-effects:* see section 8.1 and notes above; also rashes; reduce dose in severe hepatic or renal impairment; **interactions:** Appendix 1 (azathioprine)
*Dose: by mouth,* 2–2.5 mg/kg daily.
Chronic active hepatitis, 1–1.5 mg/kg daily Suppression of transplant rejection, loading dose, up to 5 mg/kg; maintenance 1–4 mg/kg daily
*By intravenous injection,* suppression of transplant rejection, loading dose, up to 5 mg/kg; maintenance dose (if oral route not possible), 1–2.5 mg/kg daily

PoM **Azathioprine** (Non-proprietary)
*Tablets,* azathioprine 50 mg. Net price 20 = £5.80
Available from APS, Ashbourne (Immunoprin®), Berk (Berkaprine®), Cox, Evans, Kerfoot, Penn (Azamune®)
PoM **Imuran**® (Wellcome)
*Tablets,* both f/c, azathioprine 25 mg (orange), net price 100-tab pack = £39.35; 50 mg (yellow), 100-tab pack = £65.61
*Injection,* powder for reconstitution, azathioprine (as sodium salt). Net price 50-mg vial = £16.54

## 8.2.2 Corticosteroids and other immunosuppressants
**Prednisolone** is widely used in oncology. It has a marked antitumour effect in acute lymphoblastic leukaemia, Hodgkin's disease, and the non-Hodgkin lymphomas. It is also active in hormone-sensitive breast cancer and may cause useful disease regression. Finally, it has a role in the palliation of symptomatic end-stage malignant disease when it may produce a sense of well-being.

The corticosteroids are also powerful immunosuppressants. They are used to prevent organ transplant rejection, and in high dose to treat rejection episodes. For notes on corticosteroids see section 6.3.

**Cyclosporin** is a fungal metabolite and potent immunosuppressant which is virtually non-myelotoxic but markedly nephrotoxic. It has found particular use in the field of organ and tissue transplantation, for prevention of graft rejection following bone marrow, kidney, liver, pancreas, heart, and heart-lung transplantation, and for prophylaxis of graft-versus-host disease.

**Antilymphocyte immunoglobulin,** obtained from immunised horses, has mainly been used to prevent transplant rejection. It is no longer available in the UK.

## CYCLOSPORIN
*Indications:* see notes above
*Cautions:* monitor liver and kidney function; other immunosuppressants; over-suppression may increase susceptibility to infection and lymphoma; avoid during pregnancy, breast-feeding; avoid in porphyria (see section 9.8.2); **interactions:** Appendix 1 (cyclosporin)
*Side-effects:* hepatic and renal impairment; tremor, gastro-intestinal disturbances, hypertrichosis; gum hyperplasia; hyperkalaemia;

*occasionally* facial oedema, hypertension, fluid retention, and convulsions; serum creatinine, urea, bilirubin, and liver enzymes may be increased; burning sensation in hands and feet during first week of oral administration

*Dose:* organ transplantation, used alone, 14–17.5 mg/kg as a single dose *by mouth* 4–12 hours before transplantation followed by 14–17.5 mg/kg daily for 1–2 weeks post-operatively then reduced in steps of about 2 mg/kg daily at intervals of 1 month to 6–8 mg/kg daily for maintenance (dose may be adjusted by monitoring blood concentrations); maintenance dose lower and reached sooner with concomitant corticosteroid therapy; if necessary one-third oral dose can be given *by intravenous infusion* over 2–6 hours (3–5 mg/kg daily if initiating therapy)

Bone-marrow transplantation, prevention of graft-versus-host disease, 3–5 mg/kg daily *by intravenous infusion* over 2–6 hours from day before transplantation to 2 weeks post-operatively (or 12.5–25 mg/kg daily *by mouth* for about 5 days) then 12.5 mg/kg daily *by mouth* for 3–6 months (up to 25 mg/kg daily and 1 year recorded) then tailed off or maintained at low dosage for mild chronic graft-versus-host disease; if necessary one-third oral dose can be given *by intravenous infusion* over 2–6 hours

COUNSELLING. Total daily dose may be taken as a single dose or in 2 divided doses. To mask taste, mix with milk, chocolate drink, or fruit juice immediately before taking

PoM **Sandimmun**® (Sandoz)

*Capsules*, cyclosporin 25 mg (pale pink), net price 30-cap pack = £21.07; 50 mg (yellow), 30-cap pack = £41.25; 100 mg (dusky pink), 30-cap pack = £78.29

*Oral solution*, oily, yellow, sugar-free, cyclosporin 100 mg/mL. Net price 50 mL = £117.31. Counselling, administration

*Concentrate for intravenous infusion* (oily), cyclosporin 50 mg/mL. To be diluted before use. Net price 1-mL amp = £1.82; 5-mL amp = £8.60

*Note.* Contains polyethoxylated castor oil which has been associated with anaphylaxis

**PREDNISOLONE**
See section 6.3.4

## 8.2.3   Immunostimulants

A suspension of inactivated *Corynebacterium parvum* organisms may be used by the intracavitary route to treat malignant effusions.

### CORYNEBACTERIUM PARVUM VACCINE

*Indications:* see notes above

*Cautions:* avoid within 10 days of thoracotomy

*Side-effects:* pyrexia common; abdominal pain, nausea and vomiting

*Dose: by intrapleural or intraperitoneal injection*, 7–14 mg

PoM **Coparvax**® (Wellcome)

*Injection*, powder for reconstitution, *Corynebacterium parvum* (inactivated). Net price 7-mg vial = £63.09

## 8.2.4   Interferons

The interferons (alfa, beta, and gamma) are naturally occurring proteins with complex effects on immunity and cell function. Recently alfa interferon (formerly called lymphoblastoid interferon) has shown some antitumour effect in certain lymphomas and solid tumours. Side-effects are dose-related, but commonly include influenza-like symptoms, lethargy, and depression. Myelosuppression may also occur, particularly affecting granulocyte counts. Finally, cardiovascular problems (hypotension, hypertension, and arrhythmias) have been reported. Avoid in pregnancy unless compelling reasons for use (see Appendix 4); **interactions:** Appendix 1 (interferons).

PoM **Intron A**® (Schering-Plough)

*Injection*, powder for reconstitution, interferon alfa-2b (rbe). Net price 3-million unit vial = £16.96; 5-million unit vial = £28.26; 10-million unit vial = £56.52; 30-million unit vial = £169.56

For use in AIDS-related Kaposi's sarcoma, hairy cell leukaemia, chronic myelogenous leukaemia, condyloma acuminata, chronic active hepatitis B, and maintenance of remission in multiple myeloma

PoM **Roferon-A**® (Roche)

*Injection*, powder for reconstitution, interferon alfa-2a (rbe). Net price 3 million-unit vial = £16.96; 9 million-unit vial = £50.88; 18 million-unit vial = £101.77; all with syringe, needles, and water for injection

For use in AIDS-related Kaposi's sarcoma, hairy cell leukaemia, recurrent or metastatic renal cell carcinoma, and chronic active hepatitis B

PoM **Wellferon**® (Wellcome)

*Injection*, interferon alfa-N1 (lns) 3 million units/mL, net price 1-mL vial = £19.93; 10 million units/mL, net price 1-mL vial = £64.55

For hairy cell leukaemia and chronic active hepatitis B

# 8.3   Sex hormones and hormone antagonists in malignant disease

8.3.1   Oestrogens
8.3.2   Progestogens
8.3.3   Androgens
8.3.4   Hormone antagonists

Hormonal manipulation has an important role in the treatment of metastatic breast, prostate, and endometrial cancer, and a more marginal role in the treatment of hypernephroma. These treatments are not curative, but may provide excellent palliation of symptoms in selected patients, sometimes for a period of years. Tumour response, and treatment toxicity should be carefully monitored and treatment changed if progression occurs or side-effects exceed benefit.

## 8.3.1    Oestrogens

**Stilboestrol** may be used in low dosage to treat symptomatic metastases from prostate cancer. It is less commonly used in postmenopausal women with breast cancer. Toxicity is common and dose-related side-effects include nausea, fluid retention, and venous and arterial thrombosis. Impotence and gynaecomastia always occur in men, and withdrawal bleeding may be a problem in women. Hypercalcaemia and bone pain may also occur in breast cancer.

**Fosfestrol** is also used for prostate cancer; it is activated by the enzyme acid phosphatase to produce stilboestrol. Side-effects are as for stilboestrol; in addition, perineal pain may complicate intravenous use.

**Ethinyloestradiol** is the most potent oestrogen available; unlike other oestrogens it is only slowly metabolised in the liver. It is used in breast cancer.

**Polyestradiol** is a long-acting oestrogen.

## STILBOESTROL

*Indications:* see notes above
*Cautions; Side-effects:* cardiovascular disease (sodium retention with oedema, thromboembolism), hepatic impairment (jaundice), feminising effects in men; see also notes above
*Dose:* breast cancer, 10–20 mg daily
    Prostate cancer, 1–3 mg daily

PoM **Stilboestrol Tablets,** stilboestrol 1 mg, net price 20 = 87p; 5 mg, 20 = £1.63

## ETHINYLOESTRADIOL

*Indications:* see notes above; other indications, see section 6.4.1.1
*Cautions; Side-effects:* see under Stilboestrol and notes above
*Dose:* breast cancer, 1–3 mg daily

**Preparations**
See section 6.4.1.1

## FOSFESTROL TETRASODIUM

*Indications:* prostate cancer
*Cautions; Contra-indications; Side-effects:* see under Stilboestrol and notes above; nausea and vomiting; after intravenous injection, perineal irritation and pain in bony metastases
*Dose:* by slow intravenous injection, 552–1104 mg daily for at least 5 days; maintenance 276 mg 1–4 times weekly
*By mouth,* maintenance 100–200 mg 3 times daily, reducing to 100–300 mg daily in divided doses

PoM **Honvan**® (ASTA Medica)
*Tablets,* fosfestrol tetrasodium 100 mg. Net price 20 = £1.87
*Injection,* fosfestrol tetrasodium 55.2 mg/mL. Net price 5-mL amp = 92p

## POLYESTRADIOL PHOSPHATE

*Indications:* prostate cancer
*Cautions; Side-effects:* see under Stilboestrol and notes above
*Dose:* by deep intramuscular injection, 80–160 mg every 4 weeks; maintenance 40–80 mg

PoM **Estradurin**® (Kabi Pharmacia)
*Injection,* powder for reconstitution, polyestradiol phosphate (with mepivacaine and nicotinamide). Net price 40-mg vial = £2.18; 80-mg vial = £3.51 (both with diluent)

## 8.3.2    Progestogens

Progestogens are used largely as second- or third-line therapy in breast cancer. They are also used to treat endometrial cancer and hypernephroma, but are little used for prostate cancer. **Medroxyprogesterone** or **megestrol** are usually chosen and can be given orally; high-dose or parenteral treatment cannot be recommended. Side-effects are mild but may include nausea, fluid retention, and weight gain.

## GESTRONOL HEXANOATE

*Indications:* see notes above; benign prostatic hypertrophy
*Cautions; Contra-indications; Side-effects:* see under Progesterone (section 6.4.1.2) and notes above
*Dose:* endometrial cancer, *by intramuscular injection,* 200–400 mg every 5–7 days
    Benign prostatic hypertrophy, *by intramuscular injection,* 200 mg every week, increased to 300–400 mg every week if necessary

PoM **Depostat**® (Schering Health Care)
*Injection* (oily), gestronol hexanoate 100 mg/mL. Net price 2-mL amp = £4.28

## MEDROXYPROGESTERONE ACETATE

*Indications:* see notes above; other indications, see section 6.4.1.2
*Cautions; Contra-indications; Side-effects:* see under Progesterone (section 6.4.1.2) and notes above; glucocorticoid effects at high dose may lead to a cushingoid syndrome
*Dose:* by mouth, endometrial, prostate, and renal cancer, 100–500 mg daily; breast cancer, various doses in range 0.4–1.5 g daily
*By deep intramuscular injection* into the gluteal muscle, various doses in range 1 g daily down to 250 mg weekly

PoM **Depo-Provera**® (Upjohn)
*Injection,* medroxyprogesterone acetate 150 mg/mL. Net price 3.3-mL (500-mg) vial = £12.49
PoM **Farlutal**® (Farmitalia Carlo Erba)
*Tablets,* both scored, medroxyprogesterone acetate 100 mg, net price 20 = £8.32; 250 mg, 50 = £52.03
*Tablets,* scored, medroxyprogesterone acetate 500 mg. Net price 56 = £116.54. Label: 27
*Injection,* medroxyprogesterone acetate 200 mg/mL. Net price 2.5-mL vial = £14.24; 5-mL vial = £23.73

PoM **Provera**® (Upjohn)
*Tablets*, medroxyprogesterone acetate 100 mg (scored), net price 20 = £8.32; 200 mg (scored), 20 = £16.47; 400 mg, 30 = £48.89
*Tablets*, medroxyprogesterone acetate 5 mg and 10 mg, see section 6.4.1.2

## MEGESTROL ACETATE

*Indications:* see notes above
*Cautions; Contra-indications; Side-effects:* see under Progesterone (section 6.4.1.2) and notes above
*Dose:* breast cancer, 160 mg daily in single or divided doses; endometrial cancer, 40–320 mg daily in divided doses

PoM **Megace**® (Bristol-Myers)
*Tablets*, both scored, megestrol acetate 40 mg, net price 20 = £5.08; 160 mg (off-white), 30-tab pack = £29.30

## NORETHISTERONE

*Indications:* see notes above; other indications, see section 6.4.1.2
*Cautions; Contra-indications; Side-effects:* see section 6.4.1.2 and notes above
*Dose:* breast cancer, 40 mg daily, increased to 60 mg daily if required

**Preparations**
See section 6.4.1.2

## NORETHISTERONE ACETATE

*Indications:* see notes above
*Cautions; Contra-indications; Side-effects:* see under Norethisterone (section 6.4.1.2) and notes above
*Dose:* breast cancer, 10 mg 3 times daily, increased to 60 mg daily if required

PoM **SH 420**® (Schering Health Care)
*Tablets*, scored, norethisterone acetate 10 mg. Net price 20 = £4.95

## 8.3.3 Androgens

The androgens are given parenterally and are predominantly used as second- or third-line therapy for metastatic breast cancer.

## TESTOSTERONE ESTERS

*Indications:* see notes above; other indications, see section 6.4.2
*Cautions; Contra-indications; Side-effects:* see under Testosterone and Esters (section 6.4.2)
*Dose:* see under Preparations

PoM **Primoteston Depot**® : see section 6.4.2
PoM **Virormone**® : see section 6.4.2

## 8.3.4 Hormone antagonists

### SEX HORMONE DEPENDENT TUMOURS

BREAST CANCER. **Tamoxifen** is an oestrogen receptor antagonist and at a dose of 20 mg daily is the hormonal treatment of choice for breast cancer in postmenopausal women with metastatic disease; it is also increasingly commonly used as a first-line treatment for premenopausal women in whom it is equivalent in effect to oophorectomy. Overall, approximately 30% of patients with metastatic breast cancer respond to hormonal manipulation. This figure is increased to 60% in patients with oestrogen receptor positive tumours; receptor negative tumours respond in less than 10%.

Adjuvant hormonal treatment with tamoxifen is also the treatment of choice in postmenopausal patients with high-risk breast cancer after treatment of the primary. Such treatment has consistently prolonged the period between diagnosis and the development of metastases; a modest increase in survival has been reported in some studies.

Side-effects are unusual with tamoxifen but patients with bony metastases may experience an exacerbation of pain, sometimes associated with hypercalcaemia. This reaction commonly precedes tumour response. Amenorrhoea commonly develops in premenopausal women.

Patients with non-threatening metastases unresponsive to tamoxifen may still respond to a secondary hormonal treatment. Certainly patients who initially respond to tamoxifen should receive second-line hormone treatment. No clear guidelines are available; for premenopausal patients oophorectomy or a progestogen (section 8.3.2) may be used; for postmenopausal patients a progestogen or aminoglutethimide (see below) may be used. Patients who respond can be given further hormones on relapse; refractory patients are better treated with chemotherapy or palliative therapy.

**Aminoglutethimide** has largely replaced adrenalectomy in postmenopausal women with breast cancer; it acts predominantly by inhibiting the conversion of androgens to oestrogens in the peripheral tissues. Corticosteroid replacement therapy is necessary (see section 6.3.1). Early toxicity is common and may include drowsiness, drug fever, and a morbilliform eruption; these side-effects generally settle spontaneously. The dose of aminoglutethimide is usually increased to 500 mg daily over 2 to 4 weeks. Hepatic enzyme induction occurs, and may require modification of the doses of other drugs (e.g. oral anticoagulants).

PROSTATE CANCER. Metastatic cancer of the prostate is commonly responsive to hormonal treatment designed to deprive the cancer of androgen. Treatment is probably best reserved for symptomatic metastatic disease. The standard treatment is bilateral subcapsular orchidectomy, which commonly results in responses lasting 12–18 months. Alternatively, a gonadotrophin-releasing hormone (GnRH) analogue such as **buserelin**, **goserelin**, or **leuprorelin** may be given. These are as effective as orchidectomy or **stilboestrol** (section 8.3.1) but are expensive and require parenteral administration, at least initially. They cause initial stimulation of luteinising hormone release by the pituitary, which in turn causes testosterone secretion by the testis; this is followed by inhibition of luteinising hormone release with achievement of an anorchic state. During the first 1 to 2 weeks of treatment a number of patients develop a tumour 'flare' which may cause spinal cord compression or increased bone pain. When such problems are anticipated, alternative treatments (e.g. orchidectomy) or the additional use of an anti-androgen such as cyproterone acetate or flutamide (see below) are recommended; anti-androgen treatment should be started 3 days before the GnRH analogue and continued for at least 3 weeks. Other side-effects of GnRH analogues are similar to those of orchidectomy.

**Cyproterone acetate** is an anti-androgen which has been used as first-line therapy; it has a number of theoretical advantages, but is expensive. **Flutamide** is also an anti-androgen; it is being studied alone and in combination for prostate cancer and may have a role in preventing and treating the 'flare' which can occur in patients treated with gonadotrophin-releasing hormone analogues.

Alternatives after orchidectomy include cyproterone acetate or prednisolone. Such second-line treatment may palliate symptoms, but rarely results in appreciable disease regression.

## AMINOGLUTETHIMIDE

*Indications:* see notes above and under Dose
*Cautions:* see notes above; avoid in porphyria (see section 9.8.2); **interactions:** Appendix 1 (aminoglutethimide)
*Side-effects:* see notes above; dizziness, somnolence, lethargy; unsteadiness at higher doses; less frequently nausea, vomiting, diarrhoea; rash (sometimes with fever) reported; allergic alveolitis and blood disorders (regular blood counts) also reported; altered thyroid function
*Dose:* breast or prostate cancer, 250 mg daily, increased once a week to max. 250 mg 4 times daily (lower doses may be adequate, see notes above); given with a glucocorticoid (and sometimes with a mineralocorticoid as well)
Cushing's syndrome due to malignant disease, 250 mg daily, increased gradually to 1 g daily in divided doses (occasionally 1.5–2 g daily); glucocorticoid given only if necessary

PoM**Orimeten**® (Ciba)
*Tablets,* scored, aminoglutethimide 250 mg. Net price 56-tab pack = £18.38

## BUSERELIN

*Indications:* prostate cancer
*Cautions:* during first month monitor patients at risk of ureteric obstruction or spinal cord compression, see notes above
*Side-effects:* initial increase in bone pain (due to transient increases in plasma testosterone); hot flushes, decreased libido, infrequent gynaecomastia, urticaria
*Dose: by subcutaneous injection,* 500 micrograms every 8 hours for 7 days, then *intranasally,* 1 spray into each nostril 6 times daily

PoM**Suprefact**® (Hoechst)
*Injection,* buserelin 1 mg (as acetate)/mL. Net price treatment pack of 2 × 5.5-mL vial = £30.37
*Nasal spray,* buserelin 100 micrograms (as acetate)/metered spray. Net price treatment pack of 4 × 10-g bottle with spray pump = £99.92

## CYPROTERONE ACETATE

*Indications:* prostate cancer, see notes above; other indications, see section 6.4.2
*Cautions:* hepatic disease; risk of recurrence of thrombo-embolic disease; severe depression; see also section 6.4.2
*Contra-indications:* none in prostate cancer; for contra-indications relating to other indications see section 6.4.2
*Side-effects:* see section 6.4.2
*Dose:* prostate cancer, 300 mg daily in 2–3 divided doses after food

PoM**Cyprostat**® (Schering Health Care)
*Tablets,* scored, cyproterone acetate 50 mg. Net price 84-tab pack = £48.35 (hosp. only); 168-tab pack = £96.70. Label: 3, 21

## FLUTAMIDE

*Indications:* prostate cancer, see notes above
*Cautions:* cardiac disease (sodium retention with oedema); monitor hepatic function; **interactions:** Appendix 1 (flutamide)
*Side-effects:* gynaecomastia (sometimes with galactorrhoea); nausea, vomiting, diarrhoea, increased appetite, insomnia, tiredness; other side-effects reported include decreased libido, inhibition of spermatogenesis, gastric and chest pain, headache, dizziness, cholestatic jaundice, oedema, blurred vision, thirst, rashes, pruritus, haemolytic anaemia, systemic lupus erythematosus-like syndrome, and lymphoedema
*Dose:* 250 mg 3 times daily (see also notes above)

▼ PoM**Drogenil**® (Schering-Plough)
*Tablets,* yellow, scored, flutamide 250 mg, net price 100-tab pack = £110.00

## GOSERELIN

*Indications:* prostate cancer
*Cautions; Side-effects:* see under Buserelin; also
rashes (reversible without stopping therapy);
bruising at injection site
*Dose:* see below

PoM **Zoladex**® (ICI)
*Implant*, goserelin 3.6 mg (as acetate) in syringe
applicator. Net price each = £125.40
*Dose: by subcutaneous injection* into anterior
abdominal wall, 3.6 mg every 28 days (local
anaesthetic if desired)

## LEUPRORELIN ACETATE

*Indications:* prostate cancer
*Cautions; Side-effects:* see under Buserelin; also,
infrequently, peripheral oedema, fatigue,
nausea, irritation at injection site; rotate injection site periodically
*Dose: by subcutaneous or by intramuscular injec-
tion,* 3.75 mg every 4 weeks (see also notes
above)

▼ PoM **Prostap SR**® (Lederle)
*Injection* (microcapsule powder for aqueous suspension), leuprorelin acetate, net price 3.75-mg
vial with 2-mL vehicle-filled syringe, needles and
swabs = £125.40

## TAMOXIFEN

*Indications:* breast cancer, see notes above
*Cautions:* interactions: Appendix 1 (tamoxifen)
*Contra-indications:* pregnancy; porphyria (see
section 9.8.2)
*Side-effects:* hot flushes, vaginal bleeding (but
suppression of menstruation in some pre-meno-
pausal women), gastro-intestinal disturbances,
dizziness; rarely fluid retention, visual disturbances; see also notes above
*Dose:* breast cancer, 20–40 mg daily as a single
dose or in 2 divided doses
Anovulatory infertility, 20 mg daily on second to
fifth days of cycle inclusive; if necessary
increased to 40 mg daily then 80 mg daily for subsequent courses; if cycles irregular, start initial
course on any day, with subsequent course starting 45 days later *or* on second day of cycle if
menstruation occurs

PoM **Tamoxifen** (Non-proprietary)
*Tablets*, tamoxifen (as citrate) 10 mg, net price 30-
tab pack = £6.60; 20 mg, 30-tab pack = £9.60;
40 mg, 30-tab pack = £21.90
Various strengths available from APS, Ashbourne (Oes-
trifen®), Berk (Emblon®), Cox, CP, Evans, Farmitalia
Carlo Erba, Kerfoot, Lederle (Noltam®), Tillotts (Tam-
ofen®)
PoM **Nolvadex**® (ICI)
*Tablets*, tamoxifen (as citrate) 10 mg, net price 30-
tab pack = £6.20; 20 mg (Nolvadex-D®), 30-tab
pack = £9.35;   40 mg   (scored,   Nolvadex-
Forte®), 30-tab pack = £22.20

## GASTRO-ENTEROPANCREATIC TUMOURS

**Octreotide** is a long-acting analogue of the hypothalamic release-inhibiting hormone somato-
statin; it is indicated for the relief of symptoms
associated with gastro-enteropancreatic endocrine tumours and for the short-term treatment of
acromegaly before intervention.

## OCTREOTIDE

*Indications:* see under Dose
*Cautions:* occasional sudden escape from symptomatic control with rapid recurrence of severe
symptoms; in insulinoma may increase depth
and duration of hypoglycaemia (close observation initially and with dose changes; marked
fluctuations may be reduced by increasing
administration frequency); in diabetes mellitus
may reduce insulin or oral antidiabetic requirements; monitor thyroid function on long-term
therapy; ultrasonic examination of gall bladder
before and at intervals of 6–12 months during
treatment; **interactions:** Appendix 1 (octreotide)
*Contra-indications:* pregnancy (unless compelling reasons) and breast-feeding
*Side-effects:* gastro-intestinal disturbances including anorexia, nausea, vomiting, abdominal
pain and bloating, flatulence, diarrhoea, and
steatorrhoea; symptoms may be reduced by
injecting between meals or at bedtime; impairment of postprandial glucose tolerance (rarely
persistent hyperglycaemia on chronic administration); hepatic disturbance reported; gall
stone formation reported after long-term treatment; pain and irritation at injection site (rotate
sites)
*Dose:* symptoms associated with carcinoid
tumours with features of carcinoid syndrome,
VIPomas, glucagonomas, *by subcutaneous
injection,* initially 50 micrograms once or twice
daily, gradually increased according to response
to 200 micrograms 3 times daily (higher doses
required exceptionally); maintenance doses
variable; in carcinoid tumours discontinue after
1 week if no effect; if rapid response required,
initial dose *by intravenous injection* (with ECG
monitoring and after dilution to a concentration
of 10–50% with sodium chloride 0.9% injection)
Acromegaly, *by subcutaneous injection,* 100–
200 micrograms 3 times daily

PoM **Sandostatin**® (Sandoz)
*Injection*, octreotide (as acetate) 50 micrograms/
mL, net price  1-mL  amp = £2.98;   100
micrograms/mL,   1-mL   amp = £5.60;   200
micrograms/mL,   5-mL   vial = £55,78;   500
micrograms/mL, 1-mL amp = £27.13

# 9: Drugs affecting
# NUTRITION and BLOOD

In this chapter drugs and preparations are discussed under the following headings:

**9.1** Anaemias and some other blood disorders
**9.2** Electrolyte and water replacement
**9.3** Intravenous nutrition
**9.4** Oral nutrition
**9.5** Minerals
**9.6** Vitamins
**9.7** Bitters and tonics
**9.8** Metabolic disorders

## 9.1 Anaemias and some other blood disorders

**9.1.1** Iron-deficiency anaemias
**9.1.2** Megaloblastic anaemias
**9.1.3** Hypoplastic and haemolytic anaemias
**9.1.4** Autoimmune thrombocytopenic purpura
**9.1.5** G6PD deficiency
**9.1.6** Drugs used in neutropenia

Before initiating treatment for anaemia it is essential to determine which type is present. Iron salts may be harmful and result in iron overload if given alone to patients with anaemias other than those due to iron deficiency.

### 9.1.1 Iron-deficiency anaemias

**9.1.1.1** Oral iron
**9.1.1.2** Parenteral iron

*Treatment* is only justified in the presence of a demonstrable iron-deficiency state.
*Prophylaxis* is justifiable in pregnancy, menorrhagia, after subtotal or total gastrectomy, and in the management of low birth-weight infants such as premature babies, twins, and in infants delivered by caesarean section.

#### 9.1.1.1 ORAL IRON

Iron salts should be given by mouth unless there are good reasons for using another route.

Ferrous salts show only marginal differences in efficiency of absorption of iron, but ferric salts are much less well absorbed. Haemoglobin regeneration rate is little affected by the type of salt used provided sufficient iron is given, and in most patients the time factor is not critical. Choice of preparation is thus usually decided by incidence of side-effects and cost.

The oral dose of elemental iron should be 100 to 200 mg daily; it is customary to give this as dried **ferrous sulphate**, 200 mg three times daily. If side-effects arise, dosage can be reduced or a change made to an alternative iron salt. It should be remembered, however, that an apparent improvement in tolerance on changing to another salt may be due to its lower content of elemental iron. The incidence of side-effects due to ferrous sulphate is no greater than with other iron salts

when compared on the basis of equivalent amounts of elemental iron.

Iron content of different iron salts

| Iron salt | Amount | Content of ferrous iron |
|---|---|---|
| Ferrous fumarate | 200 mg | 65 mg |
| Ferrous gluconate | 300 mg | 35 mg |
| Ferrous glycine sulphate | 225 mg | 40 mg |
| Ferrous succinate | 100 mg | 35 mg |
| Ferrous sulphate | 300 mg | 60 mg |
| Ferrous sulphate, dried | 200 mg | 60 mg[1] |

1. Good quality dried ferrous sulphate 200 mg may now contain approximately 65 mg ferrous iron

THERAPEUTIC RESPONSE. The haemoglobin concentration should rise by about 100–200 mg per 100 mL (1–2 g per litre) per day. After the haemoglobin has risen to normal, treatment should be continued for a further three months in an attempt to replenish the iron stores. Epithelial tissue changes such as atrophic glossitis and koilonychia are usually improved although the response is often slow.

COMPOUND PREPARATIONS. Some oral preparations contain ascorbic acid to aid absorption, or the iron is in the form of a chelate, which can be shown experimentally to produce a modest increase in absorption of iron. However, the therapeutic advantage is minimal and cost may be increased.

There is neither theoretical nor clinical justification for the inclusion of other therapeutically active ingredients, such as the B group of vitamins (except folic acid for pregnant women, see Iron and Folic Acid below).

MODIFIED-RELEASE CAPSULES AND TABLETS. These are designed to release iron gradually as the capsule or tablet passes along the gut so that a smaller amount of iron is present in the lumen at any one time. It is claimed that each dose unit contains enough iron for 24 hours, thus permitting once daily dosage.

These preparations are likely to carry the iron past the first part of the duodenum into an area of the gut where conditions for iron absorption are poor. The low incidence of side-effects may well be because of the small amounts of iron available under these conditions and so the preparations have no therapeutic advantage and should not be used.

SIDE-EFFECTS. Because iron salts are astringent, gastro-intestinal irritation may occur. Nausea and epigastric pain are dose-related but the relationship between dose and altered bowel habit (constipation or diarrhoea) is less clear. Oral iron, particularly modified-release preparations may exacerbate diarrhoea in patients with inflammatory bowel disease; care is also needed in patients with intestinal strictures and diverticulae.

Iron preparations taken orally may have a constipating effect particularly in older patients, occasionally leading to faecal impaction.

## FERROUS SULPHATE

*Indications:* iron-deficiency anaemia
*Cautions:* interactions: Appendix 1 (iron)
*Side-effects:* see notes above
*Dose:* ferrous iron, therapeutic, 120–180 mg daily in divided doses; prophylactic, 60 mg daily; CHILD, therapeutic, daily in divided doses, up to 1 year 36 mg, 1–5 years 72 mg, 6–12 years 120 mg

See also under Preparations

COUNSELLING. Although iron preparations are best absorbed on an empty stomach they may be taken after food to reduce gastro-intestinal side-effects; they may discolour stools

**Ferrous Sulphate** (Non-proprietary)
*Tablets*, coated, dried ferrous sulphate 200 mg (60 mg[1] iron), net price 20 = 8p
*Dose:* prophylactic, 1 tablet daily; therapeutic, 1 tablet 2–3 times daily
1. Good quality dried ferrous sulphate 200 mg may now contain approximately 65 mg iron

**Ferrous Sulphate Oral Solution, Paediatric, BP**
(Paediatric Ferrous Sulphate Mixture)
*Mixture*, ferrous sulphate 1.2% and a suitable antioxidant in a suitable vehicle with an orange flavour. Extemporaneous preparations should be recently prepared according to the following formula: ferrous sulphate 60 mg, ascorbic acid 10 mg, orange syrup 0.5 mL, double-strength chloroform water 2.5 mL, water to 5 mL
*Dose:* therapeutic, CHILD up to 1 year, 5 mL 3 times daily; 1–5 years, 10 mL 3 times daily; 6–12 years, 15 mL 3 times daily *or* 25 mL twice daily. To be taken well diluted with water

Modified-release preparations
**Feospan**® (SK&F)
*Spansule*® ( = capsules m/r), clear/red, enclosing green and red pellets, dried ferrous sulphate 150 mg (47 mg iron). Net price 30-cap pack = 90p. Label: 25
*Dose:* 1–2 capsules daily; CHILD over 1 year 1 capsule daily; can be opened and sprinkled on food
**Ferrograd**® (Abbott)
*Filmtabs*® ( = tablets f/c), m/r, red, dried ferrous sulphate 325 mg (105 mg iron). Net price 5 × 30-tab pack = £3.94. Label: 25
*Dose:* 1 tablet daily before food
**Slow-Fe**® (Ciba)
*Tablets*, m/r, dried ferrous sulphate 160 mg (50 mg iron). Net price 28-tab pack = 43p. Label: 25
*Dose:* prophylactic, 1 tablet daily; therapeutic, 2 tablets daily; CHILD over 6 years, 1 tablet daily

## FERROUS FUMARATE

*Indications; Cautions; Side-effects:* see under Ferrous Sulphate
*Dose:* see under preparations below

**Fersaday**® (DF)
*Tablets*, orange, f/c, ferrous fumarate 304 mg (100 mg iron). Net price 28-tab pack = 45p
*Dose:* prophylactic, 1 tablet daily; therapeutic, 1 tablet twice daily

**Fersamal**® (DF)
*Tablets*, brown, ferrous fumarate 200 mg (65 mg iron). Net price 20 = 14p
*Dose:* 1–2 tablets 3 times daily
*Syrup*, brown, ferrous fumarate 140 mg (45 mg iron)/5 mL. Net price 200 mL = £1.47
*Dose:* 10–20 mL twice daily; PREMATURE INFANT 0.6–2.4 mL/kg daily; CHILD up to 6 years 2.5–5 mL twice daily
**Galfer**® (Galen)
*Capsules*, red/green, ferrous fumarate 290 mg (100 mg iron). Net price 20 = 50p
*Dose:* 1 capsule 1–2 times daily before food
*Syrup*, brown, ferrous fumarate 140 mg (45 mg iron)/5 mL. Net price 100 mL = £2.54
*Dose:* 10 mL 1–2 times daily before food; CHILD (full-term infant and young child) 2.5–5 mL 1–2 times daily

Modified-release preparations
**Ferrocap**® (Consolidated)
*Capsules*, m/r, green/orange, enclosing brown and white granules, ferrous fumarate 330 mg (110 mg iron). Net price 30-cap pack = 79p. Label: 25
*Dose:* 1 capsule daily

## FERROUS GLUCONATE

*Indications; Cautions; Side-effects:* see under Ferrous Sulphate
*Dose:* see under preparations below

**Ferrous Gluconate** (Non-proprietary)
*Tablets*, red, coated, ferrous gluconate 300 mg (35 mg iron). Net price 20 = 12p
*Dose:* prophylactic, 2 tablets daily before food; therapeutic, 4–6 tablets daily in divided doses before food; CHILD 6–12 years, prophylactic and therapeutic, 1–3 tablets daily
**Fergon**® (Sanofi Winthrop)
*Tablets*, red, s/c, ferrous gluconate 300 mg (35 mg iron). Net price 20 = 44p
*Dose:* see above

## FERROUS GLYCINE SULPHATE

*Indications; Cautions; Side-effects:* see under Ferrous Sulphate
*Dose:* see under preparations below

**Plesmet**® (Napp)
*Syrup*, ferrous glycine sulphate 141 mg (25 mg iron)/5 mL. Net price 100 mL = 74p
*Dose:* 5–10 mL 3 times daily; CHILD 2–5 mL 2–3 times daily, according to age

Modified-release preparations
**Ferrocontin Continus**® (ASTA Medica)
*Tablets*, m/r, red, f/c, ferrous glycine sulphate 562.5 mg (100 mg iron). Net price 30-tab pack = 79p. Label: 25
*Dose:* 1 tablet daily

## FERROUS SUCCINATE

*Indications; Cautions; Side-effects:* see under Ferrous Sulphate
*Dose:* see under preparations below

**Ferromyn®** (Wellcome)

*Elixir*, brown, ferrous succinate 106 mg (37 mg iron)/5 mL. Net price 100 mL = £3.19

*Dose:* 5 mL 3 times daily; CHILD up to 2 years max. 1 mL twice daily, 2–5 years 2.5 mL 3 times daily, 5–10 years 5 mL twice daily

## POLYSACCHARIDE-IRON COMPLEX

*Indications; Cautions; Side-effects:* see under Ferrous Sulphate

**Niferex®** (Tillotts)

*Elixir*, brown, polysaccharide-iron complex equivalent to 100 mg of iron/5 mL. Net price 100 mL = £2.10; 30-mL dropper bottle for paediatric use = £1.80. Counselling, use of dropper

*Dose:* prophylactic, 2.5 mL daily; therapeutic, 5 mL daily; INFANT, 1 drop (from dropper bottle) per pound body-weight 3 times daily; CHILD 2–6 years, 2.5 mL daily, 6–12 years 5 mL daily

**Niferex-150®** (Tillotts)

*Capsules*, brown/orange, polysaccharide-iron complex equivalent to 150 mg of iron. Net price 20 = £1.90

*Dose:* 1–2 capsules daily

## SODIUM IRONEDETATE

*Indications; Cautions; Side-effects:* see under Ferrous Sulphate

**Sytron®** (P-D)

*Elixir*, sugar-free, sodium ironedetate 190 mg equivalent to 27.5 mg of iron/5 mL. Net price 100 mL = 34p

*Dose:* 5 mL increasing gradually to 10 mL 3 times daily; INFANT and PREMATURE INFANT 2.5 mL twice daily (smaller doses should be used initially); CHILD 1–5 years 2.5 mL 3 times daily, 6–12 years 5 mL 3 times daily

## IRON AND FOLIC ACID

These preparations are used for the prevention of iron and folic acid deficiencies in pregnancy. The prophylactic dose in pregnancy is the equivalent of approximately 100 mg of iron with folic acid 200–500 micrograms daily.

It is important to note that the small doses of folic acid contained in these preparations are inadequate for the treatment of megaloblastic anaemias.

**Fefol®** (SK&F)

*Spansule®* (=capsules m/r), clear/green, enclosing red, yellow, and white pellets, dried ferrous sulphate 150 mg (47 mg iron), folic acid 500 micrograms. Net price 30-cap pack = £1.00. Label: 25

*Dose:* 1 capsule daily

**Ferrocap-F 350®** (Consolidated)

*Capsules*, m/r, pink, enclosing brown, white, and yellow granules, ferrous fumarate 330 mg (110 mg iron), folic acid 350 micrograms. Net price 30-cap pack = £1.09. Label: 25

*Dose:* 1 capsule daily

**Ferrocontin Folic Continus®** (ASTA Medica)

*Tablets*, orange, f/c, ferrous glycine sulphate 562.5 mg (100 mg iron) for sustained release, folic acid 500 micrograms. Net price 30-tab pack = 79p. Label: 25

*Dose:* 1 tablet daily

**Ferrograd Folic®** (Abbott)

*Filmtabs®* ( = tablets f/c), red/yellow, dried ferrous sulphate 325 mg (105 mg iron) for sustained release, folic acid 350 micrograms. Net price 150-tab pack = £4.03. Label: 25

*Dose:* 1 tablet daily before food

**Folex-350®** (Rybar)

*Tablets*, pink, s/c, ferrous fumarate 308 mg (100 mg iron), folic acid 350 micrograms. Net price 20 = 44p

*Dose:* 1 tablet daily

**Galfer FA®** (Galen)

*Capsules*, red/yellow, ferrous fumarate 290 mg (100 mg iron), folic acid 350 micrograms. Net price 20 = 51p

*Dose:* 1 capsule daily before food

PoM **Lexpec with Iron-M®** (RP Drugs)

*Syrup*, brown, sugar-free, ferric ammonium citrate equivalent to 80 mg iron, folic acid 500 micrograms/5 mL. Net price 125 mL = £5.30

*Dose:* 5–10 mL daily before food

*Note.* Lexpec with Iron-M® contains five times less folic acid than Lexpec with Iron®

PoM **Meterfolic®** (Sinclair)

*Tablets*, grey, f/c, ferrous fumarate equivalent to 100 mg iron, folic acid 350 micrograms. Net price 20 = 46p

*Dose:* 1 tablet 1–2 times daily

PoM **Pregaday®** (DF)

*Tablets*, brown, f/c, ferrous fumarate 304 mg (100 mg iron), folic acid 350 micrograms. Net price 28-tab pack = 51p

*Dose:* 1 tablet daily

**Pregnavite Forte F**, see compound iron preparations

PoM **Slow-Fe Folic®** (Ciba)

*Tablets*, m/r, ivory, f/c, dried ferrous sulphate 160 mg (50 mg iron), folic acid 400 micrograms. Net price 30-tab pack = 46p. Label: 25

*Dose:* 1–2 tablets daily

Higher folic acid content

The daily dose of folic acid in these preparations is unnecessarily high for the prevention of folate deficiency; it also has the theoretical disadvantage of masking anaemia due to vitamin-$B_{12}$ deficiency (which could allow vitamin-$B_{12}$ neuropathy to develop).

PoM **Ferfolic SV®** (Sinclair)

*Tablets*, pink, ferrous gluconate 250 mg (30 mg iron), folic acid 5 mg, ascorbic acid 10 mg. Net price 20 = 69p

*Dose:* anaemia, 1–3 tablets daily after food; prophylaxis of neural tube defects in women known to be at risk, 1 tablet daily started before conception and continued for at least first trimester

PoM **Lexpec with Iron®** (RP Drugs)

*Syrup*, brown, sugar-free, ferric ammonium citrate equivalent to 80 mg iron, folic acid 2.5 mg/5 mL. Net price 125 mL = £5.50

*Dose:* 5–10 mL daily before food

*Note.* Lexpec with Iron® contains five times as much folic acid as Lexpec with Iron-M®

## COMPOUND IRON PREPARATIONS

There is no justification for prescribing compound iron preparations, except for preparations of iron and folic acid for prophylactic use in pregnancy (see above).

**Ferrous Sulphate Tablets, Compound,** green, s/c, dried ferrous sulphate equivalent to 170 mg of $FeSO_4$, copper sulphate 2.5 mg, manganese sulphate 2.5 mg. Net price 20 tabs = 9p
*Dose:* 1–2 tablets daily

NHS **BC 500 with Iron**® (Whitehall)
*Tablets,* red, f/c, ferrous fumarate 200 mg (65 mg iron) with vitamins B group and C. Net price 30-tab pack = £1.45
*Dose:* 1 tablet daily

NHS **Fefol-Vit**® (SK&F)
*Spansule*® ( = capsules m/r), clear/white, enclosing red, orange, yellow, and white pellets, dried ferrous sulphate 150 mg (47 mg iron) with vitamins B group (including folic acid 500 micrograms) and C. Net price 30-cap pack = £1.82. Label: 25
*Dose:* 1 capsule daily during pregnancy

**Fefol Z**® (SK&F)
*Spansule*® ( = capsules m/r), blue/clear, enclosing red, yellow, and white pellets, dried ferrous sulphate 150 mg (47 mg iron), folic acid 500 micrograms, zinc sulphate monohydrate 61.8 mg (22.5 mg zinc). Net price 30-cap pack = £1.79. Label: 25
*Dose:* 1 capsule daily during pregnancy

NHS **Ferrograd C**® (Abbott)
*Filmtabs*® ( = tablets f/c), red, dried ferrous sulphate 325 mg (105 mg iron) for sustained release, ascorbic acid 500 mg (as sodium salt). Net price 30-tab pack = £1.40. Label: 25
*Dose:* 1 tablet daily before food

NHS **Fesovit**® (Smith Kline Beecham Brands)
*Spansule*® ( = capsules m/r), colourless/yellow, enclosing red, orange, and white pellets, dried ferrous sulphate 150 mg (47 mg iron) with vitamins B group and C. Net price 30-cap pack = £1.82. Label: 25
*Dose:* 1–2 capsules daily; CHILD over 1 year 1 capsule daily

NHS **Fesovit Z**® (SK&F)
*Spansule*® ( = capsules m/r), orange/clear, enclosing red, orange, and white pellets, dried ferrous sulphate 150 mg (47 mg iron), zinc sulphate monohydrate 61.8 mg (22.5 mg zinc) with vitamins B group and C. Net price 30-cap pack = £2.80. Label: 25
*Dose:* 1–2 capsules daily; CHILD over 1 year 1 capsule daily

PoM **Folicin**® (Paines & Byrne)
*Tablets,* s/c, dried ferrous sulphate 200 mg (60 mg iron), folic acid 2.5 mg with minerals. Net price 20 = 20p
*Dose:* 1–2 tablets daily during pregnancy

NHS **Givitol**® (Galen)
*Capsules,* red/maroon, ferrous fumarate 305 mg (100 mg iron) with vitamins B group and C. Net price 20 = 82p
*Dose:* 1 capsule daily before food

NHS **Glykola**® (Sinclair)
*Elixir,* red, ferric chloride solution 0.01 mL (500 micrograms iron), caffeine 20 mg, calcium glycerophosphate 30 mg, kola liquid extract 0.12 mL/5 mL. Net price 100 mL = 70p
*Dose:* 5–10 mL 3 times daily after food

NHS **Octovit**® (SK&F)
*Tablets,* maroon, f/c, dried ferrous sulphate (10 mg iron) with vitamins A, B group, C, D, E, and minerals. Net price 14-tab pack = £2.03
*Dose:* 1 tablet daily

NHS ***Pregnavite Forte F**® (Bencard)
*Tablets,* lilac, s/c, dried ferrous sulphate 84 mg (25.2 mg iron), folic acid 120 micrograms, vitamin A 1333 units, thiamine hydrochloride 500 micrograms, riboflavine 500

micrograms, nicotinamide 5 mg, pyridoxine hydrochloride 330 micrograms, ascorbic acid 13.3 mg, vitamin D 133 units, calcium phosphate 160 mg. Net price 84-tab pack = £1.96
* except to reduce the risk of spina bifida or anencephaly in babies born to women who have previously given birth to one or more babies (or aborted a fetus) with a neural tube defect and endorsed 'S3B' ('S2B' in Scotland)
*Dose:* 1 tablet 3 times daily during or after food
*Note.* For prophylaxis of neural tube defects in pregnancy, dosage should be started not less than 28 days prior to conception and continue uninterrupted at least until the date of the second missed period

### 9.1.1.2 PARENTERAL IRON

The only valid reason for administering iron **parenterally** is failure of oral therapy. Such failure may be due to lack of patient co-operation with oral treatment, gastro-intestinal side-effects, continuing severe blood loss or malabsorption. Provided that the oral iron preparation is taken reliably and is absorbed, then with equivalent doses of iron the rate of haemoglobin response is not significantly faster when the intramuscular or intravenous instead of the oral route is used. The need for a rapid cure of the anaemia is therefore not met by parenteral administration of iron.

It is customary to give a course of *deep intramuscular* injections. The manufacturer's dosage schedules should be consulted; these usually include a supplement for reconstitution of iron stores.

**Iron dextran** (Imferon®) may also be administered as a single dose by *slow intravenous infusion* over 6 to 8 hours provided that there is no reaction to administration of a test dose. Although the incidence of side-effects is low, disquieting adverse reactions may occur, especially in allergic subjects, and intravenous infusion is contraindicated in asthmatic patients. Iron dextran should only be administered *intravenously* in selected cases where proper indications exist for its use, that is, when continuing blood loss is likely to be permanent and oral prophylaxis cannot keep pace, when a patient requiring parenteral iron has a small muscle mass or a haemostatic defect contra-indicating intramuscular injection, or when psychological or social pressures make iron treatment by other means impracticable.

Preparations suitable for parenteral use contain iron either in the form of **Iron Dextran Injection**, containing a complex of ferric hydroxide with dextrans of high molecular weight, or as **Iron Sorbitol Injection** (Jectofer®), containing a complex of iron, sorbitol and citric acid. The latter preparation is **not** suitable for intravenous injection and, although the low mean molecular weight allows rapid absorption from the injection site, excretion in the saliva and substantial urinary losses from each dose also occur.

To prevent leakage along the needle track with subsequent staining of the skin, intramuscular injections should be deep for both preparations.

## IRON DEXTRAN INJECTION

Contains 5% (50 mg/mL) of iron

*Indications:* iron deficiency anaemia (see notes above)

*Cautions:* risk of anaphylaxis especially in patients with history of allergy; test dose essential when given by intravenous infusion; patient should be under observation for entire period of infusion and 1 hour after; facilities to control allergic reactions including adrenaline should be available (see section 3.4.3)

*Contra-indications:* cardiac abnormalities (e.g. angina or arrhythmia), severe liver disease, acute kidney infections; intravenous infusion in asthmatic patients

*Side-effects:* staining of the skin if leakage along needle track occurs, transient nausea, vomiting, flushing; occasionally severe dyspnoea; rarely severe anaphylaxis (see Cautions)

*Dose:* see notes above and manufacturer's literature

PoM **Imferon**® (Fisons)

*Injection*, iron dextran injection. Net price 2-mL amp = 67p; 5-mL amp = £1.35

*Intravenous infusion*, iron dextran injection. Net price 20-mL amp = £4.48 (hosp. only)

## IRON SORBITOL INJECTION

Contains 5% (50 mg/mL) of iron

*Indications:* iron-deficiency anaemia

*Cautions:* oral administration of iron should be stopped at least 24 hours before giving iron sorbitol injection; administration of other injectable iron preparations should be stopped a week beforehand; urine may darken on standing

*Contra-indications:* cardiac abnormalities (e.g. angina or arrhythmia), liver disease, kidney disease (particularly pyelonephritis), untreated urinary-tract infections

*Side-effects:* occasionally severe arrhythmias

*Dose: by intramuscular injection*, see notes above and manufacturer's literature

PoM **Jectofer**® (Astra)

*Injection*, iron sorbitol injection. Net price 2-mL amp = 47p

## 9.1.2  Drugs used in megaloblastic anaemias

Most megaloblastic anaemias are due to lack of either vitamin $B_{12}$ or folate and it is essential to establish in every case which deficiency is present and the underlying cause. In emergencies, where delay might be dangerous, it is sometimes necessary to administer both substances after the bone marrow test while plasma assay results are awaited. Normally, however, appropriate treatment should be instituted only when the results of tests are available.

The most common cause of megaloblastic anaemia in the UK is *pernicious anaemia* in which lack of gastric intrinsic factor due to an auto-immune gastritis causes malabsorption of vitamin $B_{12}$.

Vitamin $B_{12}$ is also needed in the treatment of megaloblastosis due to *prolonged nitrous oxide anaesthesia*, which inactivates the vitamin, and in the rare syndrome of *congenital transcobalamin II deficiency*.

Vitamin $B_{12}$ should be given prophylactically after *total gastrectomy* or *total ileal resection* (or after *partial gastrectomy* if a vitamin $B_{12}$ absorption test shows vitamin $B_{12}$ malabsorption).

Apart from dietary deficiency, all other causes of vitamin-$B_{12}$ deficiency are attributable to *malabsorption* so there is little place for the use of vitamin $B_{12}$ orally and none for vitamin $B_{12}$ intrinsic factor complexes given by mouth.

**Hydroxocobalamin** has completely replaced cyanocobalamin as the form of vitamin $B_{12}$ of choice for therapy; it is retained in the body longer than cyanocobalamin and thus for maintenance therapy need only be given at intervals of 3 months. Although a haematological response in vitamin-$B_{12}$ deficiency may be obtained by small doses, it is customary to start treatment with 1 mg by intramuscular injection repeated 5 times at intervals of 2 to 3 days to replenish the depleted body stores. Thereafter, maintenance treatment, which is usually for life, can be instituted. There is no evidence that larger doses provide any additional benefit in vitamin-$B_{12}$ neuropathy.

**Folic acid** has few indications for long-term therapy since most causes of folate deficiency are self-limiting or will yield to a short course of treatment. It should not be used in undiagnosed megaloblastic anaemia unless vitamin $B_{12}$ is administered concurrently otherwise neuropathy may be precipitated (see above).

In *folate-deficient megaloblastic anaemia* (e.g. due to poor nutrition, pregnancy, or antiepileptics), standard treatment to bring about a haematological remission and replenish body stores, is oral administration of folic acid 5 mg daily for 4 months; up to 15 mg daily may be necessary in malabsorption states.

For *prophylaxis in chronic haemolytic states or in renal dialysis*, it is sufficient to give folic acid 5 mg daily or even weekly, depending on the diet and the rate of haemolysis.

For *prophylaxis in pregnancy* the dose of folic acid is 200–500 micrograms daily (see Iron and Folic Acid, section 9.1.1.1).

> There is **no** justification for prescribing multiple-ingredient vitamin preparations containing vitamin $B_{12}$ or folic acid.

## HYDROXOCOBALAMIN

*Indications:* Pernicious anaemia, other causes of vitamin-$B_{12}$ deficiency, subacute combined degeneration of the spinal cord

*Cautions:* should not be given before diagnosis fully established but see also notes above

*Dose: by intramuscular injection*, initially 1 mg repeated 5 times at intervals of 2–3 days; maintenance dose 1 mg every 3 months; CHILD, dosage as for adult

PoM **Hydroxocobalamin Injection,** hydroxocobalamin 1 mg/mL. Net price 1-mL amp = 36p
Note. The BP directs that when vitamin B_{12} injection is prescribed or demanded hydroxocobalamin injection shall be dispensed or supplied
The brand names NHS Cobalin-H® (Paines & Byrne) and NHS Neo-Cytamen® (DF) are used for hydroxocobalamin injection

CYANOCOBALAMIN

Indications: see notes above
Dose: *by intramuscular injection*, initially 1 mg repeated 10 times at intervals of 2–3 days, maintenance 1 mg every month, but see notes above

PoM **Cyanocobalamin Injection,** cyanocobalamin 1 mg/mL. Net price 1 mL amp = 34p
Note. The BP directs that when vitamin B_{12} injection is prescribed or demanded hydroxocobalamin injection shall be dispensed or supplied
The brand name NHS Cytamen® (DF) is used for cyanocobalamin injection

NHS **Cytacon®** (DF)
Tablets, f/c, cyanocobalamin 50 micrograms. Net price 50-tab pack = £1·59
Liquid, red, cyanocobalamin 35 micrograms/5 mL. Net price 200 mL = £1.59

FOLIC ACID

Indications: see notes above
Cautions: should never be given alone in the treatment of Addisonian pernicious anaemia and other vitamin B_{12}-deficiency states because it may precipitate the onset of subacute combined degeneration of the spinal cord. Do not use in malignant disease unless megaloblastic anaemia due to folate deficiency is an important complication (some malignant tumours are folate-dependent); **interactions:** Appendix 1 (vitamins)
Dose: initially, 5 mg daily for 4 months (see notes above); maintenance, 5 mg every 1–7 days depending on underlying disease; CHILD up to 1 year, 500 micrograms/kg daily; over 1 year, as adult dose

PoM [1] **Folic Acid Tablets,** folic acid 5 mg, net price 20 = 7p; 100-microgram tablets also available
1. Can be sold to the public provided daily doses do not exceed 500 micrograms

PoM **Lexpec®** (RP Drugs)
Syrup, sugar-free, folic acid 2.5 mg/5 mL. Diluent sorbitol solution, life of syrup diluted to 50% 7 days. Net price 125 mL = £4.85

9.1.3 Drugs used in hypoplastic, haemolytic, and renal anaemias

Anabolic steroids, pyridoxine, antilymphocyte immunoglobulin, and various corticosteroids are used in hypoplastic and haemolytic anaemias.

The place of **anabolic steroids** in the therapy of *aplastic anaemia* remains somewhat controversial and their effectiveness is unclear. There is a wide variation in the reported successful responses. Occasional patients, however, do seem to derive benefit. Since nandrolone decanoate requires intramuscular injection it is unsuitable in aplastic anaemia or cytotoxic aplasia because of the low platelet count; it is customary to prescribe oxymetholone in doses of the order of 2–3 mg/kg daily, and to continue therapy for at least 3 to 6 months. At these dose levels, virilising side-effects may be expected in female patients and in children. Controlled trials have shown that antilymphocyte immunoglobulin produces a response in 50% of acquired cases; higher response rates have been reported when cyclosporin is given as well.

It is unlikely that dietary deprivation of **pyridoxine** (section 9.6.2) produces haematological effects in man. However, certain forms of *sideroblastic anaemia* respond to pharmacological doses, possibly reflecting its role as a co-enzyme during haemoglobin synthesis. Pyridoxine is indicated in both *idiopathic acquired* and *hereditary sideroblastic anaemias*. Although complete cures have not been reported, some increase in haemoglobin may occur; the dose required is usually high, up to 400 mg daily. *Reversible sideroblastic anaemias* respond to treatment of the underlying cause but in pregnancy, haemolytic anaemias, and alcohol dependence, or during isoniazid treatment, pyridoxine is also indicated.

Corticosteroids (see section 6.3) have an important place in the management of a wide variety of haematological disorders. They include conditions with an immune basis such as *autoimmune haemolytic anaemia, immune thrombocytopenias* and *neutropenias*, and *major transfusion reactions*. They are also used in chemotherapy schedules for many types of lymphoma, *lymphoid leukaemias,* and *paraproteinaemias*, including *myelomatosis*. Corticosteroids are used in *aplastic anaemias*, where their value is more debatable.

NANDROLONE

Indications: aplastic anaemia but see notes above; postmenopausal osteoporosis, see section 6.4.3
Cautions; Contra-indications; Side-effects: see section 6.4.3
Dose: *by deep intramuscular injection*, aplastic anaemia (but not recommended, see notes above), nandrolone decanoate 50–100 mg weekly

PoM **Deca-Durabolin 100®** (Organon)
Injection (oily), nandrolone decanoate 100 mg/mL. Net price 1-mL amp = £6.68

OXYMETHOLONE

Indications: aplastic anaemia; see notes above
Cautions: cardiac and renal impairment, circulatory failure, hypertension, diabetes mellitus, epilepsy, migraine; monitor skeletal maturation in children for 6 months after treatment; **interactions:** Appendix 1 (anabolic steroids)

*Contra-indications:* hepatic impairment, prostatic carcinoma, pregnancy, breast-feeding, porphyria (see section 9.8.2)

*Side-effects:* acne, oedema, jaundice and liver dysfunction, virilism with high doses, hypercalcaemia, menstrual irregularities; hyperglucagonaemia has also been reported with oxymetholone

*Dose:* aplastic anaemia, 2–3 mg/kg daily in divided doses; CHILD 2–3 mg/kg daily (less in Fanconi's anaemia)

See also notes above

PoM **Anapolon 50**® (Syntex)
*Tablets,* scored, oxymetholone 50 mg. Net price 20 = £14.83

---

## ERYTHROPOIETIN

**Epoetin** (recombinant human erythropoietin) is used for the anaemia associated with chronic renal failure in patients on dialysis. The clinical efficacy of epoetin alfa and epoetin beta is similar and they can be used interchangeably.

Other factors which contribute to the anaemia of chronic renal failure such as iron or folate deficiency should be corrected; aluminium toxicity, concurrent infection or other inflammatory disease may also impair the response to epoetin.

## EPOETIN

Recombinant human erythropoietin

*Indications:* anaemia associated with erythropoietin deficiency in chronic renal failure patients on dialysis

*Cautions:* uncontrolled hypertension (monitor closely for changes in haemoglobin, blood pressure and electrolytes—hypertensive episodes may be more likely with rapid haemoglobin response), history of convulsions, chronic hepatic failure, malignant disease, ischaemic vascular disease (monitor platelets for first 8 weeks); exclude other causes of anaemia and give iron supplements if needed; increase in dialysis heparin may be required (monitor dialyser)

*Side-effects:* increased blood pressure (treat as appropriate), moderately increased platelet count (rarely significant), influenza-like symptoms, convulsions, skin reactions and palpebral oedema (possibly allergic); shunt thrombosis, isolated side-effects reported include increased creatinine, urea and phosphate serum concentrations, acne-like symptoms, myocardial infarction, and anaphylaxis

*Dose:* (aimed at increasing haemoglobin concentration at rate not exceeding 2 g/100 mL/month to stable level of 10–12 g/100 mL): *by intravenous injection* over 2 minutes, initially 40–50 units/kg 3 times weekly, increased as necessary in steps of 20–25 units/kg at intervals of 4 weeks (usual max. 600–720 units/kg weekly in 2–3 divided doses); maintenance: 90–300 units/kg weekly in 2–3 divided doses

Severe anaemia of renal origin in predialysis patients, preferably *by subcutaneous injection* (max. 1 mL per injection site), 50 units/kg 3 times weekly increased as necessary in steps of 25 units/kg; max. 600 units/kg weekly in 3 divided doses; maintenance: 50–100 units/kg weekly in 3 divided doses

▼ PoM **Eprex**® (Cilag)
*Injection,* epoetin alfa 2000 units/mL, net price 1-mL amp = £18.00; 4000 units/mL, 1-mL amp = £36.00

▼ PoM **Recormon**® (Boehringer Mannheim)
*Injection,* powder for reconstitution, epoetin beta. Net price 1000-unit vial = £9.00; 2000-unit vial = £18.00; 5000-unit vial = £45.00 (all with water for injection)
*Note.* Avoid contact of reconstituted injection with glass; use only plastic materials

---

## IRON OVERLOAD

Severe tissue iron overload may occur in aplastic and other refractory anaemias, mainly as the result of repeated blood transfusions. It is a particular problem in refractory anaemias with hyperplastic bone marrow, especially *thalassaemia major,* where excessive iron absorption from the gut and inappropriate iron therapy may add to the tissue siderosis.

Venesection therapy is contra-indicated, but the long-term administration of the iron chelating compound **desferrioxamine mesylate** is useful. Subcutaneous infusions of desferrioxamine (20–40 mg/kg over 12 hours) are given on 5 to 7 nights each week. Desferrioxamine (up to 2 g per unit of blood) may also be given through the infusion line at the time of blood transfusion.

Iron excretion induced by desferrioxamine is enhanced by administration of vitamin C (section 9.6.3) in a dose of 200 mg daily (100 mg in infants); it should be given separately from food since it also enhances iron absorption. In patients with cardiac abnormalities vitamin C should be avoided for 1–2 weeks after starting desferrioxamine treatment.

Infusion of desferrioxamine may be used to treat *aluminium overload* in dialysis patients; theoretically 100 mg of desferrioxamine binds with 4.1 mg of aluminium.

Orally active iron chelators are under clinical study but are not available for general use.

## DESFERRIOXAMINE MESYLATE

*Indications:* see notes above; iron poisoning, see Emergency Treatment of Poisoning

*Cautions:* renal impairment, eye and ear examinations; aluminium-related encephalopathy (may exacerbate neurological dysfunction), pregnancy, breast-feeding; **interactions:** Appendix 1 (desferrioxamine)

*Side-effects:* gastro-intestinal disturbances; arrhythmias, hypotension (especially when given too rapidly by intravenous injection);

---

anaphylaxis; dizziness, convulsions; Yersinia infection more frequent; disturbances of hearing and vision (including lens opacity and retinopathy); skin reactions; pain on intramuscular injection

*Dose:* see notes above; iron poisoning, see Emergency Treatment of Poisoning

*Note.* For full details and warnings relating to administration, consult data sheet

**Preparations**
See under Emergency Treatment of Poisoning

## 9.1.4   Drugs used in autoimmune thrombocytopenic purpura

It is usual to commence the treatment of autoimmune (idiopathic) thrombocytopenic purpura with corticosteroids, e.g. prednisolone of the order of 1 mg/kg daily, gradually reducing the dosage over the subsequent weeks. In patients who fail to achieve a satisfactory platelet count or relapse when corticosteroid dosage is reduced or withdrawn, splenectomy is considered.

Other therapy that has been tried in refractory cases includes azathioprine (see section 8.2.1), cyclophosphamide (see section 8.1.1), vincristine or vinblastine (see section 8.1.4) (or vinblastine-loaded platelets), cyclosporin (see section 8.2.2), and danazol (section 6.7.3). Intravenous immunoglobulins (see section 14.5), have also been used in refractory cases or where a temporary rapid rise in platelets is needed, as in pregnancy or pre-operatively. For patients with chronic severe thrombocytopenia refractory to other therapy, tranexamic acid (see section 2.11) may be given to reduce the severity of haemorrhage.

## 9.1.5   G6PD deficiency

Glucose 6-phosphate dehydrogenase (G6PD) deficiency is highly prevalent in populations originating from most parts of Africa, from most parts of Asia, from Oceania, and from Southern Europe; it can also be encountered, rarely, in any other population.

When prescribing drugs for patients who are G6PD deficient, the following three points should be kept in mind:
1. G6PD deficiency is genetically heterogeneous; different genetic variants entail different susceptibility to the haemolytic risk from drugs; thus, a drug found to be safe in some G6PD-deficient subjects may not be equally safe in others;
2. no test specifically designed to identify potential risk in G6PD-deficient subjects is currently carried out by manufacturers;
3. the risk and severity of haemolysis is almost always dose-related.

The table below should be read with these points in mind. Whenever possible, a test for G6PD deficiency should be done before prescribing a drug in the list, especially if the patient belongs to a population group in which G6PD deficiency is common.

A very small group of G6PD-deficient individuals, with chronic non-spherocytic hae-

molytic anaemia, have haemolysis even in the absence of an exogenous trigger. These patients must be regarded as being at high risk of severe exacerbation of haemolysis following administration of any of the drugs listed below.

---

Drugs with definite risk of haemolysis in most G6PD-deficient subjects

---

Dapsone and other sulphones (higher doses for dermatitis herpetiformis more likely to cause problems)
Methylene blue
Niridazole [not on UK market]
Nitrofurantoin
Pamaquin [not on UK market]
Primaquine (30 mg weekly for 8 weeks has been found to be without undue harmful effects in Afro and Asian people, see section 5.4.1)
4-Quinolones (including ciprofloxacin and nalidixic acid)
Sulphonamides (including co-trimoxazole; some sulphonamides, e.g. sulphadiazine, have been tested and found not to be haemolytic in many G6PD-deficient subjects)

---

Drugs with possible risk of haemolysis in some G6PD-deficient subjects

---

Aspirin (acceptable in a dose of at least 1 g daily in most G6PD-deficient subjects)
Chloroquine (acceptable in acute malaria)
Menadione, water-soluble derivatives (e.g. menadiol sodium phosphate)
Probenecid
Quinidine (acceptable in acute malaria)
Quinine (acceptable in acute malaria)

---

*Note.* Mothballs may contain naphthalene which also causes haemolysis in subjects with G6PD-deficiency.

## 9.1.6   Drugs used in neutropenia

**Filgrastim** (recombinant human granulocyte-colony stimulating factor) may reduce the duration of neutropenia associated with the use of cancer chemotherapy and thereby reduce the incidence of associated sepsis. Filgrastim has, however, no routine indication at present and is expensive; it should only be administered by those experienced in its use.

### FILGRASTIM

(Human granulocyte-colony stimulating factor, G-CSF)

*Indications:* reduction in duration of neutropenia and incidence of febrile neutropenia in cytotoxic chemotherapy of non-myeloid malignancy (specialist use only)

*Cautions:* tumours with myeloid characteristics (risk of tumour growth), pre-malignant myeloid conditions; reduced myeloid precursors (e.g. following extensive radiotherapy or chemotherapy); monitor leucocyte count (discontinue treatment if leucocytosis, see data sheet); monitor platelet count and haemoglobin; osteoporotic bone disease (monitor bone density if given for more than 6 months); does not prevent other toxic effects of high-dose chemotherapy; pregnancy, breast-feeding

*Side-effects:* musculoskeletal pain, transient hypotension, disturbances in liver enzymes and serum uric acid; urinary abnormalities including dysuria

*Dose:* by subcutaneous injection or by intravenous infusion, 500 000 units/kg daily started not less than 24 hours after cytotoxic chemotherapy, continued until neutrophil count in normal range, usually for up to 14 days

▼ PoM **Neupogen**® (Roche)
*Injection*, filgrastim 30 million units (300 micrograms)/mL; net price 1-mL vial = £79.00, 1.6-mL (48 million-unit) vial = £126.00

# 9.2   Fluids and electrolytes

9.2.1 Oral administration
9.2.2 Intravenous administration
9.2.3 Plasma and plasma substitutes

The following tables give a selection of useful electrolyte values:

Electrolyte concentrations—intravenous fluids

| Intravenous infusion | Millimoles per litre | | | | |
|---|---|---|---|---|---|
| | Na$^+$ | K$^+$ | HCO$_3^-$ | Cl$^-$ | Ca$^{2+}$ |
| *Normal Plasma Values* | 142 | 4.5 | 26 | 103 | 2.5 |
| Sodium Chloride 0.9% | 150 | — | — | 150 | — |
| Compound Sodium Lactate (Hartmann's) | 131 | 5 | 29 | 111 | 2 |
| Sodium Chloride 0.18% and Glucose 4% | 30 | — | — | 30 | — |
| Potassium Chloride 0.3% and Glucose 5% | — | 40 | — | 40 | — |
| Potassium Chloride 0.3% and Sodium Chloride 0.9% | 150 | 40 | — | 190 | — |
| *To correct metabolic acidosis* | | | | | |
| Sodium Bicarbonate 1.26% | 150 | — | 150 | — | — |
| Sodium Bicarbonate 8.4% for cardiac arrest | 1000 | — | 1000 | — | — |
| Sodium Lactate (M/6) | 167 | — | 167 | — | — |

Millimoles of each ion in 1 gram of salt

| Electrolyte | mmol/g approx. |
|---|---|
| Ammonium chloride | 18.7 |
| Calcium chloride (CaCl$_2$,2H$_2$O) | Ca 6.8   Cl 13.6 |
| Potassium bicarbonate | 10 |
| Potassium chloride | 13.4 |
| Sodium bicarbonate | 11.9 |
| Sodium chloride | 17.1 |
| Sodium lactate | 8.9 |

Electrolyte content—gastro-intestinal secretions

| Type of fluid | Millimoles per litre | | | | |
|---|---|---|---|---|---|
| | H$^+$ | Na$^+$ | K$^+$ | HCO$_3^-$ | Cl$^-$ |
| Gastric | 40–60 | 20–80 | 5–20 | — | 100–150 |
| Biliary | — | 120–140 | 5–15 | 30–50 | 80–120 |
| Pancreatic | — | 120–140 | 5–15 | 70–110 | 40–80 |
| Small bowel | — | 120–140 | 5–15 | 20–40 | 90–130 |

Faeces, vomit, or aspiration should be saved and analysed where possible if abnormal losses are suspected; where this is impracticable the approximations above may be helpful in planning replacement therapy.

## 9.2.1   Oral administration

9.2.1.1 Oral potassium
9.2.1.2 Oral sodium and water
9.2.1.3 Oral bicarbonate

Sodium and potassium salts, which may be given by mouth to prevent deficiencies or to treat established deficiencies of mild or moderate degree, are discussed in this section. Oral preparations for removing excess potassium and preparations for oral rehydration therapy are also included here. Oral bicarbonate, for metabolic acidosis, is also described in this section.

For reference to calcium, magnesium, and phosphate, see section 9.5.

### 9.2.1.1   ORAL POTASSIUM

Compensation for potassium loss is especially necessary:
1. in those taking digoxin or anti-arrhythmic drugs, where potassium depletion may induce arrhythmias;
2. in patients in whom secondary hyperaldosteronism occurs, e.g. renal artery stenosis, cirrhosis of the liver, the nephrotic syndrome, and severe heart failure;
3. in patients with excessive losses of potassium in the faeces, e.g. chronic diarrhoea associated with intestinal malabsorption or laxative abuse.

Measures to compensate for potassium loss may also be required in the elderly since they frequently take inadequate amounts of potassium in the diet (but see below for warning on renal insufficiency). Measures may also be required during long-term administration of drugs known to induce potassium loss (e.g. corticosteroids). Potassium supplements are seldom required with the small doses of diuretics given to treat hypertension; potassium-sparing diuretics (rather than potassium supplements) are recommended for prevention of hypokalaemia due to diuretics such as frusemide or the thiazides when these are given to eliminate oedema.

DOSAGE. If potassium salts are used for the *prevention of hypokalaemia*, then doses of potassium chloride 2 to 4 g (approx. 25 to 50 mmol) daily by mouth are suitable in patients taking a normal diet. Smaller doses must be used if there is renal insufficiency (common in the elderly) otherwise there is danger of hyperkalaemia. Potassium salts cause nausea and vomiting therefore poor compliance is a major limitation to their effectiveness; where appropriate, potassium-sparing diuretics are preferable.

When there is *established potassium depletion* or when the plasma-potassium concentration is less than 3.5mmol/litre, larger doses of 10 to 15 g (approx. 135 to 200 mmol) daily of potassium chloride may be required over periods of days or weeks. Potassium depletion is frequently associated with chloride depletion and with metabolic alkalosis, and these disorders require correction.

ADMINISTRATION. Potassium salts are preferably given as a liquid (or effervescent) preparation, rather than modified-release tablets; they should be given as the chloride (the use of effervescent potassium tablets BPC 1968 should be restricted to *hyperchloraemic states*, section 9.2.1.3).

**Salt substitutes.** A number of salt substitutes which contain significant amounts of potassium chloride are readily available as health food products (e.g. Losalt and Ruthmol). These should not be used by patients with renal failure as potassium intoxication may result.

## POTASSIUM BICARBONATE
Section 9.2.1.3

## POTASSIUM CHLORIDE
*Indications:* potassium depletion (see notes above)
*Cautions:* intestinal stricture, history of peptic ulcer, hiatus hernia (for sustained-release preparations); **interactions:** Appendix 1 (potassium salts)
*Contra-indications:* renal failure, plasma potassium concentrations above 5 mmol/litre
*Side-effects:* nausea and vomiting (severe symptoms may indicate obstruction), oesophageal or small bowel ulceration
*Dose:* see notes above
Note. Do not confuse Effervescent Potassium Tablets BPC 1968 (section 9.2.1.3) with effervescent potassium chloride tablets. Effervescent Potassium Tablets BPC 1968 do not contain chloride ions and their use should be restricted to hyperchloraemic states (section 9.2.1.3). Effervescent Potassium Chloride Tablets BP are usually available in two strengths, one containing 6.7 mmol each of $K^+$ and $Cl^-$ (corresponding to Kloref®), the other containing 12 mmol $K^+$ and 8 mmol $Cl^-$ (corresponding to Sando-K®). Generic prescriptions must specify the strength required.

**Kay-Cee-L®** (Geistlich)
*Syrup*, red, sugar-free, potassium chloride 7.5% (1 mmol/mL each of $K^+$ and $Cl^-$). Net price 200 mL = £1.95; 500 mL = £2.74. Label: 21
**Kloref®** (Cox)
*Tablets*, effervescent, betaine hydrochloride, potassium benzoate, bicarbonate, and chloride, equivalent to potassium chloride 500 mg (6.7 mmol each of $K^+$ and $Cl^-$). Net price 50 = £1.59. Label: 13, 21

**Kloref-S®** (Cox)
*Granules*, effervescent, sugar-free, betaine hydrochloride, potassium bicarbonate and chloride equivalent to potassium chloride 1.5 g (20 mmol each of $K^+$ and $Cl^-$)/sachet. Net price 30 sachets = £2.84. Label: 13, 21
**Sando-K®** (Sandoz)
*Tablets*, effervescent, potassium bicarbonate and chloride equivalent to potassium 470 mg (12 mmol of $K^+$) and chloride 285 mg (8 mmol of $Cl^-$). Net price 20 = 35p. Label: 13, 21

Modified-release preparations
Avoid unless effervescent tablets or liquid preparations inappropriate
**Leo K®** (Leo)
*Tablets*, m/r, f/c, potassium chloride 600 mg (8 mmol each of $K^+$ and $Cl^-$). Net price 20 = 20p. Label: 25, 27, counselling, swallow whole with fluid during meals while sitting or standing
**Nu-K®** (Consolidated)
*Capsules*, m/r, blue, potassium chloride 600 mg (8 mmol each of $K^+$ and $Cl^-$). Net price 20 = 35p. Label: 25, 27, counselling, swallow whole with fluid during meals while sitting or standing *or* open capsule and swallow enclosed granules with fluid or soft food
**Slow-K®** (Ciba)
*Tablets*, m/r, orange, s/c, potassium chloride 600 mg (8 mmol each of $K^+$ and $Cl^-$). Net price 20 = 10p. Label: 25, 27, counselling, swallow whole with fluid during meals while sitting or standing

## POTASSIUM CITRATE
See section 7.4.3

### POTASSIUM REMOVAL

Ion-exchange resins may be used to remove excess potassium in *mild hyperkalaemia* or in *moderate hyperkalaemia* when there are not ECG changes; intravenous therapy is required in emergencies (section 9.2.2).

## POLYSTYRENE SULPHONATE RESINS
*Indications:* hyperkalaemia associated with anuria or severe oliguria, and in dialysis patients
*Cautions:* children (impaction of resin with excessive dosage or inadequate dilution)
*Contra-indications:* avoid calcium-containing resin in hyperparathyroidism, multiple myeloma, sarcoidosis, or metastatic carcinoma; avoid sodium-containing resin in congestive heart failure and severe renal impairment
*Side-effects:* rectal ulceration following rectal administration
*Dose: by mouth*, 15 g 3–4 times daily in water (not fruit juice which has a high $K^+$ content)
*By rectum*, as an enema, 30 g in methylcellulose solution, retained for 9 hours
CHILD, either route, 0.5–1 g/kg daily

**Calcium Resonium®** (Sanofi Winthrop)
*Powder*, buff, calcium polystyrene sulphonate. Net price 300 g = £44.34. Label: 13
**Resonium A®** (Sanofi Winthrop)
*Powder*, buff, sodium polystyrene sulphonate. Net price 454 g = £54.57. Label: 13

## 9.2.1.2   ORAL SODIUM AND WATER

Sodium chloride is indicated in states of sodium depletion and usually needs to be given intravenously (section 9.2.2). In chronic conditions associated with mild or moderate degrees of sodium depletion, e.g. in salt-losing bowel or renal disease, oral supplements of sodium chloride or bicarbonate (section 9.2.1.3), according to the acid-base status of the patient, may be sufficient.

## SODIUM BICARBONATE
Section 9.2.1.3

## SODIUM CHLORIDE
**Indications:** sodium depletion; see also section 9.2.2.

**Sodium Chloride Tablets,** sodium chloride 300 mg (approx 5 mmol each of $Na^+$ and $Cl^-$). Net price 20 = 20p. Label: 13
**Slow Sodium**® (Ciba)
*Tablets,* m/r, sodium chloride 600 mg (approx. 10 mmol each of $Na^+$ and $Cl^-$). Net price 20 = 11p. Label: 25

## SODIUM CITRATE
See section 7.4.3

## ORAL REHYDRATION THERAPY (ORT)

As a worldwide problem *diarrhoea* is by far the most important indication for fluid and electrolyte replacement. Intestinal absorption of sodium and water is enhanced by glucose, therefore replacement of fluid and electrolytes lost through diarrhoea can be achieved by giving solutions containing sodium, potassium, and glucose.

Oral rehydration solutions should:
enhance optimally the absorption of water and electrolytes;
replace the electrolyte deficit adequately and safely;
contain an alkalising agent to counter acidosis;
be simple to use in hospital and at home;
be palatable and acceptable, especially to children;
be readily available.

It is the policy of the World Health Organization (WHO) to promote a single oral rehydration solution but use it flexibly (e.g. by giving extra water between drinks of oral rehydration solution to moderately dehydrated infants).

Oral rehydration solutions used in the UK are lower in sodium (35–60 mmol/litre) and higher in glucose (up to 200 mmol/litre) than the WHO formulation. They are of benefit for *mild to moderate diarrhoea*, when the body's homoeostatic mechanisms are still working and will not be harmful, but they may be suboptimal in correction of fluid loss and electrolyte imbalance. In the *more severe diarrhoeas* the WHO formulation is marginally more effective in correcting dehydration; it carries no danger of hypernatraemia if used correctly.

For intravenous rehydration see section 9.2.2

## ORAL REHYDRATION SALTS (ORS)
**Indications:** fluid and electrolyte loss in diarrhoea, see notes above
**Dose:** according to fluid loss, usually 200–400 mL solution after every loose motion; INFANT 1–1½ times usual feed volume; CHILD 200 mL after every loose motion

UK formulations
*Note.* After reconstitution any unused solution should be discarded no later than 1 hour after preparation unless stored in a refrigerator when it may be kept for up to 24 hours.
**Dextrolyte**® (Cow & Gate)
*Oral solution,* glucose, potassium chloride, sodium chloride, sodium lactate, providing $Na^+$ 35 mmol, $K^+$ 13.4 mmol, $Cl^-$ 30.5 mmol, lactate 17.7 mmol, and glucose 200 mmol/litre. 100 mL (hosp. only)
**Diocalm Junior**® (SmithKline Beecham Brands)
*Oral powder,* sodium chloride 350 mg, potassium chloride 300 mg, sodium citrate 590 mg, anhydrous glucose 4 g/sachet. Net price 5-sachet pack (orange-flavoured) = £1.10. Label: 13
Reconstitute one sachet with 200 mL of water (freshly boiled and cooled for infants)
*Note.* Five sachets reconstituted with 1 litre of water provide $Na^+$ 60 mmol, $K^+$ 20 mmol, $Cl^-$ 50 mmol, citrate 10 mmol, and glucose 111 mmol
**Dioralyte**® (Rhône-Poulenc Rorer)
*Effervescent tablets,* sodium chloride 117 mg, sodium bicarbonate 336 mg, potassium chloride 186 mg, citric acid anhydrous 384 mg, anhydrous glucose 1.62 g. Net price 10-tab pack (blackcurrant- or citrus-flavoured) = £1.20. Label: 13
Reconstitute 2 tablets with 200 mL of water (only for adults and for children over 1 year)
*Note.* Ten tablets when reconstituted with 1 litre of water provide $Na^+$ 60 mmol, $K^+$ 25 mmol, $Cl^-$ 45 mmol, citrate 20 mmol, and glucose 90 mmol
*Oral powder,* sodium chloride 470 mg, potassium chloride 300 mg, disodium hydrogen citrate 530 mg, glucose 3.56 g/sachet. Net price 20 sachet-pack (blackcurrant- or citrus-flavoured or plain) = £4.17. Label: 13
Reconstitute one sachet with 200 mL of water (freshly boiled and cooled for infants).
*Note.* Five sachets reconstituted with 1 litre of water provide $Na^+$ 60 mmol, $K^+$ 20 mmol, $Cl^-$ 60 mmol, citrate 10 mmol, and glucose 90 mmol
**Electrolade**® (Nicholas)
*Oral powder,* sodium chloride 236 mg, potassium chloride 300 mg, sodium bicarbonate 500 mg, anhydrous glucose 4 g/sachet (banana- and melon-flavoured). Net price 4-sachet pack = 80p; 20-sachet pack = £3.99. Label: 13
Reconstitute one sachet with 200 mL of water (freshly boiled and cooled for infants)
*Note.* Five sachets when reconstituted with 1 litre of water provide $Na^+$ 50 mmol, $K^+$ 20 mmol, $Cl^-$ 40 mmol, $HCO_3^-$ 30 mmol, and glucose 111 mmol

**Gluco-lyte®** (Cupal)

*Oral powder*, sodium chloride 200 mg, potassium chloride 300 mg, sodium bicarbonate 300 mg, glucose 8 g/sachet. Net price 6 sachets = £1.35. Label: 13

Reconstitute one sachet with 200 mL of water (freshly boiled and cooled for infants)

Note. Five sachets when reconstituted with 1 litre of water provide $Na^+$ 35 mmol, $K^+$ 20 mmol, $Cl^-$ 37 mmol, $HCO_3^-$ 18 mmol, and glucose 200 mmol (corresponds to Oral Rehydration Salts—Formula A, BP)

**Rapolyte®** (Janssen)

*Oral powder*, sodium chloride 350 mg, potassium chloride 300 mg, sodium citrate 600 mg, anhydrous glucose 4 g/sachet. Net price 5-sachet pack (raspberry-flavoured) = £1·01. Label: 13

Reconstitute one sachet with 200 mL of water (freshly boiled and cooled for infants)

Note. Five sachets reconstituted with 1 litre of water provide $Na^+$ 60 mmol, $K^+$ 20 mmol, $Cl^-$ 50 mmol, citrate 10 mmol, and glucose 111 mmol)

**Rehidrat®** (Searle)

*Oral powder*, sodium chloride 440 mg, potassium chloride 380 mg, sodium bicarbonate 420 mg, citric acid 440 mg, glucose 4.09 g, sucrose 8.07 g, fructose 70 mg/sachet. Net price 24-sachet pack (orange, blackcurrant or lemon and lime flavour) = £5.85; 16-sachet pack (mixed flavours) = £3.90. Label: 13

Note. Lemon and lime version stains vomit green

Reconstitute one sachet with 250 mL of water (freshly boiled and cooled for infants)

Note. Four sachets when reconstituted with one litre of water provide $Na^+$ 50 mmol, $K^+$ 20 mmol, $Cl^-$ 50 mmol, $HCO_3^-$ 20 mmol, citrate 9 mmol, glucose 91 mmol, sucrose 94 mmol, and fructose 2 mmol

WHO formulations
**WHO Oral Rehydration Salts**

*Oral powder*, sodium chloride 3.5 g, potassium chloride 1.5 g, sodium citrate 2.9 g, anhydrous glucose 20 g. To be dissolved in sufficient water to produce 1 litre (providing $Na^+$ 90 mmol, $K^+$ 20 mmol, $Cl^-$ 80 mmol, citrate 10 mmol, glucose 111 mmol/litre)

Note. Recommended by the WHO and the United Nations Childrens Fund but not commonly used in the UK. Corresponds to Oral Rehydration Salts—Citrate (Formula C) BP; the alternative WHO formulation corresponds to Oral Rehydration Salts—Bicarbonate (Formula B) BP and is less stable

## 9.2.1.3 ORAL BICARBONATE

**Sodium bicarbonate** is given by mouth for *chronic acidotic states* such as uraemic acidosis or renal tubular acidosis. The dose for correction of metabolic acidosis is not predictable and the response must be assessed; 4.8 g daily (57 mmol each of $Na^+$ and $HCO_3^-$) or more may be required. For severe metabolic acidosis, sodium bicarbonate can be given intravenously (section 9.2.2).

Sodium bicarbonate may also be used to make the pH of the urine alkaline (see section 7.4.3); for use in dyspepsia see section 1.1.2.

Sodium supplements may increase blood pressure or cause fluid retention and pulmonary oedema in those at risk; hypokalaemia may be exacerbated.

Where *hyperchloraemic acidosis* is associated with potassium deficiency, as in some renal tubular and gastro-intestinal disorders it may be appropriate to give oral **potassium bicarbonate**, although acute or severe deficiency should be managed by intravenous therapy.

## SODIUM BICARBONATE

*Indications:* see notes above
*Cautions:* see notes above; avoid in respiratory acidosis; **interactions:** Appendix 1 (antacids and adsorbents)
*Dose:* see notes above

**Sodium Bicarbonate** (Non-proprietary)

*Capsules*, sodium bicarbonate usual strengths 300 mg (approx. 3.6 mmol each of $Na^+$ and $HCO_3^-$), 500 mg (approx. 6 mmol each of $Na^+$ and $HCO_3^-$), 600 mg (approx. 7.1 mmol each of $Na^+$ and $HCO_3^-$)

Available from Martindale, Penn, etc (special order)

*Tablets*, sodium bicarbonate 300 mg, net price 20 tabs = 12p; 600 mg, 20 = 41p

## POTASSIUM BICARBONATE

*Indications:* see notes above
*Cautions:* cardiac disease, renal impairment; **interactions:** Appendix 1 (potassium salts)
*Contra-indications:* hypochloraemia; plasma potassium concentration above 5 mmol/litre
*Side-effects:* nausea and vomiting
*Dose:* see notes above

**Potassium Tablets, Effervescent,** potassium bicarbonate 500 mg, potassium acid tartrate 300 mg, each tablet providing 6.5 mmol of $K^+$. To be dissolved in water before administration. Net price 100 = £2.71. Label: 13, 21

Note. These tablets do not contain chloride; for effervescent tablets containing potassium and chloride, see under Potassium Chloride, section 9.2.1.1

## WATER

The term water used without qualification means either potable water freshly drawn direct from the public supply and suitable for drinking or freshly boiled and cooled purified water. The latter should be used if the public supply is from a local storage tank or if the potable water is unsuitable for a particular preparation. (Water for injections, section 9.2.2.)

## 9.2.2 Intravenous administration

Solutions of electrolytes are given intravenously, to meet normal fluid and electrolyte requirements or to replenish substantial deficits or continuing losses, when the patient is nauseated or vomiting and is unable to take adequate amounts by mouth.

In an individual patient the nature and severity of the electrolyte imbalance must be assessed from the history and clinical and biochemical examination. Sodium, potassium, chloride, magnesium, phosphate, and water depletion can occur singly and in combination with or without disturbances of acid-base balance; for reference to the use of magnesium and phosphates, see section 9.5.

Isotonic solutions may be infused safely into a peripheral vein. Solutions more concentrated than plasma, for example 20% glucose are best given through an indwelling catheter positioned in a large vein.

## INTRAVENOUS SODIUM

**Sodium chloride** in isotonic solution provides the most important extracellular ions in near physiological concentration and is indicated in *sodium depletion* which may arise from such conditions as gastro-enteritis, diabetic ketoacidosis, ileus, and ascites. In a severe deficit of from 4 to 8 litres, 2 to 3 litres of isotonic sodium chloride may be given over 2 to 3 hours; thereafter infusion can usually be at a slower rate.

Excessive administration should be avoided; the jugular venous pressure should be assessed, the bases of the lungs should be examined for crepitations, and in elderly or seriously ill patients it is often helpful to monitor the right atrial (central) venous pressure.

**Sodium chloride and glucose** solutions are indicated when there is combined *water and sodium depletion*. A 1:1 mixture of isotonic sodium chloride and 5% glucose allows some of the water (free of sodium) to enter body cells which suffer most from dehydration while the sodium salt with a volume of water determined by the normal plasma Na$^+$ remains extracellular. An example of combined sodium chloride and water depletion occurs in persistent vomiting.

## SODIUM CHLORIDE

*Indications:* electrolyte imbalance, also section 9.2.1.2

*Cautions:* restrict intake in impaired renal function, cardiac failure, hypertension, peripheral and pulmonary oedema, toxaemia of pregnancy

*Side-effects:* administration of large doses may give rise to sodium accumulation and oedema

*Dose:* see notes above

PoM **Sodium Chloride Intravenous Infusion,** usual strength sodium chloride 0.9% (9 g, 150 mmol each of Na$^+$ and Cl$^-$/litre), this strength being supplied when normal saline for injection is requested. Net price 2-mL amp = 23p; 5-mL amp = 30p; 10-mL amp = 34p; 20-mL amp = 62p; 50-mL amp = £1.52

In hospitals, 500- and 1000-mL packs, and sometimes other sizes, are available

*Note.* The term 'normal saline' should **not** be used to describe sodium chloride intravenous infusion 0.9%; the term 'physiological saline' is acceptable but it is preferable to give the composition (i.e. sodium chloride intravenous infusion 0.9%).

PoM **Sodium Chloride and Glucose Intravenous Infusion,** usual strength sodium chloride 0.18% (1.8 g, 30 mmol each of Na$^+$ and Cl$^-$/litre) and 4% of anhydrous glucose

In hospitals, 500- and 1000-mL packs, and sometimes other sizes are available

PoM **Ringer's Solution for Injection,** calcium chloride (dihydrate) 322 micrograms, potassium chloride 300 micrograms, sodium chloride 8.6 mg/mL, providing the following ions (in mmol/litre), Ca$^{2+}$ 2.2, K$^+$ 4, Na$^+$ 147, Cl$^-$ 156

In hospitals, 500- and 1000-mL packs, and sometimes other sizes, are available

## INTRAVENOUS GLUCOSE

**Glucose** solutions (5%) are mainly used to replace water deficits and should be given alone when there is no significant loss of electrolytes. Average water requirements in a healthy adult are 1.5 to 2.5 litres daily and this is needed to balance unavoidable losses of water through the skin and lungs and to provide sufficient for urinary excretion. Water depletion (dehydration) tends to occur when these losses are not matched by a comparable intake, as for example may occur in coma or dysphagia or in the aged or apathetic who may not drink water in sufficient amount on their own initiative.

Excessive loss of water without loss of electrolytes is uncommon, occurring in fevers, hyperthyroidism, and in uncommon water-losing renal states such as diabetes insipidus or hypercalcaemia. The volume of glucose solution needed to replenish deficits varies with the severity of the disorder, but usually lies within the range of 2 to 10 litres.

Glucose solutions are also given in regimens with calcium, bicarbonate, and insulin for the emergency management of *hyperkalaemia*. They are also given, after correction of hyperglycaemia, during treatment of diabetic ketoacidosis when they must be accompanied by continuing insulin infusion.

## GLUCOSE

(Dextrose Monohydrate)

*Note.* Glucose BP is the monohydrate but Glucose Intravenous Infusion BP is a sterile solution of anhydrous glucose or glucose monohydrate, potency being expressed in terms of anhydrous glucose

*Indications:* fluid replacement (see notes above), provision of energy (section 9.3)

*Side-effects:* glucose injections especially if hypertonic may have a low pH and may cause venous irritation and thrombophlebitis

*Dose:* water replacement, see notes above; energy source, 1–3 litres daily of 20–50% solution

PoM **Glucose Intravenous Infusion,** glucose or anhydrous glucose (potency expressed in terms of anhydrous glucose), usual strength 5% (50 mg/mL). 20% solution, net price 20-mL amp = £1.30; 25% solution, 25-mL amp = £2.21; 50% solution, price 20-mL amp = £1.50; 25-mL amp = £3.11; 50-mL amp = £2.66
In hospitals, 500- and 1000-mL packs, and sometimes other sizes, are available; also available from IMS (Min-I-Jet® Glucose, 50% in 50-ml disposable syringe).

---

## INTRAVENOUS POTASSIUM

**Potassium chloride and sodium chloride** intravenous infusion and **potassium chloride and glucose** intravenous infusion are used to correct severe *hypokalaemia* and depletion and when sufficient potassium cannot be taken by mouth. Potassium chloride, as ampoules containing 1.5 g (20 mmol $K^+$) in 10 mL[1], may be added to 500 mL of sodium chloride or glucose intravenous infusion; the solution then contains 40mmol/litre and may be given slowly over 2 to 3 hours with ECG monitoring in difficult cases[2]. Repeated measurements of plasma potassium are necessary to determine whether further infusions are required and to avoid the development of hyperkalaemia; this is especially liable to occur in renal failure.

1. **Important**: mix infusion solution **thoroughly** after adding potassium chloride; use ready-prepared solutions when possible
2. Higher concentrations may be given in severe cases but require infusion pump control

## POTASSIUM CHLORIDE

*Indications:* electrolyte imbalance; see also oral potassium supplements, section 9.2.1.1
*Cautions:* for intravenous infusion the concentration of solution should not usually exceed 3.2 g (43 mmol)/litre
*Side-effects:* rapid infusion toxic to heart
*Dose: by slow intravenous infusion,* depending on the deficit or the daily maintenance requirements, see also notes above

PoM **Potassium Chloride and Glucose Intravenous Infusion,** usual strength potassium chloride 0.3% (3 g, 40 mmol each of $K^+$ and $Cl^-$/litre) with 5% of anhydrous glucose
In hospitals, 500- and 1000-mL packs, and sometimes other sizes, are available

PoM **Potassium Chloride and Sodium Chloride Intravenous Infusion,** usual strength potassium chloride 0.3% (3 g/litre) and sodium chloride 0.9% (9 g/litre), containing 40 mmol of $K^+$, 150 mmol of $Na^+$, and 190 mmol of $Cl^-$/litre
In hospitals, 500- and 1000-mL packs, and sometimes other sizes, are available

PoM **Potassium Chloride, Sodium Chloride, and Glucose Intravenous Infusion,** sodium chloride 0.18% (1.8 g, 30 mmol of $Na^+$/litre) with 4% of anhydrous glucose and usually sufficient potassium chloride to provide 10–40 mmol of $K^+$/litre (to be specified by the prescriber)
In hospitals, 500- and 1000-mL packs, and sometimes other sizes, are available

PoM **Potassium Chloride Solution, Strong** (sterile), potassium chloride 15% (150 mg, approximately 2 mmol each of $K^+$ and $Cl^-$/mL). Net price 10-mL amp = 81p
IMPORTANT. Must be diluted with **not less** than 50 times its volume of sodium chloride intravenous infusion 0.9% or other suitable diluent and **mixed well**
Solutions containing 10 and 20% of potassium chloride are also available in both 5- and 10-mL ampoules.

---

## BICARBONATE AND LACTATE

**Sodium bicarbonate** is used to control severe *metabolic acidosis* (as in renal failure or diabetic ketoacidosis). Since this condition is usually attended by sodium depletion, it is reasonable to correct this first by the administration of isotonic sodium chloride intravenous infusion, provided the kidneys are not primarily affected and the degree of acidosis is not so severe as to impair renal function. In these circumstances, isotonic sodium chloride alone is usually effective as it restores the ability of the kidneys to generate bicarbonate. In renal acidosis or in severe metabolic acidosis of any origin (for example blood pH<7.1) sodium bicarbonate (1.26%) may be infused with isotonic sodium chloride; a total volume of up to 6 litres (4 litres of sodium chloride and 2 litres of sodium bicarbonate) may be necessary in the adult. In severe shock due for example to cardiac arrest (see section 2.7), metabolic acidosis may develop without sodium depletion; in these circumstances sodium bicarbonate is best given in a small volume of hypertonic solution, such as 50 mL of 8.4% solution intravenously; plasma pH should be monitored (ensuring adequate pulmonary ventilation and effective circulation to the lungs).

Sodium bicarbonate infusion is also used in the emergency management of *hyperkalaemia* (see also under Glucose).

**Sodium lactate** intravenous infusion is obsolete in metabolic acidosis, and carries the risk of producing lactic acidosis, particularly in seriously ill patients with poor tissue perfusion or impaired hepatic function.

## SODIUM BICARBONATE

*Indications:* metabolic acidosis
*Dose: by slow intravenous injection,* a strong solution (up to 8.4%), or *by continuous intravenous infusion,* a weaker solution (usually 1.26%), an amount appropriate to the body base deficit (see notes above)

PoM **Sodium Bicarbonate Intravenous Infusion,** usual strength sodium bicarbonate 1.26% (12.6 g, 150 mmol each of $Na^+$ and $HCO_3^-$/litre); various other strengths available
In hospitals, 500- and 1000-mL packs, and sometimes other sizes, are available

PoM **Min-I-Jet® Sodium Bicarbonate** (IMS)
*Intravenous injection,* sodium bicarbonate in disposable syringe, net price 4.2%, 10 mL = £3.81; 8.4%, 10 mL = £3.97, 50 mL = £5.87

---

## SODIUM LACTATE

*Indications:* diabetic coma, diminished alkali reserve (but see notes above)

PoM **Sodium Lactate Intravenous Infusion,** sodium lactate M/6, contains the following ions (in mmol/litre), Na$^+$ 167, HCO$_3^-$ (as lactate) 167

PoM **Sodium Lactate Intravenous Infusion, Compound,** (Hartmann's Solution for Injection; Ringer-Lactate Solution for Injection), contains the following ions (in mmol/litre), Na$^+$ 131, K$^+$ 5, Ca$^{2+}$ 2, HCO$_3^-$ (as lactate) 29, Cl$^-$ 111

In hospitals, 500- and 1000-mL packs, and sometimes other sizes, are available

---

## WATER

PoM **Water for Injections.** Net price 1-mL amp = 12p; 2-mL amp = 11p; 5-mL amp = 16p; 20-mL amp = 45p; 50-mL amp = £1·01

---

## 9.2.3   Plasma and plasma substitutes

**Plasma and albumin solutions,** prepared from whole blood, contain soluble proteins and electrolytes but no clotting factors, blood group antibodies, or pseudocholinesterases; they may be given without regard to the recipient's blood group.

Plasma and albumin solutions are used for the treatment of hypoproteinaemia and the low plasma volume associated with conditions such as burns, the complications of surgery, and pancreatitis. Plasma substitutes are more appropriate for acute blood loss (e.g. haematemesis).

---

## ALBUMIN SOLUTION
(Human Albumin Solution)

A solution containing protein derived from plasma, serum, or normal placentas; at least 95% of the protein is albumin. The solution may be isotonic (containing 4–5% protein) or concentrated (containing 15–25% protein).

*Indications:* see under preparations, below

*Cautions:* history of cardiac or circulatory disease (administer slowly to avoid rapid rise in blood pressure and cardiac failure; risk of further haemorrhage or shock due to rise in blood pressure; correct dehydration when administering concentrated solution

*Contra-indications:* cardiac failure; severe anaemia

*Side-effects:* nausea, fever, and chills particularly with rapid infusion

Isotonic solutions

*Indications:* acute or sub-acute loss of plasma volume e.g. in burns, pancreatitis, trauma, and complications of surgery; plasma exchange

Available as: *Human Albumin Solution 4.5%* (50-, 100-, 250-, and 400-mL bottles—Immuno); *Albuminar-5*® (250-mL, 500-mL, and 1-litre vials—Armour); *Albutein*® 5% (250- and 500-mL vials—Alpha); *Buminate*® 5.0% (250- and 500-mL bottles—Baxter); *Zenalb*® 4.5 (50-, 100-, 250-, and 500-mL bottles—BPL)

Concentrated solutions (20–25%)

*Indications:* severe hypoalbuminaemia associated with low plasma volume and generalised oedema where salt and water restriction with plasma volume expansion are required; adjunct in the treatment of hyperbilirubinaemia by exchange transfusion in the newborn

Available as: *Albumin Solution 20%* (5- and 100-mL vials—SNBTS); *Human Albumin Solution 20%* (10-, 50- and 100-mL vials—Immuno); *Albuminar-20*® (50- and 100-mL vials—Armour); *Albuminar-25*® (20-, 50-, and 100-mL vials—Armour); *Albutein*® 20% (50- and 100-mL vials—Alpha); *Albutein*® 25% (20-, 50-, and 100-mL vials—Alpha); *Buminate*® 20% (50- and 100-mL vials—Baxter); *Zenalb*® 20 (50- and 100-mL bottles—BPL)

---

## PLASMA PROTEIN SOLUTION
(Plasma Protein Fraction, PPF)

An isotonic solution containing 4–5% protein derived from plasma or serum; at least 85% of the protein is albumin.

*Indications:* see notes above

*Cautions; Contra-indications; Side-effects:* see under Albumin Solution

Available as: *Plasma Protein Solution 4.5%* (100- and 500-mL bottles—SNBTS); *Plasmatein*® 5% (250- and 500-mL vials—Alpha)

---

## PLASMA SUBSTITUTES

**Dextrans, gelatin,** and **hetastarch** are macromolecular substances which are slowly metabolised; they may be used at the outset to expand and maintain blood volume in shock arising from conditions such as burns or septicaemia. They are rarely needed when shock is due to sodium and water depletion as, in these circumstances, the shock responds to water and electrolyte repletion. They should not be used to maintain plasma volume in conditions such as burns or peritonitis where there is loss of plasma protein, water and electrolytes over periods of several days or weeks. In these situations, plasma or plasma protein fractions containing large amounts of albumin should be given. Plasma substitutes should be used in haemorrhage if blood is not available as an immediate short-term measure until it is.

Dextrans may interfere with blood group crossmatching or biochemical measurements and these should be carried out before infusion is begun. Dextran 70 by intravenous infusion is used predominantly for volume expansion. Dextran 40 intravenous infusion is used in an attempt to improve peripheral blood flow in ischaemic disease of the limbs and peripheral thromboembolism.

**Gelatin** and **hetastarch** are also used for short-term volume expansion.

---

                    Prices are **net**, see p. 1

Dosage. Because of the complex requirements relating to blood volume expansion and the primary significance of blood, plasma protein, and electrolyte replacement, detailed dose statements have been omitted. *In all cases specialist literature should be consulted.*

## DEXTRAN 40 INTRAVENOUS INFUSION

Dextrans of weight average molecular weight about '40000' 10% in glucose intravenous infusion 5% or in sodium chloride intravenous infusion 0.9%

*Indications:* conditions associated with peripheral local slowing of the blood flow; prophylaxis of post-surgical thrombo-embolic disease

*Cautions; Contra-indications; Side-effects:* see under Dextran 70 Intravenous Infusion; correct dehydration before infusion and give adequate fluids during therapy; very special care in those at risk of vascular overloading

*Dose:* by intravenous infusion, initially 500–1000 mL; further doses are given according to the patient's condition (see notes above)

PoM **Gentran 40**® (Baxter)
*Intravenous infusion,* dextran 40 intravenous infusion in glucose intravenous infusion 5% or in sodium chloride intravenous infusion 0.9%. 500-mL bottle (both)

PoM **Lomodex 40**® (CP)
*Intravenous infusion,* dextran 40 intravenous infusion in glucose intravenous infusion 5% or in sodium chloride intravenous infusion 0.9%. Net price 500-mL bottle (both) = £5.77

PoM **Rheomacrodex**® (Kabi Pharmacia)
*Intravenous infusion,* dextran 40 intravenous infusion in glucose intravenous infusion 5% or in sodium chloride intravenous infusion 0.9%. Net price 500-mL bottle (both) = £6.51

## DEXTRAN 70 INTRAVENOUS INFUSION

Dextrans of weight average molecular weight about '70000' 6% in glucose intravenous infusion 5% or in sodium chloride intravenous infusion 0.9%

*Indications:* short-term blood volume expansion; prophylaxis of post-surgical thrombo-embolic disease

*Cautions:* congestive heart failure, renal impairment; blood samples for cross-matching should ideally be taken before infusion

*Contra-indications:* severe congestive heart failure; renal failure; bleeding disorders such as thrombocytopenia and hypofibrinogenaemia

*Side-effects:* rarely anaphylactoid reactions

*Dose:* by intravenous infusion, after moderate to severe haemorrhage, 500–1000 mL rapidly initially followed by 500 mL later if necessary; severe burns, up to 3000 mL in the first few days with electrolytes (see also notes above)

PoM **Gentran 70**® (Baxter)
*Intravenous infusion,* dextran 70 intravenous infusion in glucose intravenous infusion 5% or in sodium chloride intravenous infusion 0.9%. 500-mL bottle (both)

PoM **Lomodex 70**® (CP)
*Intravenous infusion,* dextran 70 intravenous infusion in glucose intravenous infusion 5% or in sodium chloride intravenous infusion 0.9%. Net price 500-mL bottle (both) = £3.66

PoM **Macrodex**® (Kabi Pharmacia)
*Intravenous infusion,* dextran 70 intravenous infusion in glucose intravenous infusion 5% or in sodium chloride intravenous infusion 0.9%. Net price 500-mL bottle (both) = £4.11

## DEXTRAN 110 INTRAVENOUS INFUSION

Dextrans of weight average molecular weight about '110000' 6% in glucose intravenous infusion 5% or in sodium chloride intravenous infusion 0.9%

*Indications:* see under Dextran 70 Intravenous Infusion

*Cautions; Contra-indications; Side-effects:* see under Dextran 70 Intravenous Infusion; blood samples for cross-matching should be taken before infusion

*Dose:* by intravenous infusion, see under Dextran 70 Intravenous Infusion

PoM **Dextraven 110**® (CP)
*Intravenous infusion,* dextran 110 intravenous infusion in sodium chloride intravenous infusion 0.9%. Net price 500-mL bottle = £5.77

## GELATIN

*Note.* The gelatin is partially degraded

*Indications:* low blood volume

*Cautions; Contra-indications; Side-effects:* see under Dextran 70 Intravenous Infusion

*Dose:* by intravenous infusion, initially 500–1000 mL of a 3.5–4% solution (see notes above)

PoM **Gelofusine**® (Braun)
*Intravenous infusion,* succinylated gelatin (modified fluid gelatin, average molecular weight 30000) 4%, sodium chloride 0.9%. Net price 500-mL bottle = £3.56

PoM **Haemaccel**® (Hoechst)
*Intravenous infusion,* polygeline (degraded and modified gelatin, average molecular weight 35000) 35 g, Na$^+$145 mmol, K$^+$ 5.1 mmol, Ca$^{2+}$ 6.25 mmol, Cl$^-$ 145 mmol/litre. Net price 500-mL bottle = £3.81

## HETASTARCH

*Indications:* low blood volume (expansion)

*Cautions; Contra-indications; Side-effects:* see under Dextran 70 Intravenous Infusion

*Dose:* by intravenous infusion, 500–1000 mL; usual max. 1500 mL daily (see notes above)

PoM **Elohes**® **6%** (Oxford Nutrition)
*Intravenous infusion,* hetastarch (weight average molecular weight 200000) 6% in sodium chloride intravenous infusion 0.9%. Net price 500-mL bottle = £9.75

PoM **Hespan**® (Du Pont)
*Intravenous infusion,* hetastarch (weight average molecular weight 450000) 6% in sodium chloride intravenous infusion 0.9%. Net price 500-mL Steriflex® bag = £16.72

# 9.3   Intravenous nutrition

When adequate feeding via the alimentary tract is not possible, nutrients may be given by intravenous infusion. This may be in addition to ordinary oral or tube feeding—**supplemental parenteral nutrition**, or may be the sole source of nutrition—**total parenteral nutrition** (TPN). Indications for this method include preparation of undernourished patients for surgery, chemotherapy, or radiation therapy; severe or prolonged disorders of the gastro-intestinal tract; major surgery, trauma, or burns; prolonged coma or refusal to eat; and some patients with renal or hepatic failure. The composition of proprietary preparations available is in the table below.

**Protein** is given as mixtures of essential and non-essential synthetic L-amino acids. Ideally, all essential amino acids should be included with a wide variety of non-essential ones to provide sufficient nitrogen together with electrolytes (see also section 9.2.2). Available solutions vary in their composition of amino acids; they often contain an energy source (usually glucose) and electrolytes.

**Energy** is provided in a ratio of 0.6 to 1.1 megajoules (150–250 kcals) per gram of protein nitrogen. Energy requirements must be met if amino acids are to be utilised for tissue maintenance. Although it has long been held that carbohydrate has a greater nitrogen-sparing effect than fat, recent studies have shown that a mixture of both energy sources, usually 30 to 50% as fat, gives better utilisation of amino acid solutions than glucose alone.

**Glucose** is the preferred source of carbohydrate, but if more than 180 g is given per day frequent monitoring of blood glucose is required, and insulin may be necessary. Glucose in various strengths from 10 to 50% must be infused through a central venous catheter to avoid thrombosis. Preparations are available with useful added ions and trace elements, e.g. Glucoplex®.

Fructose and sorbitol have been used in an attempt to avoid the problem of hyperosmolar hyperglycaemic non-ketotic acidosis but other metabolic problems may occur, as with xylitol and ethanol which are now rarely used.

**Fat** emulsions have the advantages of a high energy to fluid volume ratio, neutral pH, and iso-osmolarity with plasma, and provide essential fatty acids. Available preparations are soya bean oil emulsions. Several days of adaptation may be required to attain maximal utilisation. Reactions include occasional febrile episodes (usually only with 20% emulsions) and rare anaphylactic responses. Interference with biochemical measurements such as those for blood gases and calcium may occur if samples are taken before fat has been cleared. Daily checks are necessary to ensure complete clearance from the plasma in conditions where fat metabolism may be disturbed. **Additives may only be mixed with fat emulsions where compatibility is known.**

**Total parenteral nutrition** (TPN) requires the use of a solution containing amino acids, glucose, fat, electrolytes, trace elements, and vitamins. This is now commonly provided by the pharmacy in the form of the 3-litre bag. The solution is infused through a central venous catheter inserted under full surgical precautions. Only nutritional fluids should be given by this line. Loading doses of vitamin $B_{12}$ and folic acid are advised and other vitamins are given parenterally twice weekly.

Before starting, the patient should be well oxygenated with a near normal circulating blood volume, renal function, and acid-base status. Appropriate biochemical tests should have been carried out beforehand and serious deficits corrected. Nutritional and electrolyte status must be monitored throughout treatment.

## SUPPLEMENTARY PREPARATIONS

PoM **Addamel**® (Kabi Pharmacia)
*Solution*, electrolytes and trace elements for addition to Vamin® solutions except Vamin 18®, $Ca^{2+}$ 5 mmol, $Mg^{2+}$ 1.5 mmol, $Cl^-$ 13.3 mmol/10 mL; traces of $Fe^{3+}$, $Zn^{2+}$, $Mn^{2+}$, $Cu^{2+}$, $F^-$, $I^-$. For adult use. Net price 10-mL amp = £1.59

PoM **Addiphos**® (Kabi Pharmacia)
*Solution*, sterile, phosphate 40 mmol, $K^+$ 30 mmol, $Na^+$ 30 mmol/20 mL. For addition to Vamin® solutions and glucose intravenous infusions. Net price 20-mL vial = £1.18

PoM **Additrace**® (Kabi Pharmacia)
*Solution*, trace elements for addition to Vamin® solutions traces of $Fe^{3+}$, $Zn^{2+}$, $Mn^{2+}$, $Cu^{2+}$, $Cr^{3+}$, $Se^{4+}$, $Mo^{6+}$, $F^-$, $I^-$. For adult use. Net price 10-mL amp = £1.79

PoM **Multibionta**® (Merck)
*Solution*, ascorbic acid 500 mg, dexpanthenol 25 mg, nicotinamide 100 mg, pyridoxine hydrochloride 15 mg, riboflavine sodium phosphate 10 mg, thiamine hydrochloride 50 mg, tocopheryl acetate 5 mg, vitamin A 10 000 units. For addition to infusion solutions. Net price 10-mL amp = £1.47

PoM **Ped-El**® (Kabi Pharmacia)
*Solution*, sterile, $Ca^{2+}$, $Cu^{2+}$, $Fe^{3+}$, $Mg^{2+}$, $Mn^{2+}$, $Zn^{2+}$, $Cl^-$, $F^-$, $I^-$, P. For addition to Vamin® solutions. For paediatric use. Net price 20-mL vial = £1.59

PoM **Solivito N**® (Kabi Pharmacia)
*Solution*, powder for reconstitution, biotin 60 micrograms, cyanocobalamin 5 micrograms, folic acid 400 micrograms, glycine 100 mg, nicotinamide 40 mg, pyridoxine hydrochloride 4.9 mg, riboflavine sodium phosphate 4.9 mg, sodium ascorbate 113 mg, sodium pantothenate 16.5 mg, thiamine mononitrate 3.1 mg. Dissolve in water for injections or glucose intravenous infusion for adding to glucose intravenous infusion or Intralipid®; dissolve in Vitlipid N® or Intralipid® for adding to Intralipid® only. Net price per vial = £1.80

PoM **Vitlipid N**® (Kabi Pharmacia)
*Emulsion, adult*, vitamin A 330 units, ergocalciferol 20 units, dl-alpha tocopherol 1 unit, phytomenadione 15 micrograms/mL. For addition to Intralipid®. Net price 10-mL amp = £1.75
*Emulsion, infant*, vitamin A 230 units, ergocalciferol 40 units, dl-alpha tocopherol 0.7 unit, phytomenadione 20 micrograms/mL. For addition to Intralipid®. Net price 10-mL amp = £1.75

---

Proprietary Infusion Fluids for Parenteral Feeding

| Preparation | Nitrogen g/litre | [1]Energy kJ/litre | Electrolytes mmol/litre | | | | | Other components/litre |
|---|---|---|---|---|---|---|---|---|
| | | | K+ | Mg2+ | Na+ | Acet- | Cl- | |
| Aminoplasmal L5 (Braun) | 8.03 | | 25 | 2.5 | 48 | 59 | 31 | acid phosphate 9 mmol, malate 7.5 mmol |
| Net price 500 mL = £7.50 | | | | | | | | |
| Aminoplasmal L10 (Braun) | 16.06 | | 25 | 2.5 | 48 | 59 | 62 | acid phosphate 9 mmol, malate 7.5 mmol |
| Net price 500 mL = £14.20 | | | | | | | | |
| Aminoplasmal Ped (Braun) | 7.4 | | 25 | 2.5 | 50 | 27 | 15 | |
| Net price 100 mL = £5.25; 250 mL = £6.50 | | | | | | | | |
| Aminoplex 5 (Geistlich) | 5.0 | 3600 | 28 | 4 | 35 | 28 | 43 | ethanol 5%, sorbitol 125 g, malic acid 1.85 g |
| Net price 1000 mL = £11.95 | | | | | | | | |
| Aminoplex 12 (Geistlich) | 12.44 | | 30 | 2.5 | 35 | 5 | 67 | malic acid 4.6 g |
| Net price 500 mL = £11.31; 1000 mL = £19.08 | | | | | | | | |
| Aminoplex 14 (Geistlich) | 13.4 | | 30 | | 35 | | 79 | vitamins, malic acid 5.36 g |
| Net price 500 mL = £10.36 | | | | | | | | |
| Aminoplex 24 (Geistlich) | 24.9 | | 30 | 2.5 | 35 | 5 | 67 | malic acid 4.5 g |
| Net price 250 mL = £9.79; 500 mL = £17.28 | | | | | | | | |
| Branched Chain Amino Acids (Clintec) | 4.4 | | | | | | | |
| 500-mL Viaflex® pack | | | | | | | | |
| FreAmine III 8.5% (Kendall) | 13.0 | | | | 10 | 72 | <3 | phosphate 10 mmol |
| Net price 500 mL = £10.20; 1000 mL = £18.95 | | | | | | | | |
| FreAmine III 10% (Kendall) | 15.3 | | | | 10 | 88 | <2 | phosphate 20 mmol |
| 1000 mL | | | | | | | | |
| Glucoplex 1000 (Geistlich) | | 4200 | 30 | 2.5 | 50 | | 67 | acid phosphate 18mmol, Zn2+ 0.046 mmol, anhydrous glucose 240 g |
| Net price 500 mL = £2.76; 1000 mL = £3.10 | | | | | | | | |
| Glucoplex 1600 (Geistlich) | | 6700 | 30 | 2.5 | 50 | | 67 | acid phosphate 18mmol, Zn2+ 0.046 mmol, anhydrous glucose 400 g |
| Net price 500 mL = £2.90; 1000 mL = £3.35 | | | | | | | | |
| Hepanutrin (Geistlich) | 15.6 | | | | | | | |
| Net price 500 mL = £15.74 | | | | | | | | |
| Intralipid 10% (Kabi Pharmacia) | | 4600 | | | | | | fractionated soya oil 100 g, glycerol 22.5 g |
| Net price 100 mL = £4.35; 500 mL = £9.65 | | | | | | | | |
| Intralipid 20% (Kabi Pharmacia) | | 8400 | | | | | | fractionated soya oil 200 g, glycerol 22.5 g |
| Net price 100 mL = £6.55; 500 mL = £14.40 | | | | | | | | |
| [2]Lipofundin MCT/LCT 10% (Braun) | | 4430 | | | | | | soya oil 50 g, medium chain triglycerides 50 g |
| Net price 100 mL = £6.40; 500 mL = £10.50 | | | | | | | | |
| [2]Lipofundin MCT/LCT 20% (Braun) | | 8000 | | | | | | soya oil 100 g, medium chain triglycerides 100 g |
| Net price 100 mL = £7.30; 500 mL = £16.00 | | | | | | | | |
| Lipofundin S 10% (Braun) | | 4470 | | | | | | soya oil 100 g |
| Net price 100 mL = £6.00; 500 mL = £9.80 | | | | | | | | |
| Lipofundin S 20% (Braun) | | 8520 | | | | | | soya oil 200 g |
| Net price 100 mL = £7.00; 500 mL = £15.30 | | | | | | | | |
| Nephramine 5.4% (Kendall) | 6.4 | | | | 5 | 44 | <3 | essential amino acids only |
| Net price 250 mL = £24.99 | | | | | | | | |
| Nutracel 400 (Clintec) | | 3400 | | 18 | | 0.16 | 66 | Ca2+ 15 mmol, Mn2+ 0.08mmol, Zn2+ 0.08mmol, anhydrous glucose 200 g |
| Net price 500 mL = £2.60 | | | | | | | | |
| Nutracel 800 (Clintec) | | 3400 | | 9 | | 0.08 | 33 | Ca2+ 7.5 mmol, Mn2+ 0.04 mmol, Zn2+ 0.04 mmol, anhydrous glucose 200 g |
| Net price 1000 mL = £4.50 | | | | | | | | |
| Perifusin (Kabi Pharmacia) | 5.0 | | 30 | 5 | 40 | 10 | 9 | malate 22.5 mmol |
| Net price 1000 mL = £7.20 | | | | | | | | |
| Plasma-Lyte 148 (water) (Baxter) | | | 5 | 1.5 | 140 | 27 | 98 | gluconate 23 mmol |
| 1000 mL | | | | | | | | |
| Plasma-Lyte 148 (dextrose 5%) (Baxter) | | 840 | 5 | 1.5 | 140 | 27 | 98 | gluconate 23 mmol, anhydrous glucose 50 g |
| 500 mL and 1000 mL | | | | | | | | |
| Plasma-Lyte M (dextrose 5%) (Baxter) | | 840 | 16 | 1.5 | 40 | 12 | 40 | Ca2+ 2.5 mmol, lactate 12 mmol, anhydrous glucose 50 g |
| 1000 mL | | | | | | | | |
| [3]Primene 10% (Clintec) | 15 | | | | | 25 | 15.6 | |
| Net price 100 mL = £6.20; 250 mL = £8.50 | | | | | | | | |
| Soyacal 10% (Alpha) | | 4600 | | | | | | purified soya oil 100 g, glycerol 22.1 g |
| Net price 50 mL = £2.75; 100 mL = £4.25; 250 mL = £7.25; 500 mL = £9.50 | | | | | | | | |

1. Excludes protein-derived energy
2. Treatment with Lipofundin MCT/LCT should be limited to up to 10 days
3. For use in neonates and children only

*Note.* 1000 kcal = 4.1868 MJ; 1 MJ (1000 kJ) = 238.8 kcal. All entries are PoM

Proprietary Infusion Fluids for Parenteral Feeding (*continued*)

| Preparation | Nitrogen g/litre | [1]Energy kJ/litre | Electrolytes mmol/litre K+ | Mg$^{2+}$ | Na+ | Acet$^-$ | Cl$^-$ | Other components/litre |
|---|---|---|---|---|---|---|---|---|
| Soyacal 20% (Alpha) | | 8400 | | | | | | purified soya oil 200 g, glycerol 22.1 g |
| Net price 50 mL = £4.25; 100 mL = £6.50; 250 mL = £10.75; 500 mL = £14.00 | | | | | | | | |
| Synthamin 9 (Clintec) | 9.1 | | 60 | 5 | 70 | 100 | 70 | acid phosphate 30 mmol |
| Net price 500 mL = £7.15; 1000 mL = £13.25 | | | | | | | | |
| Synthamin 14 (Clintec) | 14.0 | | 60 | 5 | 70 | 140 | 70 | acid phosphate 30 mmol |
| Net price 500 mL = £10.35; 1000 mL = £18.40 | | | | | | | | |
| Synthamin 14 without electrolytes (Clintec) | 14.0 | | | | | 68 | 34 | |
| Net price 500 mL = £10.60; 1000 mL = £18.80 | | | | | | | | |
| Synthamin 17 (Clintec) | 16.5 | | 60 | 5 | 70 | 150 | 70 | acid phosphate 30 mmol |
| Net price 500 mL = £13.60; 1000 mL = £24.70 | | | | | | | | |
| Synthamin 17 without electrolytes (Clintec) | 16.5 | | | | | 82 | 40 | |
| Net price 500 mL = £13.60; 1000 mL = £24.70 | | | | | | | | |
| Synthamix 9/800X (Clintec) | 4.55 | 1680 | 30 | 7 | 35 | 50 | 51.5 | acid phosphate 15 mmol, Zn$^{2+}$ 0.02 mmol, Ca$^{2+}$ 3.75 mmol, Mn$^{2+}$ 0.02 mmol, anhydrous glucose 100 g |
| Net price 2000 mL = £35.00 | | | | | | | | |
| Synthamix 9/1800X (Clintec) | 3.64 | 3024 | 24 | 5.6 | 28 | 40 | 41.2 | acid phosphate 12 mmol, Zn$^{2+}$ 0.016 mmol, Ca$^{2+}$ 3 mmol, Mn$^{2+}$ 0.016 mmol, anhydrous glucose 180 g |
| Net price 2500 mL = £36.50 | | | | | | | | |
| Synthamix 14/1200X (Clintec) | 7 | 2520 | 30 | 7 | 35 | 70 | 51.5 | acid phosphate 15 mmol, Zn$^{2+}$ 0.02 mmol, Ca$^{2+}$ 3.75 mmol, Mn$^{2+}$ 0.02 mmol, anhydrous glucose 150 g |
| Net price 2000 mL = £38.50 | | | | | | | | |
| Synthamix 14/2200X (Clintec) | 5.6 | 3696 | 24 | 5.6 | 28 | 56 | 41.2 | acid phosphate 12 mmol, Zn$^{2+}$ 0.016 mmol, Ca$^{2+}$ 3 mmol, Mn$^{2+}$ 0.016 mmol, anhydrous glucose 220 g |
| Net price 2500 mL = £40.00 | | | | | | | | |
| Vamin 9 (Kabi Pharmacia) | 9.4 | | 20 | 1.5 | 50 | | 55 | Ca$^{2+}$ 2.5 mmol |
| Net price 500 mL = £6.60; 1000 mL = £11.90 | | | | | | | | |
| Vamin 9 glucose (Kabi Pharmacia) | 9.4 | 1700 | 20 | 1.5 | 50 | | 55 | Ca$^{2+}$ 2.5 mmol, anhydrous glucose 100 g |
| Net price 100 mL = £3.40; 500 mL = £7.10; 1000 mL = £12.80 | | | | | | | | |
| Vamin 14 (Kabi Pharmacia) | 13.5 | | 50 | 8 | 100 | 135 | 100 | Ca$^{2+}$ 5 mmol, SO$_4^{2-}$ 8 mmol |
| Net price 500 mL = £9.55; 1000 mL = £16.95 | | | | | | | | |
| Vamin 14 (electrolyte-free) (Kabi Pharmacia) | 13.5 | | | | | | | |
| Net price 500 mL = £9.55; 1000 mL = £16.95 | | | | | | | | |
| Vamin 18 (electrolyte-free) (Kabi Pharmacia) | 18.0 | | | | | | | |
| Net price 500 mL = £12.70; 1000 mL = £22.80 | | | | | | | | |
| Vamin Infant (Kabi Pharmacia) | 9.3 | | | | | | | |
| Net price 100 mL = £3.80; 500 mL = £8.70 | | | | | | | | |
| Vitrimix KV (Kabi Pharmacia) | 7.0 | 3340 | 15 | 1.1 | 38 | | 38 | Ca$^{2+}$ 1.9 mmol, anhydrous glucose 75 g |
| Net price (combined pack of Intralipid 20% 250 mL and Vamin 9 glucose 750 mL) = £19.90 | | | | | | | | |

1. Excludes protein-derived energy

*Note.* 1000 kcal = 4.1868 MJ; 1 MJ (1000 kJ) = 238.8 kcal. All entries are PoM

# 9.4   Oral nutrition

**9.4.1** Foods for special diets
**9.4.2** Enteral nutrition

## 9.4.1   Foods for special diets

These are preparations that have been modified to eliminate a particular constituent from a food or are nutrient mixtures formulated as substitutes for the food. They are for patients who either cannot tolerate or cannot metabolise certain common constituents of food. An example is the coeliac patient who cannot tolerate gluten which is present in wheat (and to a lesser extent other cereals). In other cases, for example, in patients with phenylketonuria who cannot metabolise phenylalanine, a small amount, sufficient for tissue building and repair, must be incorporated in the formulation.

---

Prices are **net**, see p. 1

**Preparations**
See Appendix 7

## 9.4.2 Enteral nutrition

The body's reserves of protein rapidly become exhausted in severely ill patients, especially during chronic illness or in those with severe burns, extensive trauma, pancreatitis, or intestinal fistula. Much can be achieved by frequent meals and by persuading the patient to take supplementary snacks of ordinary food between the meals.

However, extra calories, protein, other nutrients, and vitamins are often best given by supplementing ordinary meals with sip or tube feeds of one of the nutritionally complete foods.

When patients cannot feed normally at all, for example patients with severe facial injury, oesophageal obstruction, or coma, a diet composed solely of nutritionally complete foods must be given. This is planned by a dietitian who will take into account the protein and total energy requirement of the patient and decide on the form and relative contribution of carbohydrate and fat to the energy requirements.

There are a number of nutritionally complete foods available and their use reduces an otherwise heavy workload in hospital or in the home. Most contain protein derived from milk or soya. Some contain protein hydrolysates or free amino acids and are only appropriate for patients who have diminished ability to break down protein, as may be the case in inflammatory bowel disease or pancreatic insufficiency.

Even when nutritionally complete feeds are being given it may be important to monitor water and electrolyte balance. Extra minerals (e.g. magnesium and zinc) may be needed in patients where gastro-intestinal secretions are being lost. Additional vitamins may also be needed. Regular haematological and biochemical tests may be needed particularly in the unstable patient.

Some feeds are supplemented with vitamin K; for drug interactions of vitamin K see Appendix 1 (vitamins).

CHILDREN. Infants and young children have special requirements and in most situations liquid feeds prepared for adults are totally unsuitable and should not be given. Expert advice should be sought.

**Preparations**
See Appendix 7

# 9.5 Minerals

**9.5.1** Calcium and magnesium
**9.5.2** Phosphorus
**9.5.3** Fluoride
**9.5.4** Zinc
See section 9.1.1 for iron salts.

## 9.5.1 Calcium and magnesium

**9.5.1.1** Calcium supplements
**9.5.1.2** Hypercalcaemia
**9.5.1.3** Magnesium

### 9.5.1.1 CALCIUM SUPPLEMENTS

Calcium supplements are usually only required where dietary calcium intake is deficient. This dietary requirement varies with age and is relatively greater in childhood, pregnancy, and lactation, due to an increased demand, and in old age, due to impaired absorption. In osteoporosis a daily supplement of 800 mg (20 mmol) calcium may reduce the rate of bone loss, but larger doses have not been shown to be more effective. Patients with hypoparathyroidism rarely require calcium supplements after the early stages of stabilisation on vitamin D (section 9.6.4).

In hypocalcaemic tetany an initial intravenous injection of 10 mL (2.25 mmol) of calcium gluconate injection 10% may be followed by the continuous infusion of about 40 mL (9 mmol) daily, but plasma calcium should be monitored. This regimen can also be used, immediately but temporarily, to reduce the toxic effects of hyperkalaemia.

Calcium may also be used in cardiac resuscitation (see section 2.7).

### CALCIUM SALTS

*Indications:* see notes above; calcium deficiency
*Cautions:* **interactions:** Appendix 1 (calcium salts)
*Side-effects:* bradycardia, arrhythmias, and irritation after intravenous injection
*Dose: by mouth,* daily in divided doses, as calcium gluconate or lactate, see notes above
*By intramuscular or slow intravenous injection,* acute hypocalcaemia, calcium gluconate 1–2 g (2.25–4.5 mmol of $Ca^{2+}$); avoid intramuscular route in children

Oral preparations
**Calcium Gluconate Tablets,** calcium gluconate 600 mg (1.35 mmol $Ca^{2+}$). To be chewed before swallowing. Net price 20 = 44p. Label: 24
**Calcium Gluconate Tablets, Effervescent,** calcium gluconate 1 g (2.25 mmol $Ca^{2+}$). Net price 100 = £5.06. Label: 13
*Note.* Each tablet usually contains sodium 102.6 mg (4.46 mmol $Na^+$)
**Calcium Lactate Tablets,** calcium lactate 300 mg (1 mmol $Ca^{2+}$), net price 20 = 25p

---

**Cacit**® (Norwich Eaton)

*Tablets*, effervescent, pink, calcium carbonate 1.25 g, providing calcium citrate when dispersed in water (500 mg calcium or 12.6 mmol $Ca^{2+}$). Net price 76-tab pack = £19.64. Label: 13

**Calcichew**® (Shire)

*Tablets* (chewable), calcium carbonate 1.26 g (500 mg calcium or 12.6 mmol $Ca^{2+}$). Net price 100 = £11.25. Label: 24

**Calcidrink**® (Shire)

*Granules*, effervescent, calcium carbonate 2.52 g (1 g calcium or 25 mmol $Ca^{2+}$). Net price 30-sachet pack = £8.70. Label: 13

**Calcium-500** (Martindale)

*Tablets*, pink, f/c, calcium carbonate 1.25 g (500 mg calcium or 12.5 mmol $Ca^{2+}$). Net price 100-tab pack = £3.49. Label: 25

**Calcium-Sandoz**® (Sandoz)

*Syrup*, calcium glubionate 1.09 g, calcium lactobionate 723 mg (108.3 mg calcium or 2.7 mmol $Ca^{2+}$)/5 mL. Net price 100 mL = 49p

**Citrical**® (Shire)

*Granules*, calcium carbonate 1.26 g (500 mg or 12.6 mmol $Ca^{2+}$)/sachet. Net price 90-sachet pack = £24.00. Label: 13

**Ossopan**® (Sanofi Winthrop)

*Tablets*, buff, f/c, hydroxyapatite 830 mg (4.4 mmol $Ca^{2+}$). Net price 50 = £10.35

*Granules*, brown, hydroxyapatite 3.32 g (17.8 mmol $Ca^{2+}$). Net price 28-sachet pack = £18.50

**Sandocal**® (Sandoz)

*Sandocal-400 tablets*, effervescent, calcium lactate gluconate 930 mg, calcium carbonate 700 mg, anhydrous citric acid 1.189 g, providing calcium 400 mg (10 mmol $Ca^{2+}$). Net price 5 × 20-tab pack = £7.37. Label: 13

*Sandocal-1000 tablets*, effervescent, calcium lactate gluconate 2.327 g, calcium carbonate 1.75 g, anhydrous citric acid 2.973 g providing 1 g calcium (25 mmol $Ca^{2+}$). Net price 3 × 10-tab pack = £6.63. Label: 13

**Titralac**®: section 9.5.2.2

Parenteral preparations

PoM**Calcium Gluconate Injection,** calcium gluconate 10%. Net price 5-mL amp = 43p; 10-mL amp = 50p

**Calcium Sandoz**® (Sandoz)

PoM*Injection*, calcium glubionate equivalent to 10% of calcium gluconate (93 mg calcium or 2.32 mmol $Ca^{2+}$/10 mL). Net price 10-mL amp = 27p

PoM**Min-I-Jet**® **Calcium Chloride 10%** (IMS)

*Injection*, calcium chloride 100 mg/mL. Net price 10-mL disposable syringe = £3.03

9.5.1.2   HYPERCALCAEMIA

*Severe hypercalcaemia* calls for urgent treatment before detailed investigation of the cause. After rehydration (if necessary with intravenous infusion of **sodium chloride 0.9%**) a **loop diuretic** may be given to increase urinary calcium excretion. Drugs (such as thiazides and vitamin D compounds) which promote hypercalcaemia, should be discontinued and dietary calcium should be restricted.

If *severe hypercalcaemia persists* drugs which inhibit mobilisation of calcium from the skeleton may be required. The **bisphosphonates** are useful and disodium pamidronate (see section 6.6.2) is probably the most effective; it is probably as effective as plicamycin, yet is less toxic and has a much longer effect. **Plicamycin** (see section 8.1.2) is probably the most rapidly effective drug but cannot be given continuously for more than a few days because of marrow toxicity; the duration of its hypocalcaemic effect is unpredictable but can last several days.

**Corticosteroids** (see section 6.3) are widely given, but may only be useful where hypercalcaemia is due to sarcoidosis or vitamin D intoxication; they often take several days to achieve the desired effect.

**Calcitonin** (see section 6.6.1) is relatively non-toxic but is expensive and its effect can wear off after a few days despite continued use; it is rarely effective where bisphosphonates have failed to reduce serum calcium adequately.

Intravenous chelating drugs such as **trisodium edetate** are rarely used; they usually cause pain in the limb receiving the infusion and may cause renal damage.

After treatment of severe hypercalcaemia the underlying cause must be established. *Further treatment* is governed by the same principles as for initial therapy. Salt and water depletion and drugs promoting hypercalcaemia should be avoided; oral administration of a bisphosphonate may be useful. **Sodium cellulose phosphate**, which binds calcium in the gut, is rarely helpful, and any associated increase in serum phosphate may be harmful. Similarly, oral and intravenous phosphate may only achieve a reduction in serum calcium by precipitating calcium phosphate in the tissues, resulting in nephrocalcinosis and impairment of renal function. Parathyroidectomy may be indicated for hyperparathyroidism.

# BISPHOSPHONATES
See section 6.6.2

# CALCITONIN
See section 6.6.1

# CORTICOSTEROIDS
See section 6.3.4

# PLICAMYCIN
See section 8.1.2

# SODIUM CELLULOSE PHOSPHATE

*Indications:* hypercalcaemia (but see notes above), reduction of calcium absorption from food (in conjunction with low-calcium diet)

*Contra-indications:* congestive heart failure, renal impairment

*Side-effects:* occasional diarrhoea
*Dose:* 5 g 3 times daily with meals; CHILD 10 g daily in 3 divided doses with meals

**Calcisorb®** (3M)
*Sachets*, sodium cellulose phosphate 5 g. Net price 90-sachet pack = £19.71. Label: 13, 21, counselling, may be sprinkled on food

## TRISODIUM EDETATE
*Indications:* hypercalcaemia (but see notes above); removal of lime burns in the eye (see under Preparations)
*Cautions:* plasma-calcium determinations required; caution in tuberculosis
*Contra-indications:* impaired renal function
*Side-effects:* nausea, diarrhoea, cramp; in overdosage renal damage
*Dose:* hypercalcaemia, *by slow intravenous infusion*, up to 70 mg/kg daily over 2–3 hours

PoM **Limclair®** (Sinclair)
*Injection*, trisodium edetate 200 mg/mL. Net price 5-mL amp = £8.31
For topical use in the eye, dilute 1 mL to 50 mL with sterile purified water

## 9.5.1.3   MAGNESIUM

Magnesium is an essential constituent of a vast number of enzyme systems, in particular those involved in energy generation. Most of it is found in the skeleton in the calcium apatite crystal lattice.

Magnesium salts are not well absorbed from the gastro-intestinal tract which explains the use of magnesium sulphate (section 1.6.4) as an osmotic laxative.

Magnesium is mainly excreted by the kidneys and is therefore retained in renal failure.

The effects of hypermagnesaemia and of hypomagnesaemia are similar to those of hyperkalaemia and hypokalaemia; hypocalcaemia is usually associated with hypomagnesaemia.

Oral magnesium salts are occasionally required on a long-term basis in patients with malabsorption.

Parenteral magnesium chloride or sulphate is occasionally needed to correct magnesium deficiency in alcoholism or that has arisen from prolonged diarrhoea or vomiting which has been treated with parenteral fluid and nutrition without magnesium supplements; 35–50 mmol of magnesium chloride (or sulphate) may be added to 1 litre of 5% glucose or other isotonic solution and given over a period of 12 to 24 hours. Repeated measurements of plasma magnesium are advisable to determine the rate and duration of the infusion. The dose should be reduced in renal failure. For maintenance (e.g. for intravenous nutrition) parenteral doses of magnesium are of the order of 10–20 mmol daily (often about 12 mmol daily).

## 9.5.2   Phosphorus
9.5.2.1   Phosphate supplements
9.5.2.2   Phosphate-binding agents

### 9.5.2.1   PHOSPHATE SUPPLEMENTS

Oral phosphate supplements may be required in addition to vitamin D in a small minority of patients with hypophosphataemic vitamin D-resistant rickets. Diarrhoea is a common side-effect and should prompt a reduction in dosage.

Phosphate infusion is occasionally needed in alcohol dependence or phosphate deficiency arising from parenteral fluid and nutrition deficient in phosphate supplements; phosphate depletion also occurs in severe diabetic ketoacidosis. A solution containing up to 50 mmol/litre can be infused in sodium chloride or glucose over 12 to 24 hours. Since potassium depletion is also commonly present the phosphate may be given as a mixture of the sodium and potassium salts.

**Phosphate-Sandoz®** (Sandoz)
*Tablets*, effervescent, anhydrous sodium acid phosphate 1.936 g, sodium bicarbonate 350 mg, potassium bicarbonate 315 mg, equivalent to phosphorus 500 mg (16.1 mmol phosphate), sodium 468.8 mg (20.4 mmol Na$^+$), potassium 123 mg (3.1 mmol K$^+$). Net price 20 = 75p. Label: 13

### 9.5.2.2   PHOSPHATE-BINDING AGENTS

Aluminium-containing and calcium-containing antacids are used as phosphate-binding agents in the management of hyperphosphataemia complicating renal failure. Calcium-containing phosphate-binding agents are contra-indicated in hypercalcaemia or hypercalciuria. Phosphate-binding agents which contain aluminium may increase plasma aluminium in dialysis patients.

## ALUMINIUM HYDROXIDE
*Indications:* hyperphosphataemia
*Cautions:* hyperaluminaemia; see also notes above; **interactions:** Appendix 1 (antacids and adsorbents)

**Aluminium Hydroxide** (Non-proprietary)
*Mixture* (gel), about 4% w/w Al$_2$O$_3$ in water. Net price 200 mL = 36p
*Dose:* hyperphosphataemia, 20–100 mL according to requirements of patient; antacid, see section 1.1.1
*Note:* The brand name NHS Aludrox® (Charwell) is used for aluminium hydroxide mixture, net price 200 mL = 69p. For NHS Aludrox® tablets see preparations with magnesium, section 1.1.1

**Alu-Cap®** (3M)
*Capsules*, green/red, dried aluminium hydroxide 475 mg (low Na$^+$). Net price 120-cap pack = £3.84
*Dose:* phosphate-binding agent in renal failure, 4–20 capsules daily in divided doses with meals; antacid, see section 1.1.1

## CALCIUM CARBONATE

*Indications:* hyperphosphataemia
*Cautions:* see notes above; **interactions:** Appendix 1 (calcium salts)
*Side-effects:* hypercalcaemia

**Calcichew**®, section 9.5.1.1
**Calcium-500**, section 9.5.1.1
**Titralac**® (3M)
*Tablets*, calcium carbonate 420 mg, glycine 180 mg. Net price 180-tab pack = £2.23
*Dose:* calcium supplement, or phosphate-binding agent (with meals) in renal failure, according to the requirements of the patient

## 9.5.3   Fluoride

Availability of adequate fluoride confers significant resistance to dental caries. It is now considered that the topical action of fluoride on enamel and plaque is more important than the systemic effect.

Where the natural fluoride content of the drinking water is significantly less than 1 mg per litre (one part per million) artificial fluoridation is the most economical method of supplementing fluoride intake.

Daily administration of tablets or drops is a suitable alternative, but systemic fluoride supplements should not be prescribed without prior reference to the fluoride content of the local water supply; they are not advisable when the water contains more than 700 micrograms per litre (0.7 parts per million). In addition, the British Association for the Study of Community Dentistry now recommends that infants need not receive fluoride supplements until the age of 6 months.

Use of dentifrices which incorporate sodium fluoride and/or monofluorophosphate is also a convenient source of fluoride.

Individuals who are either particularly caries prone or medically compromised may be given additional protection by use of fluoride rinses or by application of fluoride gels. Rinses may be used daily or weekly; daily use of a less concentrated rinse is more effective than weekly use of a more concentrated one. Gels must be applied on a regular basis under professional supervision; extreme caution is necessary to prevent the child from swallowing any excess. Less concentrated gels have recently become available for home use. Varnishes are also available and are particularly valuable for young or handicapped children since they adhere to the teeth and set in the presence of moisture.

There are arrangements for health authorities to supply fluoride tablets in the course of pre-school dental schemes, and they may also be supplied in school dental schemes.

## SODIUM FLUORIDE

*Note.* Sodium fluoride 2.2 mg provides approx. 1 mg fluoride ion
*Indications:* prophylaxis of dental caries—see notes above
*Contra-indications:* not for areas where drinking water is fluoridated
*Side-effects:* occasional white flecks on teeth with recommended doses; rarely yellowish-brown discoloration if recommended doses are exceeded
*Dose:* CHILD, as fluoride ion:
Water content less than 300 micrograms/litre, up to 6 months, none; 6 months–2 years, 250 micrograms daily; 2–4 years, 500 micrograms daily; over 4 years, 1 mg daily
Water content between 300 and 700 micrograms/litre, up to 2 years, none; 2–4 years, 250 micrograms daily; over 4 years, 500 micrograms daily

### Tablets

COUNSELLING. Tablets should be sucked or dissolved in the mouth and taken preferably in the evening

**En-De-Kay**® (Stafford-Miller)
*Fluotabs 2–4 years*, natural orange-flavoured, scored, sodium fluoride 1.1 mg (500 micrograms F⁻). Net price 200-tab pack = £1.73
*Fluotabs 4+ years*, natural orange-flavoured, scored, sodium fluoride 2.2 mg (1 mg F⁻). Net price 200-tab pack = £1.73
**Fluor-a-day**® (Dental Health)
*Tablets*, buff, scored, sodium fluoride 2.2 mg (1 mg F⁻). Net price 200-tab pack = £1.40
**Fluorigard**® (RMT)
*Tablets 0.5*, purple, scored, sodium fluoride 1.1 mg (500 micrograms F⁻). Net price 120-tab pack = £1.18
*Tablets 1.0*, sodium fluoride 2.2 mg (1 mg F⁻). Net price 120-tab pack = £1.18 (available in 4 colours and flavours)
**Oral-B Fluoride**® (Oral-B Labs)
*Tablets*, sodium fluoride 1.1 mg (500 micrograms F⁻), net price 200-tab pack = £1.80; 2.2 mg (1 mg F⁻) (pink), 12-tab pack = £1.80
**Zymafluor**® (Zyma)
*Tablets*, sodium fluoride 550 micrograms (250 micrograms F⁻), net price 400-tab pack = 75p; 2.2 mg (1 mg F⁻) (yellow-grey), 100-tab pack = 55p

### Oral drops

*Note.* Fluoride supplements no longer considered necessary below 6 months of age (see notes above)
**En-De-Kay**® (Stafford-Miller)
*Fluodrops*® (= paediatric drops), sugar-free, sodium fluoride 500 micrograms (250 micrograms F⁻)/0.15 mL. Net price 60 mL = £1.31
**Fluorigard**® (RMT)
*Paediatric drops*, sodium fluoride 275 micrograms (125 micrograms F⁻)/drop. Net price 30 mL = £1.27
**Oral-B Fluoride**® (Oral-B Labs)
*Drops*, sodium fluoride 0.15% (250 micrograms F⁻/8 drops). Net price 48.7 mL = £1.43

Mouthwashes

Rinse mouth for 1 minute and spit out

COUNSELLING. Avoid eating, drinking, or rinsing mouth for 15 minutes after use

PoM **En-De-Kay**® (Stafford-Miller)

*Fluorinse* (= mouthwash), red, sodium fluoride 2%. Net price 100 mL = £2.50. Counselling, see above

CHILD 8 years and over, for *daily* use, dilute 5 drops to 10 mL of water; for *weekly* use, dilute 20 drops to 10 mL

**Fluorigard**® (RMT)

*Daily dental rinse* (= mouthwash), blue, sodium fluoride 0.05%. Net price 500 mL = £2.52. Counselling, see above

CHILD 6 years and over, for *daily* use, rinse with 5–10 mL

*Weekly dental rinse* (= mouthwash), blue, sodium fluoride 0.2%. Net price 150 mL = £1.68. Counselling, see above

CHILD 6 years and over, for *weekly* use, rinse with 5–10 mL

## 9.5.4 Zinc

Oral zinc therapy should only be given when there is good evidence of deficiency (hypoproteinaemia spuriously lowers plasma-zinc concentrations). Zinc deficiency can occur in individuals on inadequate diets, in malabsorption, with increased body loss due to trauma, burns and protein-losing conditions, and during intravenous feeding. Therapy should continue until clinical improvement occurs and be replaced by dietary measures unless there is severe malabsorption, metabolic disease, or continuing zinc loss. Side-effects of zinc salts are abdominal pain and dyspepsia.

## ZINC SALTS

*Indications; Cautions; Side-effects:* see notes above; **interactions**: Appendix 1 (zinc)

**Solvazinc**® (Thames)

*Effervescent tablets*, yellow-white, zinc sulphate 200 mg (45 mg zinc). Net price 30 = £3.60. Label: 13, 21

*Dose:* 1 tablet in water 1–3 times daily after food

**Zincomed**® (Medo)

*Capsules*, blue/white, zinc sulphate 220 mg. Net price 30-cap pack = 99p. Label: 21

*Dose:* 1 capsule 3 times daily after food

**Z Span**® (SK&F)

*Spansule*® (= capsules m/r), blue/clear, enclosing white and grey pellets, zinc sulphate monohydrate 61.8 mg (22.5 mg zinc). Net price 30-cap pack = £1.38. Label: 25

*Dose:* adults and children over 1 year, 1–3 capsules daily as required; can be opened and pellets sprinkled on cool food; not to be chewed

# 9.6 Vitamins

Vitamins are used for the prevention and treatment of specific deficiency states or where the diet is known to be inadequate; they may be prescribed in the NHS to prevent or treat deficiency but not as dietary supplements.

Their use as general 'pick-me-ups' is of unproven value and, in the case of preparations containing vitamin A or D, may actually be harmful if patients take more than the prescribed dose. The 'fad' for mega-vitamin therapy with water-soluble vitamins, such as ascorbic acid and pyridoxine, is unscientific and can be harmful.

## 9.6.1 Vitamin A

Deficiency of vitamin A (retinol) is rare in Britain even in disorders of fat absorption.

Massive overdose can cause rough skin, dry hair, an enlarged liver, and a raised erythrocyte sedimentation rate and raised serum calcium and serum alkaline phosphatase concentrations. Use of excessive doses should be **avoided** in pregnancy (see below).

The Department of Health has advised that:

1. The recommended daily amount of vitamin A in the UK is 2250 units daily for adults, including pregnant women, increased to 4000 units daily for nursing mothers;
2. Several national and international organisations have proposed a maximum intake of vitamin A during pregnancy of 8000 to 10000 units daily;
3. Reports in the USA suggest that birth defects may follow an intake of vitamin A of 24000 to 30000 units daily.

In view of evidence suggesting that high levels of vitamin A may cause birth defects, women who are (or may become) pregnant are advised not to take vitamin A supplements (including tablets and fish-liver oil drops), except on the advice of a doctor or an antenatal clinic; nor should they eat liver or products such as liver paté or liver sausage.

## VITAMIN A

(Retinol)

*Indications; Cautions; Side-effects:* see notes above

*Dose:* see notes above and under preparations

PoM **Ro-A-Vit**® (Roche)

*Injection*, vitamin A (retinol) 50000 units (as palmitate)/mL. Net price 2-mL amp = 88p

*Dose: by deep intramuscular injection*, deficiency, 100000 units monthly, increased to weekly in acute deficiency states; courses no longer than 6 weeks with 2-week interval; Liver disease, 100000 units every 2–4 months; INFANT under 1 year and CHILD 50000 units monthly

*Note.* Contains polyethoxylated castor oil which has been associated with anaphylaxis; do **not** mix or dilute

**Cautions:** children, liver disease (specialist use); considerably enhanced bioavailability compared with previous formulation (dosage adjustment may be needed)

Vitamins A and D
**Halibut-liver Oil Capsules,** vitamin A 4000 units
[also contains vitamin D]. Net price 20 = 13p
NHS **Halycitrol**® (LAB)
*Emulsion*, vitamin A 4600 units, vitamin D 380
units/5 mL. Net price 114 mL = £1.20
*Dose:* 5 mL daily but see notes above

Vitamins A, D, and C for children
**Children's Vitamin Drops** (Hough)
*Oral drops*, ascorbic acid (as sodium ascorbate)
20 mg, vitamin A 700 units, vitamin D 300 units/
5 drops.
Recommended by Department of Health for routine
supplementation in young children. Available direct to
public under the Welfare Food Scheme from maternity
and child health clinics and welfare food distribution
centres; not available on prescription
*Dose:* CHILD 1 month–5 years, 5 drops daily
*Note.* The Department of Health recommends these
drops for children aged 6 months to 2 years (preferably
5 years particularly in winter and early spring); some
infants from 1 month of age may also benefit (for details
see *Present Day Practice in Infant Feeding* 3rd Report)
**Adexolin**® (Seven Seas)
*Oral drops*, ascorbic acid 15 mg, vitamin A 750
units, vitamin D 200 units/0.14 mL. Net price
25-mL pack with pipette = £1.02, 50-mL pack
with pipette = £1.80
*Dose:* INFANT and CHILD under 5 years, 0.28 mL
(upper level on graduated pipette) daily; INFANT
fed on vitamin D-fortified milk, CHILD over 5
years and ADULT, 0.14 mL (lower level on gradu-
ated pipette) daily

## 9.6.2  Vitamin B group

Deficiency of the B vitamins, other than deficiency
of vitamin $B_{12}$ (section 9.1.2) is rare in Britain
and is usually treated by preparations containing
thiamine ($B_1$), riboflavine ($B_2$), and nicotinamide,
which is used in preference to nicotinic acid, as it
does not cause vasodilatation. Other members (or
substances traditionally classified as members) of
the vitamin B complex such as aminobenzoic acid,
biotin, choline, inositol, and pantothenic acid or
panthenol may be included in vitamin B preparations but there is no evidence of their value.

The severe deficiency states Wernicke's
encephalopathy and Korsakoff's psychosis,
especially as seen in chronic alcoholism, are best
treated by the parenteral administration of B vitamins (Parentrovite®); anaphylaxis has been
reported with these preparations (see CSM
advice, below).

As with other vitamins of the B group, pyridoxine ($B_6$) deficiency is rare, but it may occur
during isoniazid therapy and is characterised by
peripheral neuritis. High doses of pyridoxine are
given in some metabolic disorders, such as hyp-
eroxaluria, and it is also used in sideroblastic
anaemia (section 9.1.3). Pyridoxine has been tried
in a wide variety of other disorders, including the
premenstrual syndrome, but there is little sound
evidence to support the claims, and overdosage
induces toxic effects.

## THIAMINE
(Vitamin $B_1$)
*Indications:* see notes above
*Cautions:* anaphylactic shock may occasionally
follow injection (see CSM advice below)
*Dose:* mild chronic deficiency, 10–25 mg daily;
severe deficiency, 200–300 mg daily

**Thiamine Hydrochloride Tablets,** thiamine
hydrochloride 25 mg, net price 20 = 15p; 50 mg,
20 = 24p; 100 mg, 20 = 42p; 300 mg, 20 = 68p
NHS **Benerva**® (Roche)
*Tablets*, thiamine hydrochloride 25 mg, net price
20 = 15p; 50 mg, 20 = 24p; 100 mg, 20 = 42p;
300 mg, 20 = 68p

Vitamins B and C injection

---

**CSM advice**
Since potentially serious allergic adverse reactions
may occur during, or shortly after, administration,
the CSM has recommended that:
1. Use be restricted to patients in whom parenteral
treatment is essential;
2. Intravenous injections should be administered
slowly (over 10 minutes);
3. Facilities for treating anaphylaxis should be available when administered.

---

PoM **Parentrovite**® (Bencard)
Parenteral vitamins B and C for confirmed or
imminent acute Wernicke's encephalopathy and
Korsakoff's psychosis when oral intake is impossible or inadequate
*Dose:* by intravenous injection (see CSM advice
above) or infusion, 2–4 pairs of *IVHP* ampoules
every 4–8 hours for up to 2 days, followed by 1
pair of *IMHP* ampoules by intramuscular injection *or* 1 pair of *IVHP* ampoules by intravenous
injection or infusion daily for 5–7 days
*IMHP Injection*, for intramuscular use only,
ascorbic acid 500 mg, nicotinamide 160 mg,
pyridoxine hydrochloride 50 mg, riboflavine 4
mg, thiamine hydrochloride 250 mg/7 mL. Net
price 7 mL (in 2 amps) = 43p
*IVHP Injection*, for intravenous use only, ascorbic acid 500 mg, anhydrous glucose 900 mg,
nicotinamide 160 mg, pyridoxine hydrochloride
50 mg, riboflavine 4 mg, thiamine hydrochloride
250 mg/10 mL. Net price 10 mL (in 2 amps) =
43p

Oral vitamin B complex preparations, see below

## RIBOFLAVINE
(Vitamin $B_2$)
*Indications:* see notes above

### Preparations
Injections of vitamins B and C, see under Thiamine

Oral vitamin B complex preparations, see below

---

# PYRIDOXINE HYDROCHLORIDE

(Vitamin B$_6$)

*Indications:* see under Dose

*Cautions:* interactions: Appendix 1 (vitamins)

*Dose:* deficiency states, 20–50 mg up to 3 times daily

Isoniazid neuropathy, prophylaxis 10 mg daily; therapeutic, 50 mg three times daily

Idiopathic sideroblastic anaemia, 100–400 mg daily in divided doses

Premenstrual syndrome, 50–100 mg daily (but see notes above)

**Pyridoxine Tablets,** pyridoxine hydrochloride 10 mg, net price 20 = 32p; 20 mg, 20 = 33p; 50 mg, 20 = 57p

NHS **Benadon**® (Roche)

*Tablets,* pyridoxine hydrochloride 20 mg. Net price 20 = 33p

*Tablets,* scored, pyridoxine hydrochloride 50 mg. Net price 20 = 66p

NHS **Complement Continus**® (Napp)

*Tablets,* m/r, yellow, pyridoxine hydrochloride 100 mg. Net price 28-tab pack = £1.68. Label: 25

Injections of vitamins B and C, see under Thiamine

## NICOTINAMIDE

*Indications:* see notes above

**Nicotinamide Tablets,** nicotinamide 50 mg. Net price 20 = 13p

Injections of vitamins B and C, see under Thiamine

Oral vitamin B complex preparations, see below

## NICOTINIC ACID

See section 2.12

## FOLIC ACID

See section 9.1.2

## FOLINIC ACID

See section 8.1.3

## VITAMIN B$_{12}$

See section 9.1.2

## ORAL VITAMIN B COMPLEX PREPARATIONS

*Note.* Other multivitamin preparations are in section 9.6.7.

**Vitamin B Tablets, Compound,** nicotinamide 15 mg, riboflavine 1 mg, thiamine hydrochloride 1 mg. Net price 20 = 7p

*Dose:* prophylactic, 1–2 tablets daily

**Vitamin B Tablets, Compound, Strong,** brown, f/c or s/c, nicotinamide 20 mg, pyridoxine hydrochloride 2 mg, riboflavine 2 mg, thiamine hydrochloride 5 mg. Net price 20 = 9p

*Dose:* treatment of vitamin-B deficiency, 1–2 tablets 3 times daily

NHS **Becosym**® (Roche)

*Tablets,* brown, f/c, vitamin B tablets, compound, strong. Net price 20 = 15p

*Forte tablets,* brown, f/c, thiamine hydrochloride 15 mg, riboflavine 15 mg, nicotinamide 50 mg, pyridoxine hydrochloride 10 mg. Net price 25-tab pack = £1.14

*Syrup,* orange, thiamine hydrochloride 5 mg, riboflavine 2 mg, nicotinamide 20 mg, pyridoxine hydrochloride 2 mg/5 mL. Net price 100 mL = £1.10

NHS **Benerva Compound**® (Roche)

*Tablets,* yellow, vitamin B tablets, compound. Net price 20 = 11p

NHS **Vigranon B**® (Wallace Mfg)

*Syrup,* thiamine hydrochloride 5 mg, riboflavine 2 mg, nicotinamide 20 mg, pyridoxine hydrochloride 2 mg, panthenol 3 mg/5 mL. Net price 150 mL = £1.18

## OTHER COMPOUNDS

**Potassium aminobenzoate** has been used in the treatment of various disorders associated with excessive fibrosis such as scleroderma but its therapeutic value is **doubtful**.

**Potaba**® (Glenwood)

*Capsules,* red/white, potassium aminobenzoate 500 mg. Net price 20 = 92p. Label: 21

*Tablets,* potassium aminobenzoate 500 mg. Net price 20 = 72p. Label: 21

*Dose:* Peyronie's disease, scleroderma, 12 g daily in divided doses after food

*Envules*® ( = powder in sachets), potassium aminobenzoate 3 g. Net price 40 sachets = £11.05. Label: 13, 21

## 9.6.3 Vitamin C

(Ascorbic acid)

Vitamin C therapy is essential in scurvy, but less florid manifestations of vitamin C deficiency are commonly found, especially in the elderly. It is rarely necessary to prescribe more than 100 mg daily except early in the treatment of scurvy.

Claims that vitamin C ameliorates colds or promotes wound healing have not been proved.

## ASCORBIC ACID

*Indications:* prevention and treatment of scurvy

*Dose:* prophylactic, 25–75 mg daily; therapeutic, not less than 250 mg daily in divided doses

**Ascorbic Acid Tablets,** ascorbic acid 25 mg, net price 20 = 9p; 50 mg, 20 = 7p; 100 mg, 20 = 24p; 200 mg, 20 = 28p; 500 mg (label: 24), 20 = 68p

PoM **Ascorbic Acid Injection,** ascorbic acid 100 mg/mL. Net price 5-mL amp = 65p

NHS **Redoxon**® (Roche)

*Tablets,* ascorbic acid 25 mg, net price 20 = 9p; 50 mg, 20 = 7p; 200 mg, 20 = 28p; 500 mg (label: 24), 50 = £1.69

*Tablets,* effervescent, ascorbic acid 1 g. Net price 10-tab pack = 81p. Label: 13

For children's welfare vitamin drops containing vitamin C with A and D, see vitamin A

## 9.6.4   Vitamin D

*Note.* The term Vitamin D is used for a range of compounds which possess the property of preventing or curing rickets. They include ergocalciferol (calciferol, vitamin $D_2$), cholecalciferol (vitamin $D_3$), dihydrotachysterol, alfacalcidol (1α-hydroxycholecalciferol), and calcitriol (1,25-dihydroxycholecalciferol).

Simple vitamin D *deficiency*, which is not uncommon in Asians consuming unleavened bread and in the elderly living alone, can be prevented by taking an oral supplement of only 10 micrograms (400 units) of **ergocalciferol** (calciferol, vitamin $D_2$) daily. Since there is no plain tablet of this strength available **calcium and ergocalciferol tablets** can be given (although the calcium is unnecessary).

Vitamin D deficiency caused by *intestinal malabsorption* or *chronic liver disease* usually requires vitamin D in pharmacological doses, such as **calciferol tablets** up to 1 mg (40 000 units) daily; the hypocalcaemia of *hypoparathyroidism* often requires doses of up to 2.5 mg (100 000 units) daily in order to achieve normocalcaemia. The newer vitamin D derivatives, **alfacalcidol** and **calcitriol**, have a shorter duration of action, and therefore have the advantage that problems associated with hypercalcaemia due to excessive dosage are shorter lasting and easier to treat.

Vitamin D requires hydroxylation by the kidney to its active form therefore the hydroxylated derivatives **alfacalcidol** or **calcitriol** should be prescribed if patients with *severe renal impairment* require vitamin D therapy.

**Important.** All patients receiving pharmacological doses of vitamin D should have the plasma calcium concentration checked at intervals (initially weekly) and whenever nausea or vomiting are present. Breast milk from women taking pharmacological doses of vitamin D may cause hypercalcaemia if given to an infant.

## ERGOCALCIFEROL
(Calciferol, Vitamin $D_2$)

*Indications:* see notes above

*Cautions:* take care to ensure correct dose in infants; monitor plasma calcium in patients receiving high doses

*Contra-indications:* hypercalcaemia

*Side-effects:* symptoms of overdosage include anorexia, lassitude, nausea and vomiting, diarrhoea, weight loss, polyuria, sweating, headache, thirst, vertigo, and raised concentrations of calcium and phosphate in plasma and urine

*Dose:* see notes above

### Daily supplements

*Note.* There is no plain vitamin D tablet available for treating simple deficiency (see notes above). Alternatives include vitamins capsules (see 9.6.7), preparations of vitamins A and D (see 9.6.1), and calcium and ergocalciferol tablets (see below).

**Calcium and Ergocalciferol Tablets[1]**
(Calcium and Vitamin D Tablets)

*Tablets,* calcium lactate 300 mg, calcium phosphate 150 mg (97 mg calcium or 2.4 mmol $Ca^{2+}$), ergocalciferol 10 micrograms (400 units). Net price 20 = 22p. Counselling, crush before administration or may be chewed

1. Calcium with Vitamin D Tablets (BPC) which contained ergocalciferol 12.5 micrograms (500 units) are being replaced by Calcium and Ergocalciferol Tablets

Pharmacological strengths (see notes above)
**Calciferol Tablets, BP**

*Tablets,* cholecalciferol or ergocalciferol 250 micrograms (10 000 units), net price 20 = 45p; 1.25 mg (50 000 units), 20 = 59p

*Note.* The BP directs that when high-strength calciferol tablets are prescribed or demanded, tablets containing 250 micrograms shall be dispensed or supplied, and when strong calciferol tablets are prescribed or demanded it should be **confirmed** that tablets containing 1.25 mg are intended. To avoid **errors** arising from the use of these titles prescribers should **abandon** them and **specify strength required**

PoM **Calciferol Injection,** cholecalciferol or ergocalciferol, 7.5 mg (300 000 units)/mL in oil. Net price 1-mL amp = £2.96; 2-mL amp = £3.54

## ALFACALCIDOL
(1α-Hydroxycholecalciferol)

*Indications:* see notes above

*Cautions; Contra-indications; Side-effects:* see under Ergocalciferol

*Dose:* see under preparations

PoM **One-alpha**® (Leo)

*Capsules,* alfacalcidol 250 nanograms, net price 20 = £2.42; 1 microgram (brown), 20 = £7.20

*Solution,* sugar-free, alfacalcidol 200 nanograms/mL. Net price 60 mL = £15.58 (with oral syringe)

*Dose:* ADULTS and CHILDREN over 20 kg, initially 1 microgram daily (elderly 500 nanograms), adjusted to avoid hypercalcaemia; maintenance 0.25–1 microgram daily; CHILD under 20 kg, initially 50 nanograms/kg daily; NEONATES and premature infants 50–100 nanograms/kg daily. *Note.* This solution replaces the drops which were more concentrated and required dilution

## CALCITRIOL
(1,25-Dihydroxycholecalciferol)

*Indications:* see notes above

*Cautions; Contra-indications; Side-effects:* see under Ergocalciferol

*Dose:* see under preparation

PoM **Rocaltrol**® (Roche)
*Capsules*, calcitriol 250 nanograms (red/white),
net price 20 = £3.92; 500 nanograms (red),
20 = £7.01
*Dose:* initially 1–2 micrograms daily, gradually
increased to 2–3 micrograms daily

## CHOLECALCIFEROL
(Vitamin D₃)
*Indications; Cautions; Contra-indications; Side-
effects:* see under Ergocalciferol—alternative to
ergocalciferol in calciferol tablets and injection

## DIHYDROTACHYSTEROL
*Cautions; Contra-indications; Side-effects:* see
under Ergocalciferol

**AT 10**® (Sanofi Winthrop)
*Oral solution*, dihydrotachysterol 250 micro-
grams/mL. Net price 15-mL dropper bottle =
£19.84
*Dose:* acute, chronic, and latent forms of hypocalcaemic
tetany due to hypoparathyroidism, consult data sheet
**Tachyrol**® (Duphar)
Product discontinued

## 9.6.5   Vitamin E
(Tocopherols)

The daily requirement of vitamin E has not been
well defined but is probably about 3 to 15 mg daily.
There is little evidence that oral supplements of
vitamin E are essential in adults, even where there
is fat malabsorption secondary to cholestasis. In
young children with congenital cholestasis,
abnormally low vitamin E concentrations may be
found in association with neuromuscular abnormalities, which usually respond only to the parenteral administration of vitamin E.

Vitamin E has been tried for various other
conditions but there is no scientific evidence of
its value. High doses have been associated with
adverse effects.

## ALPHA TOCOPHERYL ACETATE
*Indications:* see notes above

**Ephynal**® (Roche)
*Suspension*, alpha tocopheryl acetate 500 mg/
5 mL. Net price 100 mL = £3.64
*Dose:* cystic fibrosis, 100–200 mg daily; CHILD
under 1 year 50 mg daily; 1 year and over
100 mg daily
Abetalipoproteinaemia, ADULT and CHILD 50–
100 mg/kg daily
**Vita-E**® (Bioglan)
*Gels* (= capsules), *d*-α-tocopheryl acetate 75 units
(yellow), net price 20 = 58p; 200 units (yellow), 20 =
£1.37; 400 units (red), 20 = £2.19
*Gelucaps*® (= tablets), chewable, yellow, *d*-α-toco-
pheryl acetate 75 units. Net price 20 = 68p. Label: 24
*Succinate tablets*, yellow, *d*-α-tocopheryl succinate 50
units, net price 20 = 48p; 200 units, 20 = £1.44

## 9.6.6   Vitamin K

Vitamin K is necessary for the production of blood
clotting factors and proteins necessary for the
normal calcification of bone.

Because vitamin K is fat soluble, patients with
*fat malabsorption*, especially if due to biliary
obstruction or hepatic disease, may become deficient. For oral administration to prevent vitamin-
K deficiency in malabsorption syndromes, a
water-soluble preparation, **menadiol sodium phosphate** must be used; the usual dose is about 10 mg
daily.

In *neonates* deficiency of vitamin K may occur
because the gut is sterile and there is no synthesis
of the vitamin by *Escherichia coli*. It may be
treated with **phytomenadione** (vitamin K₁), 1 mg
by intramuscular injection.

Oral coumarin *anticoagulants* act by interfering
with vitamin K metabolism in the hepatic cells
and their effects can be antagonised by giving
vitamin K; for British Society for Haematology
Guidelines, see section 2.8.2.

## MENADIOL SODIUM PHOSPHATE
*Indications: Dose:* see notes above
*Cautions:* pregnancy; **interactions:** Appendix 1
(vitamins)

**Synkavit**® (Roche)
*Tablets*, scored, menadiol sodium phosphate
equivalent to 10 mg of menadiol phosphate.
Net price 20 = 41p

## PHYTOMENADIONE
(Vitamin K₁)
*Indications; Dose:* see notes above
*Cautions:* intravenous injections (see section
2.8.2) should be given very slowly; **interactions:**
Appendix 1 (vitamins)

**Konakion**® (Roche)
*Tablets*, s/c, phytomenadione 10 mg. Net price
25 = £4.20. Label: 24
PoM *Injection*, phytomenadione 2 mg/mL, net
price 0.5-mL amp = 22p; 10 mg/mL, 1-mL
amp = 41p
*Note.* Contains polyethoxylated castor oil which has
been associated with anaphylaxis

## 9.6.7   Multivitamin preparations

There are many preparations available. The proprietary
preparations have no advantage over the non-proprietary
preparations given separately and many are expensive.

**Children's Vitamin Drops** available under the Welfare
Food Scheme, see section 9.6.1
**Vitamins Capsules**, ascorbic acid 15 mg, nicotinamide
7.5 mg, riboflavine 500 micrograms, thiamine hydro-
chloride 1 mg, vitamin A 2500 units, vitamin D 300 units.
Net price 20 = 18p
**Abidec**® (W-L)
NHS *Capsules*, vitamins A, B group, C, and D. Net price
20 = 30p
*Drops*, vitamins A, B group, C, and D. Net price
2 × 25 mL (with dropper) = £2.32

NHS **Allbee with C**<sup>⊗</sup> (Robins)

*Capsules*, yellow/green, vitamins B group and C. Net price 20 = £1.30

NHS **BC 500**® (Whitehall)

*Tablets*, orange, f/c, vitamins B group and C. Net price 30 = £1.45

NHS **Calcimax**® (Wallace Mfg)

*Syrup*, brown, vitamins B group, C, and D. Net price 150 mL = £1.41

NHS **Concavit**® (Wallace Mfg)

*Capsules*, vitamins A, B group, C, D, and E. Net price 20 = 93p

*Drops* and *syrup*, vitamins A, B group, C, and D. Net price drops 15 mL = £1.36; syrup 150 mL = £1.58

**Dalivit**® (Paines & Byrne)

NHS *Capsules*, red, vitamins A, B group, C, and D. Net price 20 = 31p

*Oral drops*, vitamins A, B group, C, and D. Net price 2 × 15 mL = £1.26

NHS **Orovite**® (SmithKline Beecham Brands)

*Tablets*, maroon, s/c, vitamins B group and C. Net price 25-tab pack = £1.52

*Syrup*, vitamins B group and C. Net price 200 mL = £1.69

NHS **Orovite 7**® (SmithKline Beecham Brands)

*Granules*, orange, vitamins A, B group, C, and D. Net price 10-sachet pack = £1.06, 30-sachet pack = £3.03. Label: 13

NHS **Surbex T**® (Abbott)

*Tablets*, orange, vitamins B group and C. Net price 20 = 58p

---

## VITAMIN AND MINERAL SUPPLEMENTS AND ADJUNCTS TO SYNTHETIC DIETS

**Forceval**® (Unigreg)

*Capsules*, brown/red, vitamins (ascorbic acid 60 mg, biotin 100 micrograms, cyanocobalamin 3 micrograms, folic acid 300 micrograms, nicotinamide 18 mg, pantothenic acid 4 mg, pyridoxine 2 mg, riboflavine 1.6 mg, thiamine 1.2 mg, vitamin A 2500 units, vitamin $D_2$ 400 units, vitamin E 10 mg, vitamin $K_1$ 70 micrograms), minerals and trace elements (calcium 100 mg, chromium 200 micrograms, copper 2 mg, iodine 140 micrograms, iron 12 mg, magnesium 30 mg, manganese 3 mg, molybdenum 250 micrograms, phosphorus 77 mg, potassium 4 mg, selenium 50 micrograms, zinc 15 mg). Net price 15-cap pack = £2.57; 45-cap pack = £7.00

*Dose:* vitamin and mineral deficiency and as adjunct to synthetic diets, 1 capsule daily

*Junior capsules*, brown, vitamins (ascorbic acid 25 mg, biotin 50 micrograms, cyanocobalamin 2 micrograms, folic acid 100 micrograms, nicotinamide 7.5 mg, pantothenic acid 2 mg, pyridoxine 1 mg, riboflavine 1 mg, thiamine 1.5 mg, vitamin A 1250 units, vitamin $D_2$ 200 units, vitamin E 5 mg, vitamin $K_1$ 25 micrograms), minerals and trace elements (chromium 50 micrograms, copper 1 mg, iodine 75 micrograms, iron 5 mg, magnesium 1 mg, manganese 1.25 mg, molybdenum 50 micrograms, selenium 25 micrograms, zinc 5 mg). Net price 60-cap pack = £7.00

*Dose:* vitamin and mineral deficiency and as adjunct in synthetic diets, CHILD over 5 years, 2 capsules daily

**Ketovite**® (Paines & Byrne)

PoM *Tablets*, yellow, ascorbic acid 16.6 mg, riboflavine 1 mg, thiamine hydrochloride 1 mg, pyridoxine hydrochloride 330 micrograms, nicotinamide 3.3 mg, calcium pantothenate 1.16 mg, alpha tocopheryl acetate 5 mg, inositol 50 mg, biotin 170 micrograms, folic acid 250 micrograms, acetomenaphthone 500 micrograms. Net price 100-tab pack = £4.17

*Dose:* prevention of deficiency in disorders of carbohydrate or amino acid metabolism, 1 tablet 3 times

daily; with Ketovite® Liquid as vitamin supplement with synthetic diets

*Liquid*, pink, sugar-free, vitamin A 2500 units, ergocalciferol 400 units, choline chloride 150 mg, cyanocobalamin 12.5 micrograms/5 mL. Net price 150-mL pack = £2.70

*Dose:* prevention of deficiency in disorders of carbohydrate or amino acid metabolism, 5 mL daily; with Ketovite® Tablets as vitamin supplement with synthetic diets

**Supplementary Vitamin Tablets for Infants** (Cow & Gate)

*Tablets*, ferrous sulphate 4.21 mg (850 micrograms iron), folic acid 63 micrograms, thiamine hydrochloride 250 micrograms, nicotinamide 830 micrograms, riboflavine 250 micrograms, pyridoxine hydrochloride 83 micrograms, cyanocobalamin 1 microgram, ascorbic acid 10 mg, d-α-tocopheryl acetate 1.24 mg, acetomenaphthone 125 micrograms, biotin 8 micrograms, calcium pantothenate 500 micrograms, copper 34 micrograms (as sulphate), iodine 12 micrograms (as potassium iodate), manganese 5 micrograms (as sulphate), molybdenum 6 micrograms (as ammonium molybdate), zinc 620 micrograms (as sulphate). Contains sucrose. Net price 100 = £3.88

*Note.* For infants on nutritionally incomplete synthetic foods

*Dose:* consult manufacturer's literature

# 9.7    Bitters and tonics

Mixtures containing simple and aromatic bitters, such as alkaline gentian mixture, are traditional remedies for loss of appetite. All depend on suggestion.

**Gentian Mixture, Acid, BP**

*Mixture*, concentrated compound gentian infusion 10%, dilute hydrochloric acid 5% in a suitable vehicle. Extemporaneous preparations should be recently prepared according to the following formula: concentrated compound gentian infusion 1 mL, dilute hydrochloric acid 0.5 mL, double-strength chloroform water 5 mL, water to 10 mL

**Gentian Mixture, Alkaline, BP**

(Alkaline Gentian Oral Solution)

*Mixture*, concentrated compound gentian infusion 10%, sodium bicarbonate 5% in a suitable vehicle. Extemporaneous preparations should be recently prepared according to the following formula: concentrated compound gentian infusion 1 mL, sodium bicarbonate 500 mg, double-strength chloroform water 5 mL, water to 10 mL

NHS **Effico**® (Pharmax)

*Tonic*, green, thiamine hydrochloride 180 micrograms, nicotinamide 2.1 mg, caffeine 20.2 mg, compound gentian infusion 0.31 mL/5 mL. Net price 300-mL pack = £1.47, 500-ml pack = £2.12

NHS **Labiton**® (LAB)

*Tonic*, brown, thiamine hydrochloride 375 micrograms, caffeine 3.5 mg, kola nut dried extract 3.025 mg, alcohol 1.4 mL/5 mL. Net price 200 mL = £1.63

NHS **Metatone**® (W-L)

*Tonic*, thiamine hydrochloride 500 micrograms, calcium glycerophosphate 45.6 mg, manganese glycerophosphate 5.7 mg, potassium glycerophosphate 45.6 mg, sodium glycerophosphate 22.8 mg/5 mL. Net price 300 mL = £1.43

---

# 9.8  Metabolic disorders

9.8.1  Wilson's disease
9.8.2  Acute porphyrias
This section covers drugs used in metabolic disorders and not readily classified elsewhere.

## 9.8.1  Wilson's disease

**Penicillamine** (see also section 10.1.3) is used in Wilson's disease (hepatolenticular degeneration) to aid the elimination of copper ions. For use in copper and lead poisoning, see p. 21.

**Trientine** is used for the treatment of Wilson's disease only, in patients intolerant of penicillamine; it is **not** an alternative to penicillamine for rheumatoid arthritis or cystinuria.

### PENICILLAMINE

*Indications:* see under Dose below
*Cautions; Contra-indications; Side-effects:* see section 10.1.3
*Dose:* Wilson's disease, 1.5–2 g daily in divided doses before food; max. 2 g daily for 1 year; maintenance 0.75–1 g daily; ELDERLY, 20 mg/kg daily in divided doses; CHILD, up to 20 mg/kg daily in divided doses, min. 500 mg daily
Chronic active hepatitis (after disease is controlled), 500 mg daily in divided doses slowly increased over 3 months; usual maintenance dose 1.25 g daily
Cystinuria, therapeutic, 1–3 g daily in divided doses before food, adjusted to maintain urinary cystine below 200 mg/litre. Prophylactic (maintain urinary cystine below 300 mg/litre) 0.5–1 g at bedtime; maintain adequate fluid intake (at least 3 litres daily); CHILD minimum dose to maintain urinary cystine below 200 mg/litre

**Preparations**
See section 10.1.3

### TRIENTINE DIHYDROCHLORIDE

*Indications:* Wilson's disease in patients intolerant of penicillamine
*Cautions:* see notes above; pregnancy; **interactions:** Appendix 1 (trientine)
*Side-effects:* nausea; penicillamine-induced systemic lupus erythematosus may not resolve on transfer to trientine
*Dose:* 1.2–2.4 g daily in 2–4 divided doses before food

▼ PoM **Trientine Dihydrochloride Capsules,** trientine dihydrochloride 300 mg. Label: 6, 22
Available from K & K Greeff

*Note.* The CSM has requested that in addition to the usual CSM reporting request special records should also be kept by the pharmacist

## 9.8.2  Acute porphyrias

The acute porphyrias (acute intermittent porphyria, variegate porphyria, hereditary coproporphyria and plumboporphyria) are hereditary disorders of haem biosynthesis; they have a prevalence of about 1 in 10 000 of the population.

Great care must be taken when prescribing for patients with acute porphyria since many drugs can induce acute porphyric crises. Since acute porphyrias are hereditary, relatives of affected individuals should be screened and advised about the potential danger of certain drugs.

The following list contains drugs on the UK market that have been classified as 'unsafe' in porphyria because they have been shown to be porphyrinogenic in animals or *in vitro*, or have been associated with acute attacks in patients.

Further information may be obtained from:

Porphyria Research Unit
Western Infirmary
Glasgow G11 6NT
Telephone 041-339 8822 Extn 4150

For a list of drugs unsafe for use in acute porphyrias, see next page.

## Drugs unsafe for use in acute porphyrias

*Note.* Quite modest changes in chemical structure can lead to changes in porphyrinogenicity but where possible general statements have been made about groups of drugs; these should be checked first

### Drug groups (please check **first**)

| | | | |
|---|---|---|---|
| Amphetamines | Barbiturates[3] | Diuretics[6] | Menopausal Steroids[5] |
| Anabolic Steroids | Benzodiazepines[4] | Ergot Derivatives[7] | Progestogens |
| Antidepressants[1] | Cephalosporins | Hormone Replacement | Sulphonamides[8] |
| Antihistamines[2] | Contraceptives, steroid[5] | Therapy[5] | Sulphonylureas[9] |

### Individual Drugs (please check groups above **first**)

| | | | |
|---|---|---|---|
| Alcohol | Dexfenfluramine | Ketoconazole | Oxymetazoline |
| Alcuronium | Dextropropoxyphene[12] | Lignocaine | Oxyphenbutazone |
| Aluminium-containing | Diclofenac | Lisinopril | Oxytetracycline |
| Antacids[10] | Diethylpropion | Loxapine | Pentazocine[12] |
| Aminoglutethimide | Diltiazem | Mebeverine | Phenoxybenzamine |
| Amiodarone | Doxycycline | Mefenamic Acid | Phenylbutazone |
| Azapropazone | Econazole | Meprobamate | Phenytoin |
| Baclofen | Enalapril | Mercaptopurine | Piroxicam |
| Bromocriptine | Enflurane | Mercury Compounds | Pivampicillin[13] |
| Busulphan | Erythromycin | Methotrexate | Prilocaine |
| Captopril | Ethamsylate | Methyldopa | Probenecid |
| Carbamazepine | Ethionamide | Metoclopramide | Pyrazinamide |
| Carisoprodol | Ethosuximide | Metyrapone | Rifampicin |
| Chlorambucil | Etomidate | Miconazole | Simvastatin |
| Chloramphenicol | Fenfluramine | Mifepristone | Sulphinpyrazone |
| Chlormezanone | Flucloxacillin | Minoxidil | Sulpiride |
| Chloroform[11] | Flupenthixol | Nalidixic Acid | Tamoxifen |
| Clonidine | Gold salts | Natamycin | Theophylline |
| Cocaine | Griseofulvin | Nifedipine | Thioridazine |
| Colistin | Guaiphenesin | Nikethamide | Tinidazole |
| Cyclophosphamide | Halothane | Nitrofurantoin | Trimethoprim |
| Cycloserine | Hydralazine | Orphenadrine | Valproate[4] |
| Cyclosporin | Hyoscine Butylbromide | Oxpentifylline | Verapamil |
| Danazol | Isometheptene Mucate | Oxycodone | Zuclopenthixol |
| Dapsone | Isoniazid | | |

1. Includes tricyclic (and related) and MAOIs.
2. Most antihistamines should be avoided but chlorpheniramine and cyclizine thought to be safe.
3. Includes methohexitone, primidone, and thiopentone.
4. Status epilepticus has been treated successfully with intravenous diazepam; where essential, seizure prophylaxis has been undertaken with clonazepam or valproate.
5. Includes both progestogen-only and combined (progestogen content probably more hazardous than oestrogen).
6. Acetazolamide, amiloride, bumetanide, and triamterene have been used.
7. Includes ergometrine (oxytocin probably safe), lysuride and pergolide.
8. Includes co-trimoxazole and sulphasalazine.
9. Glipizide is now also considered unsafe.
10. Absorption limited but magnesium-containing antacids preferable.
11. Small amounts in medicines probably safe.
12. Morphine, diamorphine, codeine, dihydrocodeine, and pethidine are thought to be safe.
13. Ampicillin and amoxycillin probably safe.

Prices are **net**, see p. 1

# 10: Drugs used in the treatment of

# MUSCULOSKELETAL and JOINT DISEASES

In this chapter, drug treatment is discussed under the following headings:

**10.1** Drugs used in rheumatic diseases and gout
**10.2** Drugs used in neuromuscular disorders
**10.3** Drugs for the relief of soft-tissue inflammation

For treatment of septic arthritis see section 5.1, Table 1.

## 10.1 Drugs used in rheumatic diseases and gout

**10.1.1** Non-steroidal anti-inflammatory drugs (NSAIDs)
**10.1.2** Corticosteroids
**10.1.3** Drugs which suppress the rheumatic disease process
**10.1.4** Drugs used in the treatment of gout

Most rheumatic diseases require symptomatic treatment to relieve pain and stiffness. This applies to inflammatory diseases both in the adult and in the juvenile age group (juvenile arthritis—Still's disease). Suitable non-steroidal anti-inflammatory drugs (NSAIDs) are described in section 10.1.1; reference should also be made to section 10.1.4 for the treatment of acute gout.

In certain circumstances corticosteroids (section 10.1.2) may be used to suppress inflammation.

Drugs are also available which may affect the disease process itself and favourably influence the outcome. For *rheumatoid arthritis* these include penicillamine, gold salts; antimalarials (chloroquine and hydroxychloroquine), immunosuppressants (azathioprine, chlorambucil, cyclophosphamide, and methotrexate), and sulphasalazine; they are sometimes known as second-line or disease-modifying antirheumatic drugs. For *psoriatic arthritis* they include gold salts, azathioprine, and methotrexate, and for *gout* they include uricosuric drugs and allopurinol.

## 10.1.1 Non-steroidal anti-inflammatory drugs (NSAIDs)

In *single doses* NSAIDs have analgesic activity comparable to that of paracetamol (see section 4.7.1) and can therefore be taken on demand for mild or intermittent pain or as a supplement to regular treatment. In regular *full dosage* they have both a lasting analgesic and an anti-inflammatory effect. This combination makes them particularly useful for the treatment of continuous or regular pain associated with inflammation. NSAIDs are,

therefore, more appropriate than paracetamol or the opioid analgesics in the inflammatory arthritides (e.g. rheumatoid arthritis) and in advanced osteoarthrosis (also termed osteoarthritis). They may also be of benefit in the less well defined conditions of back pain and soft-tissue disorders.

Differences in anti-inflammatory activity between different NSAIDs are small, but there is considerable variation in individual patient response. About 60% of patients will respond to any NSAID. Among the rest, those who do not respond to one may well respond to another. Therefore it is often necessary to try several drugs before finding one to suit a particular patient. Most NSAIDs should produce an effect within a few days. If used for analgesia alone they should be changed if no response is obtained after a week; if an anti-inflammatory action is also required they should be changed if no response is obtained after three weeks.

The main differences between NSAIDs are in the incidence and type of side-effects. Before treatment is started the prescriber should weigh efficacy against possible side-effects.

### ASPIRIN AND THE SALICYLATES

**Aspirin**[1] was the traditional first choice but most physicians now prefer to start treatment with another NSAID which may be better tolerated and more convenient for the patient.

In regular high dosage aspirin has about the same anti-inflammatory effect as other NSAIDs. The required dose for active inflammatory joint disease is 3.6 g or more daily. There is little anti-inflammatory effect with less than 3 g daily. Gastro-intestinal side-effects such as nausea, dyspepsia, and gastro-intestinal bleeding may occur with any dosage of aspirin but anti-inflammatory doses are associated with a much higher incidence of side-effects. Gastro-intestinal side-effects may be minimised by taking the dose after food. Numerous formulations are available which improve gastric tolerance and minimise occult bleeding, including buffered, dispersible, and enteric-coated preparations.

Anti-inflammatory doses of aspirin may also cause mild chronic salicylate intoxication (salicylism) characterised by dizziness, tinnitus, and deafness; these symptoms may be controlled by reducing the dosage.

---

1. Owing to an association with Reye's syndrome the CSM has recommended that aspirin-containing preparations should no longer be given to children under the age of 12 years, unless specifically indicated, e.g. for juvenile arthritis (Still's disease).

---

**Benorylate**[1], an aspirin-paracetamol ester, is broken down after absorption from the gastro-intestinal tract. It need only be given twice daily and gastric tolerance is slightly better than with aspirin.

## ASPIRIN

*Indications:* pain and inflammation in rheumatic disease and other musculoskeletal disorders (including juvenile arthritis); see also section 4.7.1; antiplatelet, see section 2.9

*Cautions:* asthma, allergic disease, hepatic or renal impairment (avoid if severe), dehydration, pregnancy (particularly at term), elderly, concurrent anticoagulant therapy; G6PD-deficiency (see section 9.1.5); **interactions:** Appendix 1 (aspirin)

*Contra-indications:* gastro-intestinal ulceration; children under 12 years (except for juvenile arthritis) and breast-feeding (association with Reye's syndrome, see section 4.7.1); not for treatment of gout

*Side-effects:* common with anti-inflammatory doses; gastro-intestinal discomfort, ulceration, bleeding, or nausea, hearing disturbances such as tinnitus (leading rarely to deafness), vertigo, mental confusion, hypersensitivity reactions (angioedema, bronchospasm and rashes); increased bleeding time; rarely oedema, myocarditis, blood disorders, particularly thrombocytopenia; overdosage: see Emergency Treatment of Poisoning, p. 17

*Dose:* 0.3–1 g every 4 hours; max. in acute conditions 8 g daily; CHILD, juvenile arthritis, up to 80 mg/kg daily in 5–6 divided doses, increased in acute exacerbations to 130 mg/kg. Doses should be taken after food

**Preparations**
See section 4.7.1

## BENORYLATE

(Aspirin-paracetamol ester; 2 g benorylate is equivalent to approximately 1.15 g aspirin and 970 mg paracetamol)
*Indications:* pain and inflammation in rheumatic disease and other musculoskeletal disorders; see also section 4.7.1

*Cautions; Contra-indications; Side-effects:* see under Aspirin (above) and Paracetamol (section 4.7.1)

*Dose:* 4–8 g daily divided into 2–3 doses

**Benorylate** (Non-proprietary)
*Tablets*, benorylate 750 mg. Net price 100 = £8.60. Label: 21, 31
Available from APS, Sterwin
*Suspension*, benorylate 2 g/5 mL. Net price 100 mL = £4.10. Label: 21, 31
Available from APS, Berk, Sterwin

1. Owing to an association with Reye's syndrome the CSM has recommended that aspirin-containing preparations should no longer be given to children under the age of 12 years, unless specifically indicated, e.g. for juvenile arthritis (Still's disease).

**Benoral®** (Sanofi Winthrop)
*Tablets*, benorylate 750 mg. Net price 20 = £1.72. Label: 21, 31
*Granules*, benorylate 2 g/sachet. Net price 60 sachet-pack = £14.12. Label: 13, 21, 31
*Suspension*, sugar-free, benorylate 2 g/5 mL. Net price 300 mL = £12.16. Label: 21, 31

## SALICYLATE COMPOUNDS

*Indications:* pain and inflammation in rheumatic disease and other musculoskeletal disorders
*Cautions; Contra-indications; Side-effects:* see under Aspirin (above)

PoM **Disalcid®** (3M)
*Capsules*, orange/grey, salsalate 500 mg, net price 120-cap pack = £6.88. Label: 21, 33
*Dose:* 2–4 g daily in 3–4 divided doses
**Trilisate®** (Napp)
*Tablets*, orange, scored, choline magnesium tri-salicylate ≡ salicylate 500 mg, net price 60-tab pack = £4.95. Label: 21, 33
*Dose:* 0.5–1.5 g of salicylate twice daily; for maintenance, total daily dose may be taken once daily

## OTHER NSAIDs

**Ibuprofen** is a propionic acid derivative with anti-inflammatory, analgesic, and antipyretic properties. It has fewer side-effects than other NSAIDs but its anti-inflammatory properties are weaker. Doses of 1.6 to 2.4 g daily are needed for rheumatoid arthritis and it is unsuitable for conditions where inflammation is prominent such as acute gout.

Other propionic acid derivatives:
**Naproxen** has emerged as one of the first choices as it combines good efficacy with a low incidence of side-effects and administration is only twice daily.

**Fenbufen** is claimed to be associated with less gastro-intestinal bleeding, but there is a high risk of rashes (see p. 351).

**Fenoprofen** is as effective as naproxen, and **flurbiprofen** may be slightly more effective. Both are associated with slightly more gastro-intestinal side-effects than ibuprofen.

**Ketoprofen** has anti-inflammatory properties similar to ibuprofen and has more side-effects. A modified-release preparation is claimed to cause less gastro-intestinal irritation.

**Tiaprofenic acid** is as effective as naproxen; it has more side-effects than ibuprofen.

Drugs with properties similar to those of propionic acid derivatives:
**Azapropazone** is similar in effect to naproxen; it has a tendency to cause rashes.

**Diclofenac** has an action similar to that of naproxen; its side-effects are also similar. Diclofenac is also available as suppositories and as a modified-release preparation.

**Diflunisal** is an aspirin derivative but its clinical effect more closely resembles that of the propionic acid derivatives than that of its parent compound. Its long duration of action allows twice-daily administration.

**Etodolac** is comparable in effect to naproxen; side-effects appear to be comparable to those of ibuprofen but long-term data are awaited.

**Indomethacin** has an action equal to or superior to that of naproxen, but with a high incidence of side-effects including headaches, dizziness, and gastro-intestinal disturbances. It can also be used for acute gout.

**Mefenamic acid** is a related analgesic but its anti-inflammatory properties are minor and side-effects differ in that diarrhoea and occasionally haemolytic anaemia may occur which necessitate discontinuation of treatment.

**Nabumetone** is comparable in effect to naproxen; side-effects appear to be comparable to those of ibuprofen but long-term data are awaited.

**Phenylbutazone** is a potent anti-inflammatory drug but because of occasional serious side-effects its use is limited to the hospital treatment of ankylosing spondylitis. In addition to its gastric side-effects it has two rare but dangerous side-effects. It causes fluid retention and, in pre-disposed patients, may precipitate cardiac failure. It also causes agranulocytosis (which may occur within the first few days of treatment) and aplastic anaemia. In ankylosing spondylitis prolonged administration may be necessary but it should not be used unless other drugs have failed.

**Piroxicam** is as effective as naproxen and has a prolonged duration of action which permits once-daily administration. It has more gastro-intestinal side-effects than ibuprofen, especially in the elderly; suppositories or dispersible tablets are available.

**Sulindac** is similar in tolerance to naproxen.

**Tenoxicam** is similar in effectiveness and tolerance to naproxen. Its long half-life allows once-daily administration.

**Tolmetin** is comparable in effect to ibuprofen.

CAUTIONS. NSAIDs should be used with caution in the *elderly*, in *allergic disorders* (particularly salicylate hypersensitivity and asthma, see **CSM warning** below), and during *pregnancy*.

In patients with *renal, cardiac, or hepatic impairment* caution is required since the use of NSAIDs may result in deterioration of renal function (see also under Side-effects, below); the dose should be kept as **low as possible** and renal function should be **monitored**.

NSAIDs should not be given to patients with *active peptic ulceration*, see also **CSM advice** below. While it is preferable to avoid them in patients with current or previous peptic ulceration, and to withdraw them if gastro-intestinal lesions develop, nevertheless patients with serious rheumatic diseases (e.g. rheumatoid arthritis) are usually dependent on NSAIDs for effective relief of pain and stiffness. Administration of histamine $H_2$-receptor blocking drugs or misoprostol (see section 1.3.4) may permit recommencement of a

NSAID without further gastro-intestinal problems.

SIDE-EFFECTS. Side-effects are variable in severity and frequency. Gastro-intestinal discomfort, nausea, diarrhoea, and occasionally bleeding and ulceration occur; dyspepsia may be minimised by taking these drugs with food or milk. Other side-effects include hypersensitivity reactions (particularly angioedema, asthma, and rashes), headache, dizziness, vertigo, hearing disturbances such as tinnitus, and haematuria. Blood disorders have also occurred. Fluid retention may occur (rarely precipitating congestive heart failure in elderly patients). Reversible acute renal failure may be provoked by NSAIDs especially in patients with pre-existing renal impairment (**important**, see also under Cautions above). Rarely, papillary necrosis or interstitial fibrosis associated with NSAIDs may lead to renal failure. Aseptic meningitis has been reported rarely with NSAIDs; patients with connective tissue disorders such as systemic lupus erythematosus may be especially susceptible.

Overdosage: see Emergency Treatment of Poisoning, p. 18.

---

**CSM advice (peptic ulceration).**
1. NSAIDs should not be given to patients with active peptic ulceration.
2. In patients with a history of peptic ulcer disease and in the elderly they should be given only after other forms of treatment have been carefully considered.
3. In all patients it is prudent to start at the bottom end of the dose range.

**CSM warning (asthma).**
Any degree of worsening of asthma may be related to the ingestion of NSAIDs, either prescribed or (in the case of ibuprofen and others) purchased over the counter.

---

## IBUPROFEN

*Indications:* pain and inflammation in rheumatic disease (including juvenile arthritis) and other musculoskeletal disorders; see also section 4.7.1

*Cautions; Side-effects:* see notes above; **interactions:** Appendix 1 (NSAIDs)

*Dose:* initially 1.2–1.8 g daily in 3–4 divided doses preferably after food; increased if necessary to max. of 2.4 g daily; maintenance dose of 0.6–1.2 g daily may be adequate; CHILD 20 mg/kg daily in divided doses (juvenile arthritis, up to 40 mg/kg daily), not recommended for children under 7 kg

PoM **Ibuprofen** (Non-proprietary)
*Tablets*, coated, ibuprofen 200 mg, net price 20 = 26p; 400 mg, 20 = 51p; 600 mg, 20 = £1.36. Label: 21
Various strengths available from APS (Apsifen®), Ashbourne (Arthrofen®), Berk (Lidifen®), Cox, DDSA (Ebufac®), Evans, Kerfoot, Lagap (Ibular®), Rima (Rimafen®), Upjohn (Motrin®)
*Note.* Proprietary brands of ibuprofen tablets are on sale to the public; brand names include Contrapain Femafen®, Cuprofen®, Ibrufhalal®, Inoven®, Librofem®, Migrafen®, Novaprin®, Nurofen®, Pacifene®, Proflex®, Relcofen®, Seclodin®

PoM **Brufen®** (Boots)

*Tablets*, all magenta, ibuprofen 200 mg (s/c), net price 20 = 61p; 400 mg (s/c), 20 = £1.21; 600 mg (f/c), 20 = £1.93. Label: 21

*Syrup*, orange, ibuprofen 100 mg/5 mL. Net price 200 mL = £1.85. Label: 21

*Granules*, effervescent, ibuprofen 600 mg/sachet. Net price 20-sachet pack = £4.68. Label: 13, 21.

Not recommended for children under 12 years

*Note.* Contains sodium approx. 9 mmol/sachet

PoM **Brufen Retard®** (Boots)

*Tablets*, m/r, f/c, ibuprofen 800 mg, net price 56-tab pack = £11.76. Label: 25, 27

*Dose:* 2 tablets daily, preferably in the early evening, increased in severe cases to 3 tablets daily in 2 divided doses. Not recommended for children under 12 years

PoM **Fenbid®** (SK&F)

*Spansule®* (= capsule m/r), maroon/pink, enclosing off-white pellets, ibuprofen 300 mg. Net price 120-cap pack = £7.14. Label: 25

*Dose:* 1–3 capsules every 12 hours

PoM **Junifen®** : see section 4.7.1

**Topical preparations**, section 10.3.2

---

## ACEMETACIN

(Glycolic acid ester of indomethacin)

*Indications:* pain and inflammation in rheumatic disease and postoperatively

*Cautions; Side-effects:* see under Indomethacin

*Dose:* 120 mg daily in divided doses with food, increased if necessary to 180 mg daily

▼ PoM **Emflex®** (Merck)

*Capsules*, yellow/orange, acemetacin 60 mg, net price 90-cap pack = £22.50. Label: 21, counselling, driving

---

## AZAPROPAZONE

*Indications:* pain and inflammation in rheumatic disease and other musculoskeletal disorders; gout

*Cautions; Side-effects:* see notes above; photosensitivity may occur. Avoid in porphyria (see section 9.8.2); **important:** recent reports of serious enhancement of effect of warfarin; other **interactions:** Appendix 1 (NSAIDs)

*Dose:* 1.2 g daily in 2 or 4 divided doses (elderly 300 mg twice daily, max. 900 mg daily)

Acute gout, initially 2.4 g in divided doses over 24 hours, then 1.8 g reducing to 1.2 g daily in divided doses

Chronic gout, 600 mg twice daily (elderly 300 mg twice daily, max. 900 mg daily)

PoM **Rheumox®** (Wyeth)

*Capsules*, orange, azapropazone 300 mg. Net price 20 = £3.37. Label: 21, counselling: in some patients direct sunlight may lead to a rash

*Tablets*, orange, f/c, scored, azapropazone 600 mg. Net price 20 = £5.85. Label: 21, counselling: in some patients direct sunlight may lead to a rash

## DICLOFENAC SODIUM

*Indications:* pain and inflammation in rheumatic disease (including juvenile arthritis) and other musculoskeletal disorders; acute gout

*Cautions; Side-effects:* see notes above. Avoid in porphyria (see section 9.8.2); pain may occur at the injection site; suppositories may cause irritation; **interactions:** Appendix 1 (NSAIDs)

*Dose: by mouth*, 75–150 mg daily in 2–3 divided doses, preferably after food

*By deep intramuscular injection* into the gluteal region, acute exacerbations and post-operative, 75 mg once daily (twice daily in severe cases) for max. of 2 days

Ureteric colic, 75 mg then a further 75 mg after 30 minutes if necessary

*By rectum* in suppositories, 100 mg, usually at night

Max. total daily dose by any route 150 mg

CHILD 1 year or over, juvenile arthritis, *by mouth or by rectum*, 1–3 mg/kg daily in divided doses

PoM **Diclofenac Sodium** (Non-proprietary)

*Tablets*, both e/c, diclofenac sodium 25 mg, net price 20 = £1.88; 50 mg, 20 = £3.65. Label: 5, 25

Available from APS, Ashbourne (Diclozip®), Cox, Eastern (Volraman®), Evans, Kerfoot, Lagap (Rhumalgan®), Shire (Valenac®), Sterwin

PoM **Voltarol®** (Geigy)

*Tablets*, both e/c, diclofenac sodium 25 mg (yellow), net price 84-tab pack = £7.88; 50 mg (brown), 84-tab pack = £15.32. Label: 5, 25

*Dispersible tablets*, pink, diclofenac, equivalent to diclofenac sodium 50 mg, net price 21-tab pack = £4.68. Label: 13, 21

*Injection*, diclofenac sodium 25 mg/mL. Net price 3-mL amp = 79p

*Suppositories*, diclofenac sodium 100 mg. Net price 10 = £3.11

*Paediatric suppositories*, diclofenac sodium 12.5 mg. Net price 10 = 59p

*Emulgel®* gel, section 10.3.2

PoM **Voltarol® 75 mg SR** (Geigy)

*Tablets*, m/r, pink, diclofenac sodium 75 mg. Net price 56-tab pack = £18.74. Label: 21, 25

*Dose:* 1–2 tablets daily preferably with food

PoM **Voltarol® Retard** (Geigy)

*Tablets*, m/r, red, diclofenac sodium 100 mg. Net price 28-tab pack = £12.49. Label: 21, 25

*Dose:* 100 mg once daily preferably with food

---

## DIFLUNISAL

*Indications:* pain and inflammation in rheumatic disease and other musculoskeletal disorders; see also section 4.7.1

*Cautions; Side-effects:* see notes above; breast-feeding; **interactions:** Appendix 1 (NSAIDs)

*Dose:* initially 1 g daily in 2 divided doses, then 0.5–1 g daily; max. 1.5 g daily

Osteoarthrosis, rheumatoid arthritis, 0.5–1 g daily as a single daily dose *or* in 2 divided doses

---

PoM **Diflunisal** (Non-proprietary)
*Tablets*, coated, diflunisal 250 mg, net price 20 = £1.80; 500 mg, 20 = £3.61. Label: 21, 25, counselling, avoid aluminium hydroxide
Available from APS

PoM **Dolobid**® (Morson)
*Tablets*, both f/c, diflunisal 250 mg (peach), net price 20 = £1.80; 500 mg (orange), 20 = £3.61. Label: 21, 25, counselling, avoid aluminium hydroxide

## ETODOLAC
*Indications:* pain and inflammation in rheumatoid arthritis and osteoarthrosis
*Cautions; Side-effects:* see notes above; **interactions:** Appendix 1 (NSAIDs)
*Dose:* 200 mg or 300 mg twice daily *or* 400 mg or 600 mg once daily; max. 600 mg daily

PoM **Lodine**® (Wyeth)
*Capsules*, etodolac 200 mg (light- and dark-grey), net price 20 = £4.08; 300 mg (light-grey), 60-cap pack = £16.89. Label: 21
*Tablets*, brown, f/c, etodolac 200 mg. Net price 20 = £4.06. Label: 21

## FENBUFEN
*Indications:* pain and inflammation in rheumatic disease and other musculoskeletal disorders
*Cautions; Side-effects:* see notes above, but high risk of rashes (discontinue immediately); erythema multiforme and Stevens-Johnson syndrome reported; also allergic interstitial lung disorders (may follow rashes); **interactions:** Appendix 1 (NSAIDs)
*Dose:* 300 mg in the morning and 600 mg at bedtime *or* 450 mg twice daily

PoM **Lederfen**® (Lederle)
*Capsules*, dark blue, fenbufen 300 mg. Net price 84-cap pack = £19.61. Label: 21
*Tablets*, both light blue, f/c, fenbufen 300 mg, net price 84-tab pack = £19.61; 450 mg, 56-tab pack = £19.61. Label: 21

PoM **Lederfen F**® (Lederle)
*Effervescent tablets*, fenbufen 450 mg. Net price 14-tab pack = £6.21. Label: 13, 21

## FENOPROFEN
*Indications:* pain and inflammation in rheumatic disease and other musculoskeletal disorders; see also section 4.7.1
*Cautions; Side-effects:* see notes above; upper respiratory infection and nasopharyngitis reported; **interactions:** Appendix 1 (NSAIDs)
*Dose:* 300–600 mg 3–4 times daily with food; max. 3 g daily

PoM **Fenopron**® (Dista)
*Fenopron 300 tablets*, orange, fenoprofen 300 mg (as calcium salt). Net price 20 = £1.57. Label: 21
*Fenopron 600 tablets*, orange, scored, fenoprofen 600 mg (as calcium salt). Net price 20 = £3.03. Label: 21

PoM **Progesic**®: see section 4.7.1

## FLURBIPROFEN
*Indications:* pain and inflammation in rheumatoid arthritis, osteoarthrosis, and ankylosing spondylitis
*Cautions; Side-effects:* see notes above; local irritation on rectal administration; **interactions:** Appendix 1 (NSAIDs)
*Dose: by mouth or by rectum* in suppositories, 150–200 mg, daily in divided doses, increased in acute conditions to 300 mg daily

PoM **Froben**® (Boots)
*Tablets*, both yellow, s/c, flurbiprofen 50 mg, net price 20 = £1.77; 100 mg, 20 = £3.68. Label: 21
*Suppositories*, flurbiprofen 100 mg. Net price 12 = £2.90

PoM **Froben SR**® (Boots)
*Capsules*, m/r, yellow, enclosing white, off-white beads, flurbiprofen 200 mg. Net price 30-cap pack = £12.80. Label: 21, 25
*Dose:* 1 capsule daily, preferably in the evening

## INDOMETHACIN
*Indications:* pain and moderate to severe inflammation in rheumatic disease and other acute musculoskeletal disorders; acute gout; dysmenorrhoea
*Cautions:* see notes above; breast-feeding, epilepsy, parkinsonism, psychiatric disturbances; during prolonged therapy ophthalmic and blood examinations are particularly advisable; avoid rectal administration in proctitis and haemorrhoids; **interactions:** Appendix 1 (NSAIDs)
DRIVING. Dizziness may affect performance of skilled tasks (e.g. driving)
*Side-effects:* see notes above; frequently gastro-intestinal disturbances (including diarrhoea), headache, dizziness, and light-headedness; gastro-intestinal ulceration and bleeding; rarely, drowsiness, confusion, insomnia, convulsions, psychiatric disturbances, depression, syncope, blood disorders (particularly thrombocytopenia), hypertension, hyperglycaemia, blurred vision, corneal deposits, peripheral neuropathy. On rectal administration pruritus, discomfort, bleeding
*Dose: by mouth*, 50–200 mg daily in divided doses, with food
Dysmenorrhoea, up to 75 mg daily
*By rectum* in suppositories, 100 mg at night and in the morning if required
Combined oral and rectal treatment, max. total daily dose 150–200 mg

PoM **Indomethacin** (Non-proprietary)
*Capsules*, indomethacin 25 mg, net price 20 = 18p; 50 mg, 20 = 55p. Label: 21, counselling, driving, see above
Available from APS, Ashbourne (Indomax®), Berk (Imbrilon®), Cox, DDSA (Artracin®), Evans, Galen (Mobilan®), Kerfoot, Rima (Rimacid®)
*Suppositories*, indomethacin 100 mg. Net price 10 = £1.83. Counselling, driving, see above
Available from Berk (Imbrilon®), Cox, Evans

PoM **Flexin**® (Napp)

*Flexin-25 Continus*®, *tablets*, m/r, green, indomethacin 25 mg, net price 56-tab pack = £7.33. Label: 21, 25, counselling, driving, see above

*Flexin-LS Continus*®, *tablets*, m/r, red, indomethacin 50 mg, net price 28-tab pack = £7.33. Label: 21, 25, counselling, driving, see above

*Flexin Continus*®, *tablets*, m/r, yellow, indomethacin 75 mg, net price 28-tab pack = £10.47. Label: 21, 25, counselling, driving, see above

*Dose:* initially 75 mg daily, adjusted in steps of 25–50 mg; range 25–200 mg daily in 1–2 divided doses

Dysmenorrhoea, up to 75 mg daily

PoM **Indocid**® (Morson)

*Capsules*, indomethacin 25 mg, net price 20 = 99p; 50 mg, 20 = £1.78. Label: 21, counselling, driving, see above

*Suspension*, sugar-free, indomethacin 25 mg/5 mL. Net price 200 mL = £3.12. Label: 21, counselling, driving, see above

*Suppositories*, indomethacin 100 mg. Net price 10 = £2.43. Counselling, driving, see above

PoM **Indocid-R**® (Morson)

*Capsules*, m/r, ivory/clear, enclosing white and blue pellets, indomethacin 75 mg. Net price 20 = £5.71. Label: 21, 25, counselling, driving, see above

*Dose:* 1–2 capsules daily

PoM **Indomax 75 SR**® (Ashbourne)

*Capsules*, m/r, blue/clear, enclosing white pellets, indomethacin 75 mg. Net price 28-cap pack = £7.20. Label: 21, 25, counselling, driving, see above

*Dose:* 1 capsule 1–2 times daily

PoM **Indolar SR**® (Lagap)

*Capsules*, m/r, blue/clear, enclosing white pellets, indomethacin 75 mg. Net price 20 = £4.02. Label: 21, 25, counselling, driving, see above

*Dose:* 1 capsule 1–2 times daily

PoM **Indomod**® (Kabi Pharmacia)

*Capsules*, both m/r, enclosing e/c pellets, indomethacin 25 mg (orange), net price 20 = £2.24; 75 mg (brown), 30-cap pack = £7.71. Label: 25, counselling, driving, see above

PoM **Rheumacin LA**® (CP)

*Capsules*, m/r, yellow/blue, enclosing off-white pellets, indomethacin 75 mg. Net price 20 = £3.34. Label: 21, 25, counselling, driving, see above

*Dose:* 1–2 capsules daily

PoM **Slo-Indo**® (Generics)

*Capsules*, m/r, red/yellow enclosing off-white pellets, indomethacin 75 mg. Net price 20 = £4.47. Label: 21, 25, counselling, driving, see above

*Dose:* 1–2 capsules daily

PoM **Indocid PDA**® : see section 7.1.1

## KETOPROFEN

*Indications:* pain and mild inflammation in rheumatic disease and other musculoskeletal disorders, and after orthopaedic surgery; acute gout; dysmenorrhoea

*Cautions; Side-effects:* see notes above; suppositories may cause rectal irritation; **interactions:** Appendix 1 (NSAIDs)

*Dose: by mouth*, 100–200 mg daily in 2–4 divided doses with food

*By rectum* in suppositories, 100 mg at bedtime Combined oral and rectal treatment, max. total daily dose 200 mg

*By deep intramuscular injection* into the gluteal muscle, 50–100 mg every 4 hours (max. 200 mg in 24 hours) for up to 3 days

PoM **Ketoprofen** (Non-proprietary)

*Capsules*, ketoprofen 50 mg, net price 20 = £1.05; 100 mg, 20 = £2.89. Label: 21

PoM **Alrheumat**® (Bayer)

*Capsules*, off-white, ketoprofen 50 mg. Net price 20 = £1.22. Label: 21

PoM **Orudis**® (Rhône-Poulenc Rorer)

*Capsules*, ketoprofen 50 mg (green/purple), net price 112-cap pack = £8.07; 100 mg (pink), 56-cap pack = £8.09. Label: 21

*Suppositories*, ketoprofen 100 mg. Net price 10 = £3.54

PoM **Oruvail**® (Rhône-Poulenc Rorer)

*Capsules*, both m/r, enclosing white pellets, ketoprofen 100 mg (pink/purple), net price 56-cap pack = £16.14; 200 mg (pink/white), 28-cap pack = £16.41. Label: 21, 25

*Dose:* 100–200 mg once daily with food

*Injection*, ketoprofen 50 mg/mL. Net price 2-mL amp = 75p

*Gel*, section 10.3.2

## MEFENAMIC ACID

*Indications:* mild to moderate pain in rheumatoid arthritis (including juvenile arthritis), osteoarthrosis, and related conditions; see also section 4.7.1

*Cautions:* see notes above; blood tests required during long-term treatment; avoid in porphyria (see section 9.8.2); **interactions:** Appendix 1 (NSAIDs)

*Side-effects:* see notes above; drowsiness; diarrhoea or rashes (withdraw treatment); thrombocytopenia, haemolytic anaemia; convulsions in overdosage

*Dose:* 500 mg 3 times daily preferably after food; CHILD over 6 months, 25 mg/kg daily in divided doses for not longer than 7 days, except in juvenile arthritis

PoM **Mefenamic Acid** (Non-proprietary)

*Capsules*, mefenamic acid 250 mg. Net price 20 = £1.32. Label: 21

Available from APS, Ashbourne (Dysman 250®), Cox, Kerfoot, Sterwin

*Tablets*, mefenamic acid 500 mg, net price 20 = £2.76. Label: 21

Available from Ashbourne (Dysman 500®), Cox, Kerfoot

---

PoM **Ponstan**® (P-D)
*Capsules*, ivory/blue, mefenamic acid 250 mg.
Net price 20 = £1.51. Label: 21
*Dispersible tablets*, blue, mefenamic acid 250 mg.
Net price 20 = £1.71. Label: 13, 21
*Tablets forte*, yellow, f/c, mefenamic acid
500 mg. Net price 20 = £2.76. Label: 21
*Paediatric suspension*, mefenamic acid 50 mg/
5 mL. Net price 125 mL = £3.37. Label: 21

## NABUMETONE
*Indications:* pain and inflammation in
osteoarthrosis and rheumatoid arthritis
*Cautions; Side-effects:* see notes above; **interactions:** Appendix 1 (NSAIDs)
*Dose:* 1 g at night, in severe conditions 0.5–1 g in
morning as well; elderly 0.5–1 g daily

PoM **Relifex**® (Bencard)
*Tablets*, red, f/c, nabumetone 500 mg. Net price
56-tab pack = £15.68. Label: 21, 25
*Suspension*, nabumetone 500 mg/5 mL. Net
price 300-mL pack = £21.84. Label: 21

## NAPROXEN
*Indications:* pain and inflammation in rheumatic
disease (including juvenile arthritis) and other
musculoskeletal disorders; acute gout; see also
Naproxen Sodium, section 4.7.1
*Cautions; Side-effects:* see notes above; **interactions:** Appendix 1 (NSAIDs)
*Dose: by mouth*, 0.5–1 g daily in 2 divided doses
*or* 1 g once daily; CHILD (over 5 years), juvenile
arthritis, 10 mg/kg daily in 2 divided doses
Acute musculoskeletal disorders, 500 mg
initially, then 250 mg every 6–8 hours as
required; max. dose after first day 1.25 g daily
Acute gout, 750 mg initially, then 250 mg every
8 hours until attack has passed
*By rectum* in suppositories, 500 mg at bedtime;
if necessary 500 mg in morning as well

PoM **Naproxen** (Non-proprietary)
*Tablets*, naproxen 250 mg, net price 20 = £1.65;
500 mg, 20 = £3.30. Label: 21
Available from Ashbourne (Arthrosin®), BHR
(Prosaid®), Cox, CP (Arthroxen®), Evans, Goldcrest
(Rheuflex®), Kerfoot, Lagap (Laraflex®), Shire (Val-
rox®), Sterwin
PoM **Naprosyn**® (Syntex)
*Tablets*, all scored, naproxen 250 mg (buff), net
price 20 = £2.50; 375 mg (pink), 60-tab pack =
£11.25; 500 mg (buff), 60-tab pack = £14.98.
Label: 21
*Suspension*, orange, naproxen 125 mg/5 mL. Net
price 100 mL = £2.18. Label: 21
*Granules*, naproxen 500 mg/sachet. Net price 60
sachets = £19.47. Label: 13, 21
*Suppositories*, naproxen 500 mg. Net price 10 =
£3.26
PoM **Naprosyn**® **EC** (Syntex)
*Tablets*, all e/c, naproxen 250 mg, net price 56-
tab pack = £7.00; 375 mg, 56-tab pack =
£10.50; 500 mg, 56-tab pack = £14.00. Label:
5, 25

PoM **Nycopren**® (Lundbeck)
*Tablets*, both e/c, naproxen 250 mg (scored), net
price 20 = £2.07; 500 mg, 60-tab pack = £12.41.
Label: 5, 25
PoM **Synflex**® : see section 4.7.1

**With misoprostol**
For cautions, contra-indications, and side-effects of
misoprostol, see section 1.3.4
PoM **Napratec**® (Searle)
*Calendar pack*, 56 yellow scored tablets, naproxen 500 mg; 56 white scored tablets, misoprostol 200 micrograms. Net price = £18.00.
Label: 21
*Dose:* patients requiring naproxen for rheumatoid arthritis, osteoarthritis, or ankylosing
spondylitis, with prophylaxis against NSAID-
induced gastroduodenal ulceration, 1 naproxen
500-mg tablet and 1 misoprostol 200-microgram
tablet taken together twice daily with food

## PHENYLBUTAZONE
*Indications:* ankylosing spondylitis (in hospital)
*Cautions:* blood counts before and during treatment if for
more than 7 days; elderly (reduce dose); breast-feeding;
withdraw treatment if acute pulmonary syndrome
including fever and dyspnoea occurs; see also notes
above; **interactions:** Appendix 1 (NSAIDs)
*Contra-indications:* cardiovascular disease, renal and
hepatic impairment; pregnancy; history of peptic ulceration, gastro-intestinal haemorrhage, or blood
disorders; porphyria (see section 9.8.2); thyroid
disease; children under 14
*Side-effects:* see notes above; parotitis, stomatitis, goitre,
pancreatitis, hepatitis, nephritis, visual disturbances;
rarely leucopenia, thrombocytopenia, agranulocytosis,
aplastic anaemia, erythema multiforme, toxic epidermal necrolysis
*Dose:* initially 200 mg 2–3 times daily for 2 days, with or
after food, then reduced to minimum effective, usually
100 mg 2–3 times daily
Not for children under 14 years

PoM **Butacote**® (Geigy)
*Tablets*, violet, e/c, s/c, phenylbutazone 100 mg, net
price 20 = 40p. Label: 5, 21, 25

## PIROXICAM
*Indications:* pain and inflammation in rheumatic
disease (including juvenile arthritis) and other
musculoskeletal disorders; acute gout
*Cautions:* see notes above; avoid in porphyria
(see section 9.8.2); **interactions:** Appendix 1
(NSAIDs)
*Side-effects:* see notes above
*Dose: by mouth or by rectum*, initially 20 mg
daily, maintenance 10–30 mg daily, in single or
divided doses
Acute musculoskeletal disorders, 40 mg daily
in single or divided doses for 2 days, then 20 mg
daily for 7–14 days
Acute gout, 40 mg initially, then 40 mg daily in
single or divided doses for 4–6 days
CHILD (over 6 years) *by mouth*, juvenile
arthritis, less than 15 kg, 5 mg daily; 16–25 kg,
10 mg; 26–45 kg, 15 mg; over 46 kg, 20 mg

PoM **Piroxicam** (Non-proprietary)
*Capsules*, piroxicam 10 mg, net price 20 = £2.86; 20 mg, 20 = £5.80. Label: 21
Available from APS, Ashbourne (Pirozip®), Cox, Evans, Kerfoot, Lagap (Larapam®)

PoM **Feldene**® (Pfizer)
*Capsules*, piroxicam 10 mg (maroon/blue), net price 56-cap pack = £8.87; 20 mg (maroon), 28-cap pack = £8.87. Label: 21
*Dispersible tablets*, piroxicam 10 mg (scored), net price 56-tab pack = £9.75; 20 mg, 28-tab pack = £9.75. Label: 13, 21
*Suppositories*, piroxicam 20 mg. Net price 10 = £5.20
*Gel*, section 10.3.2

## SULINDAC
*Indications:* pain and inflammation in rheumatic disease and other musculoskeletal disorders; acute gout
*Cautions; Side-effects:* see notes above; caution if history of renal stones; **interactions:** Appendix 1 (NSAIDs)
*Dose:* 200 mg twice daily with food (may be reduced according to response); max. 400 mg daily; acute gout should respond within 7 days; limit treatment of peri-articular disorders to 7–10 days

PoM **Clinoril**® (MSD)
*Tablets*, both yellow, scored, sulindac 100 mg, net price 20 = £2.24; 200 mg, 20 = £4.11. Label: 21

## TENOXICAM
*Indications:* pain and inflammation in rheumatoid arthritis and osteoarthrosis
*Cautions; Side-effects:* see notes above; **interactions:** Appendix 1 (NSAIDs)
*Dose:* 20 mg daily

PoM **Mobiflex**® (Roche)
*Tablets*, red-brown, f/c, tenoxicam 20 mg. Net price 28-tab pack = £16.52. Label: 21

## TIAPROFENIC ACID
*Indications:* pain and inflammation in rheumatic disease and other musculoskeletal disorders
*Cautions; Side-effects:* see notes above; bladder irritation reported; **interactions:** Appendix 1 (NSAIDs)
*Dose:* 600 mg daily in 2–3 divided doses

PoM **Tiaprofenic Acid** (Non-proprietary)
*Tablets*, tiaprofenic acid 200 mg, net price 84-tab pack = £13.77; 300 mg, 56-tab pack = £15.13. Label: 21
Available from Cox

PoM **Surgam**® (Roussel)
*Tablets*, tiaprofenic acid 200 mg, net price 84-tab pack = £15.89; 300 mg, 56-tab pack = £15.89. Label: 21

PoM **Surgam SA**® (Roussel)
*Capsules*, m/r, maroon/pink enclosing white pellets, tiaprofenic acid 300 mg. Net price 56-cap pack = £15.89. Label: 21, 25
*Dose:* 2 capsules once daily

## TOLMETIN
*Indications:* pain and inflammation in rheumatic disease (including juvenile arthritis) and other musculoskeletal disorders
*Cautions; Side-effects:* see notes above; **interactions:** Appendix 1 (NSAIDs)
*Dose:* 0.6–1.8 g daily in 2–4 divided doses; max. 30 mg/kg daily up to 1.8 g
CHILD, juvenile arthritis, 20–25 mg/kg daily in 3–4 divided doses; max. 30 mg/kg daily up to 1.8 g

PoM **Tolectin**® (Cilag)
*Capsules*, tolmetin (as sodium salt) 200 mg (ivory/orange), net price 90-cap pack = £15.97; 400 mg (orange), 90-cap pack = £23.97. Label: 21

## 10.1.2 Corticosteroids
**10.1.2.1** Systemic corticosteroids
**10.1.2.2** Local corticosteroid injections

### 10.1.2.1 SYSTEMIC CORTICOSTEROIDS

The general actions and uses of the corticosteroids are described in section 6.3. Treatment with corticosteroids in rheumatic diseases should be reserved for specific indications, e.g. when other anti-inflammatory drugs are unsuccessful.

In severe, possibly life-threatening, situations a high initial dose of corticosteroid is given to induce remission and the dose then gradually reduced to the lowest maintenance dose that will control the disease or, if possible, discontinued altogether. A major problem is that relapse may occur as dosage reduction is made, particularly if this is carried out too rapidly. The tendency is therefore to increase and maintain dosage and consequently the patient becomes dependent on corticosteroids. For this reason pulse doses of corticosteroids (e.g. methylprednisolone up to 1 g intravenously on three consecutive days) is in current use to suppress highly active inflammatory disease while longer term and slower acting medication is being commenced.

**Prednisolone** is used for most purposes; it has the advantage over the more potent corticosteroids (see section 6.3.2) of permitting finer dosage adjustments. To minimise side-effects the maintenance dose of prednisolone should be kept as low as possible, usually 7.5 mg daily and seldom exceeding 10 mg daily.

*Polymyalgia rheumatica* and *temporal (giant cell) arteritis* are always treated with corticosteroids. The usual initial dose of prednisolone in polymyalgia rheumatica is 10 to 15 mg daily and in temporal arteritis 40 to 60 mg daily (the higher dose being used if visual symptoms occur). Treatment should be continued until remission occurs and doses then gradually reduced. Relapse is common if therapy is stopped within 3 years but most patients can discontinue treatment after approximately 3 to 6 years after which recurrences become rare.

*Polyarteritis nodosa* and *polymyositis* are usually treated with corticosteroids. An initial dose of 60 mg of prednisolone daily is often used and reduced to a maintenance dose of 10 to 15 mg daily.

*Systemic lupus erythematosus* is treated with corticosteroids when necessary using a similar dosage regimen to that for polyarteritis nodosa and polymyositis (above). Patients with pleurisy, pericarditis, or other systemic manifestations will respond to corticosteroids. It may then be possible to reduce the dosage; alternate-day treatment is sometimes adequate, and the drug may be gradually withdrawn. In some mild cases corticosteroid treatment may be stopped after a few months. Many mild cases of systemic lupus erythematosus do not require corticosteroid treatment. Alternative treatment with anti-inflammatory analgesics, and possibly chloroquine, should be considered.

Since effective doses of systemic corticosteroids may cause Cushing's syndrome these drugs should **not** be used to suppress symptoms of *rheumatoid arthritis* unless alternative anti-inflammatory drugs and drugs which may affect the disease process (section 10.1.3) have proved unsuccessful, with increasing disability due to the inflammatory process. The smallest effective dose should be used and increased if necessary, but should not exceed the equivalent of prednisolone 7.5 to 10 mg daily. Attempts should always be made gradually to reduce the dose. Corticosteroids in low dosage may be useful in the elderly patient, and similar nocturnal doses may relieve morning stiffness.

*Ankylosing spondylitis* should not be treated with long-term corticosteroids; rarely, pulse doses may be needed and may be useful in extremely active disease that does not respond to conventional treatment.

## 10.1.2.2 LOCAL CORTICOSTEROID INJECTIONS

Corticosteroids are injected locally for an anti-inflammatory effect. In inflammatory conditions of the joints, particularly in rheumatoid arthritis, they are given by *intra-articular injection* to relieve pain, increase mobility, and reduce deformity in one or a few joints. Full aseptic precautions are essential. Infected areas should be avoided. An almost insoluble, long-acting compound such as triamcinolone hexacetonide is preferred for intra-articular injection.

Smaller amounts of corticosteroids may also be injected directly into soft tissues for the relief of inflammation in conditions such as *tennis* or *golfer's elbow* or *compression neuropathies*. In *tendinitis*, injections should be made into the tendon sheath and not directly into the tendon. A soluble, short-acting compound such as betamethasone is preferred for injection into the carpal tunnel.

Cortisone acetate is **not** effective for local injection and hydrocortisone acetate or one of the synthetic analogues such as triamcinolone hexacetonide is generally used. The risk of necrosis and muscle wasting may be slightly increased with triamcinolone; flushing has been reported with intra-articular corticosteroid injections.

Corticosteroid injections are also injected into soft tissues for the treatment of skin lesions (see section 13.4).

## DEXAMETHASONE SODIUM PHOSPHATE

*Indications:* local inflammation of joints and soft tissues

*Cautions; Contra-indications; Side-effects:* see notes above and section 6.3.3

*Dose:* by intra-articular, intralesional, or soft-tissue injection, dexamethasone 0.4–4 mg, according to size of joint or amount of soft-tissue, at intervals of 3–21 days according to response

Note. 1.3 mg dexamethasone sodium phosphate ≡ 1.2 mg dexamethasone phosphate ≡ 1 mg dexamethasone

PoM **Dexamethasone** (Organon)
*Injection*, dexamethasone sodium phosphate 5 mg/mL (= 4 mg dexamethasone/mL). Net price 1-mL amp = 83p; 2-mL vial = £1.27
PoM **Decadron**® (MSD)
*Injection*, dexamethasone phosphate 4 mg/mL (as sodium salt) (≡ 3.33 mg/mL dexamethasone). Net price 2-mL vial = £1.76

## HYDROCORTISONE ACETATE

*Indications:* local inflammation of joints and soft tissues

*Cautions; Contra-indications; Side-effects:* see notes above and section 6.3.3

*Dose:* by intra-articular, intrasynovial, or soft-tissue injection, 5–50 mg, according to joint size or amount of soft tissue; not more than 3 joints should be treated on any one day; CHILD, 5–30 mg daily (divided)

PoM **Hydrocortisone Acetate Injection** (aqueous suspension), hydrocortisone acetate 25 mg/mL. Net price 1-mL amp = 88p
PoM **Hydrocortistab**® (Boots)
*Injection* (aqueous suspension), hydrocortisone acetate 25 mg/mL. Net price 1-mL amp = 88p

## METHYLPREDNISOLONE ACETATE

*Indications:* local inflammation of joints and soft-tissues

*Cautions; Contra-indications; Side-effects:* see notes above and section 6.3.3

*Dose:* by intra-articular, intrasynovial, intra-lesional, or soft-tissue injection, 4–80 mg, according to joint size or amount of soft tissue, repeated every 1–5 weeks according to response

PoM **Depo-Medrone**® (Upjohn)
*Injection* (aqueous suspension), methyl-prednisolone acetate 40 mg/mL. Net price 1-mL vial = £2.59; 2-mL vial = £4.65; 3-mL vial = £6.75

PoM **Depo-Medrone**® **with Lidocaine** (Upjohn)
*Injection* (aqueous suspension), methyl-prednisolone acetate 40 mg, lignocaine hydrochloride 10 mg/mL. For injection into joints, bursae, or tendon sheaths. Net price 1-mL vial = £2.56; 2-mL vial = £4.65

## PREDNISOLONE ACETATE
*Indications:* local inflammation of joints and soft tissues
*Cautions; Contra-indications; Side-effects:* see notes above and section 6.3.3
*Dose: by intra-articular, intrasynovial, or soft-tissue injection*, 5–25 mg according to joint size or amount of soft tissue; not more than 3 joints should be treated on any one day

PoM **Deltastab**® (Boots)
*Injection* (aqueous suspension), prednisolone acetate 25 mg/mL. Net price 1-mL amp = 88p

## TRIAMCINOLONE ACETONIDE
*Indications:* local inflammation of joints and soft tissues
*Cautions; Contra-indications; Side-effects:* see notes above and section 6.3.3; not recommended for children under 6 years
*Dose: by intra-articular injection*, 2.5–40 mg according to joint size, to a max. of 80 mg in multiple injections
*By intralesional injection*, 2–3 mg; max. 30 mg (5 mg at any one site). Doses are repeated every 1–2 weeks according to response

PoM **Adcortyl**®    **Intra-articular / Intradermal** (Squibb)
*Injection* (aqueous suspension), triamcinolone acetonide 10 mg/mL. Net price 1-mL amp = £1.02; 5-mL vial = £4.14

PoM **Kenalog**®    **Intra-articular / Intramuscular** (Squibb)
*Injection* (aqueous suspension), triamcinolone acetonide 40 mg/mL. Net price 1-mL vial = £1.70

## TRIAMCINOLONE HEXACETONIDE
*Indications:* local inflammation of joints and soft tissues
*Cautions; Contra-indications; Side-effects:* see notes above and section 6.3.3
*Dose: by intra-articular, intrasynovial, or soft-tissue injection*, 2–30 mg, according to joint size or amount of soft tissue, repeated at intervals of not less than 3–4 weeks according to the response
*By intracutaneous injection* of a suspension containing not more than 5 mg/mL, up to 500 micrograms/square inch of affected skin

PoM **Lederspan**® (Lederle)
*Injection* (aqueous suspension), triamcinolone hexacetonide 5 mg/mL. For intralesional or sublesional injection. Net price 5-mL vial = £2.92
*Injection* (aqueous suspension), triamcinolone hexacetonide 20 mg/mL. For intra-articular or intrasynovial injection. Net price 1-mL vial = £2.54; 5-mL vial = £9.90

## 10.1.3    Drugs which suppress the rheumatic disease process

Certain drugs such as gold, penicillamine, hydroxychloroquine, chloroquine, immunosuppressants, and sulphasalazine may affect the disease process in *rheumatoid arthritis*, as may gold and immunosuppressants in *psoriatic arthritis*. Unlike NSAIDs they do not produce an immediate therapeutic effect but require 4 to 6 months of treatment for a full response. If one of these drugs does not lead to objective benefit within 6 months, it should be discontinued.

These drugs may improve not only the symptoms and signs of inflammatory joint disease but also extra-articular manifestations such as vasculitis. They reduce the erythrocyte sedimentation rate and sometimes the titre of rheumatoid factor. Some (e.g. the immunosuppressants) may retard erosive damage as judged radiologically.

These drugs are used in rheumatoid arthritis where treatment with NSAIDs has been unsuccessful, so that there is evidence of disease progression including continuing active joint inflammation and worsening radiological changes. Since, in the first few months, the course of rheumatoid arthritis is unpredictable, it is usual to delay treatment for about 6 months depending on the progress of the disease, but treatment should be initiated before joint damage becomes irreversible.

Penicillamine and immunosuppressants are also sometimes used in rheumatoid arthritis where there are troublesome extra-articular features such as vasculitis, and in patients who are taking excessive doses of corticosteroids. Where the response is satisfactory there is often a striking reduction in requirements of both corticosteroids and other drugs. Gold, penicillamine, and related drugs may also be used to treat *juvenile arthritis* (Still's disease) when indications are similar.

Gold and penicillamine are effective in *palindromic rheumatism* and chloroquine is sometimes used to treat *systemic* and *discoid lupus erythematosus*.

### GOLD

**Gold** may be given by intramuscular injection as sodium aurothiomalate or by mouth as auranofin.
**Sodium aurothiomalate** must be given by deep intramuscular injection and the area gently massaged. A test dose of 10 mg must be given followed by doses of 50 mg at weekly intervals until there is definite evidence of remission. Benefit is not to

be expected until about 300 to 500 mg has been given; if there is no remission after 1 g has been given it should be discontinued. In patients who do respond, the interval between injections is then gradually increased to 4 weeks and treatment is continued for up to 5 years after complete remission. If relapse occurs dosage may be immediately increased to 50 mg weekly and only once control has been obtained again should the dosage be reduced. It is important to avoid complete relapse since second courses of gold are not usually effective. Children may be given 1 mg/kg weekly to a maximum of 50 mg weekly, the intervals being gradually increased to 4 weeks according to response; an initial test dose is given corresponding to one-tenth to one-fifth of the calculated dose.

Auranofin is given by mouth. If there is no response after 9 months treatment should be discontinued.

Gold therapy should be discontinued in the presence of blood disorders or proteinuria (associated with immune complex nephritis) which is repeatedly above 300 mg/litre without other cause (such as urinary-tract infection). Urine tests and full blood counts (including total and differential white cell and platelet counts) must therefore be performed before each intramuscular injection; in the case of oral treatment the urine and blood tests should be carried out monthly. Rashes with pruritus often occur after 2 to 6 months of intramuscular treatment and may necessitate discontinuation of treatment; the most common side-effect of oral therapy, diarrhoea with or without nausea or abdominal pain, may respond to bulking agents (such as bran) or temporary reduction in dosage.

## SODIUM AUROTHIOMALATE

*Indications:* active progressive rheumatoid arthritis, juvenile arthritis

*Cautions:* see notes above; patients should report pruritus, metallic taste, fever, sore throat or tongue, buccal ulceration, purpura, epistaxis, bleeding gums, bruising, menorrhagia, diarrhoea; renal and hepatic impairment, elderly, breast-feeding, history of urticaria, eczema, colitis, drugs which cause blood disorders; annual chest x-ray

*Contra-indications:* severe renal and hepatic disease (see notes above); history of blood disorders or bone marrow aplasia, exfoliative dermatitis, systemic lupus erythematosus, necrotising enterocolitis, pulmonary fibrosis; pregnancy (see Appendix 4); porphyria (see section 9.8.2)

*Side-effects:* severe reactions (occasionally fatal) in up to 5% of patients; mouth ulcers, skin reactions, proteinuria, blood disorders (sometimes sudden and fatal); rarely colitis, peripheral neuritis, pulmonary fibrosis, hepatotoxicity with cholestatic jaundice, alopecia

*Dose:* by deep intramuscular injection, administered on expert advice, see notes above

PoM **Myocrisin**® (Rhône-Poulenc Rorer)
*Injection 10 mg*, sodium aurothiomalate 20 mg/mL. Net price 0.5-mL amp = £1.34
*Injection 20 mg*, sodium aurothiomalate 40 mg/mL. Net price 0.5-mL amp = £1.95
*Injection 50 mg*, sodium aurothiomalate 100 mg/mL. Net price 0.5-mL amp = £3.97

## AURANOFIN

*Indications:* active progressive rheumatoid arthritis when NSAIDs inadequate alone

*Cautions; Contra-indications:* see under Sodium Aurothiomalate

*Side-effects:* diarrhoea most common (reduced by bulking agents such as bran); see also under Sodium Aurothiomalate

*Dose:* administered on expert advice, 6 mg daily (initially in 2 divided doses then if tolerated as single dose), if response inadequate after 6 months, increase to 9 mg daily (in 3 divided doses), discontinue if no response after a further 3 months

PoM **Ridaura**® (Bencard)
*Tablets*, pale yellow, f/c, auranofin 3 mg. Net price 60-tab pack = £28.00. Label: 21

## PENICILLAMINE

**Penicillamine** has a similar action to gold, and more patients are able to continue treatment than with gold but side-effects occur frequently. An initial dose of 125 to 250 mg daily before food is given for 1 month, increased by this amount every 4 to 12 weeks until remission occurs. Penicillamine should be discontinued if there is no improvement within 1 year. The usual maintenance dose is 500 to 750 mg daily, but up to 1.5 g may rarely be required.

Patients should be warned not to expect improvement for at least 6 to 12 weeks after treatment is initiated. If remission has been sustained for 6 months, reduction of dosage by 125 to 250 mg every 12 weeks may be attempted.

Blood counts, including platelets, and urine examinations should be carried out every 1 or 2 weeks for the first 2 months then every 4 weeks to detect blood disorders and proteinuria. A reduction in platelet count indicates that treatment with penicillamine should be stopped, subsequently re-introduced at a lower dosage level and then, if possible, gradually increased. Proteinuria, associated with immune complex nephritis, occurs in up to 30% of patients, but may resolve despite continuation of treatment; treatment may be continued provided that renal function tests remain normal, oedema is absent, and the 24-hour urinary excretion of protein does not exceed 2 g.

Nausea may occur but is not usually a problem provided that penicillamine is taken before food or on retiring and that low initial doses are used and only gradually increased. Loss of taste may occur about 6 weeks after treatment is started but usually returns 6 weeks later irrespective of whether or not treatment is discontinued; mineral supplements are not recommended. Rashes are a common side-effect. Those which occur in the first few months of treatment disappear when the drug is stopped and treatment may then be re-introduced at a lower dose level and gradually increased. Late rashes are more resistant and often necessitate discontinuation of treatment.

## PENICILLAMINE

*Indications:* severe active or progressive rheumatoid arthritis, juvenile arthritis. For use in Wilson's disease, see section 9.8
For use in copper and lead poisoning, see Emergency Treatment of Poisoning
*Cautions:* see notes above; renal impairment, pregnancy, and portal hypertension; avoid concurrent gold, chloroquine, hydroxychloroquine, or immunosuppressive treatment; **interactions:** Appendix 1 (penicillamine)
*Contra-indications:* lupus erythematosus
*Side-effects:* hypersensitivity reactions (may necessitate discontinuation of treatment); nausea, anorexia, taste loss, mouth ulcers, skin reactions (see notes above), oedema, proteinuria, agranulocytosis or severe thrombocytopenia (sometimes fatal); rarely myasthenia, febrile reactions, lupus erythematosus
*Dose:* rheumatoid arthritis, administered on expert advice, ADULT, see notes above; CHILD initial dose, 50 mg daily before food for 1 month, increased at 4-week intervals to a maintenance dose of 15–20 mg/kg daily

PoM **Penicillamine** (Non-proprietary)
*Tablets*, coated, penicillamine 125 mg, net price 20 = £2.70; 250 mg, 20 = £4.67. Label: 6, 22
Available from Cox, Evans
PoM **Distamine**® (Dista)
*Tablets*, all f/c, penicillamine 50 mg (scored), net price 20 = £1.09; 125 mg, 20 = £2.17; 250 mg, 20 = £3.74. Label: 6, 22
PoM **Pendramine**® (ASTA Medica)
*Tablets*, both scored, f/c, penicillamine 125 mg, net price 20 = £2.98; 250 mg, 20 = £5.13. Label: 6, 22

## ANTIMALARIALS

**Chloroquine** and **hydroxychloroquine** have a similar action to, and are better tolerated than, gold or penicillamine but their use is limited by their ocular toxicity. However, retinopathy is rare provided the doses given below are not exceeded. Nevertheless, all patients should have a full ophthalmic examination before starting treatment and then subsequently at intervals of 3 to 6 months. Ocular toxicity is also reduced if the drug is not given continuously for longer than 2 years and some physicians advise their patients to stop treatment for 2 months of each year.

These drugs should not be used for psoriatic arthritis and are best **avoided** in elderly patients as it is difficult to distinguish ageing changes from drug-induced retinopathy.

They are also used in systemic lupus erythematosus (section 10.1.2.1).
**Mepacrine** (see section 5.4.4) is sometimes used in discoid lupus erythematosus.

## CHLOROQUINE

*Indications:* active rheumatoid arthritis (including juvenile arthritis), systemic and discoid lupus erythematosus; malaria, see section 5.4.1
*Cautions:* hepatic and renal impairment, pregnancy (but for malaria benefit outweighs risk, see Appendix 4, Antimalarials), porphyria, may exacerbate psoriasis, neurological disorders (especially history of epilepsy), severe gastro-intestinal disorders, G6PD deficiency (see section 9.1.5); elderly (see notes above); regular ophthalmic examinations required (see notes above); avoid concurrent therapy with hepatotoxic drugs—other **interactions:** Appendix 1 (chloroquine)
*Side-effects:* gastro-intestinal disturbances, headache, visual disturbances, irreversible retinal damage, corneal opacities, depigmentation or loss of hair, skin reactions; rarely blood disorders (thrombocytopenia, agranulocytosis and aplastic anaemia)
*Dose:* administered on expert advice, chloroquine 150 mg daily preferably after food; CHILD, 3 mg/kg daily
*Note.* Chloroquine base 150 mg ≡ chloroquine sulphate 200 mg ≡ chloroquine phosphate 250 mg (approx.).

**Preparations**
See section 5.4.1

## HYDROXYCHLOROQUINE SULPHATE

*Indications:* active rheumatoid arthritis (including juvenile arthritis), systemic and discoid lupus erythematosus
*Cautions; Side-effects:* see under Chloroquine and notes (above)
*Dose:* administered on expert advice, initially 400 mg daily in divided doses; maintenance 200–400 mg daily; max. 6.5 mg/kg daily; CHILD, up to 6.5 mg/kg daily (dosage form not suitable for children who weigh less than 33 kg)

PoM **Plaquenil**® (Sanofi Winthrop)
*Tablets*, orange, s/c, hydroxychloroquine sulphate 200 mg. Net price 56-tab pack = £19.36. Label: 5

## IMMUNOSUPPRESSANTS

When used in *rheumatoid arthritis* **immunosuppressants** have a similar action to gold and are useful alternatives in cases that have failed to respond to gold, penicillamine, chloroquine, or hydroxychloroquine.

**Azathioprine** (see section 8.2.1) is usually chosen and is given in a dose of 1.5 to 2.5 mg/kg daily in divided doses. Blood counts should be carried out every 4 weeks to detect possible neutropenia and/or thrombocytopenia which is usually resolved by reducing the dose. Nausea, vomiting, and diarrhoea may occur, usually starting early during the course of treatment, and may necessitate withdrawal of the drug; herpes zoster infection may also occur.

**Methotrexate** (see section 8.1.3) has also been shown to be effective. It is usually given in an initial dose of 2.5 mg by mouth once a week, increased slowly to a maximum of 15 mg once a week, subject to regular full blood counts (including differential white cell count and platelet count) and liver-function tests initially weekly and monthly thereafter.

**Chlorambucil** (see section 8.1.1) is another immunosuppressant which is used in rheumatoid arthritis; a dose of 100 to 200 micrograms/kg daily is usually given initially; most patients require between 2.5 and 7.5 mg daily. Regular blood counts including platelets should be carried out.

**Cyclophosphamide** (see section 8.1.1) is more toxic but may be used at a dose of 1 to 1.5 mg/kg daily for rheumatoid arthritis with severe systemic manifestations.

Immunosuppressants are also used in the management of severe cases of *systemic lupus erythematosus* and other connective tissue disorders. They are often given in conjunction with corticosteroids for patients with severe or progressive renal disease though the evidence for their benefit is doubtful. They may be used in cases of *polymyositis* which are resistant to corticosteroids. They are used for their corticosteroid-sparing effect in patients whose corticosteroid requirements are excessive. **Azathioprine** is usually used but **chlorambucil** is an alternative.

Azathioprine and methotrexate are used in the treatment of *psoriatic arthropathy* for severe or progressive cases which are not controlled with anti-inflammatory drugs. There is an impression that **azathioprine** is the more effective for psoriatic arthritis and that **methotrexate** is the more effective for skin manifestations. Methotrexate is usually given in a dose of 10–25 mg once a week by mouth. Regular full blood counts and liver-function tests should be carried out initially weekly and monthly thereafter.

SULPHASALAZINE

**Sulphasalazine** was initially introduced for the treatment of rheumatoid arthritis. Recent re-evaluation has confirmed that it has a beneficial effect in suppressing the inflammatory activity of rheumatoid arthritis. Side-effects include rashes, gastro-intestinal intolerance and, especially in patients with rheumatoid arthritis, occasional leucopenia, neutropenia, and thrombocytopenia. These haematological abnormalities occur usually in the first 3 to 6 months of treatment and are reversible on cessation of treatment. Close monitoring of full blood counts (including differential white cell count and platelet count) is necessary throughout treatment of rheumatoid arthritis, monthly during the first 6 months and 3-monthly thereafter, liver function tests being performed at the same time.

## SULPHASALAZINE

**Indications:** active rheumatoid arthritis; ulcerative colitis, see section 1.5

**Cautions; Contra-indications; Side-effects:** see section 1.5

**Dose:** *by mouth*, administered on expert advice, as enteric-coated tablets, initially 500 mg daily, increased by 500 mg at intervals of 1 week to a max. of 2–3 g daily in divided doses

PoM **Salazopyrin EN-tabs**® (Kabi Pharmacia)
Tablets, e/c, yellow, f/c, sulphasalazine 500 mg. Net price 125-tab pack = £12.75. Label: 5, 14, 25, counselling, see lenses section 1.5

## 10.1.4 Drugs used in the treatment of gout

It is important to distinguish drugs used for the treatment of acute attacks of gout from those used in the long-term control of the disease. The latter exacerbate and prolong the acute manifestations if started during an attack.

ACUTE ATTACKS

Acute attacks of gout are usually treated with high doses of **NSAIDs** such as azapropazone, diclofenac, indomethacin, ketoprofen, naproxen, piroxicam, and sulindac (section 10.1.1). Colchicine is an alternative. Aspirin is **contra-indicated** in gout. Allopurinol and uricosurics are not effective in treating an acute attack and may prolong it indefinitely if started during the acute episode.

**Indomethacin** is often chosen in acute attacks. High doses are usually well tolerated for short periods (50 to 100 mg repeated after a few hours if necessary and followed by reducing doses every 6 hours as the patient improves). If courses of treatment last for less than one week side-effects are unusual despite the high doses used.

**Colchicine** is probably as effective as indomethacin. Its use is limited by the development of toxicity at higher doses, but it is of value in patients with heart failure since, unlike NSAIDs, it does not induce fluid retention; moreover it can be given to patients receiving anticoagulants.

## COLCHICINE

**Indications:** acute gout, short-term prophylaxis during initial therapy with allopurinol and uricosuric drugs

**Cautions:** gastro-intestinal disease, renal impairment, pregnancy and breast-feeding

**Side-effects:** most common are nausea, vomiting, and abdominal pain; excessive doses may also cause profuse diarrhoea, gastro-intestinal haemorrhage, rashes, and renal damage. Rarely peripheral neuritis, alopecia, and with prolonged treatment blood disorders

*Dose:* 1 mg initially, followed by 500 micrograms every 2–3 hours until relief of pain is obtained or vomiting or diarrhoea occurs, or until a total dose of 10 mg has been reached. The course should not be repeated within 3 days

Prevention of attacks during initial treatment with allopurinol or uricosuric drugs, 500 micrograms 2–3 times daily

PoM **Colchicine** (Non-proprietary)
*Tablets*, colchicine 500 micrograms, net price 20 = 66p

---

## INTERVAL TREATMENT

For long-term ('interval') control of gout the formation of uric acid from purines may be reduced with the **xanthine-oxidase inhibitor** allopurinol, or the **uricosuric drugs** probenecid or sulphinpyrazone may be used to increase the excretion of uric acid in the urine. Treatment should be continued indefinitely once the decision has been made to prevent further attacks of gout by correcting the hyperuricaemia. These drugs should never be started during an acute attack. The initiation of treatment may precipitate an acute attack therefore colchicine or an anti-inflammatory analgesic should be used as a prophylactic and continued for at least one month after the hyperuricaemia has been corrected (usually about 3 months of prophylaxis).

**Allopurinol** is a convenient well tolerated drug which is now widely used. It is especially useful in patients with renal impairment or urate stones where uricosuric drugs cannot be used. It is usually given once daily, as the active metabolite of allopurinol has a long half-life, but doses over 300 mg daily should be divided. Allopurinol treatment should not be started until an acute attack of gout has completely subsided, as further attacks may be precipitated. It is well tolerated in most patients but may occasionally cause rashes.

The uricosuric drugs include **probenecid** and **sulphinpyrazone**. They can be used instead of allopurinol, or in conjunction with it in cases that are resistant to treatment.

If an acute attack develops in a patient taking allopurinol or a uricosuric the treatment should continue at the same dosage while the acute attack is treated in its own right.

**Azapropazone** (section 10.1.1) also has a uricosuric effect and may be useful in the long-term treatment of chronic gout.

Aspirin and salicylates antagonise the uricosuric drugs; they do not antagonise allopurinol but are nevertheless **contra-indicated** in gout.

Crystallisation of urate in the urine may occur with the uricosuric drugs and it is important to ensure that there is an adequate urine output especially in the first few weeks of treatment. As an additional precaution the urine may be rendered alkaline.

The **NSAIDs** are described in section 10.1.1.

## ALLOPURINOL

*Indications:* gout prophylaxis, hyperuricaemia
*Cautions:* administer prophylactic colchicine or NSAID (*not* aspirin or salicylates) until at least 1 month after hyperuricaemia corrected; ensure adequate fluid intake (2 litres/day); hepatic and renal impairment. In neoplastic conditions treatment with allopurinol (if required) should be commenced before cytotoxic drugs are given; **interactions:** Appendix 1 (allopurinol)
*Contra-indications:* not a treatment for acute gout but continue if attack develops when already receiving allopurinol, and treat attack separately (see notes above)
*Side-effects:* rashes, sometimes with fever (withdraw therapy; if rash mild re-introduce cautiously but discontinue immediately if recurrence); gastro-intestinal disorders. Rarely malaise, headache, vertigo, drowsiness, taste disturbances, hypertension, symptomless xanthine deposits in muscle, alopecia, hepatotoxicity
*Dose:* initially 100 mg daily as a single dose, after food, gradually increased over 1–3 weeks according to the plasma or urinary uric acid concentration, to about 300 mg daily; usual maintenance dose 200–600 mg, rarely 900 mg daily, divided into doses of not more than 300 mg; CHILD (in neoplastic conditions, enzyme disorders) 10–20 mg/kg daily

PoM **Allopurinol** (Non-proprietary)
*Tablets*, allopurinol 100 mg, net price 20 = 50p; 300 mg, 20 = £1.74. Label: 8, 21, 27
Available from APS, Ashbourne (Xanthomax®), Berk (Caplenal®), Cox, DDSA (Cosuric®), Evans, Kerfoot, Lagap (Aloral®), Nicholas (Hamarin®), Rima (Rimapurinol®)

PoM **Zyloric®** (Wellcome)
*Tablets*, allopurinol 100 mg, net price 20 = £4.06; 300 mg, 28-tab pack = £14.56. Label: 8, 21, 27

---

## PROBENECID

*Indications:* gout prophylaxis, hyperuricaemia; reduction of tubular excretion of penicillins and certain cephalosporins, see section 5.1
*Cautions:* during initial gout therapy administer prophylactic colchicine or NSAID (*not* aspirin or salicylates), ensure adequate fluid intake (about 2 litres daily), render urine alkaline if uric acid overload is high; peptic ulceration, renal impairment (avoid if severe); transient false-positive Benedict's test; G6PD-deficiency (see section 9.1.5); **interactions:** Appendix 1 (probenecid)
*Contra-indications:* history of blood disorders, nephrolithiasis, porphyria (see section 9.8.2), acute gout attack and 3 weeks after; avoid aspirin and salicylates
*Side-effects:* infrequent; occasionally nausea and vomiting, urinary frequency, headache, flushing, dizziness, rashes; rarely hypersensitivity, nephrotic syndrome, hepatic necrosis, aplastic anaemia

---

*Dose:* uricosuric therapy, initially 250 mg twice daily after food, increased after a week to 500 mg twice daily then up to 2 g daily in 2–4 divided doses according to plasma-uric acid concentration and reduced for maintenance

PoM **Benemid**® (MSD)
*Tablets*, scored, probenecid 500 mg. Net price 20 = 55p. Label: 12, 21, 27

## SULPHINPYRAZONE

*Indications:* gout prophylaxis, hyperuricaemia
*Cautions; Contra-indications:* see under Probenecid; regular blood counts advisable; avoid in hypersensitivity to NSAIDs; **interactions:** Appendix 1 (sulphinpyrazone)
*Side-effects:* gastro-intestinal disturbances, occasionally allergic skin reactions; rarely blood disorders, gastro-intestinal ulceration and bleeding, acute renal failure, raised liver enzymes, jaundice and hepatitis
*Dose:* initially 100–200 mg daily with food (or milk) increasing over 2–3 weeks to 600 mg daily (rarely 800 mg daily), continued until serum uric acid concentration normal then reduced for maintenance

PoM **Anturan**® (Geigy)
*Tablets*, both yellow, s/c, sulphinpyrazone 100 mg, net price 20 = 94p; 200 mg, 84-tab pack = £7.82. Label: 12, 21

# 10.2  Drugs used in neuromuscular disorders

## 10.2.1  Drugs which enhance neuromuscular transmission

Anticholinesterases are used as first-line treatment in *myasthenia gravis*.

Corticosteroids are only given concomitantly if anticholinesterase treatment is failing.

Plasmapheresis may produce temporary remission in otherwise unresponsive patients.

## ANTICHOLINESTERASES

Anticholinesterase drugs are used to enhance neuromuscular transmission in voluntary and involuntary muscle in myasthenia gravis. They prolong the action of acetylcholine by inhibiting the action of the enzyme acetylcholinesterase. Excessive dosage of these drugs may impair neuromuscular transmission and precipitate 'cholinergic crises' by causing a depolarising block. This may be difficult to distinguish from a worsening myasthenic state.

Side-effects of anticholinesterases are due to their parasympathomimetic action. Muscarinic effects include increased sweating, salivary, and gastric secretion, also increased gastro-intestinal and uterine motility, and bradycardia. These effects are antagonised by atropine.

**Edrophonium** has a very brief action and is therefore used mainly for the diagnosis of myas-

thenia gravis. A single test-dose usually causes substantial improvement in muscle power (lasting about 5 minutes) in patients with the disease (if respiration already impaired, *only* in conjunction with someone skilled at intubation).

It can also be used to determine whether a patient with myasthenia is receiving inadequate or excessive treatment with cholinergic drugs. If treatment is excessive an injection of edrophonium will either have no effect or will intensify symptoms (if respiration already impaired, *only* in conjunction with someone skilled at intubation). Conversely, transient improvement may be seen if the patient is being inadequately treated. The test is best performed just before the next dose of anticholinesterase.

**Neostigmine** produces a therapeutic effect for up to 4 hours. Its pronounced muscarinic action is a disadvantage, and simultaneous administration of an antimuscarinic drug such as atropine or propantheline may be required to prevent colic, excessive salivation, or diarrhoea. In severe disease neostigmine may be given every 2 hours. The maximum that most patients can tolerate is 180 mg daily.

**Pyridostigmine** is less powerful and slower in action than neostigmine but it has a longer duration of action. It is preferable to neostigmine because of its smoother action and the need for less frequent dosage. It is particularly preferred in patients whose muscles are weak on wakening. It has a comparatively mild gastro-intestinal effect but an antimuscarinic drug may still be required. It is inadvisable to exceed a daily dose of 720 mg.

**Distigmine** has the most protracted action but the danger of a 'cholinergic crisis' caused by accumulation of the drug is greater than with shorter-acting drugs.

Neostigmine and edrophonium are also used to reverse the actions of the non-depolarising muscle relaxants (see section 15.1.6).

## NEOSTIGMINE

*Indications:* myasthenia gravis; other indications, see section 15.1.6
*Cautions:* asthma, bradycardia, recent myocardial infarction, epilepsy, hypotension, parkinsonism, vagotonia, peptic ulceration, pregnancy. Atropine or other antidote to muscarinic effects may be necessary (particularly when neostigmine is given by injection), but it should not be given routinely as it may mask signs of overdosage; **interactions:** Appendix 1 (cholinergics)
*Contra-indications:* intestinal or urinary obstruction
*Side-effects:* nausea, vomiting, increased salivation, diarrhoea, abdominal cramps (more marked with higher doses). Signs of overdosage are increased gastro-intestinal discomfort, bronchial secretions, and sweating, involuntary defaecation and micturition, miosis, nystagmus, bradycardia, hypotension, agitation, excessive dreaming, and weakness eventually leading to fasciculation and paralysis

*Dose: by mouth,* neostigmine bromide 15–30 mg at suitable intervals throughout day, total daily dose 75–300 mg (but see also notes above); NEONATE 1–5 mg every 4 hours, half an hour before feeds; CHILD up to 6 years initially 7.5 mg, 6–12 years initially 15 mg, usual total daily dose 15–90 mg

*By subcutaneous or intramuscular injection,* neostigmine methylsulphate 1–2.5 mg at suitable intervals throughout day (usual total daily dose 5–20 mg); NEONATE 50–250 micrograms every 4 hours; CHILD 200–500 micrograms as required

PoM **Prostigmin**® (Roche)
*Tablets,* scored, neostigmine bromide 15 mg. Net price 20 = 53p
*Injection,* neostigmine methylsulphate 500 micrograms/mL, net price 1-mL amp = 16p; 2.5 mg/mL, 1-mL amp = 16p

## DISTIGMINE BROMIDE
*Indications:* myasthenia gravis; urinary retention and other indications, see section 7.4.1
*Cautions; Contra-indications; Side-effects:* see under Neostigmine
*Dose:* initially 5 mg daily half an hour before breakfast, increased at intervals of 3–4 days if necessary to a max. of 20 mg daily; CHILD up to 10 mg daily according to age

**Preparations**
See section 7.4.1

## EDROPHONIUM CHLORIDE
*Indications:* see under Dose and notes above; surgery, see section 15.1.6
*Cautions; Contra-indications; Side-effects:* see under Neostigmine; *great* caution in respiratory distress (see notes above)
*Note.* Severe cholinergic reactions can be counteracted by injection of atropine sulphate (which should always be available)
*Dose:* diagnosis of myasthenia gravis, *by intravenous injection,* 2 mg followed after 30 seconds (if no adverse reaction has occurred) by 8 mg; in adults without suitable veins, *by intramuscular injection,* 10 mg
Detection of overdosage or underdosage of cholinergic drugs, *by intravenous injection,* 2 mg (best before next dose of anticholinesterase, see notes above)
CHILD *by intravenous injection* 20 micrograms/ kg followed after 30 seconds (if no adverse reaction has occurred) by 80 micrograms/kg

PoM **Tensilon**® (Roche)
*Injection,* edrophonium chloride 10 mg/mL. Net price 1-mL amp = 27p

## PYRIDOSTIGMINE BROMIDE
*Indications:* myasthenia gravis
*Cautions; Contra-indications; Side-effects:* see under Neostigmine; weaker muscarinic action

*Dose: by mouth,* 30–120 mg at suitable intervals throughout day, total daily dose 0.3–1.2 g (but see also notes above); NEONATE 5–10 mg every 4 hours, ½–1 hour before feeds; CHILD up to 6 years initially 30 mg, 6–12 years initially 60 mg, usual total daily dose 30–360 mg

PoM **Mestinon**® (Roche)
*Tablets,* scored, pyridostigmine bromide 60 mg. Net price 20 = £1.01

## IMMUNOSUPPRESSANT THERAPY

**Corticosteroids** (see section 6.3) are established as treatment for myasthenia gravis where *thymectomy* is inadvisable or to reduce the risk of surgery beforehand. The initial dose may be high (up to 100 mg **prednisolone** daily) but most advise starting with a smaller dose (20 mg prednisolone daily) and gradually increasing it. There is grave risk of exacerbation of the myasthenia during the initial stages of therapy, particularly in the first 2–3 weeks, therefore inpatient supervision is essential. Improvement usually begins after about 2 weeks on the high-dose regimen. In some patients a prolonged remission may be induced, but often patients need a maintenance dose of 10–40 mg of prednisolone daily; alternate-day therapy is popular. Patients who need a corticosteroid may benefit from the addition of **azathioprine** (see section 8.2.1) in a dose of 2 mg/kg daily which may allow a reduction in corticosteroid dosage.

## 10.2.2   Skeletal muscle relaxants
Drugs described below are used for the relief of chronic muscle spasm or spasticity; they are not indicated for spasm associated with minor injuries. They act principally on the central nervous system with the exception of dantrolene which has a peripheral site of action. They differ in action from the muscle relaxants used in anaesthesia (see section 15.1.5) which block transmission of impulses at the neuromuscular junction.

The underlying cause of spasticity should be treated and any aggravating factors (e.g. pressure sores, infection) remedied. Skeletal muscle relaxants are effective in most forms of spasticity except the rare alpha variety. The major disadvantage of treatment with these drugs is that reduction in muscle tone can cause a loss of splinting action of the spastic leg and trunk muscles and sometimes lead to an increase in disability.

**Dantrolene** acts directly on skeletal muscle and produces fewer central adverse effects making it a drug of choice. The dose should be increased slowly.

**Baclofen** inhibits transmission at spinal level and also depresses the central nervous system. The dose should be increased slowly to avoid the major side-effects of sedation and hypotonia (other adverse events are uncommon).

**Diazepam** may also be used. Sedation and, occasionally, extensor hypotonus are disadvantages. Other benzodiazepines also have muscle-relaxant properties. Muscle-relaxant doses of benzodiazepines are similar to anxiolytic doses (see section 4.1.2).

**Clonazepam** (see section 4.8) may sometimes help in myoclonus.

**Quinine** salts (see section 5.4.1) 200 to 300 mg at bedtime are effective in relieving nocturnal leg cramps. They are toxic in overdosage and accidental fatalities have occurred in children.

## BACLOFEN

*Indications:* chronic severe spasticity of voluntary muscle

*Cautions:* psychiatric illness, cerebrovascular disease, elderly; respiratory, hepatic, or renal impairment; epilepsy; hypertonic bladder sphincter; pregnancy; avoid abrupt withdrawal; avoid in peptic ulceration and in porphyria (see section 9.8.2); **interactions:** Appendix 1 (muscle relaxants)

DRIVING. Drowsiness may affect performance of skilled tasks (e.g. driving); effects of alcohol enhanced

*Side-effects:* frequently sedation, drowsiness, nausea; occasionally lightheadedness, lassitude, confusion, dizziness, ataxia, hallucinations, headache, euphoria, insomnia, depression, tremor, nystagmus, paraesthesias, convulsions, muscular pain and weakness, respiratory or cardiovascular depression, hypotension, gastro-intestinal and urinary disturbances; rarely visual disorders, taste alterations, increased sweating, rash, altered liver function, and paradoxical increase in spasticity

*Dose:* 5 mg 3 times daily, preferably after food, gradually increased; max. 100 mg daily; CHILD 0.75–2 mg/kg daily (over 10 years, max. 2.5 mg/kg daily) *or* 2.5 mg 4 times daily increased gradually according to age to maintenance: 1–2 years 10–20 mg daily, 2–6 years 20–30 mg daily, 6–10 years 30–60 mg daily

PoM **Baclofen** (Non-proprietary)
*Tablets,* baclofen 10 mg. Net price 20 = £2.43. Label: 2, 8
Available from APS, Ashbourne (Baclospas®), Cox, Evans, Kerfoot

PoM **Lioresal**® (Geigy)
*Tablets,* scored, baclofen 10 mg. Net price 20 = £2.34. Label: 2, 8
Additives: include gluten
*Liquid,* sugar-free, baclofen 5 mg/5 mL. Diluent purified water, freshly boiled and cooled, life of diluted liquid 14 days. Net price 300 mL = £6.16. Label: 2, 8

## DANTROLENE SODIUM

*Indications:* chronic severe spasticity of voluntary muscle

*Cautions:* impaired cardiac, pulmonary, and liver function; test liver function before and at intervals during therapy. Therapeutic effect may take a few weeks to develop but if treatment is ineffective it should be discontinued after 4–6 weeks. Avoid in children or when spasticity is useful, for example, locomotion; **interactions:** Appendix 1 (muscle relaxants).

DRIVING. Drowsiness may affect performance of skilled tasks (e.g. driving); effects of alcohol enhanced

*Side-effects:* transient drowsiness, dizziness, weakness, malaise, fatigue, diarrhoea (withdraw if severe, discontinue treatment if recurs on re-introduction), anorexia, nausea, headache, rash; less frequently constipation, dysphagia, speech and visual disturbances, confusion, nervousness, insomnia, depression, seizures, chills, fever, increased urinary frequency; rarely, tachycardia, erratic blood pressure, dyspnoea, haematuria, possible crystalluria, urinary incontinence or retention, pleural effusion, pericarditis, dose-related hepatotoxicity (occasionally fatal) may be more common in women over 30 especially those taking oestrogens

*Dose:* initially 25 mg daily, may be increased at weekly intervals to max. of 100 mg 4 times daily; usual dose 75 mg 3 times daily

PoM **Dantrium**® (Norwich Eaton)
*Capsules,* both orange/brown, dantrolene sodium 25 mg, net price 20 = £3.11; 100 mg, 20 = £10.88. Label: 2
*Injection*—see section 15.1.8

## DIAZEPAM

*Indications:* muscle spasm of varied aetiology, including tetanus; other indications, see sections 4.1.2, 4.8, 15.1.4.2

*Cautions; Contra-indications; Side-effects:* see section 4.1.2; also hypotonia; special precautions for intravenous injection (see section 4.8.2)

*Dose: by mouth,* 2–15 mg daily in divided doses, increased if necessary in spastic conditions to 60 mg daily according to response
Cerebral spasticity in selected cases, CHILD 2–40 mg daily in divided doses

*By intramuscular or slow intravenous injection,* in acute muscle spasm, 10 mg repeated if necessary after 4 hours; CHILD, 100–200 micrograms/kg, repeated if necessary
Tetanus, *by intravenous injection,* 100–300 micrograms/kg repeated every 1–4 hours; *by intravenous infusion (or by nasoduodenal tube),* 3–10 mg/kg over 24 hours, adjusted according to response

**Preparations**
See section 4.1.2

## OTHER MUSCLE RELAXANTS

The clinical efficacy of carisoprodol, chlormezanone and meprobamate (see section 4.1.2), methocarbamol, and orphenadrine as muscle relaxants is **not** well established although they have been included in compound analgesic preparations.

## CARISOPRODOL

*Indications:* short-term symptomatic relief of muscle spasm (but see notes above)

*Cautions; Contra-indications; Side-effects:* see under Meprobamate, section 4.1.2. Drowsiness is common; avoid in porphyria (see section 9.8.2)

*Dose:* 350 mg 3 times daily; ELDERLY half adult dose or less

PoM **Carisoma®** (Pharmax)
*Tablets,* carisoprodol 125 mg, net price 20 = 76p; 350 mg, 20 = 84p. Label: 2

## METHOCARBAMOL

*Indications:* short-term symptomatic relief of muscle spasm (but see notes above)

*Cautions:* hepatic and renal impairment (avoid injection in renal impairment)

DRIVING. Drowsiness may affect performance of skilled tasks (e.g. driving); effects of alcohol enhanced

*Contra-indications:* coma or pre-coma, brain damage, epilepsy, myasthenia gravis

*Side-effects:* lassitude, light-headedness, dizziness, restlessness, anxiety, confusion, drowsiness, nausea, allergic rash or angioedema, convulsions

*Dose:* by mouth, 1.5 g 4 times daily (elderly 750 mg or less); may be reduced to 750 mg 3 times daily

*By slow intravenous injection or by infusion,* 1–3 g (max. rate 300 mg/min.); max. dose 3 g (elderly, 1.5 g) daily for 3 days

PoM **Robaxin®** (Wyeth)
*750 Tablets,* scored, methocarbamol 750 mg. Net price 20 = £2.36. Label: 2
*Injection,* methocarbamol 100 mg/mL in aqueous macrogol '300'. Net price 10-mL amp = £1.39
PoM **Robaxisal Forte®**: see section 4.7.1.1

## ORPHENADRINE CITRATE

*Indications:* short-term symptomatic relief of muscle spasm (but see notes above)

*Cautions:* see under Benzhexol Hydrochloride, section 4.9.2. Avoid in children and in porphyria (see section 9.8.2); reduce dose in elderly

*Side-effects:* dry mouth and other antimuscarinic side-effects; see also Orphenadrine Hydrochloride, section 4.9.2

*Dose:* by intramuscular or by slow intravenous injection (over 5 minutes), 60 mg repeated after 12 hours if necessary

PoM **Norflex®** (3M)
*Injection,* orphenadrine citrate 30 mg/mL. Net price 2-mL amp = 60p

# 10.3   Drugs for the relief of soft-tissue inflammation

10.3.1   Enzymes
10.3.2   Rubefacients and other topical antirheumatics

## 10.3.1   Enzymes

**Hyaluronidase** is used to render the tissues more easily permeable to injected fluids, e.g. for introduction of fluids by subcutaneous infusion (termed hypodermoclysis).

## HYALURONIDASE

*Indications:* enhance permeation of subcutaneous or intramuscular injections; promote resorption of excess fluids and blood

*Contra-indications:* intravenous route, bites or stings, infection or malignancy at site

*Dose:* to enhance tissue permeability, *by subcutaneous or intramuscular injection,* usually 1500 units, either mixed with the injection fluid or injected into the site before injection is administered

*By subcutaneous infusion,* 1500 units administered before 500–1000 mL infusion fluid

PoM **Hyalase®** (CP)
*Injection,* powder for reconstitution, hyaluronidase (ovine). Net price 1500-unit amp = £1.98

## 10.3.2   Rubefacients and other topical antirheumatics

**Rubefacients** act by counter-irritation. Pain, whether superficial or deep-seated, is relieved by any method which itself produces irritation of the skin. Counter-irritation is comforting in painful lesions of the muscles, tendons, and joints, and in non-articular rheumatism. Rubefacients probably all act through the same essential mechanism and differ mainly in intensity and duration of action.

Topical **NSAIDs** (e.g. benzydamine, felbinac, ibuprofen, salicylamide) may provide some slight relief of pain.

**Adrenaline** is inactive when applied topically.

CAUTIONS. Apply with gentle massage. Avoid contact with eyes, mucous membranes, and inflamed or broken skin. Not generally suitable for children. Liniments are very toxic if taken by mouth.

### COUNTER-IRRITANTS

**Algesal®** (Duphar)
*Cream,* diethylamine salicylate 10%. Net price 50 g = 75p. Apply 3 times daily

**Algipan®** (Whitehall)
*Cream,* methyl nicotinate 1%, capsicin oleoresin 0.1%, glycol salicylate 10%. Net price 40 g = 77p; 80 g = £1.23
*Spray application,* methyl nicotinate 1.5%, glycol salicylate 10%. Net price 120-mL aerosol spray = £1.15

**Aradolene®** (Fisons)
*Cream,* diethylamine salicylate 5%, 'capsicin water-soluble' 0.4%, menthol 2.5%, rectified camphor oil 1.4% in a lanolin basis. Net price 40 g = 76p

**Aspellin®** (Fisons)
*Liniment,* ammonium salicylate 1%, camphor 0.6%, menthol 1.4%, ethyl and methyl salicylate 0.54%. Net price 100 mL = 52p; 500 mL = £3.06; 150-mL spray can = 96p

**Balmosa®** (Pharmax)
*Cream,* camphor 4%, capsicin oleoresin 0.035%, menthol 2%, methyl salicylate 4%. Net price 40 g = 47p

---

**Bayolin®** (Bayer)

*Cream*, benzyl nicotinate 2.5%, glycol salicylate 10%, heparinoid 50 units/g. Net price 35 g = 70p. Apply 2–3 times daily

**Bengué's Balsam®** (Bengué)

*Ointment*, menthol 20%, methyl salicylate 20% in a lanolin basis. Net price 25 g = 82p

**Bengué's Balsam SG®** (Bengué)

*Cream*, menthol 10%, methyl salicylate 15% in a vanishing cream basis. Net price 25 g = 82p

**Cremalgin®** (Rhône-Poulenc Rorer)

*Balm* (= cream), capsicin 0.1%, glycol salicylate 10%, methyl nicotinate 1%. Net price 30 g = 57p. Apply 2–3 times daily

**Dubam®** (Norma)

*Spray application*, glycol salicylate 5%, methyl nicotinate 1.6%, methyl salicylate 1%, ethyl salicylate 4%. Net price 113-g aerosol spray = £2.68

**Transvasin®** (Seton)

*Cream*, benzocaine 2%, ethyl nicotinate 2%, hexyl nicotinate 2%, tetrahydrofurfuryl salicylate 14%. Net price 30 g = 68p. Apply at least twice daily

## POULTICES

**Kaolin Poultice,** heavy kaolin 52.7%, thymol 0.05%, boric acid 4.5%, peppermint oil 0.05%, methyl salicylate 0.2%, glycerol 42.5%. Net price 200 g = £1.35

Warm and apply directly or between layers of muslin; avoid application of overheated poultice

**Kaolin Poultice K/L Pack®** (K/L)

*Kaolin poultice.* Net price 4 × 100-g pouches = £3.62

## TOPICAL NSAIDs

*Note.* For NSAID asthma warning, see p. 349.

**Difflam®** (3M)

*Cream*, benzydamine hydrochloride 3%. Net price 15 g = £1.29; 50 g = £4.83; 100 g = £8.86. Apply 1–2.5 g (3.5–8.5 cm) 3–6 times daily for up to 10 days

PoM **Feldene® Gel** (Invicta)

*Gel*, piroxicam 0.5%. Net price 60 g = £7.77

Apply 1 g (3 cm) 3–4 times daily; therapy should be reviewed after 4 weeks; 30-g tube for short-term use, net price £3.89; starter pack, 7.5-g tube = 97p

**Intralgin®** (3M)

*Gel*, benzocaine 2%, salicylamide 5% in an alcoholic vehicle. Net price 50 g = 51p

**Movelat®** (Panpharma)

*Cream*, heparinoid 0.2%, salicylic acid 2%. Net price 100 g = £3.90. Apply up to 4 times daily

*Gel*, ingredients as for cream but in a colourless alcoholic basis. Net price 100 g = £3.90. Apply up to 4 times daily

PoM **Oruvail® Gel** (Rhône-Poulenc Rorer)

*Gel*, ketoprofen 2.5%. Net price 100 g = £6.95

Apply 2–4 times daily for up to 7 days (usual recommended dose 15 g daily)

**Proflex®** (Zyma)

*Cream*, ibuprofen 5%. Net price 100 g = £8.70. Apply 4–10 cm 3–4 times daily

*Note.* Proprietary brands of topical ibuprofen (Ibugel®, Ibuleve®) are on sale to the public

PoM **Traxam®** (Lederle)

*Gel*, felbinac 3%. Net price 50 g = £8.72.

Apply 2–4 times daily; max. 25 g daily; therapy should be reviewed after 14 days

*Note.* Felbinac is an active metabolite of the NSAID fenbufen

PoM **Voltarol® Emulgel** (Geigy)

*Gel*, diclofenac diethylammonium salt 1.16% (equivalent to diclofenac sodium 1%). Net price 20 g (hosp. only) = £1.55; 100 g = £7.75. Apply 2–4 g 3–4 times daily; therapy should be reviewed after 14 days

---

# 11: Drugs acting on the
# EYE

In this chapter, drug treatment is discussed under the following headings:

**11.1** Administration of drugs to the eye
**11.2** Control of microbial contamination
**11.3** Anti-infective eye preparations
**11.4** Corticosteroids and other anti-inflammatory preparations
**11.5** Mydriatics and cycloplegics
**11.6** Treatment of glaucoma
**11.7** Local anaesthetics
**11.8** Miscellaneous ophthalmic preparations
**11.9** Contact lenses

The entries in this chapter generally relate only to local eye treatment. Systemic indications and side-effects of many of the drugs are given elsewhere (see index).

## 11.1 Administration of drugs to the eye

EYE-DROPS AND EYE OINTMENTS. When administered in the form of eye-drops, drugs penetrate the globe, probably through the cornea. However, systemic effects, which are usually undesirable, may well arise from absorption of drugs into the general circulation via conjunctival vessels or from the nasal mucosa after the excess of the preparation has drained down through the tear ducts. For example, timolol (a beta-blocker), administered as eye-drops may induce bronchospasm or bradycardia in susceptible individuals.

Eye ointments are often applied to lid margins for blepharitis. They may also be used in the conjunctival sac for other conditions especially where a prolonged action is required.

When two different preparations in the form of eye-drops are required at the same time of day, for example pilocarpine and timolol in glaucoma, dilution and overflow may occur when one immediately follows the other. The patient should therefore leave an interval of a few minutes. At night, an eye ointment for the second drug will reduce the problem.

Generally it is inadvisable for patients to continue to wear hydrophilic (soft) contact lenses when receiving eye-drops. For warnings relating to eye-drops and contact lenses, see section 11.9.

EYE LOTIONS. These are solutions for the irrigation of the conjuctival sac. They act mechanically to flush out irritants or foreign bodies as a first-aid treatment. Sterile sodium chloride 0.9% solution (section 11.8.2) is usually used. It should be used only once from a previously unopened container for first aid, while for treatment it should be used for no longer than 24 hours after the container is first opened. Single-application containers are

available. In emergency, tap water drawn freshly from the main (not stored water) will suffice.

OTHER PREPARATIONS. Subconjunctival injection may be used to administer anti-infective drugs, mydriatics, or corticosteroids for conditions not responding to topical therapy. The drug diffuses through the sclera to the anterior and posterior chambers and vitreous humour in higher concentration than can be achieved by absorption from eye-drops. However, because the dose-volume is limited (usually not more than 1 mL), this route is suitable only for drugs which are readily soluble.

Drugs such as antibiotics and corticosteroids may be administered systemically to treat an eye condition.

Suitable plastic devices which gradually release a specified amount of drug over a period of, say, 1 week are also used (e.g. Ocuserts®).

## 11.2 Control of microbial contamination

Preparations for the eye should be sterile when issued. For routine domiciliary use they are supplied in multiple-application containers for individual use. Eye-drops contain a suitable preservative and provided that contamination is avoided they may be used for not more than one month after which a new container should be opened (if treatment is to be continued) and the old one discarded.

In eye surgery it is wise to use single-application containers. Preparations used during intra-ocular procedures and others that may penetrate into the anterior chamber must be isotonic and without preservatives and buffered if necessary to a neutral pH. Large volume intravenous infusion preparations are not suitable for this purpose. For all surgical procedures, a previously unopened container is used for each patient.

## 11.3 Anti-infective eye preparations

**11.3.1** Antibacterials
**11.3.2** Antifungals
**11.3.3** Antivirals

Most acute eye infections can be treated topically. Ideally, eye-drops should be instilled very frequently (at least every 2 hours).

A useful addition for night-time use is an eye ointment because of its longer action. It will also soften crusts which cause the lids and eye lashes to adhere together when the patient is asleep. A small quantity of eye ointment is applied to the eye or inside the lower lid.

In severe infections, *subconjunctival injection* of a suitable drug may help to achieve a high intra-ocular concentration. *Systemic* treatment is indicated in infective endophthalmitis and may also help in gonococcal conjunctivitis in the newborn. The blood-aqueous barrier usually breaks down in the latter case allowing intra-ocular penetration of systemically administered drugs.

## 11.3.1   Antibacterials

When prescribing antibiotics, in general, it is preferable to use topically in the eye antibiotics that are seldom or never used for systemic infections. However, the possibility of systemic absorption (section 11.1) must be taken into consideration. Examples of antibiotics with a wide spectrum of activity are **chloramphenicol, framycetin, gentamicin**, and **neomycin**. Gentamicin and tobramycin are effective for treating infections due to *Pseudomonas aeruginosa*; that **norfloxacin** has a spectrum of activity similar to that of gentamicin. **Fusidic acid** is useful for staphylococcal infections.

**Sulphacetamide** should no longer be used topically to treat eye infections, since it is rarely of any value.

**Propamidine isethionate** eye-drops are of little value in bacterial infections but are specific for the rare but devastating condition of acanthamoeba keratitis.

The use of **mercuric oxide** eye ointment, even for short periods, is **not** recommended.

WITH CORTICOSTEROIDS. Many antibiotic preparations also incorporate a corticosteroid but such mixtures should **not** be used unless a patient is under close specialist supervision. In particular they should not be prescribed for undiagnosed 'red eye' which is sometimes caused by the herpes simplex virus and may be difficult to diagnose (section 11.4).

ADMINISTRATION
*Eye-drops.* Apply at least every 2 hours then reduce frequency as infection is controlled and continue for 48 hours after healing.
*Eye ointment.* Apply *either* at night (if eye-drops used during the day) *or* 3–4 times daily (if eye ointment used alone).

## CHLORAMPHENICOL
*Indications; Administration:* see notes above
*Side-effects:* transient stinging; rare reports of aplastic anaemia

PoM **Chloramphenicol** (Non-proprietary)
*Eye-drops*, chloramphenicol 0.5%. Net price 10 mL = 67p
*Eye ointment*, chloramphenicol 1%. Net price 4 g = 68p
PoM **Chloromycetin**® (P-D)
*Ophthalmic ointment* (= eye ointment), chloramphenicol 1%. Net price 4 g = 67p

*Redidrops*   (= eye-drops),   chloramphenicol 0.5%. Net price 5 mL = £1.10; 10 mL = £1.18
*Additives: include* phenylmercuric acetate
PoM **Sno Phenicol**® (S&N Pharm.)
*Eye-drops*, chloramphenicol 0.5%, in a viscous vehicle. Net price 10 mL = £1.11
*Additives: include* chlorhexidine acetate

Single use
PoM **Minims**® **Chloramphenicol** (S&N Pharm.)
*Eye-drops*, chloramphenicol 0.5%. Net price 20 × 0.5 mL = £5.05

## CHLORTETRACYCLINE
*Indications:* local treatment of infections, including trachoma (see notes above and under Tetracycline)
*Administration:* see notes above

PoM **Aureomycin**® (Lederle)
*Ophthalmic ointment* ( = eye ointment), chlortetracycline hydrochloride 1%. Net price 3.5 g = 94p

## FRAMYCETIN SULPHATE
*Indications; Administration:* see notes above

PoM **Soframycin**® (Roussel)
*Eye-drops*, framycetin sulphate 0.5%. Net price 8 mL = £2.97
*Additives: include* phenylmercuric nitrate
*Eye ointment*, framycetin sulphate 0.5%. Net price 5 g = £1.20
*Ophthalmic powder*, framycetin sulphate (sterile) for preparing subconjunctival injections. Net price 500-mg vial = £3.85

## FUSIDIC ACID
*Indications:* see notes above

PoM **Fucithalmic**® (Leo)
*Eye-drops*, m/r, fusidic acid 1% in gel basis (liquifies on contact with eye). Net price 5 g = £2.25
*Additives: include* benzalkonium chloride
Apply twice daily

## GENTAMICIN
*Indications; Administration:* see notes above

PoM **Cidomycin**® (Roussel)
*Drops* (for ear or eye), gentamicin 0.3% (as sulphate). Net price 8 mL = £1.34
*Additives: include* benzalkonium chloride, disodium edetate
*Eye ointment*, gentamicin 0.3% (as sulphate). Net price 3 g = £1.21
PoM **Garamycin**® (Schering-Plough)
*Drops* (for ear or eye), gentamicin 0.3% (as sulphate). Net price 10 mL = £1.79
*Additives: include* benzalkonium chloride
PoM **Genticin**® (Nicholas)
*Eye-drops*, gentamicin 0.3% (as sulphate). Net price 10 mL = £2.06
*Additives: include* benzalkonium chloride
*Eye ointment*, gentamicin 0.3% (as sulphate). Net price 3 g = £1.43
*Additives: include* hydroxybenzoates

---

Single use
PoM **Minims**® **Gentamicin** (S&N Pharm.)
*Eye-drops*, gentamicin 0.3% (as sulphate). Net
price 20 × 0.5 mL = £5.90

## NEOMYCIN SULPHATE
*Indications; Administration:* see notes above

PoM **Neomycin** (Non-proprietary)
*Eye-drops*, neomycin sulphate 0.5% (3500 units/
mL). Net price 10 mL = £1.46
*Eye ointment*, neomycin sulphate 0.5%
(3500 units/g). Net price 3 g = 64p
PoM **Neosporin**® (Cusi)
*Eye-drops*, gramicidin 25 units, neomycin
sulphate 1700 units, polymyxin B sulphate 5000
units/mL. Net price 5 mL = £5.50
*Additives: include* thiomersal
Apply 2–4 times daily or more frequently if
required

Single use
PoM **Minims**® **Neomycin Sulphate** (S&N
Pharm.)
*Eye-drops*, neomycin sulphate 0.5%. Net price
20 × 0.5 mL = £5.90

## NORFLOXACIN
*Indications; Administration:* see notes above
*Side-effects:* local burning and smarting; rarely
conjunctival hyperaemia, chemosis (conjunctival oedema) and photophobia, bitter taste

▼ PoM **Noroxin**® (MSD)
*Ophthalmic solution* (= eye-drops), norfloxacin
0.3%. Net price 5 mL = £1.97
*Additives: include* benzalkonium chloride

## POLYMYXIN B SULPHATE
*Indications; Administration:* see notes above

PoM **Polyfax**® (Cusi)
*Eye ointment*, polymyxin B sulphate 10 000 units,
bacitracin zinc 500 units/g. Net price 4 g =
£3.50
PoM **Polytrim**® (Cusi)
*Eye-drops*, trimethoprim 0.1%, polymyxin B
sulphate 10000 units/mL. Net price 5 mL =
£3.27
*Additives: include* thiomersal
*Eye ointment*, trimethoprim 0.5%, polymyxin B
sulphate 10000 units/g. Net price 4 g = £3.27

## PROPAMIDINE ISETHIONATE
*Indications:* local treatment of infections (but see
notes above)

**Brolene**® (Rhône-Poulenc Rorer)
*Eye-drops*, propamidine isethionate 0.1%. Net
price 10 mL = £1.47
Apply 4 times daily
*Eye ointment*, dibromopropamidine isethionate
0.15%. Net price 5 g = £1.47
Apply 1–2 times daily

## SULPHACETAMIDE SODIUM
*Indications:* not recommended, see notes above
*Administration:* apply eye-drops every 2–6 hours

PoM **Albucid**® (Nicholas)
*Eye-drops*, sulphacetamide sodium 10%, net price
10 mL = 85p
*Additives: include* cetrimide

Single use
PoM **Minims**® **Sulphacetamide Sodium** (S&N Pharm.)
*Eye-drops*, sulphacetamide sodium 10%. Net price
20 × 0.5 mL = £5.90

## TETRACYCLINE HYDROCHLORIDE
*Indications; Administration:* see notes above

TRACHOMA. For mass antitrachoma treatment, the
World Health Organization recommends **tetracycline
hydrochloride** eye ointment applied to both eyes twice
daily for 5 days in each month for 6 months. Chlortetracycline eye ointment may also be used but chloramphenicol is not as effective.
For active trachoma in the individual, one or both
of the following are effective. (i) For adults, orally
administered sulphonamides for 2 weeks or the long-
acting sulphadimethoxine (no longer on UK market)
1 g initially followed by 500 mg daily for 10 days (see
section 5.1.8). For children, erythromycin should be
used (see section 5.1.5). (ii) Tetracycline eye ointment
three times daily for 6 weeks.

PoM **Achromycin**® (Lederle)
*Ointment* (for ear or eye), tetracycline hydrochloride 1%. Net price 3.5 g = 70p

## TOBRAMYCIN
*Indications; Administration:* see notes above

PoM **Tobralex**® (Alcon)
*Eye-drops*, tobramycin 0.3%. Net price 5 mL =
£1.43
*Additives: include* benzalkonium chloride

## 11.3.2  Antifungals
Fungal infections of the cornea are rare but tend
to occur after agricultural injuries, especially in
hot and humid climates. Orbital mycosis is rare,
and when it occurs is usually due to direct spread
of infection from the paranasal sinuses. Increasing
age, debility, or immunosuppression by drugs,
for example, following renal transplantation, may
encourage fungal proliferation in many parts of
the body. The spread of infection via the bloodstream occasionally produces a metastatic
endophthalmitis.
A wide range of fungi are capable of producing
ocular mycosis and may be identified by appropriate laboratory procedures.
Antifungal preparations for the eye are not
generally available. Treatment will normally be
carried out at specialist centres, but requests for
information about supplies of preparations not
available commercially should be addressed to the
District Pharmaceutical Officer (or equivalent in
Scotland or Northern Ireland) or to Moorfields
Eye Hospital, City Road, London EC1V 2PD
(071-253 3411).

## 11.3.3   Antivirals

Herpes simplex infections producing, for example, dendritic corneal ulcer can be treated with **acyclovir**; alternatively **idoxuridine** may be used.

### ACYCLOVIR

*Indications:* local treatment of herpes simplex infections

*Administration:* apply 5 times daily (continue for at least 3 days after complete healing)

PoM **Zovirax**® (Wellcome)
*Eye ointment*, acyclovir 3%. Net price 4.5 g = £10.67
*Tablets* and *injection*, see section 5.3

### IDOXURIDINE

*Indications:* local treatment of herpes simplex infections

*Contra-indications:* pregnancy (toxicity in *animal* studies)

*Administration:* apply eye-drops every hour during the day and every 2 hours at night; eye ointment every 4 hours
Max. period of treatment 21 days

PoM **Idoxene**® (Spodefell)
*Eye ointment*, idoxuridine 0.5%. Net price 3 g = £1.35

# 11.4   Corticosteroids and other anti-inflammatory preparations

**11.4.1** Corticosteroids
**11.4.2** Other anti-inflammatory preparations

## 11.4.1   Corticosteroids

Corticosteroids administered topically, by subconjunctival injection, and systemically have an important place in treating uveitis and scleritis; they are also used to reduce post-operative inflammation following eye operations.

*Topical corticosteroids* should normally only be used under expert supervision; they should not be prescribed for undiagnosed 'red eye'. There are two main dangers from topical corticosteroids. First the 'red eye' may be caused by herpes simplex virus which produces a dendritic ulcer; corticosteroids aggravate the condition which may lead to loss of vision or even loss of the eye. Second, again arising from the use of eye-drop formulations, a 'steroid glaucoma' may be produced, after a few weeks treatment, in patients predisposed to chronic simple glaucoma. Use of a combination product containing a corticosteroid with an anti-infective is rarely justified.

*Systemic corticosteroids* can usefully be given on an alternate-day basis to minimise side-effects.

The risk of producing glaucoma is not great, but 'steroid cataract' is a very high risk (75%) if more than 15 mg of prednisolone or equivalent is given daily for several years. The longer the duration, the greater is the risk. A dose of less then 10 mg per day is usually safe.

### BETAMETHASONE

*Indications:* local treatment of inflammation (short-term)

*Cautions; Side-effects:* see notes above

*Administration:* apply eye-drops every 1–2 hours until controlled then reduce frequency, eye ointment 2–4 times daily or at night when used with eye-drops

PoM **Betnesol**® (Glaxo)
*Drops* (for ear, eye, or nose), betamethasone sodium phosphate 0.1%. Net price 10 mL = £1.31
*Additives: include* benzalkonium chloride
*Eye ointment*, betamethasone sodium phosphate 0.1%. Net price 3 g = 56p
PoM **Betnesol-N**® (Glaxo)
*Drops* (for ear, eye, or nose), see section 12.1.1
*Eye ointment*, betamethasone sodium phosphate 0.1%, neomycin sulphate 0.5%. Net price 3 g = 64p
PoM **Vista-Methasone**® (Daniel)
*Drops* (for ear, eye, or nose), betamethasone sodium phosphate 0.1%. Net price 5 mL = 84p; 10 mL = £1.12
*Additives: include* benzalkonium chloride
PoM **Vista-Methasone N**® (Daniel)
*Drops* (for ear, eye, or nose), see section 12.1.1

### CLOBETASONE BUTYRATE

*Indications:* local treatment of inflammation (short-term)

*Cautions; Side-effects:* see notes above; reduced tendency to raise intra-ocular pressure

*Administration:* apply eye-drops 4 times daily; severe conditions every 1–2 hours until controlled then reduce frequency

PoM **Eumovate**® (Glaxo)
*Eye-drops*, clobetasone butyrate 0.1%. Net price 10 mL = £3.04
*Additives: include* benzalkonium chloride
PoM **Eumovate-N**® (Glaxo)
*Eye-drops*, clobetasone butyrate 0.1%, neomycin sulphate 0.5%. Net price 10 mL = £2.70
*Additives: include* benzalkonium chloride

### DEXAMETHASONE

*Indications:* local treatment of inflammation (short-term)

*Cautions; Side-effects:* see notes above

*Administration:* apply eye-drops 4–6 times daily; severe conditions every hour until controlled then reduce frequency

PoM **Maxidex**® (Alcon)
*Eye-drops*, dexamethasone 0.1%, hypromellose 0.5%. Net price 5 mL = £1.53; 10 mL = £3.03
*Additives: include* benzalkonium chloride

---

PoM **Maxitrol**® (Alcon)
*Eye-drops*, dexamethasone 0.1%, hypromellose 0.5%, neomycin 0.35% (as sulphate), polymyxin B sulphate 6000 units/mL. Net price 5 mL = £1.81
*Additives: include* benzalkonium chloride
*Eye ointment*, dexamethasone 0.1%, neomycin 0.35% (as sulphate), polymyxin B sulphate 6000 units/g. Net price 3.5 g = £1.56
*Additives: include* hydroxybenzoates
PoM **Sofradex**® (Roussel)
*Drops and ointment* (for ear or eye), see section 12.1.1

## FLUOROMETHOLONE

*Indications:* local treatment of inflammation (short-term)
*Cautions; Side-effects:* see notes above; reduced tendency to raise intra-ocular pressure
*Administration:* apply eye-drops 2–4 times daily (initially every hour for 24–48 hours then reduce frequency)

PoM **FML**® (Allergan)
*Ophthalmic suspension* ( = eye-drops), fluorometholone 0.1%, polyvinyl alcohol (Liquifilm®) 1.4%. Net price 5 mL = £1.78; 10 mL = £2.83
*Additives: include* benzalkonium chloride, disodium edetate, polysorbate 80
PoM **FML-Neo**® (Allergan)
*Eye-drops*, fluorometholone 0.1%, neomycin sulphate 0.5%, polyvinyl alcohol (Liquifilm®) 1.4%. Net price 5 mL = £1.90
*Additives: include* benzalkonium chloride, disodium edetate, polysorbate 80

## HYDROCORTISONE ACETATE

*Indications:* local treatment of inflammation (short-term)
*Cautions; Side-effects:* see notes above

PoM **Hydrocortisone** (Non-proprietary)
*Eye-drops*, hydrocortisone acetate 1%. Net price 10 mL = £1.47
*Eye ointment*, hydrocortisone acetate 0.5%, net price 3 g = 85p; 1%, 3 g = £1.00; 2.5%, 3 g = 75p
PoM **Chloromycetin Hydrocortisone**® (P-D)
*Eye ointment*, chloramphenicol 1%, hydrocortisone acetate 0.5%. Net price 4 g = 70p
PoM **Neo-Cortef**® (Cusi)
*Drops and ointment* (for ear or eye), see section 12.1.1
*Note.* Eye-drops containing hydrocortisone acetate 1.5% and neomycin sulphate 0.5% also available from CP

## PREDNISOLONE

*Indications:* local treatment of inflammation (short-term)
*Cautions; Side-effects:* see notes above
*Administration:* apply eye-drops every 1–2 hours until controlled then reduce frequency

PoM **Pred Forte**® (Allergan)
*Eye-drops*, prednisolone acetate 1%. Net price 5 mL = £1.55; 10 mL = £3.09
*Additives: include* benzalkonium chloride, disodium edetate, polysorbate 80
Apply 2–4 times daily

PoM **Predsol**® (Glaxo)
*Drops* (for ear or eye), prednisolone sodium phosphate 0.5%. Net price 10 mL = £1.31
*Additives: include* benzalkonium chloride
PoM **Predsol-N**® (Glaxo)
*Drops* (for ear or eye), see section 12.1.1

Single use
PoM **Minims**® **Prednisolone** (S&N Pharm.)
*Eye-drops*, prednisolone sodium phosphate 0.5%. Net price 20 × 0.5 mL = £5.90

## 11.4.2   Other anti-inflammatory preparations

Other preparations used for the topical treatment of inflammation and allergic conjunctivitis include antihistamines, oxyphenbutazone, and sodium cromoglycate

**Oxyphenbutazone** eye ointment does not have the disadvantages of corticosteroids and has been used in the treatment of episcleritis.

Topical preparations of **antihistamines** such as eye-drops containing antazoline sulphate (with xylometazoline hydrochloride as Otrivine-Antistin®) may be used for short-term treatment of allergic conjunctivitis.

**Sodium cromoglycate** eye-drops may be useful for vernal catarrh and other allergic forms of conjunctivitis.

## ANTAZOLINE
*Indications:* allergic conjunctivitis

**Otrivine-Antistin**® (Zyma)
*Eye-drops*, antazoline sulphate 0.5%, xylometazoline hydrochloride 0.05%. Net price 10 mL = £1.40
*Additives: include* benzalkonium chloride, disodium edetate
Apply 2–3 times daily
PoM **Vasocon A**® (Iolab)
*Eye-drops*, antazoline phosphate 0.5%, naphazoline hydrochloride 0.05%. Net price 10 mL = £2.41
*Additives: include* benzalkonium chloride, disodium edetate
Apply every 3–4 hours

## OXYPHENBUTAZONE
*Indications:* local treatment of inflammation
*Administration:* apply eye ointment 2–5 times daily (discontinue if no improvement after 8 days)

PoM **Tanderil**® (Zyma)
*Eye ointment*, oxyphenbutazone 10%. Net price 5 g = 63p
*Additives: include* wool fat
PoM **Tanderil Chloramphenicol**® (Zyma)
*Eye ointment*, chloramphenicol 1%, oxyphenbutazone 10%. Net price 5 g = £1.02
*Additives: include* wool fat

## SODIUM CROMOGLYCATE
*Indications:* allergic conjunctivitis
*Administration:* apply eye-drops 4 times daily, eye ointment 2–3 times daily

PoM **Opticrom**® (Fisons)
[1]*Aqueous eye-drops*, sodium cromoglycate 2%.
Net price 13.5 mL = £5.59
  *Additives: include* benzalkonium chloride, disodium edetate
1. Formerly called *Opticrom*® *Eye-drops*
*Eye ointment*, sodium cromoglycate 4%. Net
price 5 g = £5.99
  *Additives: include* wool fat

# 11.5   Mydriatics and cycloplegics

Antimuscarinics dilate the pupil and paralyse the
ciliary muscle; they vary in potency and duration
of action. The relative potencies and durations of
action of the principal drugs, in ascending order,
are:
  tropicamide (3 hours)
  cyclopentolate, hyoscine, homatropine (all up to 24
  hours)
  atropine (7 days or longer)
  Short-acting, relatively weak mydriatics, such
as **tropicamide 0.5%**, facilitate the examination
of the fundus of the eye.
  **Cyclopentolate** 1% or **atropine** are preferable
for producing cycloplegia for refraction in young
children. Atropine 1% (in ointment form) is
sometimes preferred for children under 5 years of
age. Atropine is also used for the treatment of
iridocyclitis mainly to prevent posterior synechiae, often with phenylephrine 10% eye-drops
(2.5% in children and those with cardiac disease).

CAUTIONS AND SIDE-EFFECTS. Contact dermatitis is
not uncommon with the antimuscarinic mydriatic
drugs, especially atropine. In addition, toxic systemic reactions to atropine (and hyoscine) and
cyclopentolate may occur in the very young and
the very old.
  Darkly pigmented iris is more resistant to pupillary dilatation and caution should be exercised to
avoid overdosage.
  Mydriasis may precipitate acute closed-angle
('congestive') glaucoma in a few patients, usually
aged over 60 years, who are predisposed to the
condition because of a shallow anterior chamber.
  **Interactions**. Phenylephrine may interact with
systemically administered monoamine-oxidase
inhibitors; see also Appendix 1 (sympathomimetics).

DRIVING. Patients should be warned not to drive
for 1 to 2 hours after mydriasis.

ANTIMUSCARINICS

## ATROPINE SULPHATE

*Indications:* refraction procedures in young children; see also notes above
*Cautions:* action persistent, may precipitate glaucoma; see also notes above

PoM **Atropine Eye-drops,** atropine sulphate 1%.
Net price 10 mL = 68p
PoM **Atropine Eye Ointment,** atropine sulphate
1%. Net price 3 g = £1.01
PoM **Isopto Atropine**® (Alcon)
*Eye-drops*, atropine sulphate 1%, hypromellose
0.5%. Net price 5 mL = £1.02
  *Additives: include* benzalkonium chloride

Single use
PoM **Minims**® **Atropine Sulphate** (S&N Pharm.)
*Eye-drops*, atropine sulphate 1%. Net price
20 × 0.5 mL = £5.05

## CYCLOPENTOLATE HYDROCHLORIDE

*Indications:* see notes above
*Cautions:* patients with raised intra-ocular
pressure; see notes above

PoM **Mydrilate**® (Boehringer Ingelheim)
*Eye-drops*, cyclopentolate hydrochloride 0.5%,
net price 5 mL = 67p; 1%, 5 mL = 90p
  *Additives: include* benzalkonium chloride

Single use
PoM **Minims**® **Cyclopentolate** (S&N Pharm.)
*Eye-drops*, cyclopentolate hydrochloride 0.5 and
1%. Net price 20 × 0.5 mL (both) = £5.05

## HOMATROPINE HYDROBROMIDE

*Indications; Cautions:* see notes above

PoM **Homatropine Eye-drops,** homatropine hydrobromide 1%, net price 10 mL = £1.68; 2%,
10 mL = £1.79

Single use
PoM **Minims**®   **Homatropine   Hydrobromide**
(S&N Pharm.)
*Eye-drops*, homatropine hydrobromide 2%. Net
price 20 × 0.5 mL = £5.90

## HYOSCINE HYDROBROMIDE

*Indications; Cautions:* see notes above

PoM **Hyoscine Eye-drops,** usual strength hyoscine
hydrobromide 0.25%. Net price 10 mL = 85p

## LACHESINE CHLORIDE

*Indications:* see notes above; useful in patients
hypersensitive to other mydriatics
*Cautions:* see notes above

**Lachesine Eye-drops,** lachesine chloride 1%.
Net price 10 mL = £3.60

## TROPICAMIDE

*Indications; Cautions:* see notes above

PoM **Mydriacyl**® (Alcon)
*Eye-drops*, tropicamide 0.5%, net price 5 mL =
£1.39; 1%, 5 mL = £1.72
  *Additives: include* benzalkonium chloride

Single use
PoM **Minims® Tropicamide** (S&N Pharm.)
*Eye-drops*, tropicamide 0.5 and 1%. Net price
20 × 0.5 mL (both) = £5.90

SYMPATHOMIMETICS

## ADRENALINE
Section 11.6

## PHENYLEPHRINE HYDROCHLORIDE
*Indications; Cautions:* see notes above

**Phenylephrine Eye-drops,** phenylephrine
hydrochloride 10%. Net price 10 mL = £1.75
See also under Hypromellose (section 11.8.1)

Single use
**Minims® Phenylephrine Hydrochloride** (S&N
Pharm.)
*Eye-drops*, phenylephrine hydrochloride 2.5%,
net price 20 × 0.5 mL = £5.90; 10%, 20 ×
0.5 mL = £5.90

# 11.6   Treatment of glaucoma

An abnormally high intra-ocular pressure, glaucoma, may result in blindness. In virtually all
cases, rise in pressure is due to reduced outflow of
aqueous humour, the inflow remaining constant.

Glaucoma is treated by the application of eye-
drops containing beta-blockers, miotics, or adrenaline (and guanethidine). Acetazolamide and
dichlorphenamide are given by mouth and, in
emergency or before surgery, mannitol may be
given by intravenous infusion.

Probably the commonest condition is *chronic
simple glaucoma* where the obstruction is in the
trabecular meshwork. It is commonly first treated
with a topical beta-blocker and other drugs added
as necessary to control the intra-ocular pressure
e.g. adrenaline or pilocarpine.

If supplementary topical treatment is required
after *iridectomy* or a drainage operation in either
open-angle or closed-angle glaucoma, a beta-
blocker is preferred to pilocarpine. This is because
of the risk that posterior synechiae will be formed
as a result of the miotic effect of pilocarpine,
especially in closed-angle glaucoma. It is then also
advantageous to utilise the mydriatic side-effect
of adrenaline.

MIOTICS

The small pupil is an unfortunate side-effect of
these drugs (except when pilocarpine is used temporarily prior to operation for *closed-angle
glaucoma*). The key factor is the opening up of
the inefficient drainage channels in the trabecular
meshwork resulting from contraction or spasm of
the ciliary muscle. This also produces accommodation spasm that may result in blurring of
vision and browache (a particular disadvantage in
patients under 40 years of age).

**Pilocarpine** has a duration of action of 3 to 4
hours. **Physostigmine** is more potent; it is still used
with pilocarpine but is not usually used alone.
**Carbachol** is sometimes used to lower intra-ocular
pressure, usually in conjunction with other miotics
such as physostigmine.

**Demecarium bromide** (as *Tosmilen®*, Sinclair)
and **ecothiopate iodide** (as *Phospholine Iodide®*,
Cusi) are no longer on the UK market but are
still available on a named-patient basis for use
under expert supervision.

Generalised parasympathomimetic side effects
such as sweating, bradycardia and intestinal colic
may follow systemic absorption of these eye-
drops; other effects may include hypersalivation
and bronchospasm.

## CARBACHOL
*Indications:* see notes above
*Administration:* apply eye-drops up to 4 times
daily

PoM **Isopto Carbachol®** (Alcon)
*Eye-drops*, carbachol 3%, hypromellose 1%.
Net price 10 mL = £1.80
*Additives:* include benzalkonium chloride

## PHYSOSTIGMINE SULPHATE
(Eserine)
*Indications; Side-effects:* see notes above
*Administration:* apply eye-drops 2–6 times daily

PoM **Physostigmine** (Non-proprietary)
*Eye-drops*, physostigmine sulphate 0.25 and
0.5%. Net price 10 mL (both) = £1.90
PoM **Physostigmine and Pilocarpine** (Non-proprietary)
*Eye-drops*, physostigmine sulphate 0.25%, pilocarpine hydrochloride 2%. Net price 10 mL =
£1.72
*Eye-drops*, physostigmine sulphate 0.25%, pilocarpine hydrochloride 4%. Net price 10 mL =
£1.92
*Eye-drops*, physostigmine sulphate 0.5%, pilocarpine hydrochloride 4%. Net price 10 mL =
£2.20

## PILOCARPINE
*Indications; Side-effects:* see notes above
*Administration:* apply eye-drops 3–6 times daily

PoM **Pilocarpine** (Non-proprietary)
*Eye-drops*, pilocarpine hydrochloride 0.5 and
1%, net price 10 mL = £1.11; 2%, 10 mL =
£1.20; 3%, 10 mL = £1.36; 4%, 10 mL = £1.51
PoM **Isopto Carpine®** (Alcon)
*Eye-drops*, all with hypromellose 0.5%; pilocarpine hydrochloride 0.5%, net price 10 mL =
75p; 1%, 10 mL = 83p; 2%, 10 mL = 92p; 3%,
10 mL = 99p; 4%, 10 mL = £1.07
*Additives:* include benzalkonium chloride
PoM **Sno Pilo®** (S&N Pharm.)
*Eye-drops*, in a viscous vehicle, pilocarpine
hydrochloride 1%, net price 10 mL = £1·07;
2%, 10 mL = £1.17; 4%, 10 mL = £1.39
*Additives:* include benzalkonium chloride

Single use
PoM **Minims® Pilocarpine Nitrate** (S&N Pharm.)
*Eye-drops*, pilocarpine nitrate 1, 2, and 4%. Net price 20 × 0.5 mL (all) = £5.05

Modified release
PoM **Ocusert®** (Cusi)
*Pilo-20 ocular insert*, m/r, pilocarpine 20 micrograms released per hour for 1 week. Net price pack of 8 inserts = £35.98. Counselling, method of use
*Pilo-40 ocular insert*, m/r, pilocarpine 40 micrograms released per hour for 1 week. Net price pack of 8 inserts = £41.95. Counselling, method of use

---

## ADRENALINE/GUANETHIDINE

Adrenaline probably acts both by reducing the rate of production of aqueous humour and by increasing the outflow through the trabecular meshwork. It is contra-indicated in closed-angle glaucoma because it is a mydriatic, unless an iridectomy has been carried out. Side-effects include severe smarting and redness of the eye; adrenaline should be used with caution in patients with hypertension and heart disease.

**Dipivefrine** is a prodrug of adrenaline. It is stated to pass more rapidly through the cornea and is then converted to the active form.

**Guanethidine** enhances and prolongs the effects of adrenaline. It is also used alone and produces initial mydriasis with increased aqueous outflow followed by miosis with reduced aqueous secretion. Prolonged use, particularly of the higher strengths may result in conjunctival fibrosis with secondary corneal changes; the conjunctiva and cornea should be examined at least every six months.

## ADRENALINE

*Indications; Contra-indications:* see notes above
*Administration:* apply eye-drops 1–2 times daily

**Epifrin®** (Allergan)
*Eye-drops*, adrenaline 1% (as hydrochloride). Net price 10 mL = £2.24
*Additives: include* benzalkonium chloride, disodium edetate
**Eppy®** (S&N Pharm.)
*Eye-drops*, adrenaline 1%. Net price 7.5 mL = £4.16
*Additives: include* phenylmercuric acetate
PoM **Simplene®** (S&N Pharm.)
*Eye-drops*, adrenaline, in a viscous vehicle, 0.5%, net price 7.5 mL = £3.54; 1%, 7.5 mL = £3.89
*Additives: include* benzalkonium chloride

## DIPIVEFRINE HYDROCHLORIDE

*Indications; Contra-indications:* as for Adrenaline, see notes above
*Administration:* apply 1 drop twice daily

PoM **Propine®** (Allergan)
*Eye-drops*, dipivefrine hydrochloride 0.1%. Net price 5 mL = £4.29, 10 mL = £4.89
*Additives: include* benzalkonium chloride, disodium edetate

## GUANETHIDINE MONOSULPHATE

*Indications; Cautions:* see notes above
*Administration:* apply eye-drops 1–2 times daily

PoM **Ganda®** (S&N Pharm.)
*Eye-drops* '1 + 0.2', guanethidine monosulphate 1%, adrenaline 0.2% in a viscous vehicle. Net price 7.5 mL = £4.60
*Additives: include* benzalkonium chloride
*Eye-drops* '3 + 0.5', guanethidine monosulphate 3%, adrenaline 0.5% in a viscous vehicle. Net price 7.5 mL = £6.01
*Additives: include* benzalkonium chloride
PoM **Ismelin®** (Zyma)
*Eye-drops*, guanethidine monosulphate 5%. Net price 5 mL = £1.87
*Additives: include* benzalkonium chloride

---

## BETA-BLOCKERS

Topical application of a beta-blocker to the eye reduces intra-ocular pressure effectively in *chronic simple glaucoma*, probably by reducing the rate of production of aqueous humour. Administration by mouth also reduces intra-ocular pressure but this route is not used (see comment under Systemic Drugs).

Beta-blockers used as eye-drops include **timolol** and, more recently, **betaxolol**, **carteolol**, **levobunolol**, and **metipranolol**.

SIDE-EFFECTS. Systemic absorption may follow topical application, therefore beta-blocker eye-drops are contra-indicated in patients with asthma or a history of obstructive airways disease; the CSM has advised that both cardioselective *and* non-cardioselective beta-blocker eye-drops should be avoided.

Consider also other cautions, contra-indications and side-effects of beta-blockers (p. 71).

> **CSM advice.** The CSM has advised that beta-blockers, even those with apparent cardioselectivity, should not be used in patients with asthma or a history of obstructive airways disease, unless no alternative treatment is available. In such cases the risk of inducing bronchospasm should be appreciated and appropriate precautions taken.

Eye-drops containing a beta-blocker are also contra-indicated in patients with bradycardia, heart block, or heart failure.

Local side-effects of eye-drops containing a beta-blocker include transitory dry eyes and allergic blepharoconjunctivitis.

INTERACTIONS. Since systemic absorption may follow topical application the possibility of interactions, in particular, with drugs such as verapamil should be borne in mind. See also section 2.3.2 and Appendix 1 (beta-blockers).

## BETAXOLOL HYDROCHLORIDE

*Indications; Cautions; Contra-indications; Side-effects:* see notes above
*Administration:* apply eye-drops twice daily

PoM **Betoptic**® (Alcon)
*Eye-drops,* betaxolol 0.5% (as hydrochloride).
Net price 5 mL = £5.30
*Additives: include* benzalkonium chloride

## CARTEOLOL HYDROCHLORIDE

*Indications; Cautions; Contra-indications; Side-effects:* see notes above
*Administration:* apply eye-drops twice daily

PoM **Teoptic**® (Dispersa)
*Eye-drops,* carteolol hydrochloride 1%, net price 5 mL = £5.05; 2%, 5 mL = £5.67
*Additives: include* benzalkonium chloride

## LEVOBUNOLOL HYDROCHLORIDE

*Indications; Cautions; Contra-indications; Side-effects:* see notes above
*Administration:* apply eye-drops once or twice daily

PoM **Betagan**® (Allergan)
*Eye-drops,* levobunolol hydrochloride 0.5%, polyvinyl alcohol (Liquifilm®) 1.4%. Net price 5 mL = £5.05
*Additives: include* benzalkonium chloride, disodium edetate

## METIPRANOLOL

*Indications; Cautions; Contra-indications; Side-effects:* see notes above; granulomatous anterior uveitis reported
*Administration:* apply eye-drops twice daily

PoM **Minims**® **Metipranolol** (S&N Pharm.)
*Eye-drops,* metipranolol 0.1%, net price 20 × 0.5 mL = £10.45; 0.3%, 20 × 0.5 mL = £11.37; 0.6%, 20 × 0.5 mL = £11.99

## TIMOLOL MALEATE

*Indications; Cautions; Contra-indications; Side-effects:* see notes above
*Administration:* apply eye-drops twice daily

PoM **Timoptol**® (MSD)
*Eye-drops,* in Ocumeter® metered-dose unit, timolol (as maleate) 0.25%, net price 5 mL = £5.18; 0.5%, 5 mL = £5.82
*Additives: include* benzalkonium chloride

---

### SYSTEMIC DRUGS

---

The side-effects of beta-blockers are probably sufficient to prevent their being prescribed by the ophthalmologist for administration by mouth. Hence **acetazolamide** will retain a significant place in treatment. It inhibits carbonic anhydrase, thus reducing the bicarbonate in aqueous humour and the water secreted with it, resulting in a fall in the intra-ocular pressure. **Dichlorphenamide** has a similar but more prolonged action. Both these drugs have a diuretic action and a moderate incidence of side-effects, giving rise, especially in the elderly, to paraesthesia, hypokalaemia, lack of appetite, drowsiness and depression; rashes and blood disorders occur rarely. Intravenous hypertonic **mannitol**, or **glycerol** by mouth, are useful short-term ocular hypotensive drugs. Acetazolamide by intramuscular or preferably intravenous injection is also useful in the pre-operative treatment of closed-angle glaucoma.

## ACETAZOLAMIDE

*Indications; Side-effects:* see notes above
*Cautions;* avoid in severe renal impairment; pregnancy; not generally recommended for prolonged administration but if given blood counts needed; **interactions:** Appendix 1 (acetazolamide)
*Dose: by mouth or by intravenous injection,* 0.25–1 g daily in divided doses
*By intramuscular injection,* as for intravenous injection but preferably avoided because of alkaline pH

PoM **Diamox**® (Lederle)
*Tablets,* acetazolamide 250 mg. Net price 20 = £1.96. Label: 3
*Sustets*® (= capsules m/r), orange, acetazolamide 500 mg. Net price 20 = £5.49. Label: 3, 25
*Dose:* 1 capsule twice daily
*Sodium Parenteral* (= injection), powder for reconstitution, acetazolamide (as sodium salt). Net price 500-mg vial = £15.14

## DICHLORPHENAMIDE

*Indications; Cautions; Side-effects:* see under Acetazolamide and notes above
*Dose:* initially 100–200 mg, then 100 mg every 12 hours, adjusted according to the patient's response

PoM **Daranide**® (MSD)
*Tablets,* yellow, scored, dichlorphenamide 50 mg. Net price 20 = 79p

# 11.7　Local anaesthetics

Oxybuprocaine and amethocaine are probably the most widely used topical local anaesthetics. Proxymetacaine causes less initial stinging and is useful for children. Cocaine, by potentiating noradrenaline, produces useful vasoconstriction, but is now much less used in surgery. Oxybuprocaine or a combined preparation of lignocaine and fluorescein is used for tonometry. Lignocaine, with or without adrenaline, is injected into the eyelids for minor surgery, while a retrobulbar injection may be used for major eye surgery.

---

## AMETHOCAINE HYDROCHLORIDE

*Indications:* local anaesthetic

PoM **Amethocaine Eye-drops,** amethocaine hydrochloride 0.5%, net price, 10 mL = £1.65; 1%, 10 mL = £1.46

Single use
PoM **Minims® Amethocaine Hydrochloride** (S&N Pharm.)
*Eye-drops*, amethocaine hydrochloride 0.5 and 1%. Net price 20 × 0.5 mL (both) = £5.90

## COCAINE HYDROCHLORIDE

*Indications:* local anaesthetic

CD **Cocaine Eye-drops,** cocaine hydrochloride 4%. Net price 10 mL = £3.20
CD **Cocaine and Homatropine Eye-drops,** cocaine hydrochloride 2%, homatropine hydrobromide 2%.

## LIGNOCAINE HYDROCHLORIDE

*Indications:* local anaesthetic

PoM **Minims® Lignocaine and Fluorescein** (S&N Pharm.)
*Eye-drops*, lignocaine hydrochloride 4%, fluorescein sodium 0.25%. Net price 20 × 0.5 mL = £7.11

## OXYBUPROCAINE HYDROCHLORIDE

*Indications:* local anaesthetic

PoM **Minims® Benoxinate (Oxybuprocaine) Hydrochloride** (S&N Pharm.)
*Eye-drops*, oxybuprocaine hydrochloride 0.4%. Net price 20 × 0.5 mL = £5.05

## PROXYMETACAINE HYDROCHLORIDE

*Indications:* local anaesthetic

PoM **Ophthaine®** (Squibb)
*Eye-drops*, proxymetacaine hydrochloride 0.5%. Net price 15 mL = £4.49
*Additives: include* benzalkonium chloride, chlorbutol

# 11.8  Miscellaneous ophthalmic preparations

## 11.8.1  Preparations for tear deficiency

Chronically sore eyes associated with reduced tear secretion, usually in cases of rheumatoid arthritis (Sjögren's syndrome), often respond to hypromellose eye-drops and mucolytic agents.

## ACETYLCYSTEINE

*Indications:* tear deficiency, impaired mucus production
*Administration:* apply eye-drops 3–4 times daily

PoM **Ilube®** (Cusi)
*Eye-drops*, acetylcysteine 5%, hypromellose 0.35%. Net price 10 mL = £4.75
*Additives: include* benzalkonium chloride

## HYDROXYETHYLCELLULOSE

*Indications:* tear deficiency

**Minims® Artifical Tears** (S&N Pharm.)
*Eye-drops*, hydroxyethylcellulose 0.44%. Net price 20 × 0.5 mL = £5.90

## HYPROMELLOSE

*Indications:* tear deficiency

**Hypromellose Eye-drops,** hypromellose '4000' (or '4500' or '5000') 0.3%. Net price 10 mL = 75p
**BJ6®** (Martindale; Thornton & Ross)
*Eye-drops*, hypromellose 0.25%. Net price 10 mL = 90p and 85p, respectively
*Additives: include* chlorhexidine (as acetate or gluconate), polysorbate 80
**Isopto Alkaline®** (Alcon)
*Eye-drops*, hypromellose 1%. Net price 10 mL = £1.02
*Additives: include* benzalkonium chloride
**Isopto Plain®** (Alcon)
*Eye-drops*, hypromellose 0.5%. Net price 10 mL = 87p
*Additives: include* benzalkonium chloride
**Tears Naturale®** (Alcon)
*Eye-drops*, dextran '70' 0.1%, hypromellose 0.3%. Net price 15 mL = £1.72
*Additives: include* benzalkonium chloride, disodium edetate

With phenylephrine
**Isopto Frin®** (Alcon)
*Eye-drops*, phenylephrine hydrochloride 0.12%, hypromellose 0.5%. Net price 10 mL = £1.17
*Additives: include* benzethonium chloride

## LIQUID PARAFFIN

*Indications:* tear deficiency

**Lacri-Lube®** (Allergan)
*Eye ointment*, white soft paraffin, liquid paraffin. Net price 3.5 g = £1.97, 5 g = £2.49
*Additives: include* wool fat derivatives

## POLYVINYL ALCOHOL

*Indications:* tear deficiency

**Hypotears®** (Iolab)
*Eye-drops*, macrogol '8000' 2%, polyvinyl alcohol 1%. Net price 10 mL = £1.85
*Additives: include* benzalkonium chloride, disodium edetate
**Liquifilm Tears®** (Allergan)
*Eye-drops*, polyvinyl alcohol 1.4%. Net price 15 mL = £1.72
*Additives: include* benzalkonium chloride, disodium edetate
**Sno Tears®** (S&N Pharm.)
*Eye-drops*, polyvinyl alcohol 1.4%. Net price 10 mL = £1.13
*Additives: include* benzalkonium chloride, disodium edetate

## 11.8.2   Other preparations

**Zinc sulphate** is a traditional astringent which has been used in eye-drops for treatment of excessive lachrymation.

Simple eye ointment is a bland sterile preparation which may be used to soften crusts in blepharitis or as a bland lubricant at night.

**Fluorescein sodium** and **rose bengal** are used in diagnostic procedures and for locating damaged areas of the cornea due to injury or disease. Rose bengal is much more efficient for the diagnosis of conjunctival epithelial damage.

Certain eye-drops, e.g. benzylpenicillin, colistin, desferrioxamine, and trisodium edetate (see also section 9.5.1.2), may be prepared aseptically from material supplied for injection.

## ACETYLCHOLINE CHLORIDE

*Indications:* cataract surgery, penetrating keratoplasty, iridectomy, and other anterior segment surgery requiring rapid miosis

PoM **Miochol**® (Iolab)
*Solution for intra-ocular irrigation*, acetylcholine chloride 1%, mannitol 3% when reconstituted. Net price 2 mL-vial = £7.78

## CHYMOTRYPSIN

*Indications:* zonulolysis in intracapsular cataract extraction

PoM **Zonulysin**® (Henleys)
*Injection*, powder for reconstitution, alphachymotrypsin 300 USP units (≡ 1.5 microkatals). Net price per vial (with diluent) = £3.42

## PARAFFIN, YELLOW, SOFT

*Indications:* see notes above

**Simple Eye Ointment,** liquid paraffin 10%, wool fat 10%, in yellow soft paraffin. Net price 4 g = 96p

## SODIUM CHLORIDE

*Indications:* irrigation, including first-aid removal of harmful substances

**Balanced Salt Solution**
*Solution* (sterile), sodium chloride 0.64%, sodium acetate 0.39%, sodium citrate 0.17%, calcium chloride 0.048%, magnesium chloride 0.03%, potassium chloride 0.075%.
Available from Alcon (15 mL and 30 mL) and from Iolab (15 mL)

**Normasol**® (Seton Prebbles)
*Solution* (sterile), sodium chloride 0.9%. Net price 25 mL sachet = 16p

Single use
**Minims**® **Sodium Chloride** (S&N Pharm.)
*Eye-drops*, sodium chloride 0.9%. Net price 20 × 0.5 mL = £5.05

## SODIUM HYALURONATE

(a visco-elastic polymer normally present in the aqueous and vitreous humour)
*Indications:* used during surgical procedures on the eye
*Side-effects:* occasional hypersensitivity (avian origin); occasional transient rise in intra-ocular pressure

PoM **Healonid**® (Kabi Pharmacia)
*Injection*, sodium hyaluronate 10 mg/mL in disposable syringes, net price 0.5 mL = £41.10, 0.75 mL = £61.62

## ZINC SULPHATE

*Indications; Cautions:* see notes above

**Zinc Sulphate Eye-drops,** zinc sulphate 0.25%. Net price 10 mL = £1.64

DIAGNOSTIC PREPARATIONS

## FLUORESCEIN SODIUM

*Indications:* detection of lesions and foreign bodies

**Minims**® **Fluorescein Sodium** (S&N Pharm.)
*Eye-drops*, fluorescein sodium 1 or 2%. Net price 20 × 0.5 mL (both) = £5.05

## ROSE BENGAL

*Indications:* detection of lesions and foreign bodies

**Minims**® **Rose Bengal** (S&N Pharm.)
*Eye-drops*, rose bengal 1%. Net price 20 × 0.5 mL = £5.90

# 11.9   Contact lenses

Many patients wear these lenses and special care is required in prescribing eye preparations for them. Unless medically indicated the lenses should not be worn during treatment. If the patient is wearing hard lenses the use of eye-drops containing anti-inflammatory drugs over long periods of time is to be deprecated. Some drugs can spoil hydrophilic soft lenses. Therefore unless eye-drops are specifically indicated as safe to use with hydrophilic contact lenses, the lenses should be removed before instillation and not worn during the period of treatment.

Hydrophilic plastic used for many soft contact lenses will selectively bind certain preservatives and could then be a source of irritation. Thiomersal is usually satisfactory. Chlorhexidine acetate is satisfactory in some cases, while phenylmercuric acetate or nitrate is usually satisfactory but is not recommended for long-term treatment. Benzalkonium chloride is unsuitable in all cases.

# 12: Drugs used in the treatment of diseases of the
# EAR, NOSE, and OROPHARYNX

In this chapter, drug treatment is discussed under the following headings:

**12.1** Drugs acting on the ear
**12.2** Drugs acting on the nose
**12.3** Drugs acting on the oropharynx

## 12.1 Drugs acting on the ear

**12.1.1** Otitis externa
**12.1.2** Otitis media
**12.1.3** Removal of ear wax

For treatment of labyrinthine disorders see section 4.6.

### 12.1.1 Otitis externa

Otitis externa is an inflammatory reaction of the meatal skin. It is important to exclude an underlying chronic otitis media before treatment is commenced. Many cases recover after thorough cleansing of the external ear canal by suction, dry mopping, or gentle syringing. A frequent problem in resistant cases is the difficulty in applying lotions and ointments satisfactorily to the relatively inaccessible affected skin. The most effective method is to introduce a ribbon gauze dressing soaked with **corticosteroid** ear drops or with an astringent such as **aluminium acetate** solution. When this is not practical, the ear should be gently cleaned with a probe covered in cotton wool and the patient encouraged to lie with the affected ear uppermost for ten minutes after the canal has been filled with a liberal quantity of the appropriate solution.

If infection is present, a topical anti-infective which is not used systemically (such as **framycetin**, **neomycin**, or **clioquinol**) may be used, but for only about a week as excessive use may result in fungal infections; these may be difficult to treat and require expert advice. Sensitivity to the anti-infective or solvent may occur and resistance to antibacterials is a possibility with prolonged use. **Chloramphenicol** may also be used but the ear drops contain propylene glycol and cause sensitivity in about 10% of patients (the eye ointment can be used instead). Solutions containing an anti-infective and a corticosteroid (such as Locorten-Vioform®) are used for treating cases where infection is present with inflammation and eczema. The CSM has warned that when otitis externa is treated topically with preparations containing chlorhexidine, aminoglycosides (e.g. neomycin, framycetin), or polymyxins in patients who have a perforation of the tympanic membrane, there is an increased risk of drug-induced deafness. It is therefore important to ensure that there is no perforation in such patients before prescription of these preparations. In the presence of a perforation many specialists, however, do use these

drops cautiously in patients with *otitis media*, see section 12.1.2.

An acute infection may cause severe pain and a systemic antibiotic is required with a simple analgesic such as paracetamol. When a resistant staphylococcal infection (a boil) is present in the external auditory meatus, **flucloxacillin** is the drug of choice (see section 5.1, Table 1).

The skin of the pinna adjacent to the ear canal is often affected by eczema, and topical corticosteroid creams and ointments (see section 13.4) are then required and should be applied five or six times daily. Prolonged use should be avoided.

**Ear drops** or **ointment** should be applied using 3–4 drops of a liquid preparation or a similar quantity of ointment, warmed if necessary, inserted into the affected ear. If discharge is profuse, ear drops applied directly may be washed away; in these circumstances the ear canal should be carefully cleaned and a 1 cm gauze wick impregnated with the ear drops should be introduced into it.

---

ASTRINGENT PREPARATIONS

---

## ALUMINIUM ACETATE

*Indications:* inflammation in otitis externa

**Aluminium Acetate Ear drops (13%)** consists of aluminium acetate solution, BP.
Insert into the meatus or apply on a gauze wick which should be kept saturated with the ear-drops
Available from Martindale and Penn (special order)

**Aluminium Acetate Ear drops (8%),** prepared by diluting 8 parts of aluminium acetate solution, BP, with 5 parts of purified water, freshly boiled and cooled. It must be freshly prepared.
Directions as above

---

ANTI-INFLAMMATORY PREPARATIONS

---

## BETAMETHASONE SODIUM PHOSPHATE

*Indications:* eczematous inflammation in otitis externa
*Cautions:* avoid prolonged use
*Contra-indications:* untreated infection

PoM **Betnesol®** (Glaxo)
*Drops* (for ear, eye, or nose), betamethasone sodium phosphate 0.1%. Net price 10 mL = £1.31
*Additives: include* benzalkonium chloride
Apply every 2–3 hours; reduce frequency of application when relief is obtained

---

PoM **Vista-Methasone®** (Daniel)
*Drops* (for ear, eye, or nose), betamethasone
sodium phosphate 0.1%. Net price 5 mL = 84p;
10 mL = £1.12
*Additives: include* benzalkonium chloride
Apply every 3–4 hours; reduce frequency of
application when relief is obtained

## PREDNISOLONE SODIUM PHOSPHATE

*Indications:* eczematous inflammation in otitis
externa
*Cautions:* avoid prolonged use
*Contra-indications:* untreated infection

PoM **Predsol®** (Glaxo)
*Drops* (for ear or eye), prednisolone sodium
phosphate 0.5%. Net price 10 mL = £1.31
*Additives: include* benzalkonium chloride
Apply every 2–3 hours; reduce frequency of
application when relief is obtained

---

ANTI-INFECTIVE PREPARATIONS

## CHLORAMPHENICOL

*Indications:* bacterial infection in otitis externa
*Cautions:* avoid prolonged use (see notes above)
*Side-effects:* high incidence of sensitivity reac-
tions to vehicle
*Administration:* apply 2–3 times daily

PoM **Chloramphenicol Ear drops 5%** and **10%**, chloramphenicol in propylene glycol. Net price 10 mL
(5%) = 95p; 10 mL (10%) = £1.00

## CLIOQUINOL

*Indications:* mild bacterial or fungal infections in
otitis externa
*Cautions:* avoid prolonged use (see notes above)
*Side-effects:* local sensitivity; stains skin and
clothing

PoM **Locorten-Vioform®** (Zyma)
*Ear drops*, clioquinol 1%, flumethasone pivalate
0.02%. Net price 7.5 mL = £1.05
Apply 2–3 drops twice daily

## CLOTRIMAZOLE

*Indications:* fungal infection in otitis externa
*Side-effects:* occasional skin irritation or sensitivity

**Canesten®** (Baypharm)
*Solution*, clotrimazole 1% in polyethylene
glycol. Net price 20 mL = £2.38
Apply 2–3 times daily continuing for at least 14
days after disappearance of infection

## FRAMYCETIN SULPHATE

*Indications; Cautions; Side-effects:* see under
Gentamicin

**Preparations**
Ingredient of compound anti-infective ear preparations (see below)

## GENTAMICIN

*Indications:* bacterial infection in otitis externa
*Cautions:* avoid prolonged use; slight risk of oto-
toxicity increased if perforated eardrum (see
notes above)
*Side-effects:* local sensitivity
*Administration:* apply 3–4 times daily and at night

PoM **Cidomycin®** (Roussel)
*Drops* (for ear or eye), gentamicin 0.3% (as
sulphate). Net price 8 mL = £1.34
*Additives: include* benzalkonium chloride, disodium edetate
PoM **Garamycin®** (Schering-Plough)
*Drops* (for ear or eye), gentamicin 0.3% (as
sulphate). Net price 10 mL = £1.79
*Additives: include* benzalkonium chloride
PoM **Genticin®** (Nicholas)
*Drops* (for ear or eye), gentamicin 0.3% (as
sulphate). Net price 10 mL = £2.06
*Additives: include* benzalkonium chloride
PoM **Gentisone HC®** (Nicholas)
*Ear drops*, gentamicin 0.3% (as sulphate),
hydrocortisone acetate 1%. Net price 10 mL =
£4.27

## NEOMYCIN SULPHATE

*Indications:* bacterial infection in otitis externa
*Cautions:* avoid prolonged use; slight risk of ototoxicity increased if perforated eardrum (see
notes above)
*Side-effects:* local sensitivity
*Administration:* apply ear drops every 2–3 hours;
ear ointment 2–4 times daily. Reduce frequency
of application when relief is obtained

PoM **Audicort®** (Lederle)
*Ear drops*, neomycin (as neomycin undecenoate)
0.35%, triamcinolone acetonide 0.1%. Net
price 10 mL = £7.50
Apply 3–4 times daily
PoM **Betnesol-N®** (Glaxo)
*Drops* (for ear, eye, or nose), betamethasone
sodium phosphate 0.1%, neomycin sulphate
0.5%. Net price 10 mL = £1.35
*Additives: include* thiomersal
PoM **Neo-Cortef®** (Cusi)
*Drops* (for ear or eye), hydrocortisone acetate
1.5%, neomycin sulphate 0.5%. Net price
5 mL = £3.98
*Ointment* (for ear or eye), hydrocortisone acet-
ate 1.5%, neomycin sulphate 0.5%. Net price
3.9 g = £2.98
PoM **Otomize®** (Stafford-Miller)
*Ear spray*, dexamethasone 0.1%, neomycin
sulphate 3250 units/mL. Net price 5-mL pump-
action aerosol unit = £3.95
Apply 1 metered spray 3 times daily
PoM **Predsol-N®** (Glaxo)
*Drops* (for ear or eye), neomycin sulphate 0.5%,
prednisolone sodium phosphate 0.5%. Net
price 10 mL = £1.20
*Additives: include* thiomersal
PoM **Vista-Methasone N®** (Daniel)
*Drops* (for ear, eye, or nose), betamethasone
sodium phosphate 0.1%, neomycin sulphate
0.5%. Net price 5 mL = 92p; 10 mL = £1.18

## TETRACYCLINE HYDROCHLORIDE

*Indications:* susceptible bacterial infection in otitis externa

*Cautions:* avoid prolonged use

*Side-effects:* local sensitivity; stains skin and clothing

*Administration:* apply every 2 hours

PoM **Achromycin®** (Lederle)
*Ointment* (for ear or eye), tetracycline hydrochloride 1%. Net price 3.5 g = 70p

---

## COMPOUND ANTI-INFECTIVE PREPARATIONS

PoM **Otosporin®** (Wellcome)
*Ear drops,* hydrocortisone 1%, neomycin sulphate 0.439%, polymyxin B sulphate 0.119%. Net price 5 mL = £4.58; 10 mL = £7.83
Apply 3–4 times daily

PoM **Sofradex®** (Roussel)
*Drops* (for ear or eye), dexamethasone (as sodium metasulphobenzoate) 0.05%, framycetin sulphate 0.5%, gramicidin 0.005%. Net price 10 mL = £5.50
Apply 3–4 times daily
*Ointment* (for ear or eye), dexamethasone 0.05%, framycetin sulphate 0.5%, gramicidin 0.005%. Net price 5 g = £3.64
Apply 2–3 times daily and at bedtime

PoM **Soframycin®** (Roussel)
*Cream,* framycetin sulphate 1.5%, gramicidin 0.005% in a water-miscible basis. Net price 15 g = £1.72
*Ointment,* ingredients as for cream, but in a greasy basis. Net price 15 g = £1.72
Apply 1–3 times daily

PoM **Terra-Cortril®** (Pfizer)
*Ear suspension* ( = ear drops), hydrocortisone acetate 1.5%, oxytetracycline 0.5% (as hydrochloride), polymyxin B sulphate 0.119%. Net price 5 mL = £2.06
Apply 3 times daily

PoM **Tri-Adcortyl Otic®** (Squibb)
*Ear ointment,* gramicidin 0.025%, neomycin 0.25% (as sulphate), nystatin 3.33%, triamcinolone acetonide 0.1% in Plastibase®. Net price 10 g = £1.58
Apply 2–4 times daily

---

## OTHER AURAL PREPARATIONS

Choline salicylate is a mild analgesic but it is of doubtful value when applied topically. There is no place for the use of local anaesthetics in ear drops.

**Audax®** (Napp)
*Ear drops,* choline salicylate 20%, glycerol 10%. Net price 8 mL = £1.45

---

## 12.1.2 Otitis media

Acute otitis media is the commonest cause of severe pain in small children and recurrent attacks, especially in infants, are particularly distressing. *Sero-mucinous otitis media* ('glue ear') is present in about 10% of the child population and in 90% of children with cleft palates; this condition should be referred to hospital because of the risk of permanent damage to middle ear function and impaired language development. Chronic otitis media is thought to be a legacy from untreated or resistant cases of sero-mucinous otitis media.

Local treatment of *acute otitis media* is ineffective and there is no place for drops containing a local anaesthetic. Many attacks are viral in origin and need only treatment with a **simple analgesic** such as paracetamol for pain. Severe attacks of bacterial origin should be treated with **systemic antibiotics**; bacterial examination of any discharge is helpful in selecting the appropriate treatment (see section 5.1, Table 1). Again, simple analgesics such as paracetamol are used to relieve pain. In *recurrent acute otitis media* a daily dose of a prophylactic antibiotic (trimethoprim or erythromycin) during the winter months can be tried.

The organisms recovered from patients with *chronic otitis media* are often opportunists living in the debris, keratin, and necrotic bone present in the middle ear and mastoid. Thorough cleansing with an aural suction tube may completely control infection of many years duration. Acute exacerbations of chronic infection may require systemic antibiotics (see section 5.1, Table 1). A swab should be taken to determine the organism present and its antibiotic sensitivity. Unfortunately the culture often produces *Pseudomonas aeruginosa* and *Proteus* spp, sensitive only to parenteral antibiotics. Local debridement of the meatal and middle ear contents may then be followed by topical treatment with ribbon gauze dressings as for otitis externa (section 12.1.1). This is particularly true with infections in mastoid cavities when dusting powders can also be tried.

In the presence of a perforation, however, many specialists use ear drops containing **aminoglycosides** (e.g. neomycin, framycetin) or **polymyxins**, if the otitis media has failed to settle with systemic antibiotics; it is considered that the pus in the middle ear associated with otitis media carries a higher risk of ototoxicity than the drops themselves.

## 12.1.3 Removal of ear wax

Wax is a normal bodily secretion which provides a protective film on the meatal skin and need only be removed if it causes deafness or interferes with a proper view of the eardrum. As a general rule syringing is best avoided in patients with a history of recurring otitis externa, a perforated ear drum, or previous ear surgery. A person who has hearing only in one ear should not have that ear syringed because even a very slight risk of damage is unacceptable in this situation.

Wax may be removed by syringing with warm water. If necessary, wax can be softened before syringing with simple remedies such as **olive oil** and **almond oil.** The patient should lie with the affected ear uppermost for 5 to 10 minutes after a generous amount of the solution has been introduced into the ear. Some proprietary preparations containing organic solvents can cause irritation of the meatal skin, and in most cases the simple remedies which are indicated above are just as effective and less likely to cause irritation. **Docu-**

---

**sate sodium** is an ingredient in a number of proprietary preparations.

**Almond Oil** (warm before use)
**Olive Oil** (warm before use)
**Sodium Bicarbonate Ear Drops, BP**
*Ear drops*, sodium bicarbonate 5%. Extemporaneous preparations should be recently prepared according to the following formula: sodium bicarbonate 500 mg, glycerol 3 mL, freshly boiled and cooled purified water to 10 mL
**Audinorm®** (Carlton)
*Ear drops*, docusate sodium 5%, glycerol 10%. Net price 12 mL = 30p
**Cerumol®** (LAB)
*Ear drops*, chlorbutol 5%, paradichlorobenzene 2%, arachis oil 57%. Net price 11 mL = £1.07
**Dioctyl®** (Medo)
*Ear drops*, docusate sodium 5% in macrogol. Net price 10 mL = 79p
**Exterol®** (Dermal)
*Ear drops*, urea-hydrogen peroxide complex 5% in glycerol. Net price 12 mL = £2.75
**Molcer®** (Wallace Mfg)
*Ear drops*, docusate sodium 5%. Net price 15 mL = 90p
**Waxsol®** (Norgine)
*Ear drops*, docusate sodium 0.5%. Net price 10 mL = 98p

# 12.2    Drugs acting on the nose

12.2.1 Drugs used in nasal allergy
12.2.2 Topical nasal decongestants
12.2.3 Anti-infective nasal preparations

Rhinitis is often self-limiting and sinusitis is best treated with antibiotics (see section 5.1, Table 1). There are few indications for the use of sprays and drops except in allergic rhinitis where topical preparations of corticosteroids or sodium cromoglycate have much to offer. Most other preparations contain sympathomimetic drugs which may damage the nasal cilia and their prolonged use causes mucosal oedema and severe nasal obstruction (rhinitis medicamentosa). Symptomatic relief in chronic nasal obstruction may be obtained with **systemic nasal decongestants** (see section 3.10). Douching the nose with salt and water is **not** recommended.

## 12.2.1    Drugs used in nasal allergy

Mild cases are controlled by **oral antihistamines** and **systemic nasal decongestants** (see sections 3.4.1 and 3.10). Many patients with severe symptoms can now expect relief from topical preparations of **corticosteroids** or **sodium cromoglycate**. Although sodium cromoglycate is less effective than a topical corticosteroid, it is often the first choice in children. Treatment should begin 2 to 3 weeks before the hay fever season commences and may have to be continued for months or even years in some patients. No significant side-effects have been reported. Very disabling symptoms occasionally justify the use

of **systemic corticosteroids** for short periods (see section 6.3), for example in students taking important examinations. They may also be used at the beginning of a course of treatment with a corticosteroid spray to relieve severe mucosal oedema and allow the spray to penetrate the nasal cavity.

For reference to injections of **allergen extracts** see section 3.4.2.

## AZELASTINE HYDROCHLORIDE
*Indications:* allergic rhinitis
*Side-effects:* irritation of nasal mucosa; taste disturbance
*Administration:* apply 140 micrograms (1 spray) into each nostril twice daily; CHILD not yet recommended

▼ PoM **Rhinolast®** (ASTA Medica)
*Nasal spray*, azelastine hydrochloride 140 micrograms (0.14 mL)/metered spray. Net price 10 mL (with metered pump) = £6.40

## BECLOMETHASONE DIPROPIONATE
*Indications:* allergic and vasomotor rhinitis
*Cautions:* untreated nasal infection, prolonged use in children, previous treatment with corticosteroids by mouth
*Side-effects:* sneezing after administration; rarely dryness and irritation of nose and throat, epistaxis
*Administration:* adults and children over 6 years, apply 100 micrograms (2 sprays) into each nostril twice daily *or* 50 micrograms (1 spray) 3–4 times daily; max. 8 sprays daily

PoM **Beconase®** (A&H)
*Beconase® nasal spray (aerosol)*, beclomethasone dipropionate 50 micrograms/metered inhalation. Net price 200-spray unit with applicator = £5.01
*Beconase® aqueous nasal spray (aqueous suspension)*, beclomethasone dipropionate 50 micrograms/metered spray. Net price 200-spray unit with applicator = £5.01

## BETAMETHASONE SODIUM PHOSPHATE
*Indications; Cautions; Side-effects:* see under Beclomethasone Dipropionate
*Administration:* apply 2–3 drops into each nostril 2–3 times daily

PoM **Betnesol®** (Glaxo)
*Drops (for ear, eye, or nose)*, betamethasone sodium phosphate 0.1%. Net price 10 mL = £1.31
*Additives: include* benzalkonium chloride
PoM **Vista-Methasone®** (Daniel)
*Drops (for ear, eye, or nose)*, betamethasone sodium phosphate 0.1%. Net price 5 mL = 84p; 10 mL = £1.12
*Additives: include* benzalkonium chloride

## BUDESONIDE

*Indications:* allergic and vasomotor rhinitis

*Cautions:* see under Beclomethasone Dipropionate; also patients with pulmonary tuberculosis

*Side-effects:* see under Beclomethasone Dipropionate

PoM **Rhinocort**® (Astra)

*Rhinocort*® *nasal aerosol*, budesonide 50 micrograms/metered inhalation, 200-puff unit with nasal adaptor. Net price complete unit = £5.66

*Administration:* apply 100 micrograms (2 puffs) into each nostril twice daily, reducing to 50 micrograms (1 puff) twice daily

*Rhinocort Aqua*® *nasal spray*, budesonide 100 micrograms/metered spray. Net price 100-spray unit = £6.00

*Administration:* adults and children over 12 years, apply 200 micrograms (2 sprays) into each nostril once daily in the morning *or* 100 micrograms (1 spray) into each nostril twice daily, reduced for maintenance

## FLUNISOLIDE

*Indications; Cautions; Side-effects:* see under Beclomethasone Dipropionate

*Administration:* apply 50 micrograms (2 sprays) into each nostril 2–3 times daily; CHILD over 5 years 25 micrograms (1 spray) into each nostril 3 times daily, reduced for maintenance

PoM **Syntaris**® (Syntex)

*Nasal spray*, flunisolide 25 micrograms/0.1 mL metered spray. Net price 240-spray unit with pump and applicator = £5.47

## FLUTICASONE PROPIONATE

*Indications:* allergic rhinitis

*Cautions; Side-effects:* see under Beclomethasone Dipropionate

*Administration:* adults and children over 12 years, 100 micrograms (2 sprays) into each nostril daily in the morning, increased to twice daily if required; max. 8 sprays daily

▼ PoM **Flixonase**® (A&H)

*Aqueous nasal spray*, fluticasone propionate 50 micrograms/metered spray. Net price 120-spray unit with applicator = £11.43

## SODIUM CROMOGLYCATE

*Indications:* prophylaxis of allergic rhinitis (see notes above)

*Side-effects:* local irritation, particularly during initial treatment with insufflations; rarely transient bronchospasm

**Rynacrom**® (Fisons)

*Nasal insufflation*, cartridges, pink, sodium cromoglycate 10 mg for use with insufflator. Net price 20 cartridges = 78p; insufflator = £1.66

Adults and children, insufflate 10 mg into each nostril up to 4 times daily

*Nasal drops*, sodium cromoglycate 2%. Net price 15 mL = £4.31

Adults and children, instil 2 drops into each nostril 6 times daily

*4% nasal spray*, sodium cromoglycate 4% (5.2 mg/squeeze). Net price 22 mL with pump = £5.36

Adults and children, apply 1 squeeze into each nostril 2–4 times daily

**Rynacrom Compound**® (Fisons)

*Nasal spray*, sodium cromoglycate 2% (2.6 mg/metered spray) and xylometazoline hydrochloride 0.025% (32.5 micrograms/metered spray). Net price 26 mL with pump = £5.94

Apply 1 spray into each nostril 4 times daily

*Note.* A proprietary brand of sodium cromoglycate 2% and xylometazoline hydrochloride 0.025% (Resiston One®) is on sale to the public

## 12.2.2 Topical nasal decongestants

The nasal mucosa is sensitive to changes in the atmospheric temperature and humidity and these alone may cause slight nasal congestion. The nose and nasal sinuses produce a litre of mucus in 24 hours and much of this finds its way silently into the stomach via the nasopharynx. Slight changes in the nasal airway, accompanied by an awareness of mucus passing along the nasopharynx causes some patients to be inaccurately diagnosed as suffering from chronic sinusitis. These symptoms are particularly noticeable in the later stages of the common cold for which there is no effective treatment at the moment; the temptation to use nasal drops should be resisted. **Sodium chloride** 0.9% given as nasal drops may relieve nasal congestion by helping to liquefy mucous secretions.

Symptomatic relief from the nasal congestion associated with vasomotor rhinitis, nasal polypi, and the common cold can be obtained by the short-term use of decongestant nasal drops and sprays. These all contain sympathomimetic drugs which exert their effect by vasoconstriction of the mucosal blood vessels which in turn reduces the thickness of the nasal mucosa. They are of limited value as they can give rise to a rebound phenomenon as their effects wear off, due to a secondary vasodilatation with a subsequent temporary increase in nasal congestion. This in turn tempts the further use of the decongestant, leading to a vicious circle of events. **Ephedrine nasal drops** is the safest sympathomimetic preparation and can give relief for several hours. The more potent sympathomimetic drugs oxymetazoline, phenylephrine, and xylometazoline are more likely to cause a rebound effect. **All** of these preparations may cause a hypertensive crisis if used during treatment with a monoamine-oxidase inhibitor.

Non-allergic watery rhinorrhoea often responds well to treatment with **ipratropium bromide**.

Inhalations of **warm moist air** are useful in the treatment of symptoms of acute infective conditions, and the use of compounds containing volatile substances such as menthol and eucalyptus may encourage their use (see section 3.8).

Cautionary label wordings, see inside back cover

Prices are **net**, see p. 1

There is no evidence that nasal preparations containing antihistamines and anti-infective agents have any therapeutic effect.

Systemic nasal decongestants—see section 3.10.

## SYMPATHOMIMETICS

### EPHEDRINE HYDROCHLORIDE
*Indications:* nasal congestion
*Cautions:* avoid excessive use; caution in infants under 3 months (no good evidence of value—if irritation occurs might narrow nasal passage); **interactions:** Appendix 1 (sympathomimetics)
*Side-effects:* local irritation; after excessive use tolerance with diminished effect, rebound congestion
*Administration:* instil 1–2 drops (see below) into each nostril when required

**Ephedrine Nasal Drops, BP**
*Nasal drops*, ephedrine hydrochloride in a suitable aqueous vehicle
*Note.* The BP directs that if no strength is specified 0.5% drops should be supplied; net price 10 mL = 80p

### OXYMETAZOLINE HYDROCHLORIDE
*Indications:* nasal congestion
*Cautions; Side-effects:* see under Ephedrine Hydrochloride; avoid in porphyria (see section 9.8.2)

**NHS Afrazine®** (Schering-Plough)
*Nasal spray*, oxymetazoline hydrochloride 0.05%. Net price 15 mL = 87p
Adults and children over 5 years, apply 2–3 times to each nostril every 12 hours when required

### PHENYLEPHRINE HYDROCHLORIDE
*Indications:* nasal congestion
*Cautions; Side-effects:* see under Ephedrine Hydrochloride

Compound preparations
Section 12.2.3

### XYLOMETAZOLINE HYDROCHLORIDE
*Indications:* nasal congestion
*Cautions; Side-effects:* see under Ephedrine Hydrochloride

**Xylometazoline Nasal Drops,** xylometazoline hydrochloride 0.1%, net price 10 mL = 97p
Instil 2–3 drops into each nostril 2–3 times daily when required; not recommended for children under 12 years
**Xylometazoline Nasal Drops, Paediatric** xylometazoline hydrochloride 0.05%, net price 10 mL = 97p
CHILD over 3 months instil 1–2 drops into each nostril 1–2 times daily when required (not recommended for infants under 3 months of age)
*Note.* The brand name **NHS** Otrivine® (Ciba Consumer) is used for xylometazoline adult nasal drops 0.1%, children's nasal drops 0.05%, and adult nasal spray 0.1%.

## ANTIMUSCARINIC

### IPRATROPIUM BROMIDE
*Indications:* watery rhinorrhoea associated with perennial rhinitis
*Cautions; Side-effects:* see section 3.1.2; avoid spraying near eyes
*Administration:* apply 20–40 micrograms (1–2 puffs) into affected nostril up to 4 times daily; not recommended for children under 12 years

PoM **Rinatec®** (Boehringer Ingelheim)
*Nasal spray*, ipratropium bromide 20 micrograms/metered spray. Net price 200-dose unit = £4.21

## 12.2.3   Anti-infective nasal preparations

There is **no** evidence that topical anti-infective nasal preparations have any therapeutic value; for elimination of nasal staphylococci, see below.

Systemic treatment of sinusitis—see section 5.1, Table 1.

PoM **Betnesol-N®** (Glaxo)
*Drops* (for ear, eye, or nose), section 12.1.1
PoM **Dexa-Rhinaspray®** (Boehringer Ingelheim)
*Nasal inhalation*, dexamethasone 21-isonicotinate 20 micrograms, neomycin sulphate 100 micrograms, tramazoline hydrochloride 120 micrograms/metered inhalation. Net price 125-dose unit = £1.79
PoM **Locabiotal®** (Servier)
*Nasal inhalation*, fusafungine 125 micrograms/metered inhalation. Net price 200-dose unit = £1.59
PoM **Vibrocil®** (Zyma)
*Nasal drops*, dimethindene maleate 0.025%, neomycin sulphate 0.35%, phenylephrine 0.25%. Net price 15 mL = 52p
*Nasal gel*, dimethindene maleate 0.025%, neomycin sulphate 0.35%, phenylephrine 0.25%. Net price 12 g = 52p
*Nasal spray*, dimethindene maleate 0.025%, neomycin sulphate 0.35%, phenylephrine 0.25%. Net price 10 mL = 52p
PoM **Vista-Methasone N®** (Daniel)
*Drops* (for ear, eye, or nose), section 12.1.1

## NASAL STAPHYLOCOCCI

Elimination of organisms such as staphylococci from the nasal vestibule can be achieved by the use of a cream containing **chlorhexidine and neomycin** (Naseptin®), but re-colonisation frequently occurs. Coagulase-positive staphylococci can be obtained from the noses of 40% of the population.

A nasal ointment containing **mupirocin** is also available; it should probably be kept in reserve for resistant cases.

---

PoM **Bactroban**® **Nasal** (Beecham)
*Nasal ointment*, mupirocin 2% in white soft paraffin basis. Net price 3 g = £5.15
Apply 2–3 times daily to the inner surface of each nostril

PoM **Naseptin**® (ICI)
*Cream*, chlorhexidine hydrochloride 0.1%, neomycin sulphate 0.5%. Do not dilute. Net price 15 g = £1.02
For treatment of staphylococcal infections apply to nostrils 4 times daily for 10 days; for preventing nasal carriage of staphylococci apply to nostrils twice daily

# 12.3 Drugs acting on the oropharynx

12.3.1 Drugs for oral ulceration and inflammation
12.3.2 Oropharyngeal anti-infective drugs
12.3.3 Antiseptic lozenges, sprays, and gels
12.3.4 Mouthwashes, gargles, and dentifrices

## 12.3.1 Drugs for oral ulceration and inflammation

Ulceration of the oral mucosa may be caused by trauma (physical or chemical), recurrent aphthae, infections, carcinoma, dermatological disorders, nutritional deficiencies, gastro-intestinal disease, haematopoietic disorders, and drug therapy. It is important to establish the diagnosis in each case as the majority of these lesions require specific management in addition to local treatment. Local treatment aims at protecting the ulcerated area, or at relieving pain or reducing inflammation.

SIMPLE MOUTHWASHES. A **saline** or **compound thymol glycerin** mouthwash may relieve the pain of traumatic ulceration. The mouthwash is made up with warm water and used at frequent intervals until the discomfort and swelling subsides.

ANTISEPTIC MOUTHWASHES. Secondary bacterial infection may be a feature of any mucosal ulceration; it can increase discomfort and delay healing. Use of a **chlorhexidine** or **povidone-iodine** mouthwash is often beneficial and may accelerate healing of recurrent aphthae.

MECHANICAL PROTECTION. **Carmellose gelatin paste** may relieve some discomfort arising from ulceration by protecting the ulcer site. The paste adheres to the mucosa, but is difficult to apply effectively to some parts of the mouth.

ZINC SULPHATE. Zinc sulphate mouthwash is an astringent. Some patients find it beneficial in recurrent aphthae.

CORTICOSTEROIDS. Topical corticosteroid therapy may be used for different forms of oral ulceration. In the case of aphthous ulcers it is most effective if applied in the 'prodromal' phase.
Thrush or other types of candidiasis are recognised complications of corticosteroid treatment.

**Hydrocortisone lozenges** are allowed to dissolve next to an ulcer and are useful in recurrent aphthae, erosive lichen planus, discoid lupus erythematosus, and benign mucous membrane pemphigoid.

**Triamcinolone dental paste** is designed to keep the corticosteroid in contact with the mucosa for long enough to permit penetration of the lesion, but is difficult for patients to apply properly.

Systemic corticosteroid therapy is reserved for severe conditions such as pemphigus vulgaris (see section 6.3.4).

LOCAL ANALGESICS. Local analgesics have a limited role in the management of oral ulceration. When applied topically their action is of a relatively short duration so that analgesia cannot be maintained continuously throughout the day. The main indication for a topical local analgesic is to relieve the pain of otherwise intractable oral ulceration particularly when it is due to major aphthae. For this purpose lignocaine 5% ointment or lozenges containing a local anaesthetic are applied to the ulcer. When local anaesthetics are used in the mouth care must be taken not to produce anaesthesia of the pharynx before meals as this might lead to choking.

**Benzydamine** mouthwash or spray may be useful in palliating the discomfort associated with a variety of ulcerative conditions. It has also been found to be effective in reducing the discomfort of post-irradiation mucositis. Some patients find the full-strength mouthwash causes some stinging and, for them, it should be diluted with an equal volume of water.

**Choline salicylate** dental gel has some analgesic action and may provide relief for recurrent aphthae, but excessive application or confinement under a denture irritates the mucosa and can itself cause ulceration. Benefit in teething may merely be due to pressure of application (comparable with biting a teething ring); excessive use can lead to salicylate poisoning.

OTHER PREPARATIONS. **Carbenoxolone** gel or mouthwash may be of some value. **Tetracycline** rinsed in the mouth may also be of value.

## BENZYDAMINE HYDROCHLORIDE

*Indications:* painful inflammatory conditions of oropharynx
*Side-effects:* occasional numbness or stinging

**Difflam**® (3M)
*Oral rinse*, green, benzydamine hydrochloride 0.15%. Net price 300 mL = £4.25
Rinse or gargle, using 15 mL (diluted if stinging occurs) every 1½–3 hours as required, usually for not more than 7 days; not suitable for children under 12 years
*Spray*, benzydamine hydrochloride 0.15%. Net price 30-mL unit = £3.39
4–8 puffs onto affected area every 1½–3 hours; CHILD 6–12 years 4 puffs every 1½–3 hours

## CARBENOXOLONE SODIUM

*Indications:* mild oral and perioral lesions

**Bioral Gel®** (Sterling Health)
*Gel,* carbenoxolone sodium 2% in adhesive basis. Net price 5 g = £1.83
Apply after meals and at bedtime

PoM **Bioplex®** (Thames)
*Mouthwash granules,* carbenoxolone sodium 1%. Net price 24 × 2-g sachets = £9.60
For mouth ulcers, rinse with 2 g in 30–50 mL of warm water 3 times daily and at bedtime

## CARMELLOSE SODIUM

*Indications:* mechanical protection of oral and perioral lesions

**Orabase®** (Squibb)
*Oral paste,* carmellose sodium 16.58%, pectin 16.58%, gelatin 16.58%, in Plastibase®. Net price 30 g = £1.50; 100 g = £3.32
Apply a thin layer when necessary after meals

**Orahesive®** (Squibb)
*Powder,* carmellose sodium, pectin, gelatin, equal parts. Net price 25 g = £1.72
Sprinkle on the affected area

## CORTICOSTEROIDS

*Indications:* oral and perioral lesions
*Contra-indications:* untreated oral infection

PoM **Adcortyl in Orabase®** (Squibb)
*Oral paste,* triamcinolone acetonide 0.1% in adhesive basis. Net price 10 g = £1.27
Apply a thin layer 2–4 times daily

PoM **Corlan®** (Glaxo)
*Pellets* (= lozenges), hydrocortisone 2.5 mg (as sodium succinate). Net price 20 = £1.40
One lozenge 4 times daily, allowed to dissolve slowly in the mouth in contact with the ulcer; if ulcers recur rapidly treatment may be continued for a period at reduced dosage

## LOCAL ANAESTHETICS

*Indications:* relief of pain in oral lesions
*Cautions:* avoid prolonged use; hypersensitivity may occur

Standard strength lozenges
Available with antiseptics, section 12.3.3

High strength lozenges
**Benzocaine Lozenges, Compound,** benzocaine 100 mg, menthol 3 mg
*Note.* It is **essential** not to confuse these with benzocaine lozenges which contained one-tenth the amount of benzocaine and are no longer available
Available from Penn (**special order**, bulk quantities only)

## SALICYLATES

*Indications:* mild oral and perioral lesions
*Cautions:* frequent application, especially in children, may give rise to salicylate poisoning
*Note.* CSM warning on aspirin and Reye's syndrome does not apply to non-aspirin salicylates or to topical preparations such as teething gels

Choline salicylate
**Bonjela®** (R&C)
*Oral gel,* sugar-free, choline salicylate dental gel containing choline salicylate 8.7%. Net price 15 g = £1.11

**Teejel®** (Napp)
*Oral gel,* choline salicylate dental gel containing choline salicylate 8.7%. Net price 10 g = 66p

Salicylic acid
**Pyralvex®** (Norgine)
*Oral paint,* brown, anthraquinone glycosides 5%, salicylic acid 1%. Net price 10 mL with brush = £1.27. Apply 3–4 times daily

## TETRACYCLINE

*Indications:* severe recurrent aphthous ulceration; oral herpes (section 12.3.2)
*Side-effects:* fungal superinfection

PoM **Tetracycline Mixture**[1], tetracycline hydrochloride 125 mg (as tetracycline)/5 mL
*Administration:* 10 mL to be held in the mouth for 2–3 minutes 3 times daily for not longer than 3 days followed by a break of at least 3 days before treatment is recommenced (to avoid oral thrush); it should preferably not be swallowed
*Note.* Tetracycline stains teeth; avoid in children under 12 years of age
1. A suitable proprietary preparation is no longer available; alternatively the contents of a 250-mg tetracycline capsule (see section 5.1.3) can be stirred in a small amount of water and used in the same way as the mixture

## 12.3.2 Oropharyngeal anti-infective drugs

The most common cause of a sore throat is a viral infection which does not benefit from anti-infective treatment. Streptococcal sore throats require systemic **penicillin** therapy (see section 5.1.1). Acute ulcerative gingivitis (Vincent's infection) responds to systemic **metronidazole** 200 mg 3 times daily for 3 days (see section 5.1.11) or **nimorazole** 500 mg twice daily for 2 days (see section 5.4.3).

### FUNGAL INFECTIONS

*Candida albicans* may cause thrush and other forms of stomatitis which are sometimes a sequel to the use of broad-spectrum antibiotics or cytotoxics; withdrawing the causative drug may lead to rapid resolution. Otherwise, **nystatin**, **amphotericin**, or **miconazole** may be effective.

### AMPHOTERICIN

*Indications:* oral and perioral fungal infections

PoM **Fungilin®** (Squibb)
*Lozenges,* yellow, amphotericin 10 mg. Net price 6 × 10 lozenge-pack = £3.95. Label: 9, 24, counselling, after food
Dissolve 1 lozenge slowly in the mouth 4 times daily, may require 10–15 days' treatment; increase to 8 daily if infection severe

*Suspension*, yellow, sugar-free, amphotericin 100 mg/mL. Net price 12 mL with pipette = £2.31. Label: 9, counselling, use of pipette, hold in mouth, after food
Place 1 mL in the mouth after food and retain near lesions 4 times daily for 14 days

## MICONAZOLE
*Indications:* oral fungal infections
*Cautions:* pregnancy; **interactions:** Appendix 1 (miconazole)

PoM[1] **Daktarin**® (Janssen)
*Oral gel*, sugar-free, miconazole 25 mg/mL. Net price 80 g = £5.00. Label: 9, counselling, hold in mouth, after food
Place 5–10 mL in the mouth after food and retain near lesions before swallowing, 4 times daily; CHILD under 2 years 2.5 mL twice daily, 2–6 years 5 mL twice daily, over 6 years 5 mL 4 times daily
Localised lesions, smear affected area with clean finger; a 15-g tube (net price £1.70) also available
1. 15-g tube can be sold to the public
*Tablets*—see section 5.2

## NYSTATIN
*Indications:* oral and perioral fungal infections
*Dose:* (as pastilles or as suspension) 100 000 units 4 times daily after food, continued for 48 hours after lesions have resolved
*Note.* Immunosuppressed patients may require higher doses (e.g. 500 000 units 4 times daily)

PoM **Nystan**® (Squibb)
*Pastilles*, yellow/brown, nystatin 100 000 units. Net price 28 pastille-pack = £3.95. Label: 9, 24, counselling, after food
*Suspension*, yellow, nystatin 100 000 units/mL. Net price 30 mL with pipette = £2.50. Label: 9, counselling, use of pipette, hold in mouth, after food
*Suspension*, gluten-, lactose-, and sugar-free, nystatin 100 000 units/mL when reconstituted with water. Measure with pipette. Net price 24 mL with pipette = £1.67. Label: 9, counselling, use of pipette, hold in mouth, after food
PoM **Nystatin-Dome**® (Lagap)
*Suspension*, yellow, nystatin 100 000 units/mL. Net price 30 mL with 1-mL spoon = £2.86. Label: 9, counselling, use of 1-mL spoon, hold in mouth, after food

## VIRAL INFECTIONS

The management of herpes infections of the mouth is a soft diet, adequate fluid intake, analgesics as required, and the use of **chlorhexidine** mouthwash (Corsodyl®, section 12.3.4) to control plaque accumulation if toothbrushing is painful. In the case of severe herpetic stomatitis, systemic **acyclovir** is required (see section 5.3).

Herpes infections of the mouth may also respond to **tetracycline** (section 12.3.1) rinsed in the mouth.
**Idoxuridine** 0.1% paint has been superseded by more effective preparations.

## ACYCLOVIR
See section 5.3

## TETRACYCLINE
Section 12.3.1

## 12.3.3 Lozenges, sprays, and gels
There is no convincing evidence that antiseptic lozenges and sprays have a beneficial action and they sometimes irritate and cause sore tongue and sore lips. Some of these preparations also contain local anaesthetics which relieve pain but may cause sensitisation.
In particular preparations containing clioquinol are not recommended.

**Benzalkonium Lozenges,** benzalkonium chloride 500 micrograms. Net price 20 lozenges = 48p
**Bradosol**® (Ciba Consumer)
*Lozenges*, domiphen bromide 500 micrograms. Net price 24 lozenges = 66p
**Dequadin**® (Crookes)
*Lozenges*, orange, dequalinium chloride 250 micrograms. Net price 20 lozenges = 54p
Dissolve 1 lozenge slowly in the mouth when required
**Labosept**® (LAB)
*Pastilles*, red, dequalinium chloride 250 micrograms. Net price 20 pastilles = 68p
Suck 1 pastille slowly when required
PoM **Locabiotal**® (Servier)
*Aerosol spray*, fusafungine 125 micrograms/metered inhalation. Net price 200-dose unit with nasal and oral adaptor = £1.59
**Merocets**® (Merrell)
*Lozenges*, yellow, cetylpyridinium chloride 0.066%. Net price 24 lozenges = 78p

### Clioquinol
**Oralcer**® (Vitabiotics)
*Lozenges*, ivory, ascorbic acid 6 mg, clioquinol 35 mg. Net price 20 lozenges = 73p

### With local anaesthetic
**AAA**® (Rhône-Poulenc Rorer)
*Mouth and throat spray*, benzocaine 1.5 mg/metered dose. Net price 60-dose unit = £2.46
2 sprays every 2–3 hours (max. 16 sprays daily); CHILD 6–12 years, 1 spray every 2–3 hours (max. 8 sprays daily)
**Bradosol Plus**® (Ciba Consumer)
*Lozenges*, pink, lignocaine hydrochloride 5 mg, domiphen bromide 500 micrograms. Net price 24 = 89p
Adults and children over 12 years, 1 lozenge sucked every 2–3 hours; max. 8 lozenges daily
**Dequacaine**® (Crookes)
*Lozenges*, amber, benzocaine 10 mg, dequalinium chloride 250 micrograms. Net price 24 lozenges = 98p
Adults and children over 12 years, 1 lozenge sucked every 2 hours or as required; max. 8 lozenges daily
**Eludril**® (Fabre)
*Aerosol spray*, amethocaine hydrochloride 0.015%, chlorhexidine gluconate 0.05%. Net price 55 mL = £1.37
1 spray 3–4 times daily, increased to up to every hour in acute conditions

**Medilave®** (Martindale)

*Gel*, benzocaine 1%, cetylpyridinium chloride 0.01%. Net price 10 g = 61p

Adults, apply thin layer 3–4 times daily; no longer recommended for children under 12 years

**Merocaine®** (Merrell)

*Lozenges*, green, benzocaine 10 mg, cetylpyridinium chloride 1.4 mg. Net price 24 lozenges = 85p

Adults and children over 12 years, 1 lozenge sucked every 2 hours or as required; max. 8 lozenges daily

**Tyrozets®** (MSD)

*Lozenges*, pink, benzocaine 5 mg, tyrothricin 1 mg. Net price 24 lozenges = 66p

1 lozenge sucked every 3 hours (max. 8 lozenges daily); reduce dose in children (not for children under 3 years)

**Vicks Ultra Chloraseptic®** (Procter & Gamble)

*Throat spray*, benzocaine 1 mg/metered spray. Net price 15 mL = £2.47

Adults and children over 13 years, 3 sprays every 2–3 hours (max. 24 sprays daily); child 6–12 years, 1 spray every 2–3 hours (max. 8 sprays daily)

For teething

**Calgel®** (Wellcome)

*Teething gel*, lignocaine hydrochloride 0.33%, cetylpyridinium chloride 0.1%. Net price 10 g = 72p

Apply small quantity to gum up to 6 times daily

## 12.3.4 Mouthwashes, gargles, and dentifrices

Mouthwashes have a mechanical cleansing action and freshen the mouth. Warm **compound sodium chloride mouthwash** or **compound thymol glycerin** is as useful as any.

**Hydrogen peroxide mouthwash** has a mechanical cleansing effect due to frothing when in contact with oral debris. **Sodium perborate** is similar in effect to hydrogen peroxide.

There is evidence that **chlorhexidine** has a specific effect in inhibiting the formation of plaque on teeth. A chlorhexidine mouthwash may be useful as an adjunct to other oral hygiene measures in cases of oral infection or when toothbrushing is not possible.

There is no convincing evidence that gargles are effective.

## CETYLPYRIDINIUM CHLORIDE

*Indications:* oral hygiene

**Merocet®** (Merrell)

*Solution* ( = mouthwash or gargle), yellow, cetylpyridinium chloride 0.05%. Net price 200 mL = £1.12

To be used undiluted or diluted with an equal volume of warm water

## CHLORHEXIDINE GLUCONATE

*Indications:* oral hygiene; inhibition of plaque formation

*Side-effects:* idiosyncratic mucosal irritation; reversible brown staining of teeth

**Corsodyl®** (ICI)

*Dental gel*, chlorhexidine gluconate 1%. Net price 50 g = 83p

Brush on the teeth once or twice daily

*Mouthwash*, chlorhexidine gluconate 0.2% (original or mint-flavoured). Net price 300 mL = £1.25

Rinse the mouth with 10 mL for about 1 minute twice daily

**Eludril®** (Fabre)

*Mouthwash*, red, chlorhexidine gluconate 0.1%, chlorbutol 0.5%. Net price 90 mL = 67p; 250 mL = £1.46; 500 mL = £2.74

Use 10–15 mL in a third of a tumblerful of warm water 2–3 times daily

## HEXETIDINE

*Indications:* oral hygiene

**Oraldene®** (W-L)

*Mouthwash* or *gargle*, red, hexetidine 0.1%. Net price 100 mL = 83p; 200 mL = £1.34

Use 15 mL undiluted 2–3 times daily

## OXIDISING AGENTS

*Indications:* oral hygiene, see notes above

**Hydrogen Peroxide Mouthwash, DPF**, consists of hydrogen peroxide solution (6% ≡ approx. 20 volume)

Rinse the mouth for 2–3 minutes with 15 mL in half a tumblerful of warm water 2–3 times daily

**Bocasan®** (Oral-B Labs)

*Mouthwash*, sodium perborate 70% (buffered). Net price 20 × 1.7-g sachet-pack = £1.34

Use 1 sachet in 30 mL of water

*Cautions:* Do not use for longer than 7 days because of possible absorption of borate; not recommended in renal impairment or for children under 5 years

## PHENOL

*Indications:* oral hygiene

**Chloraseptic®** (Procter & Gamble)

*Mouthwash/gargle*, green, phenol 1.4%. Net price 150 mL = £1.85

Use every 2 hours if necessary, undiluted or diluted with an equal volume of water as a mouthwash or gargle (CHILD 6–12 years on doctor's advice only; under 6 years not recommended)

**Vicks Ultra Chloraseptic**, see section 12.3.3

## POVIDONE-IODINE

*Indications:* oral hygiene

*Cautions:* pregnancy; breast-feeding

*Side-effects:* idiosyncratic mucosal irritation and hypersensitivity reactions

**Betadine®** (Napp)

*Mouthwash* or *gargle*, amber, povidone-iodine 1%. Net price 250 mL = 82p

Adults and children over 6 years, up to 10 mL undiluted or diluted with an equal quantity of warm water up to 4 times daily for up to 14 days

## SODIUM CHLORIDE

*Indications:* oral hygiene, see notes above

**Sodium Chloride Mouthwash, Compound, BP**
*Mouthwash,* sodium bicarbonate 1%, sodium chloride 1.5% in a suitable vehicle with a peppermint flavour.
Extemporaneous preparations should be prepared according to the following formula: sodium chloride 1.5 g, sodium bicarbonate 1 g, concentrated peppermint emulsion 2.5 mL, double-strength chloroform water 50 mL, water to 100 mL
To be diluted with an equal volume of warm water

## THYMOL

*Indications:* oral hygiene, see notes above

**Compound Thymol Glycerin,** glycerol 10%, thymol 0.05% with colouring and flavouring
To be used undiluted or diluted with 3 volumes of warm water

**Mouthwash Solution-tablets,** consist of tablets which may contain antimicrobial, colouring, and flavouring agents in a suitable soluble effervescent basis to make a mouthwash suitable for dental purposes. Net price 20 solution-tablets = 32p
Dissolve 1 tablet in a tumblerful of warm water

## ZINC SULPHATE

*Indications:* see notes above

**Zinc Sulphate Lotion** (BP)
(Zinc Sulphate Mouthwash, DPF)
*Mouthwash,* zinc sulphate 1 g, amaranth solution 1 mL, water to 100 mL
Dilute 1 part with 4 parts warm water before use

## OTHER PREPARATIONS FOR OROPHARYNGEAL USE

**Artificial saliva** may be indicated for dry mouth. Proprietary preparations are available.

**Artificial Saliva, DPF**
A suitable inert, slightly viscous, aqueous liquid; it may contain an antimicrobial preservative, normal salivary constituents, small amounts of fluoride, and colouring and flavouring agents.
Extemporaneous preparations may be prepared according to the following formula: sodium chloride 100 mg, hypromellose '4500' 1.3 g, saccharin sodium 10 mg, thymol 10 mg, peppermint oil 0.02 mL, spearmint oil 0.03 mL, amaranth solution 0.1 mL, water to 100 mL
*Dose:* up to 5 mL as required; max. 20 mL daily

**Glandosane®** (Fresenius)
*Aerosol spray,* carmellose sodium 500 mg, sorbitol 1.5 g, potassium chloride 60 mg, sodium chloride 42.2 mg, magnesium chloride 2.6 mg, calcium chloride 7.3 mg, and dipotassium hydrogen phosphate 17.1 mg/50 g. Net price 50-mL unit (neutral or flavoured) = £3.65. ACBS: patients suffering from dry mouth as a result of having or having undergone radiotherapy, or sicca syndrome.
Spray onto oral and pharyngeal mucosa as required to provide artificial saliva

**Luborant®** (Antigen)
*Oral spray,* pink, sorbitol 1.8 g, carmellose sodium (sodium carboxymethylcellulose) 390 mg, dibasic potassium phosphate 48.23 mg, potassium chloride 37.5 mg, monobasic potassium phosphate 21.97 mg, calcium chloride 9.972 mg, magnesium chloride 3.528 mg, sodium fluoride 258 micrograms/60 mL, with preservatives and colouring agents. Net price 60-mL unit = £3.96
Saliva deficiency, 2–3-sprays onto oral mucosa up to 4 times daily, or as directed
*Note.* Excessive use of preparations containing fluoride has resulted in mottling of dental enamel

**Saliva Orthana®** (Nycomed)
*Aerosol spray,* gastric mucin (porcine) 3.5%, with preservatives and flavouring agents. Net price 450-mL spray bottle = £25.10 (hosp. only)
ACBS: patients suffering from dry mouth as a result of having, or undergone, radiotherapy, or sicca syndrome, spray 2–3 times onto oral and pharyngeal mucosa, when required

# 13: Drugs acting on the

# SKIN

In this chapter, drug treatment is discussed under the following headings:

13.1 Vehicles
13.2 Emollient and barrier preparations
13.3 Local anaesthetics and antipruritics
13.4 Topical corticosteroids
13.5 Preparations for psoriasis and eczema
13.6 Preparations for acne
13.7 Preparations for warts and calluses
13.8 Sunscreens and camouflagers
13.9 Shampoos and some other scalp preparations
13.10 Anti-infective skin preparations
13.11 Disinfectants and cleansers
13.12 Antiperspirants
13.13 Wound management products
13.14 Topical circulatory preparations

Suitable quantities of dermatological preparations to be prescribed for specific areas of the body are:

|  | Creams and Ointments | Lotions |
|---|---|---|
| Face | 5 to 15 g | 100 mL |
| Both hands | 25 to 50 g | 200 mL |
| Scalp | 50 to 100 g | 200 mL |
| Both arms or both legs | 100 to 200 g | 200 mL |
| Body | 200 g | 500 mL |
| Groins and genitalia | 15 to 25 g | 100 mL |
| Dusting powders | 50 to 100 g |  |
| Paints | 10 to 25 mL |  |

These amounts are usually suitable for 2 to 4 weeks.
The recommendations do not apply to corticosteroid preparations which should be applied thinly. Corticosteroid creams and ointments are available in various pack sizes, commonly 15 g or 30 g, while corticosteroid lotions are usually packed in 20- or 100-mL sizes.

## 13.1 Vehicles

Both vehicle and active ingredients are important in the treatment of skin conditions; it is being increasingly recognised that the vehicle alone may have more than a mere placebo effect. The vehicle affects the degree of hydration of the skin, has a mild anti-inflammatory effect, and aids the penetration of active drug in the preparation.

The vehicle may take the form of a cream, ointment, lotion, paste, dusting powder, application, collodion, or paint basis.

DILUTION. The BP directs that creams and ointments should **not** normally be diluted but that should dilution be necessary care should be taken, in particular, to prevent microbial contamination. The appropriate diluent should be used and heating should be avoided during mixing; excessive dilution may affect the stability of some creams. Diluted creams should normally be used within 2 weeks of their preparation.

ADDITIVES. The following additives in topical preparations may be associated with sensitisation, particularly of eczematous skin. Details of whether they are contained in preparations listed in the BNF are given after the preparation entry.

| Most commonly | Less commonly | Rarely[1] |
|---|---|---|
| Wool fat and related substances | Benzyl alcohol | Beeswax |
| Chlorocresol | Butylated hydroxyanisole | Edetic acid (EDTA) |
| Ethylenediamine | Butylated hydroxytoluene | Isopropyl palmitate |
| Fragrances | Hydroxybenzoates (parabens) | |
| | Polysorbates | |
| | Propylene glycol | |
| | Sorbic acid | |

1. Non-dermatologists can reasonably disregard the substances in this category

APPLICATIONS are usually viscous solutions, emulsions, or suspensions for application to the skin.

COLLODIONS are painted on the skin and allowed to dry to leave a flexible film over the site of application. Flexible collodion may be used to seal minor cuts and wounds. Collodions may also be used to provide a means of holding a dissolved drug in contact with the skin for a long period, e.g. salicylic acid collodion (section 13.7).

CREAMS are essentially miscible with the skin secretion. They may contain an antimicrobial preservative unless the active ingredient or basis has sufficient intrinsic bactericidal or fungicidal activity. Generally, creams are cosmetically more acceptable than ointments as they are less greasy and easier to apply.

DUSTING POWDERS are finely divided powders that contain one or more active ingredients with or without auxiliary substances. They are intended to be applied to skin for therapeutic, prophylactic or lubricant purposes. If dusting powder is intended for large open wounds or severely injured skin it should be sterile.

LINIMENTS are liquid preparations for external application and may contain analgesics and rubefacients, see section 10.3.2.

LOTIONS are usually aqueous solutions or suspensions which cool diffusely inflamed unbroken skin. They cool by evaporation and should be reapplied frequently. Volatile solvents increase the cooling effect but are liable to cause stinging. Lotions are also used to apply drugs to the skin and may be preferred to ointments or creams when it is intended to apply a thin layer of the

---

preparation over a large or hairy area. *Shake lotions* (such as calamine lotion) containing insoluble powders are applied to less acute, scabbed, dry lesions. In addition to cooling they leave a deposit of inert powder on the skin surface.

OINTMENTS are greasy preparations which are normally anhydrous and insoluble in water, and are more occlusive than creams. The most commonly used ointment bases consist of soft paraffin or a combination of soft paraffin with liquid paraffin and hard paraffin. Some modern ointment bases have both hydrophilic and lipophilic properties; they may have occlusive properties on the skin surface, encourage hydration, and be miscible with water; they often have a mild anti-inflammatory effect. Water-soluble ointments contain macrogols which are freely soluble in water and are therefore readily washed off; they have a limited but useful application in circumstances where ready removal is desirable. Ointments are particularly suitable for chronic, dry lesions.

PAINTS are liquid preparations intended for application with a brush to the skin or mucous surfaces.

PASTES are stiff preparations containing a high proportion of finely powdered solids such as zinc oxide and starch. They are used for circumscribed lesions such as those which occur in lichen simplex, chronic eczema, or psoriasis. They are less occlusive than ointments and can be used to protect sub-acute, lichenified, or excoriated skin.

# 13.2 Emollient and barrier preparations

13.2.1 Emollients
13.2.2 Barrier preparations
13.2.3 Dusting powders

BORDERLINE SUBSTANCES. The preparations marked 'ACBS' are regarded as drugs when prescribed in accordance with the advice of the Advisory Committee on Borderline Substances for the clinical conditions listed. Prescriptions issued in accordance with this advice and endorsed 'ACBS' will normally not be investigated. See Appendix 7 for listing by clinical condition.

## 13.2.1 Emollients

**Emollients** soothe, smooth and hydrate the skin and are indicated for all dry scaling disorders (such as ichthyosis). Their effects are short-lived and they should be applied frequently even after improvement occurs. They are useful in dry eczematous disorders, and to a lesser extent in psoriasis (section 13.5). Simple preparations such as **aqueous cream** are often as effective as the more complex proprietary formulations; sprays offer little advantage but, in general, the choice depends on patient preference. Some ingredients may cause sensitisation, notably hydrous wool fat (lanolin) or antibacterials and this should be suspected if an eczematous reaction occurs.

Camphor, menthol, and phenol have a mild antipruritic effect when used in emollient preparations. Calamine and zinc oxide may also be included as they slightly enhance therapeutic efficacy; they are particularly useful in dry eczema. Zinc and titanium preparations have mild astringent properties. Thickening agents such as talc and kaolin may also be included. Preparations containing an antibacterial should be avoided unless infection is present (section 13.10).

**Urea** is employed as a hydrating agent. It is used in scaling conditions and may be useful in elderly patients and infantile eczemas. It is often used with other topical agents such as corticosteroids to enhance penetration.

**Aqueous Cream, BP,** emulsifying ointment 30%, phenoxyethanol 1%, in freshly boiled and cooled purified water. Net price 100 g = 27p
Available from APS, Cox, Evans
**Emulsifying Ointment, BP,** emulsifying wax 30%, white soft paraffin 50%, liquid paraffin 20%. Net price 100 g = 30p
Available from APS, Cox, CP, Evans
**Hydrous Ointment, BP** (oily cream), dried magnesium sulphate 0.5%, phenoxyethanol 1%, wool alcohols ointment 50%, in freshly boiled and cooled purified water. Net price 100 g = 33p
Available from CP, Evans
**Paraffin, White Soft, BP** (white petroleum jelly). Net price 100 g = 34p
Available from APS, CP, Evans
**Paraffin, Yellow Soft, BP** (yellow petroleum jelly). Net price 100 g = 35p
Available from CP, Evans
**Zinc Cream, BP,** zinc oxide 32%, arachis oil 32%, calcium hydroxide 0.045%, oleic acid 0.5%, wool fat 8%, in freshly boiled and cooled purified water. Net price 50 g = 44p. For napkin and urinary rash and eczematous conditions
Available from Evans
**Zinc Ointment, BP,** zinc oxide 15%, in simple ointment. Net price 25 g = 20p. For napkin and urinary rash and eczematous conditions
Available from Evans
**Zinc and Castor Oil Ointment, BP,** zinc oxide 7.5%, castor oil 50%, arachis oil 30.5%, white beeswax 10%, cetostearyl alcohol 2%. Net price 25 g = 20p. For napkin and urinary rash
Available from CP, Evans

**Alcoderm®** (Galderma)
*Cream*, containing liquid paraffin, cetyl alcohol, stearyl alcohol, sodium lauryl sulphate, carbomer, triethanolamine, sorbitan monosterate, sorbitol, spermaceti, silicone fluid. Net price 60 g = £2.40
*Additives:* hydroxybenzoates (parabens), isopropyl palmitate
*Lotion*, water-miscible, ingredients as above. Net price 120 mL = £2.86
**Aveeno®** (Bioglan)
*Cream*, colloidal oat fraction in emollient basis containing allantoin. Net price 75 mL = £1.94.
ACBS: For endogenous and exogenous eczema, xeroderma, ichthyosis, and senile pruritus associated with dry skin
*Additives:* benzyl alcohol

**Diprobase®** (Schering-Plough)

*Cream*, cetomacrogol 2.25%, cetostearyl alcohol 7.2%, liquid paraffin 6%, white soft paraffin 15%, water-miscible basis used for Diprosone® cream. Net price 50 g = £1.65; 500-g dispenser = £7.10
*Additives:* chlorocresol

*Ointment*, liquid paraffin 5%, white soft paraffin 95%, basis used for Diprosone® ointment. Net price 50 g = £1.65
*Additives:* none as listed in section 13.1

**Dermacare®** (Elida Gibbs)

*Cream*, dimethicone 1%, while soft paraffin 15%. Net price 100 mL = £1.45. ACBS: for endogenous and exogenous eczema, xeroderma, ichthyosis and senile pruritus associated with dry skin
*Additives:* hydroxybenzoates (parabens)

*Lotion*, dimethicone 1%, liquid paraffin 4%, white soft paraffin 5% in an emollient basis. Net price 75 mL = 94p; 200 mL = £1.86. ACBS: for endogenous and exogenous eczema, xeroderma, ichthyosis and senile pruritus associated with dry skin
*Additives:* disodium edetate, hydroxybenzoates (parabens), wool fat

**Dermalex®** and **Drapolene®**—section 13.10.5

**E45®** (Crookes)

*Cream*, light liquid paraffin 11.6%, white soft paraffin 14.5%, wool fat 1% self-emulsifying monostearin, stearic acid, triethanolamine. Net price 50 g = 96p; 125 g = £1.91; 500 g = £4.46
*Additives:* hydroxybenzoates (parabens)

*Wash E45*, soap substitute, zinc oxide 5% in an emollient basis. Net price 150 mL = £2.01. ACBS: endogenous and exogenous eczema, xeroderma, ichthyosis and senile pruritus associated with dry skin
*Additives:* butylated hydroxytoluene

**Eczederm®**—section 13.3

**Hewletts Cream®** (Astra)

*Cream*, hydrous wool fat 4%, zinc oxide 8%. Net price 35 g = 56p; 400 g = £3.14. For nursing hygiene and care of skin
*Additives:* fragrance

**Humiderm®** (BritCair)

*Cream*, pyrrolidone carboxylic acid 5% (as sodium salt). Net price 60 g = £3.50. For dry skin conditions
*Additives:* hydroxybenzoates (parabens), propylene glycol

**Hydromol®** (Quinoderm Ltd)

*Cream*, arachis oil 10%, isopropyl myristate 5%, liquid paraffin 10%, sodium pyrrolidone carboxylate 2.5%, sodium lactate 1%. Net price 50 g = £1.96; 100 g = £3.24; 500 g = £10.43. For dry skin conditions
*Additives:* hydroxybenzoates (parabens)

**Kamillosan®** (Norgine)

*Ointment*, chamomile extracts 10.5%. Net price 5 g = 57p (hosp. only); 24 g = £1.43. For napkin rash, cracked nipples and chapped hands
*Additives:* beeswax, hydroxybenzoates (parabens), wool fat

**Keri®** (Bristol-Myers)

*Lotion*, mineral oil 16%, with lanolin oil. Net price 190-mL pump pack = £3.65; 380-mL pump pack = £5.96. For dry skin conditions and napkin rash
*Additives:* hydroxybenzoates (parabens), propylene glycol, fragrance

**Lacticare®** (Stiefel)

*Lotion*, lactic acid 5%, sodium pyrrolidone carboxylate 2.5%, in an emulsion basis. Net price 150 mL = £3.19. For dry skin conditions
*Additives:* isopropyl palmitate, fragrance

**Lipobase®** (Brocades)

*Cream*, fatty cream basis used for Locoid Lipocream®. Net price 50 g = £2.05
*Additives:* hydroxybenzoates (parabens)

**Massé Breast Cream®** (Cilag)

*Cream* (water-miscible), containing arachis oil, cetyl alcohol, glycerol, glyceryl monostearate, wool fat, polysorbate 60, potassium hydroxide, sorbitan monostearate, stearic acid. Net price 28 g = £1.40. For pre- and postnatal nipple care
*Additives:* hydroxybenzoates (parabens)

**Morhulin®** (Napp)

*Ointment*, cod-liver oil 11.4%, zinc oxide 38%, in a basis containing wool fat and paraffin. Net price 50 g = 82p; 350 g = £4.20. For minor wounds, varicose ulcers, and pressure sores

**Morsep®** (Napp)

*Cream*, cetrimide 0.5%, ergocalciferol 10 units/g, vitamin A 70 units/g. Net price 40 g = 87p; 300 g = £3.47. For urinary rash
*Additives:* wool fat derivative, fragrance

**Natuderm®** (Burgess)

*Cream* (hydrophilic and lipophilic), free fatty acids 5%, glycerides 15.5%, glycerol 3.7%, phospholipids 0.2%, polysorbate '60' 1.1%, sorbitan monostearate 1%, squalane 0.5%, squalene 3.3%, free sterols 0.8%, sterol esters 1.3%, α-tocopherol 0.003%, waxes 7%, butylated hydroxyanisole 0.003%. Net price 100 g = £2.08; 450 g = £8.19

**Noratex®** (Norton)

*Cream*, cod-liver oil 2.15%, light kaolin 3.5%, talc 7.4%, wool fat 1.075%, zinc oxide 21.8%. Net price 40 g = 38p; 500 g = £2.52. For napkin and urinary rash and pressure sores

**Oilatum®** (Stiefel)

*Cream*, arachis oil 21%, povidone (polyvinylpyrrolidone) 1%, in a water-miscible basis. Net price 40 g = £1.79; 80 g = £2.78
*Additives:* fragrance

**Sudocrem®** (Tosara)

*Cream*, benzyl alcohol 0.39%, benzyl benzoate 1.01%, benzyl cinnamate 0.15%, wool fat 4%, zinc oxide 15.25%. Net price 30 g = 60p; 60 g = 67p; 125 g = £1.15; 250 g = £2.07; 400 g = £2.98. For napkin rash and pressure sores
*Additives:* beeswax (synthetic), polysorbates, propylene glycol, fragrance

**Thovaline®** (Ilon)

*Ointment*, cod-liver oil 1.5%, light kaolin 2.5%, talc 3.3%, wool fat 2.5%, zinc oxide 19.8%. Net price 15 g = 36p; 40 g = 39p; 50 g = 46p; 90 g = 75p; 125 g = 90p; 500 g = £2.78. For napkin and urinary rash and pressure sores
*Additives:* fragrance

*Spray application*, ingredients as for ointment in pressurised aerosol pack. Net price 142 g = £1.73

---

**Ultrabase®** (Schering Health Care)
*Cream*, water-miscible, containing liquid paraffin and white soft paraffin. Net price 50 g = £1.05; 500 g = £5.70
*Additives:* hydroxybenzoates (parabens), disodium edetate, fragrance

**Unguentum Merck®** (Merck)
*Cream* (hydrophilic and lipophilic), cetostearyl alcohol 9%, glyceryl monostearate 3%, saturated neutral oil 2%, liquid paraffin 3%, white soft paraffin 32%, propylene glycol 5%, polysorbate '40' 8%, silicic acid 0.1%, sorbic acid 0.2%. Net price 50 g = £1.63; 100 g = £3.21; 200 mL = £6.35; 500 g = £9.80

**Vita-E®** (Bioglan)
*Ointment*, d-α-tocopheryl acetate 30 units/g in yellow soft paraffin. Net price 50 g = £1.74. For pressure sores and related conditions
*Additives:* none as listed in section 13.1

Preparations containing urea
**Aquadrate®** (Norwich Eaton)
*Cream*, urea 10% in a powder-in-cream basis. Net price 30 g = £1.63; 100 g = £4.91
*Additives:* none as listed in section 13.1
Apply thinly and rub into area when required

**Calmurid®** (Kabi Pharmacia)
*Cream*, urea 10%, lactic acid 5%, in a water-miscible basis. Diluent aqueous cream, life of diluted cream 14 days. Net price 100 g = £3.49; 400-g dispenser = £12.50
*Additives:* none as listed in section 13.1
Apply a thick layer for 3–5 minutes, massage into area, and remove excess, usually twice daily. Use half-strength cream for 1 week if stinging occurs with undiluted preparation

**Nutraplus®** (Galderma)
*Cream*, urea 10% in a water-miscible basis. Net price 60 g = £2.62
*Additives:* hydroxybenzoates (parabens), propylene glycol
Apply 2–3 times daily

**Sential E®** (Kabi Pharmacia)
*Cream*, urea 4%, sodium chloride 4%. Net price 100 g = £2.97
*Additives:* hydroxybenzoates (parabens)
For dry, scaling and itching skin, apply twice daily after washing

### 13.2.1.1 EMOLLIENT BATH ADDITIVES

For bath additives containing tar, see section 13.5 and for antiseptic bath additives, see section 13.11.

**Alpha Keri Bath®** (Bristol-Myers)
*Bath oil*, liquid paraffin 91.7%, oil-soluble fraction of wool fat 3%. Net price 240 mL = £3.54; 480 mL = £6.59
*Additives:* fragrance
Add 10–20 mL/bath (infants 5 mL)

**Aveeno Oilated®** (Bioglan)
*Bath additive*, oat (protein fraction) 41%, liquid paraffin 35%. Net price 10 × 50-g sachets = £4.94. ACBS: for endogenous and exogenous eczema, xeroderma, ichthyosis, and senile pruritus associated with dry skin
*Additives:* none as listed in section 13.1
Add 1 sachet/bath

**Aveeno Regular®** (Bioglan)
*Bath additive*, oat (protein fraction). Net price 10 × 50-g sachets = £4.94. ACBS: as for Aveeno Oilated
*Additives:* none as listed in section 13.1
Add 1 sachet/bath

**Balmandol®** (S&N Pharm.)
*Bath oil*, almond oil 30%, light liquid paraffin 69.6%. Net price 225 mL = £3.68; 500 mL = £7.36
*Additives:* butylated hydroxyanisole, fragrance
Add 15–30 mL/bath

**Balneum®** (Merck)
*Bath oil*, soya oil 84.75%. Net price 200 mL = £2.86; 500 mL = £6.22; 1 litre = £12.00
*Additives:* butylated hydroxytoluene, propylene glycol, fragrance
Add 20 mL/bath

*Balneum Plus®* *bath oil*, soya oil 82.95%, mixed lauromacrogols 15%. Net price 500 mL = £8.55
*Additives:* butylated hydroxytoluene, propylene glycol, fragrance
Add 20 mL/bath

**Balneum with Tar®**—section 13.5

**Bath E45®** (Crookes)
*Bath oil*, cetyl dimethicone 5% in an emollient basis. Net price 150 mL = £2.01. ACBS: for endogenous and exogenous eczema, xeroderma, ichthyosis, and senile pruritus associated with dry skin
*Additives:* butylated hydroxyanisole
Add 15 mL/bath

**Emmolate®** (Bio-Medical)
*Bath oil*, acetylated wool alcohols 5%, liquid paraffin 65%. Net price 200 mL = £1.95 (hosp. only)
*Additives:* none as listed in section 13.1
Add 15–30 mL/bath

**Emulsiderm®** (Dermal)
*Liquid emulsion*, liquid paraffin 25%, isopropyl myristate 25%, benzalkonium chloride 0.5%. Net price 250 mL (with 10-mL measure) = £4.44; 1 litre (with 30-mL measure) = £11.87
*Additives:* polysorbate 60
Add 30 mL/bath (infants 15 mL)

**Hydromol Emollient®** (Quinoderm Ltd)
*Bath additive*, isopropyl myristate 13%, light liquid paraffin 37.8%. Net price 150 mL = £1.54; 350 mL = £2.89; 1 litre = £6.74
Add 1–3 capfuls/bath (infants ½–2 capfuls)

**Oilatum Emollient®** (Stiefel)
*Bath additive* (emulsion), acetylated wool alcohols 5%, liquid paraffin 63.7%. Net price 150 mL = £1.65; 350 mL = £3.20
*Additives:* isopropyl palmitate, fragrance
Add 5–15 mL/bath

## 13.2.2 Barrier preparations

Barrier preparations often contain water-repellent substances such as **dimethicone** or other silicones. They are used to give protection against irritation or repeated hydration (areas around stomata, sore areas in the elderly, bedsores, etc.). They are no substitute for adequate nursing care, and it is doubtful if they are any more effective than the traditional compound **zinc ointments**.

For stoma care preparations, see section 1.8.

NAPKIN RASH. Barrier creams and ointments are also used to give protection against napkin rash which is usually a local dermatitis. The first line of treatment is to ensure that napkins are changed frequently, and that tightly fitting rubber pants are avoided. The rash may clear when left exposed to the air and an emollient, or antimicrobial preparations (e.g. miconazole cream), may be helpful. A mild corticosteroid such as hydrocortisone may be useful but treatment should be limited to a week or less and it should be remembered that napkins and plastic pants may act as an occlusive dressing and increase absorption (for cautions see hydrocortisone p. 394).

**Conotrane®** (Boehringer Ingelheim)
*Cream*, benzalkonium chloride 0.1%, dimethicone '350' 22%. Net price 50 g = 59p; 100 g = 96p; 500 g = £3.66. For napkin and urinary rash and pressure sores
*Additives:* fragrance

**Metanium®** (Bengué)
*Ointment*, titanium dioxide 20%, titanium peroxide 5%, titanium salicylate 3%, titanium tannate 0.1%, in a silicone basis. Net price 25 g = 69p. For napkin rash and related disorders
*Additives:* none as listed in section 13.1

**Rikospray Silicone®** (3M)
*Spray application*, aldioxa 0.5%, cetylpyridinium chloride 0.02%, in a water-repellent basis containing dimethicone 1000. Net price 200-g pressurised aerosol pack = £2.45. For urinary rash, pressure sores, and colostomy care
*Additives:* none as listed in section 13.1

**Siopel®** (ICI)
*Barrier cream*, dimethicone '1000' 10%, cetrimide 0.3%. Net price 50 g = 57p. For dermatoses, colostomy and ileostomy care, urinary rash, and related conditions
*Additives:* butylated hydroxytoluene, hydroxybenzoates (parabens)

**Sprilon®** (Kabi Pharmacia)
*Spray application*, dimethicone 1.04%, zinc oxide 12.5%, in a basis containing wool fat, wool alcohols, cetostearyl alcohol, dextran, white soft paraffin, liquid paraffin, propellants. Net price 115-g pressurised aerosol unit = £3.81. For urinary rash, pressure sores, and ileostomy
*Caution:* flammable

**Vasogen®** (Pharmax)
*Barrier cream*, dimethicone 20%, calamine 1.5%, zinc oxide 7.5%. Net price 50 g = 63p; 100 g = £1.07. For napkin and urinary rash, pressure sores, and pruritus ani
*Additives:* hydroxybenzoates (parabens), wool fat

## 13.2.3  Dusting powders

Dusting powders are used in folds where friction may occur between opposing skin surfaces. They should not be applied in areas that are very moist as they tend to cake and abrade the skin. **Talc** acts as a lubricant powder but does not absorb moisture whereas **starch** is less lubricant but absorbs water. Other inert powders such as kaolin or zinc oxide may also be used in the formulation of dusting powders.

See also section 13.11 for antiseptic dusting powders.

**Talc Dusting Powder, BP,** starch 10% in sterilised purified talc. Net price 100 g = 33p
**Zinc, Starch and Talc Dusting-powder, BPC,** zinc oxide 25%, starch 25%, sterilised purified talc 50%. Net price 50 g = 16p
**ZeaSORB®** (Stiefel)
*Dusting powder*, aldioxa 0.2%, chloroxylenol 0.5%, pulverised maize core 45%. Net price 50 g = £2.15
*Additives:* fragrance

# 13.3  Local anaesthetics and antipruritics

Pruritus may be caused by systemic disease (such as drug hypersensitivity, obstructive jaundice, endocrine disease, and certain malignant diseases) as well as by skin disease (e.g. psoriasis, eczema, urticaria, and scabies). Where possible the underlying causes should be treated.

There is no really effective antipruritic. **Calamine** preparations are widely prescribed. **Emollient** preparations (section 13.2.1) may also be of value. **Oral antihistamines** (section 3.4.1) should be used in allergic rashes.

Some topical antihistamines and local anaesthetics may cause sensitisation. Topical antihistamines are only marginally effective. Insect bites and stings, though often treated with such preparations, are best treated with calamine preparations or emollients.

**Crotamiton** shows little evidence of greater effectiveness than calamine in the relief of pruritus.

For preparations used in pruritus ani, see section 1.7.1.

## CALAMINE
*Indications:* pruritus

**Calamine Cream, Aqueous, BP,** calamine 4%, zinc oxide 3%, liquid paraffin 20%, self-emulsifying glyceryl monostearate 5%, cetomacrogol emulsifying wax 5%, phenoxyethanol 0.5%, freshly boiled and cooled purified water 62.5%. Net price 50 g = 28p
**Calamine Lotion, BP,** calamine 15%, zinc oxide 5%, glycerol 5%, bentonite 3%, sodium citrate 0.5%, liquefied phenol 0.5%, in freshly boiled and cooled purified water. Net price 200 mL = 48p
**Calamine Lotion, Oily, BP1980,** calamine 5%, arachis oil 50%, oleic acid 0.5%, wool fat 1% in calcium hydroxide solution. Net price 200 mL = 78p
**Calamine Ointment, BP,** calamine 15%, in white soft paraffin
**Eczederm®** (Quinoderm Ltd)
*Cream*, calamine 20.88%, arachis oil 12.5%, in an emollient basis. Net price 30 g = £1.04; 60 g = £1.79; 500 g = £9.57. For mild dermatoses including eczema
*Additives:* hydroxybenzoates (parabens), fragrance

## CROTAMITON

*Indications:* pruritus (including pruritus after scabies)
*Cautions:* avoid use near eyes and broken skin
*Contra-indications:* acute exudative dermatoses

**Eurax**® (Ciba Consumer)
*Cream*, crotamiton 10%. Net price 30 g = £1.49; 100 g = £2.58
Additives: beeswax, hydroxybenzoates (parabens), fragrance
*Lotion*, crotamiton 10%. Net price 100 mL = £1.82
Additives: propylene glycol, sorbic acid, fragrance

## LOCAL ANAESTHETICS

*Indications:* relief of local pain, see notes above. See section 15.2 for use in surface anaesthesia
*Cautions:* may cause hypersensitivity
Note. Topical local anaesthetic preparations may be absorbed, especially through mucosal surfaces, therefore excessive application should be avoided, particularly in infants and children.

**Anethaine**® (Crookes)
*Cream*, amethocaine hydrochloride 1%, in a water-miscible basis. Net price 25 g = £1.14
Additives: fragrance
**Solarcaine**® (Schering-Plough)
*Cream*, benzocaine 1%, triclosan 0.2%. Net price 25 mL = £1.26
Additives: benzyl alcohol, disodium edetate
*Lotion*, benzocaine 0.5%, triclosan 0.2%. Net price 75 mL = £1.70
Additives: disodium edetate, hydroxybenzoates (parabens)
*Spray* ( = application), benzocaine 5%, triclosan 0.1%, pressurised aerosol unit. Net price 100 g = £2.20
Additives: propylene glycol
**Xylocaine**® (Astra)
*Ointment*, see section 15.2

## TOPICAL ANTIHISTAMINES

*Indications:* pruritus, urticaria, see notes above
*Cautions:* may cause hypersensitivity; avoid in eczema; photosensitivity (diphenhydramine)

**Anthisan**® (Rhône-Poulenc Rorer)
*Cream*, mepyramine maleate 2%. Net price 25 g = £1.18
Additives: hydroxybenzoates (parabens), fragrance
Apply 2–3 times daily for up to 3 days
**Caladryl**® (W-L)
*Cream*, diphenhydramine hydrochloride 1%, calamine 8%, camphor 0.1%, in a water-miscible basis. Net price 42 g = £1.37
Additives: hydroxybenzoates (parabens), polysorbate 60, propylene glycol
*Lotion*, ingredients as for cream. Net price 125 mL = £1.37
Additives: fragrance
Apply 3–4 times daily for up to 3 days
**R.B.C.**® (Rybar)
*Cream*, antazoline hydrochloride 1.8%, calamine 8%, camphor 0.1%, cetrimide 0.5%. Net price 25 g = £1.09
Additives: propylene glycol
Apply when required for up to 3 days

# 13.4 Topical corticosteroids

Topical corticosteroids are used for the treatment of inflammatory conditions of the skin other than those due to an infection, in particular the eczematous disorders. Corticosteroids suppress various components of the inflammatory reaction while in use; they are in no sense curative, and when treatment is discontinued a rebound exacerbation of the condition may occur. They are indicated for the relief of symptoms and for the suppression of signs of the disorder when potentially less harmful measures are ineffective.

Corticosteroids are of no value in the treatment of urticaria and are **contra-indicated** in rosacea and in ulcerative conditions as they worsen the condition. They should not be used indiscriminately in pruritus.

CHOICE OF PREPARATION. The preparation containing the **least potent** drug at the **lowest strength** which is effective is the one of choice, but extemporaneous dilution should be avoided whenever possible.

There is no good evidence that it is of any benefit to prescribe a potent corticosteroid for initial treatment; it is probably just as useful to 'ascend' in potency as it is to 'descend'. It should be noted that if a patient ceases to respond to a particular corticosteroid another of similar potency ought to be prescribed, not a more potent one. In general, the most potent corticosteroids should be reserved for recalcitrant dermatoses such as *chronic discoid lupus erythematosus, lichen simplex chronicus, hypertrophic lichen planus*, and *palmar plantar pustulosis*. With rare exceptions, potent corticosteroids should not be used on the face as they may precipitate a rosacea-like disorder and aggravate pre-existing rosacea.

Considerable caution must be exercised in the use of potent corticosteroids in children (see below).

Topical corticosteroid preparations are divided into four groups in respect of potency. In ascending order these are:

| | Potency | Examples |
|---|---|---|
| IV | Mild | Hydrocortisone 1% |
| III | Moderately potent | Clobetasone butyrate 0.05% (Eumovate®) |
| II | Potent | Betamethasone 0.1% (as valerate) (Betnovate®); hydrocortisone butyrate (Locoid®) |
| I | Very potent | Clobetasol propionate 0.05% (Dermovate®) |

Intradermal corticosteroid injections (see section 10.1.2.2) are more effective than the very potent topical corticosteroid preparations and they should be reserved for severe cases where there are localised lesions and topical treatment has failed. Their effects last for several weeks.

SIDE-EFFECTS. Unlike groups I and II, groups III and IV are rarely associated with side-effects. The more potent the preparation the more care is required, as absorption through the skin can cause severe pituitary-adrenal-axis suppression and hypercorticism (see section 6.3.3), both of which depend on the area of the body treated and the duration of the treatment. It must also be remembered that absorption is greatest from areas of thin skin, raw surfaces, and intertriginous areas, and is increased by occlusion.

Local side-effects from the use of corticosteroids topically include:

(a) spread and worsening of untreated infection;
(b) thinning of the skin which may be restored over a period of time although the original structure may never return;
(c) irreversible striae atrophicae;
(d) increased hair growth;
(e) perioral dermatitis, an inflammatory papular disorder on the face of young women;
(f) acne at the site of application in some patients;
(g) mild depigmentation and vellus hair.

CHOICE OF FORMULATION. Water-miscible creams are suitable for moist or weeping lesions whereas ointments are generally chosen for dry, lichenified or scaly lesions or where a more occlusive effect is required. Lotions may be useful when minimal application to a large area is required. Occlusive polythene dressings have been used to increase the effect, but also increase the risk of side-effects. The inclusion of urea increases the penetration of the corticosteroid.

USE IN CHILDREN. Children, especially babies, are particularly susceptible to side-effects. The more potent corticosteroids should be **avoided** in paediatric treatment or if necessary used with great care for short periods; a mild corticosteroid such as hydrocortisone is useful for treating napkin rash and infantile eczemas (but see caution below). Napkins and plastic pants may however act as an occlusive dressing and increase absorption.

COMPOUND PREPARATIONS. The advantages of including other substances with corticosteroids in topical preparations are debatable. The commonest ones are the **antibacterials**.

## HYDROCORTISONE

*Indications:* mild inflammatory skin disorders
*Cautions:* see notes above and in section 13.5 (psoriasis); also avoid prolonged use in infants and children (extreme caution in dermatoses of infancy including napkin rash—where possible treatment should be limited to 5–7 days), and on the face; more potent corticosteroids contra-indicated in infants and young children
*Contra-indications:* untreated bacterial, fungal, or viral skin lesions
*Side-effects:* see notes above
*Administration:* apply thinly 2–3 times daily, reducing strength and frequency as condition responds

Creams
PoM **Hydrocortisone** (Non-proprietary)
*Cream,* hydrocortisone in a suitable basis. Net price 0.5%, 15 g = 36p; 30 g = 60p; 1%, 15 g = 47p. Label: 28. Potency IV
When hydrocortisone cream is prescribed and no strength is stated, the 1% strength should be supplied

PoM **Cobadex®** (Cox Pharmaceuticals)
*Cream,* hydrocortisone 0.5 or 1%, dimethicone '350' 20%, in a water-miscible basis, net price 20 g (0.5%) = £1.17; 20 g (1%) = £1.68. Label: 28. Potency IV
*Additives:* hydroxybenzoates (parabens), polysorbate 80, propylene glycol

> **Over-the-counter sales.** Proprietary brands of hydrocortisone cream (0.1 and 1%) and ointment (1%) are on sale to the public for treatment of allergic contact dermatitis, irritant dermatitis, and insect bite reactions only
> *Cautions:* not for children under 10 years or in pregnancy, without medical advice
> *Contra-indications:* eyes/face, anogenital region, broken or infected skin (including cold sores, acne, and athlete's foot)
> *Administration:* apply sparingly over small area 1–2 times daily for max. of 1 week
> *Labelling must state.* If the condition is not improved, consult your doctor.

PoM **Dioderm®** (Dermal)
*Cream,* hydrocortisone 0.1%, in a water-miscible basis. Net price 30 g = £2.66. Label: 28. Potency IV
*Additives:* propylene glycol

PoM **Efcortelan®** (Glaxo)
*Cream,* hydrocortisone in a water-miscible basis. Net price 0.5%, 30 g = 60p; 1%, 30 g = 74p; 2.5%, 30 g = £1.66. Label: 28. Potency IV
*Additives:* chlorocresol

PoM **Hydrocortistab®** (Boots)
*Cream,* hydrocortisone acetate 1%, in a water-miscible basis. Net price 15 g = 33p. Label: 28. Potency IV
*Additives:* chlorocresol

PoM **Hydrocortisyl®** (Roussel)
*Cream,* hydrocortisone 1%, in a water-miscible basis. Net price 15 g = 28p. Label: 28. Potency IV
*Additives:* chlorocresol

PoM **Mildison®** (Brocades)
*Lipocream,* hydrocortisone 1% in a fatty cream basis. Net price 30 g = £2.19. Label: 28. Potency IV
*Additives:* hydroxybenzoates (parabens)

Ointments
PoM **Hydrocortisone** (Non-proprietary)
*Ointment,* hydrocortisone in a suitable basis. Net price 0.5%, 15 g = 36p; 30 g = 60p; 1%, 15 g = 48p. Label: 28. Potency IV
When hydrocortisone ointment is prescribed and no strength is stated, the 1% strength should be supplied

PoM **Efcortelan®** (Glaxo)
*Ointment,* hydrocortisone in a paraffin basis. Net price 0.5%, 30 g = 60p; 1%, 30 g = 74p; 2.5%, 30 g = £1.66. Label: 28. Potency IV
*Additives:* none as listed in section 13.1

PoM **Hydrocortistab®** (Boots)
*Ointment,* hydrocortisone 1%, in an anhydrous greasy basis. Net price 15 g = 33p. Label: 28. Potency IV
*Additives:* none as listed in section 13.1

**PoM Hydrocortisyl®** (Roussel)

*Ointment*, hydrocortisone 1%, in an anhydrous greasy basis. Net price 15 g = 28p. Label: 28. Potency IV
*Additives: wool fat*

Compound preparations
*Note.* Compound preparations with coal tar, section 13.5

**PoM Alphaderm®** (Norwich Eaton)

*Cream*, hydrocortisone 1%, urea 10%, in a powder-in-cream basis. Net price 30 g = £2.42; 100 g = £7.51. Label: 28. Potency III
*Additives: none as listed in section 13.1*
Apply thinly twice daily

**PoM Calmurid HC®** (Kabi Pharmacia)

*Cream*, hydrocortisone 1%, urea 10%, lactic acid 5%, in a water-miscible basis. Diluent aqueous cream, life of diluted cream 14 days. Net price 30 g = £2.33; 100 g = £6.75. Label: 28. Potency III
*Additives: none as listed in section 13.1*
Apply thinly twice daily.
*Note.* Dilute to half-strength with aqueous cream for 1 week if stinging occurs then transfer to undiluted preparation

**PoM Epifoam®** (Stafford-Miller)

*Foam* (= application), hydrocortisone acetate 1%, pramoxine hydrochloride 1%, in a muco-adherent basis (pressurised aerosol pack). Net price 12-g unit (approx. 20 applications of 5 mL) = £2.81. Label: 28. Potency IV
*Additives: hydroxybenzoates (parabens), propylene glycol*
For perineal trauma including post-episiotomy pain and dermatoses
Apply on a pad 3–4 times daily

**PoM Eurax-Hydrocortisone®** (Zyma)

*Cream*, hydrocortisone 0.25%, crotamiton 10%. Net price 30 g = 93p. Label: 28. Potency IV
*Additives: hydroxybenzoates (parabens), propylene glycol, fragrance*
Apply thinly 2–3 times daily

**PoM Hydrocal®** (Bioglan)

*Cream*, hydrocortisone acetate 1%, in a basis containing calamine. Net price 25 g = £3.69. Label: 28. Potency IV
*Additives: hydroxybenzoates (parabens), polysorbates*
Apply thinly 2–3 times daily

**PoM Sential®** (Kabi Pharmacia)

*Cream*, hydrocortisone 0.5%, urea 4%, sodium chloride 4%, in a water-miscible basis. Net price 30 g = £2.40. Label: 28. Potency IV
*Additives: sorbic acid*
Apply thinly twice daily

With antimicrobials
**PoM Barquinol HC®** (Fisons)

*Cream*, hydrocortisone acetate 0.5%, clioquinol 3%. Net price 15 g = 58p. Label: 28. Potency IV
*Additives: hydroxybenzoates (parabens), wool fat*
Apply thinly 2–3 times daily
*Caution:* stains clothing

**PoM Canesten HC®** (Baypharm)

*Cream*, hydrocortisone 1%, clotrimazole 1%. Net price 30 g = £3.18. Label: 28. Potency IV
*Additives: benzyl alcohol*
Apply thinly twice daily

**PoM Daktacort®** (Janssen)

*Cream*, hydrocortisone 1%, miconazole nitrate 2%, in a water-miscible basis. Net price 30 g = £2.24. Label: 28. Potency IV
*Additives: butylated hydroxyanisole, disodium edetate*
*Ointment*, hydrocortisone 1%, miconazole nitrate 2%, in a greasy basis. Net price 30 g = £3.10. Label: 28. Potency IV
*Additives: none as listed in section 13.1*
Apply thinly 2–3 times daily

**PoM Econacort®** (Squibb)

*Cream*, hydrocortisone 1%, econazole nitrate 1%. Net price 30 g = £2.85. Label: 28. Potency IV
*Additives: butylated hydroxyanisole*
Apply thinly twice daily

**PoM Fucidin H®** (Leo)

*Cream*, hydrocortisone acetate 1%, fusidic acid 2%. Net price 15 g = £3.30; 30 g = £5.69. Label: 28. Potency IV
*Additives: butylated hydroxyanisole, potassium sorbate*
*Gel*, hydrocortisone acetate 1%, fusidic acid 2%, in a water-miscible basis. Net price 15 g = £2.91; 30 g = £5.06. Label: 28. Potency IV
*Additives: hydroxybenzoates (parabens), polysorbate 80*
*Ointment*, hydrocortisone acetate 1%, sodium fusidate 2%. Net price 15 g = £2.70; 30 g = £4.68. Label: 28. Potency IV
*Additives: wool fat*
Apply thinly 3–4 times daily

**PoM Gentisone® HC** (Nicholas)

*Cream*, hydrocortisone acetate 1%, gentamicin 0.3% (as sulphate), in a water-miscible basis. Net price 15 g = £2.05. Label: 28. Potency IV
*Additives: hydroxybenzoates (parabens), polysorbates, propylene glycol*
*Ointment*, ingredients as for cream but greasy basis. Net price 15 g = £2.05. Label: 28. Potency IV
*Additives: none as listed in section 13.1*
Apply thinly 3–4 times daily
Formerly Genticin® HC

**PoM Gregoderm®** (Unigreg)

*Ointment*, hydrocortisone 1%, neomycin sulphate 0.4%, nystatin 100 000 units/g, polymyxin B sulphate 7250 units/g. Net price 15 g = £2.24. Label: 28. Potency IV
*Additives: none as listed in section 13.1*
Apply thinly 2–3 times daily

**PoM Nystaform-HC®** (Bayer)

*Cream*, hydrocortisone 0.5%, nystatin 100 000 units/g, chlorhexidine hydrochloride 1%, in a water-miscible basis. Net price 30 g = £2.73. Label: 28. Potency IV
*Additives: benzyl alcohol, polysorbate 60*
*Ointment*, hydrocortisone 1%, nystatin 100 000 units/g, chlorhexidine acetate 1%, in a water-repellent basis. Net price 30 g = £2.73. Label: 28. Potency IV
*Additives: none as listed in section 13.1*
Apply thinly 2–3 times daily

**PoM Quinocort®** (Quinoderm Ltd)

*Cream*, hydrocortisone 1%, potassium hydroxyquinoline sulphate 0.5% in a vanishing cream basis. Net price 30 g = £2.59. Label: 28. Potency IV
*Additives: edetic acid (EDTA), chlorocresol*
Apply thinly 2–3 times daily

---

Cautionary label wordings, see inside back cover

Prices are **net**, see p. 1

PoM **Terra-Cortril®** (Pfizer)
*Topical ointment*, hydrocortisone 1%, oxytetracycline 3% (as hydrochloride), in a paraffin basis. Net price 15 g = £1.01; 30 g = £1.82. Label: 28. Potency IV
*Additives:* none as listed in section 13.1
Apply thinly 2–4 times daily
*Spray application*, hydrocortisone 50 mg, oxytetracycline 150 mg (as hydrochloride), 30-mL pressurised aerosol unit, net price = £1.44; double these amounts in 60-mL unit, net price = £2.50. Label: 28. Potency IV
*Additives:* none as listed in section 13.1
Spray area thinly 2–4 times daily

PoM **Terra-Cortril Nystatin®** (Pfizer)
*Cream*, hydrocortisone 1%, nystatin 100 000 units/g, oxytetracycline 3% (as calcium salt). Net price 30 g = £2.01. Label: 28. Potency IV
*Additives:* hydroxybenzoates (parabens), polysorbate, propylene glycol, fragrance
Apply thinly 2–4 times daily

PoM **Timodine®** (R&C)
*Cream*, hydrocortisone 0.5%, nystatin 100 000 units/g, benzalkonium chloride solution 0.2%, dimethicone '350' 10%. Net price 30 g = £2.38. Label: 28. Potency IV
*Additives:* butylated hydroxyanisole, hydroxybenzoates (parabens), sorbic acid
Apply thinly 3 times daily (napkin rash, after each change)

PoM **Tri-Cicatrin®** (Wellcome)
*Ointment*, hydrocortisone 1%, bacitracin zinc 250 units/g, neomycin sulphate 3400 units/g, nystatin 100 000 units/g. Net price 15 g = £5.23; 30 g = £9.50. Label: 28. Potency IV
*Additives:* none as listed in section 13.1
Apply thinly 1–3 times daily

PoM **Vioform-Hydrocortisone®** (Zyma)
*Cream*, hydrocortisone 1%, clioquinol 3%. Net price 30 g = £1.57. Label: 28. Potency IV
*Additives:* none as listed in section 13.1
*Ointment*, hydrocortisone 1%, clioquinol 3%. Net price 30 g = £1.57. Label: 28. Potency IV
*Additives:* none as listed in section 13.1
Apply thinly 1–3 times daily
*Caution:* stains clothing

## HYDROCORTISONE BUTYRATE

*Indications:* severe inflammatory skin disorders such as eczema unresponsive to less potent corticosteroids
*Cautions; Contra-indications; Side-effects:* see under Hydrocortisone and notes above
*Administration:* apply thinly 2–4 times daily, reducing frequency as condition responds

PoM **Locoid®** (Brocades)
*Cream*, hydrocortisone butyrate 0.1%, in a water-miscible basis. Net price 30 g = £2.27; 100 g = £6.95. Label: 28. Potency II
*Additives:* hydroxybenzoates (parabens)
*Lipocream*, hydrocortisone butyrate 0.1% in a fatty cream basis. Net price 30 g = £2.38; 100 g = £7.29. Label: 28. Potency II
*Additives:* hydroxybenzoates (parabens)
*Note.* For bland cream basis see Lipobase®, section 13.2.1

*Ointment*, hydrocortisone butyrate 0.1%, in an anhydrous greasy basis. Net price 30 g = £2.27; 100 g = £6.95. Label: 28. Potency II
*Additives:* none as listed in section 13.1
*Scalp lotion*, hydrocortisone butyrate 0.1%, in an aqueous isopropyl alcohol basis. Net price 30 mL = £3.20; 100 mL = £9.81. Label: 15, 28. Potency II
*Additives:* none as listed in section 13.1
Apply 1–2 times daily, reducing frequency as condition responds

With antimicrobials
PoM **Locoid C®** (Brocades)
*Cream*, hydrocortisone butyrate 0.1%, chlorquinaldol 3%. Net price 30 g = £2.97. Label: 28. Potency II
*Additives:* none as listed in section 13.1
*Ointment*, ingredients as for cream, in a greasy basis. Net price 30 g = £2.97. Label: 28. Potency II
*Additives:* none as listed in section 13.1
Apply thinly 2–4 times daily.
Max. 60 g for up to 14 days

## ALCLOMETASONE DIPROPIONATE

*Indications:* inflammatory skin disorders such as eczema
*Cautions; Contra-indications; Side-effects:* see under Hydrocortisone and notes above
*Administration:* apply thinly 2–3 times daily, reducing frequency as condition responds

PoM **Modrasone®** (Schering-Plough)
*Cream*, alclometasone dipropionate 0.05%. Net price 15 g = £1.70; 50 g = £4.80. Label: 28. Potency III
*Additives:* chlorocresol, propylene glycol
*Ointment*, alclometasone dipropionate 0.05%. Net price 15 g = £1.70; 50 g = £4.80. Label: 28. Potency III
*Additives:* beeswax, propylene glycol

## BECLOMETHASONE DIPROPIONATE

*Indications:* severe inflammatory skin disorders such as eczema unresponsive to less potent corticosteroids
*Cautions; Contra-indications; Side-effects:* see under Hydrocortisone and notes above
*Administration:* apply thinly twice daily, reducing strength and frequency as condition responds

PoM **Propaderm®** (Glaxo)
*Cream*, beclomethasone dipropionate 0.025%. Net price 30 g = £1.58. Label: 28. Potency II
*Additives:* chlorocresol
*Ointment*, beclomethasone dipropionate 0.025%. Net price 30 g = £1.58. Label: 28. Potency II
*Additives:* propylene glycol

With antibacterials
**PoM Propaderm-A®** (Glaxo)
*Ointment*, beclomethasone dipropionate 0.025%, chlortetracycline hydrochloride 3%. Net price 30 g = £1.78. Label: 28. Potency II
*Additives:* none as listed in section 13.1
Initially apply thinly twice daily, reducing frequency as condition responds
*Caution:* stains clothing

---

## BETAMETHASONE ESTERS

*Indications:* severe inflammatory skin disorders such as eczema unresponsive to less potent corticosteroids
*Cautions; Contra-indications; Side-effects:* see under Hydrocortisone and notes above. Application of more than 100 g per week of 0.1% preparation is likely to cause adrenal suppression
*Administration:* apply thinly 2–3 times daily, reducing strength and frequency as condition responds

**PoM Betamethasone Valerate** (Non-proprietary)
*Cream*, betamethasone 0.1% (as valerate). Net price 15 g = £1.40; 30 g = £3.95. Label: 28. Potency II
*Ointment*, betamethasone 0.1% (as valerate). Net price 15 g = £1.40; 30 g = £3.95. Label: 28. Potency II

**PoM Betnovate®** (Glaxo)
*Cream*, betamethasone 0.1% (as valerate), in a water-miscible basis. Net price 30 g = £1.40; 100 g = £3.95; 100 g pump-dispenser = £4.45. Label: 28. Potency II
*Additives:* chlorocresol
*Ointment*, betamethasone 0.1% (as valerate), in an anhydrous paraffin basis. Net price 30 g = £1.40; 100 g = £3.95; 100 g pump-dispenser = £4.45. Label: 28. Potency II
*Additives:* none as listed in section 13.1
*Lotion*, betamethasone 0.1% (as valerate). Net price 100 mL = £4.75. Label: 28. Potency II
*Additives:* hydroxybenzoates (parabens)
*Scalp application*, betamethasone 0.1% (as valerate), in a thickened alcoholic basis. Net price 100 mL = £5.18. Label: 15, 28. Potency II
*Additives:* none as listed in section 13.1
Apply thinly 1–2 times daily, then reduce

**PoM Betnovate-RD®** (Glaxo)
*Cream*, betamethasone 0.025% (as valerate) in a water-miscible basis (1 in 4 dilution of Betnovate cream). Net price 100 g = £3.26. Label: 28. Potency III
*Additives:* chlorocresol
*Ointment*, betamethasone 0.025% (as valerate) in an anhydrous paraffin basis (1 in 4 dilution of Betnovate ointment). Net price 100 g = £3.26. Label: 28. Potency III
*Additives:* none as listed in section 13.1

**PoM Diprosalic®** (Schering-Plough)
*Ointment*, betamethasone 0.05% (as dipropionate), salicylic acid 3%. Net price 30 g = £3.30; 100 g = £9.50. Label: 28. Potency II
*Additives:* none as listed in section 13.1

*Scalp application*, betamethasone 0.05% (as dipropionate), salicylic acid 2%, in an alcoholic basis. Net price 30 mL = £4.20; 100 mL = £10.50. Label: 28. Potency II
*Additives:* disodium edetate
Apply thinly 1–2 times daily; max. 60 g per week

**PoM Diprosone®** (Schering-Plough)
*Cream*, betamethasone 0.05% (as dipropionate), in a water-miscible basis. Net price 30 g = £2.57; 100 g = £7.30. Label: 28. Potency II
*Additives:* chlorocresol
*Note.* For bland cream basis see Diprobase®, section 13.2.1
*Ointment*, betamethasone 0.05% (as dipropionate). Net price 30 g = £2.57; 100 g = £7.30. Label: 28. Potency II
*Additives:* none as listed in section 13.1
*Note.* For bland ointment basis see Diprobase®, section 13.2.1
Apply thinly once or twice daily
*Lotion*, betamethasone 0.05% (as dipropionate), in a thickened alcoholic basis. Net price 30 mL = £3.25; 100 mL = £9.30. Label: 28. Potency II
*Additives:* none as listed in section 13.1
Apply twice daily, then reduce

With antimicrobials
**PoM Betnovate-C®** (Glaxo)
*Cream*, betamethasone 0.1% (as valerate), clioquinol 3%, in a water-miscible basis. Net price 30 g = £1.72. Label: 28. Potency II
*Additives:* chlorocresol
*Ointment*, betamethasone 0.1% (as valerate), clioquinol 3%, in a paraffin basis. Net price 30 g = £1.72. Label: 28. Potency II
*Additives:* none as listed in section 13.1
Apply thinly 2–3 times daily
*Caution:* stains clothing

**PoM Betnovate-N®** (Glaxo)
*Cream*, betamethasone 0.1% (as valerate), neomycin sulphate 0.5%, in a water-miscible basis. Net price 30 g = £1.72; 100 g = £4.77. Label: 28. Potency II
*Additives:* chlorocresol
*Ointment*, betamethasone 0.1% (as valerate), neomycin sulphate 0.5%, in a paraffin basis. Net price 30 g = £1.72; 100 g = £4.77. Label: 28. Potency II
*Additives:* none as listed in section 13.1
Apply thinly 2–3 times daily

**PoM Fucibet®** (Leo)
*Cream*, betamethasone 0.1% (as valerate), fusidic acid 2%, in a water-miscible basis. Net price 15 g = £3.84; 30 g = £6.48. Label: 28. Potency II
*Additives:* chlorocresol
Apply thinly 2–3 times daily

**PoM Lotriderm®** (Schering-Plough)
*Cream*, betamethasone 0.05% (as dipropionate), clotrimazole 1%. Net price 15 g = £3.49. Label: 28. Potency II
*Additives:* benzyl alcohol, propylene glycol
Apply thinly twice daily

---

## BUDESONIDE

*Indications:* severe inflammatory skin disorders such as eczema

*Cautions; Contra-indications; Side-effects:* see under Hydrocortisone and notes above

*Administration:* apply thinly 2–3 times daily

PoM **Preferid**® (Brocades)

*Cream*, budesonide 0.025% in a water-miscible basis. Net price 30 g = £2.96; 100 g = £9.06. Label: 28. Potency II
*Additives:* sorbic acid

*Ointment*, budesonide 0.025% in a paraffin basis. Net price 30 g = £2.96; 100 g = £9.06. Label: 28. Potency II
*Additives:* white beeswax, propylene glycol

## CLOBETASOL PROPIONATE

*Indications:* short-term treatment only of severe resistant inflammatory skin disorders such as psoriasis (excluding widespread plaque psoriasis), recalcitrant eczemas, lichen planus, discoid lupus erythematosus unresponsive to less potent corticosteroids

*Cautions; Contra-indications; Side-effects:* see under Hydrocortisone and notes above. Not more than 50 g of 0.05% preparation should be applied per week

*Administration:* apply thinly 1–2 times daily for up to 4 weeks, reducing frequency as condition responds

PoM **Dermovate**® (Glaxo)

*Cream*, clobetasol propionate 0.05%, in a water-miscible basis. Net price 30 g = £2.56; 100 g = £7.52. Label: 28. Potency I
*Additives:* beeswax (or beeswax substitute), chlorocresol, propylene glycol

*Ointment*, clobetasol propionate 0.05%, in an anhydrous paraffin basis. Net price 30 g = £2.56; 100 g = £7.52. Label: 28. Potency I
*Additives:* propylene glycol

*Scalp application*, clobetasol propionate 0.05%, in a thickened alcoholic basis. Net price 30 mL = £2.93; 100 mL = £9.91. Label: 15, 28. Potency I
*Additives:* none as listed in section 13.1

With antimicrobials

PoM **Dermovate-NN**® (Glaxo)

*Cream*, clobetasol propionate 0.05%, neomycin sulphate 0.5%, nystatin 100 000 units/g. Net price 30 g = £3.50. Label: 28. Potency I
*Additives:* beeswax substitute

*Ointment*, ingredients as for cream, in a paraffin basis. Net price 30 g = £3.50. Label: 28. Potency I
*Additives:* none as listed in section 13.1

Apply thinly once or twice daily, for up to 4 weeks reducing as condition responds

## CLOBETASONE BUTYRATE

*Indications:* eczema and dermatitis of all types; maintenance between courses of more potent corticosteroids

*Cautions; Contra-indications; Side-effects:* see under Hydrocortisone and notes above

*Administration:* apply thinly up to 4 times daily, reducing frequency as condition responds

PoM **Eumovate**® (Glaxo)

*Cream*, clobetasone butyrate 0.05%, in a water-miscible basis. Net price 30 g = £1.76; 100 g = £5.16. Label: 28. Potency III
*Additives:* beeswax substitute, chlorocresol

*Ointment*, clobetasone butyrate 0.05%, in an anhydrous paraffin basis. Net price 30 g = £1.76; 100 g = £5.16. Label: 28. Potency III
*Additives:* none as listed in section 13.1

With antimicrobials

PoM **Trimovate**® (Glaxo)

*Cream*, clobetasone butyrate 0.05%, oxytetracycline 3% (as calcium salt), nystatin 100 000 units/g, in a water-miscible basis. Net price 30 g = £3.13. Label: 28. Potency III
*Additives:* chlorocresol

*Ointment*, clobetasone butyrate 0.05%, chlortetracycline hydrochloride 3%, nystatin 100 000 units/g, in a paraffin basis. Net price 30 g = £3.13. Label: 28. Potency III
*Additives:* none as listed in section 13.1

Apply thinly up to 4 times daily
*Caution:* stains clothing

## DESOXYMETHASONE

*Indications:* severe acute inflammatory, allergic, and chronic skin disorders

*Cautions; Contra-indications; Side-effects:* see under Hydrocortisone and notes above

*Administration:* apply thinly 2–3 times daily reducing frequency as condition responds

PoM **Stiedex**® (Stiefel)

*Oily cream*, desoxymethasone 0.25%, in an oily basis. Net price 30 g = £3.43. Label: 28. Potency II
*Additives:* wool fat

*LP Oily cream*, desoxymethasone 0.05%, in an oily basis. Net price 30 g = £2.86. Label: 28. Potency III
*Additives:* edetic acid (EDTA), wool fat

*Lotion*, desoxymethasone 0.25%, salicylic acid 1%. Net price 50 mL = £8.05. Label: 28. Potency II
*Additives:* disodium edetate, propylene glycol

## DIFLUCORTOLONE VALERATE

*Indications:* severe inflammatory skin disorders such as eczema unresponsive to less potent corticosteroids; high strength (0.3%), short-term treatment of severe exacerbations

*Cautions; Contra-indications; Side-effects:* see under Hydrocortisone and notes above; not more than 50 g of 0.3% applied per week

*Administration:* apply thinly 2–3 times daily for up to 4 weeks (0.1% preparations) or 2 weeks (0.3% preparations), reducing strength and frequency as condition responds

---

PoM **Nerisone**® (Schering Health Care)
*Cream*, diflucortolone valerate 0.1%, in a water-miscible basis. Net price 30 g = £2.56. Label: 28. Potency II
*Additives:* disodium edetate, hydroxybenzoates (parabens)
*Note.* For bland cream basis see Ultrabase®, section 13.2.1
*Oily cream*, diflucortolone valerate 0.1%, in a water-in-oil basis. Net price 30 g = £2.56. Label: 28. Potency II
*Additives:* none as listed in section 13.1
*Ointment*, diflucortolone valerate 0.1%, in an anhydrous basis. Net price 30 g = £2.56. Label: 28. Potency II
*Additives:* none as listed in section 13.1

PoM **Nerisone Forte**® (Schering Health Care)
*Oily cream*, diflucortolone valerate 0.3%, in a water-in-oil basis. Net price 15 g = £2.09. Label: 28. Potency I
*Additives:* none as listed in section 13.1
*Ointment*, diflucortolone valerate 0.3% in an anhydrous fatty basis. Net price 15 g = £2.09. Label: 28. Potency I
*Additives:* none as listed in section 13.1

## FLUCLOROLONE ACETONIDE

*Indications:* severe inflammatory skin disorders such as eczema unresponsive to less potent corticosteroids
*Cautions; Contra-indications; Side-effects:* see under Hydrocortisone and notes above
*Administration:* apply thinly twice daily, reducing frequency as condition responds

PoM **Topilar**® (Bioglan)
*Cream*, fluclorolone acetonide 0.025%, in a non-aqueous, water-miscible basis. Net price 30 g = £2.80; 100 g = £8.39. Label: 28. Potency II
*Additives:* propylene glycol
*Ointment*, fluclorolone acetonide 0.025%, in an ointment basis. Net price 30 g = £2.80; 100 g = £8.39. Label: 28. Potency II
*Additives:* propylene glycol, wool fat

## FLUOCINOLONE ACETONIDE

*Indications:* inflammatory skin disorders such as eczema, 0.0025–0.01% in milder conditions, 0.025% in severe conditions
*Cautions; Contra-indications; Side-effects:* see under Hydrocortisone and notes above
*Administration:* apply thinly 2–3 times daily, reducing strength and frequency as condition responds

PoM **Synalar**® (ICI)
*Cream*, fluocinolone acetonide 0.025%, in a water-miscible basis. Net price 15 g = 78p; 30 g = £1.40; 50 g = £2.10; Label: 28. Potency II
*Additives:* benzyl alcohol, polysorbates, propylene glycol
*Gel*, fluocinolone acetonide 0.025%, in a water-miscible basis. Net price 30 g = £1.49. For use on scalp and other hairy areas. Label: 28. Potency II
*Additives:* hydroxybenzoates (parabens), propylene glycol

*Ointment*, fluocinolone acetonide 0.025%, in a greasy basis. Net price 15 g = 78p; 30 g = £1.40; 50 g = £2.10. Potency II
*Additives:* propylene glycol, wool fat

PoM **Synalar 1 in 4 Dilution**® (ICI)
*Cream*, fluocinolone acetonide 0.00625% in a water-miscible basis. Net price 50 g = £1.60. Label: 28. Potency III
*Additives:* benzyl alcohol, polysorbates, propylene glycol
*Ointment*, fluocinolone acetonide 0.00625% in a greasy basis. Net price 50 g = £1.88. Label: 28. Potency III
*Additives:* propylene glycol, wool fat

PoM **Synalar 1 in 10 Dilution**® (ICI)
*Cream*, fluocinolone acetonide 0.0025% in a water-miscible basis. Net price 50 g = £1.52. Label: 28. Potency IV
*Additives:* benzyl alcohol, polysorbates, propylene glycol

With antibacterials
PoM **Synalar C**® (ICI)
*Cream*, fluocinolone acetonide 0.025%, clioquinol 3%, in a water-miscible basis. Net price 15 g = 96p. Label: 28. Potency II
*Additives:* disodium edetate, hydroxybenzoates (parabens), polysorbates, propylene glycol
*Ointment*, ingredients as for cream, in a greasy basis. Net price 15 g = 96p. Label: 28. Potency II. *Caution:* stains clothing
*Additives:* propylene glycol, wool fat
Apply thinly 2–3 times daily
PoM **Synalar N**® (ICI)
*Cream*, fluocinolone acetonide 0.025%, neomycin sulphate 0.5%, in a water-miscible basis. Net price 15 g = 83p; 30 g = £1.45. Label: 28. Potency II
*Additives:* hydroxybenzoates (parabens), polysorbates, propylene glycol
*Ointment*, ingredients as for cream, in a greasy basis. Net price 15 g = 83p; 30 g = £1.45. Label: 28. Potency II
*Additives:* propylene glycol, wool fat
Apply thinly 2–3 times daily

## FLUOCINONIDE

*Indications:* severe inflammatory skin disorders such as eczema unresponsive to less potent corticosteroids
*Cautions; Contra-indications; Side-effects:* see under Hydrocortisone and notes above
*Administration:* apply thinly 3–4 times daily, reducing frequency as condition responds

PoM **Metosyn**® (Stuart)
*FAPG cream*, fluocinonide 0.05%, in a non-aqueous water-miscible basis. Net price 25 g = £1.25; 100 g = £4.71. Label: 28. Potency II
*Additives:* propylene glycol
*Ointment*, fluocinonide 0.05%, in a paraffin basis. Net price 25 g = £1.25; 100 g = £4.71. Label: 28. Potency II
*Additives:* propylene glycol, wool fat
*Scalp lotion*, fluocinonide 0.05% in a propylene glycol-alcohol basis. Net price 30 mL (with applicator) = £2.59. Label: 15, 28. Potency II
*Additives:* propylene glycol
Apply 1–2 times daily, reducing frequency as condition responds

---

## FLUOCORTOLONE

*Indications:* 0.25%—severe inflammatory skin disorders such as eczema unresponsive to less potent corticosteroids; 0.1%—milder inflammatory skin disorders

*Cautions; Contra-indications; Side-effects:* see under Hydrocortisone and notes above

*Administration:* apply thinly 2–3 times daily, reducing strength and frequency as condition responds

PoM **Ultradil Plain**® (Schering Health Care)
*Cream*, fluocortolone hexanoate 0.1%, fluocortolone pivalate 0.1%, in a water-miscible basis. Net price 50 g = £2.86. Label: 28. Potency III
*Additives:* disodium edetate, hydroxybenzoates (parabens), fragrance
*Note.* For bland cream basis see Ultrabase®, section 13.2.1
*Ointment*, fluocortolone hexanoate 0.1%, fluocortolone pivalate 0.1%, in a water-in-oil emulsion basis. Net price 50 g = £2.86. Label: 28. Potency III
*Additives:* wool fat, fragrance

PoM **Ultralanum Plain**® (Schering Health Care)
*Cream*, fluocortolone hexanoate 0.25%, fluocortolone pivalate 0.25%, in a water-miscible basis. Net price 50 g = £4.65. Label: 28. Potency III
*Additives:* disodium edetate, hydroxybenzoates (parabens), fragrance
*Note.* For bland cream basis see Ultrabase®, section 13.2.1
*Ointment*, fluocortolone 0.25%, fluocortolone pivalate 0.25%, in a water-in-oil emulsion basis. Net price 50 g = £4.65. Label: 28. Potency III
*Additives:* wool fat, fragrance

## FLURANDRENOLONE

*Indications:* eczema and dermatitis of all types
*Cautions; Contra-indications; Side-effects:* see under Hydrocortisone and notes above
*Administration:* apply thinly 2–3 times daily, reducing strength and frequency as condition responds

PoM **Haelan**® (Dista)
*Cream*, flurandrenolone 0.0125%, in a water-miscible basis. Net price 60 g = £2.97. Label: 28. Potency III
*Additives:* propylene glycol
*Ointment*, flurandrenolone 0.0125%, in an anhydrous greasy basis. Net price 60 g = £2.97. Label: 28. Potency III
*Additives:* beeswax, polysorbate

With antibacterials
PoM **Haelan-C**® (Dista)
*Cream*, flurandrenolone 0.0125%, clioquinol 3%. Net price 30 g = £2.02, 60 g = £2.97. Label: 28. Potency III
*Additives:* hydroxybenzoates (parabens), disodium edetate
*Ointment*, flurandrenolone 0.0125%, clioquinol 3%. Net price 30 g = £2.02, 60 g = £2.97. Label: 28. Potency III
*Additives:* none as listed in section 13.1
Apply thinly 2–3 times daily
*Caution:* stains clothing

## HALCINONIDE

*Indications:* severe inflammatory skin disorders such as eczema unresponsive to less potent corticosteroids
*Cautions; Contra-indications; Side-effects:* see under Hydrocortisone and notes above
*Administration:* apply thinly 2–3 times daily, reducing frequency as condition responds

PoM **Halciderm Topical**® (Squibb)
*Cream*, halcinonide 0.1%, in a water-miscible basis. Net price 30 g = £3.40. Label: 28. Potency I
*Additives:* propylene glycol

## METHYLPREDNISOLONE ACETATE

*Indications:* see notes above
*Cautions; Contra-indications; Side-effects:* see under Hydrocortisone

PoM **Neo-Medrone**® (Upjohn)
*Cream*, methylprednisolone acetate 0.25%, neomycin sulphate 0.5%. Net price 15 g = £1.44. Label: 28. Potency IV
*Additives:* butylated hydroxyanisole, butylated hydroxytoluene, hydroxybenzoates (parabens), fragrance
Apply thinly 1–3 times daily

## TRIAMCINOLONE ACETONIDE

*Indications:* severe inflammatory skin disorders such as eczema unresponsive to less potent corticosteroids
*Cautions; Contra-indications; Side-effects:* see under Hydrocortisone and notes above
*Administration:* apply thinly 2–4 times daily, reducing frequency as condition responds

PoM **Adcortyl**® (Squibb)
*Cream*, triamcinolone acetonide 0.1%, in a water-miscible basis. Net price 30 g = £1.98. Label: 28. Potency II
*Additives:* benzyl alcohol, propylene glycol
*Ointment*, triamcinolone acetonide 0.1%, in an anhydrous greasy basis. Net price 30 g = £1.98. Label: 28. Potency II
*Additives:* none as listed in section 13.1

PoM **Ledercort**® (Lederle)
*Cream*, triamcinolone acetonide 0.1%, in water-miscible basis. Net price 15 g = £1.72; 250 g = £25.90. Label: 28. Potency II
*Additives:* benzyl alcohol
*Ointment*, triamcinolone acetonide 0.1%, in an anhydrous greasy basis. Net price 15 g = £1.72. Label: 28. Potency II
*Additives:* hydroxybenzoates (parabens), wool fat

With antimicrobials
PoM **Adcortyl with Graneodin**® (Squibb)
*Cream*, triamcinolone acetonide 0.1%, gramicidin 0.025%, neomycin 0.25% (as sulphate), in a vanishing-cream basis. Net price 25 g = £3.00. Label: 28. Potency II
*Additives:* benzyl alcohol, propylene glycol
Apply thinly 2–4 times daily

---

PoM **Aureocort®** (Lederle)

*Cream*, triamcinolone acetonide 0.1%, chlortetracycline hydrochloride 3% (as chlortetracycline), in a water-miscible basis. Net price 15 g = £2.77. Label: 28. Potency II

*Additives:* chlorocresol

*Ointment*, triamcinolone acetonide 0.1%, chlortetracycline hydrochloride 3%, in an anhydrous greasy basis containing wool fat and white soft paraffin. Net price 15 g = £2.77. Label: 28. Potency II

*Additives:* hydroxybenzoates (parabens), wool fat

*Caution:* stains clothing

Apply thinly 2–3 times daily

PoM **Nystadermal®** (Squibb)

*Cream*, triamcinolone acetonide 0.1%, nystatin 100 000 units/g. Net price 15 g = £2.27. Label: 28. Potency II

*Additives:* benzyl alcohol, propylene glycol, fragrance

Apply thinly 2–4 times daily on moist weeping lesions

PoM **Pevaryl TC®** (Cilag)

*Cream*, triamcinolone 0.1%, econazole nitrate 1%. Net price 15 g = £4.00. Label: 28. Potency II

*Additives:* butylated hydroxyanisole, disodium edetate, benzoic acid

Apply thinly twice daily for 14 days

PoM **Tri-Adcortyl®** (Squibb)

*Cream*, triamcinolone acetonide 0.1%, gramicidin 0.025%, neomycin 0.25% (as sulphate), nystatin 100 000 units/g. Net price 30 g = £3.23. Label: 28. Potency II

*Additives:* benzyl alcohol, ethylenediamine, propylene glycol, fragrance

*Ointment*, ingredients as for cream, in an ointment basis. Net price 30 g = £3.23. Label: 28. Potency II

*Additives:* none as listed in section 13.1

Apply thinly 2–4 times daily

# 13.5  Preparations for psoriasis and eczema

## ECZEMA

*Eczema* ('dermatitis') is due to a particular type of epidermal inflammation and is caused by a wide variety of factors; where possible the causative factors should be established and removed. In many cases no underlying factor can be identified (atopic eczema).

Dry, fissured, scaly lesions are treated with bland **emollients** (section 13.2.1) which are often all that is necessary to allay irritation and permit healing. Preparations containing zinc oxide and calamine are sometimes useful; zinc may have a weak anti-eczematous action. Preparations such as **emulsifying ointment** are used as soap substitutes and in the bath. **Keratolytics** such as salicylic acid, followed by coal tar (see p. 402) are used in chronic eczematous conditions where there is marked thickening of the skin and pronounced scaling.

*Weeping eczemas* may be treated with corticosteroids; they are, however, commonly secondarily infected. Wet dressings of **potassium permanganate** (0.01%) (section 13.11.6) are applied; if a large area is involved, potassium permanganate baths are taken. When necessary **topical antibacterials** are used (section 13.10.1) but those which are not given systemically should be chosen.

**Coal tar** is more active than salicylic acid and has anti-inflammatory, antipruritic and keratolytic properties. It is used in psoriasis and eczema. Coal tar has superseded wood tar as it is more active. The formulation and strength chosen depends on patient acceptability and severity of the condition; the 'thicker' the patch of eczema or psoriasis the stronger the concentration of coal tar required. **Coal tar paste** or **zinc and coal tar paste** are generally suitable for most cases but are limited by their unpleasant appearance and smell and they may not be used on the face. Some of the newer preparations are less unsightly and may be preferred. Preparations such as Carbo-Dome® are suitable for treating the face. **Zinc paste and coal tar bandage** (section 13.13.1) is useful for treating the limbs. **Tar shampoos** are described in section 13.9. Combinations of coal tar with zinc or salicylic acid have no advantage over the simpler preparations. Preparations containing hydrocortisone and coal tar are useful in eczemas.

**Ichthammol** has a milder action than coal tar and has been used in the less acute forms of eczema. It can be applied conveniently to flexures of the limbs as **zinc paste and ichthammol bandage** (section 13.13.1).

**Gamolenic acid** has been claimed to improve patients with eczema and in particular atopic dermatitis. However, the evidence in favour of a useful therapeutic effect is slim.

## PSORIASIS

*Psoriasis* is characterised by epidermal thickening and scaling. It has less tendency to heal spontaneously than eczema. For mild conditions, treatment, other than reassurance and an emollient, may be unnecessary. In more troublesome cases, local application of **salicylic acid**, **coal tar**, or **dithranol** may have a beneficial effect. Topical and systemic corticosteroids should be avoided or given under specialist supervision because, although they may be effective, subsequent treatment becomes more difficult, as tachyphylaxis may occur and they may induce or precipitate severe pustular psoriasis. In resistant cases an antimetabolite, usually methotrexate (see section 8.1.3), may be used for its antimitotic activity but this must always be done under hospital supervision and the dose adjusted according to severity of the condition and in accordance with haematological and biochemical measurements; the usual dose is 15 to 25 mg of methotrexate weekly, usually by mouth.

**Salicylic acid** may be used in all hyperkeratotic and scaling conditions to enhance the rate of loss of surface scale. Preparations containing salicylic acid 2% are used initially and then gradually increased to concentrations of 3 to 6%. Side-effects are few but include allergic contact sensitivity, or, when large areas are treated, salicylism (see section 10.1.1).

**Dithranol** is used in psoriasis and is the most potent topical preparation available for this condition. The preparation is applied carefully to the lesion, covered with a dressing, and left for one hour. Traditionally applications have been left on the skin overnight but this has now been shown to be unnecessary as short contact applications of one hour or less are equally effective. Usual concentrations are 0.1–2% although in individual patients 5% or more may be used. Dithranol must be used with caution as it can cause quite severe skin irritation. For this reason it must be applied only to the lesions and it is customary to start with low concentrations and gradually build up to the maximum concentration which produces a therapeutic effect without irritation. Hands should be washed thoroughly after use. Some patients are intolerant to dithranol even in low concentrations; it is important to recognise them early in treatment. Fair skin is more sensitive than dark skin. Proprietary preparations such as Dithrocream® are most commonly used as they may cause less staining and irritation than dithranol paste. Dithranol and urea combinations (Psoradrate®) may improve skin texture by rehydration. **Dithranol triacetate** has no advantage over traditional preparations.

Ingram's method of applying dithranol is used in hospital. The patient soaks in a warm bath containing coal tar solution 1 in 800 and after drying is exposed to ultraviolet radiation B (UVB) to produce a slight erythema. **Dithranol paste** is applied to the lesions and the normal skin protected by applying talc and stockinette dressings. The procedure is repeated daily.

**PUVA**, photochemotherapy using psoralens with long-wave ultraviolet irradiation (UVA), is an effective method of treating some patients with psoriasis. Special lamps are required, and a psoralen, generally methoxsalen (available on named-patient basis only) is given by mouth about 2 hours beforehand, to sensitise the skin to the effects of irradiation. A course of PUVA may last 4 to 6 weeks and requires a variable number of treatments. Treatment is only available in specialist centres; it has to be carefully regulated, owing to the short-term hazard of severe burning and the long-term hazards of cataract formation, accelerated ageing, and the development of skin cancer.

**Calcipotriol** is a vitamin D derivative that has been newly introduced for topical application for mild to moderate psoriasis affecting up to 40% of skin area.

**Etretinate** is given by mouth for the treatment of severe resistant or complicated psoriasis and some of the congenital disorders of keratinisation including Darier's disease (keratosis follicularis). It should be prescribed **only** by, or under the supervision of, a consultant dermatologist and is available to hospitals **only**. It is a retinoid compound with marked effects on keratinising epithelia. A therapeutic effect occurs after 2 to 4 weeks with maximum benefit after 4 to 6 weeks. Etretinate treats only manifestations not the ultimate causes of these diseases, but treatment should be limited to a period of 6 to 9 months with a 3- to 4-month rest period before repeating treatment, as experience with this drug is limited. Most patients suffer from dryness and cracking of the lips. Other side-effects include a mild transient increase in the rate of hair fall (reversible on withdrawal), occasional generalised pruritus, paronychia, and nose bleeds. There is a tendency for the plasma lipids to rise in some patients. Etretinate is **teratogenic** and must be **avoided** in pregnancy. Contraceptive measures must be taken at least 1 month before and during treatment by women who may become pregnant and for at least two years after a course of the drug.

## TOPICAL PREPARATIONS FOR PSORIASIS OR ECZEMA

### COAL TAR
*Indications:* chronic eczema and psoriasis
*Cautions:* avoid broken or inflamed skin
*Side-effects:* skin irritation and acne-like eruptions, photosensitivity; stains skin, hair, and fabric
*Administration:* apply 1–3 times daily starting with low-strength preparations
*Note.* For shampoo preparations see section 13.9

Ointments and similar preparations
**Calamine and Coal Tar Ointment, BP,** calamine 12.5 g, strong coal tar solution 2.5 g, zinc oxide 12.5 g, hydrous wool fat 25 g, white soft paraffin 47.5 g

**Coal Tar and Salicylic Acid Ointment, BP,** coal tar 2 g, salicylic acid 2 g, emulsifying wax 11.4 g, white soft paraffin 19 g, coconut oil 54 g, polysorbate '80' 4 g, liquid paraffin 7.6 g

**Coal Tar Paste, BP,** strong coal tar solution 7.5%, in compound zinc paste

**Zinc and Coal Tar Paste, BP,** zinc oxide 6%, coal tar 6%, emulsifying wax 5%, starch 38%, yellow soft paraffin 45%

**Alphosyl**® (Stafford-Miller)
*Cream,* coal tar extract 5%, allantoin 2%, in a vanishing-cream basis. Net price 100 g = £2.50
*Additives:* beeswax, hydroxybenzoates (parabens), isopropyl palmitate, propylene glycol
For application to skin particularly intertriginous areas, 2–4 times daily
*Lotion,* coal tar extract 5%, allantoin 2%. Net price 250 mL = £2.27. For application to skin or scalp, 2–4 times daily
*Additives:* isopropyl palmitate, propylene glycol

**Carbo-Dome**® (Lagap)
*Cream,* coal tar solution 10%, in a water-miscible basis. Net price 30 g = £1.97; 100 g = £5.95
*Additives:* beeswax, hydroxybenzoates (parabens)
Apply 2–3 times daily

**Clinitar®** (Shire)
*Cream*, coal tar extract 1%. Net price 60 g = £3.31
*Additives:* isopropyl palmitate, propylene glycol
Apply 1–2 times daily

**Cocois®** (Bioglan)
*Ointment*, coal tar solution 12%, salicylic acid 2%, precipitated sulphur 4%, and coconut oil. Net price 40 g (with applicator nozzle) = £3.41
*Additives:* none as listed in section 13.1
For dry and scaly scalp conditions, apply at night and remove by washing in the morning

**Gelcosal®** (Quinoderm Ltd)
*Gel*, strong coal tar solution 5%, pine tar 5%, salicylic acid 2% in a water-miscible basis. Net price 50 g = £2.89
*Additives:* none as listed in section 13.1
Apply twice daily

**Gelcotar®** (Quinoderm Ltd)
*Gel*, strong coal tar solution 5%, pine tar 5%, in a water-miscible basis. Net price 50 g = £2.66; 500 g = £13.90
*Additives:* none as listed in section 13.1
Apply twice daily
*Liquid*, see section 13.9

**Pragmatar®** (Bioglan)
*Cream*, cetyl alcohol-coal tar distillate 4%, salicylic acid 3%, sulphur (precipitated) 3%, in a water-miscible basis. Net price 25 g = £1.90; 100 g = £6.37
*Additives:* fragrance
Apply thinly daily; for scalp apply weekly to clean hair or in severe cases daily. Dilute with a few drops of water before application to infants

**Psoriderm®** (Dermal)
*Cream*, coal tar 6%, lecithin 0.4%. Net price 225 mL = £3.32
*Additives:* hydroxybenzoates (parabens), isopropyl palmitate, propylene glycol
Apply 1–2 times daily

**PsoriGel®** (Galderma)
*Gel*, coal tar solution USP 7.5% in an alcoholic emollient basis. Net price 90 g = £3.81
*Additives:* propylene glycol
Apply 1–2 times daily

Impregnated dressings
**Zinc Paste and Coal Tar Bandage, BP,** (Coltapaste®, Tarband®), see section 13.13.1

Bath preparations
**Coal Tar Solution, BP,** coal tar 20%, polysorbate '80' 5%, in alcohol (96%). Net price 100 mL = 49p
Use 100 mL in a bath
*Note.* Strong Coal Tar Solution BP contains coal tar 40%

**Balneum with Tar®** (Merck)
*Bath oil*, coal tar distillate 30%, soya oil 55%. Net price 225 mL = £3.72. For psoriasis and eczema
*Additives:* none as listed in section 13.1
Use 1 measure (20 mL) in bath

**Polytar Emollient®** (Stiefel)
*Bath additive*, coal tar solution 2.5%, arachis oil extract of coal tar 7.5%, tar 7.5%, cade oil 7.5%, liquid paraffin 35%. Net price 350 mL = £4.87. ACBS: for psoriasis, eczema, atopic and pruritic dermatosis
*Additives:* isopropyl palmitate
Use 2–4 capfuls in bath and soak for 20 minutes

**Psoriderm®** (Dermal)
*Bath emulsion*, coal tar 40%. Net price 200 mL = £2.95. For psoriasis
*Additives:* polysorbate 20
Use 30 mL in a bath and soak for 5 minutes

Coal tar and corticosteroid preparations
PoM **Alphosyl HC®** (Stafford-Miller)
*Cream*, coal tar extract 5%, hydrocortisone 0.5%, allantoin 2%, in aqueous-cream basis. Net price 30 g = £1.70; 100 g = £4.85. Label: 28. Potency IV
*Additives:* beeswax, hydroxybenzoates (parabens), isopropyl palmitate, wool fat
Apply thinly twice daily

PoM **Carbo-Cort®** (Lagap)
*Cream*, coal tar solution 3%, hydrocortisone 0.25%, in a water-miscible basis. Price 30 g = £3.61. Label: 28. Potency IV
*Additives:* beeswax, hydroxybenzoates (parabens)
Apply thinly 2–3 times daily

PoM **Tarcortin®** (Stafford-Miller)
*Cream*, coal tar extract 5%, hydrocortisone 0.5%, in a vanishing-cream basis. Net price 100 g = £3.88. Label: 28. Potency IV
*Additives:* hydroxybenzoates (parabens), isopropyl palmitate, propylene glycol, polysorbates, fragrance
Apply thinly 2–4 times daily

## BUFEXAMAC

*Indications:* mild inflammatory skin disorders
*Cautions:* avoid broken skin
*Side-effects:* skin irritation

PoM **Parfenac®** (Lederle)
*Cream*, bufexamac 5%, in a water-miscible basis. Net price 30 g = £2.16
*Additives:* hydroxybenzoates (parabens)
Apply thinly 2–3 times daily (not indicated for infants)

## CALCIPOTRIOL

*Indications:* mild to moderate psoriasis
*Cautions:* pregnancy; avoid use on face and inadvertent transfer to other body areas; wash hands thoroughly after application
*Contra-indications:* disorders of calcium metabolism
*Side-effects:* transient local irritation; rarely facial or perioral dermatitis
*Administration:* apply twice daily; max. 100 g weekly, period of treatment should not exceed 6 weeks

▼ PoM **Dovonex®** (Leo)
*Ointment*, calcipotriol 50 micrograms/g in a paraffin basis. Net price 30 g = £7.95; 100 g = £22.85
*Additives:* disodium edetate, propylene glycol

## DITHRANOL

*Indications:* subacute and chronic psoriasis, see notes above
*Cautions:* avoid use near eyes; see also notes above

*Contra-indications:* hypersensitivity; acute psoriasis
*Side-effects:* local burning sensation and irritation; stains skin, hair, and fabrics
*Administration:* see notes above

**\*PoM Dithranol Ointment, BP,** dithranol, in yellow soft paraffin; usual strengths 0.1–2%. Part of basis may be replaced by hard paraffin if a stiffer preparation is required. Label: 28
\*PoM if dithranol content more than 1%, otherwise P

**Dithranol Paste, BP,** dithranol in zinc and salicylic acid (Lassar's) paste. Usual strengths 0.1–1% of dithranol. Label: 28

**Alphodith®** (Stafford-Miller)
*Ointment,* dithranol 0.4%, net price 50 g = £3.50; 1%, 50 g = £4.25; PoM 2%, 50 g = £6.00; PoM 3%, 50 g = £8.50. Label: 10 patient information leaflet, 28. For application to skin or scalp
*Additives:* none as listed in section 13.1

**Anthranol®** (Stiefel)
*Ointment,* dithranol 0.4%, net price 50 g = £3.50; 1%, 50 g = £4.25; PoM 2%, 50 g = £6.00. Label: 28. For application to skin or scalp
*Additives:* contains salicylic acid 0.5% as an antioxidant

**Dithrocream®** (Dermal)
*Cream,* dithranol in a water-miscible basis, 0.1%, net price 50 g = £3.96; 0.25%, 50 g = £4.25; 0.5% (Forte), 50 g = £4.89; 1% (HP); 50 g = £5.69; PoM 2%, 50 g = £7.13. Label: 28. For application to skin or scalp
*Additives:* chlorocresol

**Dithrolan®** (Dermal)
*Ointment,* dithranol 0.5%, salicylic acid 0.5%. Net price 90 g = £5.49. Label: 28
*Additives:* none as listed in section 13.1

**Psoradrate®** (Norwich Eaton)
*Cream,* dithranol in a powder-in-cream basis containing urea. 0.1%, net price 30 g = £2.54, 100 g = £7.59; 0.2%, 30 g = £2.81, 100 g = £8.72; 0.4%, 100 g = £10.03. Label: 28
*Additives:* polysorbate 40

**Psorin®** (Thames)
*Ointment,* dithranol 0.11%, crude coal tar 1%, salicylic acid 1.6%, in an emollient basis. Net price 25 g = £2.79; 50 g = £5.30; 100 g = £10.50. Label: 28
*Additives:* beeswax, wool fat

Dithranol triacetate
**Exolan®** (Dermal)
*Cream,* dithranol triacetate 1% in a water-miscible basis. Net price 50 g = £3.00. Label: 28
*Additives:* chlorocresol
Apply daily to skin and scalp

## ICHTHAMMOL

*Indications:* chronic eczema
*Side-effects:* skin irritation and sensitisation
*Administration:* apply 1–3 times daily

**Ichthammol Ointment, BP1980,** ichthammol 10%, yellow soft paraffin 45%, wool fat 45%. Net price 25 g = 17p

**Zinc and Ichthammol Cream, BP,** ichthammol 5%, cetostearyl alcohol 3%, wool fat 10%, in zinc cream. Net price 100 g = 60p

**Zinc Paste and Ichthammol Bandage, BP** (Ichthopaste®, Icthaband®), see section 13.13.1

## SALICYLIC ACID

*Indications:* hyperkeratoses
*Cautions:* see notes above; avoid broken or inflamed skin
*Side-effects:* sensitivity, excessive drying, irritation, systemic effects after prolonged use (see section 10.1.1)

**Salicylic Acid Collodion, BP**—section 13.7

**Salicylic Acid Ointment, BP,** salicylic acid 2%, in wool alcohols ointment. Net price 25 g = 15p
Apply twice daily

**Zinc and Salicylic Acid Paste, BP** (Lassar's Paste), zinc oxide 24%, salicylic acid 2%, starch 24%, white soft paraffin 50%. Net price 25 g = 15p
Apply twice daily

## ORAL PREPARATIONS FOR PSORIASIS OR ECZEMA

## ETRETINATE

*Indications:* severe extensive psoriasis resistant to other forms of therapy; palmo-plantar pustular psoriasis; severe congenital ichthyosis; severe Darier's disease (keratosis follicularis)
*Cautions:* exclude pregnancy before starting—patients should avoid pregnancy at least 1 month before, during, and for at least 2 years after treatment, should avoid concomitant high doses of vitamin A and use of keratolytics, and should not donate blood during or for 2 years after stopping therapy (teratogenic risk); monitor hepatic function and plasma lipids (especially in hypertriglyceridaemia) at start, 1 month after initiating treatment, and then at intervals of 3 months; diabetes (can alter glucose tolerance); radiographic assessment on long-term treatment; investigate atypical musculoskeletal symptoms; avoid long-term use in children (skeletal hyperostosis and extra-osseous calcification); **interactions:** Appendix 1 (etretinate)
*Contra-indications:* hepatic and renal impairment; pregnancy (**important teratogenic risk: see** Cautions and Appendix 4); breast-feeding
*Side-effects:* (mainly dose-related) dryness of mucous membranes (sometimes erosion), of skin (sometimes scaling, thinning, erythema, and pruritus), and of conjunctiva (sometimes conjunctivitis); palmar and plantar exfoliation; epistaxis, and epidermal fragility reported, also paronychia; granulomatous lesions reported; reversible alopecia; myalgia and arthralgia; occasional nausea, headache, malaise, drowsiness and sweating; benign intracranial hypertension reported (avoid concomitant tetracyclines); raised liver enzymes, rarely jaundice and hepatitis (avoid concomitant

methotrexate); raised triglycerides; decreased night vision reported

*Dose:* administered in accordance with expert advice, adults and children, initially up to 750 micrograms/kg daily in divided doses for 2–4 weeks, increased to 1 mg/kg daily if necessary (max. daily dose 75 mg), then reduced to 500 micrograms/kg daily for a further 6–8 weeks, then intermittently as necessary; usual maintenance dose 250–500 micrograms/kg daily (**important:** see Cautions and notes above)

PoM **Tigason**® (Roche)

*Capsules*, etretinate 10 mg (yellow), net price 56-cap pack = £20.40; 25 mg (orange/yellow), 56-cap pack = £44.05 (**hosp. only**, specialist dermatological supervision). Label: 10, patient information card, 21

## GAMOLENIC ACID

*Indications:* see under preparations

*Cautions:* history of epilepsy, concomitant treatment with epileptogenic drugs e.g. phenothiazines

*Side-effects:* occasional nausea, indigestion, headache

*Dose:* see below

PoM **Epogam**® (Searle)

*Capsules*, gamolenic acid 40 mg in evening primrose oil. Net price 240-cap pack = £25.04. Counselling, see below
*Additives: include* vitamin E 10 mg as *in vivo* antoxidant
*Dose:* 4–6 capsules twice daily; CHILD 1–12 years 2–4 capsules twice daily

*Paediatric capsules*, gamolenic acid 80 mg in evening primrose oil. Net price 60-cap pack = £15.80. Counselling, see below
*Additives: include* vitamin E 20 mg as *in vivo* antoxidant
*Dose:* CHILD over 1 year, 1–2 capsules twice daily

COUNSELLING. Capsules may be cut open and contents swallowed or taken on bread; paediatric capsules have 'snip-off' neck for convenience of administration

Mastalgia

PoM **Efamast**® (Searle)

*Capsules*, gamolenic acid 40 mg in evening primrose. Net price 224-cap pack = £24.33
*Additives: include* vitamin E 10 mg as *in vivo* antoxidant
*Dose:* symptomatic relief of cyclical and noncyclical mastalgia, 3–4 capsules twice daily

# 13.6 Preparations for acne

TOPICAL TREATMENT. Most topical preparations are intended for removing follicular plugs and reducing skin flora. The skin is cleansed regularly with detergent solutions, for example cetrimide solution (section 13.11.3). Abrasive agents may also be used but their effectiveness is uncertain.

Cleansing is followed by application of **anti-septics** and **keratolytics**; thick greasy preparations should not be used. Preparations usually contain benzoyl peroxide, hydroxyquinoline, sulphur, salicylic acid, or tretinoin. Many of these irritate the skin but it is doubtful if a therapeutic effect can be obtained without some degree of irritation (which subsides with continued treatment). Topical application of **tretinoin** (Retin-A®) a vitamin A derivative has been shown to be useful in treating acne but patients should be warned that some redness and skin peeling may occur after application for several days.

Topical antibiotics are also used for mild to moderately severe acne. Topical preparations of erythromycin, tetracycline, and clindamycin seem to be quite useful for many patients with the milder forms of acne; they can produce mild irritation of the skin but rarely sensitise. It has been suggested that percutaneous absorption of clindamycin can cause pseudomembranous colitis. Chloramphenicol is included in some preparations but can sensitise the skin; topical neomycin is not suitable owing to sensitisation. Antibiotics cause resistant strains of micro-organisms to appear but as yet no adverse clinical effects have resulted.

Topical **corticosteroids** should **not** be used in acne.

SYSTEMIC TREATMENT. Systemic antibacterial treatment is useful. **Tetracycline** (see section 5.1.3), **erythromycin** (see section 5.1.5), and occasionally other antibacterials are used. The usual dosage regimen for tetracycline and erythromycin, taken before meals, is 250 mg 3 times daily for 1–4 weeks and then reduced to twice daily until improvement occurs. Higher doses are sometimes indicated when there is a poor response to the usual regimen; in general the dose of the antibiotic used should be matched to the patient's condition. Maximum improvement usually occurs after three or four months but in resistant cases treatment may need to be continued for two or more years. As there have been some reports of pseudomembranous colitis with tetracycline, caution is necessary in long-term administration.

**Cyproterone acetate** with **ethinyloestradiol** (Dianette®) contains an anti-androgen and is used to treat women with severe acne refractory to prolonged oral antibacterial therapy. Improvement of acne probably occurs because of decreased sebum secretion which is under androgen control. Some women with mild to moderate idiopathic hirsutism may also benefit as hair growth is also androgen-dependent (see also section 6.4.2). Dianette® may also be used as an oral contraceptive but should be reserved for women who are being treated for androgen-dependent skin conditions. It is contra-indicated in pregnancy and in a predisposition to thrombosis.

**Isotretinoin** (Roaccutane®) has recently been introduced for the systemic treatment of cystic and conglobate acne and severe acne which has failed to respond to an adequate course of a systemic antimicrobial agent. It should be prescribed **only** by, or under the supervision of, a consultant dermatologist, and is available to hospitals **only**. It is given in doses of 500 micrograms/kg/day for 12–16 weeks but doses may be adjusted if necessary after 4 weeks. Repeat courses should not normally be given. An exacerbation is common some 2–4 weeks after starting treatment but usually subsides after a few weeks.

Side-effects include dry lips, sore eyes, nose bleeds, mild transient hair loss, and joint pains. Plasma lipids and liver function should be checked by investigation monthly as there is a tendency for the plasma lipids to rise in some patients. The drug is **teratogenic** and must **not** be given to women who are pregnant or those who may become pregnant unless there is concomitant effective contraception and then only after detailed explanation by the physician. The contraceptive measures must continue for at least one month after ceasing treatment with the drug.

---

## TOPICAL ACNE PREPARATIONS

## ABRASIVE AGENTS

*Indications:* cleansing in acne vulgaris
*Cautions:* avoid contact with eyes; discontinue use temporarily if skin becomes irritated
*Contra-indications:* superficial venules, telangiectasia

**Brasivol**® (Stiefel)
*Paste No. 1*, aluminium oxide 38.09% in fine particles, in a soap-detergent basis. Net price 75 g = £2.49
  *Additives:* fragrance
*Paste No. 2*, aluminium oxide 52.2% in medium particles, in a soap-detergent basis. Net price 75 g = £2.49
  *Additives:* fragrance
Use instead of soap 1–3 times daily, starting with fine grade

**Ionax Scrub**® (Galderma)
*Gel*, polyethylene granules 21.9%, benzalkonium chloride 0.25% in a foaming aqueous alcoholic basis. Net price 60 g = £3.13. ACBS: for control and hygiene of acne and cleansing of the skin prior to acne treatment
  *Additives:* propylene glycol
Use instead of soap 1–2 times daily

## ANTIBIOTICS

*Indications:* acne vulgaris
*Cautions:* alcoholic preparations are not suitable for use with benzoyl peroxide; max. duration of treatment 10–12 weeks

PoM **Dalacin T**® (Upjohn)
*Topical solution*, clindamycin (as phosphate) 1%, in an aqueous alcoholic basis. Net price 30 mL (with applicator) = £6.05
  *Additives:* propylene glycol
Apply to clean skin twice daily
*Lotion*, clindamycin (as phosphate) 1% in an aqueous basis. Net price 30 mL = £6.65
  *Additives:* hydroxybenzoates (parabens)
Apply to clean skin twice daily

PoM **Stiemycin**® (Stiefel)
*Solution*, erythromycin 2% in an alcoholic basis. Net price 2 × 25 mL applicator bottles = £9.00
  *Additives:* propylene glycol
Apply to clean skin twice daily

PoM **Topicycline**® (Norwich Eaton)
*Solution*, powder for reconstitution, tetracycline hydrochloride, 4-epitetracycline hydrochloride, providing tetracycline hydrochloride 2.2 mg/mL when reconstituted with solvent containing n-decyl methyl sulphoxide and citric acid in 40% alcohol. Net price per pack of powder and solvent to provide 70 mL = £7.90
  *Additives:* none as listed in section 13.1
Apply to clean skin twice daily

PoM **Zineryt**® (Brocades)
*Topical solution*, powder for reconstitution, erythromycin 40 mg, zinc acetate 12 mg/mL when reconstituted with solvent containing ethanol. Net price per pack of powder and solvent to provide 30 mL = £8.04
  *Additives:* none as listed in section 13.1.
Apply to clean skin twice daily

---

## BENZOYL PEROXIDE

*Indications:* acne vulgaris
*Cautions:* avoid contact with eyes, mouth, and mucous membranes; may bleach fabrics
*Side-effects:* skin irritation
*Administration:* apply 1–2 times daily to clean skin, starting treatment with lower-strength preparations

**Acetoxyl**® (Stiefel)
*'2.5' Gel*, benzoyl peroxide 2.5%, in an aqueous-acetone-gel basis. Net price 40 g = £1.59
  *Additives:* propylene glycol
*'5' Gel*, benzoyl peroxide 5%, in an aqueous-acetone-gel basis. Net price 40 g = £1.76
  *Additives:* propylene glycol

**Acnegel**® (Stiefel)
*Gel*, benzoyl peroxide 5%, in an aqueous alcoholic basis. Net price 50 g = £2.17
  *Additives:* none as listed in section 13.1
*Forte gel*, benzoyl peroxide 10%, in an aqueous alcoholic basis. Net price 50 g = £2.38
  *Additives:* none as listed in section 13.1

**Acnidazil**® (Janssen)
*Cream*, benzoyl peroxide 5%, miconazole nitrate 2%. Net price 15 g = £2.10; 30 g = £3.40
  *Additives:* polysorbate 20, propylene glycol

**Benoxyl**® (Stiefel)
*'5' Cream*, benzoyl peroxide 5%, in a non-greasy basis. Net price 40 g = £1.29
  *Additives:* isopropyl palmitate, propylene glycol
*'5' Lotion*, benzoyl peroxide 5%, in a non-greasy basis. Net price 30 mL = £1.03
  *Additives:* isopropyl palmitate, propylene glycol
*'10' Lotion*, benzoyl peroxide 10%, in a water-miscible basis. Net price 30 mL = £1.09
  *Additives:* isopropyl palmitate, propylene glycol

**Benzagel**® (Bioglan)
*'5' Gel*, benzoyl peroxide 5%. Net price 40 g = £2.40
*'10' Gel*, benzoyl peroxide 10%. Net price 40 g = £2.74

**Nericur**® (Schering Health Care)
*Gel 5*, benzoyl peroxide 5%, in an aqueous gel basis. Net price 30 g = £1.45
  *Additives:* propylene glycol
*Gel 10*, benzoyl peroxide 10%, in an aqueous gel basis. Net price 30 g = £1.60
  *Additives:* propylene glycol

---

**Panoxyl®** (Stiefel)

*'2.5' Aquagel* (= aqueous gel), benzoyl peroxide 2.5%. Net price 40 g = £1.72
*Additives:* propylene glycol

*'5' Gel*, benzoyl peroxide 5%, in an aqueous alcoholic basis. Net price 40 g = £1.44
*Additives:* fragrance

*'5' Aquagel* (= aqueous gel), benzoyl peroxide 5%. Net price 40 g = £1.92
*Additives:* propylene glycol

*'10' Gel*, benzoyl peroxide 10%, in an aqueous alcoholic basis. Net price 40 g = £1.63
*Additives:* fragrance

*'10' Aquagel* (= aqueous gel), benzoyl peroxide 10%. Net price 40 g = £2.12
*Additives:* propylene glycol

*'10' Wash*, benzoyl peroxide 10%, in a detergent basis. Net price 150 mL = £3.50
*Additives:* none as listed in section 13.1

**Quinoderm®** (Quinoderm Ltd)

*Cream*, benzoyl peroxide 10%, potassium hydroxyquinoline sulphate 0.5%, in an astringent vanishing-cream basis. Net price 25 g = £1.15; 50 g = £1.73
*Additives:* edetic acid (EDTA)

*Cream 5*, benzoyl peroxide 5%, potassium hydroxyquinoline sulphate 0.5%, in an astringent vanishing-cream basis. Net price 50 g = £1.61
*Additives:* edetic acid (EDTA)

*Lotio-gel 5%*, benzoyl peroxide 5%, potassium hydroxyquinoline sulphate 0.5%, in an astringent creamy basis. Net price 30 mL = £1.38
*Additives:* edetic acid (EDTA)

Apply 1–3 times daily

---

## CORTICOSTEROIDS

*Indications:* not recommended (see notes above)
*Cautions; Contra-indications; Side-effects:* section 13.4 and notes above

PoM **Actinac®** (Roussel)

*Lotion* (powder for reconstitution), chloramphenicol 1.25%, hydrocortisone acetate 1.25%, allantoin 0.75%, butoxyethyl nicotinate 0.75%, precipitated sulphur 10%, when reconstituted with solvent. Discard after 21 days. Net price 2 × 6.25 g bottles powder with 2 × 20-mL bottles solvent = £9.54. Label: 28. Potency IV
*Additives:* fragrance

PoM **Quinoderm with Hydrocortisone®** (Quinoderm Ltd)

*Cream*, hydrocortisone 1%, benzoyl peroxide 10%, potassium hydroxyquinoline sulphate 0.5%, in an astringent vanishing-cream basis. Net price 30 g = £1.77. Label: 28. Potency IV
*Additives:* edetic acid (EDTA)

---

## SULPHUR

*Cautions:* avoid contact with eyes, mouth, and mucous membranes; causes skin irritation

With resorcinol
Prolonged application of resorcinol may interfere with thyroid function therefore not recommended

**Eskamel®** (SK&F)

*Cream*, resorcinol 2%, sulphur 8%, in a non-greasy flesh-coloured basis. Net price 25 g = £1.26
*Additives:* propylene glycol, fragrance

With salicylic acid
**Salicylic Acid and Sulphur Cream, BP 1980**, salicylic acid 2%, precipitated sulphur 2%, in aqueous cream
**Salicylic Acid and Sulphur Ointment, BPC**, salicylic acid 3%, precipitated sulphur 3%, in hydrous ointment (oily cream). Net price 25 g = 21p

---

## TRETINOIN

*Indications:* acne vulgaris
*Cautions:* avoid contact with eyes, mouth, and mucous membranes; do not use simultaneously with other peeling agents (can be alternated every 12 hours with benzoyl peroxide); do not use with ultra-violet lamps
*Contra-indications:* eczema, broken skin
*Side-effects:* irritation, erythema, peeling, with excessive use; changes in pigmentation, photosensitivity
*Administration:* apply to clean skin 1–2 times daily

PoM **Retin-A®** (Cilag)

*Cream*, tretinoin 0.025%, net price 60 g = £6.03; 0.05% (cream forte), 60 g = £6.03. For dry or fair skin
*Additives:* butylated hydroxytoluene, sorbic acid

*Gel*, tretinoin 0.01%, net price 60 g = £6.03; 0.025% (gel forte), 60 g = £6.03. For severe acne, initial treatment, or dark and oily skins
*Additives:* butylated hydroxytoluene

*Lotion*, tretinoin 0.025%. Net price 100 mL = £6.94. For application to large areas such as the back
*Additives:* butylated hydroxytoluene

---

ORAL PREPARATIONS

---

## CYPROTERONE ACETATE

*Indications:* see notes above
*Cautions; Contra-indications; Side-effects:* see under Combined Oral Contraceptives (section 7.3.1)

PoM **Dianette®** (Schering Health Care)

*Tablets*, beige, s/c, cyproterone acetate 2 mg, ethinyloestradiol 35 micrograms. Net price 21-tab pack = £4.80

*Dose:* 1 tablet daily for 21 days starting on 5th day of menstrual cycle and repeated after a 7-day interval, usually for several months

## ISOTRETINOIN

*Indications:* see notes above
*Cautions:* exclude pregnancy before starting—pregnancy must be avoided at least 1 month before, during, and for at least 1 month after treatment; avoid donating blood during and for at least 1 month after treatment; monitor hepatic function and plasma lipids at start, 1 month after initiating treatment, then at intervals; avoid high doses of vitamin A and use of keratolytics during treatment; monitor blood glucose in diabetic patients
*Contra-indications:* pregnancy (**important teratogenic risk:** see Cautions and Appendix 4); breast-feeding; renal or hepatic impairment

---

*Side-effects:* (mainly dose-related) dryness of skin (with scaling, thinning, erythema, pruritus), epidermal fragility (trauma may cause blistering); dryness of nasal mucosa (with mild epistaxis), dryness of conjunctiva (sometimes conjunctivitis), decreased tolerance to contact lenses; visual disturbances (papilloedema, optic neuritis, corneal opacities, decreased night vision, blurred vision); hair thinning (reversible on withdrawal); nausea, headache, malaise, drowsiness, sweating; benign intracranial hypertension (avoid concomitant tetracyclines); myalgia and arthralgia; raised liver enzymes; raised plasma triglycerides and cholesterol; allergic vasculitis and granulomatous lesions reported

*Dose:* initially 500 micrograms/kg daily in 1–2 divided doses with food for 4 weeks; if good response continue for further 8–12 weeks; if little response, up to 1 mg/kg daily for 8–12 weeks; if intolerant, reduce dose to 100–200 micrograms/kg daily

PoM **Roaccutane®** (Roche)
*Capsules*, isotretinoin 5 mg (red-violet/white), net price 56-cap pack = £19.08; 20 mg (red-violet/white), 56-cap pack = £54.98 (**hosp. only**, specialist dermatological supervision). Label: 10, patient information card, 21

# 13.7 Preparations for warts and calluses

The least destructive method possible should be chosen to treat these lesions as they are self-limiting and all viral warts including those on the soles of the feet (verrucas) eventually disappear spontaneously. The preparations used are keratolytics which slowly remove the hyperkeratotic layers and destroy the underlying epidermis.

**Salicylic acid** preparations are useful but can cause considerable irritation of the treated area. They are suitable for the removal of *warts and calluses.*

**Podophyllum** preparations may also be useful but again can cause considerable irritation of the treated area and podophyllum treatment may be painful. An ointment containing podophyllum resin with salicylic acid (*Posalfilin®*) is available for treating *plantar warts.* Podophyllum resin made into a paint, in concentrations of between 5 and 20% is employed for the treatment of *anogenital warts.* The paint should be allowed to stay on the treated area for not longer than 6 hours and then washed off. Care should be taken to avoid splashing the surrounding skin during application; it must be covered with soft paraffin as a protection. Where there are a large number of warts only a few should be treated at any one time as **severe toxicity** caused by absorption of podophyllin has been reported. It should also be avoided in pregnancy. Preparations containing **podophyllotoxin** (*Condyline®*, *Warticon®*) are also available for *anogenital warts.*

Preparations containing **formaldehyde**, **glutaraldehyde**, and **bromine** are also available but their effects are unpredictable. Formaldehyde and glutaraldehyde preparations may both irritate and sensitise the skin.

## SALICYLIC ACID

*Cautions:* protect surrounding skin and avoid broken skin; not suitable for application to face, anogenital region, or large areas

*Contra-indications:* diabetes or if peripheral blood circulation impaired

*Side-effects:* skin irritation, see notes above

ADMINISTRATION. Instructions in proprietary packs generally incorporate advice to remove dead skin by gentle rubbing with a pumice stone and to cover with plaster after application (unless in collodion basis)

**Salicylic Acid Collodion, BP,** salicylic acid 12%, in flexible collodion. Label: 15. For warts and calluses, apply daily or on alternate days

**Cuplex®** (S&N Pharm.)
*Gel*, salicylic acid 11%, lactic acid 4%, copper acetate (= $Cu^{2+}$ 0.0011%), in a collodion basis. Net price 5 g = £2.39. Label: 15. For plantar and mosaic warts, corns, and calluses, apply twice daily

**Duofilm®** (Stiefel)
*Paint*, salicylic acid 16.7%, lactic acid 16.7%, in flexible collodion. Net price 15 mL (with applicator) = £1.95. Label: 15. For plantar and mosaic warts, apply daily

**Salactol®** (Dermal)
*Paint*, salicylic acid 16.7%, lactic acid 16.7%, in flexible collodion. Net price 10 mL (with applicator) = £1.98. Label: 15. For warts, particularly plantar warts, verrucas, corns, and calluses, apply daily

**Salatac®** (Dermal)
*Gel*, salicylic acid 12%, lactic acid 4% in a collodion basis. Net price 8 g (with applicator) = £3.45. Label: 15. For warts, verrucas, corns, and calluses, apply daily

**Verrugon®** (Pickles)
*Ointment*, salicylic acid 50% in a paraffin basis. Net price 6 g = £1.25. For plantar warts apply daily

## BROMINE COMPLEXES

*Cautions; Contra-indications; Side-effects:* see under Salicylic Acid

**Callusolve®** (Dermal)
*Paint*, benzalkonium chloride-bromine adduct 25%. Net price 10 mL (with applicator) = £2.44. For warts, particularly plantar and mosaic warts, apply daily

## FORMALDEHYDE

*Cautions; Contra-indications; Side-effects:* see under Salicylic Acid

**Formaldehyde Lotion,** formaldehyde solution, BP, 3 mL, water to 100 mL. For plantar warts, applied at night as a soak

---

**Veracur®** (Typharm)
*Gel*, formaldehyde solution 1.5% in a water-miscible gel basis. Net price 15 g = £1.15. For warts, particularly plantar warts, apply twice daily

With salicylic acid
**Posalfilin®** (Norgine)
*Ointment*, podophyllum resin 20%, salicylic acid 25%. Net price 10 g = £3.20. For plantar warts only, apply 2–3 times weekly
*Note.* Not suitable for anogenital warts

## GLUTARALDEHYDE
*Cautions; Contra-indications; Side-effects:* see under Salicylic Acid, stains skin brown

**Glutarol®** (Dermal)
*Solution* (= application), glutaraldehyde 10%. Net price 10 mL (with applicator) = £2.25. For warts, particularly plantar warts, apply twice daily
**Novaruca®** (Bioglan)
*Gel*, glutaraldehyde 10%. Net price 15 g = £1.95. For warts, particularly plantar warts, apply twice daily
**Verucasep®** (Galen)
*Gel*, glutaraldehyde 10%. Net price 15 g = £1.95. For warts, particularly plantar warts, apply twice daily

## PODOPHYLLUM RESIN
*Cautions:* avoid normal skin and open wounds; keep away from face; very irritant to eyes; **important:** see also notes above
*Contra-indications:* pregnancy
*Side-effects:* may cause pain on application; see also notes above

PoM **Podophyllin Paint, Compound, BP,** (podophyllum resin 15% in compound benzoin tincture), podophyllum resin 1.5 g, compound benzoin tincture to 10 mL; 5 mL to be dispensed unless otherwise directed. Label: 15, counselling, application, see notes above. External anogenital warts, applied weekly in genitourinary clinic (**important cautions**, see notes above)

Podophyllotoxin
PoM **Condyline®** (Brocades)
*Solution*, podophyllotoxin 0.5% in alcoholic basis. Net price 3.5 mL (with applicators) = £16.00. Label: 15
External anogenital warts (condylomata acuminata), apply twice daily for 3 days; treatment may be repeated after 7 days if necessary; max. 5 treatment courses; direct medical supervision for lesions in the female and for lesions greater than 4 cm$^2$ in the male
PoM **Warticon®** (Kabi Pharmacia)
*Solution*, podophyllotoxin 0.5% in alcoholic basis. Net price 3 mL (with applicators) = £16.00. Label: 15
Penile warts in preputial space (condylomata acuminata), apply twice daily for 3 days; treatment may be repeated after 7 days if necessary; max. 5 treatment courses; direct medical supervision for lesions greater than 4 cm$^2$

## CRYOTHERAPY

**Histofreezer®** (Thames, direct mail), an aerosol kit consisting of ether (diethyl ether) and propane, is available as an alternative to liquid nitrogen for cryotherapy of warts. The kit includes 40 cotton bud applicators and a detailed instruction booklet. It is not available on the NHS but a claim can be made for removal of warts as a minor surgical procedure.

# 13.8  Sunscreens and camouflagers

BORDERLINE SUBSTANCES. The preparations marked 'ACBS' are regarded as drugs when prescribed for skin protection against ultraviolet radiation in photodermatoses, including those resulting from radiotherapy. Prescriptions issued in accordance with this advice and endorsed 'ACBS' will normally not be investigated. See Appendix 7 for listing by clinical condition.

## 13.8.1  Sunscreening preparations
Solar ultraviolet irradiation is harmful to the skin. It is responsible for disorders such as polymorphic light eruption, Hutchinson's summer prurigo, and the various cutaneous porphyrias. It also provokes (or at least aggravates) disorders such as rosacea and lupus erythematosus. It may also contribute to serious skin disorders in patients sensitised by drugs such as demeclocycline, phenothiazines, or amiodarone. All these conditions (as well as sunburn) may occur after relatively short periods of exposure to the sun. Exposure over longer periods may cause more serious problems. Both melanoma and non-melanoma skin cancer are now thought to be caused in many instances by solar ultraviolet irradiation. It is now also believed that exposure to the sun causes the skin to wrinkle and develop other signs associated with aging.

Solar ultraviolet radiation is approximately 200–400 nm in wavelength. The medium wavelengths (280–310 nm, known as UVB) cause sunburn and contribute to the long-term changes responsible for skin cancer and aging. The long wavelengths (310–400 nm, known as UVA) do not cause sunburn but are responsible for many photosensitivity reactions and photodermatoses; they also seem to contribute to long-term damage and to be involved in the pathogenesis of skin cancer and aging.

Sunscreen preparations that contain substances such as aminobenzoic acid protect the skin against UVB and hence against sunburn. The sun protection factor (SPF, usually indicated in the preparation title) provides guidance on the degree of protection offered against UVB; it indicates the multiples of protection provided against burning, compared with unprotected skin; for example, an SPF of 8 should enable a person to remain 8 times longer in the sun without burning. Such preparations, however, do not prevent long-term damage associated with UVA, which might not become apparent for 10 to 20 years. Preparations that also contain reflective substances, such as titanium dioxide, provide the most effective protection against UVA.

Some sunscreens, particularly aminobenzoates, may rarely cause photosensitivity reactions. Bergamot oil (which contains 5-methoxypsoralen) occasionally causes photosensitisation with subsequent pigmentation; it is suspected of increasing the incidence of skin cancers, but this has not been established.

## Almay Total Sunbloc® (Sara Lee)
*Cream*, (SPF 15), padimate-O 7%, oxybenzone 3%, titanium dioxide. Net price 50 mL = £2.41. ACBS
*Additives:* disodium edetate, hydroxybenzoates (parabens), propylene glycol
*Lip protector*, (SPF 15), padimate-O 7%, oxybenzone 3%. Net price 10 mL = £1.42. ACBS
*Additives:* butylated hydroxyanisole, hydroxybenzoates (parabens), propylene glycol

## Ambre Solaire® (Garnier)
*Additives:* butylated hydroxytoluene, edetic acid (EDTA), hydroxybenzoates (parabens), wool fat, fragrance
*High Protection Cream*, (SPF 10), water resistant, butyl methoxydibenzoylmethane 1%, benzylidene camphor 0.5%, phenylbenzimidazolesulphonic acid 0.5%, titanium dioxide 2%. Net price 100 mL = £4.38. ACBS
*High Protection Milk*, (SPF 12), water resistant, butyl methoxydibenzoylmethane 1%, benzylidene camphor 1%, phenylbenzimidazolesulphonic acid 0.5%, titanium dioxide 2%. Net price 200 mL = £4.91. ACBS
*Maximum Protection Cream*, (SPF 25), water resistant, butyl methoxydibenzoylmethane 1.5%, benzylidene camphor 3%, phenylbenzimidazolesulphonic acid 3%, titanium dioxide 4%. Net price 100 mL = £4.84. ACBS

## Coppertone® (Scholl)
*Sunstick 15*, titanium dioxide 17.6% in wax-based stick. Net price 6 g = £2.46. ACBS
*Additives:* butylated hydroxytoluene, hydroxybenzoates (parabens), wool fat, fragrance
*Supershade 15 lotion*, padimate-O 7%, oxybenzone 3%. Net price 125 mL = £4.21. ACBS
*Additives:* wool fat, fragrance
*Ultrashade 23 lotion*, ethylhexyl p-methoxycinnamate 7.5%, oxybenzone 3%, padimate-O 2.5%. Net price 150 mL = £4.53. ACBS
*Additives:* hydroxybenzoates (parabens), wool fat, fragrance

## Piz Buin® (Ciba Consumer)
*Additives:* hydroxybenzoates (parabens), propylene glycol, fragrance
*Cream No. 12*, ethylhexyl p-methoxycinnamate 7%, butyl methoxydibenzoylmethane 1.5%,

titanium dioxide 1.5%. Net price 30 mL = £3.11. ACBS
*Lotion*, (SPF 12), ethylhexyl p-methoxycinnamate 7.5%, butyl methoxydibenzoylmethane 1.5%, titanium dioxide 1.5%. Net price 125 mL = £5.03. ACBS
*Sun allergy lotion*, (SPF 12), ethylhexyl p-methoxycinnamate 7.5%, butyl methoxydibenzoylmethane 2.5%, titanium dioxide 2%. Net price 125 mL = £5.91. ACBS
*Sunblock lotion*, (SPF 24), ethylhexyl p-methoxycinnamate 7.5%, butyl methoxydibenzoylmethane 2%, titanium dioxide 3%. Net price 125 mL = £5.91. ACBS

## RoC® (RoC)
*Total sunblock cream*, (SPF over 15), colourless or tinted, ethylhexyl p-methoxycinnamate 5%, oxybenzone 4%, dibenzoylmethane 2%, titanium dioxide 4%. Net price 50 mL = £3.57. ACBS
*Additives:* beeswax, hydroxybenzoates (parabens)
*Sunscreen stick*, (SPF 10–15), cinnamic ester 7.5%, dibenzoylmethane 4%. Net price 3-g stick = £2.00. ACBS
*Additives:* none as listed in section 13.1

## Spectraban® (Stiefel)
*Lotion*, (SPF 10), ethylhexyl p-methoxycinnamate 5%, oxybenzone 5%. Net price 150 mL = £2.98. ACBS
*Additives:* propylene glycol
*Lotion*, (SPF 15) aminobenzoic acid 5%, padimate-O 3.2%, in an alcoholic basis. Net price 150 mL = £2.49. ACBS
*Additives:* fragrance
*Caution:* flammable; stains clothing
*Ultra lotion*, (SPF 17), water resistant, butyl methoxydibenzoylmethane 2%, oxybenzone 3%, padimate-O 8%, titanium dioxide 2%. Net price 150 mL = £4.32. ACBS
*Additives:* benzyl alcohol, disodium edetate, sorbic acid, fragrance

## Sun E45® (Crookes)
*Sunblock cream*, (SPF 25), water resistant, titanium dioxide 18%. Net price 75 mL = £4.30. ACBS.
*Additives:* butylated hydroxytoluene, isopropyl palmitate
*Ultra protection lotion*, (SPF 15), water resistant, titanium dioxide 13.4%. Net price 150 mL = £5.40. ACBS
*Additives:* butylated hydroxytoluene, isopropyl palmitate

## Uvistat® (Windsor)
*Cream*, (SPF 8), water-resistant, mexenone 4%, ethylhexyl p-methoxycinnamate 7.5%. Net price 100 g = £3.30. ACBS
*Additives:* hydroxybenzoates (parabens), fragrance
*Cream*, (SPF 10), mexenone 2%, ethylhexyl p-methoxycinnamate 7%, butyl methoxydibenzoylmethane 2%, titanium dioxide 2%. Net price 100 g = £3.70. ACBS
*Additives:* hydroxybenzoates (parabens), fragrance
*Cream* (SPF 15), water-resistant, mexenone 4%, ethylhexyl p-methoxycinnamate 7.5%, butyl methoxydibenzoylmethane 2%. Net price 100 g = £3.88. ACBS
*Additives:* Hydroxybenzoates (parabens), fragrance
*Lipscreen*, (SPF 15), mexenone 2%, ethylhexyl p-methoxycinnamate 6%, butyl methoxydibenzoylmethane 2%. Net price 5-g stick = £1.15.

ACBS (also sunlight-provoked chronic or recurrent herpes labialis)
*Additives:* fragrance

*Cream* (SPF 20), water-resistant, ethylhexyl *p*-methoxycinnamate 7%, mexenone 2%, butyl methoxydibenzoylmethane 2%, titanium dioxide 4.5%. Net price 50 g = £2.89, 100 g = £4.34. ACBS
*Additives:* hydroxybenzoates (parabens), fragrance

*Ultrablock cream*, (SPF 30), mexenone 2%, ethylhexyl *p*-methoxycinnamate 7.5%, butyl methoxydibenzoylmethane 4%, titanium dioxide 6%. Net price 50 g = £3.47. ACBS
*Additives:* hydroxybenzoates (parabens), fragrance

## 13.8.2 Camouflagers

Disfigurement of the skin can be very distressing to patients and have a marked psychological effect. In skilled hands, or with experience, these preparations can be very effective in concealing scars, areas of discoloration, and birthmarks.

**Boots Covering Cream®** (Boots)
*Cream* (4 shades). 20 g. ACBS
*Additives:* hydroxybenzoates (parabens)

**Covermark®** (Stiefel)
*Additives:* beeswax, hydroxybenzoates (parabens), fragrance
*Cream rouge*, (3 shades). Net price 4.5 g = £2.96. ACBS
*Grey toner* (= cream). Net price 8 g = £2.96. ACBS
*Masking cream* (covering cream, 10 shades). Net price 25 g = £4.35. ACBS
*Shading cream*. Net price 4.5 g = £2.96. ACBS
*Finishing powder*. Net price 50 g = £2.62; 250 g = £9.37. ACBS

**Dermablend®** (DDC)
*Cover creme*, (10 shades). Net price 10.7 g = £5.95; 28.4 g = £10.22. ACBS
*Additives:* beeswax, hydroxybenzoates (parabens)
*Leg cover*, (6 shades). Net price 64 g = £8.85. ACBS
*Additives:* beeswax, hydroxybenzoates (parabens)
*Setting powder*. Net price 28 g = £8.23. ACBS
*Additives:* hydroxybenzoates (parabens)

**Dermacolor®** (Fox)
*Camouflage creme*, (30 shades). Net price 30 g = £5.80. ACBS
*Additives:* beeswax, wool fat, fragrance
*Fixing powder*, (5 shades). Net price 75 g = £4.64. ACBS
*Additives:* fragrance

**Keromask®** (Network management)
*Masking cream*, (2 shades). Net price 15 mL = £3.56. ACBS
*Additives:* butylated hydroxyanisole, hydroxybenzoates (parabens), wool fat
*Finishing powder*. Net price 25 g = £3.56. ACBS
*Additives:* none as listed in section 13.1

**Veil®** (Blake)
*Cover cream*, (19 shades). Net price 19 g = £3.41; 44 g = £4.82; 70 g = £6.53. ACBS
*Additives:* hydroxybenzoates (parabens), wool fat derivative
*Finishing powder*, translucent. Net price 35 g = £3.41. ACBS
*Additives:* butylated hydroxyanisole, hydroxybenzoates (parabens)

# 13.9 Shampoos and some other scalp preparations

> BORDERLINE SUBSTANCES. The preparations marked 'ACBS' are regarded as drugs when prescribed in accordance with the advice of the Advisory Committee on Borderline Substances for the clinical conditions listed. Prescriptions issued in accordance with this advice and endorsed 'ACBS' will normally not be investigated. See Appendix 7 for listing by clinical condition.

*Dandruff (pityriasis capitis)* is believed to be caused by follicular overgrowth with pityrosporum yeasts; it often increases at puberty. The treatment of choice is the frequent use of a mild detergent shampoo generally once or twice weekly; this rids the scalp of scale but does not have a therapeutic effect in itself. Shampoos containing antimicrobial agents such as **pyrithione zinc** have beneficial effects and are on sale to the general public. Shampoos containing **tar** extracts may be useful and they are also used in *psoriasis*, both as adjunctive treatment and for the removal of pastes etc. Shampoos containing **selenium sulphide** are of no more value than the other shampoos and should not be used within 48 hours of applying hair colouring or permanent waving preparations. **Ketoconazole** is also useful as a shampoo (see section 13.10.2) and **lithium succinate** has been shown to be effective in shampoo form.

For more severe conditions, weak **corticosteroid** gels and lotions (section 13.4), applied to the scalp may be helpful.

*Cradle cap* in infants may be treated with **olive oil** or **arachis oil** applications before shampooing.

See also sections 13.5 (psoriasis and eczema), 13.10.4 (lice), and 13.10.2 (ringworm).

ADMINISTRATION. Shampoos should be used once or twice weekly

**Alphosyl®** (Stafford-Miller)
*Shampoo*, allantoin 0.2%, refined coal tar extract 5%. Net price 125 mL = £1.30; 250 mL = £2.41. ACBS: for psoriasis and other scaly disorders of the scalp
*Additives:* hydroxybenzoates (parabens), fragrance

**Baltar®** (Merck)
*Shampoo*, coal tar distillate 1.5% in soap-free basis. Net price 225 mL = £2.63; 500 mL = £4.60
*Additives:* fragrance

**Betadine®** (Napp)
*Scalp and skin cleanser*—section 13.11.4
*Shampoo solution*, povidone-iodine 4%, in a surfactant solution. Net price 250 mL = £1.74. ACBS: for seborrhoeic scalp conditions associated with excessive dandruff, pruritic scaling, seborrhoeic dermatitis, pityriasis capitis, infected lesions of the scalp, pyodermas (recurrent furunculosis, infective folliculitis, impetigo)
*Additives:* wool fat, fragrance

**Calmurid®** (Kabi Pharmacia)
*Solution*, urea 20%, lactic acid 5%, in an aqueous vehicle. Net price 125 mL = £4.10
*Additives:* polysorbate 20
Apply twice daily to scalp

**Capasal®** (Dermal)
*Shampoo*, coal tar 1%, coconut oil 1%, salicylic acid 0.5%. Net price 250 mL = £4.95
*Additives:* none as listed in section 13.1

**Capitol®** (Dermal)
*Gel*, benzalkonium chloride 0.5%. Net price 120 g = £3.13. ACBS: for pityriasis capitis and seborrhoeic dermatitis of the scalp
*Additives:* none as listed in section 13.1

**Ceanel Concentrate®** (Quinoderm Ltd)
*Shampoo*, cetrimide 10%, undecenoic acid 1%, phenethyl alcohol 7.5%. Net price 50 mL = 98p; 150 mL = £2.60; 500 mL = £7.70. ACBS: for psoriasis or seborrhoeic conditions
*Additives:* none as listed in section 13.1

**Clinitar®** (Shire)
*Shampoo solution*, coal tar extract 2%. Net price 60 g = £2.47
*Additives:* polysorbate, fragrance

PoM **Efalith®** (Scotia)
*Ointment*, lithium succinate 8%, zinc sulphate 0.05%. Net price 20 g = £12.50
*Additives:* wool fat derivative
*Cautions:* psoriasis
Seborrhoeic dermatitis, apply thinly twice daily initially, then reduce

**Gelcotar®** (Quinoderm Ltd)
*Liquid*, strong coal tar solution 1.25%, cade oil 0.5%, in a shampoo basis. Net price 150 mL = £1.33; 350 mL = £2.66. ACBS: for psoriasis of the scalp, seborrhoeic dermatitis, and dandruff
*Additives:* chlorocresol, fragrance
*Gel*, see section 13.5

**Genisol®** (Fisons)
*Liquid*, prepared coal tar 2% (as purified coal tar fractions), sodium sulphosuccinated undecylenic monoalkylolamide 1%. Net price 58 mL = £1.22; 250 mL = £3.98; 600 mL = £8.29. ACBS: for psoriasis, eczema, and scaling of the scalp (psoriasis, dandruff, or eczema)
*Additives:* fragrance

**Ionil T®** (Galderma)
*Shampoo application*, benzalkonium chloride 0.2%, coal tar solution 5%, salicylic acid 2% in an alcoholic basis. Net price 200 mL = £2.56. ACBS: for seborrhoeic dermatitis of the scalp
*Additives:* tetrasodium edetate

**Lenium®** (Janssen)
*Cream*, selenium sulphide 2.5%. Net price 42 g = 88p; 100 g = £1.50
*Additives:* fragrance

PoM **Nizoral®** shampoo—section 13.10.2

**Polytar®** (Stiefel)
*Liquid*, arachis oil extract of crude coal tar 0.3%, cade oil 0.3%, coal tar solution 0.3%, oleyl alcohol 1%, tar 0.3%. Net price 65 mL = 91p; 150 mL = £1.34; 350 mL = £2.37. ACBS: for psoriasis, eczema, and scaling of the scalp (psoriasis, dandruff, and eczema)
*Additives:* polysorbate 80, fragrance

**Polytar Plus®** (Stiefel)
*Liquid*, ingredients as above with hydrolysed animal protein 3%. Net price 350 mL = £3.29. ACBS: for scalp disorders such as scaling (psoriasis, dandruff, eczema), pruritus, and in the removal of pastes and pomades used in psoriasis
*Additives:* fragrance

**Pragmatar®**—section 13.5

**Psoriderm®** (Dermal)
*Scalp lotion* (= shampoo), coal tar 2.5%, lecithin 0.3%. Net price 250 mL = £4.97
*Additives:* disodium edetate

**Selsun®** (Abbott)
*Shampoo application*, selenium sulphide 2.5%. Net price 50 mL = 92p; 100 mL = £1.40; 150 mL = £1.91
*Additives:* fragrance

**Synogist®** (Townendale)
*Shampoo solution*, sodium sulphosuccinated undecylenic monoalkylolamide 2%. Net price 200 mL = £12.98
*Additives:* hydroxybenzoates (parabens)

**T/Gel®** (Neutrogena)
*Shampoo*, coal tar extract 2%. Net price 125 mL = £2.13. ACBS: for psoriasis, eczema, and scaling of the scalp (psoriasis, dandruff, and eczema)
*Additives:* hydroxybenzoates (parabens), tetrasodium edetate, fragrance

---

## MALE-PATTERN BALDNESS

Topical application of minoxidil may stimulate limited hair growth in a small proportion of patients but only for as long as it is used

### MINOXIDIL

*Indications:* male-pattern baldness (men and women)
*Cautions; Contra-indications; Side-effects:* see section 2.5.1 (about 1.4% absorbed); local side-effects: itching, dermatitis

NHS PoM **Regaine®** (Upjohn)
*Topical solution*, minoxidil 2% in an aqueous alcoholic basis. Net price 60-mL bottle = £20.00
*Additives:* propylene glycol
*Cautions:* flammable; wash hands after application
*Note.* The Royal Pharmaceutical Society's Law Department has reminded pharmacists that neither the safety nor the stability of mixtures of Minoxidil lotion with other products has been established, and that this fact should be drawn to the prescriber's attention before any such mixture is dispensed.

# 13.10 Anti-infective skin preparations

13.10.1 Antibacterial preparations
13.10.2 Antifungal preparations
13.10.3 Antiviral preparations
13.10.4 Parasiticidal preparations
13.10.5 Preparations for minor skin infections

---

   

## 13.10.1   Antibacterial preparations

For many skin infections such as *erysipelas* and *cellulitis* systemic antibacterial treatment is the method of choice because the infection is too deeply sited for adequate penetration of topical preparations. For details of suitable treatment see section 5.1, table 1.

*Impetigo* may be treated by local application with **chlortetracycline** or, if there is systemic toxicity, with oral administration of **flucloxacillin** or **erythromycin** (see section 5.1, table 1). Mild antiseptics such as **povidone-iodine** (section 13.11.4) are used to remove crusts and exudate.

Although there are a great many antibacterial drugs presented in topical preparations they are potentially hazardous and frequently their use is not necessary if adequate hygienic measures can be taken. Moreover not all skin conditions that are oozing, crusted, or characterised by pustules are actually infected.

To minimise the development of resistant organisms it is advisable to limit the choice of drugs applied topically to those not used systemically. Unfortunately some of these drugs, for example neomycin, may cause sensitisation and, if large areas of skin are being treated, ototoxicity may be a hazard, particularly in children and the elderly. Resistant organisms are more common in hospitals, and whenever possible swabs for examination should be taken before beginning treatment.

**Mupirocin** is not related to any other antibiotic in use. Its use should be restricted as it is particularly useful when there is resistant infection.

**Silver sulphadiazine** is used in the treatment of infected burns.

### 13.10.1.1   ANTIBACTERIAL PREPARATIONS ONLY USED TOPICALLY

### FRAMYCETIN SULPHATE
*Indications; Cautions; Side-effects:* see under Neomycin Sulphate
*Administration:* apply 3 times daily

PoM **Soframycin®** (Roussel)
*Cream*, framycetin sulphate 1.5%, gramicidin 0.005%, in a vanishing-cream basis. Net price 15 g = £1.72
*Additives:* hydroxybenzoates (parabens)
*Ointment*, ingredients as for cream, in a wool fat and paraffin basis. Net price 15 g = £1.72
*Additives:* wool fat
*Sterile powder* for preparing topical solutions, framycetin sulphate. Net price 500-mg vial = £3.85
**Sofra-Tulle®** *see* Framycetin Gauze Dressing, section 13.13.6

### MUPIROCIN
*Indications:* bacterial skin infections
*Cautions:* see below
*Administration:* apply up to 3 times daily for up to 10 days

PoM **Bactroban®** (Beecham)
*Ointment*, mupirocin 2%, in a water-miscible macrogol basis. Net price 15 g = £4.08
*Additives:* none as listed in section 13.1
Note. Contains macrogol therefore caution in renal impairment; may sting
*Nasal ointment*, see section 12.2.3

### NEOMYCIN SULPHATE
*Indications:* skin infections
*Cautions:* see notes above; large open wounds, sensitivity to other aminoglycosides
*Side-effects:* local hypersensitivity reactions

Creams and ointments
PoM **Neomycin Cream, BPC**, neomycin sulphate 0.5%, cetomacrogol emulsifying ointment 30%, chlorocresol 0.1%, disodium edetate 0.01%, in freshly boiled and cooled purified water. Net price 15 g = 52p
Apply up to 3 times daily; max. 60 g daily for 3 weeks; do not repeat for at least 3 months
PoM **Cicatrin®** (Wellcome)
*Cream*, neomycin sulphate 3300 units, bacitracin zinc 250 units, cysteine 2 mg, glycine 10 mg, threonine 1 mg/g. Net price 15 g = £4.52; 30 g = £8.22
*Additives:* wool fat derivative
Apply up to 3 times daily; max. 60 g daily for 3 weeks; do not repeat for at least 3 months
PoM **Graneodin®** (Squibb)
*Ointment*, neomycin sulphate 0.25%, gramicidin 0.025%. Net price 25 g = £1.47
*Additives:* none as listed in section 13.1
Apply 2–4 times daily

Powders and sprays
PoM **Cicatrin®** (Wellcome)
*Dusting powder*, neomycin sulphate 3300 units, bacitracin zinc 250 units, cysteine 2 mg, glycine 10 mg, threonine 1 mg/g. Net price 15 g = £4.87; 50 g = £12.31. Max. 50 g daily for 4 weeks; do not repeat for at least 3 months
*Additives:* none as listed in section 13.1
*Powder spray*, neomycin sulphate 16500 units, bacitracin zinc 1250 units, cysteine 12 mg, glycine 60 mg/g; pressurised aerosol unit. Net price 3 g = £11.74. Max. 3 g daily for 12 weeks; do not repeat for at least 3 months
*Additives:* none as listed in section 13.1
PoM **Polybactrin®** (Wellcome)
*Powder spray*, neomycin sulphate 495000 units, bacitracin zinc 37500 units, polymyxin B sulphate 150000 units/pressurised aerosol unit. Net price per unit (115 mL) = £21.51. Max. 1 unit daily for 7 days; do not repeat for at least 3 months
*Additives:* none as listed in section 13.1
PoM **Tribiotic®** (3M)
*Spray application*, neomycin sulphate 500000 units, bacitracin zinc 10000 units, polymyxin B sulphate 150000 units/pressurised aerosol unit. Net price per unit (110 g) = £5.72. Max. 1 unit daily for 7 days; do not repeat for at least 3 months
*Additives:* none as listed in section 13.1

## POLYMYXINS

(Includes colistin sulphate and polymyxin B sulphate)
*Indications:* skin infections
*Cautions:* see notes above; large open wounds
*Side-effects:* transient irritation; local hyper-
sensitivity reactions

PoM **Polyfax**® (Cusi)
*Ointment*, polymyxin B sulphate 10 000 units,
bacitracin zinc 500 units/g, in a paraffin basis.
Net price 20 g = £8.95
Apply 3 times daily
PoM **Colomycin**® (Pharmax)
*Powder*, sterile, for making topical preparations
(usually 1%), colistin sulphate. Net price 1 g
vial = £18.79

## SILVER SULPHADIAZINE

*Indications:* skin infection, particularly Gram-
negative infections such as pseudomonal infections in second- and third-degree burns,
infected leg ulcers, and pressure sores
*Cautions:* hepatic and renal impairment
*Contra-indications:* sensitivity to sulphonamides
*Side-effects:* rarely allergic reactions including
rashes

PoM **Flamazine**® (S&N Pharm.)
*Cream*, silver sulphadiazine 1%, in a water-
soluble basis. Net price 50 g = £4.41; 250 g =
£11.82; 500 g = £20.92
*Additives:* polysorbates, propylene glycol
In burns apply daily with sterile applicator; in
leg ulcers apply at least 3 times a week

13.10.1.2  ANTIBACTERIAL
PREPARATIONS ALSO USED
SYSTEMICALLY

## CHLORTETRACYCLINE
## HYDROCHLORIDE

*Indications:*  susceptible  skin  infections;
impetigo, see section 5.1, Table 1
*Cautions:* see notes above; overgrowth with non-
susceptible organisms; stains clothing
*Side-effects:* rarely local hypersensitivity reactions
*Administration:* apply 1 to 3 times daily

PoM **Aureomycin**® (Lederle)
*Cream*, chlortetracycline hydrochloride 3% (as
chlortetracycline), in a water-miscible basis.
Net price 30 g = £1.82
*Additives:* chlorocresol
*Ointment*, chlortetracycline hydrochloride 3%,
in a greasy basis. Net price 30 g = £1.82
*Additives:* hydroxybenzoates (parabens), wool fat

## FUSIDIC ACID

*Indications:* staphylococcal skin infections and
abscesses
*Cautions:* see notes above; avoid contact with
eyes
*Side-effects:* rarely local hypersensitivity reactions
*Administration:* apply 3 times daily

PoM **Fucidin**® (Leo)
*Cream*, fusidic acid 2%. Net price 15 g = £2.94;
30 g = £4.96
*Additives:* butylated hydroxyanisole
*Gel*, fusidic acid 2%, in a water-miscible basis.
Net price 15 g = £2.54; 30 g = £4.40
*Additives:* hydroxybenzoates (parabens), polysorbate 80
*Caviject gel*, fusidic acid 2%, in a single-dose
unit (7 g) fitted with elongated nozzle. For treat-
ment of abscesses. Net price 1 unit = £1.49
Inject once only into curetted abscess and apply
dressing
*Ointment*, sodium fusidate 2%, in an anhydrous
greasy basis. Net price 15 g = £2.40; 30 g =
£4.07
*Additives:* wool fat
PoM **Fucidin Intertulle**® *see* section 13.13.6

## GENTAMICIN

*Indications:* skin infections
*Cautions:* see notes above; large open wounds,
sensitivity to other aminoglycosides
*Administration:* apply 3 times daily

PoM **Cidomycin Topical**® (Roussel)
*Cream*, gentamicin 0.3% (as sulphate), in a
water-miscible basis. Do not dilute. Net price
15 g = £1.75; 30 g = £3.40
*Additives:* hydroxybenzoates (parabens), propylene glycol
*Ointment*, gentamicin 0.3% (as sulphate), in a
paraffin basis. Do not dilute. Net price 15 g =
£1.75; 30 g = £3.40
*Additives:* none as listed in section 13.1
PoM **Genticin**® (Nicholas)
*Cream*, gentamicin 0.3% (as sulphate), in
a water-miscible basis. Net price 15 g = £1.37;
100 g = £9.15
*Additives:* hydroxybenzoates (parabens)
*Ointment*, gentamicin 0.3% (as sulphate), in
an anhydrous greasy basis. Net price 15 g =
£1.37; 100 g = £9.15
*Additives:* hydroxybenzoates (parabens)

## METRONIDAZOLE

*Indications:* de-odourisation of fungating malodorous tumours
*Administration:* apply to clean wound 1 to 2 times
daily and cover (flat wounds, apply liberally;
cavities, smear on paraffin gauze and pack
loosely); use tube once only

PoM **Metrotop**® (Farmitalia Carlo Erba)
*Gel*, metronidazole 0.8% in aqueous basis. Net
price 30 g = £6.95
*Additives:* none as listed in section 13.1

## TETRACYCLINE HYDROCHLORIDE

*Indications; Cautions; Side-effects:* see under
Chlortetracycline Hydrochloride

PoM **Achromycin Topical**® (Lederle)
*Ointment*, tetracycline hydrochloride 3%, in a
wool fat and paraffin basis. Net price 30 g =
£1.48
*Additives:* hydroxybenzoates (parabens), wool fat
Apply 1–3 times daily

## 13.10.2   Antifungal preparations

Ideally skin scrapings should be examined to confirm diagnosis before treatment is begun. Widespread or intractable fungal infections are treated systemically (see section 5.2). Most localised infections are treated with the topical preparations described below.

Nail ringworm (tinea unguium) and scalp ringworm (*T. capitis*) are best treated systemically (see section 5.2). Most other ringworm infections, including tinea pedis, may be adequately treated with topical preparations. The imidazoles **clotrimazole**, **econazole**, and **miconazole** are all effective and commonly used. **Sulconazole** is a recently introduced imidazole with similar properties. Combinations of imidazoles and weak corticosteroids may be of use in the treatment of some eczematous disorders and, in the first few days only, of a severely inflamed patch of ringworm. **Compound benzoic acid ointment** (Whitfield's ointment) is also quite effective but cosmetically less acceptable than the proprietary preparations. It is generally used to treat patches of ringworm (tinea) on the trunk, limbs, palms, or soles. The **undecenoates** and **tolnaftate** are less effective in treating ringworm infections.

Candidal skin infections may also be treated by topical application with the broad-spectrum antifungals, clotrimazole, econazole, and miconazole. **Nystatin** preparations are also equally as effective in candidiasis although they are ineffective against infections due to dermatophyte fungi (tinea).

Lotions are generally chosen for application to large and hairy areas. Ointments are best avoided on moist surfaces because of their occlusive properties. Dusting-powders have no place in the treatment of fungal infections, except for toiletry or cosmetic purposes, as they are therapeutically ineffective and may cause skin irritation.

## AMOROLFINE

*Indications:* see under preparations
*Cautions:* pregnancy, breast-feeding; avoid eyes, ears, and mucous membranes
*Side-effects:* occasional transient burning sensation, erythema, pruritus

▼ PoM **Loceryl**® (Roche)
*Cream*, amorolfine (as hydrochloride) 0.25%. Net price 20 g = £4.95. Label: 10 patient information leaflet
   *Administration:* fungal skin infections, apply once daily after cleansing in the evening for at least 2–3 weeks (up to 6 weeks for foot mycoses)
*Nail lacquer*, amorolfine (as hydrochloride) 5%. Net price 5-mL pack (with nail files, spatulas and cleansing swabs) = £34.38. Label: 10 patient information leaflet
   *Administration:* fungal nail infections, apply to infected nails 1–2 times weekly after filing and cleansing; allow to dry (approx. 3 minutes); treat finger nails for 6 months, toe nails for 9–12 months (review at intervals of 3 months)

## BENZOIC ACID

*Indications:* ringworm (tinea)

**Benzoic Acid Ointment, Compound, BP** (Whitfield's ointment), benzoic acid 6%, salicylic acid 3%, in emulsifying ointment. Net price 25 g = 15p
Apply twice daily

## BENZOYL PEROXIDE

*Indications:* fungal skin infections, particularly tinea pedis

**Quinoped**® (Quinoderm Ltd)
*Cream*, benzoyl peroxide 5%, potassium hydroxyquinoline sulphate 0.5%, in an astringent basis. Net price 25 g = 92p
   *Additives:* edetic acid (EDTA)
Apply twice daily

## CLOTRIMAZOLE

*Indications:* fungal skin infections
*Side-effects:* occasional skin irritation or sensitivity
*Administration:* apply 2–3 times daily continuing for 14 days after lesions have healed

**Canesten**® (Baypharm)
*Cream*, clotrimazole 1%, in a water-miscible basis. Net price 20 g = £1.82; 50 g = £4.26
   *Additives:* benzyl alcohol, polysorbate 60
*Solution*, clotrimazole 1% in macrogol 400. Net price 20 mL = £2.38. For hairy areas
   *Additives:* none as listed in section 13.1
*Spray*, clotrimazole 1%, in 30% isopropyl alcohol. Net price 40-mL atomiser = £5.12. Label: 15. For large or hairy areas
   *Additives:* propylene glycol
*Dusting-powder*, clotrimazole 1%. Net price 30 g = £1.56
   *Additives:* none as listed in section 13.1

## ECONAZOLE NITRATE

*Indications; Side-effects:* see under Clotrimazole
*Administration:* apply 2–3 times daily continuing for 14 days after lesions have healed; nail infections, apply daily under occlusive dressing

**Ecostatin**® (Squibb)
*Cream*, econazole nitrate 1%, in a water-miscible basis. Net price 15 g = £1.49; 30 g = £2.75
   *Additives:* butylated hydroxyanisole, fragrance
*Lotion*, econazole nitrate 1%. Net price 30 mL = £2.75
   *Additives:* butylated hydroxyanisole, fragrance
*Spray solution*, econazole nitrate 1% in an alcoholic solution. Net price 150 g = £3.48. Label: 15
   *Additives:* propylene glycol, fragrance
*Dusting-powder*, econazole nitrate 1% in a talc basis. Net price 30 g = £2.90
   *Additives:* fragrance
*Spray-powder*, econazole nitrate 1% in a talc basis. Net price 200-g unit = £2.64
   *Additives:* fragrance

**Pevaryl**® (Cilag)

*Cream*, econazole nitrate 1% in a water-miscible
basis. Net price 30 g = £2.65
*Additives:* butylated hydroxyanisole, fragrance

*Lotion*, econazole nitrate 1% in a water-miscible
basis. Net price 30 mL = £3.33
*Additives:* butylated hydroxyanisole, fragrance

*Spray-powder*, econazole nitrate 1%. Net price
200-g pressurised aerosol unit (20 g
powder) = £3.33
*Additives:* fragrance

## KETOCONAZOLE

*Indications; Side-effects:* see under Clotrimazole

PoM **Nizoral**® (Janssen)

*Cream*, ketoconazole 2% in a water-miscible
basis. Net price 30 g = £3.81
*Additives:* polysorbates, propylene glycol

Apply 1–2 times daily, continuing for a few days
after lesions have healed

*Shampoo*, ketoconazole 2%. Net price 100 mL =
£8.75
*Additives:* fragrance

For seborrhoeic dermatitis and dandruff apply
twice weekly for 2–4 weeks, for pityriasis versicolor once daily for max. 5 days; avoid for 2
weeks following topical corticosteroid treatment

## MICONAZOLE NITRATE

*Indications; Side-effects:* see under Clotrimazole
*Administration:* apply twice daily continuing for
10 days after lesions have healed; nail infections, apply daily under occlusive dressing

**Daktarin**® (Janssen)

*Cream*, miconazole nitrate 2%, in a water-miscible basis. Net price 30 g = £2.07
*Additives:* butylated hydroxyanisole
*Note.* A generic version of miconazole nitrate 2% cream
is also available from Hillcross, net price 30 g = £2.04

*Dusting-powder*, miconazole nitrate 2%. Net
price 20 g = £1.50
*Additives:* none as listed in section 13.1

*Spray powder*, miconazole nitrate 0.16%, in an
aerosol basis. Net price 100 g = £1.50
*Additives:* none as listed in section 13.1

*Twin pack*, 1 × 30 g pack of cream miconazole
nitrate 2%, with 1 × 30 g dusting-powder
miconazole nitrate 2%. Net price (complete
pack) = £3.80

## NYSTATIN

*Indications:* skin infections due to *Candida* spp.
*Administration:* apply 2–4 times daily, continuing
for 7 days after lesions have healed

PoM **Nystaform**® (Bayer)

*Cream*, nystatin 100000 units/g, chlorhexidine
hydrochloride 1%. Net price 30 g = £2.69
*Additives:* benzyl alcohol, polysorbate 60

*Ointment*, nystatin 100000 units/g, chlorhex-
idine acetate 1%, in a water-repellent basis.
Net price 30 g = £2.69
*Additives:* none as listed in section 13.1

PoM **Nystan**® (Squibb)

*Cream*, nystatin 100 000 units/g, in a water-miscible basis. Net price 30 g = £2.66
*Additives:* benzyl alcohol, propylene glycol, fragrance

*Gel*, nystatin 100 000 units/g. Net price 30 g =
£2.66
*Additives:* chlorocresol, fragrance

*Ointment*, nystatin 100 000 units/g, in Pla-
stibase®. Net price 30 g = £2.14
*Additives:* none as listed in section 13.1

PoM **Tinaderm-M**® (Schering-Plough)

*Cream*, nystatin 100000 units/g, tolnaftate 1%,
in a water-miscible basis. Net price 20 g =
£1.83. For *Candida* infections and tinea
*Additives:* butylated hydroxytoluene, hydroxybenzoates
(parabens), fragrance

Apply 2–3 times daily

## SALICYLIC ACID

*Indications:* fungal skin infections, particularly
tinea
*Side-effects:* hypersensitivity reactions

**Phytex**® (Pharmax)

*Paint*, salicylic acid 1.46% (total combined), tannic acid
4.89% and boric acid 3.12% (as borotannic complex),
in a vehicle containing alcohol and ethyl acetate. Net
price 25 mL (with brush) = £1.33. For fungal nail infections (onychomycosis)
*Additives:* none as listed in section 13.1
Apply twice daily
*Caution:* flammable; avoid in pregnancy and children
under 5 years

**Phytocil**® (Fisons)

*Cream*, salicylic acid 1.5%, 2-*p*-chlorophenoxyethanol
1%, menthol 1%, 1-phenoxypropan-2-ol 2%. Net price
25 g = 66p. For tinea pedis, tinea cruris, and tinea cir-
cinata
*Additives:* none as listed in section 13.1
Apply 2–3 times daily

## SULCONAZOLE NITRATE

*Indications; Side-effects:* see under Clotrimazole
*Cautions:* avoid contact with eyes (lens changes
in *animals* after high oral doses)
*Administration:* apply 1–2 times daily continuing
for 2–3 weeks after lesions have healed

PoM **Exelderm**® (ICI)

*Cream*, sulconazole nitrate 1%, in a water-miscible basis. Net price 30 g = £3.90
*Additives:* polysorbates, propylene glycol

## TIOCONAZOLE

*Indications:* fungal nail infections
*Side-effects:* local irritation, usually during first
week of treatment; discontinue if sensitivity
reaction develops
*Administration:* apply to nails and surrounding
skin twice daily for up to 6 months (may be
extended to 12 months)

PoM **Trosyl**® (Novex)

*Nail solution*, tioconazole 28%. Net price 12 mL
(with applicator brush) = £25.00
*Additives:* none as listed in section 13.1

## TOLNAFTATE

*Indications:* skin infections, particularly tinea pedis

*Side-effects:* rarely hypersensitivity

**Timoped®** (R&C)

*Cream,* tolnaftate 1%, triclosan 0.25%. Net price 30 g = £3.10
*Additives:* none as listed in section 13.1

Apply twice daily

## UNDECENOATES

*Indications:* skin infections, particularly tinea pedis

**Monphytol®** (LAB)

*Paint,* methyl undecenoate 5%, propyl undecenoate 0.7%, salicylic acid 3%, methyl salicylate 25%, propyl salicylate 5%, chlorbutol 3%. Net price 18 mL (with brush) = £1.17. For fungal (particularly nail) infections
*Additives:* none as listed in section 13.1

Apply 4 times daily

**Mycota®** (Crookes)

*Cream,* zinc undecenoate 20%, undecenoic acid 5%. Net price 25 g = 79p
*Additives:* fragrance

*Dusting powder,* zinc undecenoate 20%, undecenoic acid 2%. Net price 70 g = £1.28
*Additives:* fragrance

*Spray application,* undecenoic acid 2.5%, dichlorophen 0.25% (pressurised aerosol pack). Net price 113 g = £1.28
*Additives:* fragrance

Apply 1–2 times daily

**Phytocil®** (Fisons)

*Dusting powder,* zinc undecenoate 5.8%, 2-*p*-chlorophenoxyethanol 1%, 1-phenoxypropan-2-ol 2%. Net price 50 g = 91p. For use with cream
*Additives:* none as listed in section 13.1

## 13.10.3   Antiviral preparations

**Acyclovir** cream is indicated for the treatment of initial and recurrent labial and genital herpes simplex infections; treatment should begin as early as possible. Systemic treatment is necessary for buccal or vaginal infections; herpes zoster (shingles) also requires systemic treatment (for details of systemic use see section 5.3).

**Idoxuridine** solution (5% in dimethyl sulphoxide) is used less frequently for herpetic infections of the skin since acyclovir is more effective. Herpes simplex seems to respond to frequent applications if started early and continued for 3 to 4 days, but may be less successful if delayed after 7 days. Evidence of its value in herpes zoster infections is conflicting.

## ACYCLOVIR

*Indications:* see notes above

*Side-effects:* transient stinging or burning on application; occasionally erythema or drying of the skin

*Cautions:* avoid contact with eyes and mucous membranes

*Administration:* apply to lesions every 4 hours (5 times daily) for 5 days, started at first sign of attack

**PoM Zovirax®** (Wellcome)

*Cream,* acyclovir 5% in an aqueous cream basis. Net price 2 g = £8.37; 10 g = £25.22
*Additives:* propylene glycol

*Eye ointment,* see section 11.3.3

*Tablets,* see section 5.3

## IDOXURIDINE IN DIMETHYL SULPHOXIDE

*Indications:* see notes above

*Cautions:* avoid contact with the eyes, mucous membranes, and textiles; breast-feeding

*Contra-indications:* pregnancy (toxicity in *animal* studies)

*Side-effects:* stinging on application, changes in taste; overuse may cause maceration

*Administration:* apply 5% solution to lesions 4 times daily for 3–4 days; in severe zoster (shingles) apply 40% solution over affected area daily for 4 days

*Note.* Not to be used in mouth

**PoM Herpid®** (Boehringer Ingelheim)

*Application,* idoxuridine 5% in dimethyl sulphoxide. Net price 5 mL (with brush) = £7.04
*Additives:* none as listed in section 13.1

**PoM Iduridin®** (Ferring)

*Application,* idoxuridine 5% in dimethyl sulphoxide. Net price 5 mL (with applicator) = £4.90
*Additives:* none as listed in section 13.1

*Application,* idoxuridine 40% in dimethyl sulphoxide. Net price 5 mL (with applicator) = £19.00; 20 mL with dropper = £39.00. For severe herpes zoster
*Additives:* none as listed in section 13.1

**PoM Virudox®** (Bioglan)

*Application,* idoxuridine 5% in dimethyl sulphoxide. Net price 5 mL (with brush) = £5.95
*Additives:* none as listed in section 13.1

## 13.10.4   Parasiticidal preparations

SCABIES (*Sarcoptes scabiei*). **Lindane** and **malathion** are the treatments of choice for scabies, but lindane should be avoided during pregnancy or breast-feeding, in young children, and in patients with low body-weight or a history of epilepsy.

Older preparations include benzyl benzoate, which is an irritant and should be avoided in children, and monosulfiram, which may induce disulfiram-like reactions with alcohol. Evidence that monosulfiram is particularly suitable for children is inconclusive; it is not appropriate for self treatment.

Aqueous lotions are preferable to creams as they give better coverage; alcoholic lotions are not recommended owing to irritation of excoriated skin and the genitalia. Although the preparations have traditionally been applied after a hot bath there is evidence that this may increase absorption of the acaricide into the bloodstream.

All members of the affected household should be treated. Treatment should be applied to the whole body paying particular attention to the webs of the fingers and toes and brushing lotion under the ends of the nails. In the case of infants and young children (up to the age of about 2 years) the lotion (preferably malathion, see notes above) should also be applied on the scalp, neck, face, and ears. Providing the application is done properly lindane and malathion need only be applied once; in the case of benzyl benzoate up to three applications on consecutive days may be needed.

The itch of scabies persists for some days after the infestation has been eliminated and anti-pruritic treatment may be required. Application of **crotamiton** can be used to control itching after treatment with more effective acaricides, but caution is necessary if the skin is excoriated. **Calamine** is probably more suitable. Oral administration of a sedative antihistamine at night may also be useful.

HEAD LICE (*Pediculus humanis capitis*). **Malathion** and **carbaryl** are the treatments of choice for *head lice*. **Lindane** is no longer recommended because of resistant strains. Lotions should be used in preference to shampoos, which are not in contact with the hair long enough and are normally diluted too much in use to be effective; aqueous lotions are preferred for asthmatic patients and small children, to avoid alcoholic fumes. A contact time of 12 hours or overnight treatment is recommended. A 2-hour treatment is no longer regarded as sufficient to ensure death of eggs. **Permethrin** and **phenothrin** are two recently introduced pyrethroids, both of which are very effective if formulated in a good carrier basis.

In general, treatment for head lice should preferably be repeated after 7 days to kill lice emerging from any eggs that might have survived the first application.

> **Rotational policies**. Most health districts operate a rotating policy for head lice treatment. Details of the drugs which are currently recommended for use in the different health districts can be obtained from District Pharmaceutical Officers.

CRAB (PUBIC) LICE (*Pthirus pubis*). **Malathion**, **lindane** and **carbaryl** are effective for *crab lice*. Aqueous lotions should be applied to all hairy parts of the body for 12 hours or overnight; a second treatment is preferable after one week to kill lice emerging from surviving eggs. Alcoholic lotions are not recommended (owing to irritation of excoriated skin and the genitalia). Aqueous malathion lotion should be used for *crab lice of the eye lashes*.

## BENZYL BENZOATE

*Indications:* scabies, pediculosis (but see notes above)

*Cautions:* children (see notes above), avoid contact with eyes and mucous membranes

*Side-effects:* skin irritation, burning sensation especially on genitalia and excoriations, occasionally rashes

**Benzyl Benzoate Application, BP,** benzyl benzoate 25% in an emulsion basis.

*Administration:* scabies—apply 25% application over the whole body, omitting the head and neck; repeat without bathing on the following day and wash off 24 hours later; a third application may be required in some cases

Note. Not recommended for children—dilution to reduce irritant effect also reduces efficacy (see notes above)

Available from Rhône-Poulenc Rorer (Ascabiol®, net price 100 mL = £1.17); generic versions available from CP and Evans

## CARBARYL

*Indications:* pediculosis

*Cautions:* avoid contact with eyes; alcoholic lotions **not** recommended for pediculosis in asthmatics or small children, or for crab lice (see notes above); do not use more than once a week for 3 weeks at a time

*Side-effects:* skin irritation

*Administration:* lotion—apply to dry hair and rub into the hair and scalp or affected areas, allow to dry, comb, and remove by washing 12 hours later (see also notes above); shampoo—shampoo in, leave on hair for 5 minutes, rinse, repeat, rinse, allow to dry, comb, repeat twice at intervals of 3 days

**Carylderm®** (Napp)

*Lotion*, carbaryl 0.5%, in an alcoholic basis. Net price 55 mL = £1.16; 110 mL = £2.21. Label: 15

Additives: none as listed in section 13.1

*Shampoo*, carbaryl 1%. Net price 100 mL = £1.86

Additives: wool fat derivative, fragrance

**Clinicide®** (De Witt)

*Lotion*, carbaryl 0.5% in an aqueous basis containing 10% alcohol. Net price 50 mL = £1.04

Additives: none as listed in section 13.1

**Derbac® C** (International Labs)

*Liquid* (= lotion), carbaryl 1% in an aqueous basis. Net price 50 mL = £1.19; 200 mL = £2.83. Label: 10 patient information leaflet

Additives: hydroxybenzoates (parabens)

*Shampoo solution*, carbaryl 0.5% in an aqueous basis. Net price 75 mL = £1.17. Label: 10 patient information leaflet

Additives: hydroxybenzoates (parabens), fragrance

**Suleo-C®** (International Labs)

*Lotion*, carbaryl 0.5%, in an alcoholic basis. Net price 55 mL = £1.14; 210 mL = £2.64. Label: 15

Additives: fragrance

*Shampoo*, carbaryl 0.5%. Net price 75 mL = £1.16

Additives: fragrance

## LINDANE

*Indications:* scabies, pediculosis (but see notes above)

*Cautions:* avoid contact with eyes and mucous membranes; do not use more than twice for one course of treatment; see also above (under Scabies)

*Side-effects:* skin irritation

*Administration:* see preparations

**Quellada®** (Stafford-Miller)

*Lotion*, lindane 1%, in a lotion basis. Net price 100 mL = 63p; 500 mL = £2.08. For scabies
*Additives:* hydroxybenzoates (parabens), fragrance
*Administration:* scabies, apply thinly over whole body, omitting head and neck, wash off using cool water after 24 hours; repeat if necessary after 7 days

*Application PC*, lindane 1%, in a shampoo basis. Net price 100 mL = 71p; 500 mL = £2.54. For pediculosis (but see notes above)
*Additives:* polysorbates
*Administration:* pediculosis (but see notes above), apply to dry hair, leave for 4 minutes, add water to produce lather, rinse, towel dry, comb

## MALATHION

*Indications:* pediculosis, scabies
*Cautions:* avoid contact with eyes; alcoholic lotions **not** recommended for pediculosis in asthmatics or small children, or for scabies or crab lice (see notes above); do not use more than once a week for 3 weeks at a time
*Side-effects:* skin irritation
*Administration:* pediculosis—rub 0.5% lotion into dry hair, scalp, and affected area, comb, allow to dry naturally, remove by washing after 12 hours (see also notes above); apply 1% shampoo to hair for 5 minutes, rinse, repeat, rinse again, comb, repeat twice at intervals of 3 days
Scabies—apply 0.5% preparation over whole body, omitting the head and neck, and wash off after 24 hours, but see also notes above

**Derbac-M®** (International Labs)
*Liquid*, malathion 0.5% in an aqueous basis. Net price 55 mL = £1.19; 200 mL = £2.83
*Additives:* hydroxybenzoates (parabens), fragrance

**Prioderm®** (Napp)
*Lotion*, malathion 0.5%, in an alcoholic basis. Net price 55 mL = £1.16; 110 mL = £2.21. Label: 15
*Additives:* fragrance
*Cream shampoo*, malathion 1%. Net price 40 g = £1.16
*Additives:* disodium edetate, hydroxybenzoates (parabens), propylene glycol, wool fat derivative, fragrance

**Suleo-M®** (International Labs)
*Lotion*, malathion 0.5%, in an alcoholic basis. Net price 55 mL = £1.14; 210 mL = £2.64. Label: 15
*Additives:* fragrance

## MONOSULFIRAM

*Indications:* scabies, but see notes above
*Cautions:* avoid contact with eyes; avoid alcohol; not appropriate for self-treatment; **interactions:** Appendix 1 (monosulfiram)
*Side-effects:* hypersensitivity, rashes
*Administration:* apply diluted solution over whole body omitting head and neck; repeat if necessary for 2–3 consecutive days

**Tetmosol®** (ICI)
*Solution*, monosulfiram 25%, in industrial methylated spirit. Dilute with 2–3 parts of water before use. Net price 100 mL = £1.20. Label: 4, 15. ACBS: for control of scabies (clinic use)
*Additives:* none as listed in section 13.1

## PERMETHRIN

*Indications:* pediculosis
*Cautions:* avoid contact with eyes; use in children under 2 years only under medical supervision
*Side-effects:* pruritus, erythema, and stinging of scalp; rarely scalp rashes and oedema

**Lyclear®** (Wellcome)
*Cream rinse*, permethrin 1% in basis containing isopropyl alcohol 20%. Net price 59 mL = £1.68
*Additives:* hydroxybenzoates (parabens), propylene glycol, fragrance
*Administration:* apply to clean damp hair, leave on for 10 minutes, rinse and dry

## PHENOTHRIN

*Indications:* pediculosis
*Cautions:* avoid contact with eyes; children under 6 months (medical supervision required)
*Side-effects:* skin irritation

**Full Marks®** (Napp)
*Shampoo*, phenothrin 0.2%. Net price 125 mL = £2.48
*Additives:* fragrance
*Administration:* shampoo hair, leave on for at least 5 minutes, rinse, repeat once, comb
*Lotion*, phenothrin 0.2% in basis containing isopropyl alcohol 69.3%. Net price 55 mL = £1.22; 110 mL = £2.33. Label: 15
*Additives:* fragrance
*Administration:* apply to dry hair, allow to dry naturally; shampoo after 2 hours, comb while still wet

## 13.10.5 Preparations for minor skin infections

Some of the preparations listed are used in minor burns, and abrasions. They are applied as necessary. Preparations containing camphor, hydrargaphen, and sulphonamides should be **avoided**. Preparations such as magnesium sulphate paste are also listed but are now rarely used to treat carbuncles and boils as these are best treated with antibiotics (see section 5.1.1.2).

**Cetrimide Cream, BP,** cetrimide 0.5% in a suitable water-miscible basis such as cetostearyl alcohol 5%, liquid paraffin 50% in freshly boiled and cooled purified water. Net price 50 g = 55p

**Chlorhexidine Cream, BP,** chlorhexidine gluconate solution usually 5% (≡ chlorhexidine gluconate 1%), cetomacrogol emulsifying wax 25%, liquid paraffin 10%, in purified water, freshly boiled and cooled

**Proflavine Cream, BPC,** proflavine hemisulphate 0.1%, yellow beeswax 2.5%, chlorocresol 0.1%, liquid paraffin 67.3%, freshly boiled and cooled purified water 25%, wool fat 5%. Net price 100 mL = 33p
*Caution:* stains clothing

**Anaflex®** (Geistlich)
*Cream*, polynoxylin 10%, in a water-miscible basis. Net price 50 g = £2.59
*Additives:* fragrance

**Betadine®** (Napp)
*Ointment*, povidone-iodine 10%, in a water-miscible basis. Net price 80 g = £2.03
*Additives:* none as listed in section 13.1

**Brulidine®** (Rhône-Poulenc Rorer)
*Cream*, dibromopropamidine isethionate 0.15%, in a water-miscible basis. Net price 25 g = 74p
*Additives:* hydroxybenzoates (parabens), fragrance

**Cetavlex®** (ICI)
*Cream*, cetrimide 0.5%, in a water-miscible basis. Net price 50 g = 50p
*Additives:* hydroxybenzoates (parabens)

**Dermalex®** (Sanofi Winthrop)
*Skin lotion*, allantoin 0.25%, hexachlorophane 0.5%, squalane 3% in an emulsion basis. Net price 100 mL = £2.05; 250 mL = £5.35. For prevention of pressure sores and prevention and treatment of urinary rash. Avoid in children under 2 years
*Additives:* butylated hydroxyanisole, edetic acid, hydroxybenzoates (parabens), wool fat, fragrance

**Drapolene®** (Wellcome)
*Cream*, benzalkonium chloride 0.01%, cetrimide 0.2% in a water-miscible basis. Net price 55 g = 70p; 100 g = £1.08. For urinary rash and minor wounds
*Additives:* chlorocresol, wool fat

**Vesagex®** (Rybar)
*Cream*, cetrimide 1%. Net price 500 g = £4.60
*Additives:* chlorocresol, fragrance

Preparations for boils
**Magnesium Sulphate Paste, BP,** dried magnesium sulphate 45 g, glycerol 55 g, phenol 500 mg
Should be stirred before use
Apply under dressing
**Secaderm®**—section 13.14

---

COLLODION

**Flexible collodion** may be used to seal minor cuts and wounds that have partially healed.

**Collodion, Flexible, BP,** castor oil 2.5%, colophony 2.5% in a collodion basis, prepared by dissolving pyroxylin (10%) in a mixture of 3 volumes of ether and 1 volume of alcohol (90%). Net price 10 mL = 12p. Label: 15

# 13.11   Disinfectants and cleansers

13.11.1   Alcohols and saline
13.11.2   Chlorhexidine salts
13.11.3   Cationic surfactants and soaps
13.11.4   Chlorine and iodine
13.11.5   Phenolics
13.11.6   Astringents, oxidisers, and dyes
13.11.7   Desloughing agents

The choice of *cleanser* is an important factor in treating skin conditions. For example, scaling disorders are best treated with **emulsifying ointment** (section 13.2.1) or other cleansers that do not irritate the skin.

**Sodium chloride solution 0.9%** is suitable for general cleansing of skin and wounds.

Useful *disinfectants* for skin cleansing include **cetrimide** (which has useful detergent properties), **chlorhexidine** and **potassium permanganate solution** 1 in 8000. **Povidone-iodine** is preferred to chlorinated solutions (such as dilute sodium hypochlorite solution) which are too irritant and are no longer recommended. Topical preparations of **hexachlorophane** should be used with caution in neonates and should **not** be used on large raw surfaces.

*Astringent* preparations, such as **potassium permanganate** solution are useful for treating eczematous reactions (section 13.5). Silver nitrate lotion is now rarely used as it stains the skin black and may cause toxic effects if used for prolonged periods.

> BORDERLINE SUBSTANCES. The preparations marked 'ACBS' are regarded as drugs when prescribed in accordance with the advice of the Advisory Committee on Borderline Substances for the clinical conditions listed. Prescriptions issued in accordance with this advice and endorsed 'ACBS' will normally not be investigated. See Appendix 7 for listing by clinical condition.

## 13.11.1   Alcohols and saline

### ALCOHOL
*Indications:* skin preparation before injection
*Cautions:* flammable; avoid broken skin; patients have suffered severe burns when diathermy has been preceded by application of alcoholic skin disinfectants.

### Industrial Methylated Spirit, BP
Mixture of 19 volumes of ethanol (absolute alcohol) of an appropriate strength with 1 volume of approved wood naphtha and is Industrial Methylated Spirit of the quality known either as '66 OP' or as '74 OP'
Net price 100 mL = 15p. Label: 15

**Surgical Spirit, BP,** methyl salicylate 0.5 mL, diethyl phthalate 2%, castor oil 2.5%, in industrial methylated spirit. Net price 100 mL = 17p. Label: 15

### SODIUM CHLORIDE
*Indications:* see notes above

**Normasol®** (Seton)
*Solution* (sterile), sodium chloride 0.9%. Net price 25 × 25-mL sachet = £3.98; 6 × 100-mL sachet = £2.97. To be used undiluted for topical irrigation of burns, wounds, and eyes
See also section 11.8.2

**Sterac® Sodium Chloride** (Galen)
*Solution* (sterile), sodium chloride 0.9%. Net price 150 mL = 83p; 1000 mL = £1.10. For irrigation of eyes and wounds

---

## 13.11.2 Chlorhexidine salts

### CHLORHEXIDINE

*Indications:* skin disinfection such as pre-operative skin preparation, obstetrics and wound cleansing; bladder irrigation (see also section 7.4.4)

*Cautions:* avoid contact with eyes, brain, meninges and middle ear; not for use in body cavities; alcoholic solutions not suitable before diathermy

*Side-effects:* occasional sensitivity may occur

*Administration:* chlorhexidine acetate or gluconate, body cavity and bladder irrigation 0.01–0.02%[1], urethral disinfection and catheter lubrication 0.05% (in glycerol), pre-operative skin preparation 0.5% (in alcohol 70%); chlorhexidine hydrochloride 1% as a dusting-powder or cream

1. Solutions containing chlorhexidine 0.01% are usually preferred for postoperative bladder instillation

**Chlorasept®** (Baxter)

*2000 Solution* (sterile), pink, chlorhexidine acetate 0.05%. Net price 500 mL = 74p; 1000 mL = 79p. For cleansing and disinfecting wounds and burns

**CX Antiseptic Dusting Powder®** (Bio-Medical)

*Dusting powder*, sterile, chlorhexidine acetate 1%. Net price 15 g = £2.00. For skin disinfection and antisepsis

*Note.* Chlorhexidine Dusting Powder BP contains chlorhexidine hydrochloride 0.5% but no preparation is available commercially

**Hibidil®** (ICI)

*Solution* (sterile), pink, chlorhexidine gluconate solution 0.25% (≡ chlorhexidine gluconate 0.05%) in sterile aqueous solution. Net price 25 × 25-mL sachets = £2.00; 6 × 100-mL sachets = £1.15; 1000 mL also available. For swabbing wounds and burns and in obstetrics

**Hibiscrub®** (ICI)

*Cleansing solution*, red, chlorhexidine gluconate solution 20% (≡ 4% chlorhexidine gluconate), perfumed, in a surfactant solution. Net price 12 × 100-mL sachets = £11.16; 250 mL = £1.13; 500 mL = £1.65. Use instead of soap for pre-operative hand and skin preparation and for general hand and skin antisepsis

**Hibisol®** (ICI)

*Solution*, chlorhexidine gluconate solution 2.5% (≡ 0.5% chlorhexidine gluconate), in isopropyl alcohol 70% with emollients. Net price 250 mL = £1.04; 500 mL = £1.72. To be used undiluted for hand and skin disinfection

**Hibitane Obstetric®** (ICI)

*Cream*, chlorhexidine gluconate solution 5% (≡ 1% chlorhexidine gluconate), in a pourable water-miscible basis. Net price 250 mL = 91p. For use in obstetrics and gynaecology as an antiseptic and lubricant (for application to skin around vulva and perineum and to hands of midwife or doctor)

**Phiso-med®** (Sanofi Winthrop)

*Solution*, chlorhexidine gluconate 4% in an emulsion basis. Net price 150 mL = £4.76. For use as a soap substitute in acne and seborrhoeic conditions; for bathing mothers and babies in maternity units (as 1 in 10 dilution) to prevent cross-infection and for pre-operative hand and skin preparation

**Rotersept®** (Roterpharma)

*Spray application*, chlorhexidine gluconate 0.2% in a pressurised aerosol unit. Net price 284-g unit = £1.99. For prevention and treatment of sore cracked nipples

**Sterexidine®** (Galen)

*Solution* (sterile), chlorhexidine gluconate 0.02%. Net price 150 mL = 83p; 1000 mL = £1.10. For disinfection and wound cleansing

**Unisept®** (Seton)

*Solution* (sterile), pink, chlorhexidine gluconate 0.05%. Net price 25 × 25-mL sachet = £2.20; 6 × 100-mL sachet = £1.26. For cleansing and disinfecting wounds and burns and swabbing in obstetrics

With cetrimide

**Savloclens®** (ICI)

*Solution* (sterile), yellow, chlorhexidine gluconate solution 0.25% (≡ chlorhexidine gluconate 0.05%), cetrimide 0.5% ≡ a dilution of 1 in 30 of Savlon Hospital Concentrate. Net price 100-mL sachet = 20p. For cleansing and disinfecting contaminated wounds and burns

**Savlodil®** (ICI)

*Solution* (sterile), yellow, chlorhexidine gluconate solution 0.075% (≡ chlorhexidine gluconate 0.015%), cetrimide 0.15% (sterile). Net price 25 × 25-mL sachets = £1.29; 6 × 100-mL sachets = 88p. For cleansing and disinfecting wounds and burns and swabbing in obstetrics

**Tisept®** (Seton)

*Solution* (sterile), yellow, chlorhexidine gluconate 0.015%, cetrimide 0.15%. Net price 25 × 25-mL sachet = £1.45; 6 × 100-mL sachet = 99p. To be used undiluted for general skin disinfection and wound cleansing

**Travasept 100®** (Baxter)

*Solution* (sterile), yellow, chlorhexidine acetate 0.015%, cetrimide 0.15%. Net price 500 mL = 74p; 1000 mL = 79p. To be used undiluted in skin disinfection such as wound cleansing and obstetrics

---

## CONCENTRATES

### Hibitane 5% Concentrate® (ICI)

*Solution*, red, chlorhexidine gluconate solution 25% (≡ 5% chlorhexidine gluconate), in a perfumed aqueous solution. Net price 5 litres = £11.75. To be used diluted 1 in 10 (0.5%) with alcohol 70% for pre-operative skin preparation, or 1 in 100 (0.05%) with water for general skin disinfection

*Note.* Alcoholic solutions not suitable before diathermy (see Alcohol, above)

---

**Hibitane Gluconate 20%®** (ICI)
*Solution*, chlorhexidine gluconate 20% in an aqueous solution. Net price 500 mL = £4.25. To be used diluted as above in body cavity and bladder irrigation, urethral disinfection and catheter lubrication

With cetrimide
**Savlon Hospital Concentrate®** (ICI)
*Solution*, orange, chlorhexidine gluconate solution 7.5% (≡ chlorhexidine gluconate 1.5%), cetrimide 15%. Net price 1 litre = £1.59. To be used diluted 1 in 100 (1%) to 1 in 30 with water for skin disinfection and wound cleansing, and diluted 1 in 30 in alcohol 70% for pre-operative skin preparation
*Note.* Alcoholic solutions not suitable before diathermy (see Alcohol, above)

## 13.11.3   Cationic surfactants and soaps

### BENZALKONIUM CHLORIDE
*Indications:* skin disinfection such as pre-operative skin preparation, obstetrics, wound cleansing and bladder irrigation
*Cautions:* avoid contact with eyes

**Roccal®** (Sterling-Winthrop)
*Solution*, blue, benzalkonium chloride 1%. Net price 250 mL = £1.22; 500 mL = £2.44. To be used diluted 1 in 10 to 1 in 200
*Additives:* fragrance
**Roccal Concentrate 10X®** (Sterling-Winthrop)
*Concentrate*, blue, benzalkonium chloride 10%. Net price 2.25 litres = £44.99. For preparation of Roccal Solution with freshly boiled and cooled purified water
*Additives:* fragrance

### CETRIMIDE
*Indications:* skin disinfection
*Cautions:* avoid contact with eyes; avoid use in body cavities
*Side-effects:* skin irritation and occasionally sensitisation

**Preparations**
Ingredient of Savloclens®, Savlodil®, Savlon Hospital Concentrate®, Tisept®, and Travasept® 100, see above

### SOFT SOAP
*Indications:* removal of adherent crusts

**Soap Spirit, BP,** soft soap 65% in alcohol (90%). Net price 100 mL = 54p

### SUBSTITUTE SOAPS
See section 13.2.1 (emulsifying ointment); section 13.2.1.1 (emollient bath additives)

## 13.11.4   Chlorine and iodine

### CHLORINATED SOLUTIONS
*Cautions:* bleaches fabric; irritant (protect surrounding tissues with soft paraffin)

**Chlorinated Lime and Boric Acid Solution, BP,** (Eusol), chlorinated lime 1.25%, boric acid 1.25%, in purified water, freshly boiled and cooled. Contains not less than 0.25% available chlorine. It must be freshly prepared. Has been used undiluted for skin disinfection, particularly in wound and ulcer cleansing but no longer recommended (too irritant)
**Chlorinated Soda Solution, Surgical, BPC,** (Dakin's Solution), boric acid, chlorinated lime, sodium carbonate, sufficient of each to provide a solution containing 0.5% of available chlorine in purified water, freshly boiled and cooled. Net price 500 mL = 68p. Has been used undiluted for cleansing wounds and ulcers but no longer recommended (too irritant)
**Chlorasol®** (Seton)
*Solution* (sterile), sodium hypochlorite, containing 0.3–0.4% available chlorine. Net price 25 × 25-mL sachets = £6.61
*Additives:* none as listed in section 13.1
Irritant therefore no longer recommended

### IODINE COMPOUNDS
*Indications:* skin disinfection
*Cautions:* pregnancy, breast-feeding; broken skin; thyroid disorders
*Side-effects:* rarely sensitivity; may interfere with thyroid function tests
**Betadine®** (Napp)
*Antiseptic paint*, povidone-iodine 10% in an alcoholic solution. Net price 8 mL (with applicator brush) = 69p. Apply undiluted to minor wounds and infections, twice daily
*Additives:* none as listed in section 13.1
*Alcoholic solution*, povidone-iodine 10%. Net price 500 mL = £1.24. To be applied undiluted in pre- and post-operative skin disinfection
*Additives:* none as listed in section 13.1
*Note.* Flammable—caution in procedures involving hot wire cautery and diathermy
*Antiseptic solution*, povidone-iodine 10% in aqueous solution. Net price 500 mL = £1.09. To be applied undiluted in pre- and post-operative skin disinfection
*Additives:* none as listed in section 13.1
*Dry powder spray*, povidone-iodine 2.5% in a pressurised aerosol unit. Net price 150-g unit = £2.36. For skin disinfection, particularly minor wounds and infections
*Scalp and skin cleanser solution*, povidone-iodine 7.5%, in a surfactant basis. Net price 250 mL = £2.06. ACBS: for infective conditions of the skin. Retain on scalp for 5 minutes before rinsing
*Skin cleanser solution*, povidone-iodine 4%, in a surfactant basis. Net price 250 mL = £1.74. ACBS: for infective conditions of the skin. Retain on skin for 3–5 minutes before rinsing; repeat twice daily
*Surgical scrub*, povidone-iodine 7.5%, in a non-ionic surfactant basis. Net price 500 mL = 96p. To be used as a pre-operative scrub for hands and skin
*Additives:* wool fat derivative

**Savlon Dry®** (Ciba)
*Dry powder spray*, povidone-iodine 0.5% in a pressurised aerosol unit. Net price 55-g unit = £1.49. For minor wounds and infections

**Videne®** (3M)
*Dusting powder*, povidone-iodine 5%. Net price 15 g = £2.60. For minor wounds and infections

**Aluminium Acetate Lotion,** aluminium acetate solution 5 mL, purified water, freshly boiled and cooled, to 100 mL. It should be freshly prepared. To be used undiluted as a wet dressing
*Note.* Aluminium acetate solution (13%) for the preparation of aluminium acetate lotion (0.65%) is available from Martindale, Penn, etc. (special order)

## 13.11.5 Phenolics

### HEXACHLOROPHANE
*Indications:* see under preparations (below)
*Contra-indications:* avoid use on badly burned or excoriated skin; pregnancy; children under 2 years except on medical advice
*Side-effects:* sensitivity; rarely photosensitivity

PoM **Ster-Zac DC Skin Cleanser®** (Hough)
*Cream*, hexachlorophane 3%. Net price 100 mL = 69p. Use 3–5 mL instead of soap as pre-operative scrub for hands
*Additives:* information not disclosed for BNF

**Ster-Zac Powder®** (Hough)
*Dusting-powder*, hexachlorophane 0.33%, zinc oxide 3%, talc 88.67%, starch 8% (sterile). Net price 30 g = 66p
*Additives:* information not disclosed for BNF
Prevention of neonatal staphylococcal sepsis, after ligature of cord sprinkle on perineum, groin, front of abdomen, and axillas; after cutting cord and spraying with plastic dressing, powder stump and adjacent skin; after every napkin change powder stump, adjacent skin, perineum, groin, axillas, buttocks, and front of abdomen; continue until stump drops away and wound healed
Adjunct for treatment of recurrent furunculosis, powder daily area of skin normally subject to furunculosis

### TRICLOSAN
*Indications:* skin disinfection
*Cautions:* avoid contact with eyes

**Manusept®** (Hough)
*Antibacterial hand rub*, blue, triclosan 0.5%, isopropyl alcohol 70%. Net price 250 mL = 96p; 500 mL = £1.47. For disinfection and pre-operative hand preparation
*Additives:* information not disclosed for BNF

**Ster-Zac Bath Concentrate®** (Hough)
*Solution*, triclosan 2%. Net price 28.5 mL = 38p; 500 mL = £3.64. ACBS: for staphylococcal skin infections. For prevention of cross-infection use 1 sachet/bath
*Additives:* information not disclosed for BNF

## 13.11.6 Astringents, oxidisers, and dyes

### ALUMINIUM ACETATE
*Indications:* exudative eczematous reactions and wounds

### CRYSTAL VIOLET
(Gentian violet)
*Indications:* see below
*Cautions:* stains clothes and skin
*Side-effects:* mucosal ulcerations

**Crystal Violet Paint, BP1980,** crystal violet 0.5%, in purified water, freshly boiled and cooled. To be used undiluted
*Note.* Licensed for topical application on unbroken skin only; no longer recommended for application to mucous membranes or open wounds; restrictions do not apply to use for skin marking prior to surgery

### HYDROGEN PEROXIDE
*Indications:* skin disinfection, particularly cleansing and deodorising wounds and ulcers
*Cautions:* large or deep wounds; avoid normal skin; bleaches fabric

**Hydrogen Peroxide Solution, BP**
*Solution* 6% (20 vols). Net price 100 mL = 20p
*Solution* 3% (10 vols). Net price 100 mL = 16p
*Note.* The BP directs that when hydrogen peroxide is prescribed, hydrogen peroxide solution 6% (20 vols) should be dispensed.
IMPORTANT. Strong solutions of hydrogen peroxide which contain 27% (90 vols) and 30% (100 vols) are only for the preparation of weaker solutions
**Hioxyl®** see Desloughing Agents (below)

### POTASSIUM PERMANGANATE
*Indications:* cleansing and deodorising suppurating eczematous reactions and wounds
*Cautions:* irritant to mucous membranes; stains skin and clothing
*Administration:* wet dressings or baths, approx. 0.01% solution

**Potassium Permanganate Solution,** potassium permanganate 0.1% (1 in 1000) in water
To be diluted 1 in 10 to provide a 0.01% (1 in 10 000) solution

**Permitabs®** (Bioglan)
*Solution tablets*, for preparation of topical solution, potassium permanganate 400 mg. Net price 30-tab pack = £2.26
1 tablet dissolved in 4 litres of water provides a 0.01% (1 in 10 000) solution

## ZINC SULPHATE
*Indications:* indolent ulcers

**Zinc Sulphate Lotion, BP** (Lotio Rubra), zinc sulphate 1 g, amaranth solution 1 mL, water to 100 mL. It must be freshly prepared. Apply undiluted as a wet dressing
*Note.* Zinc Sulphate Mouthwash DPF consists of zinc sulphate lotion BP; 1 part is diluted with 4 parts of warm water before use

### 13.11.7    Desloughing agents
Desloughing agents for ulcers are second-line treatment and the underlying causes should be treated. The main beneficial effect is removal of slough and clot and the ablation of local infection. Preparations which absorb or help promote the removal of exudate may also help (section 13.13.8). It should be noted that substances applied to an open area are easily absorbed and perilesional skin is easily sensitised. Gravitational dermatitis may be due to neomycin or lanolin sensitivity. Enzyme preparations such as streptokinase-streptodornase or alternatively dextranomer (section 13.13.8) are designed for sloughing ulcers and may help.

**Aserbine®** (Bencard)
*Cream,* benzoic acid 0.024%, malic acid 0.36%, propylene glycol 1.7%, salicylic acid 0.006%. Net price 100 g = £1.20
*Additives:* hydroxybenzoates (parabens)
*Solution,* benzoic acid 0.15%, malic acid 2.25%, propylene glycol 40%, salicylic acid 0.0375%. Net price 500 mL = £1.81
*Additives:* fragrance
**Hioxyl®** (Quinoderm Ltd)
*Cream,* hydrogen peroxide (stabilised) 1.5%. Net price 25 g = £1.68; 100 g = £5.29. For leg ulcers and pressure sores
*Additives:* none as listed in section 13.1
Apply when necessary and if necessary cover with a dressing
**Variclene®** (Dermal)
*Gel,* brilliant green 0.5%, lactic acid 0.5%, in an aqueous basis. Net price 50 g = £4.58. For venous and other skin ulcers
*Additives:* none as listed in section 13.1
Apply to cleaned and dried lesion with a sterile applicator avoiding surrounding skin; in severe ulceration apply on dressing and repeat as required at intervals of not more than 7 days
PoM **Varidase Topical®** (Lederle)
*Powder,* streptokinase 100 000 units, streptodornase 25 000 units. For preparing solutions for topical use. Net price per vial = £7.80
*Additives:* none as listed in section 13.1
Apply as wet dressing usually 1–2 times daily
Also used to dissolve clots in the bladder or urinary catheters

## 13.12    Antiperspirants
Aluminium chloride and hydroxychloride are potent antiperspirants used in the treatment of severe hyperhidrosis.
Dusting powders are described in section 13.2.3.

### ALUMINIUM CHLORIDE
*Indications:* hyperhidrosis
*Cautions:* avoid contact with eyes; do not shave axilla or use depilatories within 12 hours of use
*Side-effects:* skin irritation—may be less with hydroxychloride
*Administration:* apply at night to dry skin, wash off on following morning, initially daily then reduce frequency as condition improves—do not bathe immediately before use

PoM **Anhydrol Forte®** (Dermal)
*Solution* ( = application), aluminium chloride hexahydrate 20%. Net price 10-mL bottle with roll-on applicator = £2.75. Label: 15
*Additives:* none as listed in section 13.1
PoM **Driclor®** (Stiefel)
*Application,* aluminium chloride hexahydrate 20% in an alcoholic basis. Net price 60-mL bottle with roll-on applicator = £2.82. Label: 15
*Additives:* none as listed in section 13.1
**Hyperdrol®** (BritCair)
*Cream,* aluminium hydroxychloride 19%. Net price 60 g = £4.38
*Additives:* hydroxybenzoates (parabens), propylene glycol
*Gel,* aluminium hydroxychloride 19%. Net price 60-g roll-on applicator = £5.63
*Additives:* none as listed in section 13.1

## 13.13    Wound management products
13.13.1   Bandages
13.13.2   Surgical adhesive tapes
13.13.3   Adhesive dressings
13.13.4   Surgical absorbents
13.13.5   Wound dressing pads
13.13.6   Tulle dressings
13.13.7   Semipermeable adhesive film
13.13.8   Gel and colloid dressings
13.13.9   Foam dressings
13.13.10  Elastic hosiery

### 13.13.1    Bandages

### RETENTION BANDAGES

Non-stretch fabric retention bandages
**Open-wove Bandage, BP** (types 1, 2 and 3). Cotton cloth, plain weave, warp of cotton, weft of cotton, viscose, or combination, one continuous length. Type 1, 5 m (all): 2.5 cm, net price = 23p; 5 cm = 38p; 7.5 cm = 55p; 10 cm = 70p (most suppliers) 5 m × 5 cm supplied when size not stated
*Uses:* protection and retention of absorbent dressings; support for minor strains, sprains; securing splints
*Note.* Type 1 bandage formerly described as Open-Wove Bandage BPC 1973; Type 2 formerly described as 'medium quality'; Type 3 formerly described as 'hospital quality'

**Triangular Calico Bandage**, BP. Unbleached calico rt. angle triangle. 90 cm × 90 cm × 1.27 m, net price = 89p (most suppliers)
*Uses:* sling

NHS **Domette Bandage**, BP. Fabric, plain weave, cotton warp and wool weft (hospital quality also available, all cotton). 5 m (all): 5 cm, net price = 54p; 7.5 cm = 81p; 10 cm = £1.08; 15 cm = £1.61 (Robert Bailey, Vernon-Carus)
*Uses:* protection and support where warmth required

**Multiple Pack Dressing No. 1** (Drug Tariff). Contains absorbent cotton, absorbent cotton gauze type 13 light (sterile), open-wove bandages (banded). Net price per pack = £2.66

**Multiple Pack Dressing No. 2** (Drug Tariff). As for No. 1 (above) but with larger quantities of cotton and cotton gauze and two sizes of bandages. Net price per pack = £4.47

Stretch fabric retention bandages

**Cotton Conforming Bandage**, BP. Cotton fabric, plain weave, treated to impart some elasticity to warp and weft. 3.5 m (all):
type A, 5 cm, net price = 46p, 7.5 cm = 59p, 10 cm = 72p, 15 cm = 98p (S&N—*Crinx*®)
type B, 5 cm = 51p, 7.5 cm = 65p, 10 cm = 80p, 15 cm = £1.07 (J&J—*Kling*®)
*Uses:* retention of dressings in difficult positions (e.g. over joints)

**Polyamide and Cellulose Contour Bandage**, BP (formerly Nylon and Viscose Stretch Bandage). Fabric, plain weave, warp of polyamide filament, weft of cotton or viscose, fast edges, one continuous length. 4 m stretched (all): Robinsons—*Stayform*® (5 cm = 27p, 7.5 cm = 35p, 10 cm = 40p, 15 cm = 67p); Seton—*Slinky*® (net price 5 cm = 33p, 7.5 cm = 46p, 10 cm = 56p, 15 cm = 79p); S&N—*Easifix*® (5 cm = 25p, 7.5 cm = 32p, 10 cm = 36p, 15 cm = 60p)
*Uses:* retention of dressings

NHS **Tubular Gauze Bandage, Seamless**. Unbleached cotton yarn, positioned with applicators. 20 m roll (all): 00, net price = £1.70; 01 = £1.74; 12 = £2.33; 34 = £3.42; 56 = £4.73; 78 = £5.54; T1 = £7.98; T2 = £10.29 (Seton—*Tubegauz*®)
*Uses:* retention of dressings on limbs, abdomen, trunk

**Elasticated Tubular Bandage**, BP (formerly Elasticated Surgical Tubular Stockinette). Knitted fabric, elasticated threads of rubber-cored polyamide or polyester with cotton or cotton and viscose yarn, tubular. Lengths 50 cm and 1 m, various widths 6.25 cm–12 cm, net price 45p–£1.43 (JLB Textiles—*Textube*® (formerly called *Lastogrip*®); Salt—*Rediform*®; S&N—*Tensogrip*®; Seton—*Tubigrip*®; Texlastic—*Texagrip*®). Where no brand stated by prescriber, net price of stockinette supplied not to exceed: length 50 cm, 6.25 cm = 51p, 6.75 cm = 55p, 7.5 cm = 56p, 8.75 cm = 62p, 10 cm = 63p, 12 cm = 64p; length 1 m, 6.25 cm = 92p, 6.75 cm = 98p, 7.5 cm = £1.00, 8.75 cm = £1.05, 10 cm = £1.05, 12 cm = £1.21
*Uses:* retention of dressings on limbs, abdomen, trunk

**Foam Padded Elasticated Surgical Tubular Stockinette** (Drug Tariff). Fabric as for Elasticated Tubular Bandage with polyurethane foam lining. Heel, elbow, knee, small, net price = £1.95, medium = £2.10, large = £2.26; sacral, small, medium, and large (all) = £10.03 (Seton—*Tubipad*®)
*Uses:* relief of pressure and elimination of friction in relevant area; porosity of foam lining allows normal water loss from skin surface

**Elasticated Viscose Stockinette** (Drug Tariff). Lightweight plain-knitted elasticated tubular bandage. Length 1 m (all): net price 5 cm (medium limb) = 63p; 7.5 cm (large limb) = 83p; 10.75 cm (OS limb, head, child trunk) = £1.34; 17.5 cm (adult trunk) = £1.68 (Seton—*Tubifast*®)
*Uses:* retention of dressings

**Elastic Net Surgical Tubular Stockinette** (Drug Tariff). Lightweight elastic open-work net tubular fabric.
type A: arm/leg, 40 cm × 1.8 cm (size C), net price = 32p; thigh/head, 60 cm × 2.5 cm (size E) = 58p; trunk (adult), 60 cm × 4.5 cm (size F) = 85p; trunk (OS adult) 60 cm × 5.4 cm (size G) = £1.14 (Brevit—*Netelast*®)
type B: withdrawn
type C: arm/leg, 40 cm × 1.8 cm (size C) = 25p; thigh/head, 60 cm × 2.7 cm (size E) = 48p; trunk (adult), 60 cm × 5.5 cm (size F) = 67p; trunk (OS adult) 60 cm × 6 cm (size G) = 85p (Martindale—*Macrofix*®)
Drug Tariff requires size and type to be specified by prescriber
*Uses:* retention of dressings, particularly on awkward sites

**Cotton Stockinette**, BP (formerly Cotton Surgical Tubular Stockinette). Knitted fabric, cotton yarn, tubular. 1 m × 2.5 cm, net price = 21p; 5 cm = 32p; 7.5 cm = 38p; 5 m × 10 cm = £2.65 (J&J, Seton)
*Uses:* 1 m lengths, basis (with wadding) for Plaster of Paris bandages etc.; 6 m length, compression bandage

**Ribbed Cotton and Viscose Surgical Tubular Stockinette**, BP. Knitted fabric of 1:1 ribbed structure, singles yarn spun from blend of two-thirds cotton and one third viscose fibres, tubular. Length 5 m (all):
type A (lightweight): arm/leg (child), arm (adult) 5 cm, net price = £1.70; arm (OS adult), leg (adult) 7.5 cm = £2.05; leg (OS adult) 10 cm = £2.94; trunk (child) 15 cm = £4.23; trunk (adult) 20 cm = £4.88; trunk (OS adult) 25 cm = £5.85 (Seton)
type B (heavyweight): sizes as for type A, net price £1.58–£5.42 (Sallis—*Eesiban*®)
Drug Tariff specifies various combinations of sizes to provide sufficient material for part or full body coverage
*Uses:* protective dressings with tar-based and other non-steroid ointments

## SUPPORT AND COMPRESSION BANDAGES

### Non-adhesive woven extensible bandages

**Crepe Bandage**, BP. Fabric, plain weave, warp of wool threads and crepe-twisted cotton threads, weft of cotton threads; stretch bandage. 4.5 m stretched (all): 5 cm, net price = 69p; 7.5 cm = 97p; 10 cm = £1.29; 15 cm = £1.83 (most suppliers)
*Uses:* light support system for strains, sprains, compression over paste bandages for varicose veins

**Cotton Crepe Bandage**, BP. Fabric, plain weave, warp of crepe-twisted cotton threads, weft of cotton and/or viscose threads; stretch bandage. 4.5 m stretched (both): 7.5 cm, net price = £2.09; 10 cm = £2.70; other sizes NHS (most suppliers)
*Uses:* light support system for strains, sprains, compression over paste bandages for varicose ulcers

NHS **Cotton Stretch Bandage**, BP. Fabric, plain weave, warp of crepe-twisted cotton threads, weft of cotton threads; stretch bandage, lighter than cotton crepe. 4.5 m stretched (all): 5 cm, net price = 30p; 7.5 cm = 41p; 10 cm = 54p; 15 cm = 76p (most suppliers)
*Uses:* light support system for strains, sprains, compression over paste bandages for varicose veins

**Cotton Suspensory Bandage** (Drug Tariff). Type 1: cotton net bag with draw tapes and webbing waistband; net price small, medium, and large (all) = £1.15, extra large = £1.21. Type 2: cotton net bag with elastic edge and webbing waistband; small = £1.26, medium = £1.30, large = £1.35, extra large = £1.41. Type 3: cotton net bag with elastic edge and webbing waistband with elastic insertion; small, medium, and large (all) = £1.36; extra large = £1.42
Type supplied to be endorsed
*Uses:* support of scrotum

---

**NHS Cotton and Rubber Elastic Bandage**, BP. Fabric, plain weave, warp of combined cotton and rubber threads, weft of cotton threads (S&N)
*Uses:* provision of high compression and medium support
**Heavy Cotton and Rubber Elastic Bandage**, BP. Heavy version of above with one end folded as foot loop; fastener also supplied. 1.8 m unstretched × 7.5 cm, net price = £8.97 (Marlow, Seton, S&N—*Elastoweb®*).
*Uses:* provision of high even compression over large surface
**Elastic Web Bandage**, BP. (also termed Blue Line Webbing). Characteristic fabric woven ribbon fashion, warp threads of cotton and rubber with mid-line threads coloured blue, weft threads of cotton or combined cotton and viscose; may be dyed skin colour; with or without foot loop. Per m (both): 7.5 cm, net price = 65p; 10 cm = 90p; with foot loop 7.5 cm each = £3.46 (Marlow, Seton)
*Uses:* provision of support and high compression over large surface
**Elastic Web Bandage without Foot Loop** (also termed Red Line Webbing) (Scott-Curwen). Characteristic fabric woven ribbon fashion, warp threads of cotton and rubber with mid-line threads coloured red, weft threads of cotton or combined cotton and viscose. 7.5 cm × 2.75 m (2.5 m approx. unstretched), net price = £3.03; 7.5 cm × 3.75 m (3.5 m approx. unstretched) = £3.66
*Uses:* provision of support and high compression over large surfaces

High compression extensible bandages
**PEC High Compression Bandage** (Drug Tariff). Polymide, elastane, and cotton compression (high) extensible bandage, 3 m unstreatched (both): 7.5 cm, net price = £1.98; 10 cm = £2.56 (Seton—*Setopress®*)
*Uses:* high compression for varicose ulcers
**VEC High Compression Bandage** (Drug Tariff). Viscose, elastane, and cotton compression (high) extensible bandage, 3 m unstretched (both); 7.5 cm, net price = £2.09; 10 cm = £2.70 (S&N—*Tensopress®*)
*Uses:* high compression for varicose ulcers

Adhesive woven extensible bandages
**Titanium Dioxide Elastic Adhesive Bandage**, BP. (Drug Tariff title: Porous Flexible Adhesive Bandage). Woven fabric, elastic in warp (crepe-twisted cotton threads), weft of cotton and/or viscose threads, spread with adhesive mass containing titanium dioxide but free from rubber and zinc oxide. 4.5 m stretched × 7.5 cm, net price = £2.99 (Scholl—*Poroplast®*)
*Uses:* compression for chronic leg ulcers; continuous pressure and support in patients hypersensitive to rubber and zinc oxide.
**Elastic Adhesive Bandage**, BP. Woven fabric, elastic in warp (crepe-twisted cotton threads), weft of cotton and/or viscose threads spread with adhesive mass containing zinc oxide. 4.5 m stretched (all): 5 cm, net price = £2.45; 7.5 cm = £3.58; 10 cm = £4.77 (Robinsons—*Flexoplast®*; S&N—*Elastoplast®* Bandage). 7.5 cm width supplied when size not stated
*Uses:* compression for chronic leg ulcers; compression and support for fractured ribs, clavicles, swollen or sprained joints
**NHS Half-spread Elastic Adhesive Bandage**, BP. Fabric as for elastic adhesive bandage but only partially spread with adhesive. (S&N)
*Uses:* compression for leg ulcers; compression and support for fractured ribs, clavicles, swollen/sprained joints
**NHS Ventilated Elastic Adhesive Bandage**, BP. Fabric as for elastic adhesive bandage but adhesive spread such that there are regular strips of unspread fabric along length. (S&N)
*Uses:* compression for leg ulcers; compression and support for fractured ribs, clavicles, swollen/sprained joints

**NHS Extension Plaster**, BP. Woven fabric, elastic in weft, spread with adhesive mass containing zinc oxide, warp threads cotton and/or viscose, weft threads crepe-twisted cotton. (S&N)
*Uses:* support of light strains, joints and limbs removed from plaster casts, fractured ribs; traction bandaging

**NHS Cohesive extensible bandages.**
These elastic bandages adhere to themselves and not to the patient's skin, which prevents slipping during use. 2.25 m (both): 5 cm, 10 cm; 4.5 m (all): 5 cm, 7.5 cm, 10 cm, 15 cm (Boots, 3M—*Coban®*, J&J—*Secure®*, Seton, Steriseal—*Cohepress®*)
*Uses:* support of sprained joints

## MEDICATED BANDAGES
**Zinc Paste Bandage**, BP. Cotton fabric, plain weave, impregnated with suitable paste containing zinc oxide; requires additional bandaging. Net price 6 m × 7.5 cm = £2.48 (Seton—*Zincaband®* (15%)); £2.53 (S&N—*Viscopaste PB7®* (10%), *additives:*hydroxybenzoates)
**Zinc Paste and Calamine Bandage** (Drug Tariff). Cotton fabric, plain weave, impregnated with suitable paste containing calamine and zinc oxide; requires additional bandaging. Net price 6 m × 7.5 cm = £2.55 (Seton—*Calaband®*)
**Zinc Paste, Calamine, and Clioquinol Bandage**, BP. Cotton fabric, plain weave, impregnated with suitable paste containing calamine, clioquinol, and zinc oxide; requires additional bandaging. Net price 6 m × 7.5 cm = £2.55 (Seton—*Quinaband®*, *additives:* hydroxybenzoates)
**Zinc Paste and Coal Tar Bandage**, BP. Cotton fabric, plain weave, impregnated with a suitable paste containing coal tar and zinc oxide; requires additional bandaging. Net price 6 m × 7.5 cm = £2.58 (Seton—*Tarband®*, *additives:* hydroxybenzoates; S&N—*Coltapaste®*, *additives:* wool fat)
*Uses:* see section 13.5
**Zinc Paste and Ichthammol Bandage**, BP. Cotton fabric, plain weave, impregnated with suitable paste containing ichthammol and zinc oxide; requires additional bandaging. Net price 6 m × 7.5 cm = £2.54 (Seton—*Icthaband®* (15/2%), *additives:* hydroxybenzoates; S&N—*Ichthopaste®* (6/2%), *additives:* none as listed in section 13.1)
*Uses:* see section 13.5

## 13.13.2   Surgical adhesive tapes

### PERMEABLE SURGICAL ADHESIVE TAPES
**Zinc Oxide Surgical Adhesive Tape**, BP. (Zinc Oxide Plaster). Fabric, plain weave, warp and weft of cotton and/or viscose, spread with an adhesive containing zinc oxide. 1.25 cm, net price 1 m = 22p, 3 m = 45p, 5 m = 63p; 2.5 cm, 1 m = 30p, 3 m = 65p, 5 m = 92p; 5 cm × 5 m = £1.56; 7.5 cm × 5 m = £2.22 (most suppliers)
Drug Tariff specifies 1 m × 2.5 cm supplied when size not stated
*Uses:* securing dressings and immobilising small areas
**Permeable Woven Surgical Synthetic Adhesive Tape**, BP. Non-extensible closely woven fabric, spread with a polymeric adhesive. 5 m (all): 1.25 cm, net price = 55p; 2.5 cm = 80p; 5 cm = £1.40 (Beiersdorf—*Leukosilk®*)
*Uses:* securing dressings
For patients with skin reaction to other plasters and strapping, requiring use for long periods
**Elastic Surgical Adhesive Tape**, BP (Elastic Adhesive Plaster). Woven fabric, elastic in warp (crepe-twisted cotton threads), weft of cotton and/or viscose threads, spread with adhesive mass containing zinc oxide. 1.5 m

---

stretched × 2.5 cm, net price = 58p; 4.5 m stretched × 2.5 cm = £1.09 (Robinsons—*Flexoplast®*; S&N—*Elastoplast®*)
*Uses:* securing dressings
For 5 cm width, see Elastic Adhesive Bandage, section 13.13.1

**Permeable Non-woven Surgical Synthetic Adhesive Tape**, BP. Backing of paper-based or non-woven textile material spread with a polymeric adhesive mass. 5 m (all): Associated Hospital Supply—*Scanpor®* (net price 1.25 cm = 34p, 2.5 cm = 54p, 5 cm = 96p); Beiersdorf—*Leukopor®* (1.25 cm = 39p, 2.5 cm = 61p, 5 cm = £1.07); 3M—*Micropore®* (1.25 cm = 46p, 2.5 cm = 72p, 5 cm = £1.27); S&N—*Hypal 2®* (1.25 cm = 49p, 2.5 cm = 76p, 5 cm = £1.39)
Where no brand stated by prescriber, net price of tape supplied not to exceed 34p (1.25 cm), 54p (2.5 cm), 96p (5 cm)
*Uses:* securing dressings; skin closures for small incisions
For patients with skin reaction to other plasters and strapping, requiring use for long periods

NHS **Permeable Plastic Surgical Adhesive Tape**, BP. Extensible perforated plastic film spread with an adhesive mass; permeable to air and water (most suppliers)
*Uses:* securing dressings and appliances; covering sites of infection; allows immersion in water without loss of adhesion

## SEMIPERMEABLE SURGICAL ADHESIVE TAPES

NHS **Semipermeable Waterproof Plastic Surgical Adhesive Tape**, BP. Extensible water-impermeable, air and water-vapour permeable plastic film spread with an adhesive mass. (3M; J&J; S&N)
*Uses:* covering dressings and appliances where free passage of air and water-vapour but exclusion of water required; covering possible sites of infection; preparation of waterproof, microporous plastic wound dressings

## OCCLUSIVE SURGICAL ADHESIVE TAPES

**Impermeable Plastic Surgical Adhesive Tape**, BP. Extensible water-impermeable plastic film spread with an adhesive mass. 2.5 cm × 3 m, net price = 85p; 5 m = £1.28; 5 cm × 5 m = £1.64; 7.5 cm × 5 m = £2.36 (Robinsons; Seton; S&N)
*Uses:* securing dressings; covering site of infection where exclusion of air, water, and water vapour is required

**Impermeable Plastic Surgical Synthetic Adhesive Tape**, BP. Extensible water-impermeable plastic film spread with a polymeric adhesive mass. 5 m (both): net price, 2.5 cm = £1.20; 5 cm = £2.28 (3M—*Blenderm®*)
*Uses:* isolating wounds from external environment; covering sites where total exclusion of water and water vapour required; securing dressings and appliances

## 13.13.3 Adhesive dressings

(also termed Island dressings)

### PERMEABLE ADHESIVE DRESSINGS

NHS **Elastic Adhesive Dressing**, BP. Wound dressing or dressing strip, pad attached to piece of extension plaster, leaving suitable adhesive margin; both pad and margin covered with suitable protector; pad may be dyed yellow and may be impregnated with suitable antiseptic (see below); extension plaster may be perforated or ventilated (most suppliers)
*Uses:* general purpose wound dressing
*Note.* Permitted antiseptics are aminacrine hydrochloride, chlorhexidine hydrochloride (both 0.07–0.13%), chlorhexidine gluconate (0.11–0.20%); domiphen bromide (0.05–0.25%)

NHS **Permeable Plastic Wound Dressing**, BP. Consisting of an absorbent pad, which may be dyed and impregnated with a suitable antiseptic (see under Elastic Adhesive Dressing), attached to a piece of permeable plastic surgical adhesive tape, to leave a suitable adhesive margin; both pad and margin covered with suitable protector (most suppliers)
*Uses:* general purpose wound dressing, permeable to air and water

## SEMIPERMEABLE ADHESIVE DRESSINGS

**Semipermeable Waterproof Plastic Wound Dressing**, BP. Consists of absorbent pad, may be dyed and impregnated with suitable antiseptic (see under Elastic Adhesive Dressing), attached to piece of semipermeable waterproof surgical adhesive tape, to leave suitable adhesive margin; both pad and margin covered with suitable protector. 8.5 cm × 6 cm, net price = 26p (S&N—*Airstrip®*)
*Uses:* general purpose waterproof wound dressing, permeable to air and water vapour

## OCCLUSIVE ADHESIVE DRESSINGS

NHS **Impermeable Plastic Wound Dressing**, BP. Consists of absorbent pad, may be dyed and impregnated with suitable antiseptic (see under Elastic Adhesive Dressing), attached to piece of impermeable plastic surgical adhesive tape, to leave suitable adhesive margin; both pad and margin covered with suitable protector (most suppliers)
*Uses:* protective covering for wounds requiring an occlusive dressing

## 13.13.4 Surgical absorbents

**Absorbent Cotton**, BP. Carded cotton fibres of not less than 10 mm average staple length, available in rolls and balls. 25 g, net price = 47p; 100 g = £1.08; 500 g = £3.75 (most suppliers). 25-g pack to be supplied when weight not stated
*Uses:* general purpose cleansing and swabbing, pre-operative skin preparation, application of medicaments; supplementary absorbent pad to absorb excess wound exudate

**Absorbent Cotton, Hospital Quality.** As for absorbent cotton but lower quality materials, shorter staple length etc. 100 g, net price = 78p; 500 g = £2.56 (most suppliers)
Drug Tariff specifies to be supplied only where specifically ordered
*Uses:* suitable only as general purpose absorbent, for swabbing, and routine cleansing of incontinent patients; not for wound cleansing

**Gauze and Cotton Tissue**, BP. Consists of absorbent cotton enclosed in absorbent cotton gauze type 12 or absorbent cotton and viscose gauze type 2. 500 g, net price = £4.91 (most suppliers)
*Uses:* absorbent and protective pad, as burns dressing on non-adherent layer

**Gauze and Cotton Tissue** (Drug Tariff). Similar to above. 500 g, net price = £3.67 (most suppliers)
Drug Tariff specifies to be supplied only where specifically ordered
*Uses:* absorbent and protective pad, as burns dressing on non-adherent layer

**Absorbent Lint**, BPC. Cotton cloth of plain weave with nap raised on one side from warp yarns. 25 g, net price = 61p; 100 g = £1.87; 500 g = £7.90 (most suppliers). 25-g pack supplied where no quantity stated
*Uses:* external absorbent protective dressing

**Absorbent Cotton Gauze**, BP. Cotton fabric of plain weave, in rolls and as swabs (see below), usually Type 13 light, sterile. 90 cm (all) × 1 m, net price = 71p; 3 m = £1.49; 5 m = £2.32; 10 m = £4.48 (most suppliers). 1-m packet supplied when no size stated
*Uses:* pre-operative preparation, for cleansing and swabbing
*Note.* Drug Tariff also includes unsterilised absorbent cotton gauze, 25 m roll, net price = £10.53

**Cellulose Wadding**, BP. Delignified wood pulp bleached white, in multiple laminate form. 500 g, net price = £2.02 (most suppliers, including Robinsons—*Cellosene®*)
*Uses:* absorbing large volumes of fluid

**Gauze and Cellulose Wadding Tissue**, BP. Consists of thick layer of cellulose wadding enclosed in absorbent cotton gauze type 12 or absorbent cotton and viscose gauze type 2. 500 g, net price = £2.71 (most suppliers)
*Uses:* absorbing large volumes of fluid

**NHS Absorbent Muslin**, BP. Fabric of plain weave, warp threads of cotton, weft threads of cotton and/or viscose (most suppliers)
*Uses:* wet dressing, soaked in 0.9% sterile sodium chloride solution

**NHS Absorbent Cotton Ribbon Gauze**, BP. Cotton fabric of plain weave in ribbon form with fast selvedge edges (most suppliers)
*Uses:* post-surgery cavity packing for sinus, dental, throat cavities etc.

**Absorbent Cotton and Viscose Ribbon Gauze**, BP. Woven fabric in ribbon form with fast selvedge edges, warp threads of cotton, weft threads of viscose or combined cotton and viscose yarn, sterile. 5 m (both) × 1.25 cm, net price = 55p; 2.5 cm = 62p (most suppliers)
*Uses:* post-surgery cavity packing for sinus, dental, throat cavities etc.

**Gauze Swab**, BP. Consists of absorbent cotton gauze type 13 light or absorbent cotton and viscose gauze type 1 folded into squares or rectangles of 8-ply with no cut edges exposed. Sterile, 7.5 cm square, net price 5-pad packet = 26p; non-sterile, 10 cm square 100-pad packet = £4.37 (most suppliers)

**Filmated Gauze Swab**, BP. As for Gauze Swab, but with thin layer of Absorbent Cotton enclosed within. Non-sterile, 10 cm × 10 cm, net price 100-pad packet = £5.51 (Vernon-Carus—*Cotfil®*)
*Uses:* general swabbing and cleansing

**Non-woven Swab** (Drug Tariff). Consists of non-woven viscose fabric folded 4-ply; alternative to gauze swabs, type 13 light. Sterile, 7.5 cm square, net price 5-pad packet = 25p; non-sterile, 10 cm square, 100-pad packet = £3.20 (J&J—*Topper 8®*)
*Uses:* general purpose swabbing and cleansing; absorbs more quickly than gauze

**Non-woven Filmated Swab** (Drug Tariff). Film of viscose fibres enclosed within non-woven viscose fabric folded 8-ply. Non-sterile, 10 cm square, net price 100-pad packet = £4.38 (J&J—*Regal®*)
*Uses:* general purpose swabbing and cleansing

## 13.13.5   Wound dressing pads

**Perforated Film Absorbent Dressing**, BP. Low-adherence dressing consisting of 3 layers; wound-facing layer, film of poly-(ethylene terephthalate) perforated in regular pattern; absorbent middle layer of type 1 consists of non-woven bleached cotton and viscose fibres or mixture of these with polyacrylonitrile fibres; in type 2 (NHS ) middle layer consists of bleached cotton fibres; backing layer of type 1 is apertured non-woven cellulose material; in type 2, the backing layer is identical with wound-facing layer. Type 1, 5 cm × 5 cm, net price, each = 10p; 10 cm × 10 cm = 19p; 20 × 10 cm = 35p (S&N—*Melo-*

*lin®* (type 1); Kendall—*Telfa®* (type 2)). 5 cm size supplied where size not stated
*Uses:* dressing for post-operative and low exudate wounds; low adherence property and low absorption capacity

**Knitted Viscose Primary Dressing**, BP. (Drug Tariff title: Sterile Knitted Viscose Dressing). Warp knitted fabric manufactured from a bright viscose monofilament. 9.5 cm × 9.5 cm (both): net price = 25p (J&J—*N-A Dressing®*); net price = 20p (S&N—*Tricotex®*)
*Uses:* low adherence wound contact layer for use on ulcerative and other granulating wounds with superimposed absorbent pad

**Sterile Dressing Pack** (Drug Tariff specification 10). Contains gauze and cotton tissue pad, gauze swabs, absorbent cotton balls, absorbent paper towel, water repellent inner wrapper. Net price per pack = 63p

**Sterile Dressing Pack with Non-woven Pads** (Drug Tariff specification 35). Contains non-woven fabric covered dressing pad (*Surgipad®*), non-woven fabric swabs (*Topper 8®*), absorbent cotton wool balls, absorbent paper towel, water repellent inner wrapper. Net price per pack = 60p

**NHS* Surgipad®**. Absorbent pad of absorbent cotton and viscose in sleeve of non-woven viscose fabric (J&J )
*Uses:* for heavily exuding wounds requiring frequent dressing changes
* Except in Sterile Dressing Pack with Non-woven Pads (see above)

**NHS Perfron®**. Absorbent pad consisting of alternate layers of absorbent cotton and crepe cellulose tissue, in sleeve of non-woven viscose fabric with coating of polypropylene (J&J)
*Uses:* low adherence pad for heavily exuding wounds; laminate structure delays strike through

**NHS Melolite®**. Absorbent fabric pad covered on both sides by polyethylene net (S&N)
*Uses:* primary dressing over clean sutured wounds, lacerations, and abrasions

**NHS Mesorb®**. Cellulose wadding pad with gauze wound contact layer and non-woven water repellent backing (Molnlycke)
*Uses:* post-operative dressing for heavily exuding wounds

**NHS Ete®**. Wound pad of rayon wadding with rayon silk wound contact layer stitched in chequered pattern (Molnlycke)
*Uses:* leg wounds, decubitus ulcers, minor burns, donor sites

**NHS Release II®**. Two layered knitted construction of bright viscose in non-woven, non-adherent sleeve. Pack of 100 (all): 5 cm × 5 cm, net price = £5.23; 10 cm × 10 cm = £11.50; 10 cm × 20 cm = £18.93 (J&J)
*Uses:* high absorbency, low adherence wound contact dressing

## Charcoal cloth dressings

*Uses:* to deodorise discharging, infected, malodorous wounds and ulcers

**NHS Actisorb Plus®**. Knitted fabric of activated charcoal, with one-way stretch, with silver residues, within spun-bonded nylon sleeve. Net price (each) 10.5 cm × 10.5 cm = £1.37; 19 cm × 10.5 cm = £2.66 (J&J)

**NHS Carbonet®**. Activated charcoal dressing. 10 cm × 10 cm, net price, each = £1.56; 10 cm × 20 cm = £3.05 (S&N)

**NHS Carbosorb®**. Outer cover of non-woven polyester-nylon fabric, activated charcoal cloth layer bonded to outer cover and semipermeable polyurethane film contact layer (Seton)

**NHS CliniFlex® Odour Control Dressings**. Layer of activated charcoal cloth between viscose rayon with outer polyamide coating. Net price 10 cm × 10 cm, 10 = £12.00; 10 cm × 20 cm, 10 = £16.00; 15 cm × 25 cm, 10 = £26.00 (CliniFlex)

---

NHS **Lyofoam C**®. Lyofoam sheet with layer of activated charcoal cloth and additional outer envelope of polyurethane foam. 10 cm × 10 cm, net price, each = £1.26; 15 cm × 20 cm = £2.80 (Ultra)

## 13.13.6   Tulle dressings

### Non-medicated tulle dressings

**Paraffin Gauze Dressing**, BP. Fabric of leno weave, weft and warp threads of cotton and/or viscose yarn, impregnated with white or yellow soft paraffin; sterile. 10 cm × 10 cm, net price, each = 25p; pack of 10 pieces = £1.62 (most suppliers including Seton—*Paratulle*®; Roussel—*Unitulle*®; S&N—*Jelonet*®)

*Uses:* treatment of abrasions, burns, and other injuries of skin, and ulcerative conditions; post-operatively as penial and vaginal dressing and for sinus packing; heavier loading for skin graft transfer

### Medicated tulle dressings

**Chlorhexidine Gauze Dressing**, BP. Fabric of leno weave, weft and warp threads of cotton and/or viscose yarn, impregnated with ointment containing chlorhexidine acetate; sterile. 5 cm × 5 cm, net price = 19p; 10 cm × 10 cm = 39p (Seton—*Serotulle*®; Roussel—*Clorhexitulle*®; S&N—*Bactigras*®)

PoM **Framycetin Gauze Dressing**, BP. Fabric of leno weave, weft and warp threads of cotton, impregnated with ointment containing framycetin sulphate 1% in white soft paraffin containing 10% wool fat; sterile. 10 cm × 10 cm, net price = 24p; NHS 10 cm × 30 cm, 10 = £8.45 (Roussel—*Sofra-Tulle*®)

PoM **Sodium Fusidate Gauze Dressing**, BP. Leno weave cotton gauze impregnated with ointment containing sodium fusidate 2% in white soft paraffin and wool fat. 10 cm × 10 cm, net price = 22p (Leo—*Fucidin Intertulle*®)

**Povidone-Iodine Fabric Dressing.** Knitted viscose primary dressing impregnated with povidone-iodine ointment 10%. 5 cm × 5 cm, net price, each = 20p; 9.5 cm × 9.5 cm = 34p (J&J—*Inadine*®)

*Uses:* wound contact layer for abrasions and superficial burns; max. 4 dressings at same time

## 13.13.7   Semipermeable films and membranes

**Semipermeable Adhesive Film**, BP. Sterile, extensible, waterproof, water vapour-permeable polyurethane film coated with synthetic adhesive mass; transparent. Supplied in single-use pieces. Type 1: 10 cm × 10 cm, net price = £1.10 (S&N—*Opsite*® *Flexigrid*), Type 2: 10 cm × 12 cm, net price = £1.04 (3M—*Tegaderm*®). Type 3: 10.2 cm × 12.7 cm, net price = £1.10 (J&J—*Bioclusive*®)

*Uses:* post-operative dressing, donor sites, IV sites, superficial decubitus ulcers, amputation stumps, stoma care; protective cover to prevent skin breakdown

NHS **Dermoclude**®. Sterile, water-vapour permeable, transparent copolymer film. Supplied in single-use pieces. Pack of 25 (both): 10 cm × 10 cm, net price per pack = £22.50; 15 cm × 20 cm, £56.25 (BritCair).

*Uses:* cuts, grazes, minor burns and scalds, pressure sores, superficial leg ulcers

NHS **FlexiPore 6000**®. Sterile, water-vapour permeable double polymer membrane. Net price 10 cm × 10 cm, 50 = £92.50; 10 cm × 30 cm, 20 = £99.00; 15 cm × 20 cm, 20 = £99.00; 20 cm × 30 cm, 10 = £99.00 (CliniFlex)

*Uses:* donor sites, superficial burns, cuts, grazes, orthopaedic surgery

NHS **Omiderm**®. Sterile, adherent, water-vapour permeable polyurethane film. Net price 5 cm × 7 cm, net price 20 = £23.00; 8 cm × 10 cm, 20 = £49.00; 18 cm × 10 cm, 25 = £121.25; 60 cm × 10 cm, 10 = £138.00; 21 cm × 31 cm, 5 = £72.50 (Perstorp)

*Uses:* donor sites; superficial and partial thickness burns

NHS **Transite Film Dressing**®. Primary exudate transfer film composed of two layers which allow excess exudate to pass to secondary absorbent dressing through fine slits which narrow again when exudation decreases. Pack of 10 (all): 10 cm × 10 cm, net price = 79p; 15 cm × 20 cm = £1.24; 30 cm × 40 cm = £2.36 (S&N)

*Uses:* donor sites; partial and full thickness burns

## 13.13.8   Gel and colloid dressings

Occlusive or semi-occlusive dressings which adhere to dry skin and interact with moisture in the wound to form a gel; may remain on a wound for up to 7 days.

### Hydrogels

NHS **Bard Absorption Dressing**®. A dry polysaccharide derivative in flake form which is mixed with water and applied directly into the wound. 60-g pack

*Uses:* treatment of wounds and ulcers.

**Debrisan**®. Spherical beads of dextranomer packed in plastic castors, single-use sachets, paste or pads. Beads sprinkled onto cleansed wound and covered with a suitable non-woven, adhesive, semi-occlusive covering, or sterile dressing. Alternatively paste or pad is applied and covered in similar manner. Beads, net price 4-g sachet = £1.99, 60 g = £29.75; paste in sachets, 4 × 10 g = £20.40; pads, 3 g sachet = £2.36 (Kabi Pharmacia)

*Uses:* debriding agent to remove necrotic tissue

NHS **Geliperm**®. Gel sheets, dry and wet forms; tubed granulated gel. Dry, 11 cm × 25 cm, net price, 6 sheets = £51.23; granulate, 20 g, 6 tubes = £20.82, 50 g, 6 tubes = £52.04. Wet, 10 cm × 10 cm, net price, 20 sheets = £44.85, 12 cm × 13 cm, 6 sheets = £25.62; 12 cm × 26 cm, 6 sheets = £51.23 (Geistlich)

*Uses:* wound and ulcer dressing, burns, donor sites

PoM **Iodosorb**® Microbeads of cadexomer iodine (modified starch gel containing iodine 0.9%). Net price 3-g sachet = £2.07; also *Iodosorb*® Ointment, 4 × 10 g = £19.05; 2 × 20 g = £19.05 (Perstorp)

*Uses:* for venous leg ulcers and pressure sores apply 3 mm layer to wound surface and renew daily or when saturated with exudate

NHS **Kaltocarb**®. Dressing in 3 layers: wound-facing layer of calcium alginate fibre; absorbent middle layer of activated charcoal cloth; backing layer of bonded polyester and viscose non-woven material. Net price 7.5 cm × 12 cm, 25 = £44.75; 15 cm × 15 cm, 15 = £61.50 (BritCair)

*Uses:* discharging infected malodorous wounds and ulcers

NHS **Kaltoclude**®. Calcium alginate fibre bonded to semipermeable copolymer adhesive film. Pack of 25 (both); 10 cm × 10 cm, net price per pack = £40.00; 15 cm × 20 cm = £120.00 (BritCair)

*Uses:* light to moderately exuding wounds such as leg ulcers and pressure sores

**Kaltostat**®. (Drug Tariff title: Calcium Alginate Dressing, type 2). Calcium alginate fibre, flat non-woven pads, 5 cm × 5 cm, net price, each = 60p; 7.5 cm × 12 cm = £1.46; other sizes (NHS) 10 cm × 20 cm, 25 = £82.50; 15 cm × 25 cm, 25 = £143.75; 30 cm × 60 cm, 5 = £107.25; wound packing, 2 g, 25 = £70.00; also (NHS) Kaltostat® Fortex, 10 cm × 10 cm, 10 = £38.50 (BritCair)

*Uses:* haemostatic

**Scherisorb**® Gel. A ready-mixed hydrogel containing Graft T® starch copolymer applied directly into the wound. 15-g sachet, net price = £1.50 (S&N)

**Sorbsan®** (Drug Tariff title: Calcium Alginate Dressing, type 1). Calcium alginate fibre, highly absorbent, flat non-woven pads, 5 cm × 5 cm, net price, each = 77p; 10 cm × 10 cm = £1.22; other sizes (NHS) 10 cm × 20 cm, 5 = £18.00; surgical packing 30 cm, 5 = £19.50; ribbon, 40 cm (+12.5-cm probe), 5 = £12.50; also (bonded to a secondary absorbent viscose pad) Sorbsan® + (NHS), 7.5 cm × 10 cm, 5 = £9.95; 10 cm × 15 cm, 5 = £18.25 (Steriseal)
*Uses:* heavily to moderately exudating wounds

**NHS Sorbsan® SA** Calcium alginate fibre, highly absorbent flat non-woven pads for wound contact bonded to adhesive semipermeable polyurethane foam. Net price 9 cm × 11 cm, 5 = £9.50 (Steriseal)
*Uses:* moderately to lightly exudating shallow wounds

**NHS Vigilon®.** Semi-permeable hydrogel sheets on a polyethylene mesh support. Sterile, 3 in × 6 in, net price 10 = £35.50, 4 in × 4 in, 10 = £35.50; non-sterile, 4 in × 4 in, 10 = £24.75, 13 in × 24 in, 2 = £43.00 (Seton)

## Hydrocolloids

**NHS Biofilm®.** Hydrocolloid dressing with non-woven fibre backing; also in powder form for direct application into wound: 10 cm × 10 cm, net price 10 = £16.50; 20 cm × 20 cm, 5 = £28.50; powder, 10 sachets = £18.20 (CliniMed)

**Comfeel®.** Soft elastic pad consisting of carmellose (carboxymethylcellulose) sodium particles embedded in adhesive mass; smooth outer layer and polyurethane film backing; available as sheets, powder in plastic blister units and paste for direct application into the wound: ulcer dressing, 10 cm × 10 cm, net price each = £1.79; 15 cm × 15 cm = £3.58; 20 cm × 20 cm = £5.37; other sizes (NHS) 4 cm × 6 cm, 30 = £22.20; transparent dressing, 5 cm × 7 cm, 10 = £9.70; 9 cm × 14 cm, 10 = £28.60; 15 cm × 20 cm, 5 = £32.15; powder 6 g, 10 = £24.80; paste 12-g sachet, 10 = £10.40, 50-g tube, 10 = £36.60 (Coloplast)

**NHS Dermiflex®.** Hydrocolloid dressing bonded to PVC foam 10.2 cm × 10.2 cm, net price, each = £1.95 (J&J)

**Granuflex®.** Hydrocolloid wound contact layer bonded to plastic foam layer, with outer impermeable plastic film. 10 cm × 10 cm, net price each = £1.88; 15 cm × 20 cm = £4.00; other sizes (NHS), 20 cm × 20 cm, 3 = £18.11, 15 cm × 15 cm with adhesive foam border, 5 = £19.47; also Granuflex® Extra Thin (NHS), 7.5 cm × 7.5 cm, 5 = £5.05; 10 cm × 10 cm, 5 = £6.91; 15 cm × 15 cm, 5 = £15.58; 5 cm × 10 cm, 10 = £6.92; 5 cm × 20 cm, 10 = £13.82; also Granuflex® Compression Bandage (NHS), 10 cm × 6.5 cm, 6 = £32.62; also Granuflex Paste (NHS), net price 30 g = £2.61 (Convatec)
*Uses:* chronic ulcers, pressure sores, open wounds, debridement of wounds; powders and pastes used with sheet dressings to fill deep or heavily exudating wounds

**Tegasorb®.** Hydrocolloid dressing bordered with adhesive film edge, 10 cm × 12 cm (oval), net price each = £1.76; other sizes (NHS) 13 cm × 15 cm (oval), 5 = £23.14; 17 cm × 20 cm (oval), 3 = £20.15 (3M)
*Uses:* chronic wounds such as leg ulcers and pressure sores

## 13.13.9    Foam dressings

**Polyurethane Foam Dressing,** BP. Absorbent foam dressing of low adherence; sterile. 7.5 cm × 7.5 cm, net price, each = 69p; 10 cm × 10 cm, each = 82p; other sizes (NHS) 10 cm × 17.5 cm, 25 = £31.68; 15 cm × 20 cm, 20 = £34.46; 10 cm × 25 cm, 35 = £58.05; 25 cm × 30 cm, each = £3.91 (Ultra—Lyofoam®)
*Uses:* treatment of burns, decubitus ulcers, donor sites, granulating wounds

**NHS Allevyn®.** Hydrophilic polyurethane dressing; foam sheets with trilaminate structure, non-adherent wound contact layer, foam based central layer, bacteria and waterproof outer layer. 10 cm × 10 cm, each = £2.95 (S&N)
*Uses:* treatment of heavily exuding wounds, specifically venous leg ulcers

**NHS Silicone Foam Cavity Wound Dressing,** BP. Soft slightly absorbent wound dressing of low adherence prepared from fluid silicone elastomer base and tin (II) 2-ethylhexanoate by mixing thoroughly for 15 seconds immediately before use and allowing to expand to about 4 times its volume within the wound. Foam dressing, 20 g, net price = £5.10; 500 g = £83.43; gel sheeting, 12 cm × 15 cm, 10 = £77.50 (Dow Corning—Silastic®)
*Uses:* in the managment of open granulating wounds such as pressure sores, abdominal wall breakdown, pilonidal sinus excision

## 13.13.10    Elastic hosiery

Before elastic hosiery can be dispensed, the quantity (single or pair), article (including accessories), and compression class (I, II or III) must be specified by the prescriber; for further details see Drug Tariff

### Graduated compression hosiery

**Class 1** Light Support
*Hosiery,* compression at ankle 14–17 mm Hg, thigh length or below knee with knitted in heel. Net price per pair, circular knit (standard), thigh length = £5.50, below knee = £5.00; light weight elastic net (made-to-measure), thigh length = £13.98, below knee = £10.90
*Uses:* superficial or early varices, varicosis during pregnancy

**Class 2** Medium Support
*Hosiery,* compression at ankle 18–24 mm Hg, thigh length or below knee with knitted in heel. Net price per pair, circular knit (standard), thigh length = £8.20, below knee = £7.30, (made-to-measure), thigh length = £26.40, below knee = £16.50; net (made-to-measure), thigh length = £13.98, below knee = £10.90; flat bed (made-to-measure, only with closed heel and open toe), thigh length = £26.40, below knee = £16.50
*Uses:* varices of medium severity, ulcer treatment and prophylaxis, mild oedema, varicosis during pregnancy

**Class 3** Strong Support
*Hosiery,* compression at ankle 25–35 mm Hg, thigh length or below knee with open or knitted in heel. Net price per pair, circular knit (standard), thigh length = £9.70, below knee = £8.30, (made-to-measure) thigh length = £26.40, below knee = £16.50; one way stretch (made-to-measure, only with open heel and open toe), thigh length = £26.40, below knee = £16.50
*Uses:* gross varices, post thrombotic venous insufficiency, gross oedema, ulcer treatment and prophylaxis

### Accessories

*Suspender,* for thigh stockings, net price = 46p; belt (specification 13), = £3.50, fitted (additional price) = 46p

### Anklets

**Class 2** Medium Support
*Anklets,* compression 18–24 mm Hg, circular knit (standard and made-to-measure), net price per pair = £4.62; flat bed (standard and made-to-measure) = £9.68; net (made-to-measure) = £8.98
*Uses:* soft tissue support

**Class 3** Strong Support

*Anklets*, compression 25–35 mm Hg, circular knit (standard and made-to-measure), net price per pair = £6.42; one way stretch (standard and made-to-measure) = £6.42

*Uses:* soft tissue support

## Kneecaps

**Class 2** Medium Support

*Kneecaps*, circular knit (standard and made-to-measure), net price per pair = £4.62; flat bed (standard and made-to-measure) = £9.68; net (made-to-measure) = £7.46

*Uses:* soft tissue support

**Class 3** Strong Support

*Kneecaps*, circular knit (standard and made-to-measure), net price per pair = £6.18; one way stretch (standard and made-to-measure) = £6.18

*Uses:* soft tissue support

# 13.14   Topical circulatory preparations

These preparations are used to improve circulation in conditions such as bruising, superficial thrombophlebitis, chilblains and varicose veins but are of little value. Chilblains are best managed by avoidance of exposure to cold; neither systemic nor topical vasodilator therapy is established as being effective. Sclerotherapy of varicose veins is described in section 2.13.

Rubefacients are described in section 10.3.2.

**Hirudoid**® (Panpharma)

*Cream*, heparinoid 0.3% in a vanishing-cream basis. Net price 40 g = £1.90

*Additives:* hydroxybenzoates (parabens)

*Gel*, heparinoid 0.3%. Net price 40 g = £1.90

*Additives:* propylene glycol, fragrance

Apply up to 4 times daily in superficial soft-tissue injuries and superficial thrombophlebitis

**Lasonil**® (Bayer)

*Ointment*, heparinoid 50 units, hyaluronidase 150 units/g. Net price 14 g = 38p; 40 g = £1.08

*Additives:* wool fat derivative

Apply 2–3 times daily in superficial soft-tissue injuries

**Secaderm**® (Fisons)

*Salve* (= ointment), colophony 26%, melaleuca oil 5.6%, phenol 2.4%, terebene 5.25%, turpentine oil 6% for boils and chilblains. Net price 15 g = 85p

*Additives:* beeswax

Apply 1–2 times daily and cover with dressing

---

432

# 14: Immunological products and

# VACCINES

In this chapter, immunisation is discussed under the following headings:

**14.1** Active immunity
**14.2** Passive immunity
**14.3** Storage and use
**14.4** Vaccines and antisera
**14.5** Immunoglobulins
**14.6** International travel

## 14.1 Active immunity

**Vaccines** produce specific protection against a given disease. They may consist of:

1. an attenuated form of an infective agent, as in the vaccines which are used against virus diseases such as rubella and measles, or BCG used against tuberculosis,
2. inactivated preparations of the virus (e.g. influenza vaccine) or bacteria (e.g. typhoid vaccine), or
3. extracts of or detoxified exotoxins produced by a micro-organism (e.g. tetanus vaccine).

Vaccines stimulate the production of protective antibodies and other components of the immune mechanism.

For **live** vaccines, immunisation is generally achieved with a single dose, but 3 doses are required with oral poliomyelitis vaccine. Live virus multiplies in the body and usually produces a durable immunity but not always as long as that of the natural infection. When two live virus vaccines are required (and are not available as a combined preparation) they should be given either simultaneously at different sites or with an interval of at least 3 weeks.

**Inactivated** vaccines usually require a primary series of doses of vaccine to produce an adequate antibody response and in most cases reinforcing or 'booster' injections are required. The duration of immunity following the use of inactivated vaccines varies from months to many years.

The health departments of the UK have issued a memorandum, *Immunisation against Infectious Disease 1990* which describes the vaccines, immunoglobulins, and antisera in routine use in the UK; recommended schemes for immunisation in childhood are included and advice is given on storage, technique, and record keeping.

*Immunisation against Infectious Disease* can be obtained from:

HMSO Publications Centre
PO Box 276, London SW8 5DT
Telephone orders, 071-873 9090

*or* from HMSO bookshops and through all good booksellers.

SIDE-EFFECTS. Some vaccines (e.g. poliomyelitis vaccines) produce very few reactions, while others (e.g. measles and rubella vaccines) may produce a very mild form of the disease. Some vaccines may produce discomfort at the site of injection and mild fever and malaise. Occasionally there are more serious untoward reactions and these

should always be reported in the usual way to the CSM. Anaphylactic reactions are very rare but can be fatal (see section 3.4.3 for the management of allergic emergencies).

CONTRA-INDICATIONS. Most vaccines have some basic contra-indication to their use, and the manufacturer's leaflet should always be consulted. In general, vaccination should be postponed if the subject is suffering from an *acute illness*. Minor infections without fever or systemic upset are not contra-indications.

Some viral vaccines contain small quantities of antibiotics such as neomycin or polymyxin (or both); such vaccines may need to be withheld from individuals who are *sensitive to the antibiotic*. *Hypersensitivity to egg* contra-indicates influenza vaccine (residual egg protein present) and, if evidence of previous anaphylactic reaction, also MMR and yellow fever vaccines.

Live vaccines should not be routinely administered to *pregnant women* because of possible harm to the fetus but where there is a significant risk of exposure (e.g. to poliomyelitis or yellow fever), the need for vaccination outweighs any possible risk to the fetus. Live vaccines should not be given to individuals with *impaired immune responsiveness*, whether caused by disease (for special reference to *AIDS*, see below) or as a result of radiotherapy or treatment with high doses of corticosteroids or other immunosuppressive drugs[1,2]. They should not be given to those suffering from *malignant conditions* or other tumours of the reticulo-endothelial system[2].

VACCINES AND AIDS. The Department of Health has advised that HIV-positive subjects with or without symptoms can receive the following live vaccines as appropriate:

measles[2] (or MMR), mumps, poliomyelitis[3], rubella;

and the following inactivated vaccines:

cholera, diphtheria, hepatitis B, pertussis, poliomyelitis[3], tetanus, typhoid.

HIV-positive subjects should **not** receive:

BCG, yellow fever[4]

*Note.* The above advice differs from that for other immunocompromised patients.

---

1. Live vaccines should be postponed until at least 3 months after stopping corticosteroids and 6 months after stopping chemotherapy.
2. Consideration should be given to use of normal immunoglobulin after exposure to measles and to varicella-zoster immunoglobulin after exposure to varicella.
3. Virus may be excreted for longer periods than in normal subjects; contacts should be warned of this and of need for washing hands after changing a vaccinated infant's nappies; HIV-positive contacts are at greater risk than normal contacts. For HIV-positive symptomatic subjects inactivated poliomyelitis vaccine can be used at discretion of clinician.
4. Because insufficient evidence of safety.

# Vaccination programmes

The principal points are as follows:

1. The *basic course* is as set out below.

2. There is no contra-indication to administration of pertussis vaccine to unimmunised older children in order to protect infants and siblings. Since a course of 3 injections is required to protect against whooping cough, vaccine cannot be used to control an outbreak.

If the pertussis component has been omitted from earlier vaccinations 3 doses of pertussis vaccine can be given at monthly intervals to provide protection.

Where the basic course against diphtheria and tetanus is incomplete triple vaccine may be used to begin or complete the course against whooping-cough so that the infant is not given more injections than necessary.

3. Measles/mumps/rubella vaccine can be given at the time of the reinforcing dose of diphtheria/tetanus vaccine and poliomyelitis vaccine; because the diphtheria/tetanus vaccine can be more painful, measles/mumps/rubella vaccine should be injected first; the diphtheria/tetanus should then be given with a separate syringe and needle in the opposite limb (or a second appointment can be made).

> Vaccines for the childhood immunisation programme should be obtained via local Health Authorities rather than by FP10 prescription.

| Age | Vaccine | Interval | Notes |
|---|---|---|---|
| During the first year of life | DTPer/Vac/Ads *and* Pol/Vac (Oral) | 3 doses at intervals of 4 weeks | The first doses should be given at 2 months of age |
| During the second year of life | Meas/Mump/Rub (MMR) Vac (Live) | | |
| At school entry or entry to nursery school | DT/Vac/Ads *and* Pol/Vac (Oral) | Preferable to allow an interval of at least 3 years after completing basic course | |
| | Meas/Mump/Rub (MMR) Vac (Live) | | Unless documented history of measles/mumps/rubella vaccination *or* valid contra-indication *or* laboratory evidence of immunity to measles, mumps, and rubella |
| Between 10th and 14th birthdays | BCG | Leave an interval of not less than 3 weeks between BCG and rubella vaccination | For tuberculin-negative children. For tuberculin-negative contacts at any age |
| Between 10th and 14th birthdays (girls only) | Rub/Vac (Live) | | All girls of this age should be offered rubella vaccine regardless of a past history of an attack of rubella (unless documented history of Meas/Mump/Rub Vac) |
| On leaving school or before employment or further education | Pol/Vac (Oral) *and* Tet/Vac/Ads | | |
| Adult life | Pol/Vac (Oral) if previously unvaccinated | 3 doses at intervals of 4 weeks | No adult should remain unimmunised; reinforcing doses for travellers to countries where polio endemic and for health care workers in possible contact with polio |
| | Rub/Vac (Live) for susceptible women of child-bearing age | | Women of child-bearing age should be tested for rubella antibodies and if sero-negative offered rubella vaccination. Pregnancy must be excluded and patient warned not to become pregnant for 1 month after |
| | Tet/Vac/Ads if previously unvaccinated | For previously unvaccinated adults: 2 doses at an interval of 4 weeks followed by a third dose 4 weeks later | A reinforcing dose 10 years after primary course and again 10 years later maintains a satisfactory level of protection |
| | Hepatitis B | | Individuals in high-risk groups |
| | Influenza | | Individuals in high-risk groups |

Cautionary label wordings, see inside back cover

Prices are **net**, see p. 1

Post-immunisation pyrexia—Joint Committee on Vaccination and Immunisation recommendation. The doctor should advise the parent that if pyrexia develops after immunisation the child can be given a dose of paracetamol followed, if necessary, by a second dose 4 to 6 hours later. The dose of paracetamol for post-immunisation pyrexia in an infant aged 2–3 months is 60 mg; an oral syringe can be obtained from any pharmacy to give the small dose-volume required. The doctor should warn the parent that if the pyrexia persists after the second dose medical advice should be sought.

For full range of doses of paracetamol, see p. 167.

## 14.2   Passive immunity

Immunity with immediate protection against certain infective organisms can be obtained by injecting preparations made from the plasma of immune individuals with adequate levels of antibody to the disease for which protection is sought (see under Immunoglobulins, section 14.5). This passive immunity lasts only a few weeks; where necessary passive immunisation can be repeated.

Antibodies of human origin are usually termed *immunoglobulins*. The term *antiserum* is applied to material prepared in animals. Because of serum sickness and other allergic-type reactions that may follow injections of antisera, this therapy has been replaced wherever possible by the use of immunoglobulins. Reactions are theoretically possible after injection of human immunoglobulins but reports of such reactions are very rare.

## 14.3   Storage and use

Care must be taken to store all vaccines and other immunological products under the conditions recommended in the manufacturer's leaflet, otherwise the preparation may become denatured and totally ineffective. **Refrigerated storage** is usually necessary; many vaccines need to be stored at 2–8°C and not allowed to freeze. Opened multidose vials which have not been fully used should be discarded within one hour if no preservative is present (most live virus vaccines) or within 3 hours or at the end of a session (when vaccines containing a preservative are used but also including oral poliomyelitis vaccine).

Particular attention must be paid to the instructions on the use of diluents and ampoules of vaccine should always be adequately shaken before use to ensure uniformity of the material to be injected.

*Note.* The Department of Health has advised against the use of jet guns for vaccination owing to the risk of transmitting blood-borne infections, such as HIV.

## 14.4   Vaccines and antisera

AVAILABILITY. Anthrax, rabies, smallpox, and yellow fever vaccines, botulism antitoxin, and snake venom antitoxin are available from local designated holding centres. Details of current arrangements with names, addresses, and telephone numbers of holding centres are given in: *The Health Service Supply Purchasing Guide*, section D pp. 1101–1199

and

*The Pharmaceutical Supplies Bulletin*, volume 8, no. 5, Oct. 1985, 63/85.

For telephone numbers for information on supply of antivenom, see also p. 22.

Enquiries for vaccines not available commercially can also be made to
Department of Health
Room 222
14 Russell Square
London WC1B 5EP
telephone 071-636 6811 extn 3117/3236.

In Scotland information about availability of vaccines can be obtained from the Chief Administrative Pharmaceutical Officer of the local Health Board. In Wales enquiries should be directed to the Welsh Office, Cathays Park, Cardiff CF1 3NQ, telephone 0222 825111, extn 4658 and in Northern Ireland to the Department of Health and Social Services, Dundonald House, Belfast BT4 3FS, telephone 0232 63939 extn 2841.

For further details of availability, see under individual vaccines.

## ANTHRAX VACCINE

Anthrax vaccine is available for anyone subject to heavy exposure to anthrax, such as those exposed to infected hides and carcasses and to imported bonemeal, fishmeal, and feeding stuffs. The vaccine is the alum precipitate of an antigen from *Bacillus anthracis* and, following the primary course of injections, reinforcing doses should be given at about yearly intervals.

PoM **Anthrax Vaccine**
*Dose:* initial course 3 doses of 0.5 mL by intramuscular injection at intervals of 3 weeks followed by a 4th dose after an interval of 6 months
Reinforcing doses: 0.5 mL annually
Available from local designated centres

## BCG VACCINES

BCG (Bacillus Calmette-Guérin) is a live attenuated strain derived from bovine *Mycobacterium tuberculosis* which stimulates the development of hypersensitivity to *M. tuberculosis*. BCG vaccine should be given intradermally by operators skilled in the technique (see below); the percutaneous vaccine is **not** recommended.

Within 2–6 weeks a small swelling appears at the injection site which progresses to a papule or to a benign ulcer about 10 mm in diameter and heals in 6–12 weeks. A dry dressing may be used if the ulcer discharges, but the air should **not** be excluded. The CSM has reported that serious reactions with BCG are uncommon and most often consist of prolonged ulceration or subcutaneous abscess formation due to faulty injection technique.

BCG is recommended for the following groups if they are negative for tuberculoprotein hypersensitivity:

contacts of those with active respiratory tuberculosis (immigrants in whose communities there is a high incidence of tuberculosis may be regarded as contacts—newborn infants need not be tested for sensitivity but should be vaccinated without delay);

health service staff (including medical students, hospital medical staff, nurses, and anybody who comes into contact with patients, including physiotherapists and radiographers, technical staff in pathology departments and any others considered to be at special risk because of the likelihood of contact with infective patients or their sputum; particularly important to test staff in maternity and paediatric departments);

children between their tenth and fourteenth birthdays (see schedule, section 14.1);

students (including those in teacher training colleges);

veterinary and other staff who handle animal species known to be susceptible to tuberculosis;

those travelling to countries with a high incidence of tuberculosis (section 14.6)

Apart from newborn infants any person being considered for BCG vaccination must first be given a skin test for hypersensitivity to tuberculoprotein (see under Diagnostic agents, below).

It is recommended that an interval of at least 3 weeks should be allowed between the administration of a live vaccine and BCG. However, when BCG is given to infants, there is no need to delay the primary immunisations, including poliomyelitis.

See section 14.1 for general contra-indications. BCG is also contra-indicated in subjects with generalised septic skin conditions (in the case of eczema, a vaccination site free from lesions should be chosen).

PoM **Bacillus Calmette-Guérin Vaccine.** BCG Vaccine, Dried Tub/Vac/BCG. A freeze-dried preparation of live bacteria of a strain derived from the bacillus of Calmette and Guérin.
*Dose:* 0.1 mL (INFANT under 3 months 0.05 mL) by intradermal injection
Available from District Health Authorities (also from Evans)

INTRADERMAL INJECTION TECHNIQUE. After swabbing with spirit and allowing to dry, skin is stretched between thumb and forefinger and needle (size 25G) inserted (bevel upwards) for about 2 mm into superficial layers of dermis (almost parallel with surface). Needle should be short with short bevel (can usually be seen through epidermis during insertion). Raised blanched bleb showing tips of hair follicles is sign of correct injection; 7 mm bleb ≡ 0.1 mL injection; if considerable resistance not felt, needle is removed and reinserted before giving more vaccine.

Injection site is at insertion of deltoid muscle onto humerus (sites higher on arm more likely to lead to keloid formation); tip of shoulder should be **avoided**; in girls, for cosmetic reasons, upper and lateral surface of thigh may be preferred.

PoM **Bacillus Calmette-Guérin Vaccine, Isoniazid-Resistant.** A freeze-dried preparation of live bacteria of an isoniazid-resistant strain derived from the bacillus of Calmette and Guérin.
*Dose:* 0.1 mL (INFANT under 3 months 0.05 mL) by intradermal injection; for active immunisation of tuberculosis contacts receiving prophylactic treatment with isoniazid.
Available from Evans

PoM **Bacillus Calmette-Guérin Vaccine, Percutaneous** Tub/Vac/BCG(Perc). A preparation of live bacteria of a strain derived from the bacillus of Calmette and Guérin.
*Dose:* 0.02 mL by percutaneous administration but not recommended, see notes above.
Available from Evans

DIAGNOSTIC AGENTS. In the *Mantoux test* the initial diagnostic dose in patients in whom tuberculosis is suspected (or who are known to be hypersensitive to tuberculin) is 1 unit of tuberculin PPD in 0.1 mL by intradermal injection and in subsequent tests 10 and finally 100 units in 0.1 mL may be given. For routine pre-BCG skin-testing the 10-unit dose of tuberculin PPD is used. In the *Heaf test* (multiple puncture) a solution containing 100 000 units in 1 mL is used.

PoM **Tuberculin PPD.** Prepared from the heat-treated products of growth and lysis of the appropriate species of mycobacterium, and containing 100 000 units/mL. Net price 1-mL amp = £5.89. Also available diluted 1 in 100 (1000 units/mL), 1 in 1000 (100 units/mL), and 1 in 10000 (10 units/mL). Net price 1 mL (all) = £2.22
Available from District Health Authorities (also from Evans)

## BOTULISM ANTITOXIN

A trivalent botulism antitoxin is available for the post-exposure prophylaxis of botulism and for the treatment of persons thought to be suffering from botulism. It specifically neutralises the toxins produced by *Clostridium botulinum* types A, B, and E. It is not effective against infantile botulism as the toxin (type A) is seldom, if ever, found in the blood in this type of infection.

Hypersensitivity reactions are a problem. It is essential to read the contra-indications, warnings, and details of sensitivity tests on the package insert. Prior to treatment checks should be made regarding previous administration of any antitoxin and history of any allergic condition, e.g. asthma, hay fever, etc. All patients should be tested for sensitivity (diluting the antitoxin if history of allergy).

PoM **Botulism Antitoxin.** A preparation containing the specific antitoxic globulins that have the power of neutralising the toxins formed by types A, B, and E of *Clostridium botulinum*.
*Note.* The BP title Botulinum Antitoxin is not used because the preparation currently available has a higher phenol content (0.45% against 0.25%).
*Dose:* prophylaxis, 20 mL by intramuscular injection as soon as possible after exposure; treatment, 20 mL by slow intravenous infusion followed by 10 mL 2–4 hours later if necessary, and further doses at intervals of 12–24 hours.
Available from local designated centres

## CHOLERA VACCINE

**Cholera vaccine** contains heat-killed Inaba and Ogawa sub-types of *Vibrio cholerae*, Serovar O1. Cholera vaccine provides little protection and cannot control the spread of the disease. The Department of Health has therefore advised that:

immunisation against cholera is no longer a legal requirement for entry into any foreign country and should not be required of any traveller. However, border officials in some countries may still ask people travelling from endemic or epidemic areas for evidence of immunisation. Travellers who are likely to cross borders from such areas, especially overland, should therefore be advised to have the vaccine here before travel rather than risk injections abroad. One injection is sufficient.

Patients who travel to a country where cholera exists should be warned that attention to the hygiene of food and water is **essential**, even after vaccination.

PoM **Cholera Vaccine** Cho/Vac. Net price 1.5-mL vial = £4.51; 10-mL vial = £7.18
*Dose:* 0.5 mL by deep subcutaneous or by intramuscular injection; CHILD under 1 year, not recommended, 1–5 years 0.1 mL, 5–10 years 0.3 mL
*Note.* Department of Health (Chief Medical Officer's letter of September 1991) recommends that only 1 dose need be given, see also notes above
Available from Evans

## DIPHTHERIA VACCINES

Protection against diphtheria is essentially due to antitoxin, the production of which is stimulated by vaccines prepared from the toxin of *Corynebacterium diphtheriae*. These are more effective and cause fewer reactions if adsorbed onto a mineral carrier. Adsorbed diphtheria vaccines are recommended for the routine immunisation of babies and given in the form of a triple vaccine, **adsorbed diphtheria, tetanus, and pertussis vaccine** (see schedule, section 14.1). Adsorbed diphtheria and tetanus vaccine is used when immunisation against whooping-cough is contra-indicated.

A reinforcing dose of adsorbed diphtheria and tetanus vaccine is recommended at school entry (4–5 years of age), preferably given at least 3 years after the last dose of the basic course.

Further reinforcing doses of diphtheria vaccine are not recommended as a routine except in the case of those who work in units where there is a potentially high risk of infection such as those employed in infectious disease units or microbiology laboratories. A dilute vaccine, adsorbed diphtheria vaccine for adults, is available for this purpose. The small quantity of diphtheria toxoid present in the preparation is sufficient to recall immunity in individuals previously immunised against diphtheria but whose immunity may have diminished with time; it is insufficient to cause the serious reactions that may occur when diphtheria vaccine of conventional formulation is used in an individual who is already immune. The dilute vaccine must be used when immunising adults and children over 10 years; it may be given without prior Schick testing.

**Diphtheria antitoxin** is used for passive immunisation; it is prepared in horses therefore reactions are common after administration.

It is now only used in suspected cases of diphtheria (without waiting for bacteriological confirmation); tests for hypersensitivity should be first carried out.

It is no longer used for prophylaxis because of the risk of hypersensitivity; unimmunised contacts should be promptly investigated and given erythromycin prophylaxis (see section 5.1, table 2) and vaccine (see below).

Combined vaccines
*With tetanus and pertussis (triple vaccine)*
PoM **Adsorbed Diphtheria, Tetanus, and Pertussis Vaccine** DTPer/Vac/Ads. Prepared from diphtheria formol toxoid, tetanus formol toxoid, and pertussis vaccine with a mineral carrier (aluminium hydroxide).
*Dose:* primary immunisation of children, 0.5 mL by intramuscular or deep subcutaneous injection at 2 months followed by second dose after 4 weeks and third dose after another 4 weeks (see schedule, section 14.1)
Available as **Trivax-AD®** (Evans). Net price 0.5-mL amp = £1.32; 5-mL vial = £7.02
PoM **Diphtheria, Tetanus, and Pertussis Vaccine** DTPer/Vac. A mixture of diphtheria formol toxoid, tetanus formol toxoid, and pertussis vaccine. The adsorbed vaccine is preferred
Available as **Trivax®** (Evans). Net price 0.5-mL amp = £1.32; 5-mL vial = £7.02

*With tetanus only*
PoM **Adsorbed Diphtheria and Tetanus Vaccine** DT/Vac/Ads. Prepared from diphtheria formol toxoid and tetanus formol toxoid with a mineral carrier (aluminium hydroxide).
*Dose:* primary immunisation of children omitting pertussis component, 0.5 mL by intramuscular or deep subcutaneous injection at 2 months followed by second dose after 4 weeks and third dose after another 4 weeks (see schedule, section 14.1); reinforcement at school entry, 0.5 mL (see schedule, section 14.1)
Available from Evans (net price 0.5-mL amp = £1.14; 5-mL vial = £4.95), Merieux (net price 0.5-mL amp = £1.11; 0.5-mL pre-filled syringe = £1.95)
PoM **Diphtheria and Tetanus Vaccine** DT/Vac/FT. A mixture of diphtheria formol toxoid and tetanus formol toxoid. The adsorbed vaccine is preferred
Available from Evans. Net price 5-mL vial = £4.95

Single antigen vaccines
*For children*
PoM **Diphtheria Vaccine, Adsorbed** Dip/Vac/Ads. Prepared from diphtheria formol toxoid with a mineral carrier (aluminium hydroxide). Net price 0.5-mL amp = £1.12
*Note.* Used only for contacts of a diphtheria case or carrier; immunised children under 10 years are given one dose of 0.5 mL by intramuscular or by deep subcutaneous injection, unimmunised children under 10 years are given three doses of 0.5 mL with an interval of 4 weeks between first and second doses and another 4 weeks between second and third; adults and children over 10 years must be given diphtheria vaccine for adults, adsorbed (see below).
Available from Evans

---

*Low dose vaccine for adults*

PoM **Diphtheria Vaccine for Adults, Adsorbed.**
Dip/Vac/Ads for Adults. Net price 0.5-mL
amp = £3.00

*Dose:* primary immunisation in patients over 10
years without prior Schick testing, three doses
each of 0.5 mL by intramuscular or deep subcutaneous injection separated by intervals of 1
month; reinforcement, 0.5 mL

Note. Unimmunised adults and children over 10 years
who are contacts of a diphtheria case or carrier are given
the primary immunisation course; immunised adults and
children over 10 years are given the reinforcement dose.

Available from distributor (Regent)

Antisera

PoM **Diphtheria Antitoxin** Dip/Ser.
*Dose:* prophylactic 500 to 2000 units by intramuscular injection (but **not** used, see notes
above); therapeutic 10 000 to 30 000 units
increased to 40 000 to 100 000 units in severe
cases; doses of up to 30 000 units should be given
intramuscularly but for those over 40 000 units a
portion is given intramuscularly followed by the
bulk of the dose intravenously after an interval of
$\frac{1}{2}$–2 hours

Note. Children require the same dose as adults, depending
on the severity of the case.

Available from distributor (Regent) or stocks may
be held by hospital pharmacies

DIAGNOSTIC AGENTS. The *Schick test* is recommended for
individuals who may be exposed to diphtheria in the course
of their work. In such cases immunity to diphtheria is
confirmed by means of a Schick test carried out at least 3
months after completion of immunisation. A dose of
0.2 mL of Schick Test Toxin is injected intradermally into
the flexor surface of the left forearm and 0.2 mL of Schick
Control into the corresponding position on the right arm.
Readings are made at 24–48 hours and 5–7 days.

PoM **Schick Test Toxin** and **Control.** Sterile diluted fil-
trate from a culture of *Corynebacterium diphtheriae*. The
control is the same medium heated to inactivate the
toxin. Net price 2-mL toxin and control set = £15.71
Available from Evans

## HEPATITIS B VACCINE

**Hepatitis B vaccine** is an alum-adsorbed, inactivated hepatitis B virus surface antigen (HBsAg)
vaccine. It is made biosynthetically using recombinant DNA technology. The vaccine is used in
individuals at high risk of contracting hepatitis B.

In the UK, high-risk groups include health care
personnel and patients in units where there is a
high incidence of hepatitis B or a direct risk of
contact with contaminated human blood, and also
certain family contacts of carriers. Similar persons
in indirect contact with a source of infection and at
a lower risk would be considered a lower priority
group. Another group for whom vaccination is
recommended is infants born to mothers who are
hepatitis B carriers or HBsAg-positive (particularly if they are e antigen-positive or are without anti-e antibody). Active immunisation
combined with hepatitis B immunoglobulin is
started immediately after delivery.

It should be borne in mind that immunisation
takes up to 6 months to confer adequate protec-

tion; the duration of immunity is thought to last
for 3 to 5 years.

More detailed guidance is given in the memorandum *Immunisation against Infectious Disease
1990* (for availability see section 14.1). Vaccination does not eliminate the need for com-
monsense precautions for avoiding the risk of
infection from known carriers by the routes of
infection which have been clearly established, see
*Guidance for Clinical Health Care Workers: Pro-
tection against Infection with HIV and Hepatitis
Viruses.* Accidental inoculation of hepatitis B
virus-infected blood into a wound, incision,
needle-prick, or abrasion may lead to infection,
whereas it is unlikely that indirect exposure to a
carrier will do so.

Specific hepatitis B immunoglobulin ('HBIG')
is available for use with the vaccine in those accidentally infected and in infants (section 14.5).

See section 14.1 for general contra-indications.

PoM **Engerix B**® (SK&F)
A suspension of hepatitis B surface antigen (rby,
prepared from yeast cells by recombinant DNA
technique) 20 micrograms/mL adsorbed onto
aluminium hydroxide. Net price 1-mL vial =
£11.55

*Dose:* by intramuscular injection (see note
below), 3 doses of 1 mL, the second 1 month
and the third 6 months after the first dose; more
rapid (e.g. for travellers), third dose 2 months
after first dose with booster at 12 months; CHILD
birth to 12 years 3 doses of 0.5 mL; INFANTS
born to HBsAg-positive mothers, 3 doses of
0.5 mL, first dose at birth with hepatitis B
immunoglobulin injection (separate site)

Note. The deltoid muscle is the preferred site of injection
in adults; the anterolateral thigh is the preferred site in
infants and children; the buttock must not be used because
vaccine efficacy may be reduced. The subcutaneous route
is used for patients with haemophilia.

## INFLUENZA VACCINES

While most viruses are antigenically stable, the
influenza viruses A and B (especially A) are constantly altering their antigenic structure as indicated by changes in the haemagglutinins (H) and
neuraminidases (N) on the surface of the viruses.
It is essential that influenza vaccines in use contain
the H and N components of the prevalent strain
or strains. Every year the World Health Organization recommends which strains should be
included.

The recommended strains are grown in the
allantoic cavity of chick embryos (therefore **contra-indicated** in those hypersensitive to eggs).

Since influenza vaccines will not control epi-
demics they are recommended *only for persons at
high risk.* Immunisation is strongly recommended
for those of all ages with the following conditions:
chronic respiratory disease, including asthma;
chronic heart disease;
chronic renal failure;
diabetes mellitus, and other endocrine disorders;
immunosuppression due to disease or treatment.
Influenza vaccination is also recommended for

residents of nursing homes, old peoples homes, and other long-stay facilities.

In non-pandemic years immunisation is not recommended for Health Service staff, except for those at high risk (owing to medical disorders).

**Interactions:** Appendix 1 (influenza vaccine).

See section 14.1 for general contra-indications.

PoM **Fluvirin**® (Evans)
Inactivated influenza vaccine, surface antigen. Net price 0.5-mL disposable syringe = £5.09
*Dose:* 0.5 mL by deep subcutaneous or intramuscular injection; CHILD 4–13 years, 0.5 mL repeated once after 4–6 weeks

PoM **Fluzone**® (Servier)
Inactivated influenza vaccine (split virion vaccine). Net price 0.5-mL disposable syringe = £5.31
*Dose:* 0.5 mL by intramuscular injection; CHILD 6 months to 3 years, 0.25 mL repeated once after 4–6 weeks; 4–13 years, 0.5 mL repeated once after 4–6 weeks

PoM **Influvac Sub-unit**® (Duphar)
Inactivated influenza vaccine, surface antigen. Net price 0.5-mL disposable syringe = £5.08
*Dose:* 0.5 mL by deep subcutaneous or intramuscular injection; CHILD 4–13 years, 0.5 mL repeated once after 4–6 weeks

PoM **MFV-Ject**® (Merieux)
Inactivated influenza vaccine (split virion vaccine). Net price 0.5-mL disposable syringe = £5.10
*Dose:* 0.5 mL by deep subcutaneous or intramuscular injection; CHILD 4–13 years, 0.5 mL repeated once after 4–6 weeks
*Note.* A generic version is also available from Merieux at the same price

## MEASLES VACCINE

**Measles vaccine** has been replaced by a combined measles/mumps/rubella vaccine (MMR vaccine) for all eligible children.

Administration of a measles-containing vaccine to children may be associated with a mild measles-like syndrome with a measles-like rash and pyrexia about a week after injection. Much less commonly, convulsions and, very rarely, encephalitis have been reported. Convulsions in infants are much less frequently associated with measles vaccines than with other conditions leading to febrile episodes.

MMR vaccine may be used in the control of outbreaks of measles (see under MMR vaccine, below).

Single antigen vaccine
Available from Merieux on named patient basis

Combined vaccines
*With mumps and rubella*
See below

## MMR VACCINE

A combined measles/mumps/rubella vaccine (MMR vaccine) has been introduced with the aim of eliminating rubella (and congenital rubella syndrome), measles, and mumps. Health authorities have an obligation to ensure that every child has received MMR vaccine by entry to primary school, unless there is a valid contra-indication, parental refusal, or laboratory evidence of previous infection. Vaccination records should be checked; where there is no record of MMR vaccination or where the child has received single-antigen measles vaccine, parents should be advised that their children should receive MMR.

MMR vaccine has replaced measles vaccine for children of both sexes aged 1 to 2 years (or after this age if appointments have been missed).

MMR vaccine should be given to children of both sexes aged 4 to 5 years before starting primary school (irrespective of previous measles vaccine or of a history of measles, mumps, or rubella) unless there is:

a documented history of MMR vaccination;
a valid contra-indication (see below);
laboratory evidence of immunity to measles, mumps, and rubella.

MMR vaccine may also be used in the control of outbreaks of measles and should be offered to susceptible children within 3 days of exposure to infection (**important:** MMR vaccine is not suitable for prophylaxis following exposure to mumps or rubella since the antibody response to the mumps and rubella components is too slow for effective prophylaxis).

Children with partially or totally impaired immune responsiveness should not receive live vaccines (for advice on AIDS see section 14.1). If they have been exposed to measles infection they should be given immunoglobulin (section 14.5).

As with measles vaccine, malaise, fever and/or a rash may occur with MMR vaccine, most commonly about a week after vaccination and lasting about 2 to 3 days. Parents should be given written information and advice for reducing fever (including the use of paracetamol). Parotid swelling occasionally occurs, usually in the third week. Post-vaccination meningoencephalitis has been reported very rarely (with complete recovery). Children with post-vaccination symptoms are not infectious.

Contra-indications to MMR include:
children with untreated malignant disease or altered immunity, and those receiving immunosuppressive drugs or radiotherapy, or high-dose corticosteroids;
children who have received another live vaccine by injection within 3 weeks;
children with allergies to neomycin or kanamycin, or a history of anaphylaxis due to any cause;
children with acute febrile illness (vaccination should be deferred);
if given to adult women, pregnancy should be avoided for 1 month (as for rubella vaccine);
should not be given within 3 months of an immunoglobulin injection.

It should be noted that:
children with a personal or close family history of convulsions should be given MMR vaccine, provided the

parents understand that there may be a febrile response; immunoglobulin must not be given with MMR vaccine since the immune response to rubella and mumps may be inhibited; doctors should seek specialist paediatric advice rather than refuse vaccination;
allergy to egg is only a contra-indication if the child has had an anaphylactic reaction to food containing egg (dislike of egg or refusal to eat is not a contra-indication).

For general contra-indications to vaccines, see section 14.1

PoM **MMR Vaccine**
Live, measles, mumps, and rubella vaccine
*Dose:* 0.5 mL by deep subcutaneous or by intra-muscular injection
Available from District Health Authorities as *Immravax*® (Merieux), *MMR II*® (Wellcome), *Pluserix MMR*® (SK&F)

---

# MENINGOCOCCAL POLYSACCHARIDE VACCINE

**Meningococcal polysaccharide vaccine** is indicated for areas of the world where the risk of acquiring meningococcal infection is much higher than in the UK, particularly for travellers proposing to travel 'rough'.

These areas include New Delhi, Nepal, Mecca (see below), and the meningitis belt of Africa, which encompasses southern sub-Saharan parts of Senegal, Mali, Niger, Chad, and Sudan; all of Gambia, Guinea, Togo, and Benin; South-west Ethiopia; northern parts of Sierra Leone, Liberia, Ivory Coast, Nigeria, Cameroon, Central African Republic, Uganda, and Kenya.

Saudi Arabia requires vaccination of pilgrims to Mecca during the Haj annual pilgrimage; this may apply to others visiting Saudi Arabia in the months leading up to August.

See section 14.1 for general contra-indications.

PoM **AC Vax**® (SK&F)
Meningococcal polysaccharide vaccine prepared from *Neisseria meningitidis* (meningococcus) groups A and C. Net price single-dose vial (with diluent) = £6.86; 10-dose vial = £61.74
*Dose:* ADULT and CHILD aged 2 months and over, 0.5 mL by deep subcutaneous or intramuscular injection

PoM **Mengivac (A+C)**® (Merieux)
Meningococcal polysaccharide vaccine prepared from *Neisseria meningitidis* (meningococcus) groups A and C. Net price single-dose vial (with syringe containing diluent) = £6.86
*Dose:* ADULT and CHILD aged over 18 months, 0.5 mL by deep subcutaneous or intramuscular injection
*Note.* The lower age range for AC Vax® and Mengivac (A+C)® differ; in the case of Mengivac (A+C)® the manufacturer's literature states that clinical data has confirmed efficacy of the serogroup A component over 3 months of age, that although the response to the serogroup C component is transitory it can be of limited value during a severe epidemic, and that transient side-effects are more common below the age of 18 months

# MUMPS VACCINE

Mumps vaccine consists of a live attenuated strain of virus grown in chick-embryo tissue culture.
See under MMR vaccine and section 14.1 for contra-indications.

PoM **Mumpsvax**® (Morson)
Mumps vaccine (Jeryl Lynn strain). Net price single-dose vial (with diluent) = £4.00
*Dose:* ADULT and CHILD over 1 year, 0.5 mL by subcutaneous injection

Combined vaccines
*With measles and rubella*
See MMR Vaccine

---

# PERTUSSIS VACCINE
(Whooping-cough vaccine)

**Pertussis vaccine** is usually given combined with diphtheria and tetanus vaccine (in triple vaccine) starting at 2 months of age (see schedule, section 14.1) but may also be given as a single antigen vaccine.

With some vaccines available in the early 1960s persistent screaming and collapse were reported but these reactions are rarely observed with the vaccines now available.

Convulsions and encephalopathy have been reported as rare complications, but such conditions may arise from other causes and be falsely attributed to the vaccine. Neurological complications after whooping cough itself are considerably more common than after the vaccine.

As with any other elective immunisation procedure it is advisable to postpone vaccination if the child is suffering from any acute illness, until fully recovered. Minor infections without fever or systemic upset are not reasons to delay immunisation. Vaccination should not be carried out in children who have a history of severe local or general reaction to a preceding dose; the following reactions should be regarded as severe:

*Local*—an extensive area of redness and swelling which becomes indurated and involves most of the antero-lateral surface of the thigh or a major part of the circumference of the upper arm; this reaction may increase in severity with each subsequent injection.
*General*—fever equal to or more than 39.5°C within 48 hours of vaccine, anaphylaxis, bronchospasm, laryngeal oedema, generalised collapse, prolonged unresponsiveness, prolonged inconsolable screaming, and convulsions occurring within 72 hours.

A personal or family history of allergy is **not** a contra-indication to immunisation against whooping cough; nor are stable neurological conditions such as cerebral palsy or spina bifida.

There are certain groups of children in whom the advisability of whooping cough immunisation requires special consideration because of their own or their family histories. For these, the likelihood of febrile convulsions following vaccine may be higher, but the effects of whooping cough could be more severe. The balance of risk and benefit should be assessed in each case. Where there is doubt, appropriate advice should be sought from a consultant paediatrician, a consultant in public health medicine, or a district immunisation coordinator before a decision is made to withhold vaccine. When pertussis vaccine is given to such children, parents should be given advice on the management of pyrexia and the prevention of febrile convulsions (see also p. 434). Groups requiring special consideration are:

children with a documented history of cerebral damage in the neonatal period;

children with a personal history of convulsions;

children whose parents or siblings have a history of idiopathic epilepsy; in such children there may be a risk of developing a similar condition irrespective of vaccine.

PoM **Pertussis Vaccine** Per/Vac. A sterile suspension of killed *Bordetella pertussis*. Net price 0.5-mL amp = £1.31

*Dose:* primary immunisation if pertussis component has been omitted from earlier vaccinations, three doses each of 0.5 mL by intramuscular or deep subcutaneous injection, separated by intervals of 1 month (see section 14.1)

Available from Evans

Combined vaccines, see under Diphtheria Vaccines

## PNEUMOCOCCAL VACCINE

A polyvalent pneumococcal vaccine is available for the immunisation of persons for whom the risk of contracting pneumococcal pneumonia is unusually high, for example patients who have had a splenectomy. It is effective in a single dose if the types of pneumonia in the community are reflected in the polysaccharides contained in the vaccine. Studies with other pneumococcal vaccines suggest that protection may last for 5 years. Revaccination should not be carried out because of the risk of adverse reactions. The vaccine should not be given to children under 2 years, in pregnancy, or when there is infection. It should be used with caution in cardiovascular or respiratory disease. Hypersensitivity reactions may occur.

See section 14.1 for general contra-indications.

PoM **Pneumovax® II** (Morson)

Polysaccharide from each of 23 capsular types of pneumococcus

*Dose:* 0.5 mL by subcutaneous or intramuscular injection

## POLIOMYELITIS VACCINES

There are two types of poliomyelitis vaccine, poliomyelitis vaccine, live (oral) (Sabin) and poliomyelitis vaccine, inactivated (Salk). The oral vaccine, consisting of a mixture of attenuated strains of virus types 1, 2, and 3 is at present generally used in the UK.

INITIAL COURSE. **Poliomyelitis vaccine, live (oral)** is given on 3 occasions, usually at the same time as routine immunisation against diphtheria, tetanus, and pertussis (see schedule, section 14.1).

The initial course of 3 doses should also be given to all unimmunised adults.

REINFORCEMENT. A reinforcing dose of oral poliomyelitis vaccine is recommended at school entry at which time children should also receive a reinforcing dose of diphtheria and tetanus vaccine, and a dose of MMR vaccine if this has not already been given. Oral poliomyelitis vaccine is also recommended at school leaving.

Vaccine-associated poliomyelitis and poliomyelitis in contacts of vaccinees are both rare. In England and Wales there is an annual average of 1 recipient and 1 contact case in relation to over 2 million doses of oral vaccine. The need for strict personal hygiene must be stressed; the contacts of a recently vaccinated baby should be advised of the necessity for personal hygiene, particularly of the need to wash their hands after changing the baby's napkins.

**Contra-indications** to the use of oral poliomyelitis vaccine include vomiting and diarrhoea, and immunodeficiency disorders (or household contacts of patients with immunodeficiency disorders). See section 14.1 for further contra-indications.

**Poliomyelitis vaccine (inactivated)** may be used for those in whom poliomyelitis vaccine (oral) is contra-indicated because of immunosuppressive disorders (for advice on AIDS see section 14.1).

TRAVELLERS. Travellers to areas other than Australia, New Zealand, Europe, and North America should be given a full course of oral poliomyelitis vaccine if they have not been immunised in the past. Those who have not received immunisation within the last 10 years should be given a booster dose of oral poliomyelitis vaccine.

Live (oral) (Sabin)

PoM **Poliomyelitis Vaccine, Live (Oral)** Pol/Vac (Oral)[1]. A suspension of suitable live attenuated strains of poliomyelitis virus, types 1, 2, and 3. Available in single-dose and 10-dose containers

*Dose:* 3 drops from a multidose container or the total contents of a single-dose container; for primary immunisation 3 doses are required (see schedule, section 14.1)

Available from District Health Authorities (private purchases available from SK&F and Evans)

1. BP permits code OPV for vaccine in single doses provided it also appears on pack.

*Note.* Poliomyelitis vaccine loses potency once the container has been opened, therefore any vaccine remaining at the end of an immunisation session should be discarded; whenever possible sessions should be arranged to avoid undue wastage.

Inactivated (Salk)

PoM **Poliomyelitis Vaccine, Inactivated** Pol/Vac (Inact). An inactivated suspension of suitable strains of poliomyelitis virus, types 1, 2, and 3.

*Dose:* 0.5 mL or as stated on the label by deep subcutaneous or intramuscular injection; for primary immunisation 3 doses are required (see schedule, section 14.1)

Available from Department of Health, Room 222, 14 Russell Square, London WC1B 5EP, telephone 071-636 6811, extn 3117/3236 *and* Scottish Home and Health Department, telephone 031-552 6255, extn 2162 *and*

Welsh Health Common Services Authority, Heron House, 35–43 Newport Road, Cardiff CF2 1SB, telephone 0222 471234
*Note.* Should be ordered one dose at a time and only when required for use.

## RABIES VACCINE

A human diploid cell **rabies vaccine** is now in use. It should be offered prophylactically to those at high risk—those working in quarantine stations, animal handlers, veterinary surgeons, and field workers who may be exposed to bites of wild animals. A detailed list is given in Health Circular HC(77)29. For *prophylactic* use the vaccine produces a good antibody response when given in a 2-dose schedule with an interval of one month between doses and a reinforcing dose after an interval of 6–12 months with further reinforcing doses every 1–3 years depending on the risk of exposure, and also following exposure to possible rabies.

For *post-exposure treatment* of previously unvaccinated patients a course of injections should be started as soon as possible after exposure (days 0, 3, 7, 14, 30, and 90). The course may be discontinued if it is proved that the patient was not at risk. There are no specific contra-indications to this diploid cell vaccine and its use should be considered whenever a patient has been attacked by an animal in a country where rabies is endemic, even if there is no direct evidence of rabies in the attacking animal. Rabies immunoglobulin (section 14.5) should also be given.

*Staff in attendance* on a patient who is highly suspected of, or known to be suffering from, rabies should be offered vaccination. Four intradermal doses of 0.1 mL of human diploid cell vaccine (Merieux) given on the same day at different sites has been suggested for this purpose (ensuring correct intradermal technique).

Advice on post-exposure vaccination and treatment of rabies is available from the Virus Reference Laboratory, Central Public Health Laboratory, Colindale Avenue, Colindale, London NW9 5HT, telephone 081-200 4400.

PoM **Merieux Inactivated Rabies Vaccine** (Merieux)
Freeze-dried human diploid cell rabies vaccine prepared from Wistar strain PM/WI 38 1503-3M. Single-dose vial with syringe containing diluent
*Note.* Studies have shown that when this vaccine is injected into the gluteal region there is a poor response.
*Dose:* prophylactic, 1 mL by deep subcutaneous or intramuscular injection in the deltoid region, followed by a second dose after 1 month and a third after 6–12 months; also further reinforcing doses every 1–3 years depending on the risk of infection
Post-exposure, 1 mL on the first, third, seventh and fourteenth day and after 1 and 3 months
*Staff in attendance,* see notes above
Also available from local designated centres (special workers and post-exposure treatment)

## RUBELLA VACCINE

The selective policy of protecting women of child-bearing age from the risks of rubella (German measles) in pregnancy has been extended to a policy of eliminating the circulation of rubella among young children. The existing rubella vaccination policy will therefore be reinforced by the mass vaccination of children of both sexes, using a combined measles, mumps, and rubella vaccine (see under MMR Vaccine).

Rubella vaccine is still recommended for pre-pubertal girls between their tenth and fourteenth birthdays (unless there is documented evidence that they have received MMR) and for seronegative women of child-bearing age (see schedule, section 14.1) as well as those who might put pregnant women at risk of infection (e.g. nurses and doctors in obstetric units).

Rubella vaccination should be avoided in early pregnancy, and women of child-bearing age should be advised not to become pregnant within 1 month of vaccination. However, despite active surveillance in the UK, the USA, and Germany, no case of congenital rubella syndrome has been reported following inadvertent vaccination shortly before or during pregnancy. There is thus no evidence that the vaccine is teratogenic, and termination of pregnancy following inadvertent vaccination should not be routinely recommended; potential parents should be given this information before making a decision about termination.

Vaccine may conveniently be offered to previously unvaccinated and seronegative post-partum women. Again they must avoid pregnancy for 1 month. Immunising susceptible post-partum women a few days after delivery is important as far as the overall reduction of congenital abnormalities in the UK is concerned, for about 60% of these abnormalities occur in the babies of multiparous women.

Susceptible pregnant women who are exposed to rubella and who do not want therapeutic abortion may be offered normal immunoglobulin injection (section 14.5).

PoM **Rubella Vaccine, Live** Rub/Vac (Live). A freeze-dried suspension of a suitable live attenuated strain of rubella virus grown in suitable cell cultures.
*Dose:* 0.5 mL by deep subcutaneous or by intramuscular injection (see schedule, section 14.1 and notes above)
Available as
PoM **Almevax®** (Evans)
Rubella vaccine, live, prepared from Wistar RA 27/3 strain propagated in human diploid cells.
Net price single-dose amp with diluent = £2.61; 10-dose vial with diluent = £21.64

PoM **Ervevax®** (SK&F)

Rubella vaccine, live, prepared from Wistar RA 27/3 strain propagated in human diploid cells. Net price single-dose vial = £2.30; 10-dose vial = £19.10 (both with diluent)

PoM **Rubavax®** (Merieux)

Rubella vaccine, live, prepared from Wistar RA27/3 strain propagated in human diploid cells. Net price single-dose vial with syringe containing diluent = £2.61

Combined vaccines

*With measles and mumps*

See MMR Vaccine

## SMALLPOX VACCINE

**Smallpox vaccination** is no longer required routinely in the UK and other countries because global eradication of smallpox has now been achieved. Workers in laboratories where pox viruses (such as vaccinia) are handled, and others whose work involves an identifiable risk of exposure to pox virus, should be advised of the possible risk and vaccination should be considered. Detailed guidance for laboratory staff has been prepared by the Advisory Committee on Dangerous Pathogens and the Advisory Committee on Genetic Manipulation. There is no requirement for smallpox vaccination of travellers.

PoM **Smallpox Vaccine** Var/Vac. Consists of a suspension of live vaccinia virus grown in the skin of living animals, supplied in freeze-dried form with diluent

Advice on the need for vaccination and on contra-indications should be obtained from the Virus Reference Laboratory, Central Public Health Laboratory, Colindale (081-200 4400) who will also supply the vaccine (free of charge)

## TETANUS VACCINES

(Tetanus toxoids)

**Tetanus vaccines** stimulate the production of the protective antitoxin. In general, adsorption on aluminium hydroxide, aluminium phosphate, or calcium phosphate improves antigenicity. Adsorbed tetanus vaccine is offered routinely to babies in combination with adsorbed diphtheria vaccine (DT/Vac/Ads) and more usually also combined with killed *Bordetella pertussis* organisms as a triple vaccine, adsorbed diphtheria, tetanus, and pertussis vaccine (DT Per/Vac/Ads), see schedule, section 14.1.

Of the single antigen tetanus vaccines adsorbed tetanus vaccine is again preferred to the plain vaccine. Adsorbed vaccine must not be given intradermally.

In children, the triple vaccine not only gives protection against tetanus in childhood but also gives the basic immunity for subsequent reinforcing doses of tetanus vaccine at school entry and at school leaving and also when a potentially tetanus-contaminated injury has been received. Normally, tetanus vaccine should not be given unless more than 10 years have elapsed since the last reinforcing dose because of the possibility that hypersensitivity reactions may develop.

Active immunisation is important for persons in older age groups who may never have had a routine or complete course of immunisation when younger. In these persons a course of adsorbed tetanus vaccine may be given. Very rarely, tetanus has developed after abdominal surgery; patients awaiting elective surgery should be asked about tetanus immunisation and immunised if necessary.

See section 14.1 for general contra-indications.

For serious, potentially contaminated wounds tetanus immunoglobulin injection (section 14.5) should be selectively used in addition to wound toilet, adsorbed tetanus vaccine, and benzylpenicillin or another appropriate antibiotic.

Single antigen vaccines

The BP directs that when Tetanus Vaccine is prescribed or demanded and the form is not stated, Adsorbed Tetanus Vaccine may be dispensed or supplied.

PoM **Adsorbed Tetanus Vaccine** Tet/Vac/Ads. Prepared from tetanus formol toxoid with a mineral carrier (aluminium hydroxide).

*Dose:* 0.5 mL or as stated on the label, by intramuscular or deep subcutaneous injection followed after 4 weeks by a second dose and after a further 4 weeks by a third

Note. This dose reflects the guidelines of the Joint Committee on Vaccination and Immunisation, see *Immunisation against Infectious Disease* 1990

Available from Evans (net price 0.5-mL amp = 71p; 5-mL vial = £3.86, and as **Closet®**, net price 0.5-mL single-dose syringe = £1.40), Merieux (as **Tetavax®**, net price 0.5-mL amp = 55p; 5-mL single-dose syringe = £1.20; 5-mL vial = £2.80), and from Servier (net price 0.5-mL amp = 64p; 5-mL vial = £2.89)

PoM **Tetanus** Tet/Vac/FT. Tetanus formol toxoid. 0.5-mL amp and 5-mL vial

*Dose:* as for Adsorbed Tetanus Vaccine which is preferred (see notes above)

Available from Evans

Combined vaccines, see Diphtheria Vaccines

## TUBERCULOSIS VACCINES

See BCG Vaccines

## TYPHOID VACCINE

**Typhoid vaccine** consists of single antigen typhoid vaccine; it is no substitute for personal hygiene (see section 14.6). Normally, 2 doses should be given at 4–6 weeks interval for primary immunisation, with reinforcing doses about every 3 years on continued exposure.

Local reactions, which consist of swelling, pain, and tenderness, appear about 2–3 hours after the deep subcutaneous or intramuscular injection of the vaccine. Systemic reactions which consist of fever, malaise, and headache may also occur and usually last for about 36 hours after injection. If severe reactions are experienced after the first dose intradermal (intracutaneous) injection may be preferred for the second dose, as these reactions are virtually absent when this route is used.

See section 14.1 for general contra-indications.

PoM **Typhoid Vaccine** Typhoid/Vac. A suspension of killed *Salmonella typhi* organisms. Net price 1.5-mL vial = £4.11
*Dose:* 0.5 mL by deep subcutaneous or intramuscular injection; CHILD 1–10 years 0.25 mL
Second dose after 4–6 weeks, 0.5 mL (or 0.1 mL by intradermal injection); CHILD 1–10 years 0.25 mL (or 0.1 mL by intradermal injection)
*Note.* The Department of Health now recommends that the second dose of typhoid vaccine can be given intradermally to reduce reactions
Available from Evans

## WHOOPING-COUGH VACCINES
See Pertussis Vaccines

## YELLOW FEVER VACCINE
Yellow fever vaccine consists of a live attenuated yellow fever virus (17D strain) grown in developing chick embryos. Infants under 9 months of age should only be vaccinated if the risk of yellow fever is unavoidable since there is a small risk of encephalitis. The vaccine should not be given to those with impaired immune responsiveness, or who have had an anaphylactic reaction to egg; it should not be given during pregnancy (but where there is a significant risk of exposure the need for vaccination outweighs any risk to the fetus). See section 14.1 for further contra-indications. Reactions are few. The immunity which probably lasts for life is officially accepted for 10 years starting from 10 days after primary vaccination and for a further 10 years immediately after revaccination.

PoM **Yellow Fever Vaccine, Live** Yel/Vac. A suspension of chick embryo proteins containing attenuated 17D strain virus
*Dose:* 0.5 mL by subcutaneous injection
Available (only to designated Yellow Fever Vaccination centres) as
PoM **Arilvax**® (Evans)
Freeze-dried yellow fever vaccine, live. 1-, 5-, and 10-dose vials (with diluent)

# 14.5 Immunoglobulins

Injection of immunoglobulins produces immediate protection lasting about 4–6 weeks. Immunoglobulins of animal origin (antisera) were frequently associated with hypersensitivity which led to their virtual abandonment; human immunoglobulins took their place.

The two types of human immunoglobulin preparation are **normal immunoglobulin** and **specific immunoglobulins**.

Further information about immunoglobulins is included in *Immunisation against Infectious Disease* (see section 14.1).

AVAILABILITY. Normal immunoglobulin and the specific immunoglobulins are available from the Public Health Laboratory Service laboratories and Regional Blood Transfusion Centres in England and Wales with the exception of tetanus immunoglobulin which is distributed through Regional Blood Transfusion Centres to hospital pharmacies or blood transfusion departments and is also available to general medical practitioners. Rabies immunoglobulin is available from the Central Public Health Laboratory, London.

In Scotland all immunoglobulins are available from the Blood Transfusion Service. Tetanus immunoglobulin is distributed by the Blood Transfusion Service to hospitals and general medical practitioners on demand.

Normal immunoglobulin injection, anti-D (Rh₀) immunoglobulin injection, and tetanus immunoglobulin injection are also available commercially.

For further details of availability see under individual immunoglobulins.

## NORMAL IMMUNOGLOBULIN
(Gamma Globulin)
Human **normal immunoglobulin** ('HNIG') is prepared from pools of at least 1000 donations of human plasma; it contains antibody to measles, mumps, varicella, hepatitis A, and other viruses that are currently prevalent in the general population. It is administered by intramuscular injection for the protection of susceptible contacts against hepatitis A virus (infective hepatitis), measles and, to a lesser extent, rubella. Injection of human immunoglobulin produces immediate passive immunity lasting about 4–6 weeks. Intravenous administration is used for replacement therapy (see below).

Side-effects of immunoglobulin include malaise, chills, fever, and rarely anaphylaxis. Human normal immunoglobulin is **contra-indicated** in patients with known class specific antibody to immunoglobulin A (IgA).

HEPATITIS A. **Hepatitis A** viral vaccines are undergoing clinical trials but are not yet generally available. Control depends on good hygiene and many studies have also shown the value of normal immunoglobulin in the prevention and control of outbreaks of this disease. It is recommended for controlling infection in contacts in closed institutions and also, under certain conditions, in school and home contacts and for travellers going to areas where the disease is highly endemic (all countries excluding Northern Europe, North America, Australia, and New Zealand).

MEASLES. Normal immunoglobulin may be given for prophylaxis in children with compromised immunity (and in adults with compromised immunity who have no measles antibodies); it should be given as soon as possible after contact with measles. It should also be given to children under 12 months with recent severe illness for whom measles should be avoided; MMR vaccine should then be given (after an interval of **at least** 3 months) at around the usual age.

RUBELLA. Immunoglobulin after exposure does **not** prevent infection in non-immune contacts and is **not** recommended for protection of pregnant women exposed to rubella. It may however reduce the likelihood of a clinical attack which may possibly reduce the risk to the fetus. It should only be used when termination of pregnancy would be unacceptable when it should be given as soon as possible after exposure. Serological follow-up of recipients is essential.

For routine prophylaxis, see Rubella Vaccine.

---

**Interference with live virus vaccines**
Normal immunoglobulin may interfere with the immune response to live virus vaccines which should therefore only be given at least 3 weeks before or 3 months after an injection of normal immunoglobulin. This does not apply to yellow fever vaccine since normal immunoglobulin does not contain antibody to this virus. For travellers, if there is insufficient time, the recommended interval may have to be ignored.

---

For intramuscular use

PoM **Human Normal Immunoglobulin** Human normal immunoglobulin injection. 250-mg vial; 750-mg vial
Available from BPL and SNBTS
*Dose:* by intramuscular injection, Hepatitis A travel prophylaxis (2 months or less abroad), 250 mg; CHILD under 10 years 125 mg; longer travel prophylaxis (3–5 months abroad) and to control outbreaks, 500 mg; CHILD under 10 years 250 mg

Measles prophylaxis, CHILD under 1 year 250 mg; 1–2 years 500 mg, 3 years and over 750 mg; to allow attenuated attack, CHILD under 1 year 100 mg, 1 year and over 250 mg

Rubella in pregnancy, prevention of clinical attack, 750 mg

[1]PoM **Gammabulin**® (Immuno)
Human normal immunoglobulin injection. Net price 2-mL vial = £3.20; 5-mL vial = £6.50; 10-mL vial = £11.00; 320-mg vial with 2 mL water for injections = £3.50

[1]PoM **Kabiglobulin**® (Kabi Pharmacia)
Human normal immunoglobulin injection 16%. Net price 2-mL amp = £2.85; 5-mL amp = £6.15

1. Doses for these preparations are expressed in terms of volume:
*Dose:* by intramuscular injection,
Hepatitis A prophylaxis, ADULT and CHILD 0.02–0.04 mL/kg; greater exposure risk, 0.06–0.12 mL/kg
Measles prophylaxis, 0.2 mL/kg; to allow attenuated attack, 0.04 mL/kg
Rubella in pregnancy, prevention of clinical attack, 20 mL

---

## REPLACEMENT THERAPY

Special formulations for intravenous administration are available for replacement therapy for patients with congenital agammaglobulinaemia and hypogammaglobulinaemia, for the treatment of idiopathic thrombocytopenic purpura and Kawasaki syndrome, and for the prophylaxis of infection following bone marrow transplantation.

For intravenous use
Available as: *Endobulin*® (500 mg, 1 g, 2.5 g, 5 g, 7.5 g, 10 g—Immuno); *Gamimune-N*® (500 mg, 2.5 g, 5 g—Cutter); Human Immunoglobulin (3 g—SNBTS); *Sandoglobulin*® (1 g, 3 g, 6 g—Sandoz); *Venoglobulin*® (500 mg, 2.5 g, 5g—Alpha); *Vigam*® (2.5 g, 5 g—BPL)

## SPECIFIC IMMUNOGLOBULINS

Specific immunoglobulins are prepared by pooling the plasma of selected donors with high levels of the specific antibody required.

Although a hepatitis B vaccine is now available for those at high risk of infection, specific **hepatitis B immunoglobulin** ('HBIG') is available for use in association with the vaccine for the prevention of infection in laboratory and other personnel who have accidentally been contaminated with hepatitis B virus, and in infants born to mothers who have become infected with this virus in pregnancy or who are high-risk carriers.

Following exposure to a rabid animal, specific **rabies immunoglobulin**, if possible of human origin, should be injected at the site of the bite and also given intramuscularly. Rabies vaccine should also be given.

**Tetanus immunoglobulin** of human origin ('HTIG') should be used selectively in addition to wound toilet, vaccine, and benzylpenicillin (or another appropriate antibiotic) for the more seriously contaminated wounds; it is rarely required for those with an established immunity in whom protection may be achieved by a reinforcing dose of vaccine if considered advisable. The administration of tetanus immunoglobulin should be considered for patients not known to have received active immunisation (a) whose wound was sustained more than 6 hours before treatment was received and (b) with puncture wounds or wounds potentially heavily contaminated with tetanus spores, septic, or with much devitalised tissue. A dose of adsorbed tetanus vaccine should be given at the same time as the tetanus immunoglobulin and the course of vaccine subsequently completed.

Other specific immunoglobulins include varicella-zoster immunoglobulin ('ZIG') and are in limited supply. Others are under study, but their availability and evaluation requires the cooperation of general practitioners to provide blood from patients who are convalescent from these and other specific viral infections in order to prepare specific immunoglobulin preparations.

PoM **Hepatitis B Immunoglobulin** (Antihepatitis B Immunoglobulin). See notes above
Available from Public Health Laboratory Service (also from BPL and SNBTS)

---

PoM **Rabies Immunoglobulin** (Antirabies Immunoglobulin Injection). Used for protection of persons who have been bitten by rabid animals or otherwise exposed to infection (see notes above)
*Dose:* 20 units/kg, half by intramuscular injection and half by infiltration around wound
Available from Public Health Laboratory Service (also from BPL and SNBTS)

PoM **Tetanus Immunoglobulin** (Antitetanus Immunoglobulin Injection). Used for the protection of unimmunised persons when there is a specific risk of tetanus
*Dose:* by intramuscular injection, prophylactic 250 units, increased to 500 units if more than 24 hours have elapsed or there is risk of heavy contamination
Therapeutic, 150 units/kg (multiple sites)
Available from BPL, SNBTS, and Wellcome (as *Humotet®*; net price 1-mL vial = £18.94)

PoM **Tetanus Immunoglobulin for Intravenous Use.** Used for proven or suspected clinical tetanus
*Dose:* by intravenous infusion, 5000–10000 units
Available from SNBTS (2500-unit vial)

PoM **Varicella-Zoster Immunoglobulin** (Antivaricella-zoster Immunoglobulin). Used for protection of immunosuppressed persons and neonates at risk.
Available from Public Health Laboratory Service (also from BPL and SNBTS)

## ANTI-D (Rh$_0$) IMMUNOGLOBULIN

Anti-D immunoglobulin is available to prevent a rhesus-negative mother from forming antibodies to fetal rhesus-positive cells which may pass into the maternal circulation during childbirth or abortion. It should be injected within 72 hours of the birth or abortion but even if a longer period has elapsed it may still give protection and should be administered. The objective is to protect any subsequent child from the hazard of haemolytic disease of the newborn.

PoM **Anti-D (Rh$_0$) Immunoglobulin Injection.**
See notes above
*Dose:* for rhesus-negative women, 500 units by intramuscular injection following birth of rhesus-positive infant; 250 units if before 20 weeks gestation; after transfusion, consult literature (5000 units capable of neutralising 40–50 mL packed red cells)
*Note.* Rubella vaccine may be administered in the postpartum period simultaneously with anti-D (Rh$_0$) immunoglobulin injection providing separate syringes are used and the products are administered into contralateral limbs. A blood test should be done not sooner than 8 weeks later to ensure that rubella antibodies have been produced. If blood transfusion was necessary vaccination should be delayed for 3 months.
Available from Regional Blood Transfusion Centres and from BPL and SNBTS (also available from Immuno (*Partobulin®*)—consult data sheet for details of dose)

### MONOCLONAL ANTIBODY

The cell line used to produce the human monoclonal IgM antibody HA-1A was prepared from cells derived from a patient immunised with a heat-inactivated J5 mutant *Escherichia coli* 0111:B4 vaccine.

### HA-1A
*Indications:* sepsis syndrome and Gram-negative bacteraemia, especially with septic shock
*Cautions:* use in meningococcal septicaemia and in patients with burns not recommended; pregnancy and breast-feeding
*Contra-indications:* hypersensitivity to mouse proteins; previous exposure to HA-1A
*Side-effects:* rarely, transient flushing, localised urticaria, and hypotension
*Dose:* by intravenous infusion, 100 mg; not to be repeated

▼ PoM **Centoxin®** (Centocor)
*Intravenous solution*, HA-1A 5 mg/mL, net price 20-mL vial = £2200.00. For dilution and use as an infusion

## 14.6 International travel

*Note.* For advice on **malaria chemoprophylaxis**, see section 5.4.1.
No particular immunisation is required for travellers to the United States, Europe, Australia, or New Zealand although the traveller should have immunity to tetanus and poliomyelitis. In Non-European areas surrounding the Mediterranean, in Africa, the Middle East, Asia, and South America, certain special precautions are required.

**Typhoid vaccine** is indicated for travellers to those countries where typhoid is endemic but is no substitute for personal precautions. Green salads and uncooked vegetables should be avoided and only fruits which can be peeled should be eaten. Only suitable bottled water, or water that has been boiled, or treated with sterilising tablets should be used for drinking purposes. This advice also applies to cholera and other diarrhoeal diseases (including travellers' diarrhoea).

**Cholera vaccine** is no substitute for personal hygiene and has little value in preventing infections. For current advice, see p. 436.

Long-term travellers to areas that have a high incidence of **poliomyelitis** or **tuberculosis** should be immunised with the appropriate vaccine; in the case of poliomyelitis previously vaccinated adults may be given a reinforcing dose of oral poliomyelitis vaccine. BCG vaccination is recommended for travellers proposing to stay for longer than one month in Asia, Africa, or Central and South America; it should preferably be given three months or more before departure.

International Certificates of vaccination against **yellow fever** (section 14.4) are still required for travel to much of Africa and South America.

Vaccination against **meningococcal meningitis** is required for a number of areas of the world (for details, section 14.4).

Overland travellers to Asia and Africa and others at high risk may be given **normal immunoglobulin injection** (section 14.5) for protection against hepatitis A. It is preferable to complete active immunisation and wait 4 weeks before administering the immunoglobulin. An interval of 2 weeks is acceptable provided the immunoglobulin is given just before departure. If time is short, it can be given with any vaccine (including polio).

The Department of Health has issued 2 booklets, *Health Advice For Travellers* (code: T2 for travel inside the European Community, T3 for travel outside the European Community) which can be obtained from travel agents, post offices (booklet T2), or by telephoning 0800 555 777 (24-hour service, booklet T3); bulk copies of booklet T3 may be ordered from:

Health Publications Unit
No. 2 Site, Heywood Stores
Manchester Road
Heywood
Lancs OL10 2PZ

They provide details of vaccination requirements or recommendations country-by-country, health insurance, and reciprocal agreements. Further advice (including details of a **rapid schedule** for travellers required to go abroad at short notice) may be obtained from the Department of Health memorandum, *Immunisation against Infectious Disease* (for details, section 14.1).

*Travel Information for Medical Practitioners* is a Department of Health booklet supplementing the guidance provided by the publications mentioned above. It also contains addresses of suppliers of emergency medical travel kits which are intended to reduce the risk of transmission of blood-borne infections such as HIV and hepatitis B. The booklet is not available to the public, but medical practitioners may obtain copies from:

Health Publications Unit
No. 2 Site, Heywood Stores
Manchester Road
Heywood
Lancs OL10 2PZ

Vaccination requirements change from time to time, and information on the current requirements for any particular country may be obtained from:

Department of Health
Friars House
London SE1 8EU
telephone 071-972 2000

Communicable Disease Surveillance Centre Travel Unit
61 Colindale Avenue
London NW9 5EQ
telephone 081-200 6868

Scottish Home and Health Department
St. Andrew's House
Edinburgh EH1 3DE
telephone 031-556 8400

Welsh Office
Cathays Park,
Cardiff CF1 3NQ
telephone Cardiff 825111

Department of Health and Social Services
Dundonald House
Upper Newtownards Road
Belfast BT4 3FS
telephone 0232 63939;

or from the embassy or legation of the appropriate country.

# 15: Drugs used in
# ANAESTHESIA

This chapter describes briefly drugs used in anaesthesia; the reader is referred to other sources for more detailed information. The chapter is divided into two sections:

15.1 General anaesthesia
15.2 Local anaesthesia

## 15.1 General anaesthesia

15.1.1 Intravenous anaesthetics
15.1.2 Inhalational anaesthetics
15.1.3 Antimuscarinic premedication drugs
15.1.4 Sedative and analgesic peri-operative drugs
15.1.5 Muscle relaxants
15.1.6 Anticholinesterases used in surgery
15.1.7 Antagonists for central and respiratory depression
15.1.8 Antagonists for malignant hyperthermia

---

*Note.* The drugs in section 15.1 should be used only by experienced personnel and where adequate resuscitative equipment is available.

---

ANAESTHESIA AND DRIVING. Patients given sedatives and analgesics during minor outpatient procedures should be very carefully warned about the risk of driving afterwards. For intravenous benzodiazepines and for a short general anaesthetic the risk extends to **at least 24 hours** after administration. Responsible persons should be available to take patients home. The dangers of taking **alcohol** should also be emphasised.

MODERN ANAESTHETIC TECHNIQUE. It is now common practice to administer several drugs with different actions to produce a state of surgical anaesthesia with minimal risk of toxic effects. An intravenous anaesthetic is frequently used for induction, followed by maintenance with inhalational anaesthetics, perhaps supplemented by other drugs administered intravenously. Specific drugs are often used to produce muscular relaxation. Many of the drugs used interfere with the reflex maintenance of spontaneous respiration and intermittent positive pressure ventilation by manual or mechanical means is commonly employed.

For certain procedures controlled hypotension may be required. Labetalol (see section 2.4), sodium nitroprusside (see section 2.5.1), and trimetaphan camsylate (see section 2.5.6) are used.

Beta-blockers (see section 2.4) or verapamil (see section 2.6.2) may be used to control arrhythmias during anaesthesia.

Prazosin (see section 2.5.4) is also used to control hypertension, particularly postoperatively.

## GAS CYLINDERS

Each gas cylinder bears a label with the name of the gas contained in the cylinder. The name or chemical symbol of the gas is stencilled in paint on the shoulder of the cylinder; the letters are not less than 9 mm high on cylinders up to and including 80 mm diameter, not less than 12 mm high on cylinders over 80 mm and up to and including 105 mm diameter, and 19 mm high on cylinders above 105 mm diameter. The name or chemical symbol of the gas is also clearly and indelibly stamped on the cylinder valve. The colours applied to the valve end of the cylinder extend down the cylinder to the shoulder; in the case of mixed gases the colours for the individual gases are applied in four segments, two for each colour. See table below.

Gas cylinders should be stored in a cool well-ventilated room, free from materials of a flammable nature.

**No lubricant of any description should be used.**

| Name of gas | Symbol | Colour of cylinder body | Colour of valve end where different from body |
|---|---|---|---|
| Oxygen | $O_2$ | Black | White |
| Nitrous oxide | $N_2O$ | Blue | — |
| Cyclopropane | $C_3H_6$ | Orange | — |
| Carbon dioxide | $CO_2$ | Grey | — |
| Ethylene | $C_2H_4$ | Violet | — |
| Helium | He | Brown | — |
| Nitrogen | $N_2$ | Grey | Black |
| Oxygen and carbon dioxide mixture | $O_2 + CO_2$ | Black | White and Grey |
| Oxygen and helium mixture | $O_2 + He$ | Black | White and Brown |
| Oxygen and nitrous oxide mixture | $O_2 + N_2O$ | Blue | Blue and White |
| Air (medical) | AIR | Grey | White and Black |

British Standard 1319:1976; Medical gas cylinders, valves and yoke connections. The colours used for gas cylinders comply with specifications in British Standards 4800 and 5252.

---

SURGERY AND LONG-TERM MEDICATION. The risk of stopping long-term medication before surgery is often greater than the risk of continuing it during surgery. This applies particularly to corticosteroids, since patients with adrenal atrophy (see section 6.3.3) may experience a precipitous fall in blood pressure unless corticosteroid cover is provided during anaesthesia or in the immediate postoperative period. Anaesthetists must therefore know whether a patient is, or has been, taking corticosteroids. Other drugs that should not normally be stopped before surgery include analgesics, antiepileptics, antiparkinsonian drugs, bronchodilators, cardiovascular drugs, glaucoma drugs, and thyroid or antithyroid drugs. Although it is preferable to discontinue oral anticoagulants electively before operation, this is not possible in patients requiring long-term treatment (e.g. for valve prostheses). The haematologist or physician should be consulted for further advice.

Drugs that should be stopped before surgery include oestrogens and combined oral contraceptives, which should be discontinued (and adequate alternative contraceptive arrangements made) 4 weeks before major elective surgery (for details see Surgery, section 7.3.1). In view of their hazardous interactions MAOIs should normally be stopped 2 weeks before surgery. Tricyclic antidepressants need not be stopped, but there may be an increased risk of arrhythmias and hypotension, therefore the anaesthetist should be informed if they are not. Lithium should be stopped 2 days before major surgery but the normal dose can be continued for minor surgery (with careful monitoring of fluids and electrolytes). To avoid withdrawal symptoms antidepressants need to be withdrawn gradually (see section 4.3.1).

In all cases it is vital that the anaesthetist should know of all drugs that a patient is, or has been, taking.

## 15.1.1   Intravenous anaesthetics

Intravenous anaesthetics may be used alone to produce anaesthesia for short surgical procedures but are more commonly used for induction only. Intravenous anaesthetics are potent drugs which nearly all produce their effect in one arm-brain circulation time and can cause apnoea and hypotension, and so adequate resuscitative facilities **must** be available. Large doses should be avoided in obstetrics, as the drug may cross the placental barrier. The drugs are **contra-indicated** in any dose in patients in whom the anaesthetist is not confident to maintain the airway, for example if there are tumours in the pharynx or larynx. Extreme care is required in surgery of the mouth, pharynx, or larynx and in patients with acute cardiovascular failure (shock) or fixed cardiac output. Patients with a full stomach present a hazard during induction since there is a danger of regurgitation and pulmonary aspiration. This may cause Mendelson's syndrome, particularly in the pregnant patient. Cricoid pressure is applied until the lungs have been protected by a cuffed endotracheal tube.

Individual requirements vary considerably and the recommended dosage is only a guide. Smaller dosage is indicated in ill, shocked, or debilitated patients, while robust individuals may require more. The estimated dosage should be injected over 20 seconds and a further 20 to 30 seconds allowed to assess the effect before a supplementary dose is given. For tracheal intubation, induction should be followed by inhalational anaesthesia or by a neuromuscular blocking drug.

TOTAL INTRAVENOUS ANAESTHESIA. This is a technique in which major surgery is carried out with all anaesthetic drugs being given intravenously. Respiration is controlled, the lungs being inflated with oxygen-enriched air. Muscle relaxant drugs are used to provide relaxation and prevent reflex muscle movements. The main problem to be overcome is the assessment of depth of anaesthesia in the paralysed ventilated patient.

DRIVING. For advice on anaesthesia and driving, see previous page.

## BARBITURATES

**Thiopentone sodium** is the most widely used intravenous anaesthetic, but has no analgesic properties. Induction is generally smooth and rapid, but owing to the potency of the drug, overdosage with cardiorespiratory depression may occur. Aqueous solutions are unstable, particularly when exposed to air. The solution is alkaline and therefore irritant on misplaced injection outside the vein, while arterial injection is particularly dangerous. The usual strength used is a 2.5% solution in water for injections.

Awakening from a moderate dose of thiopentone is rapid due to redistribution of the drug in the whole body tissues. Metabolism is, however, slow and some sedative effects may persist for up to 24 hours during which time the subject is particularly susceptible to the effects of alcohol. Repeated doses have a cumulative effect.

**Methohexitone sodium** is less irritant to tissues than thiopentone; it is usually used as a 1% solution. Recovery is marginally more rapid than in the case of thiopentone. Induction is less smooth with an incidence of hiccup, tremor, involuntary movements, and pain on injection.

Both thiopentone and methohexitone are **contra-indicated** in porphyria (see section 9.8.2).

## OTHER INTRAVENOUS ANAESTHETICS

**Etomidate** is an induction agent associated with rapid recovery without hangover effect. It causes less hypotension than other drugs used for induction. There is a high incidence of extraneous muscle movement and pain on injection. These effects can be minimised by premedication with an opioid analgesic and the use of larger veins. There is evidence that repeated doses of etomidate have an undesirable suppressant effect on adrenocortical function.

**Propofol** is associated with rapid recovery without hangover effect. There is sometimes pain on intravenous injection, but significant extraneous muscle movements do not occur. The CSM have received reports of convulsions, anaphylaxis, and delayed recovery from anaesthesia after propofol administration. Propofol has been associated with bradycardia, occasionally profound; intravenous administration of an antimuscarinic may be necessary to prevent this.

**Ketamine** can be given by the intravenous or the intramuscular route, and has good analgesic properties when used in sub-anaesthetic dosage. The maximum effect occurs in more than one arm-brain circulation time. Muscle tone is increased and the airway is usually well maintained. There is cardiovascular stimulation and arterial pressure may rise with tachycardia. The main disadvantage is the high incidence of hallucinations and other transient psychotic sequelae, though it is believed that these are much less significant in children. The incidence can be reduced when drugs such as diazepam are also used. Ketamine is **contra-indicated** in patients with hypertension and is best avoided in those prone to hallucinations. It is used mainly for paediatric anaesthesia, particularly when repeated administrations are required. Recovery is relatively slow.

**Midazolam** (section 15.1.4.1) is in increasing use as an induction agent.

## THIOPENTONE SODIUM

*Indications:* induction of general anaesthesia; anaesthesia of short duration

*Cautions; Contra-indications; Side-effects:* see notes above; reduce induction dose in severe liver disease; avoid in porphyria (see section 9.8.2); **interactions:** Appendix 1 (anaesthetics)

*Dose: by intravenous injection,* in fit premedicated adults, initially 100–150 mg (4–6 mL of 2.5% solution) over 10–15 seconds, repeated if necessary according to response after 20–30 seconds; *or* up to 4 mg/kg; CHILD induction 4–8 mg/kg

PoM **Thiopentone Sodium** (Non-proprietary)
*Injection,* powder for reconstitution, thiopentone sodium. Net price 500-mg vial = £1.10

PoM **Add-A-Med**® **Thiopentone Sodium** (IMS)
*Injection,* thiopentone sodium 2.5 g with 100 mL diluent to provide a 2.5% solution, net price 1 unit = £7.75; 5 g with 200 mL diluent to provide a 2.5% solution, 1 unit = £13.25

PoM **Intraval Sodium**® (Rhône-Poulenc Rorer)
*Injection 2.5%,* powder for reconstitution, thiopentone sodium. Net price 500-mg amp = £1.49; 2.5-g vial = £4.80
*Injection 5%,* powder for reconstitution, thiopentone sodium. Net price 1-g amp = £1.79

PoM **Min-I-Mix**® **Thiopentone Sodium** (IMS)
*Injection,* thiopentone sodium 500 mg with diluent to provide a 2.5% solution on reconstitution. Net price per unit = £4.34

## ETOMIDATE

*Indications:* induction of anaesthesia

*Cautions; Contra-indications; Side-effects:* see notes above; avoid in porphyria (see section 9.8.2); **interactions:** Appendix 1 (anaesthetics)

*Dose: by slow intravenous injection,* 300 micrograms/kg; high-risk patients, 100 micrograms/kg/minute until anaesthetised (about 3 minutes)

PoM **Hypnomidate**® (Janssen)
*Injection,* etomidate 2 mg/mL in propylene glycol 35%. Net price 10-mL amp = £1.62
*Concentrate injection,* etomidate 125 mg (as hydrochloride)/mL. To be diluted before use. Net price 1-mL amp = £5.47
Note. With the concentrate use only glass syringes, avoid contact with plastics

## KETAMINE

*Indications:* induction and maintenance of anaesthesia

*Cautions; Contra-indications; Side-effects:* see notes above; **interactions:** Appendix 1 (anaesthetics)

*Dose: by intramuscular injection,* short procedures, initially 6.5–13 mg/kg (10 mg/kg usually produces 12–25 minutes of surgical anaesthesia)

Diagnostic manoeuvres and procedures not involving intense pain, initially 4 mg/kg

*By intravenous injection* over at least 60 seconds, short procedures, initially 1–4.5 mg/kg (2 mg/kg usually produces 5–10 minutes of surgical anaesthesia)

*By intravenous infusion* of a solution containing 1 mg/mL, longer procedures, induction, total dose of 0.5–2 mg/kg; maintenance (using microdrip infusion), 10–45 micrograms/kg/minute, rate adjusted according to response

PoM **Ketalar**® (P-D)
*Injection,* ketamine (as hydrochloride) 10 mg/mL, net price 20-mL vial = £3.52; 50 mg/mL, 10-mL vial = £7.31; 100 mg/mL, 5-mL vial = £6.71

## METHOHEXITONE SODIUM

*Indications:* induction and maintenance of anaesthesia for short procedures; with other anaesthetics for more prolonged anaesthesia

*Cautions; Contra-indications; Side-effects:* avoid or reduce dose in liver disease; see also under Thiopentone Sodium and notes above

*Dose: by intravenous injection,* usually as a 1% solution, 50–120 mg according to response at rate of 10 mg in 5 seconds; maintenance, 20–40 mg (2–4 mL of 1% solution) every 4–7 minutes; CHILD induction approx. 1 mg/kg

PoM **Brietal Sodium**® (Lilly)
*Injection,* powder for reconstitution, methohexitone sodium, net price 100 mg in 10-mL vial = 83p; 500 mg in 50-mL vial = £2.14

## PROPOFOL

*Indications:* induction and maintenance of general anaesthesia; sedation of ventilated patients receiving intensive care for up to 3 days

*Cautions; Contra-indications; Side-effects:* see notes above; monitor blood lipid concentrations in patients at risk of fat overload; contra-indicated if history of propofol allergy (see CSM warning above); **interactions:** Appendix 1 (anaesthetics)

*Dose:* induction, *by intravenous injection*, 2–2.5 mg/kg (less in elderly) at a rate of 20–40 mg every 10 seconds; CHILD over 3 years 2.5 mg/kg adjusted as necessary

Maintenance, *by intravenous infusion*, 4–12 mg/kg/hour; CHILD over 3 years 9–15 mg/kg/hour

Sedation during intensive care (with assisted ventilation), *by intravenous infusion*, 1–4 mg/kg/hour for up to 3 days; CHILD not recommended

PoM **Diprivan**® (ICI)

*Injection* (emulsion), propofol 10 mg/mL, net price 20-mL amp = £3.98; 50-mL vial = £9.95

---

## 15.1.2   Inhalational anaesthetics

Inhalational anaesthetics may be gases or volatile liquids. They can be used both for induction and maintenance of anaesthesia and may be used following induction with an intravenous anaesthetic (section 15.1.1).

Gaseous anaesthetics require suitable equipment for storage and administration. They may be supplied via hospital pipelines or from metal cylinders. In clinical use it is necessary to monitor flow rate. Volatile anaesthetics are usually administered using calibrated vaporisers, using air, oxygen, or nitrous oxide–oxygen mixtures as the carrier gas.

To prevent hypoxia gaseous anaesthetics must be given with adequate concentrations of oxygen.

DRIVING. For advice on outpatient anaesthesia and driving, see section 15.1.

---

## HALOGENATED ANAESTHETICS

**Halothane** is a volatile anaesthetic. Its advantages are that it is potent, induction is smooth, the vapour is non-irritant, pleasant to inhale, and seldom induces coughing or breath-holding. The incidence of postoperative vomiting is low.

It is indicated for induction and maintenance of anaesthesia in major surgery with oxygen or nitrous oxide–oxygen mixtures, but is much less widely used than previously owing to its association with severe hepatotoxicity (see CSM findings, below).

Halothane causes cardiorespiratory depression and because of its potency is administered from calibrated vaporisers. Respiratory depression results in elevation of arterial carbon dioxide tension and perhaps ventricular dysrhythmias. Intermittent positive-pressure ventilation must be carried out with care as myocardial depression may follow increase in blood concentrations. Halothane depresses the cardiac muscle fibres and may cause bradycardia. The result is diminished cardiac output and fall of arterial pressure. There is also peripheral vasodilatation. Adrenaline infiltrations should be used with care as ventricular dysrhythmias may result.

Halothane produces moderate muscle relaxation, but this may be inadequate for major abdominal surgery and specific muscle relaxants are then used.

In a publication on findings confirming that *severe hepatotoxicity* can follow halothane anaesthesia the CSM has reported that this occurs more frequently after repeated exposures to halothane and has a high mortality. The risk of severe hepatotoxicity appears to be increased by repeated exposures within a short time interval, but even after a long interval (sometimes of several years) susceptible patients have been reported to develop jaundice. Since there is no reliable way of identifying susceptible patients the CSM recommends the following precautions prior to use of halothane:

1. a careful anaesthetic history should be taken to determine previous exposure and previous reactions to halothane;
2. repeated exposure to halothane within a period of at least 3 months should be avoided unless there are overriding clinical circumstances;
3. a history of unexplained jaundice or pyrexia in a patient following exposure to halothane is an absolute **contra-indication** to its future use in that patient.

**Enflurane** is a volatile anaesthetic similar to halothane, but it is less potent, about twice the concentration being necessary for induction and maintenance. Administration from a calibrated vaporiser is recommended.

Enflurane is a powerful cardiorespiratory depressant. Shallow respiration is likely to result in a rise of arterial carbon dioxide tension, but ventricular dysrhythmias are uncommon and it is probably safe to use adrenaline infiltrations. Myocardial depression may result in a fall in cardiac output and in arterial hypotension.

Enflurane is usually given to supplement nitrous oxide–oxygen mixtures in concentrations of 1 to 3%. The drug is often used in preference to halothane when repeated anaesthesia is required.

**Isoflurane** is an isomer of enflurane. It has a potency intermediate between that of halothane and enflurane, and even less of an inhaled dose is metabolised than with enflurane. Heart rhythm is generally stable during isoflurane anaesthesia, but heart-rate may rise, particularly in younger patients. Systemic arterial pressure may fall, due to a decrease in systemic vascular resistance and with less decrease in cardiac output than occurs with halothane. Respiration is depressed. Muscle relaxation is produced and muscle relaxant drugs potentiated.

---

## ENFLURANE

*Indications; Cautions; Side-effects:* see notes above; avoid in porphyria (see section 9.8.2); **interactions:** Appendix 1 (anaesthetics)
*Dose:* using a specifically calibrated vaporiser, *induction*, increased gradually from 0.4% to max. of 4.5% in air, oxygen, or nitrous oxide–oxygen, according to response
*Maintenance*, 0.5–3% in nitrous oxide–oxygen

**Enflurane** (Abbott)
Enflurane. 250 mL

## HALOTHANE

*Indications; Cautions; Contra-indications; Side-effects:* see notes above; avoid in porphyria (see section 9.8.2); **interactions:** Appendix 1 (anaesthetics)
*Dose:* using a suitable vaporiser, *induction*, increased gradually to 2–4% in oxygen or nitrous oxide–oxygen; CHILD 1.5–2%
*Maintenance*, 0.5–2%

**Halothane** (Rhône-Poulenc Rorer)
Net price 250 mL = £10.49
**Fluothane®** (ICI)
Halothane. Net price 250 mL = £10.49

## ISOFLURANE

*Indications; Cautions; Side-effects:* see notes above; **interactions:** Appendix 1 (anaesthetics)
*Dose:* using a specifically calibrated vaporiser, *induction*, increased gradually from 0.5% to 3%, in oxygen or nitrous oxide–oxygen
*Maintenance*, 1–2.5% in nitrous oxide–oxygen; an additional 0.5–1% may be required when given with oxygen alone; caesarean section, 0.5–0.75% in nitrous oxide–oxygen

**Isoflurane** (Abbott)
Isoflurane. Net price 100 mL = £35.95

NITROUS OXIDE

**Nitrous oxide** is used for induction and maintenance of anaesthesia and, in sub-anaesthetic concentrations, for analgesia in a variety of situations. For anaesthesia it is commonly used in a concentration of 50 to 70% in oxygen as part of a balanced technique in association with other inhalational or intravenous agents. Nitrous oxide is unsatisfactory as a sole anaesthetic owing to lack of potency, but is useful as part of a sequence of drugs since it allows a significant reduction in dosage.

A mixture of nitrous oxide and oxygen containing 50% of each gas (Entonox®) is used to produce analgesia without loss of consciousness. Self-administration using a demand valve is popular and may be appropriate in obstetric practice, for changing painful dressings, as an aid to postoperative physiotherapy, and in emergency ambulances.

Nitrous oxide may have a deleterious effect if used in patients with an air-containing closed space since nitrous oxide diffuses into such a space with a resulting build up of pressure. This effect may be dangerous in the presence of a pneumothorax which may enlarge to compromise respiration. Exposure of patients to nitrous oxide for prolonged periods, either by continuous or intermittent administration, may result in megaloblastic anaemia due to interference with the action of vitamin $B_{12}$. For the same reason, exposure of anaesthetists and theatre staff to nitrous oxide should be minimised. Depression of white cell formation may also occur.

## NITROUS OXIDE

*Indications; Cautions; Side-effects:* see notes above; **interactions:** Appendix 1 (anaesthetics)
*Dose:* using a suitable anaesthetic apparatus, a mixture with 20–30% oxygen for *induction* and *maintenance* of light anaesthesia
*Analgesic*, as a mixture with 50% oxygen, according to the patient's needs

## 15.1.3 Antimuscarinic premedication drugs

Antimuscarinic premedication drugs are used (less commonly nowadays) to dry bronchial and salivary secretions which are increased by intubation and the inhalational anaesthetics. They are also used before or with neostigmine (section 15.1.6) to prevent bradycardia, excessive salivation, and other muscarinic actions of neostigmine. They are also used to prevent bradycardia and hypotension associated with agents such as halothane, propofol, and suxamethonium.

**Atropine** is the most commonly used. Intravenous administration immediately before anaesthesia or intramuscular injection (which should be given 30–60 minutes before the operation) is satisfactory.

**Hyoscine** effectively reduces secretions and also provides a degree of amnesia. It produces less tachycardia than atropine. In some patients, especially the elderly, hyoscine may cause the central anticholinergic syndrome (excitement, ataxia, hallucinations, behavioural abnormalities, and drowsiness).

**Glycopyrronium bromide** produces good drying of salivary secretions. When given intravenously it produces less tachycardia than atropine.

**Phenothiazines** have too little drying activity to be effective when used alone.

## ATROPINE SULPHATE

*Indications:* drying secretions, reversal of excessive bradycardia; with neostigmine for reversal of competitive neuromuscular block; other indications, see sections 1.2, 2.3.1, 11.5
*Cautions:* cardiovascular disease; **interactions:** Appendix 1 (antimuscarinics)
*Side-effects:* tachycardia; see also section 1.2

---

*Dose:* premedication, *by intravenous injection,* 300–600 micrograms immediately before induction of anaesthesia, and in incremental doses of 100 micrograms for the treatment of bradycardia

*By intramuscular injection,* 300–600 micrograms 30–60 minutes before induction; CHILD 20 micrograms/kg

For control of muscarinic side-effects of neostigmine in reversal of competitive neuromuscular block, *by intravenous injection,* 0.6–1.2 mg

Acute arrhythmias after myocardial infarction, see section 2.3.1; see also Cardiopulmonary Resuscitation algorithm, section 2.7

PoM **Atropine** (Non-proprietary)
*Tablets,* atropine sulphate 600 micrograms. Net price 20 = £1.70
*Injection,* atropine sulphate 600 micrograms/mL. Net price 1-mL amp = 29p
*Note.* Other strengths also available

PoM **Min-I-Jet® Atropine Sulphate** (IMS)
*Injection,* atropine sulphate 100 micrograms/mL, net price 5-mL disposable syringe = £3.20; 10-mL disposable syringe = £3.20

CD **Morphine and Atropine Injection** see under Morphine Salts (section 15.1.4.3)

## GLYCOPYRRONIUM BROMIDE
*Indications; Cautions; Side-effects:* see under Atropine Sulphate
*Dose:* premedication, *by intramuscular or intravenous injection,* 200–400 micrograms, *or* 4–5 micrograms/kg to a max. of 400 micrograms; CHILD, *by intramuscular or intravenous injection,* 4–8 micrograms/kg to a max. of 200 micrograms; intra-operative use, *by intravenous injection,* as for premedication
For control of muscarinic side-effects of neostigmine in reversal of competitive neuromuscular block, *by intravenous injection,* 10–15 micrograms/kg with 50 micrograms/kg neostigmine; CHILD, 10 micrograms/kg with 50 micrograms/kg neostigmine

PoM **Robinul®** (Wyeth)
*Injection,* glycopyrronium bromide 200 micrograms/mL. Net price 1-mL amp = 63p; 3-mL amp = £1.06
PoM **Robinul-Neostigmine®**: section 15.1.6

## HYOSCINE HYDROBROMIDE
(Scopolamine Hydrobromide)
*Indications:* drying secretions, amnesia; other indications, see sections 4.6, 11.5
*Cautions; Side-effects:* see under Atropine Sulphate; may slow heart; avoid in the elderly (see notes above)
*Dose:* premedication, *by subcutaneous or intramuscular injection,* 200–600 micrograms 30–60 minutes before induction of anaesthesia, usually with papaveretum; CHILD 15 micrograms/kg

PoM **Hyoscine** (Non-proprietary)
*Injection,* hyoscine hydrobromide 400 micrograms/mL, net price 1-mL amp = £1.34; 600 micrograms/mL, 1-mL amp = £1.08

CD **Papaveretum and Hyoscine Injection,** see under Papaveretum (section 15.1.4.3)

## 15.1.4  Sedative and analgesic perioperative drugs
15.1.4.1 Anxiolytics and neuroleptics
15.1.4.2 Non-opioid analgesics
15.1.4.3 Opioid analgesics

These drugs are given to allay the apprehension of the patient in the pre-operative period (including the night before operation), to relieve pain and discomfort when present, and to augment the action of subsequent anaesthetic agents. A number of the drugs used also provide some degree of pre-operative amnesia. The choice will vary with the individual patient, the nature of the operative procedure, the anaesthetic to be used and other prevailing circumstances such as out-patients, obstetrics, recovery facilities etc. The choice would also vary in elective and emergency operations.

PREMEDICATION IN CHILDREN. Oral or rectal administration is preferred to injections where possible but is not altogether satisfactory. Oral **trimeprazine** is still used but when given alone it may cause postoperative restlessness when pain is present. An alternative is **diazepam**. Some anaesthetists prefer the use of adult regimens, with dosage on a weight basis. (For guidelines on dose calculation in children, see Prescribing for Children.)

Atropine or hyoscine is often given orally to children, but may be given intravenously immediately before induction.

DRIVING. For advice on outpatient anaesthesia and driving, see section 15.1.

## 15.1.4.1  ANXIOLYTICS AND NEUROLEPTICS

Oral premedication is increasing in popularity using benzodiazepines such as diazepam, lorazepam, and temazepam. A short-acting oral benzodiazepine is the most common premedicant.

**Diazepam** is used to produce light sedation with amnesia. The 'sleep' dose shows too great an individual variation to recommend it for induction of anaesthesia, and while this variation exists with regard to its sedative effect, it is probably less marked with lower doses and of little clinical significance. It is particularly valuable in sub-anaesthetic doses to produce light sedation for unpleasant procedures or for operations under local anaesthesia, including dentistry; sub-anaesthetic doses allow retention of the pharyngeal reflexes while a local block is performed, and

---

the resultant amnesia is such that the patient is unlikely to have any unpleasant memories of the procedure (however, benzodiazepines, particularly when used for deep sedation, can sometimes induce sexual fantasies). Diazepam can also be used in a similar manner for endoscopy, with or without an opioid analgesic.

Preparations of diazepam in organic solvents are painful on intravenous injection and followed by a high incidence of venous thrombosis which may not be noticed until a week after the injection. They are also painful on intramuscular injection, and absorption from the injection site is erratic. An emulsion preparation of diazepam (Diazemuls®) is less irritant on intravenous injection and is followed by a negligible incidence of venous thrombosis, but it should not be given intramuscularly. Diazepam is also available as a rectal solution (Stesolid®).

Diazepam and related drugs are of particular value for sedation of patients in an intensive care unit, particularly those on ventilators. It can be given 4–6 hourly but dosage should be gradually reduced after some days to prevent delay in recovery, which can be caused by a build up of its metabolite. Since it has no analgesic action it is often given in conjunction with small doses of opioid analgesics.

Diazepam may on occasions cause marked respiratory depression and facilities for treatment of this are essential. Dental patients who are sitting in one position for a long time may develop hypotonia after diazepam and they should be warned about this possibility. Outpatients should be advised that this is a long-acting drug, and that a second period of drowsiness can occur 4–6 hours after its administration.

By virtue of its physical characteristics, diazepam can accumulate in the fetus and, particularly after the mother has been given large doses, babies can be born in a depressed state, with hypotonia and a tendency to develop hypothermia.

**Temazepam** has a shorter action and relatively more rapid onset than diazepam. Used orally as a premedicant, anxiolytic and sedative effects are produced which continue for one and a half hours. After this period patients are usually fully alert but there may be residual drowsiness. It has proved useful as a premedicant in inpatient and day-case surgery.

**Lorazepam** produces more prolonged sedation than temazepam. In addition amnesia is commonplace. It is particularly useful when used as a premedicant the night prior to major surgery; sound sleep is assured when an oral dose of 1 to 5 mg is given. A further, smaller, dose the following morning will be required if any delay in the commencement of surgery is anticipated. Alternatively the first dose may be given in the early morning of the day of operation.

**Midazolam** is a water-soluble benzodiazepine which is often used in preference to diazepam. Recovery is faster than with diazepam. The incidence of side-effects is low but the CSM has received reports of respiratory depression (some-

times associated with severe hypotension) following intravenous administration. A preparation containing 2 mg/mL is available to ensure easier titration of dosage.

**Chlormethiazole** has been used as an intravenous infusion to maintain sleep during surgery carried out under regional analgesia, including extradural block. It has no analgesic effect, little cardiac and respiratory depression, and may be used in elderly patients.

## CHLORMETHIAZOLE EDISYLATE

*Indications:* sedative during regional anaesthesia; other indications, see sections 4.1.1, 4.8.2

*Cautions; Side-effects:* see section 4.8.2

*Contra-indications:* acute pulmonary insufficiency

*Dose: by intravenous infusion,* as a 0.8% solution, induction 25 mL (200 mg)/minute for 1–2 minutes; maintenance 1–4 mL (8–32 mg)/ minute

*Note.* Special care on prolonged intravenous administration since accumulation may occur; also, contains no electrolytes

PoM **Heminevrin**® (Astra)
*Intravenous infusion 0.8%,* chlormethiazole edisylate 8 mg/mL. Net price 500-mL bottle = £5.25

## CHLORPROMAZINE HYDROCHLORIDE

*Indications:* see under Dose; other indications, see section 4.2.1

*Cautions; Contra-indications; Side-effects:* see section 4.2.1

*Dose:* induction of hypothermia (to prevent shivering), *by deep intramuscular injection,* 25–50 mg every 6–8 hours; CHILD 1–12 years, initially 0.5–1 mg/kg, maintenance 500 micrograms/kg every 4–6 hours

PoM **Chlorpromazine** (Non-proprietary)
*Injection,* chlorpromazine hydrochloride 25 mg/ mL, net price 1-mL amp = 21p; 2-mL amp = 27p

PoM **Largactil**® (Rhône-Poulenc Rorer)
*Injection,* chlorpromazine hydrochloride 25 mg/ mL. Net price 2-mL amp = 28p

## DIAZEPAM

*Indications:* premedication; sedation with amnesia, and in conjunction with local anaesthesia; other indications, see sections 4.1.2, 4.8, 10.2.2

*Cautions; Contra-indications; Side-effects:* see notes above and sections 4.1.2, 4.8.2

*Dose: by mouth,* 5 mg at night, 5 mg on waking, and 5 mg 2 hours before minor or dental surgery

*By intravenous injection,* 10–20 mg over 2–4 minutes as sedative cover for minor surgical and medical procedures; premedication 100–200 micrograms/kg

*By rectum* in solution, ADULT and CHILD over 3 years 10 mg; CHILD 1–3 years and elderly 5 mg

**Parenteral preparations**

PoM **Diazepam** (Non-proprietary)

*Injection* (solution), diazepam 5 mg/mL. See Appendix 6. Net price 2-mL amp = 25p
Available from CP

PoM **Diazemuls**® (Dumex)

*Injection* (emulsion), diazepam 5 mg/mL. For intravenous injection or infusion. See Appendix 6. Net price 2-mL amp = 69p

PoM **Valium**® (Roche)

*Injection* (solution), diazepam 5 mg/mL. See Appendix 6. Net price 2-mL amp = 30p

---

## DROPERIDOL

*Indications:* anti-emetic, pre-operative sedation; neuroleptanalgesia; other indications, see section 4.2.1

*Cautions; Contra-indications; Side-effects:* see section 4.2.1

*Dose:* premedication, *by intramuscular injection*, up to 10 mg 60 minutes before operation; CHILD 200–500 micrograms/kg

Neuroleptanalgesia, *by intravenous injection*, 5–15 mg at induction with an opioid analgesic; CHILD 200–300 micrograms/kg

PoM **Droleptan**® (Janssen)

*Injection*, droperidol 5 mg/mL. Net price 2-mL amp = 92p

CD **Thalamonal**® — see under Fentanyl (section 15.1.4.1)

---

## LORAZEPAM

*Indications:* sedation with amnesia; as pre-medication; other indications, see sections 4.1.2, 4.8.2

*Cautions; Contra-indications; Side-effects:* see under Diazepam

*Dose: by mouth*, 1–3 mg at night *or* 1–5 mg 2–6 hours before surgery

*By slow intravenous injection*, preferably diluted with an equal volume of sodium chloride intravenous infusion 0.9% or water for injections, 50 micrograms/kg 30–45 minutes before operation

*By intramuscular injection*, diluted as above, 50 micrograms/kg 1–1½ hours before operation

PoM **Ativan**® (Wyeth)

*Injection*, lorazepam 4 mg/mL. Net price 1-mL amp = 40p

*Tablets*, see section 4.1.2

---

## MIDAZOLAM

*Indications:* sedation with amnesia, and in conjunction with local anaesthesia; premedication, induction

*Cautions; Contra-indications; Side-effects:* see under Diazepam; see notes above for CSM warning; **important:** plasma concentration increased by erythromycin—profound sedation reported with oral midazolam (not on UK market); other **interactions:** Appendix 1 (benzodiazepines)

*Dose:* sedation, *by intravenous injection* over 30 seconds, 2 mg (elderly 1–1.5 mg) followed after 2 minutes by increments of 0.5–1 mg if sedation not adequate; usual range 2.5–7.5 mg (about 70 micrograms/kg), elderly 1–2 mg

Premedication, *by intramuscular injection*, 70–100 micrograms/kg 30–60 minutes before surgery; usual dose 5 mg (2.5 mg in elderly)

Induction, *by slow intravenous injection*, 200–300 micrograms/kg (elderly 100–200 micrograms/kg)

PoM **Hypnovel**® (Roche)

*Injection*, midazolam (as hydrochloride) 2 mg/mL, net price 5-mL amp = 92p; 5 mg/mL, 2-mL amp = 77p

---

## PROMETHAZINE HYDROCHLORIDE

*Indications:* anti-emetic, pre-operative sedative and antimuscarinic; other indications, see sections 3.4.1, 3.4.3

*Cautions; Side-effects:* see section 4.6

*Dose:* premedication, *by mouth,* CHILD 1–5 years 15–20 mg, 6–10 years 20–25 mg

*By deep intramuscular injection*, 25–50 mg 1 hour before operation; CHILD 5–10 years, 6.25–12.5 mg

**Preparations**

See section 3.4.1

---

## TEMAZEPAM

*Indications:* premedication before minor surgery; anxiety before investigatory procedures; hypnotic, see section 4.1.1

*Cautions; Contra-indications; Side-effects:* see under Diazepam

*Dose: by mouth*, premedication, 20–40 mg (elderly, 10–20 mg) 1 hour before operation; CHILD 1 mg/kg (max. 30 mg)

**Preparations**

See section 4.1.1

---

## TRIMEPRAZINE TARTRATE

*Indications:* pre-operative sedation, anti-emetic; other indications, see section 3.4.1

*Cautions; Side-effects:* see notes above and section 3.4.1

*Dose: by mouth*, premedication, 3 mg/kg 1–2 hours before operation; CHILD 2–7 years up to 2 mg/kg

**Preparations**

See section 3.4.1

---

15.1.4.2  NON-OPIOID ANALGESICS

---

## DICLOFENAC SODIUM

See section 10.1.1

## KETOPROFEN

See section 10.1.1

---

## KETOROLAC TROMETAMOL
*Indications:* pain associated with surgical procedures

*Cautions; Contra-indications; Side-effects:* as for other NSAIDs, see section 10.1.1; postoperative wound haemorrhage and pain at injection site reported; **interactions:** Appendix 1 (NSAIDs)

*Dose: by intramuscular injection*, initially 30 mg, then 10–30 mg every 4–6 hours when required (every 2 hours in initial postoperative period); max. 120 mg daily; max. duration of treatment 5 days; ADOLESCENT and CHILD under 16 years not recommended

▼ PoM **Toradol**® (Syntex)
*Injection*, ketorolac trometamol 30 mg/mL, net price 1-mL amp = £1.31

### 15.1.4.3  OPIOID ANALGESICS

An opioid analgesic is commonly used as a premedicant, e.g. morphine or pethidine given intramuscularly about an hour before operation, usually combined with an antisialogogue. Sometimes they are combined with a phenothiazine or droperidol. The main side-effects are respiratory depression, cardiovascular depression, and nausea and vomiting. The principal advantages are that opioid analgesics provide analgesia persisting into the operative period giving a reduced chance of awareness during anaesthesia with full doses of muscle relaxants.

INTRA-OPERATIVE ANALGESIA. Many of the conventional opioid analgesics are used to supplement general anaesthesia, usually in combination with nitrous oxide–oxygen and a muscle relaxant. Pethidine was the first to be used for this purpose but other drugs now available include alfentanil, fentanyl, meptazinol, nalbuphine, and phenoperidine. The longer-acting drugs morphine and papaveretum, although equally effective for this purpose, are not commonly used because of the problems of respiratory depression in the postoperative period.

Small doses of opioids given immediately before or with thiopentone will reduce the induction dose of the barbiturate and this is a popular technique in poor-risk patients. **Alfentanil** and **fentanyl** are particularly useful in this respect because of their short duration of action although there may be some cumulation with large doses. Alfentanil may be preferable for short operations because of its very brief duration of action; for long procedures it can be given as a continuous infusion.

Repeated doses of intra-operative analgesics should be given with care, since not only may the respiratory depression persist into the postoperative period but it may become apparent for the first time postoperatively when the patient is away from immediate nursing attention. The specific opioid antagonist, naloxone (section 15.1.7), will immediately reverse this respiratory depression but the dose may have to be repeated. In clinical doses it will also reverse most of the analgesia. An alternative and equally acceptable approach is to use the specific respiratory stimulant, doxapram (see section 3.5.1), which can be given in an infusion and which will not affect the opioid analgesia. The use of intra-operative opioids should be borne in mind when prescribing postoperative analgesics. In many instances they will delay the need for the first dose but caution is necessary since there may be some residual respiratory depression potentiated by the postoperative analgesic.

**Fentanyl** may produce severe respiratory depression, especially in patients with decreased respiratory function or when other respiratory depressant drugs have been given. Respiratory depression may be treated by artificial ventilation or be reversed by naloxone or doxapram (see above). Alfentanil may also cause severe respiratory depression, especially when other respiratory depressant drugs have already been given; this may be reversed with naloxone (see above).

**Meptazinol** can be used for analgesia during or after operation. It is associated with nausea and vomiting, but is claimed to have a reduced incidence of respiratory depression.

For general notes on analgesics see section 4.7.

## ALFENTANIL
*Indications:* analgesia especially during short operative procedure and outpatient surgery; enhancement of anaesthesia; analgesic and respiratory depressant in assisted respiration

*Cautions; Contra-indications; Side-effects:* see under Fentanyl and notes above

*Dose: by intravenous injection*, spontaneous respiration, ADULT, initially up to 500 micrograms over 30 seconds; supplemental, 250 micrograms
With assisted ventilation, ADULT and CHILD, initially 30–50 micrograms/kg; supplemental, 15 micrograms/kg

*By intravenous infusion*, with assisted ventilation, ADULT and CHILD, initially 50–100 micrograms/kg over 10 minutes *or* as a bolus, followed by maintenance of 0.5–1 micrograms/kg/minute

CD **Rapifen**® (Janssen)
*Injection*, alfentanil 500 micrograms (as hydrochloride)/mL. Net price 2-mL amp = 74p; 10-mL amp = £3.39
*Intensive care*[1] *injection*, alfentanil 5 mg (as hydrochloride)/mL. To be diluted before use. Net price 1-mL amp = £2.72
1. Formerly Rapifen® Concentrate injection

---

Cautionary label wordings, see inside back cover

Prices are **net**, see p. 1

## BUPRENORPHINE

*Indications:* peri-operative analgesia; premedication; analgesia in other situations, see section 4.7.2

*Cautions; Contra-indications; Side-effects:* see section 4.7.2

*Dose:* pain, *by slow intravenous injection*, 300–450 micrograms

Premedication, *by sublingual administration*, 400 micrograms

*By intramuscular injection*, 300 micrograms

**Preparations**
See section 4.7.2

## FENTANYL

*Indications:* analgesia during operation, neuroleptanalgesia, enhancement of anaesthesia; respiratory depressant in assisted respiration

*Cautions:* chronic respiratory disease, myasthenia gravis; reduce dose in elderly, hypothyroidism, chronic liver disease; obstetric use may cause respiratory depression in neonate; see also notes above; **interactions:** Appendix 1 (opioid analgesics)

*Contra-indications:* respiratory depression or obstructive airways disease unless patient ventilated

*Side-effects:* respiratory depression, transient hypotension, bradycardia, nausea and vomiting

*Dose: by intravenous injection*, with spontaneous respiration, 50–200 micrograms, then 50 micrograms as required; CHILD 3–5 micrograms/kg, then 1 microgram/kg as required

With assisted ventilation, 0.3–3.5 mg, then 100–200 micrograms as required; CHILD 15 micrograms/kg, then 1–3 micrograms/kg as required

CD **Fentanyl Citrate** (Non-proprietary)
*Injection*, fentanyl 50 micrograms (as citrate)/mL, net price 2-mL amp = 45p; 10-mL amp = £2.05
Available from David Bull, Evans

CD **Sublimaze**® (Janssen)
*Injection*, fentanyl 50 micrograms (as citrate)/mL. Net price 2-mL amp = 25p; 10-mL amp = £1.20

CD **Thalamonal**® (Janssen)
*Injection*, fentanyl 50 micrograms (as citrate), droperidol 2.5 mg/mL. Net price 2-mL amp = 95p

*Dose:* premedication, neuroleptanalgesia, by intramuscular injection 1–2 mL 5–15 minutes before operation; induction, by intravenous injection 6–8 mL followed by assisted ventilation; maintenance, by intravenous injection, 1–2 mL as required; CHILD premedication, neuroleptanalgesia, by intramuscular injection 0.4–1.5 mL

## MEPTAZINOL

*Indications:* analgesia during and after operation; analgesia in other situations, see section 4.7.2

*Cautions; Contra-indications; Side-effects:* see section 4.7.2 and notes above

*Dose: by mouth*, 200 mg every 3–6 hours as required

*By intramuscular injection*, 75–100 mg, repeated every 2–4 hours as required

*By slow intravenous injection*, 50–100 mg, repeated every 2–4 hours as required

See also section 4.7.2 for analgesia

PoM **Meptid**® (Wyeth)
*Tablets*, orange, f/c, meptazinol 200 mg. Net price 20 = £1.80. Label: 2
*Injection*, meptazinol 100 mg (as hydrochloride)/mL. Net price 1-mL amp = 79p

## MORPHINE SALTS

*Indications:* analgesia during and after operation; enhancement of anaesthesia; pre-operative sedation; analgesia in other situations, see section 4.7.2

*Cautions; Contra-indications; Side-effects:* see section 4.7.2 and notes above

*Dose: by subcutaneous or intramuscular injection*, up to 10 mg 1–1½ hours before operation; CHILD, *by intramuscular injection*, 150 micrograms/kg. See also section 4.7.2 for analgesia

CD **Morphine Sulphate Injection**, morphine sulphate, 10, 15 and 30 mg/mL. Net price 1- and 2-mL amp (all) = 51–86p

CD **Morphine and Atropine Injection**, morphine sulphate 10 mg, atropine sulphate 600 micrograms/mL. Net price 1-mL amp = 53p
*Dose:* premedication, by subcutaneous injection, 0.5–1 mL

## NALBUPHINE HYDROCHLORIDE

*Indications:* peri-operative analgesia; premedication; analgesia in other situations, see section 4.7.2

*Cautions; Contra-indications; Side-effects:* see section 4.7.2 and notes above; also caution in ambulant patients (impairment of mental and physical ability)

*Dose:* acute pain, *by subcutaneous, intramuscular, or intravenous injection*, 10–20 mg, adjusted according to response; CHILD up to 300 micrograms/kg repeated once or twice as necessary. See also section 4.7.2. for analgesia

Premedication, *by subcutaneous, intramuscular, or intravenous injection*, 100–200 micrograms/kg

Induction, *by intravenous injection*, 0.3–1 mg/kg over 10–15 minutes

Intra-operative analgesia, *by intravenous injection*, 250–500 micrograms/kg at 30-minute intervals

PoM **Nubain**® (Du Pont)
*Injection*, nalbuphine hydrochloride 10 mg/mL. Net price 1-mL amp = 75p; 2-mL amp = £1.16

---

## PAPAVERETUM and OTHER MIXED OPIUM ALKALOIDS

*Indications:* analgesia during and after operation; pre-medication; see also under preparations

*Cautions; Contra-indications; Side-effects:* see section 4.7.2 and notes above; noscapine in papaveretum contra-indicated in women of child-bearing potential (see Appendix 4)

Papaveretum

The hydrochlorides of alkaloids of opium, containing the equivalent of anhydrous morphine 47.5–52.5%, anhydrous codeine 2.5–5%, noscapine 16–22%, and papaverine 2.5–7%

*Note.* Papaveretum 20 mg is approximately equivalent to morphine 12.5 mg

IMPORTANT. Do **not** confuse with papaverine (see section 7.4.5)

**CD Papaveretum Injection,** papaveretum 10 mg/mL, net price 1-mL amp = 31p; 20 mg/mL, 1-mL amp = 36p

*Dose:* acute pain, *by subcutaneous or intramuscular injection,* 20 mg repeated every 4 hours if necessary (10 mg for elderly or lighter patients); CHILD up to 1 month 150 micrograms/kg, 1–12 months 200 micrograms/kg, 1–12 years 200–300 micrograms/kg

*By slow intravenous injection,* quarter to half corresponding subcutaneous or intramuscular dose

Pre-operative sedation, *by subcutaneous or intramuscular injection,* 10–20 mg 45–60 minutes before anaesthesia; CHILD single doses as above

**CD Papaveretum and Hyoscine Injection,** papaveretum 20 mg, hyoscine hydrobromide 400 micrograms/mL. Net price 1-mL amp = 36p

*Dose:* premedication, by subcutaneous or intramuscular injection, 0.5–1 mL

Other mixed opium alkaloids

*Note.* Do not contain noscapine

**CD Omnopon®** (Roche) [New formulation]

*Injection,* morphine hydrochloride 13.44 mg (≡ anhydrous morphine 10 mg), codeine hydrochloride 1.04 mg, papaverine hydrochloride 1.2 mg/mL. Net price 1-mL amp = 17p

*Dose:* postoperative analgesia, premedication, severe chronic pain, and pain in myocardial infarction, by subcutaneous, intramuscular, or intravenous[1] injection, ADULT 0.5–1 mL repeated every 4 hours if necessary in chronic pain (0.5 mL for elderly); CHILD 1–12 years 0.01–0.015 mL/kg

*Paediatric injection,* morphine hydrochloride 6.72 mg (≡ anhydrous morphine 5 mg), codeine hydrochloride 520 micrograms, papaverine hydrochloride 600 micrograms/mL. Net price 1-mL amp = 16p

*Dose:* postoperative analgesia, premedication, severe chronic pain, and pain in myocardial infarction, by subcutaneous, intramuscular, or intravenous[1] injection, ADULT 1–2 mL repeated every 4 hours if necessary in chronic pain (1 mL for elderly); CHILD up to 1 month 0.015 mL/kg, 1–12 months 0.015–0.02 mL/kg, 1–12 years 0.02–0.03 mL/kg

1. In general the intravenous dose should be quarter to half corresponding subcutaneous or intramuscular dose.

## PETHIDINE HYDROCHLORIDE

*Indications:* peri-operative analgesia, enhancement of anaesthesia, for basal narcosis with phenothiazines; premedication; analgesia in other situations, see section 4.7.2

*Cautions; Contra-indications; Side-effects:* see section 4.7.2 and notes above

*Dose:* premedication, *by intramuscular injection,* 25–100 mg 1 hour before operation; CHILD 0.5–2 mg/kg

Adjunct to nitrous oxide–oxygen, *by slow intravenous injection,* 10–25 mg repeated when required

See also section 4.7.2 for analgesia

**CD Pethidine** (Roche)

*Injection,* pethidine hydrochloride 50 mg/mL, net price 1-mL amp = 11p; 2-mL amp = 14p; 10 mg/mL, 5-mL amp = 66p; 10-mL amp = 69p

*Tablets,* see section 4.7.2

**CD Pamergan P100®** (Martindale)

*Injection,* pethidine hydrochloride 50 mg, promethazine hydrochloride 25 mg/mL. Net price 2-mL amp = 45p

*Dose:* premedication, 2 mL by intramuscular injection 1–1½ hours before operation; CHILD, by intramuscular injection, 8–12 years 0.75 mL, 13–16 years 1 mL

## PHENOPERIDINE HYDROCHLORIDE

*Indications:* analgesia during operation, neuroleptanalgesia, enhancement of anaesthetics; respiratory depressant in prolonged assisted respiration

*Cautions; Contra-indications; Side-effects:* see under Pethidine Hydrochloride and Fentanyl. Doses above 1 mg cause respiratory depression and require assisted ventilation (effects may be terminated with naloxone)

*Dose:* by intravenous injection, with spontaneous respiration, up to 1 mg, then 500 micrograms every 40–60 minutes as required; CHILD 30–50 micrograms/kg

With assisted ventilation, 2–5 mg, then 1 mg as required; CHILD 100–150 micrograms/kg

**CD Operidine®** (Janssen)

*Injection,* phenoperidine hydrochloride 1 mg/mL. Net price 2-mL amp = 77p; 10-mL amp = £4.05

## 15.1.5   Muscle relaxants

Muscle relaxants used in anaesthesia are also known as **neuromuscular blocking drugs** or **myoneural blocking drugs**. By specific blockade of the neuromuscular junction they enable light levels of anaesthesia to be employed with adequate relaxation of the muscles of the abdomen and diaphragm. They also relax the vocal cords and allow the passage of a tracheal tube. Their action differs from the muscle relaxants acting on the spinal cord or brain which are used in musculoskeletal disorders (see section 10.2.2).

Patients who have received a muscle relaxant should **always** have their respiration assisted or controlled until the drug has been inactivated or antagonised (section 15.1.6).

## NON-DEPOLARISING MUSCLE RELAXANTS

Drugs of this group (also known as competitive muscle relaxants) cause blockade by competing with acetylcholine at the receptor site at the neuromuscular junction. These drugs are best suited to the production of paralysis of long duration. They have a slower, less complete action than the depolarising muscle relaxants and should be avoided in myasthenia gravis.

These drugs may be used during surgical operations and for patients receiving long-term ventilation in intensive care units, when larger total doses will be appropriate.

The action of the competitive muscle relaxants may be reversed with anticholinesterases such as neostigmine (section 15.1.6).

**Atracurium** and **vecuronium** are much more widely employed than the other muscle relaxants, atracurium because of its non-enzymatic elimination and vecuronium because it has the fewest side-effects.

**Atracurium** has a duration of action of 15 to 35 minutes. Histamine release may occur. The drug is without vagolytic or sympatholytic properties. It has an advantage over other non-depolarising muscle relaxants in patients with renal or hepatic impairment, as it is degraded by non-enzymatic Hofmann elimination, which is independent of liver and kidney function. It is non-cumulative on repeated dosage. Its action is reversed by neostigmine. Duration of action may be prolonged in hypothermia.

**Vecuronium** has a duration of action of 20 to 30 minutes. Large doses may have a cumulative effect. The drug does not cause histamine release, sympathetic blockade, or vagolytic effects.

**Pancuronium** does not cause ganglionic blockade or significant changes in blood pressure and may therefore be favoured when it is important to maintain cardiac output.

**Tubocurarine** starts to act between 3–5 minutes and lasts for about 30 minutes after injection. It may cause an erythematous rash on the chest and neck and this is probably due to histamine release. Onset of blockade may be associated with hypotension and this, though transient, may be important in poor-risk patients.

**Gallamine** has a more rapid onset of action and recovery than tubocurarine or pancuronium. It causes undesirable tachycardia by its vagolytic action. It should be avoided in patients with severe renal disease.

**Alcuronium** appears to have no significant advantages over other muscle relaxants. Its duration of action is similar to that of tubocurarine.

## ALCURONIUM CHLORIDE

**Indications:** non-depolarising muscle relaxant of medium duration
**Cautions; Contra-indications; Side-effects:** see notes above. Reduce dose in renal impairment; avoid in porphyria (see section 9.8.2); **interactions:** Appendix 1 (muscle relaxants)
**Dose:** *by intravenous injection*, initially 200–250 micrograms/kg, then incremental doses of one-sixth to one-quarter of the initial dose, as required; CHILD over 1 month, 125–200 micrograms/kg

PoM **Alloferin®** (Roche)
*Injection*, alcuronium chloride 5 mg/mL. Net price 2-mL amp = 58p

## ATRACURIUM BESYLATE

**Indications:** non-depolarising muscle relaxant of short to medium duration
**Cautions; Contra-indications; Side-effects:** see notes above; **interactions:** Appendix 1 (muscle relaxants)
**Dose:** *by intravenous injection*, ADULT and CHILD over 1 month initially 300–600 micrograms/kg, then 100–200 micrograms/kg as required
*By intravenous infusion*, 5–10 micrograms/kg/minute (300–600 micrograms/kg/hour)

PoM **Tracrium®** (Wellcome)
*Injection*, atracurium besylate 10 mg/mL. Net price 2.5-mL amp = £1.83; 5-mL amp = £3.38; 25-mL amp = £14.53

## GALLAMINE TRIETHIODIDE

**Indications:** non-depolarising muscle relaxant of medium duration
**Cautions; Contra-indications; Side-effects:** see notes above; reduce dose in renal impairment (avoid if severe); **interactions:** Appendix 1 (muscle relaxants)
**Dose:** *by intravenous injection*, 80–120 mg, then 20–40 mg as required; CHILD, 1.5 mg/kg

PoM **Flaxedil®** (Rhône–Poulenc Rorer)
*Injection*, gallamine triethiodide 40 mg/mL. Net price 2-mL amp = 74p

## PANCURONIUM BROMIDE

**Indications:** non-depolarising muscle relaxant of medium duration
**Cautions; Contra-indications; Side-effects:** see notes above; caution in hepatic impairment; reduce dose in renal impairment; **interactions:** Appendix 1 (muscle relaxants)
**Dose:** *by intravenous injection*, initially for intubation 50–100 micrograms/kg then 10–20 micrograms/kg as required; CHILD initially 60–100 micrograms/kg, then 10–20 micrograms/kg, NEONATE 30–40 micrograms/kg initially then 10–20 micrograms/kg
Intensive care, *by intravenous injection*, 60 micrograms/kg every 1–1½ hours

PoM **Pavulon**® (Organon-Teknika)
*Injection*, pancuronium bromide 2 mg/mL. Net price 2-mL amp = 67p

## TUBOCURARINE CHLORIDE

*Indications:* non-depolarising muscle relaxant of medium to long duration

*Cautions; Contra-indications; Side-effects:* see notes above. Reduce dose in renal impairment; **interactions:** Appendix 1 (muscle relaxants)

*Dose: by intravenous injection*, initially 15–30 mg according to circumstances then 5–10 mg as required; CHILD, initially 300–500 micrograms/kg then 60–100 micrograms/kg as required; NEONATE initially 200–250 micrograms/kg then 40–50 micrograms/kg as required

PoM **Jexin**® (DF)
*Injection*, tubocurarine chloride 10 mg/mL. Net price 1.5-mL amp = 71p
PoM **Tubarine**® (Wellcome)
*Injection*, tubocurarine chloride 10 mg/mL. Net price 1.5-mL amp = £1.86

## VECURONIUM BROMIDE

*Indications:* non-depolarising muscle relaxant of short to medium duration

*Cautions; Contra-indications; Side-effects:* see notes above; reduce dose in renal impairment; **interactions:** Appendix 1 (muscle relaxants)

*Dose: by intravenous injection*, initially 80–100 micrograms/kg (max. 250 micrograms/kg), then 30–50 micrograms/kg as required; CHILD, as adult dose (onset more rapid)
*By intravenous infusion*, 50–80 micrograms/kg/hour

PoM **Norcuron**® (Organon-Teknika)
*Injection*, powder for reconstitution, vecuronium bromide. Net price 10-mg vial = £3.48 (with water for injections)

## DEPOLARISING MUSCLE RELAXANTS

**Suxamethonium** is the only commonly used drug of this group. With a 5-minute duration of action it is ideal for passage of a tracheal tube but may be used in repeated dosage for longer procedures.

It acts by mimicking acetylcholine at the neuromuscular junction but disengagement from the receptor site and subsequent breakdown is slower than for acetylcholine; depolarisation is therefore prolonged and neuromuscular blockade results.

It produces rapid, complete, and predictable paralysis, and recovery is spontaneous. Unlike the non-depolarising muscle relaxants its action cannot be reversed and clinical application is therefore limited.

Suxamethonium should be given after induction of anaesthesia because paralysis is usually preceded by painful muscle fasciculation. There is a transient rise in plasma potassium and creatine phosphokinase and there may be muscle pains postoperatively. Suxamethonium is **contra-indicated** in severe liver disease and in burned patients. Premedication with atropine is desirable.

Prolonged muscle paralysis may occur in patients with low or atypical plasma pseudocholinesterase enzymes. Prolonged paralysis may also occur in **dual block**, which occurs after repeated doses of suxamethonium have been used and is caused by the development of a non-depolarising block following the primary depolarising block. Artificial ventilation should be continued until muscle function is restored. Dual block is diagnosed by giving a short-acting anticholinesterase such as edrophonium; if an improvement occurs the block is treated with neostigmine (section 15.1.6).

## SUXAMETHONIUM CHLORIDE

*Indications:* depolarising muscle relaxant of short duration

*Cautions; Contra-indications; Side-effects:* see notes above; **interactions:** Appendix 1 (muscle relaxants)

*Dose: by intravenous injection*, 600 micrograms/kg (range 0.3–1.1 mg/kg depending on degree of relaxation required); usual range 20–100 mg
*By intravenous infusion*, as a 0.1% solution, 2–5 mg/minute (2–5 mL/minute)

PoM **Anectine**® (Wellcome)
*Injection*, suxamethonium chloride 50 mg/mL. Net price 2-mL amp = 73p
PoM **Min-I-Mix**® **Suxamethonium Chloride** (IMS)
*Injection*, suxamethonium chloride 100 mg with diluent to provide a 2% solution on reconstitution. Net price per unit = £3.55
PoM **Scoline**® (DF)
*Injection*, suxamethonium chloride 50 mg/mL. Net price 2-mL amp = 31p

## 15.1.6 Anticholinesterases used in surgery

Anticholinesterases reverse the effects of the non-depolarising (competitive) muscle relaxant drugs such as tubocurarine but they prolong the action of the depolarising muscle relaxant drug suxamethonium.

**Edrophonium** has a transient action and is used to diagnose dual block caused by suxamethonium (section 15.1.5).

**Neostigmine** has a longer duration of action than edrophonium. It is the specific drug for reversal of non-depolarising (competitive) blockade. It acts within one minute of intravenous injection and lasts for 20 to 30 minutes; a second dose may then be necessary. It is also used in the treatment of dual block. Atropine or glycopyrronium (section 15.1.3) should be given before or with neostigmine in order to prevent bradycardia, excessive salivation, and other muscarinic actions of neostigmine.

For anticholinesterases used in myasthenia gravis see section 10.2.1.

## EDROPHONIUM CHLORIDE

*Indications:* see under Dose
*Cautions; Contra-indications; Side-effects:* see section 10.2.1 and notes above. Atropine should also be given
*Dose:* brief reversal of non-depolarising neuromuscular blockade, *by intravenous injection* over several minutes, 500–700 micrograms/kg (after or with atropine sulphate 0.6–1.2 mg)
Diagnosis of dual block, *by intravenous injection*, 10 mg (with atropine)
Diagnosis of myasthenia gravis, see section 10.2.1

PoM **Tensilon**® (Roche)
*Injection*, edrophonium chloride 10 mg/mL. Net price 1-mL amp = 27p

## NEOSTIGMINE METHYLSULPHATE

*Indications:* see under Dose
*Cautions; Contra-indications; Side-effects:* see section 10.2.1 and notes above. Atropine should also be given
*Dose:* reversal of non-depolarising neuromuscular blockade, *by intravenous injection* over 1 minute, 50–70 micrograms/kg (max. 5 mg) after or with atropine sulphate 0.6–1.2 mg
Myasthenia gravis, see section 10.2.1

PoM **Prostigmin**® (Roche)
*Injection*, neostigmine methylsulphate 500 micrograms/mL, net price 1-mL amp = 16p; 2.5 mg/mL, 1-mL amp = 16p
PoM **Robinul-Neostigmine**® (Wyeth)
*Injection*, neostigmine methylsulphate 2.5 mg, glycopyrronium bromide 500 micrograms/mL. Net price 1-mL amp = £1.06
  *Dose:* by intravenous injection over 10–30 seconds, 1–2 mL *or* 0.02 mL/kg;
  CHILD 0.02 mL/kg (*or* 0.2 mL/kg of a 1 in 10 dilution using water for injections or sodium chloride injection 0.9%)

## 15.1.7  Antagonists for central and respiratory depression

The opioid antagonist **naloxone** can be used at the end of an operation to reverse respiratory depression caused by opioid analgesics. Unless the dosage is carefully adjusted, analgesia may also be reversed. For respiratory stimulants see section 3.5.1. **Doxapram** is a respiratory stimulant which does not reverse the other effects of opioid analgesics.

**Flumazenil** is a benzodiazepine antagonist for the reversal of the central sedative effects of benzodiazepines in anaesthetic and similar procedures. It is important to recognize that the half-life of flumazenil is shorter than those of diazepam and midazolam, in order to avoid the risk of patients becoming resedated.

## DOXAPRAM HYDROCHLORIDE

*Indications:* see under Dose
*Cautions; Contra-indications; Side-effects:* see section 3.5.1

*Dose:* postoperative respiratory depression, *by intravenous injection* over at least 30 seconds, 1–1.5 mg/kg repeated if necessary after intervals of 1 hour
*By intravenous infusion*, 2–3 mg/minute
  Ventilatory failure, see section 3.5.1

PoM **Dopram**® (Wyeth)
*Injection*, doxapram hydrochloride 20 mg/mL. Net price 5-mL amp = £2.14
*Intravenous infusion:* see section 3.5.1

## FLUMAZENIL

*Indications:* reversal of sedative effects of benzodiazepines in anaesthetic, intensive care, and diagnostic procedures
*Cautions:* short-acting (repeat doses may be necessary); benzodiazepine effects may persist for at least 24 hours; benzodiazepine dependence; ensure neuromuscular blockade cleared before giving; avoid rapid injection in high-risk or anxious patients and following major surgery; hepatic impairment
*Contra-indications:* epileptics who have received prolonged benzodiazepine therapy
*Side-effects:* nausea, vomiting, and flushing; if wakening too rapid, agitation, anxiety, and fear; transient increase in blood pressure and heart-rate in intensive care patients; very rarely convulsions (particularly in epileptics)
*Dose:* by intravenous injection, 200 micrograms over 15 seconds, then 100 micrograms at 60-second intervals if required; usual dose range, 300–600 micrograms; max. total dose 1 mg (2 mg in intensive care); question aetiology if no response to repeated doses
*By intravenous infusion*, if drowsiness recurs after injection, 100–400 micrograms/hour, adjusted according to level of arousal

PoM **Anexate**® (Roche)
*Injection*, flumazenil 100 micrograms/mL. Net price 5-mL amp = £16.32

## NALOXONE HYDROCHLORIDE

*Indications:* reversal of opioid-induced respiratory depression
*Cautions:* see under Emergency Treatment of Poisoning
*Dose:* by intravenous injection, 100–200 micrograms (1.5–3 micrograms/kg); if response inadequate, increments of 100 micrograms every 2 minutes; further doses *by intramuscular injection* after 1–2 hours if required
  CHILD, *by intravenous injection*, 10 micrograms/kg; subsequent dose of 100 micrograms/kg if no response; if intravenous route not possible, may be given in divided doses by *intramuscular or subcutaneous injection*
  NEONATE, *by subcutaneous, intramuscular, or intravenous injection*, 10 micrograms/kg, repeated every 2 to 3 minutes *or* 200 micrograms (60 micrograms/kg) *by intramuscular injection* as a single dose at birth (onset of action slower)

PoM **Naloxone Hydrochloride** (Non-proprietary)
*Injection*, naloxone hydrochloride 20 micrograms/mL. Net price 2-mL amp = £3.57
*Injection*, naloxone hydrochloride 400 micrograms/mL—see under Emergency Treatment of Poisoning
PoM **Narcan**® —see under Emergency Treatment of Poisoning
PoM **Narcan Neonatal**® (Du Pont)
*Injection*, naloxone hydrochloride 20 micrograms/mL. Net price 2-mL amp = £3.57

### 15.1.8 Antagonists for malignant hyperthermia

**Dantrolene** is used in the treatment of malignant hyperthermia which is a rare but lethal complication of anaesthesia. It is characterised by a rapid rise in temperature, increasing muscle rigidity, tachycardia, and acidosis and can be triggered off by volatile anaesthetics, especially halothane, and suxamethonium. Dantrolene acts on skeletal muscle by interfering with calcium efflux in the muscle cell and stopping the contractile process. Known trigger agents should be avoided during anaesthesia.

### DANTROLENE SODIUM

*Indications:* malignant hyperthermia
*Cautions:* avoid extravasation; **interactions:** Appendix 1 (muscle relaxants)
*Dose: by rapid intravenous injection*, 1 mg/kg, repeated as required to a cumulative max. of 10 mg/kg

PoM **Dantrium Intravenous**® (Norwich Eaton)
*Injection*, powder for reconstitution, dantrolene sodium. Net price 20-mg vial = £22.52 (hosp. only)

## 15.2 Local anaesthesia

The use of local anaesthetics by injection or by application to mucous membranes to produce local analgesia is discussed in this section.

See also section 1.7 (colon and rectum), section 11.7 (eye), section 12.3 (oropharynx), and section 13.3 (skin).

USE OF LOCAL ANAESTHETICS. Local anaesthetic drugs act by causing a reversible block to conduction along nerve fibres. The smaller the nerve fibre the more sensitive it is so that a differential block may occur where the smaller fibres carrying pain sensation and automatic impulses are blocked, sparing coarse touch and movement. The drugs used vary widely in their potency, toxicity, duration of action, stability, solubility in water, and ability to penetrate mucous membranes. These variations determine their suitability for use by various routes, e.g. topical (surface), infiltration, plexus, epidural (extradural) or spinal block.

ADMINISTRATION. In estimating the safe dosage of these drugs it is important to take account of the rate at which they are absorbed and excreted as well as their potency. The patient's age, weight, physique, and clinical condition, the degree of vascularity of the area to which the drug is to be applied, and the duration of administration are other factors which must be taken into account.

Local anaesthetics do not rely on the circulation to transport them to their sites of action, but uptake into the general circulation is important in terminating their action. Following most regional anaesthetic procedures, maximum arterial plasma concentrations of anaesthetic develop within about 10 to 25 minutes, so careful surveillance for toxic effects is necessary during the first 30 minutes after injection.

Epidural anaesthesia is commonly used during surgery, often combined with general anaesthesia, because of its protective effect against the stress response of surgery. It is often used when good postoperative pain relief is essential (e.g. aortic aneurysm surgery or major gut surgery).

TOXICITY. Toxic effects associated with the local anaesthetics are usually a result of excessively high plasma concentrations. The main effects are excitation of the central nervous system (nervousness, nausea, and convulsions) followed by depression. Less commonly the cardiovascular system is depressed. Hypersensitivity reactions occur mainly with the ester-type local anaesthetics such as amethocaine, benzocaine, cocaine, and procaine; reactions are less frequent with the amide types such as lignocaine, bupivacaine, and prilocaine.

USE OF VASOCONSTRICTORS. Toxicity may occur with repeated dosages due to accumulation of the drug, and reducing doses should therefore be given. Toxic effects may also occur if the injection is too rapid. Local anaesthetics should **not** be injected into inflamed or infected tissues nor should they be applied to the traumatised urethra. Under these conditions the drug may be so rapidly absorbed that a systemic rather than a local reaction is produced.

Most local anaesthetics, with the exception of cocaine, cause dilatation of blood vessels. The addition of a vasoconstrictor such as **adrenaline** diminishes local blood flow, slows the rate of absorption of the local anaesthetic, and prolongs its local effect. Care is necessary when using adrenaline for this purpose because, in excess, it may produce ischaemic necrosis.

Adrenaline should **not** be added to injections used in digits and appendages. When adrenaline is included in an injection of lignocaine or procaine the final concentration should be 1 in 200 000. In dental surgery, up to 1 in 80 000 of adrenaline is used with local anaesthetics. There is no justification for using higher concentrations.

The total dose of adrenaline should **not** exceed 500 micrograms and it is essential not to exceed a concentration of 1 in 200 000 if more than 50 mL of the mixture is to be injected. For cautions associated with the use of adrenaline, see section 2.7. For drug interactions, see Appendix 1 (sympathomimetics).

## LIGNOCAINE

Lignocaine is the most widely used local anaesthetic drug. It acts more rapidly and is more stable than most other local anaesthetics. It is effectively absorbed from mucous membranes and is a useful surface anaesthetic in concentrations of 2 to 4%. Except for surface anaesthesia, solutions should not usually exceed 1% in strength. The duration of the block (with adrenaline) is about 1½ hours. Concentrations of 1.5% are used for epidural (extradural) block, and for spinal anaesthesia a 5% solution in glucose intravenous infusion is used as a hyperbaric solution.

## LIGNOCAINE HYDROCHLORIDE

*Indications:* see under Dose; also dental anaesthesia; ventricular arrhythmias (section 2.3.2)

*Cautions:* epilepsy, hepatic or respiratory impairment, impaired cardiac conduction, bradycardia; reduce dose in elderly or debilitated; resuscitative equipment should be available; see section 2.3.2 for effects on heart

*Contra-indications:* hypovolaemia, complete heart block; avoid in porphyria (see section 9.8.2); do not use solutions containing adrenaline for anaesthesia in appendages

*Side-effects:* hypotension, bradycardia, cardiac arrest. CNS effects include agitation, euphoria, respiratory depression, convulsions. See also notes above

*Dose:* adjusted according to site of operation and response of patient

*By injection,* max. dose 200 mg, or 500 mg with solutions which also contain adrenaline. Max. dose of adrenaline 500 micrograms (see also notes above)

*Infiltration anaesthesia,* 0.25–0.5%, with adrenaline 1 in 200000, using 2–50 mL of a 0.5% solution in minor surgery and up to 60 mL in more extensive surgery

*Nerve blocks,* with adrenaline 1 in 200000, 1% to a max. of 50 mL, 2% to a max. of 25 mL

*Epidural and caudal block,* with adrenaline 1 in 200000, 1% to a max. of 50 mL, 2% to a max. of 25 mL

*Surface anaesthesia,* usual strengths 2–4%. Mouth, throat, and upper gastro-intestinal tract, max. 200 mg

Lignocaine hydrochloride injections
PoM **Lignocaine** (Non-proprietary)
*Injection 0.5%,* lignocaine hydrochloride 5 mg/mL, net price 10-mL amp = 22p
*Injection 1%,* lignocaine hydrochloride 10 mg/mL, net price 2-mL amp = 14p; 5-mL amp = 21p; 10-mL amp = 40p; 20-mL amp = 42p
*Injection 2%,* lignocaine hydrochloride 20 mg/mL, net price 2-mL amp = 22p; 5-mL amp = 25p

PoM **Min-I-Jet® Lignocaine Hydrochloride with Adrenaline** (IMS)
*Injection,* lignocaine hydrochloride 5 mg/mL, adrenaline 1 in 200000 (500 micrograms/100 mL). Net price 5-mL disposable syringe = £2.84

PoM **Xylocaine®** (Astra)
*Injection 0.5%,* anhydrous lignocaine hydrochloride 5 mg/mL. Net price 20-mL vial = 67p
*Injection 0.5% with adrenaline 1 in 200000,* anhydrous lignocaine hydrochloride 5 mg/mL, adrenaline 1 in 200000. Net price 20-mL vial = 69p
*Injection 1%,* anhydrous lignocaine hydrochloride 10 mg/mL. Net price 20-mL vial = 69p
*Injection 1% with adrenaline 1 in 200000,* anhydrous lignocaine hydrochloride 10 mg/mL, adrenaline 1 in 200000. Net price 20-mL vial = 71p
*Injection 1.5%,* for epidural use, anhydrous lignocaine hydrochloride 15 mg/mL. Net price 25-mL amp = £1.21
*Injection 2%,* anhydrous lignocaine hydrochloride 20 mg/mL. Net price 20-mL vial = 73p
*Injection 2% with adrenaline 1 in 200000,* anhydrous lignocaine hydrochloride 20 mg/mL, adrenaline 1 in 200000. Net price 20-mL vial = 75p

Lignocaine injections for dental use
A large variety of lignocaine injections, plain or with adrenaline or noradrenaline, is also available in dental cartridges under the names **Lidocaton, Lignostab, Neo-Lidocaton, Xylocaine,** and **Xylotox.**

Lignocaine for surface anaesthesia
*Note.* Local anaesthetic ointments can be absorbed through the rectal mucosa therefore excessive application should be avoided, particularly in infants and children
PoM **Emla®** (Astra)
*Drug Tariff cream,* lignocaine 2.5%, prilocaine 2.5%. Net price 5-g tube = £1.73
*Surgical pack cream,* lignocaine 2.5%, prilocaine 2.5%. Net price 30-g tube (with spatula) = £10.25
NHS *Hospital pack cream,* lignocaine 2.5%, prilocaine 2.5%. Net price 10 × 5-g tube with 25 occlusive dressings = £19.50
Anaesthesia before e.g. venepuncture (not for infants), apply a thick layer under an occlusive dressing 1–5 hours before procedure; split skin grafting, apply a thick layer under an occlusive dressing 2–5 hours before procedure; genital warts (not for children), apply up to 10 g 5–10 minutes before removal
*Cautions:* not for wounds, mucous membranes (except genital warts in adults) or atopic dermatitis; avoid use near eyes or middle ear; side-effects include transient paleness, redness, and oedema

**Instillagel®** (CliniMed)
*Gel,* lignocaine hydrochloride 2%, chlorhexidine gluconate solution 0.25%, in a sterile lubricant basis in disposable syringe. Net price 6-mL syringe = £1.05; 11-mL syringe = £1.18
*Dose:* 6–11 mL into urethra

**Xylocaine®** (Astra)

*Antiseptic gel,* lignocaine hydrochloride 2%, chlorhexidine gluconate solution 0.25% in a sterile lubricant water-miscible basis. Net price 20 g = £1.09

Dose: into urethra, men 10 mL followed by 3–5 mL; women 3–5 mL

*Gel,* anhydrous lignocaine hydrochloride 2%, in a sterile lubricant water-miscible basis. Net price 20 g = 78p; 20-g single-use syringe (Accordion®) = £1.00

Dose: into urethra, men 10 mL followed by 3–5 mL; women 3–5 mL

*Ointment,* lignocaine 5% in a water-miscible basis. Net price 15 g = 83p

Dose: max. 35 g in 24 hours

*Spray* (= pump spray), lignocaine 10% (100 mg/g) supplying 10 mg lignocaine/dose; 500 spray doses per container. Net price 50-mL bottle = £3.21

Dose: dental practice, 1–5 doses; maxillary sinus puncture, 3 doses; during delivery in obstetrics, up to 20 doses; procedures in pharynx, larynx, and trachea, up to 20 doses

*Topical 4%,* anhydrous lignocaine hydrochloride 40 mg/mL. Net price 30-mL bottle = £1.24

Dose: bronchoscopy, 2–3 mL with suitable spray; biopsy in mouth, 3–4 mL with suitable spray *or* swab (with adrenaline if necessary); max. 7.5 mL

---

## BUPIVACAINE

The great advantage of bupivacaine over other local anaesthetics is its duration of action of up to 8 hours when used for nerve blocks. It has a slow onset of action, taking up to 30 minutes for full effect. It is often used in lumbar epidural blockade and is particularly suitable for continuous epidural analgesia in labour; it then has a 2- to 3-hour duration of action. It is **contra-indicated** in intravenous regional anaesthesia (Bier's block). It is the principal drug for spinal anaesthesia in the UK.

## BUPIVACAINE HYDROCHLORIDE

*Indications:* see under Dose

*Cautions; Contra-indications; Side-effects:* see under Lignocaine Hydrochloride and notes above; myocardial depression may be more severe and more resistant to treatment; contra-indicated in intravenous regional anaesthesia (Bier's block)

*Dose:* adjusted according to site of operation and response of patient

*Local infiltration,* 0.25% (up to 60 mL)

*Peripheral nerve block,* 0.25% (max. 60 mL), 0.5% (max. 30 mL)

*Epidural block,*

Surgery, *lumbar,* 0.5–0.75% (max. 20 mL of either)

*caudal,* 0.5% (max. 30 mL)

Labour, *lumbar,* 0.25–0.5% (max. 12 mL of either)

*caudal,* 0.25% (max. 30 mL), 0.5% (max. 20 mL)

*Note.* 0.75% **contra-indicated** for epidural use in obstetrics.

PoM **Marcain Heavy®** (Astra)

*Injection,* bupivacaine hydrochloride 5 mg, glucose 80 mg/mL. Net price 4-ml amp = £1.00

Dose: spinal anaesthesia, 2–4 mL

PoM **Marcain®** (Astra)

*Injection 0.25%,* bupivacaine hydrochloride 2.5 mg/mL. Net price 10-mL amp = £1.13

*Injection 0.5%,* bupivacaine hydrochloride 5 mg/mL. Net price 10-mL amp = £1.30

*Injection 0.75%,* bupivacaine hydrochloride 7.5 mg/mL. Net price 10-mL amp = £1.95

PoM **Marcain with Adrenaline®** (Astra)

*Injection 0.25%,* bupivacaine hydrochloride 2.5 mg/mL, adrenaline 1 in 200000. Net price 10-mL amp = £1.27

*Injection 0.5%,* bupivacaine hydrochloride 5 mg/mL, adrenaline 1 in 200000. Net price 10-mL amp = £1.43

---

## PRILOCAINE

Prilocaine is a local anaesthetic of low toxicity which is similar to lignocaine. It can be used for infiltration, regional nerve block, and spinal anaesthesia and regional intravenous analgesia. If used in high doses, methaemoglobinaemia may occur which can be treated with intravenous injection of methylene blue 1% using a dose of 75–100 mg.

## PRILOCAINE HYDROCHLORIDE

*Indications:* see under Dose; also dental anaesthesia

*Cautions; Contra-indications; Side-effects:* see under Lignocaine Hydrochloride and notes above; avoid in anaemia or congenital or acquired methaemoglobinaemia

*Dose:* adjusted according to site of operation and response of patient, to max. 400 mg used alone, or 600 mg if used with adrenaline or felypressin

PoM **Citanest®** (Astra)

*Injection 0.5%,* prilocaine hydrochloride 5 mg/mL. Net price 20-mL multidose vial = 73p; 50-mL multidose vial = £1.02; 50-mL single dose vial = £1.30

*Injection 1%,* prilocaine hydrochloride 10 mg/mL. Net price 20-mL vial = 75p; 50-mL vial = £1.06

*Injection 2%,* prilocaine hydrochloride 20 mg/mL. Net price 10-mL single dose vial = 75p

*Injection 4%,* prilocaine hydrochloride 40 mg/mL. Net price 2-mL cartridge = 11p

PoM **Citanest with Octapressin®** (Astra)

*Injection 3%,* prilocaine hydrochloride 30 mg/mL, felypressin 0.03 unit/mL. Net price 2-mL cartridge and self-aspirating cartridge (both) = 13p

---

Prices are **net**, see p. 1

## PROCAINE

Procaine is now seldom used. It is as potent an anaesthetic as lignocaine but has a shorter duration of action. It provides less intense analgesia because it has less tendency to spread through the tissues. It is poorly absorbed from mucous membranes and is of no value as a surface anaesthetic. When used for infiltration or regional anaesthesia, adrenaline 1 in 200000 is generally added. Its metabolite para-aminobenzoic acid inhibits the action of the sulphonamides.

### PROCAINE HYDROCHLORIDE

*Indications:* local anaesthesia by infiltration and regional routes
*Cautions; Side-effects:* see notes above
*Dose:* adjusted according to site of operation and patient's response
*By injection*, up to 1 g (200 mL of 0.5% solution or 100 mL of 1%) with adrenaline 1 in 200000

PoM **Procaine Injection**, procaine hydrochloride 2% (20 mg/mL) in sodium chloride intravenous infusion. Net price 2-mL amp = 57p; 1% in 2-mL amp also available

## OTHER LOCAL ANAESTHETICS

**Amethocaine** is an effective local anaesthetic for topical application. It is rapidly absorbed from mucous membranes and should **never** be applied to inflamed, traumatised, or highly vascular surfaces. It should **never** be used to provide anaesthesia for bronchoscopy or cystoscopy, as lignocaine is a safer alternative. It is used in ophthalmology (see section 11.7) and in skin preparations (see section 13.3). Hypersensitivity to amethocaine has been reported.

**Benzocaine** is a local anaesthetic of low potency and toxicity. Its only use is in surface anaesthesia for the relief of pain and irritation in the oropharynx (see section 12.3.1).

**Cocaine** readily penetrates mucous membranes and is an effective surface anaesthetic but it has now been replaced by less toxic alternatives. It potentiates the action of adrenaline and possesses vasoconstrictor and mydriatic properties and should therefore **not** be used with adrenaline. It should **never** be given by injection because of its toxicity and doses not exceeding 3 mg/kg should be applied to mucous membranes. It stimulates the central nervous system and is a drug of addiction. It should be avoided in porphyria (see section 9.8.2). Concentrations of 4 to 10% (40–100 mg/mL) are applied to the nose, throat, and larynx. For the use of cocaine in ophthalmology see section 11.7.

# Appendix 1: Interactions

Two or more drugs given at the same time may exert their effects independently or may interact. The interaction may be potentiation or antagonism of one drug by another, or occasionally some other effect. Adverse drug interactions should be reported to the CSM as for other adverse drug reactions.

Drug interactions may be **pharmacodynamic** or **pharmacokinetic**.

## PHARMACODYNAMIC INTERACTIONS

These are interactions between drugs which have similar or antagonistic pharmacological effects or side-effects. They may be due to competition at receptor sites, or occur between drugs acting on the same physiological system. They are usually predictable from a knowledge of the pharmacology of the interacting drugs; in general, those demonstrated with one drug are likely to occur with related drugs. They occur to a greater or lesser extent in most patients who receive the interacting drugs.

## PHARMACOKINETIC INTERACTIONS

These occur when one drug alters the absorption, distribution, metabolism, or excretion of another, thus increasing or reducing the amount of drug available to produce its pharmacological effects. They are not easily predicted and many of them affect only a small proportion of patients taking the combination of drugs. Pharmacokinetic interactions occurring with one drug cannot be assumed to occur with related drugs unless their pharmacokinetic properties are known to be similar.

Pharmacokinetic interactions are of several types:

AFFECTING ABSORPTION. The rate of absorption or the total amount absorbed can both be altered by drug interactions. Delayed absorption is rarely of clinical importance unless high peak plasma concentrations are required (e.g. when giving an analgesic). Reduction in the total amount absorbed, however, may result in ineffective therapy.

DUE TO CHANGES IN PROTEIN BINDING. To a variable extent most drugs are loosely bound to plasma proteins. Protein-binding sites are non-specific and one drug can displace another thereby increasing its proportion free to diffuse from plasma to its site of action. This only produces a detectable increase in effect if it is an extensively bound drug (more than 90%) that is not widely distributed throughout the body. Even so displacement rarely produces more than transient

potentiation because this increased concentration of free drug results in an increased rate of elimination.

Displacement from protein binding plays a part in the potentiation of warfarin by phenylbutazone, sulphonamides, and tolbutamide but the importance of these interactions is due mainly to the fact that warfarin metabolism is also inhibited.

AFFECTING METABOLISM. Many drugs are metabolised in the liver. Induction of the hepatic microsomal enzyme system by one drug can gradually increase the rate of metabolism of another, resulting in lower plasma concentrations and a reduced effect. On withdrawal of the inducer plasma concentrations increase and toxicity may occur. Barbiturates, griseofulvin, most antiepileptics, and rifampicin are the most important enzyme inducers in man. Drugs affected include warfarin and the oral contraceptives.

Conversely when one drug inhibits the metabolism of another higher plasma concentrations are produced, rapidly resulting in an increased effect with risk of toxicity. Some drugs which potentiate warfarin and phenytoin do so by this mechanism.

AFFECTING RENAL EXCRETION. Drugs are eliminated through the kidney both by glomerular filtration and by active tubular secretion. Competition occurs between those which share active transport mechanisms in the proximal tubule. Thus probenecid delays the excretion of many drugs including penicillins, some cephalosporins, indomethacin, and dapsone; aspirin may increase the toxicity of methotrexate by a similar mechanism.

## RELATIVE IMPORTANCE OF INTERACTIONS

Many drug interactions are harmless and many of those which are potentially harmful only occur in a small proportion of patients; moreover, the severity of an interaction varies from one patient to another. Drugs with a small therapeutic ratio (e.g. phenytoin) and those which require careful control of dosage (e.g. anticoagulants, antihypertensives, and antidiabetics) are most often involved.

Patients at increased risk from drug interactions include the elderly and those with impaired renal or liver function.

HAZARDOUS INTERACTIONS. The symbol ● has been placed against interactions that are **potentially hazardous** and where combined administration of the drugs involved should be **avoided** (or only undertaken with caution and appropriate monitoring).

Interactions that have no symbol do not usually have serious consequences.

# List of drug interactions

The following is an alphabetical list of drugs and their interactions; to avoid excessive cross-referencing each drug or group is listed twice: in the alphabetical list and also against the drug or group with which it interacts; changes in the interactions lists since BNF No. 22 (September 1991) are <u>underlined</u>.
For explanation of symbol • see previous page

## ACE Inhibitors
Alcohol: enhanced hypotensive effect
• Anaesthetics: enhanced hypotensive effect
Analgesics: antagonism of hypotensive effect and increased risk of renal failure with *NSAIDs*; hyperkalaemia with *indomethacin and possibly other NSAIDs*
Antacids: absorption of *fosinopril* reduced
Antibacterials: absorption of *tetracyclines* reduced by *quinapril* (tablets contain magnesium carbonate excipient)
Antidepressants: enhanced hypotensive effect
*other* Antihypertensives: enhanced hypotensive effect
Antipsychotics: severe postural hypotension with *chlorpromazine and possibly other phenothiazines*
Anxiolytics and Hypnotics: enhanced hypotensive effect
Beta-blockers: enhanced hypotensive effect
Calcium-channel Blockers: enhanced hypotensive effect
Corticosteroids: antagonism of hypotensive effect
Cyclosporin: increased risk of hyperkalaemia
• Diuretics: enhanced hypotensive effect (can be extreme); hyperkalaemia with *potassium-sparing diuretics*
Dopaminergics: *levodopa* enhances hypotensive effect
• Lithium: *ACE inhibitors* reduce excretion of *lithium* (increased plasma-lithium concentration)
Muscle Relaxants: *baclofen* enhances hypotensive effect
Nitrates: enhance hypotensive effect
• Potassium Salts: hyperkalaemia
Sex Hormones: *oestrogens and combined oral contraceptives* antagonise hypotensive effect
Sympathomimetics: *see* Sympathomimetics (main list)
Ulcer-healing Drugs: *carbenoxolone* antagonises hypotensive effect
Uricosurics: *probenecid* reduces excretion of *captopril*

**Acebutolol** *see* Beta-blockers
**Acemetacin** *see* NSAIDs
**Acetazolamide** (general hypokalaemic interactions *as for* Diuretics)
Analgesics: *aspirin* reduces excretion of *acetazolamide* (risk of toxicity)
Anti-arrhythmics: excretion of *flecainide, mexiletine, and quinidine* reduced in alkaline urine (occasionally increased plasma-concentrations)
Antiepileptics: *phenytoin* possibly increases risk of osteomalacia
Lithium: *lithium* excretion increased

**Acrivastine** *see* Antihistamines
**Acrosoxacin** *see* 4-Quinolones
**Acyclovir**
*other* Antivirals: extreme lethargy reported on administration of *zidovudine* with *intravenous acyclovir*
Uricosurics: *probenecid* reduces *acyclovir* excretion (increased plasma concentrations and risk of toxicity)

## Adenosine
• <u>Antiplatelet Drugs: effect enhanced by *dipyridamole* (risk of toxicity)</u>
Theophylline: antagonism of anti-arrhythmic effect

**Adrenaline** *see* Sympathomimetics

## Adrenergic Neurone Blockers (*see also* Bretylium)
Alcohol: enhanced hypotensive effect
• Anaesthetics: enhanced hypotensive effect
Analgesics: *NSAIDs* antagonise hypotensive effect
Antidepressants: *tricyclics* antagonise hypotensive effect
*other* Antihypertensives: enhanced hypotensive effect
Antipsychotics: *phenothiazines* enhance hypotensive effect (antagonism of hypotensive effect with higher doses of *chlorpromazine*)
Anxiolytics and Hypnotics: enhanced hypotensive effect
Beta-blockers: enhanced hypotensive effect
Calcium-channel Blockers: enhanced hypotensive effect
Corticosteroids: antagonism of hypotensive effect
Diuretics: enhanced hypotensive effect
Dopaminergics: *levodopa* enhances hypotensive effect
Nitrates: enhance hypotensive effect
Pizotifen: antagonism of hypotensive effect
Sex Hormones: *oestrogens and combined oral contraceptives* antagonise hypotensive effect
• Sympathomimetics: *some anorectics (e.g. mazindol) and some cough and cold remedies (e.g. ephedrine)* antagonise hypotensive effect
Ulcer-healing Drugs: *carbenoxolone* antagonises hypotensive effect

## Alcohol
Antibacterials: disulfiram-like reaction with *cephamandole, metronidazole, nimorazole and tinidazole*
• Anticoagulants: anticoagulant effects of *warfarin and nicoumalone* enhanced
• Antidepressants: sedative effect of *tricyclic and related antidepressants* enhanced; *tyramine contained in some alcoholic and dealcoholised beverages* interacts with *MAOIs* (hypertensive crisis)
Antidiabetics: enhanced hypoglycaemic effect; flushing with *chlorpropamide* (in susceptible subjects); increased risk of lactic acidosis with *metformin*
Antihistamines: enhanced sedative effect
Antihypertensives: enhanced hypotensive effect; sedative effect of *indoramin* enhanced
Antipsychotics: enhanced sedative effect
Anxiolytics and Hypnotics: enhanced sedative effect
Beta-blockers: enhanced hypotensive effect
Cytotoxics: disulfiram-like reaction with *procarbazine*
Dopaminergics: reduced tolerance to *bromocriptine*
Monosulfiram: disulfiram-like reaction
Muscle Relaxants: *baclofen* enhances sedative effect
<u>Nabilone: enhanced sedative effect</u>
Nitrates: enhanced hypotensive effect

**Alcuronium** *see* Muscle Relaxants (non-depolarising)

**Alfentanil** *see* Opioid Analgesics
**Allopurinol**
  Anticoagulants: effects of *nicoumalone and warfarin* may be enhanced
  ● Cytotoxics: effects of *azathioprine, cyclophosphamide, and mercaptopurine* enhanced with increased toxicity
**Allyloestrenol** *see* Progestogens
**Alpha-blockers** (general hypotensive interactions *as for* Hydralazine)
  Alcohol: sedative effect of *indoramin* enhanced
  Anxiolytics and Hypnotics: enhanced sedative effect
  ● Beta-blockers: increased risk of first-dose hypotensive effect of *post-synaptic alpha-blockers such as prazosin and terazosin*
  ● Diuretics: increased risk of first-dose hypotensive effect of *post-synaptic alpha-blockers such as prazosin and terazosin*
**Alprazolam** *see* Benzodiazepines and other Anxiolytics and Hypnotics
**Aluminium Hydroxide** *see* Antacids and Adsorbents
**Amantadine**
  Antihypertensives: *methyldopa, metirosine, and rauwolfia alkaloids* have extrapyramidal side-effects
  Antimuscarinics: increased antimuscarinic side-effects
  Antipsychotics: all have extrapyramidal side-effects
  Domperidone and Metoclopramide: have extrapyramidal side-effects
  Tetrabenazine: has extrapyramidal side-effects
**Ambutonium** *see* Antimuscarinics
**Amikacin** *see* Aminoglycosides
**Amiloride** *see* Diuretics (potassium-sparing)
**Aminoglutethimide**
  ● Anticoagulants: metabolism of *nicoumalone and warfarin* accelerated (reduced anticoagulant effect)
  Cardiac glycosides: metabolism of *digitoxin only* accelerated (reduced effect)
  Corticosteroids: metabolism of *dexamethasone* accelerated (reduced effect)
  Theophylline: metabolism of *theophylline* accelerated (reduced effect)
**Aminoglycosides**
  *other* Antibacterials: increased risk of nephrotoxicity with *cephalosporins notably cephalothin, colistin, and polymyxin*; increased risk of ototoxicity and nephrotoxicity with *capreomycin and vancomycin*
  Anticoagulants: *see* Phenindione and Warfarin
  Antifungals: increased risk of nephrotoxicity with *amphotericin*
  Bisphosphonates: severe hypocalcaemia
  ● Cholinergics: antagonism of effect of *neostigmine and pyridostigmine*
  ● Cyclosporin: increased risk of nephrotoxicity
  ● Cytotoxics: increased risk of nephrotoxicity and possibly of ototoxicity with *cisplatin*
  Diuretics: increased risk of ototoxicity with *loop diuretics*
  ● Muscle Relaxants: effect of *non-depolarising muscle relaxants such as tubocurarine* enhanced
**Aminophylline** *see* Theophylline
**Amiodarone**
  ● *other* Anti-arrhythmics: additive effect with *disopyramide, flecainide, procainamide, and quinidine* (increased risk of ventricular arrhythmias); increased plasma concentrations of *flecainide and procainamide*; increased myocardial depression with any anti-arrhythmic

**Amiodarone** (*continued*)
  ● Anticoagulants: metabolism of *nicoumalone and warfarin* inhibited (enhanced anticoagulant effect)
  ● Antiepileptics: metabolism of *phenytoin* inhibited (increased plasma concentration)
  ● Beta-blockers: increased risk of bradycardia, AV block, and myocardial depression
  ● Calcium-channel Blockers: *diltiazem and verapamil* increase risk of bradycardia, AV block, and myocardial depression
  ● Cardiac Glycosides: increased plasma concentration of *digoxin* (halve digoxin maintenance dose)
  Diuretics: toxicity increased if hypokalaemia occurs with *acetazolamide, loop diuretics, and thiazides*
  Ulcer-healing Drugs: *cimetidine* increases plasma concentrations of *amiodarone*
**Amitriptyline** *see* Antidepressants, Tricyclic
**Amlodipine** *see* Calcium-channel Blockers
**Amoxapine** *see* Antidepressants, Tricyclic
**Amoxycillin** *see* Penicillins
**Amphetamines** *see* Sympathomimetics
**Amphotericin**
  Antibacterials: increased risk of nephrotoxicity with *aminoglycosides and cephalothin*
  *other* Antifungals: antagonises *miconazole*
  ● Cyclosporin: increased risk of nephrotoxicity
**Ampicillin** *see* Penicillins
**Amylobarbitone** *see* Barbiturates and Primidone
**Anabolic Steroids**
  ● Anticoagulants: anticoagulant effect of *nicoumalone, phenindione, and warfarin* enhanced
**Anaesthetics** (*see also* Surgery and Long-term Medication, section 15.1)
  Antibacterials: effect of *thiopentone* enhanced by *sulphonamides*
  Antidepressants: risk of arrhythmias and hypotension increased with *tricyclics*
  ● Antihypertensives: enhanced hypotensive effect
  ● Antipsychotics: enhanced hypotensive effect
  Anxiolytics and Hypnotics: enhanced sedative effect
  ● Beta-blockers: enhanced hypotensive effect
  ● Calcium-channel Blockers: enhanced hypotensive effect and AV delay with *verapamil*
  ● Dopaminergics: risk of arrhythmias if *volatile anaesthetics such as cyclopropane or halothane* given with *levodopa*
  ● Sympathomimetics: risk of arrhythmias if *adrenaline or isoprenaline* given with *volatile anaesthetics such as cyclopropane or halothane*
  Theophylline: increased risk of arrhythmias with *halothane*
**Analgesics** *see* Aspirin, Nefopam, NSAIDs, Opioid Analgesics, and Paracetamol
**Anion-exchange Resins** *see* Cholestyramine and Colestipol
**Antacids and Adsorbents**
  Analgesics: excretion of *aspirin* increased in alkaline urine; *antacids* reduce absorption of *diflunisal*
  Anti-arrhythmics: excretion of *quinidine* reduced in alkaline urine (may occasionally increase plasma concentrations)
  Antibacterials: *antacids* reduce absorption of *azithromycin, ciprofloxacin, isoniazid, norfloxacin, ofloxacin, pivampicillin, rifampicin, temafloxacin, and most tetracyclines; kaolin* reduces absorption of *lincomycin*
  Antiepileptics: *antacids* reduce *phenytoin* absorption

**Antacids and Adsorbents** (*continued*)

Antifungals: *antacids* reduce absorption of *itraconazole* and *ketoconazole*

Antihypertensives: *antacids* reduce absorption of *fosinopril*

Antiplatelet Drugs: *dipyridamole* patient information leaflet advises avoidance of *antacids*

Antimalarials: *antacids* reduce absorption of *chloroquine and hydroxychloroquine*

Antipsychotics: *antacids* reduce absorption of *phenothiazines*

Bisphosphonates: *antacids* reduce absorption

Iron: *magnesium trisilicate* reduces absorption of *oral iron*

Lithium: *sodium bicarbonate* increases excretion (reduced plasma-lithium concentration)

Penicillamine: *antacids* reduce absorption

**Antazoline** *see* Antihistamines

**Anti-arrhythmics** *see* individual drugs

**Anticholinergics** *see* Antimuscarinics

**Anticoagulants** *see* Heparin, Phenindione, and Warfarin

**Antidepressants** *see* individual entries for Antidepressants, Serotonin-uptake Inhibitor; Antidepressants, Tricyclic; MAOIs; Mianserin; Trazodone; Tryptophan; and Viloxazine

**Antidepressants, Serotonin-uptake Inhibitor**

● Anticoagulants: effect of *nicoumalone and warfarin* possibly enhanced by *fluvoxamine* and *paroxetine*

● *other* Antidepressants: CNS effects of *MAOIs* increased (risk of toxicity); avoid *MAOIs* for at least 2 weeks before *serotonin-uptake inhibitor*; avoid *fluoxetine* for at least 5 weeks and *sertraline* for at least 7 days before *MAOIs*; *fluoxetine* increases plasma concentrations of some *tricyclics*; agitation and nausea with *tryptophan*

Antiepileptics: antagonism (convulsive threshold lowered); plasma concentration of *carbamazepine* increased by *fluoxetine*; *phenytoin and possibly other antiepileptics* reduce plasma concentration of *paroxetine*

Antipsychotics: plasma concentration of *haloperidol* increased by *fluoxetine*

Beta-blockers: plasma concentration of *propranolol* increased by *fluvoxamine*

● Lithium: increased risk of CNS toxicity

● Sumatriptan: risk of CNS toxicity

**Antidepressants, Tricyclic**

● Alcohol: enhanced sedative effect

Anaesthetics: risk of arrhythmias and hypotension increased

● *other* Antidepressants: CNS excitation and hypertension with *MAOIs* (avoid for at least 2 weeks after stopping MAOIs); *fluoxetine* increases plasma concentrations of some *tricyclics*

● Antiepileptics: antagonism (convulsive threshold lowered); plasma concentrations of *tricyclics* reduced (reduced antidepressant effect)

Antihistamines: increased antimuscarinic and sedative effects

Antihypertensives: in general, hypotensive effect enhanced, but antagonism of effect of *adrenergic neurone blockers* and of *clonidine* (and increased risk of hypertension on clonidine withdrawal)

Antimuscarinics: increased antimuscarinic side-effects

Antipsychotics: increased antimuscarinic side-effects with *phenothiazines*

Anxiolytics and Hypnotics: enhanced sedative effect

Barbiturates: *see under* Antiepileptics, above

Calcium-channel Blockers: *diltiazem* and *verapamil* increase plasma concentration of *imipramine* and possibly *other tricyclics*

**Antidepressants, Tricyclic** (*continued*)

Disulfiram: inhibition of metabolism of *tricyclics* (increased plasma concentrations and increased disulfiram reaction reported with *alcohol with amitriptyline*)

Diuretics: increased risk of postural hypotension

Nitrates: reduced effect of *sublingual nitrates* (owing to dry mouth)

Sex Hormones: *oral contraceptives* antagonise antidepressant effect (but side-effects may be increased due to increased plasma concentrations of *tricyclics*)

● Sympathomimetics: hypertension and arrhythmias with *adrenaline* (but local anaesthetics with adrenaline appear to be safe); hypertension with *noradrenaline*

Ulcer-healing Drugs: plasma concentrations of *amitriptyline, desipramine, doxepin, imipramine, nortriptyline, and probably other tricyclics* increased by *cimetidine* (inhibition of metabolism)

**Antidiabetics** (includes Insulin, Metformin, and Sulphonylureas)

Alcohol: enhanced hypoglycaemic effect; flushing with *chlorpropamide* (in susceptible subjects); risk of lactic acidosis with *metformin*

● Analgesics: *azapropazone* and *phenylbutazone* enhance effect of *sulphonylureas*

● Antibacterials: *chloramphenicol, co-trimoxazole, sulphonamides,* and *trimethoprim* enhance effect of *sulphonylureas*; *rifampicin* reduces effect of *sulphonylureas* (accelerates metabolism)

Antidepressants: *MAOIs* enhance hypoglycaemic effect

Antiepileptics: *plasma-phenytoin* concentration transiently increased by *tolbutamide* (possibility of toxicity)

● Antifungals: *miconazole* and possibly *fluconazole* enhance effect of *sulphonylureas*

Antihypertensives: hypoglycaemic effect antagonised by *diazoxide*

Beta-blockers: enhanced hypoglycaemic effect (and masking of warning signs such as tremor)

Calcium-channel Blockers: *nifedipine* may occasionally impair glucose tolerance

Clofibrate Group: may improve glucose tolerance and have an additive effect

Corticosteroids: antagonism of hypoglycaemic effect

Diuretics: hypoglycaemic effect antagonised by *loop and thiazide diuretics*; *chlorpropamide* increases risk of hyponatraemia with *thiazides in combination with potassium-sparing diuretics*

Hormone Antagonists: *octreotide* may reduce *insulin and antidiabetic drug* requirements in diabetes mellitus

Lithium: may occasionally impair glucose tolerance

Sex Hormones: *oral contraceptives* antagonise hypoglycaemic effect

Ulcer-healing Drugs: *cimetidine* inhibits renal excretion of *metformin* (increased plasma-metformin concentrations)

● Uricosurics: *sulphinpyrazone* enhances effect of *sulphonylureas*

**Antiepileptics** *see* individual drugs

**Antifungals** *see* individual drugs

**Antihistamines**

*Note.* The following interactions apply to a lesser extent to the non-sedative antihistamines, and they do not appear to potentiate the effects of alcohol

Alcohol: enhanced sedative effect

Antidepressants: *tricyclics* increase antimuscarinic and sedative effects

**Antihistamines** (*continued*)

   Antifungals: *ketoconazole* inhibits *terfenadine* metabolism (cardiac toxicity reported)

   Antimuscarinics: increased antimuscarinic side-effects

   Anxiolytics and Hypnotics: enhanced sedative effect

   Betahistine: antagonism (theoretical)

**Antihypertensives** *see* individual drugs or groups

**Antimalarials** *see* individual drugs

**Antimuscarinics**

   *Note*. Many drugs have antimuscarinic effects; concomitant use of two or three such drugs can increase side-effects such as dry mouth, urine retention, and constipation; concomitant use can also lead to confusion in the elderly

   Analgesics: increased antimuscarinic effects with *nefopam*

   Anti-arrhythmics: increased antimuscarinic effects with *disopyramide; atropine* delays absorption of *mexiletine*

   Antidepressants: increased antimuscarinic side-effects with *tricyclics and MAOIs*

   Antifungals: reduced absorption of *ketoconazole*

   Antihistamines: increased antimuscarinic side-effects

   Antipsychotics: increased antimuscarinic side-effects of *phenothiazines* (but reduced plasma concentrations)

   Cisapride: antagonism of gastro-intestinal effect

   Domperidone and Metoclopramide: *antimuscarinics such as propantheline* antagonise gastro-intestinal effects

   Dopaminergics: increased antimuscarinic side-effects with *amantadine*

   Nitrates: reduced effect of *sublingual nitrates* (failure to dissolve under tongue owing to dry mouth)

**Antiplatelet Drugs** *see* Aspirin and Dipyridamole

**Antipsychotics** *see* Phenothiazines and other Antipsychotics

**Antivirals** *see* individual drugs

**Anxiolytics** *see* Benzodiazepines and other Anxiolytics and Hypnotics

**Appetite Suppressants** *see* Sympathomimetics

**Aspirin**

   Antacids and Adsorbents: excretion of *aspirin* increased in alkaline urine

   ● Anticoagulants: increased risk of bleeding due to antiplatelet effect

   Antiepileptics: enhancement of effect of *phenytoin and sodium valproate*

   ● Cytotoxics: reduced excretion of *methotrexate* (increased toxicity)

   Diuretics: antagonism of diuretic effect of *spironolactone;* reduced excretion of *acetazolamide* (risk of toxicity)

   Domperidone and Metoclopramide: *metoclopramide* enhances effect of *aspirin* (increased rate of absorption)

   Mifepristone: manufacturer recommends avoid *aspirin* until 8–12 days after *mifepristone* administration

   Uricosurics: effect of *probenecid and sulphinpyrazone* reduced

**Astemizole** *see* Antihistamines

**Atenolol** *see* Beta-blockers

**Atracurium** *see* Muscle Relaxants (non-depolarising)

**Atropine** *see* Antimuscarinics

**Azapropazone** *see* NSAIDs

**Azatadine** *see* Antihistamines

**Azathioprine**

   ● Allopurinol: enhancement of effect with increased toxicity

**Azithromycin**

   Antacids and Adsorbents: *antacids* reduce absorption of *azithromycin*

   Anticoagulants: effect of *warfarin* possibly enhanced

   Cardiac Glycosides: effect of *digoxin* possibly enhanced

   Ergotamine: ergotism possible

**Azlocillin** *see* Penicillins

**Aztreonam**

   ● Anticoagulants: anticoagulant effect of *nicoumalone and warfarin* enhanced

**Baclofen** *see* Muscle Relaxants

**Barbiturates and Primidone**

   Anti-arrhythmics: metabolism of *disopyramide and quinidine* increased (reduced plasma concentrations)

   Antibacterials: metabolism of *chloramphenicol, doxycycline, and metronidazole* accelerated (reduced effect); *sulphonamides* enhance effect of *thiopentone*

   ● Anticoagulants: metabolism of *nicoumalone and warfarin* accelerated (reduced anticoagulant effect)

   ● Antidepressants: antagonism of anticonvulsant effect (convulsive threshold lowered); metabolism of *tricyclics* accelerated (reduced plasma concentrations)

   ● Antiepileptics: concomitant administration of *phenobarbitone or primidone* with other antiepileptics may enhance toxicity without a corresponding increase in antiepileptic effect; moreover interactions can complicate monitoring of treatment; interactions include enhanced effects, increased sedation, and reductions in plasma concentrations; metabolism of *clonazepam* accelerated

   Antifungals: *phenobarbitone* accelerates metabolism of *griseofulvin* (reduced effect)

   ● Antipsychotics: antagonism of anticonvulsant effect (convulsive threshold lowered)

   ● Calcium-channel Blockers: effect of *felodipine, isradipine* and probably *nicardipine* and *nifedipine* reduced

   Cardiac Glycosides: metabolism of *digitoxin only* accelerated (reduced effect)

   ● Corticosteroids: metabolism of *corticosteroids* accelerated (reduced effect)

   ● Cyclosporin: metabolism of *cyclosporin* accelerated (reduced effect)

   ● Sex Hormones: metabolism of *gestrinone, tibolone,* and *oral contraceptives* accelerated (reduced effect)

   Theophylline: metabolism of *theophylline* accelerated (reduced effect)

   Thyroxine: metabolism of thyroxine accelerated (may increase thyroxine requirements in hypothyroidism)

**Beclomethasone** *see* Corticosteroids

**Bendrofluazide** *see* Diuretics (thiazide)

**Benorylate** *see* Aspirin *and* Paracetamol

**Benperidol** *see* Phenothiazines and other Antipsychotics

**Benzhexol** *see* Antimuscarinics

**Benzodiazepines and other Anxiolytics and Hypnotics**

   Alcohol: enhanced sedative effect

   Anaesthetics: enhanced sedative effect

   Analgesics: *opioid analgesics* enhance sedative effect

   Antibacterials: *erythromycin* inhibits metabolism of *midazolam* (increased plasma concentration, see also p. 454); *isoniazid* inhibits metabolism of *diazepam*

**Benzodiazepines and other Anxiolytics and Hypnotics** (*continued*)

Anticoagulants: *chloral hydrate* may transiently enhance effect of *nicoumalone and warfarin*

Antidepressants: enhanced sedative effect; manufacturer contra-indicates *buspirone* with *MAOIs*

Antiepileptics: metabolism of *clonazepam* accelerated (reduced effect)

Antihistamines: enhanced sedative effect

Antihypertensives: enhanced hypotensive effect; enhanced sedative effect with *alpha-blockers*

Antipsychotics: enhanced sedative effect

Disulfiram: metabolism of *diazepam and chlordiazepoxide* inhibited (enhanced sedative effect)

Dopaminergics: *benzodiazepines* occasionally antagonise effect of *levodopa*

Muscle Relaxants: *baclofen* enhances sedative effect

Nabilone: enhanced sedative effect

Ulcer-healing Drugs: *cimetidine* inhibits metabolism of *benzodiazepines and chlormethiazole* (increased plasma concentrations); *omeprazole* inhibits metabolism of *diazepam* (increased plasma concentrations)

**Benzthiazide** *see* Diuretics (thiazide)
**Benztropine** *see* Antimuscarinics
**Beta-blockers**

Alcohol: enhanced hypotensive effect
● Anaesthetics: enhanced hypotensive effect

Analgesics: *NSAIDs* antagonise hypotensive effect
● Anti-arrhythmics: increased risk of myocardial depression and bradycardia; with *amiodarone* increased risk of bradycardia and AV block; increased risk of *lignocaine* toxicity with *propranolol*

Antibacterials: *rifampicin* accelerates metabolism of *bisoprolol* and *propranolol* (reduced plasma concentration)

Antidepressants: *fluvoxamine* increases plasma concentration of *propranolol*

Antidiabetics: enhanced hypoglycaemic effect (and masking of warning signs such as tremor)
● Antihypertensives: enhanced hypotensive effect; increased risk of withdrawal hypertension with *clonidine*; increased risk of first-dose hypotensive effect with *post-synaptic alpha-blockers such as prazosin and terazosin*; increased bradycardia with *rauwolfia alkaloids*

Antimalarials: increased risk of bradycardia with *mefloquine*

Antipsychotics: plasma concentration of *chlorpromazine* increased by *propranolol*

Anxiolytics and Hypnotics: enhanced hypotensive effect
● Calcium-channel Blockers: increased risk of bradycardia and AV block with *diltiazem*; severe hypotension and heart failure occasionally with *nifedipine*; asystole, severe hypotension, and heart failure with *verapamil* (see section 2.3.2)

Cardiac Glycosides: increased AV block and bradycardia

Cholinergics: *propranolol* antagonises effect of *neostigmine and pyridostigmine*

Corticosteroids: antagonism of hypotensive effect

Diuretics: enhanced hypotensive effect; risk of ventricular arrhythmias associated with *sotalol* increased by hypokalaemia

Ergotamine: increased peripheral vasoconstriction

Muscle Relaxants: *propranolol* enhances effect

Sex Hormones: *oestrogens* and *combined oral contraceptives* antagonise hypotensive effect

**Beta-blockers** (*continued*)
● Sympathomimetics: severe hypertension with *adrenaline and noradrenaline* (especially with *non-selective beta-blockers*); severe hypertension also possible with *sympathomimetics in anorectics and cough and cold remedies*

Theophylline: *beta-blockers* should be avoided on pharmacological grounds (bronchospasm)

Thyroxine: metabolism of *propranolol* accelerated (reduced effect)

Ulcer-healing Drugs: plasma concentrations of *labetalol and propranolol* increased by *cimetidine*; hypotensive effect antagonised by *carbenoxolone*

Xamoterol: antagonism of effect of xamoterol and reduction in beta-blockade

**Betahistine**
Antihistamines: antagonism (theoretical)

**Betamethasone** *see* Corticosteroids
**Betaxolol** *see* Beta-blockers
**Bethanechol** *see* Cholinergics
**Bethanidine** *see* Adrenergic Neurone Blockers
**Bezafibrate** *see* Clofibrate Group
**Biperiden** *see* Antimuscarinics
**Bisphosphonates**

Antacids: absorption reduced

Antibacterials: severe hypocalcaemia reported with *aminoglycosides*

Calcium Salts: reduced absorption (give at least 2 hours apart)

**Bismuth Chelate**
Antibacterials: reduced absorption of *tetracyclines*

**Bisoprolol** *see* Beta-blockers
**Bretylium** (*see also* Adrenergic Neurone Blockers)
other Antiarrhythmics: increased myocardial depression with any combination of two or more anti-arrhythmics

**Bromazepam** *see* Benzodiazepines and other Anxiolytics and Hypnotics
**Bromocriptine**

Alcohol: reduced tolerance to *bromocriptine*

Antibacterials: *erythromycin* increases plasma concentration

Antipsychotics: antagonism of hypoprolactinaemic and antiparkinsonian effects

Domperidone and Metoclopramide: antagonise hypoprolactinaemic effect

**Budesonide** *see* Corticosteroids
**Bumetanide** *see* Diuretics (loop)
**Buprenorphine** *see* Opioid Analgesics
**Buspirone** (general sedative interactions as for Benzodiazepines and other Anxiolytics and Hypnotics)

Antidepressants: *MAOIs* contra-indicated by manufacturer

**Butobarbitone** *see* Barbiturates
**Butriptyline** *see* Antidepressants, Tricyclic
**Calcium Salts**

Antibacterials: reduced absorption of *tetracyclines*

Bisphosphonates: reduce absorption

Cardiac Glycosides: large intravenous doses of *calcium* can precipitate arrhythmias

Diuretics: increased risk of hypercalcaemia with *thiazides*

**Calcium-channel Blockers**
● Anaesthetics: *verapamil* increases hypotensive effect of *general anaesthetics* and risk of AV delay
● Anti-arrhythmics: *amiodarone-induced risk* of bradycardia, AV block, and myocardial depression increased by *diltiazem and verapamil*; with *verapamil* raised plasma concentration of *quinidine* (extreme hypotension may occur)

**Calcium-channel Blockers** (*continued*)

Antibacterials: *rifampicin* increases metabolism of *verapamil and possibly isradipine* (reduced plasma concentrations)

Antidepressants: *diltiazem* and *verapamil* increase plasma concentration of *imipramine and possibly other tricyclics*

Antidiabetics: *nifedipine* may occasionally impair glucose tolerance

● Antiepileptics: effect of *carbamazepine* enhanced by *diltiazem and verapamil; diltiazem* increases plasma concentration of *phenytoin*; effect of *felodipine* and *isradipine* and probably *nicardipine* and *nifedipine* reduced by *carbamazepine, phenobarbitone, phenytoin, and primidone*

Antihypertensives: enhanced hypotensive effect

Antimalarials: possible increased risk of bradycardia with some *calcium-channel blockers* and *mefloquine*

Antipsychotics: enhanced hypotensive effect

● Beta-blockers: increased risk of bradycardia and AV block with *diltiazem;* occasionally severe hypotension and heart failure with *nifedipine;* asystole, severe hypotension, and heart failure with *verapamil* (see section 2.3.2)

● Cardiac Glycosides: plasma concentration of *digoxin* increased by *diltiazem, nicardipine,* and *verapamil;* increased AV block and bradycardia with *verapamil*

Cyclosporin: plasma-cyclosporin concentrations increased by *diltiazem, nicardipine, and verapamil;* possibly increases plasma concentration of *nifedipine*

Lithium: neurotoxicity may occur without increased plasma-lithium concentrations in patients given *diltiazem* and *verapamil*

Muscle Relaxants: *nifedipine* and *verapamil* enhance effect of *non-depolarising muscle relaxants such as tubocurarine;* hypotension, myocardial depression, and hyperkalaemia with *verapamil* and intravenous *dantrolene*

Sympathomimetics: *see* Sympathomimetics (main list)

● Theophylline: *diltiazem and verapamil* enhance effect

Ulcer-healing Drugs: *cimetidine* inhibits metabolism of *some calcium-channel blockers* (increased plasma concentrations)

**Canrenoate** *see* Diuretics (*as for* spironolactone)

**Capreomycin**

*other* Antibacterials: increased risk of nephrotoxicity with *cephalothin, colistin, and polymyxin*; increased risk of nephrotoxicity and ototoxicity with *aminoglycosides and vancomycin*

Cytotoxics: increased risk of nephrotoxicity and ototoxicity with *cisplatin*

**Captopril** *see* ACE Inhibitors

**Carbachol** *see* Cholinergics

**Carbamazepine**

● Analgesics: *dextropropoxyphene* enhances effect of *carbamazepine*

● Antibacterials: metabolism of *doxycycline* accelerated (reduced effect); plasma-*carbamazepine* concentration increased by *erythromycin and isoniazid*

● Anticoagulants: metabolism of *nicoumalone and warfarin* accelerated (reduced anticoagulant effect)

**Carbamazepine** (*continued*)

● Antidepressants: antagonism of anticonvulsant effect (convulsive threshold lowered); plasma concentration of *carbamazepine* increased by *fluoxetine* and *viloxazine*; metabolism of *tricyclics* accelerated (reduced plasma concentrations); manufacturer advises avoid with *MAOIs* or within 2 weeks of *MAOIs*

● *other* Antiepileptics: concomitant administration of *two or more antiepileptics* may enhance toxicity without a corresponding increase in antiepileptic effect; moreover interactions between individual antiepileptics can complicate monitoring of treatment; interactions include enhanced effects, increased sedation, and reductions in plasma concentrations

● Antipsychotics: antagonism of anticonvulsant effect (convulsive threshold lowered); metabolism of *haloperidol* accelerated (reduced plasma-haloperidol concentration)

● Calcium-channel Blockers: *diltiazem and verapamil* enhance effect of *carbamazepine*; effect of *felodipine, isradipine* and probably *nicardipine* and *nifedipine* reduced

Cardiac Glycosides: metabolism of *digitoxin only* accelerated (reduced effect)

● Corticosteroids: metabolism accelerated (reduced effect)

● Cyclosporin: metabolism accelerated (reduced plasma-cyclosporin concentration)

● Hormone Antagonists: *danazol* inhibits metabolism of *carbamazepine* (enhanced effect)

Lithium: neurotoxicity may occur without increased plasma-lithium concentration

● Sex Hormones: *carbamazepine* accelerates metabolism of *oral contraceptives* (reduced contraceptive effect) and of *gestrinone and tibolone*

Theophylline: metabolism of *theophylline* accelerated (reduced effect)

Thyroxine: metabolism accelerated (may increase thyroxine requirements in hypothyroidism)

● Ulcer-healing Drugs: metabolism inhibited by *cimetidine* (increased plasma-carbamazepine concentration)

**Carbenicillin** *see* Penicillins

**Carbenoxolone**

*Note.* Do not apply to small amounts used topically on oral mucosa

Antihypertensives: antagonism of hypotensive effect

Cardiac Glycosides: toxicity increased if hypokalaemia occurs

Corticosteroids: increased risk of hypokalaemia

Diuretics: antagonism of diuretic effect; increased risk of hypokalaemia with *acetazolamide, thiazides, and loop diuretics*; inhibition of ulcer healing with *amiloride and spironolactone*

**Cardiac Glycosides**

Analgesics: *NSAIDs* may exacerbate heart failure, reduce GFR and increase plasma-cardiac glycoside concentrations

Anion-exchange Resins: absorption reduced by *cholestyramine and colestipol*

● Anti-arrhythmics: plasma concentration of *digoxin* increased by *amiodarone, propafenone, and quinidine* (halve maintenance dose of digoxin)

Antibacterials: *erythromycin* and possibly *azithromycin* enhance effect of *digoxin*; *rifampicin* accelerates metabolism of *digitoxin only* (reduced effect)

Antiepileptics: metabolism of *digitoxin only* accelerated (reduced effect)

**Cardiac Glycosides** (*continued*)
- Antimalarials: *quinine* (includes use of quinine for cramp) and possibly *chloroquine* raises plasma concentration of *digoxin* (halve maintenance dose of digoxin); possible increased risk of bradycardia with *mefloquine*

  Barbiturates: *see under* Antiepileptics, above

  Beta-blockers: increased AV block and bradycardia

  Calcium Salts: large intravenous doses of *calcium* can precipitate arrhythmias
- Calcium-channel Blockers: plasma concentration of *digoxin* increased by *diltiazem, nicardipine,* and *verapamil*; increased AV block and bradycardia with *verapamil*
- Diuretics: increased toxicity if hypokalaemia occurs with *acetazolamide, loop diuretics, and thiazides*; effects of *digoxin* enhanced by *spironolactone*

  Hormone Antagonists: *aminoglutethimide* accelerates metabolism of *digitoxin only* (reduced effect)

  Muscle Relaxants: arrhythmias with *suxamethonium*

  Ulcer-healing Drugs: increased toxicity if hypokalaemia occurs with *carbenoxolone*; absorption possibly reduced by *sucralfate*

**Carfecillin** *see* Penicillins

**Carteolol** *see* Beta-blockers

**Celiprolol** *see* Beta-blockers

**Cephalosporins**
  Alcohol: disulfiram-like reaction with *cephamandole*

  *other* Antibacterials: *cephalothin* increases risk of nephrotoxicity with *aminoglycosides, capreomycin,* and *vancomycin*
- Anticoagulants: anticoagulant effect of *warfarin and nicoumalone* enhanced by *cephamandole* and possibly others

  Antifungals: *cephalothin* increases risk of nephrotoxicity with *amphotericin*

  Diuretics: *loop diuretics* increase nephrotoxicity of *cephalothin*

  Probenecid: reduced excretion of *cephalosporins* (increased plasma concentrations)

**Cetirizine** *see* Antihistamines

**Chloral** (general sedative interactions *as for* Benzodiazepines and other Anxiolytics and Hypnotics)
  Anticoagulants: may transiently enhance anticoagulant effect of *nicoumalone and warfarin*

**Chloramphenicol**
  *other* Antibacterials: *rifampicin* accelerates metabolism (reduced chloramphenicol-plasma concentration)
- Anticoagulants: anticoagulant effect of *nicoumalone and warfarin* enhanced
- Antidiabetics: effect of *sulphonylureas* enhanced
- Antiepileptics: metabolism accelerated by *phenobarbitone* (reduced chloramphenicol-plasma concentration); increased plasma concentration of *phenytoin* (risk of toxicity)

  Barbiturates: *see under* Antiepileptics, above

**Chlordiazepoxide** *see* Benzodiazepines and other Anxiolytics and Hypnotics

**Chlormethiazole** (for general sedative interactions *see also* Benzodiazepines and other Anxiolytics and Hypnotics)
  Ulcer-healing Drugs: *cimetidine* inhibits metabolism (increased plasma-chlormethiazole concentration)

**Chlormezanone** *see* Benzodiazepines and other Anxiolytics and Hypnotics

**Chloroquine and Hydroxychloroquine**
  Antacids: reduced absorption
- Cardiac Glycosides: *chloroquine* possibly increases plasma concentration of *digoxin*

  Cholinergics: interaction no longer considered significant

  Ulcer-healing Drugs: *cimetidine* inhibits metabolism of *chloroquine* (increased plasma concentration)

**Chlorothiazide** *see* Diuretics (thiazide)

**Chlorpheniramine** *see* Antihistamines

**Chlorpromazine** *see* Phenothiazines and other Antipsychotics

**Chlorpropamide** *see* Antidiabetics (sulphonylurea)

**Chlorprothixene** *see* Phenothiazines and other Antipsychotics

**Chlortetracycline** *see* Tetracyclines

**Chlorthalidone** *see* Diuretics (thiazide-related)

**Cholestyramine and Colestipol**
  Analgesics: reduced absorption of *paracetamol* and *phenylbutazone*

  Antibacterials: antagonism of effect of oral *vancomycin*
- Anticoagulants: anticoagulant effect of *nicoumalone, phenindione, and warfarin* may be enhanced or reduced

  Cardiac Glycosides: reduced absorption

  Diuretics: reduced absorption of *thiazides* (give at least 2 hours apart)

  Thyroxine: reduced absorption

**Cholinergics**
  Anti-arrhythmics: *procainamide, quinidine* and possibly *propafenone* antagonise effect of *neostigmine and pyridostigmine*
- Antibacterials: *aminoglycosides, clindamycin, lincomycin,* and *polymyxins* antagonise effect of *neostigmine and pyridostigmine*

  Antimalarials: interaction no longer considered significant

  Beta-blockers: *propranolol* antagonises effect of *neostigmine and pyridostigmine*

  Lithium: antagonism of effect of *neostigmine and pyridostigmine*

  Muscle Relaxants: *demecarium and ecothiopate eye-drops, and neostigmine and pyridostigmine* enhance effect of *suxamethonium*, but antagonise effect of *non-depolarising muscle relaxants such as tubocurarine*

**Cilazapril** *see* ACE Inhibitors

**Cimetidine** *see* Histamine H2-antagonists

**Cinnarizine** *see* Antihistamines

**Cinoxacin** *see* 4-Quinolones

**Ciprofloxacin** *see* 4-Quinolones

**Cisapride**
  Analgesics: *opioid analgesics* possibly antagonise effect on gastro-intestinal motility

  Antimuscarinics: antagonism of effect on gastro-intestinal motility

**Cisplatin**
- Antibacterials: *aminoglycosides and capreomycin* increase risk of nephrotoxicity and possibly of ototoxicity

**Clarithromycin** *see* Erythromycin

**Clemastine** *see* Antihistamines

**Clindamycin**
  Cholinergics: antagonism of effect of *neostigmine and pyridostigmine*

  Muscle relaxants: enhancement of effect of *non-depolarising muscle relaxants such as tubocurarine*

**Clobazam** *see* Benzodiazepines and other Anxiolytics and Hypnotics

**Clodronate Sodium** *see* Bisphosphonates

**Clofibrate Group**
- Anticoagulants: enhancement of effect of *nicoumalone, phenindione, and warfarin*

  Antidiabetics: may improve glucose tolerance and have additive effect

  *other* Lipid-lowering Drugs: increased risk of myopathy with *pravastatin and simvastatin*

**Clomipramine** *see* Antidepressants, Tricyclic

**Clomocycline** *see* Tetracyclines

**Clonazepam** (general sedative interactions *as for* Benzodiazepines and other Anxiolytics and Hypnotics)

  *other* Antiepileptics: metabolism of *clonazepam* accelerated by *carbamazepine, phenobarbitone and phenytoin*

**Clonidine** (for general hypotensive interactions *see also* Hydralazine)
- Antidepressants: *tricyclics* antagonise hypotensive effect and also increase risk of rebound hypertension on *clonidine* withdrawal
- Beta-blockers: increased risk of hypertension on *clonidine* withdrawal

**Clopamide** *see* Diuretics (thiazide)

**Clorazepate** *see* Benzodiazepines and other Anxiolytics and Hypnotics

**Cloxacillin** *see* Penicillins

**Clozapine**

  *Note.* Clozapine should not be used concurrently with drugs associated with a substantial potential for causing agranulocytosis, such as co-trimoxazole, chloramphenicol, sulphonamides, penicillamine, or cytotoxics

  *see also* Phenothiazines and other Antipsychotics

**Codeine** *see* Opioid Analgesics

**Cold and Cough Remedies** *see* Antihistamines and Sympathomimetics

**Colestipol** *see* Cholestyramine and Colestipol

**Colistin** *see* Polymyxins

**Contraceptives, Oral**

  *Note.* Also covers oestrogens taken alone; in case of hormone replacement therapy low dose unlikely to induce interactions

- Antibacterials: *rifampicin* accelerates metabolism of both *combined and progestogen-only oral contraceptives* (possibility of reduced contraceptive effect); when *broad-spectrum antibiotics such as ampicillin and tetracycline* given with *combined oral contraceptives* possibility of reduced contraceptive effect (risk probably small)
- Anticoagulants: antagonism of anticoagulant effect of *nicoumalone, phenindione, and warfarin*

  Antidepressants: antagonism of antidepressant effect has been reported, but side-effects of *tricyclics* may be increased due to higher plasma concentrations

  Antidiabetics: antagonism of hypoglycaemic effect
- Antiepileptics: *carbamazepine, phenobarbitone, phenytoin, and primidone* accelerate metabolism (reduced contraceptive effect)
- Antifungals: *griseofulvin* accelerates metabolism (reduced contraceptive effect)

  Antihypertensives: *combined oral contraceptives* antagonise hypotensive effect

  Barbiturates: *see under* Antiepileptics, above

  Beta-blockers: *oestrogens* and *combined oral contraceptives* antagonise hypotensive effect
- Cyclosporin: increased plasma-cyclosporin concentration

  Diuretics: *combined oral contraceptives* antagonise diuretic effect

  Theophylline: *combined oral contraceptives* delay excretion (increased plasma-theophylline concentration)

**Corticosteroids**

  *Note.* Do not generally apply to corticosteroids with potent topical action such as beclomethasone

- Antibacterials: *rifampicin* accelerates metabolism of *corticosteroids* (reduced effect)

  Antidiabetics: antagonism of hypoglycaemic effect

- Antiepileptics: *carbamazepine, phenobarbitone, phenytoin, and primidone* accelerate metabolism of *corticosteroids* (reduced effect)

  Antihypertensives: antagonism of hypotensive effect

  Barbiturates: *see under* Antiepileptics, above

  Diuretics: antagonism of diuretic effect; *acetazolamide, loop diuretics, and thiazides* increase risk of hypokalaemia

  Hormone Antagonists: *aminoglutethimide* accelerates metabolism of *dexamethasone* (reduced effect)

  Sympathomimetics *see* Sympathomimetics, Beta₂ (main list)

  Ulcer-healing Drugs: *carbenoxolone* increases risk of hypokalaemia

**Co-trimoxazole and Sulphonamides**

  Anaesthetics: effect of *thiopentone* enhanced

- Anticoagulants: effect of *nicoumalone and warfarin* enhanced
- Antidiabetics: effect of *sulphonylureas* enhanced
- Antiepileptics: antifolate effect and plasma concentration of *phenytoin* increased by *co-trimoxazole*

  Antimalarials: increased risk of antifolate effect with *pyrimethamine* (includes *Fansidar®* and *Maloprim®*)

  Cyclosporin: increased risk of nephrotoxicity

  Cytotoxics: antifolate effect of *methotrexate* increased by *co-trimoxazole*

**Cyclizine** *see* Antihistamines

**Cyclobarbitone** *see* Barbiturates

**Cyclopenthiazide** *see* Diuretics (thiazide)

**Cyclopentolate** *see* Antimuscarinics

**Cyclophosphamide**
- Allopurinol: toxicity of *cyclophosphamide* increased

  Muscle Relaxants: *cyclophosphamide* enhances effect of *suxamethonium*

**Cyclopropane** *see* Anaesthetics

**Cycloserine**

  *other* Antibacterials: increased CNS toxicity with *isoniazid*
- Antiepileptics: increased plasma concentration of *phenytoin* (risk of toxicity)

**Cyclosporin**
- Analgesics: increased risk of nephrotoxicity with *NSAIDs*
- Antibacterials: *aminoglycosides, co-trimoxazole, and 4-quinolones* increase risk of nephrotoxicity; *erythromycin* increases plasma-cyclosporin concentration; *rifampicin* reduces plasma-cyclosporin concentration
- Antiepileptics: *carbamazepine, phenobarbitone, phenytoin, and primidone* accelerate metabolism (reduced plasma-cyclosporin concentration)
- Antifungals: *amphotericin* increases risk of nephrotoxicity; *itraconazole, ketoconazole* and possibly *fluconazole* inhibit metabolism (increased plasma-cyclosporin concentration)

  Antihypertensives: increased risk of hyperkalaemia with *ACE inhibitors*

  Barbiturates: *see under* Antiepileptics, above
- Calcium-channel Blockers: *diltiazem, nicardipine, and verapamil* increase plasma-cyclosporin concentration; *cyclosporin* possibly increases plasma concentration of *nifedipine*

**Cyclosporin** (*continued*)
- Diuretics: *potassium-sparing diuretics* increase risk of hyperkalaemia
- Hormone Antagonists: *danazol* inhibits metabolism (increased plasma-cyclosporin concentration); *octreotide* reduces absorption (reduced plasma-cyclosporin concentration)

  Lipid-lowering Drugs: increased risk of myopathy with *pravastatin and simvastatin*
- Potassium Salts: increased risk of hyperkalaemia
- Sex Hormones: *progestogens* inhibit metabolism (increased plasma-cyclosporin concentration)

**Cyproheptadine** *see* Antihistamines
**Cytotoxics** *see under* individual drugs
**Dalteparin** *see* Heparin
**Danazol**
- Anticoagulants: effect of *nicoumalone and warfarin* enhanced (inhibits metabolism)
- Antiepileptics: inhibits metabolism of *carbamazepine* (increased plasma-carbamazepine concentration)
- Cyclosporin: inhibits metabolism (increased plasma-cyclosporin concentration)

**Dantrolene** *see* Muscle Relaxants
**Dapsone**
  Probenecid: *dapsone* excretion reduced (increased risk of side-effects)
**Debrisoquine** *see* Adrenergic Neurone Blockers
**Demecarium** *see* Cholinergics
**Demeclocycline** *see* Tetracyclines
**Desferrioxamine**
  Antipsychotics: manufacturer advises avoid *prochlorperazine*
**Desipramine** *see* Antidepressants, Tricyclic
**Dexamethasone** *see* Corticosteroids
**Dexamphetamine** *see* Sympathomimetics
**Dexfenfluramine** *see* Sympathomimetics
**Dextromoramide** *see* Opioid Analgesics
**Dextropropoxyphene** *see* Opioid Analgesics
**Diamorphine** *see* Opioid Analgesics
**Diazepam** *see* Benzodiazepines and other Anxiolytics and Hypnotics
**Diazoxide** (general hypotensive interactions *as for* Hydralazine)
  Antidiabetics: antagonism of hypoglycaemic effect
**Dichlorphenamide** *see* Acetazolamide
**Diclofenac** *see* NSAIDs
**Dicyclomine** *see* Antimuscarinics
**Diethylpropion** *see* Sympathomimetics
**Diflunisal** *see* NSAIDs
**Digitoxin** *see* Cardiac Glycosides
**Digoxin** *see* Cardiac Glycosides
**Dihydrocodeine** *see* Opioid Analgesics
**Dihydroergotamine** *see* Ergotamine
**Diltiazem** *see* Calcium-channel Blockers
**Dimenhydrinate** *see* Antihistamines
**Dimethindene** *see* Antihistamines
**Diphenhydramine** *see* Antihistamines
**Diphenylpyraline** *see* Antihistamines
**Diphenoxylate** *see* Opioid Analgesics
**Dipipanone** *see* Opioid Analgesics
**Dipivefrine** *see* Sympathomimetics (*as for* adrenaline)
**Dipyridamole**
  Antacids: patient information leaflet advises avoidance of *antacids*
- Anti-arrhythmics: effect of *adenosine* enhanced (risk of toxicity)
- Anticoagulants: enhanced effect due to antiplatelet action of *dipyridamole*

**Disodium Etidronate** *see* Bisphosphonates
**Disodium Pamidronate** *see* Bisphosphonates

**Disopyramide**
- *other* Anti-arrhythmics: *amiodarone* increases risk of ventricular arrhythmias; increased myocardial depression with any *anti-arrhythmic*
- Antibacterials: plasma concentration of *disopyramide* reduced by *rifampicin* but increased by *erythromycin* (risk of toxicity)

  Antiepileptics: plasma concentration of *disopyramide* reduced by *phenobarbitone, phenytoin, and primidone*

  Antimuscarinics: increased antimuscarinic side-effects

  Barbiturates: *see under* Antiepileptics, above
- Diuretics: toxicity of *disopyramide* increased if hypokalaemia occurs with *acetazolamide, loop diuretics, and thiazides*

  Nitrates: reduced effect of *sublingual nitrates* (failure to dissolve under tongue owing to dry mouth)
**Distigmine** *see* Cholinergics
**Disulfiram**
  Alcohol: disulfiram reaction (*see* section 4.10)

  Antibacterials: psychotic reaction with *metronidazole* reported
- Anticoagulants: effect of *nicoumalone and warfarin* enhanced

  Antidepressants: inhibition of metabolism of *tricyclic antidepressants* (increased plasma concentrations); increased disulfiram reaction with alcohol reported if *amitriptyline* also taken
- Antiepileptics: inhibition of metabolism of *phenytoin* (increased risk of toxicity)

  Anxiolytics and Hypnotics: inhibition of metabolism of *chlordiazepoxide and diazepam* (enhanced sedative effect)

  Theophylline: inhibition of metabolism (increased risk of toxicity)
**Diuretics**
  Analgesics: *diuretics* increase risk of nephrotoxicity of *NSAIDs*; *NSAIDs* notably *indomethacin* antagonise diuretic effect; *indomethacin and possibly other NSAIDs* increase risk of hyperkalaemia with *potassium-sparing diuretics*; diuretic effect of *spironolactone* antagonised by *aspirin*; *aspirin* reduces excretion of *acetazolamide* (risk of toxicity)

  Anion-exchange Resins: *cholestyramine and colestipol* reduce absorption of *thiazides* (give at least 2 hours apart)
- Anti-arrhythmics: toxicity of *amiodarone, disopyramide, flecainide, and quinidine* increased if hypokalaemia occurs; action of *lignocaine, mexiletine, and tocainide* antagonised by hypokalaemia; *acetazolamide* reduces excretion of *quinidine* (increased plasma concentration)

  Antibacterials: *loop diuretics* increase ototoxicity of *aminoglycosides, polymyxins, and vancomycin; loop diuretics* increase nephrotoxicity of *cephalothin*

  Antidepressants: increased risk of postural hypotension with *tricyclics*

  Antidiabetics: hypoglycaemic effect antagonised by *loop and thiazide diuretics; chlorpropamide* increases risk of hyponatraemia associated with *thiazides in combination with potassium-sparing diuretics*
- Antihypertensives: enhanced hypotensive effect; enhancement of effect of *ACE inhibitors* (risk of extreme hypotension, also risk of hyperkalaemia with *potassium-sparing diuretics*); increased risk of first-dose hypotensive effect of post-synaptic *alpha-blockers* such as *prazosin and terazosin*; increased risk of hypokalaemia with *indapamide*

**Diuretics** (*continued*)

Antipsychotics: in hypokalaemia increased risk of ventricular arrhythmias with *pimozide*

Beta-blockers: in hypokalaemia increased risk of ventricular arrhythmias with *sotalol*

Calcium Salts: risk of hypercalcaemia with *thiazides*

• Cardiac Glycosides: increased toxicity if hypokalaemia occurs with *acetazolamide, loop diuretics, and thiazides;* effect enhanced by *spironolactone*

Corticosteroids: increased risk of hypokalaemia with *acetazolamide, loop diuretics, and thiazides;* antagonism of diuretic effect

• Cyclosporin: increased risk of hyperkalaemia with *potassium-sparing* diuretics

*other* Diuretics: increased risk of hypokalaemia if *acetazolamide, loop diuretics or thiazides* given together; profound diuresis possible if *metolazone* given with *frusemide* (section 2.2.1)

Hormone Antagonists: *trilostane* increases risk of hyperkalaemia with *potassium-sparing diuretics*

• Lithium: lithium excretion reduced by *loop diuretics and thiazides* (increased plasma-lithium concentration and risk of toxicity—*loop diuretics safer than thiazides);* lithium excretion increased by *acetazolamide*

• Potassium Salts: hyperkalaemia with *potassium-sparing diuretics*

Sex Hormones: *oestrogens and combined oral contraceptives* antagonise diuretic effect

Ulcer-healing Drugs: increased risk of hypokalaemia if *acetazolamide, loop diuretics, and thiazides* given with *carbenoxolone; carbenoxolone* antagonises diuretic effect; *amiloride and spironolactone* antagonise ulcer-healing effect of *carbenoxolone*

**Domperidone**

Analgesics: *opioid analgesics* antagonise effect on gastro-intestinal activity

Antimuscarinics: antagonism of effect on gastro-intestinal activity

Dopaminergics: antagonism of hypoprolactinaemic effect of *bromocriptine*

**Dopamine** *see* Sympathomimetics

**Dopaminergics** *see* Amantadine, Bromocriptine, Levodopa, and Lysuride

**Dopexamine** *see* Sympathomimetics

**Dothiepin** *see* Antidepressants, Tricyclic

**Doxapram**

Sympathomimetics: risk of hypertension

Theophylline: increased CNS stimulation

**Doxazosin** *see* Alpha-blockers (post-synaptic)

**Doxepin** *see* Antidepressants, Tricyclic

**Doxycycline** *see* Tetracyclines

**Droperidol** *see* Phenothiazines and other Antipsychotics

**Ecothiopate** *see* Cholinergics

**Edrophonium** *see* Cholinergics

**Enalapril** *see* ACE Inhibitors

**Enoxacin** *see* 4-Quinolines

**Enoxaparin** *see* Heparin

**Ephedrine** *see* Sympathomimetics

**Ergotamine**

Antibacterials: ergotism with *erythromycin* and possibly *azithromycin*

Beta-blockers: increased peripheral vasoconstriction

• Sumatriptan: risk of CNS toxicity

**Erythromycin**

Analgesics: plasma concentration of *alfentanil* increased

• Anti-arrhythmics: plasma concentration of *disopyramide* increased (risk of toxicity)

**Erythromycin** (*continued*)

• Anticoagulants: effect of *nicoumalone and warfarin* enhanced

▶ Antiepileptics: inhibition of metabolism of *carbamazepine* (increased plasma-carbamazepine concentration)

Anxiolytics and Hypnotics: inhibition of metabolism of *midazolam* (increased plasma concentration, see also p. 454)

Cardiac Glycosides: effect of *digoxin* enhanced

• Cyclosporin: inhibition of metabolism (increased plasma-cyclosporin concentration)

Dopaminergics: plasma concentration of *bromocriptine* increased

Ergotamine: ergotism reported

• Theophylline: inhibition of metabolism (increased plasma-theophylline concentration)

**Ethacrynic Acid** *see* Diuretics (loop)

**Ethosuximide**

• Antibacterials: *isoniazid* increases plasma concentrations (increased risk of toxicity)

• Antidepressants: antagonism (convulsive threshold lowered)

• *other* Antiepileptics: concomitant administration of two or more antiepileptics may enhance toxicity without a corresponding increase in antiepileptic effect; moreover interactions between individual antiepileptics can complicate monitoring of treatment; interactions include enhanced effects, increased sedation, and reductions in plasma concentrations

• Antipsychotics: antagonism (convulsive threshold lowered)

**Etidronate Disodium** *see* Bisphosphonates

**Etodolac** *see* NSAIDs

**Etretinate**

Cytotoxics: increased plasma concentration of *methotrexate*

**Famotidine** *see* Histamine H2-antagonists

**Fansidar®** *contains* Sulfadoxine and Pyrimethamine

**Felodipine** *see* Calcium-channel Blockers

**Fenbufen** *see* NSAIDs

**Fenfluramine** *see* Sympathomimetics

**Fenofibrate** *see* Clofibrate Group

**Fenoprofen** *see* NSAIDs

**Fenoterol** *see* Sympathomimetics, Beta₂

**Fentanyl** *see* Opioid Analgesics

**Ferrous Salts** *see* Iron

**Flavoxate** *see* Antimuscarinics

**Flecainide**

Antacids and Adsorbents: interaction no longer considered significant

• *other* Anti-arrhythmics: *amiodarone* increases plasma-flecainide concentration (and increases risk of ventricular arrhythmias); increased myocardial depression with any *anti-arrhythmic*

• Diuretics: toxicity increased if hypokalaemia occurs; excretion reduced by *acetazolamide* (occasionally increased plasma concentration)

Ulcer-healing Drugs: *cimetidine* inhibits metabolism of *flecainide* (increased plasma-flecainide concentration)

**Flucloxacillin** *see* Penicillins

**Fluconazole**

Antibacterials: *rifampicin* reduces plasma concentration

• Anticoagulants: effect of *nicoumalone and warfarin* enhanced

Antidiabetics: plasma concentrations of *sulphonylureas* possibly increased

**Fluconazole** (*continued*)

- Antiepileptics: effect of *phenytoin* enhanced
  Cyclosporin: possible inhibition of metabolism and increased plasma-cyclosporin concentration

**Fludrocortisone** *see* Corticosteroids

**Flunitrazepam** *see* Benzodiazepines and other Anxiolytics and Hypnotics

**Fluorouracil**
  Ulcer-healing Drugs: *cimetidine* inhibits metabolism (increased plasma-fluorouracil concentration)

**Fluoxetine** *see* Antidepressants, Serotonin-uptake Inhibitor

**Flupenthixol** *see* Phenothiazines and other Antipsychotics

**Fluphenazine** *see* Phenothiazines and other Antipsychotics

**Flurazepam** *see* Benzodiazepines and other Anxiolytics and Hypnotics

**Flurbiprofen** *see* NSAIDs

**Fluspirilene** *see* Phenothiazines and other Antipsychotics

**Flutamide**
- Anticoagulants: effect of *warfarin* enhanced

**Fluvoxamine** *see* Antidepressants, Serotonin-uptake Inhibitor

**Folic Acid** *see* Vitamins

**Fosinopril** *see* ACE Inhibitors

**Framycetin** *see* Aminoglycosides

**Frusemide** *see* Diuretics (loop)

**Gallamine** *see* Muscle Relaxants (non-depolarising)

**Ganciclovir**
  *Note:* increased risk of myelosuppression with other *myelosuppressive drugs*
  *other* Antivirals: profound myelosuppression with *zidovudine*

**Gemfibrozil** *see* Clofibrate Group

**Gentamicin** *see* Aminoglycosides

**Gestrinone**
  Antibacterials: *rifampicin* accelerates metabolism (reduced plasma concentration)
  Antiepileptics: *carbamazepine, phenobarbitone, phenytoin, and primidone* accelerate metabolism (reduced plasma concentration)

**Glibenclamide** *see* Antidiabetics (sulphonylurea)

**Gliclazide** *see* Antidiabetics (sulphonylurea)

**Glipizide** *see* Antidiabetics (sulphonylurea)

**Gliquidone** *see* Antidiabetics (sulphonylurea)

**Glyceryl Trinitrate** (general hypotensive interactions *as for* Hydralazine)
  Anti-arrhythmics: *disopyramide* may reduce effect of *sublingual nitrates* (owing to dry mouth)
  Antidepressants: *tricyclics* may reduce effect of *sublingual nitrates* (owing to dry mouth)
  Antimuscarinics: *antimuscarinics such as atropine and propantheline* may reduce effect of *sublingual nitrates* (owing to dry mouth)

**Griseofulvin**
- Anticoagulants: metabolism of *nicoumalone and warfarin* accelerated (reduced anticoagulant effect)
  Antiepileptics: metabolism accelerated by *phenobarbitone* (reduced effect)
- Sex Hormones: metabolism of *oral contraceptives* accelerated (reduced effect)

**Guanethidine** *see* Adrenergic Neurone Blockers

**Guar Gum**
  Antibacterials: absorption of *phenoxymethylpenicillin* reduced

**Haloperidol** *see* Phenothiazines and other Antipsychotics

**Halothane** *see* Anaesthetics (volatile)

**Heparin**
  Analgesics: *aspirin* enhances anticoagulant effect
  Antiplatelet Drugs: *aspirin and dipyridamole* enhance anticoagulant effect

**Hexamine**
  Potassium Citrate: urine should be acid

**Histamine H1-antagonists** *see* Antihistamines

**Histamine H2-antagonists**
  Analgesics: *cimetidine* inhibits metabolism of *opioid analgesics notably pethidine* (increased plasma concentrations)
- Anti-arrhythmics: *cimetidine* increases plasma concentrations of *amiodarone, flecainide, lignocaine, procainamide, propafenone, and quinidine*
  Antibacterials: *rifampicin* accelerates metabolism of *cimetidine* (reduced plasma-cimetidine concentration); *cimetidine* inhibits metabolism of *metronidazole* (increased plasma-metronidazole concentration)
- Anticoagulants: *cimetidine* enhances anticoagulant effect of *nicoumalone and warfarin* (inhibits metabolism)
  Antidepressants: *cimetidine* inhibits metabolism of *amitriptyline, desipramine, doxepin, imipramine, and nortriptyline* (increased plasma concentrations)
  Antidiabetics: *cimetidine* inhibits renal excretion of *metformin* (increased plasma concentration)
- Antiepileptics: *cimetidine* inhibits metabolism of *carbamazepine and phenytoin* (increased plasma concentrations)
  Antifungals: absorption of *itraconazole and ketoconazole* reduced
  Antimalarials: *cimetidine* inhibits metabolism of *chloroquine and quinine* (increased plasma concentrations)
  Antipsychotics: *cimetidine* may enhance effect of *chlorpromazine, clozapine, and possibly other antipsychotics*
  Anxiolytics and Hypnotics: *cimetidine* inhibits metabolism of *benzodiazepines and chlormethiazole* (increased plasma concentrations)
  Beta-blockers: *cimetidine* inhibits metabolism of *beta-blockers such as labetalol and propranolol* (increased plasma concentrations)
  Calcium-channel Blockers: *cimetidine* inhibits metabolism of *some calcium-channel blockers* (increased plasma concentrations)
  Cytotoxics: *cimetidine* increases plasma concentration of *fluorouracil*
- Theophylline: *cimetidine* inhibits metabolism (increased plasma-theophylline concentration)

**Homatropine** *see* Antimuscarinics

**Hydralazine**
  Alcohol: enhanced hypotensive effect
- Anaesthetics: enhanced hypotensive effect
  Analgesics: *NSAIDs* antagonise hypotensive effect
  Antidepressants: enhanced hypotensive effect
  *other* Antihypertensives: additive hypotensive effect
  Antipsychotics: enhanced hypotensive effect
  Anxiolytics and Hypnotics: enhanced hypotensive effect
  Beta-blockers: enhanced hypotensive effect
  Calcium-channel Blockers: enhanced hypotensive effect
  Corticosteroids: antagonism of hypotensive effect
  Diuretics: enhanced hypotensive effect
  Dopaminergics: *levodopa* enhances hypotensive effect
  Muscle Relaxants: *baclofen* enhances hypotensive effect

**Hydralazine** (*continued*)

Nitrates: enhance hypotensive effect

Sex Hormones: *oestrogens and combined oral contraceptives* antagonise hypotensive effect

Ulcer-healing Drugs: *carbenoxolone* antagonises hypotensive effect

**Hydrochlorothiazide** *see* Diuretics (thiazide)

**Hydrocortisone** *see* Corticosteroids

**Hydroflumethiazide** *see* Diuretics (thiazide)

**Hydroxychloroquine** *see* Chloroquine and Hydroxychloroquine

**Hydroxyzine** *see* Antihistamines

**Hyoscine** *see* Antimuscarinics

**Hypnotics** *see* Benzodiazepines and other Anxiolytics and Hypnotics

**Ibuprofen** *see* NSAIDs

**Ifosfamide**

● Anticoagulants: effect of *warfarin* possibly enhanced

**Imipramine** *see* Antidepressants, Tricyclic

**Indapamide** *see* Diuretics (thiazide-related)

**Indomethacin** *see* NSAIDs

**Indoramin** *see* Alpha-blockers

**Influenza Vaccine**

Anticoagulants: effect of *warfarin* occasionally enhanced

Antiepileptics: effect of *phenytoin* enhanced

Theophylline: effect occasionally enhanced

**Insulin** *see* Antidiabetics

**Interferons**

Theophylline: metabolism of *theophylline* inhibited (enhanced effect)

**Iprindole** *see* Antidepressants, Tricyclic

**Iron**

Antacids: *magnesium trisilicate* reduces absorption of *oral iron*

Antibacterials: *tetracyclines* reduce absorption of *oral iron* (and *vice versa*); absorption of *ciprofloxacin, norfloxacin,* and *ofloxacin* reduced by *oral iron*

Dopaminergics: absorption of *levodopa* may be reduced

Penicillamine: reduced absorption of *penicillamine*

Trientine: reduced absorption of *oral iron*

Zinc: reduced absorption of *oral iron* (and *vice versa*)

**Isocarboxazid** *see* MAOIs

**Isometheptene** *see* Sympathomimetics

**Isoniazid**

Antacids and Adsorbents: *antacids* reduce absorption

*other* Antibacterials: increased CNS toxicity with *cycloserine*

● Antiepileptics: metabolism of *carbamazepine, ethosuximide, and phenytoin* inhibited (enhanced effect)

Anxiolytics and Hypnotics: metabolism of *diazepam* inhibited

Theophylline: *isoniazid* possibly increases plasma-theophylline concentration

**Isoprenaline** *see* Sympathomimetics

**Isosorbide Dinitrate** *see* Glyceryl Trinitrate

**Isosorbide Mononitrate** *see* Glyceryl Trinitrate

**Isradipine** *see* Calcium-channel Blockers

**Itraconazole**

Antacids and Adsorbents: *antacids* reduce absorption

Antibacterials: metabolism accelerated by *rifampicin* (reduced plasma-itraconazole concentration)

● Anticoagulants: effect of *warfarin* enhanced

**Itraconazole** (*continued*)

● Cyclosporin: metabolism inhibited (increased plasma-cyclosporin concentration)

Ulcer-healing Drugs: *histamine H2-antagonists* reduce absorption

**Kanamycin** *see* Aminoglycosides

**Kaolin** *see* Antacids and Adsorbents

**Ketoconazole**

Antacids and Adsorbents: *antacids* reduce absorption

Antibacterials: metabolism accelerated by *rifampicin* (reduced plasma-ketoconazole concentration)

● Anticoagulants: effect of *nicoumalone and warfarin* enhanced

● Antiepileptics: plasma-ketoconazole concentration reduced by *phenytoin* and effect of *phenytoin* enhanced

Antihistamines: *terfenadine* metabolism inhibited (risk of cardiac toxicity)

Antimuscarinics: reduced absorption

● Cyclosporin: metabolism inhibited (increased plasma-cyclosporin concentration)

Ulcer-healing Drugs: *histamine H2-antagonists* reduce absorption

**Ketoprofen** *see* NSAIDs

**Ketorolac** *see* NSAIDs

**Ketotifen** *see* Antihistamines

**Labetalol** *see* Beta-blockers

**Lamotrigine**

● *other* Antiepileptics: concomitant administration of *two or more antiepileptics* may enhance toxicity without a corresponding increase in antiepileptic effect; moreover interactions between individual antiepileptics can complicate monitoring of treatment; interactions include enhanced effects, increased sedation, and reductions in plasma concentrations

**Lanatoside C** *see* Cardiac Glycosides

**Levodopa**

● Anaesthetics: risk of arrhythmias with *volatile anaesthetics such as cyclopropane and halothane*

● Antidepressants: hypertensive crisis with *MAOIs*

Antihypertensives: enhanced hypotensive effect; effect of *levodopa* antagonised by *rauwolfia alkaloids*

Antipsychotics: antagonism of effect

Anxiolytics and Hypnotics: occasional antagonism of effect by *chlordiazepoxide, diazepam, lorazepam and possibly other benzodiazepines*

Domperidone and Metoclopramide: levodopa-plasma concentrations increased by *metoclopramide*

Iron: absorption of *levodopa* may be reduced

Vitamins: effect of *levodopa* antagonised by *pyridoxine* unless a *dopa decarboxylase inhibitor* also given

**Lignocaine**

*other* Anti-arrhythmics: increased myocardial depression

Beta-blockers: increased risk of myocardial depression; increased risk of *lignocaine* toxicity with *propranolol*

Diuretics: effect of *lignocaine* antagonised by hypokalaemia with *acetazolamide, loop diuretics, and thiazides*

Ulcer-healing Drugs: *cimetidine* inhibits metabolism of *lignocaine* (increased risk of toxicity)

**Lincomycin**

Antacids and Adsorbents: *kaolin* reduces absorption

- Cholinergics: antagonism of effect of *neostigmine and pyridostigmine*
- Muscle Relaxants: enhancement of effect of *non-depolarising muscle relaxants such as tubocurarine*

**Lisinopril** *see* ACE Inhibitors

**Lithium**

- Analgesics: *NSAIDs* reduce excretion of *lithium* (possibility of toxicity)

Antacids and Adsorbents: *sodium bicarbonate* increases excretion of *lithium* (reduced plasma-lithium concentrations)

Antibacterials: *lithium* toxicity reported with *metronidazole* and *spectinomycin*

- Antidepressants: *fluoxetine, fluvoxamine, paroxetine, and sertraline* increase risk of CNS toxicity

Antidiabetics: *lithium* may occasionally impair glucose tolerance

Antiepileptics: neurotoxicity may occur with *carbamazepine and phenytoin* without increased plasma-lithium concentration

- Antihypertensives: *ACE inhibitors* reduce excretion of *lithium* (increased plasma-lithium concentration); neurotoxicity may occur with *methyldopa* without increased plasma-lithium concentration

Antipsychotics: increased risk of extrapyramidal effects and possibility of neurotoxicity (notably with *haloperidol*)

Calcium-channel Blockers: neurotoxicity may occur with *diltiazem and verapamil* without increased plasma-lithium concentration

Cholinergics: *lithium* antagonises effect of *neostigmine and pyridostigmine*

- Diuretics: *lithium* excretion reduced by *loop diuretics and thiazides* (increased plasma-lithium concentration and risk of toxicity—*loop diuretics* safer than *thiazides*); *lithium* excretion increased by *acetazolamide*

Domperidone and Metoclopramide: increased risk of extrapyramidal effects and possibility of neurotoxicity with *metoclopramide*

Muscle Relaxants: muscle relaxant effect enhanced

- Sumatriptan: risk of CNS toxicity

Theophylline: *lithium* excretion increased (reduced plasma-lithium concentration)

**Lofepramine** *see* Antidepressants, Tricyclic

**Loprazolam** *see* Benzodiazepines and other Anxiolytics and Hypnotics

**Loratadine** *see* Antihistamines

**Lorazepam** *see* Benzodiazepines and other Anxiolytics and Hypnotics

**Lormetazepam** *see* Benzodiazepines and other Anxiolytics and Hypnotics

**Loxapine** *see* Phenothiazines and other Antipsychotics

**Lymecycline** *see* Tetracyclines

**Lysuride**

Antipsychotics: antagonism of effect

**Magnesium Salts** (*see also* Antacids and Adsorbents)

Muscle Relaxants: effect of *non-depolarising muscle relaxants such as tubocurarine* enhanced by *parenteral magnesium salts*

**Magnesium Trisilicate** *see* Antacids and Adsorbents

**Maloprim®** *contains* Dapsone and Pyrimethamine

**MAOIs**

- Alcohol: some *alcoholic and dealcoholised beverages contain tyramine* which interacts with *MAOIs* (hypertensive crisis); foods, *see* MAOI card, section 4.3.2

**MAOIs** (*continued*)

- Analgesics: CNS excitation or depression (hypertension or hypotension) with *pethidine and possibly other opioid analgesics;* manufacturer advises avoid *nefopam*

Anorectics: *see* Sympathomimetics, below

- *other* Antidepressants: enhancement of CNS effects and toxicity with *other MAOIs* (avoid for at least a week after stopping *previous MAOIs* then start with reduced dose); CNS excitation and hypertension with most *tricyclics and related antidepressants* (avoid for at least 2 weeks after stopping MAOIs); enhancement of CNS effects and toxicity possible with *serotonin-uptake inhibitors* (avoid MAOIs for at least 2 weeks before *serotonin-uptake inhibitors* and avoid *fluoxetine* for at least 5 weeks and *sertraline* for 7 days before MAOIs); CNS excitation and confusion with *tryptophan* (reduce tryptophan dose)

Antidiabetics: effect of *insulin, metformin, and sulphonylureas* enhanced

- Antiepileptics: antagonism of anticonvulsant effect (convulsive threshold lowered); manufacturer advises avoid *carbamazepine* with or within 2 weeks of MAOIs
- Antihypertensives: hypotensive effect enhanced; CNS excitation and hypertension with *rauwolfia alkaloids*

Antimuscarinics: increased side-effects

- Antipsychotics: CNS excitation and hypertension with *oxypertine*

Anxiolytics and Hypnotics: manufacturer advises avoidance of *buspirone*

- Dopaminergics: hypertensive crisis with *levodopa*
- Sumatriptan: risk of CNS toxicity
- Sympathomimetics: hypertensive crisis with *sympathomimetics such as dexamphetamine and other amphetamines, dexfenfluramine, diethylpropion, dopamine, dopexamine, ephedrine, fenfluramine, isometheptene, mazindol, pemoline, phentermine, phenylephrine, phenylpropanolamine, and pseudoephedrine*
- Tetrabenazine: CNS excitation and hypertension

**Maprotiline** *see* Antidepressants, Tricyclic

**Mazindol** *see* Sympathomimetics

**Mebhydrolin** *see* Antihistamines

**Medazepam** *see* Benzodiazepines and other Anxiolytics and Hypnotics

**Mefenamic Acid** *see* NSAIDs

**Mefloquine**

*other* Antimalarials: increased risk of side-effects with *quinine*, but should not prevent use of intravenous quinine in severe cases; for full precautions see p. 236 (also applies to *quinidine*)

Cardioactive drugs: possible increased risk of bradycardia with *beta-blockers*, *digoxin*, and *some calcium-channel blockers*

**Mefruside** *see* Diuretics (thiazide)

**Mepacrine**

*other* Antimalarials: increased plasma concentration of *primaquine* (risk of toxicity)

**Mepenzolate** *see* Antimuscarinics

**Meprobamate** *see* Benzodiazepines and other Anxiolytics and Hypnotics

**Meptazinol** *see* Opioid Analgesics

**Mequitazine** *see* Antihistamines

**Mercaptopurine**

- Allopurinol: enhancement of effect (increased toxicity)

**Metaraminol** *see* Sympathomimetics (*as* noradrenaline)

**Metformin** *see* Antidiabetics

**Methadone** *see* Opioid Analgesics

**Methixene** see Antimuscarinics
**Methocarbamol** see Muscle Relaxants
**Methotrexate**
- Analgesics: excretion reduced by *aspirin, aza-propazone, diclofenac, indomethacin, keto-profen, naproxen, phenylbutazone, and probably other NSAIDs* (increased risk of toxicity)
Antibacterials: antifolate effect increased by *co-trimoxazole and trimethoprim*
Antiepileptics: *phenytoin* increases antifolate effect
Antimalarials: antifolate effect increased by *pyri-methamine* (ingredient of *Fansidar®* and *Malo-prim®*)
Etretinate: increased plasma concentration of *methotrexate*
- Uricosurics: excretion reduced by *probenecid* (increased risk of toxicity)

**Methotrimeprazine** see Phenothiazines and other Antipsychotics
**Methoxamine** see Sympathomimetics (*as* noradrena-line)
**Methyclothiazide** see Diuretics (thiazide)
**Methyldopa**
Alcohol: enhanced hypotensive effect
- Anaesthetics: enhanced hypotensive effect
Analgesics: *NSAIDs* antagonise hypotensive effect
*other* Antihypertensives: enhanced hypotensive effect
Antidepressants: enhanced hypotensive effect
Antipsychotics: increased risk of extrapyramidal effects; enhanced hypotensive effect
Anxiolytics and Hypnotics: enhanced hypotensive effect
Beta-blockers: enhanced hypotensive effect
Calcium-channel Blockers: enhanced hypotensive effect
Corticosteroids: antagonism of hypotensive effect
Diuretics: enhanced hypotensive effect
Dopaminergics: antagonism of antiparkinsonian effect; *levodopa* enhances hypotensive effect
Lithium: neurotoxicity may occur without increased plasma-lithium concentration
Nitrates: enhance hypotensive effect
Sex Hormones: *oestrogens and combined oral con-traceptives* antagonise hypotensive effect
Sympathomimetics: *see* Sympathomimetics (main list)
Ulcer-healing Drugs: *carbenoxolone* antagonises hypotensive effect

**Methylphenobarbitone** see Barbiturates
**Methylprednisolone** see Corticosteroids
**Metipranolol** see Beta-blockers
**Metirosine**
Antipsychotics: increased risk of extrapyramidal effects
Dopaminergics: antagonism

**Metoclopramide**
Analgesics: increased absorption of *aspirin and par-acetamol* (enhanced effect); *opioid analgesics* antagonise effect on gastro-intestinal activity
Antihypertensives: increased risk of extrapyramidal effects with *rauwolfia alkaloids*
Antimuscarinics: antagonism of effect on gastro-intestinal activity
Antipsychotics: increased risk of extrapyramidal effects
Dopaminergics: antagonism of hypoprolactinaemic effect of *bromocriptine*; increased plasma con-centration of *levodopa*
Lithium: increased risk of extrapyramidal effects and possibility of neurotoxicity
Tetrabenazine: increased risk of extrapyramidal effects

**Metolazone** see Diuretics (thiazide-related)
**Metoprolol** see Beta-blockers
**Metronidazole**
Alcohol: disulfiram-like reaction
- Anticoagulants: effect of *nicoumalone and warfarin* enhanced
- Antiepileptics: *metronidazole* inhibits metabolism of *phenytoin* (increased plasma-phenytoin con-centration); *phenobarbitone* accelerates metab-olism of *metronidazole* (reduced plasma-metronidazole concentration)
Disulfiram: psychotic reactions reported
Lithium: increased toxicity reported
Ulcer-healing Drugs: *cimetidine* inhibits metab-olism of *metronidazole* (increased plasma-metronidazole concen-tration)

**Mexiletine**
Analgesics: *opioid analgesics* delay absorption
Antacids and Adsorbents: interaction no longer considered significant
- *other* Anti-arrhythmics: increased myocardial depression with any combination of *anti-arrhythmics*
Antibacterials: *rifampicin* accelerates metabolism (reduced plasma-mexiletine concentration)
Anti-epileptics: *phenytoin* accelerates metabolism (reduced plasma-mexiletine concentration)
Antimuscarinics: *atropine* delays absorption
Diuretics: action of *mexiletine* antagonised by hypo-kalaemia due to *acetazolamide, loop diuretics, and thiazides;* excretion of mexiletine reduced by *acetazolamide* (plasma-mexiletine concentrations occasionally increased)
Theophylline: plasma-theophylline concentration increased

**Mezlocillin** see Penicillins
**Mianserin**
Alcohol: enhanced effect
Antiepileptics: antagonism of anticonvulsant effect
Anxiolytics and Hypnotics: enhanced effect

**Miconazole**
- Anticoagulants: effect of *nicoumalone and warfarin* enhanced
- Antidiabetics: effect of *sulphonylureas* enhanced
- Antiepileptics: effect of *phenytoin* enhanced
*other* Antifungals: *amphotericin* antagonises effect

**Mifepristone**
Analgesics: manufacturer recommends avoid *aspirin* and *NSAIDs* until 8–12 days after *mifep-ristone* administration

**Minocycline** see Tetracyclines
**Minoxidil** see Hydralazine for general hypotensive interactions
**Monoamine-oxidase Inhibitors** see MAOIs
**Monosulfiram**
Alcohol: disulfiram-like reaction
**Morphine** see Opioid Analgesics
**Muscle Relaxants**
Alcohol: enhanced sedative effect with *baclofen*
- Anti-arrhythmics: *procainamide* and *quinidine* enhance muscle relaxant effect
- Antibacterials: effect of *non-depolarising muscle relaxants* such as *tubocurarine* enhanced by *aminoglycosides, azlocillin, clindamycin, linco-mycin, mezlocillin, and polymyxins*
Antihypertensives: enhanced hypotensive effect with *baclofen*
Anxiolytics and Hypnotics: enhanced sedative effect with *baclofen*
Beta-blockers: *propranolol* enhances muscle relax-ant effect

**Muscle Relaxants** (*continued*)

Calcium-channel Blockers: *nifedipine* and *verapamil* enhance effect of *non-depolarising muscle relaxants such as tubocurarine*; hypotension, myocardial depression, and hyperkalaemia reported with intravenous *dantrolene* and *verapamil*

Cardiac Glycosides: arrhythmias if *suxamethonium* given with *digoxin*

Cholinergics: *demecarium* and *ecothiopate* eyedrops, and *neostigmine*, and *pyridostigmine* enhance effect of *suxamethonium* but antagonise effect of *non-depolarising muscle relaxants such as tubocurarine*

Cytotoxics: *cyclophosphamide* and *thiotepa* enhance effect of *suxamethonium*

Lithium: *lithium* enhances muscle relaxant effect

Magnesium Salts: *parenteral magnesium* enhances effect of *non-depolarising muscle relaxants such as tubocurarine*

**Nabilone**

Alcohol: sedative effect of *nabilone* enhanced

Anxiolytics and Hypnotics: enhanced sedative effect

**Nabumetone** see NSAIDs

**Nadolol** see Beta-blockers

**Nalbuphine** see Opioid Analgesics

**Nalidixic Acid** see 4-Quinolones

**Nandrolone** see Anabolic Steroids

**Naproxen** see NSAIDs

**Nefopam**

• Antidepressants: manufacturer recommends avoid *MAOIs*

Antimuscarinics: increased side-effects

**Neomycin** see Aminoglycosides

**Neostigmine** see Cholinergics

**Netilmicin** see Aminoglycosides

**Nicardipine** see Calcium-channel Blockers

**Nicoumalone** see Warfarin

**Nifedipine** see Calcium-channel Blockers

**Nimodipine** see Calcium-channel Blockers

**Nimorazole** alcohol interaction *as for* Metronidazole

**Nitrates** see Glyceryl Trinitrate

**Nitrazepam** see Benzodiazepines and other Anxiolytics and Hypnotics

**Nitrofurantoin**

Uricosurics: *probenecid* reduces excretion of *nitrofurantoin* (risk of toxicity)

**Nitroprusside** *as for* Hydralazine

**Nizatidine** see Histamine H2-antagonists

**Noradrenaline** see Sympathomimetics

**Norfloxacin** see 4-Quinolones

**Nortriptyline** see Antidepressants, Tricyclic

**NSAIDs** (*see also* Aspirin)

Anion-exchange Resins: *cholestyramine* reduces absorption of *phenylbutazone*

Antacids and Adsorbents: *antacids* reduce absorption of *diflunisal*

Anticoagulants: *see* Warfarin

• Antidiabetics: effect of *sulphonylureas* enhanced by *azapropazone* and *phenylbutazone*

• Antiepileptics: effect of *phenytoin* enhanced by *azapropazone* and *phenylbutazone*

Antihypertensives: antagonism of hypotensive effect; hyperkalaemia and increased risk of renal failure on administration of *ACE inhibitors* with *indomethacin* and possibly other *NSAIDs*

Cardiac Glycosides: *NSAIDs* may exacerbate heart failure, reduce GFR, and increase plasma-cardiac glycoside concentration

• Cyclosporin: increased risk of nephrotoxicity

• Cytotoxics: excretion of *methotrexate* reduced by *aspirin, azapropazone, diclofenac, indomethacin, ketoprofen, naproxen, phenylbutazone* and probably other *NSAIDs* (increased risk of toxicity)

**NSAIDs** (*continued*)

Diuretics: risk of nephrotoxicity of *NSAIDs* increased; *NSAIDs* notably indomethacin antagonise diuretic effect; *indomethacin* and possibly other *NSAIDs* increase risk of hyperkalaemia with *potassium-sparing diuretics*; occasional reports of decreased renal function when *indomethacin* given with *triamterene*

• Lithium: excretion of *lithium* reduced by *diclofenac, ibuprofen, indomethacin, mefenamic acid, naproxen, phenylbutazone, piroxicam,* and probably other *NSAIDs* (possibility of toxicity)

Mifepristone: manufacturer recommends avoid *aspirin* and *NSAIDs* until 8–12 days after *mifepristone* administration

Thyroxine: false low total plasma-thyroxine concentration with *phenylbutazone*

Uricosurics: *probenecid* delays excretion of *indomethacin, ketoprofen,* and *naproxen* (raised plasma concentrations)

**Octreotide**

Antidiabetics: reduces *insulin and antidiabetic drug* requirements in diabetes mellitus

Cyclosporin: absorption of *cyclosporin* reduced (reduced plasma concentration)

**Oestrogens** see Contraceptives, Oral

**Ofloxacin** see 4-Quinolones

**Omeprazole**

• Anticoagulants: effects of *warfarin* enhanced

• Antiepileptics: effects of *phenytoin* enhanced

Anxiolytics and Hypnotics: metabolism of *diazepam* inhibited (increased effect possible)

**Opioid Analgesics**

Anti-arrhythmics: delayed absorption of *mexiletine*

Antibacterials: *rifampicin* accelerates metabolism of *methadone* (reduced effect); *erythromycin* increases plasma concentration of *alfentanil*

• Anticoagulants: *dextropropoxyphene* may enhance effect of *nicoumalone and warfarin*

• Antidepressants: CNS excitation or depression (hypertension or hypotension) if *pethidine and possibly other opioid analgesics* given to patients receiving *MAOIs*

• Antiepileptics: *dextropropoxyphene* enhances effect of *carbamazepine*

Anxiolytics and Hypnotics: enhanced sedative effect

Cisapride: possible antagonism of gastro-intestinal effect

Domperidone and Metoclopramide: antagonism of gastro-intestinal effects

Dopaminergics: hyperpyrexia and CNS toxicity reported with *selegiline*

Ulcer-healing Drugs: *cimetidine* inhibits metabolism of opioid analgesics notably *pethidine* (increased plasma concentration)

**Orciprenaline** see Sympathomimetics

**Orphenadrine** see Antimuscarinics

**Oxatomide** see Antihistamines

**Oxazepam** see Benzodiazepines and other Anxiolytics and Hypnotics

**Oxprenolol** see Beta-blockers

**Oxybutynin** see Antimuscarinics

**Oxymetazoline** see Sympathomimetics

**Oxymetholone** see Anabolic Steroids

**Oxypertine** see Phenothiazines and other Antipsychotics

**Oxytetracycline** see Tetracyclines

**Pamidronate Sodium** see Bisphosphonates

**Pancuronium** see Muscle Relaxants (non-depolarising)

**Papaveretum** see Opioid Analgesics

**Paracetamol**

Anion-exchange Resins: *cholestyramine* reduces absorption of *paracetamol*

Anticoagulants: prolonged regular use of *paracetamol* possibly enhances *warfarin*

Antivirals: regular use of *paracetamol* possibly reduces metabolism of *zidovudine* (increased risk of neutropenia)

Domperidone and Metoclopramide: *metoclopramide* accelerates absorption of *paracetamol* (enhanced effect)

**Paroxetine** see Antidepressants, Serotonin-uptake Inhibitor

**Pemoline** see Sympathomimetics

**Penbutolol** see Beta-blockers

**Penicillamine**

Antacids and Adsorbents: *antacids* reduce absorption

Iron: reduced absorption of *penicillamine*

Zinc: reduced absorption of *penicillamine*

**Penicillins**

Antacids: reduced absorption of *pivampicillin*

Anticoagulants: see Phenindione and Warfarin

Guar Gum: reduced absorption of *phenoxymethylpenicillin*

Muscle Relaxants: effects of *non-depolarising muscle relaxants* such as *tubocurarine* enhanced by *azlocillin and mezlocillin*

Probenecid: reduced excretion of *penicillins*

Sex Hormones: see Contraceptives, Oral

**Pentaerythritol Tetranitrate** see Glyceryl Trinitrate

**Pentazocine** see Opioid Analgesics

**Pergolide**

Antipsychotics: antagonism of effect

**Pericyazine** see Phenothiazines and other Antipsychotics

**Perindopril** see ACE Inhibitors

**Perphenazine** see Phenothiazines and other Antipsychotics

**Pethidine** see Opioid Analgesics

**Phenazocine** see Opioid Analgesics

**Phenelzine** see MAOIs

**Phenindamine** see Antihistamines

**Phenindione**

● Anabolic Steroids: anticoagulant effect enhanced by *oxymetholone, stanozolol and others*

● Analgesics: anticoagulant effect enhanced by *aspirin*

Anion-exchange Resins: anticoagulant effect enhanced or reduced by *cholestyramine*

Antibacterials: although studies have failed to demonstrate interaction common experience in anticoagulant clinics is that prothrombin time can be prolonged by course of *oral broad-spectrum antibiotic such as ampicillin* (may also apply to antibiotics given for local action on gut such as *neomycin*)

● Antiplatelet Drugs: anticoagulant effect enhanced by *aspirin and dipyridamole*

● Clofibrate Group: enhanced anticoagulant effect

● Sex Hormones: anticoagulant effect antagonised by *oral contraceptives*

● Thyroxine: enhanced anticoagulant effect

● Vitamins: anticoagulant effect antagonised by vitamin K (present in some enteral feeds)

**Pheniramine** see Antihistamines

**Phenobarbitone** see Barbiturates

**Phenoperidine** see Opioid Analgesics

**Phenothiazines and other Antipsychotics**

Alcohol: enhanced sedative effect

● Anaesthetics: enhanced hypotensive effect

Antacids: reduced absorption of *phenothiazines*

**Phenothiazines and other Antipsychotics** (*continued*)

Anti-arrhythmics: increased risk of ventricular arrhythmias with drugs which prolong QT interval

Antibacterials: *rifampicin* accelerates metabolism of *haloperidol* (reduced plasma-haloperidol concentration)

● Antidepressants: increased antimuscarinic effects notably on administration of *tricyclics* with *phenothiazines; fluoxetine* increases plasma concentration of *haloperidol*; oxypertine causes CNS excitation and hypertension with *MAOIs*

● Antiepileptics: antagonism (convulsive threshold lowered); *carbamazepine* accelerates metabolism of *haloperidol* (reduced plasma concentration); *phenytoin* accelerates metabolism of *clozapine*

Antihypertensives: enhanced hypotensive effect; higher doses of *chlorpromazine* antagonise hypotensive effect of *adrenergic neurone blockers*; severe postural hypotension on administration of *ACE inhibitors* with *chlorpromazine and possibly other antipsychotics*; increased risk of extrapyramidal effects on administration of *methyldopa, metirosine, and rauwolfia alkaloids*

Antimuscarinics: antimuscarinic side-effects of *phenothiazines* increased (but reduced plasma concentrations)

Anxiolytics and Hypnotics: enhanced sedative effect

Beta-blockers: *propranolol* increases plasma concentration of *chlorpromazine*

Calcium-channel Blockers: enhanced hypotensive effect

Desferrioxamine: manufacturer advises avoid *prochlorperazine*

Diuretics: hypokalaemia increases risk of ventricular arrhythmias with *pimozide*

Domperidone and Metoclopramide: increased risk of extrapyramidal effects with *metoclopramide*

Dopaminergics: antagonism of hypoprolactinaemic and antiparkinsonian effects of *bromocriptine*; antagonism of effect of *levodopa, lysuride,* and *pergolide*

Lithium: increased risk of extrapyramidal effects and possibility of neurotoxicity with *haloperidol and phenothiazines*

Tetrabenazine: increased risk of extrapyramidal effects

Ulcer-healing Drugs: *cimetidine* may enhance effects of *chlorpromazine, clozapine,* and possibly *other antipsychotics*

**Phenoxymethylpenicillin** see Penicillins

**Phentermine** see Sympathomimetics

**Phenylbutazone** see NSAIDs

**Phenylephrine** see Sympathomimetics

**Phenylpropanolamine** see Sympathomimetics

**Phenytoin**

● Analgesics: plasma-phenytoin concentration increased by *aspirin, azapropazone, and phenylbutazone*

Antacids: reduced *phenytoin* absorption

● Anti-arrhythmics: *amiodarone* increases plasma-phenytoin concentration; *phenytoin* reduces plasma concentrations of *disopyramide, mexiletine, and quinidine*

● Antibacterials: plasma-phenytoin concentration increased by *chloramphenicol, cycloserine, isoniazid, and metronidazole*; plasma-phenytoin concentration and antifolate effect increased by *cotrimoxazole* and *trimethoprim*; plasma phenytoin concentration reduced by *rifampicin*; plasma concentration of *doxycycline* reduced by *phenytoin*

**Phenytoin** (*continued*)

- Anticoagulants: metabolism of *nicoumalone and warfarin* accelerated (possibility of reduced anticoagulant effect, but enhancement also reported)
- Antidepressants: antagonism of anticonvulsant effect (convulsive threshold lowered); *viloxazine* increases plasma-phenytoin concentration; *phenytoin* reduces plasma concentrations of *paroxetine and tricyclics*

  Antidiabetics: plasma-phenytoin concentration transiently increased by *tolbutamide* (possibility of toxicity)

- *other* Antiepileptics: concomitant administration of *two or more antiepileptics* may enhance toxicity without a corresponding increase in antiepileptic effect; moreover interactions between individual antiepileptics can complicate monitoring of treatment; interactions include enhanced effects, increased sedation, and reductions in plasma concentrations
- Antifungals: plasma-phenytoin concentration increased by *fluconazole, ketoconazole, and miconazole*; plasma concentration of *ketoconazole and possibly others* reduced

  Antimalarials: increased risk of antifolate effect with *pyrimethamine* (includes *Fansidar®* and *Maloprim®*)

  Antiplatelet Drugs: plasma-phenytoin concentration increased by *aspirin*

- Antipsychotics: antagonism of anticonvulsant effect (convulsive threshold lowered); *phenytoin* accelerates metabolism of *clozapine*

  Calcium-channel Blockers: *diltiazem* increases plasma concentration of *phenytoin*; effect of *felodipine, isradipine* and probably *nicardipine* and *nifedipine* reduced

  Cardiac Glycosides: metabolism of *digitoxin only* accelerated (reduced effect)

- Corticosteroids: metabolism of *corticosteroids* accelerated (reduced effect)
- Cyclosporin: metabolism of *cyclosporin* accelerated (reduced plasma concentration)

  Cytotoxics: reduced absorption of *phenytoin*; increased anti-folate effect with *methotrexate*

- Disulfiram: plasma-phenytoin concentration increased

  Diuretics: increased risk of osteomalacia with *carbonic anhydrase inhibitors*

  Food: some *enteral foods* may interfere with absorption of *phenytoin*

  Lithium: neurotoxicity may occur without increased plasma-lithium concentration

- Sex Hormones: metabolism of *gestrinone, tibolone, and oral contraceptives* accelerated (reduced contraceptive effect)

  Theophylline: metabolism of *theophylline* accelerated (reduced plasma-theophylline concentration)

  Thyroxine: metabolism of *thyroxine* accelerated (may increase thyroxine requirements in hypothyroidism)

- Ulcer-healing Drugs: *cimetidine* inhibits metabolism (increased plasma-phenytoin concentration); *sucralfate* reduces absorption; *omeprazole* enhances effect of *phenytoin*
- Uricosurics: plasma-phenytoin concentration increased by *sulphinpyrazone*

  Vaccines: effect enhanced by *influenza vaccine*

  Vitamins: plasma-phenytoin concentration occasionally reduced by *folic acid*

**Physostigmine** *see* Cholinergics

**Phytomenadione** *see* Vitamins (Vitamin K)

**Pimozide** *see* Phenothiazines and other Antipsychotics (CSM: *see also* p. 145)

**Pindolol** *see* Beta-blockers

**Pipenzolate** *see* Antimuscarinics

**Piperazine**

other Anthelmintics: antagonism of *pyrantel*

**Pipothiazine** *see* Phenothiazines and other Antipsychotics

**Pirbuterol** *see* Sympathomimetics, Beta$_2$

**Piretanide** *see* Diuretics (loop)

**Piroxicam** *see* NSAIDs

**Pivampicillin** *see* Penicillins

**Pizotifen**

Antihypertensives: hypotensive effect of *adrenergic neurone blockers* antagonised

**Poldine** *see* Antimuscarinics

**Polymyxins** (*see also* Aminoglycosides)

Muscle Relaxants: enhanced muscle relaxant effect

**Polythiazide** *see* Diuretics (thiazides)

**Potassium Salts**

- Antihypertensives: hyperkalaemia with *ACE inhibitors*
- Cyclosporin: increased risk of hyperkalaemia
- Diuretics: hyperkalaemia with *potassium-sparing diuretics*

**Pravastatin**

Clofibrate Group: increased risk of myopathy

Cyclosporin: increased risk of myopathy

**Prazosin** *see* Alpha-blockers (post-synaptic)

**Prednisolone** *see* Corticosteroids

**Prednisone** *see* Corticosteroids

**Primaquine**

other Antimalarials: *mepacrine* increases plasma concentration of *primaquine* (risk of toxicity)

**Primidone** *see* Barbiturates and Primidone

**Probenecid**

Analgesics: *aspirin* antagonises effect; excretion of *indomethacin, ketoprofen, and naproxen* delayed (increased plasma concentrations)

Antibacterials: reduced excretion of *cephalosporins, cinoxacin, dapsone, nalidixic acid, nitrofurantoin, and penicillins* (increased plasma-concentrations); antagonism by *pyrazinamide*

Antihypertensives: reduced excretion of *captopril*

Antivirals: reduced excretion of *acyclovir and zidovudine* (increased plasma concentrations and risk of toxicity)

- Cytotoxics: reduced excretion of *methotrexate* (increased risk of toxicity)

**Procainamide**

- *other* Anti-arrhythmics: *amiodarone* increases procainamide-plasma concentrations; increased myocardial depression with any anti-arrhythmic

  Antibacterials: *trimethoprim* increases plasma concentration of *procainamide*

  Cholinergics: antagonism of effect of *neostigmine* and *pyridostigmine*

- Muscle Relaxants: muscle relaxant effect enhanced
- Ulcer-healing Drugs: *cimetidine* inhibits metabolism (increased plasma-procainamide concentration)

**Procarbazine**

Alcohol: disulfiram-like reaction

**Prochlorperazine** *see* Phenothiazines and other Antipsychotics

**Procyclidine** *see* Antimuscarinics

**Progestogens** (*see also* Contraceptives, Oral)

- Cyclosporin: increased plasma-cyclosporin concentration (inhibition of metabolism)

**Proguanil**

- Anticoagulants: effect of warfarin possibly enhanced

**Promazine** see Phenothiazines and other Antipsychotics

**Promethazine** see Antihistamines

**Propafenone**

other Anti-arrhythmics: *quinidine* increases plasma concentration of *propafenone*; increased myocardial depression with any *anti-arrhythmic*

Antibacterials: *rifampicin* reduces plasma concentration of *propafenone*

● Anticoagulants: increased plasma concentration of *warfarin and nicoumalone* (enhanced effect)

● Cardiac Glycosides: increased plasma concentrations of *digoxin* (halve maintenance dose of digoxin)

Cholinergics: possible antagonism of effect of *neostigmine* and *pyridostigmine*

● Ulcer-healing Drugs: *cimetidine* increases plasma-propafenone concentration

**Propantheline** see Antimuscarinics

**Propranolol** see Beta-Blockers

**Protriptyline** see Antidepressants, Tricyclic

**Pyrantel**

other Anthelmintics: antagonism of *piperazine*

**Pyrazinamide**

Uricosurics: antagonism of effect of *probenecid* and *sulphinpyrazone*

**Pyridostigmine** see Cholinergics

**Pyridoxine** see Vitamins

**Pyrimethamine**

Antibacterials: increased antifolate effect with *co-trimoxazole* and *trimethoprim*

Antiepileptics: increased antifolate effect with *phenytoin*

Cytotoxics: increased antifolate effect with *methotrexate*

**Quinalbarbitone** see Barbiturates and Primidone

**Quinapril** see ACE Inhibitors

**Quinidine**

Antacids: reduced excretion in alkaline urine (plasma-quinidine concentration occasionally increased)

● other Anti-arrhythmics: *amiodarone* increases plasma-quinidine concentrations (and increases risk of ventricular arrhythmias); plasma concentration of *propafenone* increased; increased myocardial depression with *any anti-arrhythmic*

Antibacterials: *rifampicin* accelerates metabolism (reduced plasma-quinidine concentration)

Anticoagulants: effect of *nicoumalone and warfarin* may be enhanced

Antiepileptics: *phenobarbitone, phenytoin, and primidone* accelerate metabolism (reduced plasma-quinidine concentration)

Barbiturates: see under Antiepileptics, above

● Calcium-channel Blockers: *verapamil* increases plasma-quinidine concentration (possibility of extreme hypotension)

● Cardiac Glycosides: plasma concentration of *digoxin* increased (halve digoxin maintenance dose)

Cholinergics: antagonism of effect of *neostigmine and pyridostigmine*

● Diuretics: *acetazolamide* reduces excretion (plasma-quinidine concentration occasionally increased); quinidine toxicity increased if hypokalaemia occurs with *acetazolamide, loop diuretics, and thiazides*

● Muscle Relaxants: muscle relaxant effect enhanced

● Ulcer-healing Drugs: *cimetidine* inhibits metabolism (increased plasma-quinidine concentration)

**Quinine**

other Antimalarials: see Mefloquine

● Cardiac Glycosides: plasma concentration of *digoxin* increased (halve digoxin maintenance dose); includes use of quinine for cramps

Ulcer-healing Drugs: *cimetidine* inhibits metabolism (increased plasma-quinine concentration)

**4-Quinolones**

Antacids and Adsorbents: *antacids* reduce absorption of *ciprofloxacin, norfloxacin, ofloxacin* and *temafloxacin*

● Anticoagulants: anticoagulant effect of *nicoumalone and warfarin* enhanced by *ciprofloxacin, enoxacin, nalidixic acid, and norfloxacin*

Cyclosporin: increased risk of nephrotoxicity

Iron: absorption of *ciprofloxacin, norfloxacin, and ofloxacin* reduced by *oral iron*

● Theophylline: *ciprofloxacin, enoxacin, and norfloxacin* increase plasma-theophylline concentration

Ulcer-healing Drugs: *sucralfate* reduces absorption of *ciprofloxacin, norfloxacin, and ofloxacin*

Uricosurics: *probenecid* reduces excretion of *cinoxacin* and *nalidixic acid* (increased side-effects)

Zinc Salts: *zinc* reduces absorption of *ciprofloxacin*

**Ramipril** see ACE Inhibitors

**Ranitidine** see Histamine H2-antagonists

**Remoxipride**

Domperidone and Metoclopramide: increased risk of extrapyramidal effects with *metoclopramide*

Dopaminergics: antagonism of hypoprolactinaemic and antiparkinsonian effects of *bromocriptine*; antagonism of effect of *levodopa, lysuride* and *pergolide*

Tetrabenazine: increased risk of extrapyramidal effects

**Rauwolfia Alkaloids**

Alcohol: enhanced hypotensive effect

Anaesthetics: enhanced hypotensive effect

Analgesics: *NSAIDs* antagonise hypotensive effect

● Antidepressants: CNS excitation and hypertension with *MAOIs*

other Antihypertensives: additive hypotensive effect

Antipsychotics: increased risk of extrapyramidal effects

Anxiolytics and Hypnotics: enhanced hypotensive effect

Beta-blockers: increased bradycardia

Calcium-channel Blockers: enhanced hypotensive effect

Corticosteroids: antagonism of hypotensive effect

Diuretics: enhanced hypotensive effect

Domperidone and Metoclopramide: increased risk of extrapyramidal effects with *metoclopramide*

Dopaminergics: *levodopa* enhances hypotensive effect; antagonism of *amantadine* and *levodopa*

Nitrates: *nitrates* enhance hypotensive effect

Sex Hormones: *oestrogens and combined oral contraceptives* antagonise hypotensive effect

Sympathomimetics: see Sympathomimetics (main list)

Ulcer-healing Drugs: *carbenoxolone* antagonises hypotensive effect

**Reproterol** see Sympathomimetics, Beta2

**Rifampicin**

Analgesics: metabolism of *methadone* accelerated (reduced effect)

Antacids: reduced absorption of *rifampicin*

Anti-arrhythmics: metabolism accelerated—reduced plasma concentrations of *disopyramide, mexiletine, propafenone, and quinidine*

**Rifampicin** (*continued*)

*other* Antibacterials: metabolism of *chloramphenicol* accelerated (reduced plasma concentration)

● Anticoagulants: metabolism of *nicoumalone and warfarin* accelerated (reduced anticoagulant effect)

● Antidiabetics: metabolism of *chlorpropamide, tolbutamide and possibly other sulphonylureas* accelerated (reduced effect)

● Antiepileptics: metabolism of *phenytoin* accelerated (reduced plasma concentration)

Antifungals: metabolism of *fluconazole, itraconazole and ketoconazole* accelerated (reduced plasma concentrations)

Antipsychotics: metabolism of *haloperidol* accelerated (reduced plasma concentration)

Beta-blockers: metabolism of *bisoprolol* and *propranolol* accelerated (reduced plasma concentration)

Calcium-channel Blockers: metabolism of *verapamil and possibly isradipine* accelerated (reduced plasma concentration)

Cardiac glycosides: metabolism of *digitoxin only* accelerated (reduced effect)

● Corticosteroids: metabolism of *corticosteroids* accelerated (reduced effect)

● Cyclosporin: metabolism accelerated (reduced plasma-cyclosporin concentration)

● Sex Hormones: metabolism accelerated (contraceptive effect of *both combined and progestogen-only oral contraceptives* reduced)

Theophylline: metabolism accelerated (reduced plasma-theophylline concentration)

Thyroxine: metabolism of *thyroxine* accelerated (may increase requirements in hypothyroidism)

Ulcer-healing Drugs: metabolism of *cimetidine* accelerated (reduced plasma concentration)

**Rimiterol** *see* Sympathomimetics, Beta₂

**Ritodrine** *see* Sympathomimetics, Beta₂

**Rowachol®**

Anticoagulants: effect of *nicoumalone and warfarin* may be reduced

**Salbutamol** *see* Sympathomimetics, Beta₂

**Salmeterol** *see* Sympathomimetics, Beta₂

**Selegiline**

Analgesics: hyperpyrexia and CNS toxicity with *pethidine*

**Sertraline** *see* Antidepressants, Serotonin-uptake Inhibitor

**Simvastatin**

● Anticoagulants: effect of *nicoumalone and warfarin* may be enhanced

Cyclosporin: increased risk of myopathy

*other* Lipid-lowering Drugs: increased risk of myopathy with *clofibrate group*

**Sodium Bicarbonate** *see* Antacids and Adsorbents

**Sodium Clodronate** *see* Bisphosphonates

**Sodium Valproate** *see* Valproate

**Sotalol** *see* Beta-blockers

**Spectinomycin**

Lithium: increased toxicity reported

**Spironolactone** *see* Diuretics (potassium-sparing)

**Stanozolol** *see* Anabolic Steroids

**Streptomycin** *see* Aminoglycosides

**Sucralfate**

Antibacterials: reduced absorption of *ciprofloxacin, norfloxacin, ofloxacin,* and *tetracycline*

● Anticoagulants: absorption of *warfarin* possibly reduced

● Antiepileptics: reduced absorption of *phenytoin*

Cardiac Glycosides: absorption of *cardiac glycosides* possibly reduced

**Sulfadoxine** *see* Co-trimoxazole and Sulphonamides

**Sulfametopyrazine** *see* Co-trimoxazole and Sulphonamides

**Sulindac** *see* NSAIDs

**Sulphadiazine** *see* Co-trimoxazole and Sulphonamides

**Sulphadimidine** *see* Co-trimoxazole and Sulphonamides

**Sulphinpyrazone**

Analgesics: *aspirin* antagonises uricosuric effect

Antibacterials: *pyrazinamide* antagonises effect

● Anticoagulants: anticoagulant effect of *nicoumalone and warfarin* enhanced

● Antidiabetics: effect of *sulphonylureas* enhanced

● Antiepileptics: plasma concentration of *phenytoin* increased

Theophylline: plasma-theophylline concentration reduced

**Sulphonamides** *see* Co-trimoxazole and Sulphonamides

**Sulphonylureas** *see* Antidiabetics

**Sulpiride** *see* Phenothiazines and other Antipsychotics

**Sumatriptan**

● Antidepressants: risk of CNS toxicity with *MAOIs* and *serotonin-uptake inhibitors*

● Ergotamine: risk of CNS toxicity

● Lithium: risk of CNS toxicity

**Suxamethonium** *see* Muscle Relaxants

**Sympathomimetics** (*see below* for Beta₂-Sympathomimetics)

● Anaesthetics: risk of arrhythmias if *adrenaline and isoprenaline* given with *volatile anaesthetics*

● Antidepressants: with *tricyclics* administration of *adrenaline and noradrenaline* may cause hypertension and arrhythmias (but local anaesthetics with adrenaline appear to be safe); with *MAOIs* administration of inotropics such as *dopamine* and *dopexamine* may cause hypertensive crisis; also with *MAOIs* administration of *dexamphetamine and other amphetamines, dexfenfluramine, diethylpropion, ephedrine, fenfluramine, isometheptene, mazindol, pemoline, phentermine, phenylephrine, phenylpropanolamine, and pseudoephedrine* may cause hypertensive crisis (these drugs are contained in anorectics or cold and cough remedies)

Antihypertensives: sympathomimetics in *anorectics and cold and cough remedies* (*see* above) antagonise hypotensive effect of *adrenergic neurone blockers;* hypotensive effect of some other antihypertensives may be enhanced by *dexfenfluramine and fenfluramine*

● Beta-blockers: severe hypertension with *adrenaline and noradrenaline* (especially with non-selective beta-blockers); severe hypertension also possible with sympathomimetics in *anorectics and cold and cough remedies, see* above

Respiratory Stimulants: risk of hypertension with *doxapram*

*other* Sympathomimetics: *dopexamine* possibly potentiates effect of *adrenaline* and *noradrenaline*

**Sympathomimetics, Beta₂**

Corticosteroids: increased risk of hypokalaemia if high doses of *corticosteroids* given with high doses of *fenoterol, pirbuterol, reproterol, rimiterol, ritodrine, salbutamol, salmeterol, terbutaline* and *tulobuterol*

Theophylline: increased risk of hypokalaemia if given with high doses of *fenoterol, pirbuterol, reproterol, rimiterol, ritodrine, salbutamol, salmeterol, terbutaline,* and *tulobuterol*

**Tamoxifen**
- Anticoagulants: anticoagulant effect of *nicoumalone and warfarin* enhanced

**Temafloxacin** *see* 4-Quinolones

**Temazepam** *see* Benzodiazepines and other Anxiolytics and Hypnotics

**Tenoxicam** *see* NSAIDs

**Terazosin** *see* Alpha-blockers (post-synaptic)

**Terbutaline** *see* Sympathomimetics, Beta₂

**Terfenadine** *see* Antihistamines

**Tetrabenazine** (general extrapyramidal interactions *as for* phenothiazines)
- Antidepressants: CNS excitation and hypertension with *MAOIs*

**Tetracyclines**
Antacids: reduced absorption
Anticoagulants: *see* Phenindione and Warfarin
Antiepileptics: *carbamazepine, phenobarbitone, phenytoin, and primidone* increase metabolism of *doxycycline* (reduced plasma concentration)
Antihypertensives: *quinapril* reduces absorption (tablets contain magnesium carbonate excipient)
Barbiturates: *see under* Antiepileptics, above
Calcium Salts: reduced absorption of *tetracyclines*
Dairy products: reduced absorption (except *doxycycline* and *minocycline*)
Iron: absorption of *oral iron* reduced by *tetracyclines* and *vice versa*
Sex Hormones: *see* Contraceptives, Oral (main list)
Ulcer-healing Drugs: *bismuth chelate and sucralfate* reduce absorption
Zinc Salts: reduced absorption (and *vice versa*)

**Theophylline**
Anaesthetics: increased risk of arrhythmias with *halothane*
Anthelmintics: *thiabendazole* may increase plasma-theophylline concentration
Anti-arrhythmics: antagonism of anti-arrhythmic effect of *adenosine*; plasma-theophylline concentration increased by *mexiletine*
- Antibacterials: plasma-theophylline concentration increased by *ciprofloxacin, enoxacin, erythromycin, and norfloxacin* and possibly increased by *isoniazid*; plasma-theophylline concentration reduced by *rifampicin*
Antidepressants: plasma-theophylline concentration increased by *viloxazine*
Antiepileptics: plasma-theophylline concentration reduced by *carbamazepine, phenobarbitone, phenytoin, and primidone*
Barbiturates: *see under* Antiepileptics, above
Beta-blockers: should be avoided on pharmacological grounds (bronchospasm)
- Calcium-channel Blockers: plasma-theophylline concentration increased by *diltiazem and verapamil*
Disulfiram: increases plasma-theophylline concentration
Hormone Antagonists: plasma-theophylline concentration reduced by *aminoglutethimide*
Interferons: plasma-theophylline concentration increased
Lithium: *lithium* excretion accelerated (reduced plasma-lithium concentration)
Respiratory Stimulants: increased CNS stimulation
Sex Hormones: plasma-theophylline concentration increased by *combined oral contraceptives*
Sympathomimetics: increased risk of hypokalaemia if *theophylline* given with high doses of *fenoterol, pirbuterol, reproterol, rimiterol, ritodrine, salbutamol, salmeterol, terbutaline, and tulobuterol*

**Theophylline** (*continued*)
- Ulcer-healing Drugs: plasma-theophylline concentration increased by *cimetidine*
Uricosurics: plasma-theophylline concentration reduced by *sulphinpyrazone*
Vaccines: plasma-theophylline concentration occasionally increased by *influenza vaccine*

**Thiabendazole**
Theophylline: plasma concentration may be increased

**Thiazides** *see* Diuretics

**Thiethylperazine** *see* Phenothiazines and other Antipsychotics

**Thiopentone** *see* Barbiturates and Primidone

**Thioridazine** *see* Phenothiazines and other Antipsychotics

**Thiotepa**
Muscle Relaxants: effect of *suxamethonium* enhanced

**Thyroxine**
Analgesics: false low total plasma-thyroxine concentration with *phenylbutazone*
Anion-exchange Resins: absorption of *thyroxine* reduced by *cholestyramine*
Antibacterials: *rifampicin* accelerates metabolism of thyroxine (may increase requirements in hypothyroidism)
- Anticoagulants: effect of *nicoumalone, phenindione, and warfarin* enhanced
Antiepileptics: *carbamazepine, phenobarbitone, phenytoin, and primidone* accelerate metabolism of *thyroxine* (may increase requirements in hypothyroidism)
Barbiturates: *see under* Antiepileptics, above
Beta-blockers: metabolism of propranolol accelerated (reduced effect)

**Tiaprofenic Acid** *see* NSAIDs

**Tibolone**
Antibacterials: *rifampicin* accelerates metabolism (reduced plasma concentration)
Antiepileptics: *carbamazepine, phenobarbitone, phenytoin, and primidone* accelerate metabolism (reduced plasma concentration)

**Timolol** *see* Beta-blockers

**Tinidazole** alcohol interaction *as for* Metronidazole

**Tobramycin** *see* Aminoglycosides

**Tocainide**
*other* Anti-arrhythmics: increased myocardial depression with any anti-arrhythmic
Beta-blockers: increased risk of bradycardia and myocardial depression
Diuretics: effect of *tocainide* antagonised by hypokalaemia with *acetazolamide, loop diuretics, and thiazides*

**Tolazamide** *see* Antidiabetics (sulphonylurea)

**Tolbutamide** *see* Antidiabetics (sulphonylurea)

**Tolmetin** *see* NSAIDs

**Tranylcypromine** *see* MAOIs

**Trazodone**
Alcohol: enhanced sedative effect
- *other* Antidepressants: interaction with *MAOIs* possible (avoid for at least 2 weeks after stopping MAOI)
Antiepileptics: antagonism of anticonvulsant effect
Anxiolytics and Hypnotics: enhanced sedative effect

**Triamcinolone** *see* Corticosteroids

**Triamterene** *see* Diuretics (potassium-sparing)

**Triclofos** *see* Chloral

**Trientine**
Iron: absorption of *oral iron* reduced

**Trifluoperazine** *see* Phenothiazines and other Anti-psychotics
**Trifluperidol** *see* Phenothiazines and other Anti-psychotics
**Trilostane**
Diuretics: increased risk of hyperkalaemia with *pot-assium-sparing diuretics*
**Trimeprazine** *see* Antihistamines
**Trimethoprim**
Anti-arrhythmics: plasma concentration of *pro-cainamide* increased
Anticoagulants: effect of *nicoumalone* and *warfarin* possibly enhanced
Antidiabetics: effect of *sulphonylureas* enhanced
Antiepileptics: antifolate effect of *phenytoin* increased
Antimalarials: increased risk of antifolate effect with *pyrimethamine* (ingredient of *Fansidar®* and *Maloprim®*)
Cytotoxics: antifolate effect of *methotrexate* increased
**Trimipramine** *see* Antidepressants, Tricyclic
**Triprolidine** *see* Antihistamines
**Tropicamide** *see* Antimuscarinics
**Tryptophan**
● *other* Antidepressants: CNS excitation and confusion with *MAOIs* (reduce tryptophan dose); agitation and nausea with *fluoxetine, fluvox-amine, paroxetine,* and *sertraline*
**Tubocurarine** *see* Muscle Relaxants (non-depolarising)
**Tulobuterol** *see* Sympathomimetics, Beta₂
**Ulcer-healing Drugs** *see* individual drugs
**Uricosurics** *see* individual drugs
**Vaccines** *see* Influenza Vaccine
**Valproate**
Analgesics: *aspirin* enhances effect
● Antidepressants: antagonism of anticonvulsant effect (convulsive threshold lowered)
● *other* Antiepileptics: concomitant administration of two or more antiepileptics may enhance toxicity without a corresponding increase in antiepileptic effect; moreover, interactions between individual antiepileptics can complicate monitoring of treatment; interactions include enhanced effects, increased sedation, and reductions in plasma concentrations
● Antipsychotics: antagonism of anticonvulsant effect (convulsive threshold lowered)
**Vancomycin**
Anion-exchange Resins: antagonism of *oral van-comycin* by *cholestyramine*
*other* Antibacterials: increased risk of ototoxicity and nephrotoxicity with *aminoglycosides and cap-reomycin;* increased risk of nephrotoxicity with *cephalosporins notably cephalothin*
Diuretics: increased risk of ototoxicity with *loop diuretics*
**Vecuronium** *see* Muscle Relaxants (non-depolarising)
**Verapamil** *see* Calcium-channel blockers
**Vigabatrin**
*other* Antiepileptics: *vigabatrin* lowers plasma concentration of *phenytoin*
**Viloxazine**
● Antiepileptics: increased plasma concentrations of *carbamazepine* and *phenytoin*
Theophylline: increased plasma-theophylline concentration

**Vitamins**
● Anticoagulants: anticoagulant effect of *nicoum-alone, phenindione, and warfarin* antagonised by *vitamin K* (present in some enteral feeds)
Antiepileptics: *folic acid* occasionally reduces plasma-phenytoin concentration
Dopaminergics: effect of *levodopa* antagonised by *pyridoxine* (unless a dopa decarboxylase inhibitor also given)
**Warfarin**
● Alcohol: enhanced anticoagulant effect
Allopurinol: anticoagulant effect possibly enhanced
● Anabolic Steroids: *oxymetholone, stanozolol and others* enhance anticoagulant effect
● Analgesics: *aspirin* increases risk of bleeding due to antiplatelet effect; anticoagulant effect seriously enhanced by *azapropazone (see also* p. 330) and *phenylbutazone,* and possibly enhanced by *diflu-nisal, flurbiprofen, mefenamic acid, piroxicam, sulindac, and possibly other NSAIDs;* anticoagulant effect possibly also enhanced by *dex-tropropoxyphene* and by prolonged regular use of *paracetamol*
● Anion-exchange Resins: *cholestyramine* may enhance or reduce anticoagulant effect
● Anti-arrhythmics: *amiodarone and propafenone* enhance anticoagulant effect; *quinidine* may enhance anticoagulant effect
● Antibacterials: anticoagulant effect reduced by *rif-ampicin;* anticoagulant effect enhanced by *aztreonam, cephamandole, chloramphenicol, ciprofloxacin, co-trimoxazole, erythromycin, metronidazole,* and *sulphonamides;* anticoagulant effect possibly also enhanced by *azithro-mycin, enoxacin, nalidixic acid, neomycin, norfloxacin, tetracyclines,* and *trimethoprim;* although studies have failed to demonstrate interaction, common experience in anticoagulant clinics is that prothrombin time can be prolonged by few seconds following course of oral broad-spectrum antibiotic, such as ampicillin (may also apply to antibiotics given for local action on gut such as neomycin)
● Antidepressants: *fluvoxamine and paroxetine* may enhance anticoagulant effect
● Antiepileptics: reduced anticoagulant effect with *carbamazepine, phenobarbitone, and primidone;* both reduced and enhanced effects reported with *phenytoin*
● Antifungals: anticoagulant effect reduced by *gri-seofulvin;* anticoagulant effect enhanced by *flu-conazole, itraconazole, ketoconazole, and miconazole*
● Antimalarials: anticoagulant effect possibly enhanced by *proguanil*
● Antiplatelet Drugs: *aspirin and dipyridamole* increase risk of bleeding due to antiplatelet effect
Anxiolytics and Hypnotics: *chloral* may transiently enhance anticoagulant effect
● Barbiturates: anticoagulant effect reduced
● Clofibrate Group: enhanced anticoagulant effect
● Cytotoxics: anticoagulant effect possibly enhanced by *ifosfamide*
● Disulfiram: enhanced anticoagulant effect
● Hormone Antagonists: *aminoglutethimide* reduces anticoagulant effect; *danazol, flutamide, and tamoxifen* enhance anticoagulant effect
*Rowachol®:* may reduce anticoagulant effect
● Sex Hormones: *oral contraceptives* reduce anticoagulant effect
● Simvastatin: may enhance anticoagulant effect
● Thyroxine: enhanced anticoagulant effect

**Warfarin** (*continued*)

- Ulcer-healing Drugs: *sucralfate* possibly reduces anticoagulant effect (reduced absorption); *cimetidine and omeprazole* enhance anticoagulant effect
- Uricosurics: *sulphinpyrazone* enhances anticoagulant effect

  Vaccines: influenza vaccine occasionally enhances anticoagulant effect
- Vitamins: *vitamin K* reduces anticoagulant effect; major changes in diet (especially involving vegetables) may affect control; vitamin K also present in some enteral feeds

**Xamoterol**

Beta-blockers: antagonism of effect of *xamoterol* and reduction in beta-blockade

**Xipamide** *see* Diuretics (thiazide-related)

**Xylometazoline** *see* Sympathomimetics

**Zidovudine**

*Note.* Increased risk of toxicity with other nephrotoxic and myelosuppressive drugs

Analgesics: regular use of *paracetamol* possibly reduces metabolism of *zidovudine* (increased risk of neutropenia

*other* Antivirals: extreme lethargy reported on administration of *intravenous acyclovir*; profound myelosuppression with *ganciclovir*

Uricosurics: *probenecid* increases plasma-zidovudine concentration and risk of toxicity

**Zinc**

Antibacterials: reduced absorption of *ciprofloxacin*; *tetracyclines* reduce absorption of *zinc* (and *vice versa*)

Iron: reduced absorption of *oral iron* (and *vice versa*)

Penicillamine: reduced absorption of *penicillamine*

**Zopiclone** (general sedative interactions *as for* Benzodiazepines and other Anxiolytics and Hypnotics)

**Zuclopenthixol** *see* Phenothiazines and other Antipsychotics

# Appendix 2: Liver Disease

Liver disease may alter the response to drugs in several ways as indicated below, and drug prescribing should be kept to a minimum in all patients with severe liver disease. The main problems occur in patients with jaundice, ascites, or evidence of encephalopathy.

IMPAIRED DRUG METABOLISM. Metabolism by the liver is the main route of elimination for many drugs, but the hepatic reserve appears to be large and liver disease has to be severe before important changes in drug metabolism occur. Routine liver-function tests are a poor guide to the capacity of the liver to metabolise drugs, and in the individual patient it is not possible to predict the extent to which the metabolism of a particular drug may be impaired.

A few drugs, e.g. rifampicin and fusidic acid, are excreted in the bile unchanged and may accumulate in patients with intrahepatic or extrahepatic obstructive jaundice.

HYPOPROTEINAEMIA. The hypoalbuminaemia in severe liver disease is associated with reduced protein binding and increased toxicity of some highly protein-bound drugs such as phenytoin and prednisolone.

REDUCED CLOTTING. Reduced hepatic synthesis of blood-clotting factors, indicated by a prolonged prothrombin time, increases the sensitivity to oral anticoagulants such as warfarin and phenindione.

HEPATIC ENCEPHALOPATHY. In severe liver disease many drugs can further impair cerebral function and may precipitate hepatic encephalopathy. These include all sedative drugs, opioid analgesics, those diuretics that produce hypokalaemia, and drugs that cause constipation.

FLUID OVERLOAD. Oedema and ascites in chronic liver disease may be exacerbated by drugs that give rise to fluid retention, e.g. NSAIDs, corticosteroids, and carbenoxolone.

HEPATOTOXIC DRUGS. Hepatotoxicity is either dose-related or unpredictable (idiosyncratic). Drugs causing dose-related toxicity may do so at lower doses than in patients with normal liver function, and some drugs producing reactions of the idiosyncratic kind do so more frequently in patients with liver disease. These drugs should be avoided.

## Table of drugs to be avoided or used with caution in liver disease

The list of drugs given below is not comprehensive and is based on current information concerning the use of these drugs in therapeutic dosage. Products introduced or amended since publication of BNF No. 22 (September 1991) are underlined.

| Drugs | Comment | Drugs | Comment |
|---|---|---|---|
| Acemetacin see NSAIDs | | Antidepressants, Tricyclic (and related) | Tricyclics preferable to MAOIs but sedative effects increased; iprindole may cause idiosyncratic hepatotoxicity; lofepramine contra-indicated |
| Acrivastine see Antihistamines | | | |
| Alfentanil see Opioid Analgesics | | | |
| Alprazolam see Anxiolytics and Hypnotics | | | |
| Aminophylline see Theophylline | | | |
| Amitriptyline see Antidepressants, Tricyclic | | | |
| Amlodipine | Reduce dose | | |
| Amoxapine see Antidepressants, Tricyclic | | Antihistamines | Avoid—may precipitate coma |
| Anabolic Steroids | Preferably avoid—dose-related toxicity | Antipsychotics | All can precipitate coma; phenothiazines are hepatotoxic |
| Analgesics see NSAIDs and Opioid Analgesics | | | |
| Androgens | Preferably avoid—dose-related toxicity with some, and produce fluid retention | Anxiolytics and Hypnotics | All can precipitate coma; small dose of oxazepam or temazepam probably safest; reduce oral dose of chlormethiazole |
| Antacids | In patients with fluid retention, avoid those containing large amounts of sodium, e.g. magnesium trisilicate mixture, Gaviscon®. Avoid those causing constipation—can precipitate coma | Aspirin | Avoid—increased risk of gastro-intestinal bleeding |
| | | Astemizole see Antihistamines | |
| | | Auranofin see Gold | |
| | | Aurothiomalate see Gold | |
| | | Azapropazone see NSAIDs | |
| | | Azatadine see Antihistamines | |
| | | Azathioprine | May need dose reduction |
| Anticoagulants, Oral | Avoid, especially if prothrombin time is already prolonged | Bendrofluazide see Thiazides | |
| | | Benorylate [aspirin-paracetamol ester] see Aspirin | |
| | | Benperidol see Antipsychotics | |
| Antidepressants, MAOI see MAOIs | | Benzodiazepines see Anxiolytics and Hypnotics | |
| Antidepressants, Serotonin-uptake Inhibitor | Reduce dose in severe liver disease | Beta-blockers see individual drugs | |
| | | Bezafibrate | Avoid in severe liver disease |
| | | Bromazepam see Anxiolytics and Hypnotics | |

Table of drugs to be avoided or used with caution in liver disease (*continued*)

| Drugs | Comment | Drugs | Comment |
|-------|---------|-------|---------|
| Brompheniramine *see* Antihistamines | | Dimenhydrinate *see* Antihistamines | |
| Bumetanide *see* Loop Diuretics | | Dimethindene *see* Antihistamines | |
| Bupivacaine *see* Lignocaine | | Diphenoxylate *see* Opioid Analgesics | |
| Buprenorphine *see* Opioid Analgesics | | Diphenylpyraline *see* Antihistamines | |
| Butriptyline *see* Antidepressants | | Dipipanone *see* Opioid Analgesics | |
| Carbenoxolone | Produces sodium and water retention and hypokalaemia | Dothiepin *see* Antidepressants, Tricyclic | |
| Cetirizine *see* Antihistamines | | Doxepin *see* Antidepressants, Tricyclic | |
| Chenodeoxycholic Acid | Avoid in chronic liver disease; patients with non-functioning gall-bladder do not respond | Doxorubicin | Reduce dose according to bilirubin concentration |
| | | Droperidol *see* Antipsychotics | |
| Chloral Hydrate *see* Anxiolytics and Hypnotics | | Epirubicin | Reduce dose according to bilirubin concentration |
| Chloramphenicol | Avoid—increased risk of bone-marrow depression | Ergotamine | Avoid in severe liver disease—risk of toxicity increased |
| Chlordiazepoxide *see* Anxiolytics and Hypnotics | | | |
| Chlormethiazole | Reduce oral dose; *see* Anxiolytics and Hypnotics | Erythromycin | May cause idiosyncratic hepatotoxicity |
| Chlormezanone *see* Anxiolytics and Hypnotics | | Ethacrynic acid *see* Loop Diuretics | |
| Chlorothiazide *see* Thiazides | | Etodolac *see* NSAIDs | |
| Chlorpheniramine *see* Antihistamines | | Etretinate | Avoid—further impairment of liver function may occur |
| Chlorpromazine *see* Antipsychotics | | | |
| Chlorpropamide *see* Sulphonylureas | | Felodipine | Reduce dose |
| Chlorthalidone *see* Thiazides | | Fenbufen *see* NSAIDs | |
| Cholestyramine | Interferes with absorption of fat-soluble vitamins and may aggravate malabsorption in primary biliary cirrhosis | Fenofibrate *see* Clofibrate | |
| | | Fenoprofen *see* NSAIDs | |
| | | Fentanyl *see* Opioid Analgesics | |
| | | Flecainide | Avoid (or reduce dose) in severe liver disease |
| Choline Magnesium Trisalicylate *see* Aspirin | | | |
| Choline Theophyllinate *see* Theophylline | | Flunitrazepam *see* Anxiolytics and Hypnotics | |
| Cimetidine | Increased risk of confusion; reduce dose | Fluoxetine *see* Antidepressants, Serotonin-uptake Inhibitor | |
| Cinnarizine *see* Antihistamines | | Flupenthixol *see* Antipsychotics | |
| Cisapride | Halve dose initially | Fluphenazine *see* Antipsychotics | |
| Clemastine *see* Antihistamines | | Flurazepam *see* Anxiolytics and Hypnotics | |
| Clindamycin | Reduce dose | Flurbiprofen *see* NSAIDs | |
| Clobazam *see* Anxiolytics and Hypnotics | | Fluspirilene *see* Antipsychotics | |
| Clofibrate | Avoid in severe liver disease | Fluvoxamine *see* Antidepressants, Serotonin-uptake Inhibitor | |
| Clomiphene | Avoid in severe liver disease | Frusemide *see* Loop Diuretics | |
| Clomipramine *see* Antidepressants, Tricyclic | | Fusidic Acid | Impaired biliary excretion; may be increased risk of hepatotoxicity; avoid or reduce dose |
| Clopamide *see* Thiazides | | | |
| Clorazepate *see* Anxiolytics and Hypnotics | | | |
| Clozapine *see* Antipsychotics | | | |
| Codeine *see* Opioid Analgesics | | Gemfibrozil | Avoid in severe liver disease |
| Contraceptives, Oral | Avoid in cholestatic liver disease and in patients with a history of pruritus or cholestasis during pregnancy | Glibenclamide *see* Sulphonylureas | |
| | | Gliclazide *see* Sulphonylureas | |
| | | Glipizide *see* Sulphonylureas | |
| | | Gliquidone *see* Sulphonylureas | |
| Cyclizine *see* Antihistamines | | Gold (auranofin, aurothiomalate) | Avoid in severe liver disease—hepatotoxicity may occur |
| Cyclofenil | Avoid in severe liver disease | | |
| Cyclopenthiazide *see* Thiazides | | | |
| Cyproheptadine *see* Antihistamines | | Haloperidol *see* Antipsychotics | |
| Cyproterone Acetate | Avoid—dose-related toxicity | Hydrochlorothiazide *see* Thiazides | |
| Dantrolene | Avoid—may cause severe liver damage | Hydroflumethiazide *see* Thiazides | |
| | | Hydroxyzine *see* Antihistamines | |
| Dehydrocholic Acid | Avoid in intra-hepatic cholestasis or complete biliary obstruction | Hypnotics *see* Anxiolytics and Hypnotics | |
| | | Ibuprofen *see* NSAIDs | |
| Desipramine *see* Antidepressants, Tricyclic | | Idarubicin | Reduce dose according to bilirubin concentration |
| Dextromethorphan *see* Opioid Analgesics | | | |
| Dextromoramide *see* Opioid Analgesics | | Imipramine *see* Antidepressants, Tricyclic | |
| Dextropropoxyphene *see* Opioid Analgesics | | Indapamide *see* Thiazides | |
| Diamorphine *see* Opioid Analgesics | | Indomethacin *see* NSAIDs | |
| Diazepam *see* Anxiolytics and Hypnotics | | Iprindole *see* Antidepressants, Tricyclic (and related) | |
| Diclofenac *see* NSAIDs | | | |
| Diflunisal *see* NSAIDs | | Isocarboxazid *see* MAOIs | |
| Dihydrocodeine *see* Opioid Analgesics | | Isoniazid | Avoid—idiosyncratic hepatotoxicity more common |
| Diltiazem | Reduce dose | | |
| | | Isotretinoin | Avoid—*see* Etretinate |

Table of drugs to be avoided or used with caution in liver disease (*continued*)

| Drugs | Comment | Drugs | Comment |
|---|---|---|---|
| Isradipine | Reduce dose | Nandrolone *see* Anabolic Steroids | |
| Itraconazole | Avoid—toxicity with related drugs | Naproxen *see* NSAIDs | |
| | | Narcotic Analgesics *see* Opioid Analgesics | |
| Ketoconazole | Induces hepatitis-like reaction; may accumulate in severe liver disease; contra-indicated unless no alternative | Nicardipine | Reduce dose |
| | | Nifedipine | Reduce dose |
| | | Niridazole | Increased CNS toxicity in patients with cirrhosis or portal-systemic shunts |
| Ketoprofen *see* NSAIDs | | Nitrazepam *see* Anxiolytics and Hypnotics | |
| Ketorolac *see* NSAIDs | | Nitroprusside | Avoid in severe liver disease |
| Ketotifen *see* Antihistamines | | Nortriptyline *see* Antidepressants, Tricyclic | |
| Labetalol | Avoid—severe hepatocellular injury reported | NSAIDs | Increased risk of gastro-intestinal bleeding and can cause fluid retention |
| Lignocaine | Avoid (or reduce dose) in severe liver disease | | |
| | | Oestrogens | Avoid; *see also* Contraceptives, oral |
| Lincomycin | Avoid if possible | | |
| Lofepramine *see* Antidepressants, Tricyclic | | Omeprazole | In severe liver disease not more than 20 mg daily should be needed |
| Loop diuretics | Hypokalaemia may precipitate coma; potassium-sparing diuretic should be used to prevent this; increased risk of hypomagnesaemia in alcoholic cirrhosis | | |
| | | Ondansetron | Reduce dose; not more than 8 mg daily in severe liver disease |
| | | Opioid Analgesics | Avoid—may precipitate coma |
| | | Oral Contraceptives *see* Contraceptives, Oral | |
| Loprazolam *see* Anxiolytics and Hypnotics | | Oxatomide *see* Antihistamines | |
| Lorazepam *see* Anxiolytics and Hypnotics | | Oxazepam *see* Anxiolytics and Hypnotics | |
| Lormetazepam *see* Anxiolytics and Hypnotics | | Oxprenolol | Reduce oral dose |
| Loxapine *see* Antipsychotics | | Oxymetholone *see* Anabolic Steroids | |
| Magnesium Salts | Avoid in hepatic coma if risk of renal failure | Oxypertine *see* Antipsychotics | |
| | | Papaveretum *see* Opioid Analgesics | |
| MAOIs | May cause idiosyncratic hepatotoxicity | Paracetamol | Dose-related toxicity—avoid large doses |
| Maprotiline *see* Antidepressants, Tricyclic (and related) | | Paroxetine *see* Antidepressants, Serotonin-uptake Inhibitor | |
| Mebhydrolin *see* Antihistamines | | Pentazocine *see* Opioid Analgesics | |
| Medazepam *see* Anxiolytics and Hypnotics | | Pericyazine *see* Antipsychotics | |
| Mefenamic Acid *see* NSAIDs | | Perphenazine *see* Antipsychotics | |
| Mefruside *see* Thiazides | | Pethidine *see* Opioid Analgesics | |
| Meprobamate *see* Anxiolytics and Hypnotics | | Phenazocine *see* Opioid Analgesics | |
| Meptazinol *see* Opioid Analgesics | | Phenelzine *see* MAOIs | |
| Mequitazine *see* Antihistamines | | Phenindamine *see* Antihistamines | |
| Metformin | Avoid—increased risk of lactic acidosis | Pheniramine *see* Antihistamines | |
| | | Phenobarbitone | May precipitate coma |
| Methadone *see* Opioid Analgesics | | Phenoperidine *see* Opioid Analgesics | |
| Methohexitone | Avoid or reduce dose | Phenothiazines *see* Antipsychotics | |
| Methotrexate | Dose-related toxicity—avoid in non-malignant conditions (e.g. psoriasis) | Phenylbutazone *see* NSAIDs | |
| | | Phenytoin | Reduce dose to avoid toxicity |
| | | Pholcodine *see* Opioid Analgesics | |
| Methotrimeprazine *see* Antipsychotics | | Pimozide *see* Antipsychotics | |
| Methoxsalen | Avoid or reduce dose | Pipothiazine *see* Antipsychotics | |
| Methyclothiazide *see* Thiazides | | Piretanide *see* Loop Diuretics | |
| Methyldopa | Avoid—increased risk of hepatotoxicity | Piroxicam *see* NSAIDs | |
| | | Plicamycin | Avoid if possible (increased risk of toxicity) |
| Metoclopramide | Reduce dose in severe liver disease | | |
| | | Polythiazide *see* Thiazides | |
| Metolazone *see* Thiazides | | Prednisolone | Side-effects more common |
| Metoprolol | Reduce oral dose | Prednisone | Prednisolone is preferable (prednisone needs conversion to prednisolone by liver before active) |
| Metronidazole | Reduce dose in severe liver disease | | |
| Mexiletine | Avoid (or reduce dose) in severe liver disease | | |
| | | Primidone | May precipitate coma |
| Mianserin *see* Antidepressants, Tricyclic (and related) | | Procainamide | Avoid or reduce dose |
| | | Prochlorperazine *see* Antipsychotics | |
| Monoamine-oxidase Inhibitors *see* MAOIs | | Progestogens | Avoid; *see also* Contraceptives, Oral |
| Morphine *see* Opioid Analgesics | | | |
| Nabumetone *see* NSAIDs | | Promazine *see* Antipsychotics | |
| Nalbuphine *see* Opioid Analgesics | | Promethazine *see* Antihistamines | |
| Nalidixic Acid | Partially conjugated in liver | Propafenone | Reduce dose |

Table of drugs to be avoided or used with caution in liver disease (*continued*)

| Drugs | Comment | Drugs | Comment |
|---|---|---|---|
| Propranolol | Reduce oral dose | Thiazides | Hypokalaemia may precipitate coma (potassium-sparing diuretic can prevent); increased risk of hypomagnesaemia in alcoholic cirrhosis |
| Protriptyline *see* Antidepressants, Tricyclic | | | |
| Pyrazinamide | Avoid—idiosyncratic hepatotoxicity more common | | |
| Ranitidine | Increased risk of confusion; reduce dose | | |
| | | Thiethylperazine *see* Antipsychotics | |
| Rifampicin | Impaired elimination; may be increased risk of hepatotoxicity; avoid or do not exceed 8 mg/kg daily | Thiopentone | Reduce dose for induction in severe liver disease |
| | | Thioridazine *see* Antipsychotics | |
| | | Tiaprofenic acid *see* NSAIDs | |
| Salsalate *see* Aspirin | | Tibolone | Avoid in severe liver disease |
| Sertraline *see* Antidepressants, Serotonin-uptake Inhibitor | | Tocainide | Avoid (or reduce dose) in severe liver disease |
| Simvastatin | Avoid—hepatotoxic | | |
| Sodium Aurothiomalate *see* Gold | | Tolazamide *see* Sulphonylureas | |
| Sodium Fusidate *see* Fusidic Acid | | Tolbutamide *see* Sulphonylureas | |
| Sodium Nitroprusside *see* Nitroprusside | | Tolmetin *see* NSAIDs | |
| Sodium Valproate *see* Valproate | | Tranylcypromine *see* MAOIs | |
| Stanozolol *see* Anabolic Steroids | | Trazodone *see* Antidepressants, Tricyclic (and related) | |
| Sulindac *see* NSAIDs | | Triclofos *see* Anxiolytics and Hypnotics | |
| Sulphonylureas | Increased risk of hypoglycaemia in severe liver disease; avoid or use small dose; can produce jaundice | Trifluoperazine *see* Antipsychotics | |
| | | Trifluperidol *see* Antipsychotics | |
| | | Trimeprazine *see* Antihistamines | |
| Suxamethonium | Prolonged apnoea may occur in severe liver disease due to reduced hepatic synthesis of pseudocholinesterase | Trimipramine *see* Antidepressants, Tricyclic | |
| | | Triprolidine *see* Antihistamines | |
| | | Valproate | Avoid if possible—hepatotoxicity and liver failure may occasionally occur (usually in first 6 months) |
| Temazepam *see* Anxiolytics and Hypnotics | | | |
| Tenoxicam *see* NSAIDs | | | |
| Terbinafine | Reduce dose | Verapamil | Reduce oral dose |
| Terfenadine *see* Antihistamines | | Zidovudine | Accumulation may occur |
| Testosterone *see* Androgens | | Zopiclone | Reduce dose |
| Tetracyclines | Avoid—dose-related toxicity by i/v route | Zuclopenthixol *see* Antipsychotics | |
| Theophylline | Reduce dose | | |

# Appendix 3: Renal Impairment

The use of drugs in patients with reduced renal function can give rise to problems for several reasons:

> failure to excrete a drug or its metabolites may produce toxicity;
> sensitivity to some drugs is increased even if elimination is unimpaired;
> many side-effects are tolerated poorly by patients in renal failure;
> some drugs cease to be effective when renal function is reduced.

Many of these problems can be avoided by reducing the dose or by using alternative drugs.

## Principles of dose adjustment in renal impairment

The level of renal function below which the dose of a drug must be reduced depends on whether the drug is eliminated entirely by renal excretion or is partly metabolised, and on how toxic it is.

For many drugs with only minor or no dose-related side-effects very precise modification of the dose regimen is unnecessary and a simple scheme for dose reduction is sufficient.

For more toxic drugs with a small safety margin dose regimens based on glomerular filtration rate should be used. For those where both efficacy and toxicity are closely related to plasma concentrations recommended regimens should be seen only as a guide to initial treatment; subsequent treatment must be adjusted according to clinical response and plasma concentration.

The total daily maintenance dose of a drug can be reduced either by reducing the size of the individual doses or by increasing the interval between doses. For some drugs, if the size of the maintenance dose is reduced it will be important to give a loading dose if an immediate effect is required. This is because when a patient is given a regular dose of any drug it takes more than five times the half-life to achieve steady-state plasma concentrations. As the plasma half-life of drugs excreted by the kidney is prolonged in renal failure it may take many days for the reduced dosage to achieve a therapeutic plasma concentration. The loading dose should usually be the same size as the initial dose for a patient with normal renal function.

**Nephrotoxic drugs** should, if possible, be avoided in patients with renal disease because the consequences of nephrotoxicity are likely to be more serious when the renal reserve is already reduced.

## Use of dosage table

Dose recommendations are based on the severity of renal impairment. This is expressed in terms of glomerular filtration rate (GFR), usually measured by the **creatinine clearance**. The serum-creatinine concentration can be used instead as a measure of renal function but is only a rough guide unless corrected for age, weight, and sex. Nomograms are available for making the correction and should be used where accuracy is important.

Renal impairment is arbitrarily divided into 3 grades:

| Grade | GFR | Serum creatinine (approx.) |
|---|---|---|
| Mild | 20–50 mL/min | 150–300 μmol/litre |
| Moderate | 10–20 mL/min | 300–700 μmol/litre |
| Severe | < 10 mL/min | > 700 μmol/litre |

*Note.* Conversion factors are:
Litres/24 hours = mL/minute × 1.44
mL/minute = Litres/24 hours × 0.69

Renal function declines with age; many elderly patients have a glomerular filtration rate below 50 mL/minute which, because of reduced muscle mass, may not be indicated by a raised serum creatinine. It is wise to assume at least mild impairment of renal function when prescribing for the elderly.

The following table may be used as a guide to drugs which are known to require a reduction in dose in renal impairment, and to those which are potentially harmful or are ineffective. Drug prescribing should be kept to the minimum in all patients with severe renal disease.

If renal impairment is considered likely on clinical grounds renal function should be checked before prescribing **any** drug which requires dose modification even when renal impairment is mild.

## Table of drugs to be avoided or used with caution in renal impairment
Products introduced or amended since publication of BNF No. 22 (September 1991) are underlined.

| Drug and Degree of impairment | Comment | Drug and Degree of impairmant | Comment |
|---|---|---|---|
| Acebutolol | | Acipimox | |
| Moderate | Start with small dose; active metabolite accumulates | Mild | Reduce dose |
| Acemetacin *see* NSAIDs | | Acrivastine | |
| Acetazolamide | | Moderate | Avoid; excreted by kidney |
| Mild | Avoid; metabolic acidosis | | |

Table of drugs to be avoided or used with caution in renal impairment (*continued*)

| Drug and Degree of impairment | Comment | Drug and Degree of impairmant | Comment |
|---|---|---|---|
| **Acyclovir** | | **Bacampicillin** | |
| Mild | Reduce dose; possible transient increase in plasma urea | Severe | Reduce dose; rashes more common |
| Alcuronium *see* Tubocurarine | | **Baclofen** | |
| Alfentanil *see* Opioid Analgesics | | Mild | Use smaller doses; excreted by kidney |
| **Allopurinol** | | Bendrofluazide *see* Thiazides | |
| Moderate | Max. 200 mg daily; increased toxicity; rashes | Benorylate [aspirin-paracetamol ester] *see* Aspirin | |
| Severe | Max. 100 mg daily | Benperidol *see* Antipsychotics | |
| Alprazolam *see* Anxiolytics and Hypnotics | | Benzodiazepines *see* Anxiolytics and Hypnotics | |
| **Alteplase** | | **Benzylpenicillin** | |
| Moderate | Risk of hyperkalaemia | Severe | Max. 6 g daily; neurotoxicity—high doses may cause convulsions |
| **Aluminium Salts** | | | |
| Severe | Aluminium may accumulate | **Beta-blockers** | |
| **Amantadine** | | Severe | Start with small dose; higher plasma concentrations after oral administration; may reduce renal blood flow and adversely affect renal function in severe impairment |
| Mild to moderate | Reduce dose; excreted by kidney | | |
| Severe | Avoid | | |
| Amikacin *see* Aminoglycosides | | | |
| Amiloride *see* Potassium-sparing Diuretics | | | |
| **Aminoglycosides** | | | |
| Mild | Reduce dose; monitor plasma concentrations; ototoxic; nephrotoxic | Betaxolol *see* Beta-blockers | |
| | | **Bethanidine** | |
| **Amiodarone** | | Moderate | Avoid; increased postural hypotension; decrease in renal blood flow |
| Moderate | Accumulation of iodine may increase risk of thyroid dysfunction | | |
| | | **Bezafibrate** | |
| **Amoxycillin** | | Mild to moderate | Reduce dose; further deterioration in renal function |
| Severe | Reduce dose; rashes more common | | |
| | | Severe | Avoid |
| **Amphotericin** | | Bicarbonate *see* Sodium Bicarbonate | |
| Mild | Use only if no alternative; nephrotoxic | Bisoprolol *see* Beta-blockers | |
| | | **Bleomycin** | |
| **Ampicillin** | | Moderate | Reduce dose |
| Severe | Reduce dose; rashes more common | Bromazepam *see* Anxiolytics and Hypnotics | |
| | | **Bumetanide** | |
| **Amylobarbitone** | | Moderate | May need high doses |
| Severe | Reduce dose; active metabolite accumulates | Buprenorphine *see* Opioid Analgesics | |
| | | **Capreomycin** | |
| Analgesics *see* Opioid Analgesics and NSAIDs | | Mild | Reduce dose; nephrotoxic; ototoxic |
| **Antipsychotics** | | | |
| Severe | Start with small doses; increased cerebral sensitivity; *see also* Sulpiride | **Captopril** | |
| | | Mild | Reduce dose and monitor response; avoid if possible; excreted by kidney; hyperkalaemia and other side-effects more common (but specialised role in some forms of renal disease) |
| **Anxiolytics and Hypnotics** | | | |
| Severe | Start with small doses; increased cerebral sensitivity | | |
| **Aspirin** | | | |
| Severe | Avoid; fluid retention; deterioration in renal function; increased risk of gastro-intestinal bleeding | | |
| | | **Carbenicillin** | |
| | | Moderate | Reduce dose; neurotoxic; may produce bleeding diathesis; 1 g contains 5.4 mmol sodium |
| **Atenolol** | | | |
| Moderate | Reduce dose; excreted unchanged | | |
| Auranofin *see* Gold | | **Carbenoxolone** | |
| Aurothiomalate *see* Gold | | Moderate | Avoid; fluid retention |
| Azapropazone *see* NSAIDs (excreted by kidney) | | Carboplatin *see* Cisplatin | |
| **Azathioprine** | | Cartelol *see* Beta-blockers | |
| Severe | Reduce dose | **Cefadroxil** | |
| **Azlocillin** | | Moderate | Reduce dose |
| Moderate | Reduce dose | **Cefixime** | |
| **Aztreonam** | | Moderate | Reduce dose |
| Moderate | Reduce dose | **Cefotaxime** | |
| | | Severe | Use half dose |

Table of drugs to be avoided or used with caution in renal impairment (*continued*)

| Drug and Degree of impairment | Comment | Drug and Degree of impairment | Comment |
|---|---|---|---|
| Cefoxitin | | Clofibrate | |
| Mild | Reduce dose | Mild to moderate | Reduce dose; further deterioration in renal function; myopathy |
| Cefsulodin | | | |
| Moderate | Reduce dose | Severe | Avoid |
| Ceftazidime | | Clopamide *see* Thiazides | |
| Mild | Reduce dose | Clorazepate *see* Anxiolytics and Hypnotics | |
| Ceftizoxime | | Clozapine *see* Antipsychotics | |
| Mild | Reduce dose | Co-amoxiclav | |
| Cefuroxime | | Moderate | Reduce dose |
| Mild | Reduce parenteral dose | Codeine | |
| Celiprolol *see* Beta-blockers | | Moderate | Avoid; increased and prolonged effect; *see also* Opioid Analgesics |
| Cephalexin | | | |
| Severe | Max. 500 mg daily | | |
| Cephamandole | | Colchicine | |
| Mild | Reduce dose | Severe | Avoid or reduce dose if no alternative |
| Cephazolin | | | |
| Mild | Reduce dose | Colistin | |
| Cephradine | | Mild | Reduce dose; nephrotoxic; neurotoxic |
| Mild | Reduce dose | | |
| Cetirizine | | *Colven*® | |
| Moderate | Use half dose | Severe | Avoid; high sodium content |
| Chloral Hydrate *see* Anxiolytics and Hypnotics | | Co-trimoxazole | |
| Chloramphenicol | | Moderate | Reduce dose; rashes and blood disorders; may cause further deterioration in renal function |
| Severe | Avoid unless no alternative; dose-related depression of haematopoiesis | | |
| Chlordiazepoxide *see* Anxiolytics and Hypnotics | | Cyclopenthiazide *see* Thiazides | |
| Chlormethiazole *see* Anxiolytics and Hypnotics | | Cyclophosphamide | |
| Chlormezanone *see* Anxiolytics and Hypnotics | | Moderate | Reduce dose |
| Chloroquine | | Cycloserine | |
| Mild to moderate | Reduce dose; only on prolonged use | Mild to moderate | Reduce dose |
| | | Severe | Avoid |
| Severe | Avoid | Cyclosporin *see* section 8.2.2 | |
| Chlorothiazide *see* Thiazides | | Debrisoquine | |
| Chlorpromazine *see* Antipsychotics | | Moderate | Avoid; increased postural hypotension; decrease in renal blood flow |
| Chlorpropamide | | | |
| Mild | Avoid; tolbutamide and gliquidone suitable alternatives | | |
| | | *De-Nol*®, *De-Noltab*® | |
| | | Severe | Avoid |
| Chlorthalidone *see* Thiazides | | Dextromethorphan *see* Opioid Analgesics | |
| Choline Magnesium Trisalicylate *see* Aspirin | | Dextromoramide *see* Opioid Analgesics | |
| Cilazapril | | Dextropropoxyphene | |
| Mild | Reduce dose and monitor response; avoid if possible; *see also* Captopril | Severe | Avoid; increased CNS toxicity |
| | | Diamorphine *see* Opioid Analgesics | |
| | | Diazepam *see* Anxiolytics and Hypnotics | |
| Cimetidine | | Diazoxide | |
| Moderate | 400–600 mg daily; occasional risk of confusion | Severe | 75–150 mg i/v; increased sensitivity to hypotensive effect |
| Severe | 400 mg daily | | |
| Cinoxacin | | *Dicapen*® | |
| Moderate | Avoid; nausea, rashes | Severe | Reduce dose |
| Ciprofloxacin | | Diclofenac *see* NSAIDs | |
| Moderate | Use half dose | Diflunisal *see* NSAIDs (excreted by kidney) | |
| Cisapride | | Digitoxin | |
| Moderate | Start with half dose | Severe | Max. 100 micrograms daily; *see also* Digoxin |
| Cisplatin | | | |
| Mild | Avoid if possible; nephrotoxic | Digoxin | |
| | | Mild | 250 micrograms daily; toxicity increased by electrolyte disturbances |
| Clarithromycin | | | |
| Moderate | Reduce dose | | |
| Clavulanic acid [ingredient] *see* Co-amoxiclav, *Timentin*® | | Moderate | 125–250 micrograms daily |
| Clobazam *see* Anxiolytics and Hypnotics | | Severe | Up to 125 micrograms daily |
| Clodronate sodium | | | |
| Moderate | Avoid | | |

Table of drugs to be avoided or used with caution in renal impairment (*continued*)

| Drug and Degree of impairment | Comment | Drug and Degree of impairmant | Comment |
|---|---|---|---|
| **Dihydrocodeine** | | **Fluvoxamine** | |
| Moderate | Avoid; increased and prolonged effect; *see also* Opioid Analgesics | Moderate | Start with smaller dose |
| | | **Foscarnet** | |
| **Diphenoxylate** *see* Opioid Analgesics | | Mild | Reduce dose; consult data sheet |
| **Dipipanone** *see* Opioid Analgesics | | **Fosinopril** | |
| **Disopyramide** | | Mild | Start with 10 mg daily; *see also* Captopril |
| Mild | 100 mg every 8 hours *or* 150 mg every 12 hours | **Frusemide** | |
| Moderate | 100 mg every 12 hours | Moderate | May need high doses; deafness may follow rapid i/v injection |
| Severe | 150 mg every 24 hours | | |
| **Domperidone** | | *Fybogel®* | |
| Severe | Reduce dose by 30–50% | Severe | Avoid; contains 7 mmol potassium per sachet |
| **Droperidol** *see* Antipsychotics | | **Gallamine** | |
| **Enalapril** | | Moderate | Avoid; prolonged paralysis |
| Mild | Reduce dose and monitor response; avoid if possible; *see also* Captopril | **Ganciclovir** | |
| | | Mild | Reduce dose; consult data sheet |
| **Enoxacin** | | *Gaviscon®* | |
| Moderate | Max. 400 mg daily | Severe | Avoid; high sodium content |
| **Ephedrine** | | **Gemfibrozil** | |
| Severe | Avoid; increased CNS toxicity | Severe | Start with 900 mg daily |
| | | **Gentamicin** *see* Aminoglycosides | |
| **Ergotamine** | | **Glibenclamide** | |
| Moderate | Avoid; nausea and vomiting; risk of renal vasoconstriction | Severe | Avoid; increased risk of prolonged hypoglycaemia |
| **Erythromycin** | | **Gliclazide** | |
| Severe | Max. 1.5 g daily (ototoxicity) | Severe | Start with small dose; increased risk of hypoglycaemia |
| **Ethacrynic Acid** | | | |
| Severe | Avoid; ototoxic | **Glipizide** | |
| **Ethambutol** | | Severe | Start with small dose; increased risk of hypoglycaemia |
| Mild | Avoid; optic nerve damage | | |
| **Etidronate Disodium** | | **Gliquidone** | |
| Mild | Max. 5 mg/kg daily; excreted by kidney | Severe | May need dose reduction; increased risk of hypoglycaemia |
| Moderate | Avoid | | |
| **Etodolac** *see* NSAIDs | | **Gold (auranofin, aurothiomalate)** | |
| **Etoposide** | | Mild | Avoid; nephrotoxic |
| Mild | Reduce dose | **Guanethidine** | |
| **Etretinate** | | Moderate | Avoid; increased postural hypotension and decrease in renal blood flow |
| Mild | Avoid; increased risk of toxicity | | |
| **Famotidine** | | **Haloperidol** *see* Antipsychotics | |
| Severe | Reduce dose | **Hexamine** | |
| **Fenbufen** *see* NSAIDs | | Mild | Avoid; ineffective |
| **Fenofibrate** | | **Hydralazine** | |
| Mild | 200 mg daily | Moderate | Start with small dose; increased hypotensive effect |
| Moderate | 100 mg daily | | |
| **Fenoprofen** *see* NSAIDs | | **Hydrochlorothiazide** *see* Thiazides | |
| **Fentanyl** *see* Opioid Analgesics | | **Hydroflumethiazide** *see* Thiazides | |
| **Flecainide** | | **Hydroxychloroquine** | |
| Mild | Reduce dose | Mild to moderate | Reduce dose; only on prolonged use |
| **Fluconazole** | | | |
| Mild | Reduce dose for multiple dose therapy | Severe | Avoid |
| **Flucytosine** | | **Hypnotics** *see* Anxiolytics and Hypnotics | |
| Mild | Reduce dose | **Ibuprofen** *see* NSAIDs | |
| **Flunitrazepam** *see* Anxiolytics and Hypnotics | | **Idarubicin** | |
| **Fluoxetine** | | Mild | Reduce dose |
| Moderate | Start with smaller dose | **Ifosfamide** | |
| Severe | Avoid | Moderate | Reduce dose |
| **Flupenthixol** *see* Antipsychotics | | **Indapamide** *see* Thiazides | |
| **Fluphenazine** *see* Antipsychotics | | | |
| **Flurazepam** *see* Anxiolytics and Hypnotics | | | |
| **Flurbiprofen** *see* NSAIDs | | | |
| **Fluspirilene** *see* Antipsychotics | | | |

Table of drugs to be avoided or used with caution in renal impairment (*continued*)

| Drug and Degree of impairment | Comment | Drug and Degree of impairmant | Comment |
|---|---|---|---|
| Indomethacin *see* NSAIDs | | Methyldopa | |
| Inosine Pranobex | | Moderate | Start with small dose; increased sensitivity to hypotensive and sedative effect |
| Mild | Avoid; metabolised to uric acid | | |
| Insulin | | Metoclopramide | |
| Severe | May need dose reduction; insulin requirements fall; compensatory response to hypoglycaemia is impaired | Severe | Avoid or use small dose; increased risk of extrapyramidal reactions |
| | | Metolazone *see* Thiazides | |
| Isoniazid | | Metoprolol *see* Beta-blockers | |
| Severe | Max. 200 mg daily; peripheral neuropathy | Mezlocillin | |
| | | Severe | Reduce dose |
| Isotretinoin | | Milrinone | |
| Mild | Avoid; increased risk of toxicity | Mild | Reduce dose and monitor response |
| Kanamycin *see* Aminoglycosides | | Morphine | |
| Ketoprofen *see* NSAIDs | | Moderate | Avoid; increased and prolonged effect; *see also* Opioid Analgesics |
| Ketorolac *see* NSAIDs | | | |
| Lincomycin | | | |
| Moderate | Use clindamycin instead | Nabumetone *see* NSAIDs | |
| Lisinopril | | Nadolol | |
| Mild | Reduce dose and monitor response; *see also* Captopril | Moderate | Reduce dose; excreted unchanged |
| Lithium | | Nalbuphine *see* Opioid Analgesics | |
| Mild | Avoid if possible or reduce dose and monitor plasma concentration carefully | Nalidixic Acid | |
| | | Moderate | Avoid; increased risk of nausea, vomiting, rashes, photosensitivity; ineffective because of inadequate urine concentration |
| Moderate | Avoid | | |
| Loprazolam *see* Anxiolytics and Hypnotics | | | |
| Lorazepam *see* Anxiolytics and Hypnotics | | | |
| Lormetazepam *see* Anxiolytics and Hypnotics | | Naproxen *see* NSAIDs | |
| Loxapine *see* Antipsychotics | | Narcotic Analgesics *see* Opioid Analgesics | |
| Magnesium Salts | | Neomycin | |
| Moderate | Avoid or reduce dose; increased risk of toxicity; magnesium carbonate mixture and magnesium trisilicate mixture also have high sodium content | Mild | Avoid; ototoxic; nephrotoxic |
| | | Netilmicin *see* Aminoglycosides | |
| | | Nicardipine | |
| | | Moderate | Start with small dose |
| | | Nifedipine | |
| Medazepam *see* Anxiolytics and Hypnotics | | Moderate | Start with small dose; reversible deterioration in renal function has been reported |
| Mefenamic Acid *see* NSAIDs | | | |
| Mefruside *see* Thiazides | | | |
| Melphalan | | | |
| Moderate | Reduce dose | Nitrazepam *see* Anxiolytics and Hypnotics | |
| Meprobamate *see* Anxiolytics and Hypnotics | | Nitrofurantoin | |
| Meptazinol *see* Opioid Analgesics | | Mild | Avoid; peripheral neuropathy; ineffective because of inadequate urine concentrations |
| Mercaptopurine | | | |
| Moderate | Reduce dose | | |
| Mesalazine | | | |
| Mild | Avoid; nephrotoxic | Nitroprusside | |
| Metformin | | Moderate | Avoid prolonged use |
| Mild | Avoid; increased risk of lactic acidosis | Nizatidine | |
| | | Mild | 150 mg daily |
| Methadone *see* Opioid Analgesics | | Moderate | 150 mg on alternate days |
| Methocarbamol | | Norfloxacin | |
| Mild | Avoid; increased plasma urea and acidosis due to solvent in injection | Moderate | Use half dose |
| | | Severe | Avoid |
| | | NSAIDs | |
| Methotrexate | | Mild | Avoid if possible; deterioration in renal function (**important**: see section 10.1.1); sodium and water retention |
| Mild | Reduce dose; accumulates; nephrotoxic | | |
| Moderate | Avoid | | |
| Methotrimeprazine *see* Antipsychotics | | Ofloxacin | |
| Methyclothiazide *see* Thiazides | | Mild | Use half dose |
| | | Moderate | 100 mg every 48 hours |

Table of drugs to be avoided or used with caution in renal impairment (*continued*)

| Drug and Degree of impairment | Comment | Drug and Degree of impairment | Comment |
|---|---|---|---|
| **Opioid Analgesics** | | **Potassium-sparing Diuretics** | |
| Moderate | Use small doses—avoid codeine, dihydrocodeine, morphine; increased cerebral sensitivity; *see also* individual entries | Mild | Monitor plasma K$^+$; high risk of hyperkalaemia in renal impairment; amiloride excreted by kidney unchanged |
| Severe | Avoid dextropropoxyphene, pethidine | Moderate | Avoid |
| Oxazepam *see* Anxiolytics and Hypnotics | | **Povidone-iodine** | |
| Oxprenolol *see* Beta-blockers | | Severe | Avoid regular application to inflamed or broken mucosa |
| Oxypertine *see* Antipsychotics | | **Prazosin** | |
| **Pamidronate Disodium** | | Severe | Start with small dose; increased sensitivity to hypotensive effect and possible CNS toxicity |
| Severe | Divide daily dose | | |
| Pancuronium *see* Tubocurarine | | ***Primaxin*®** | |
| Papaveretum *see* Opioid Analgesics | | Mild | Reduce dose |
| **Paroxetine** | | **Primidone** | |
| Moderate | Start with smaller dose | Severe | Avoid large doses |
| Penbutolol *see* Beta-blockers | | **Probenecid** | |
| **Penicillamine** | | Moderate | Avoid; ineffective and toxicity increased |
| Mild | Avoid if possible or reduce dose; nephrotoxic | **Procainamide** | |
| **Pentamidine** | | Mild | Avoid or reduce dose |
| Mild | Reduce dose; consult data sheet | **Procarbazine** | |
| | | Moderate | Reduce dose |
| Pentazocine *see* Opioid Analgesics | | Prochlorperazine *see* Antipsychotics | |
| Pericyazine *see* Antipsychotics | | **Proguanil** | |
| **Perindopril** | | Severe | Avoid or reduce dose; increased risk of haematological toxicity |
| Mild | Reduce dose and monitor response; *see also* Captopril | | |
| Perphenazine *see* Antipsychotics | | Promazine *see* Antipsychotics | |
| **Pethidine** | | Propranolol *see* Beta-blockers | |
| Severe | Avoid; increased CNS toxicity; *see also* Opioid Analgesics | **Propylthiouracil** | |
| | | Mild | Reduce dose |
| Phenazocine *see* Opioid Analgesics | | **Pseudoephedrine** | |
| **Phenobarbitone** | | Severe | Avoid; increased CNS toxicity |
| Severe | Avoid large doses | | |
| Phenoperidine *see* Opioid Analgesics | | **Quinapril** | |
| Phenothiazines *see* Antipsychotics | | Mild | Start with 2.5 mg daily; *see also* Captopril |
| Phenylbutazone *see* NSAIDs | | | |
| Pholcodine *see* Opioid Analgesics | | **Ramipril** | |
| Pimozide *see* Antipsychotics | | Mild | Start with 1.25 mg daily; *see also* Captopril |
| **Pindolol** | | | |
| Moderate | Reduce dose; excreted unchanged | **Ranitidine** | |
| **Piperacillin** | | Severe | Use half normal dose; occasional risk of confusion |
| Moderate | Reduce dose | ***Regulan*®** | |
| **Piperazine** | | Severe | Avoid; contains 6.4 mmol potassium per sachet |
| Severe | Reduce dose; neurotoxic | | |
| Pipothiazine *see* Antipsychotics | | Remoxipride *see* Antipsychotics | |
| Piroxicam *see* NSAIDs | | Salicylates *see* Aspirin | |
| **Pivampicillin** | | Salsalate *see* Aspirin | |
| Severe | Reduce dose; rashes more common | **Salt substitutes** | |
| | | Moderate | Avoid routine use; high risk of hyperkalaemia |
| **Plicamycin** | | **Sertraline** | Manufacturer recommends avoid |
| Moderate | Avoid if possible | | |
| Polythiazide *see* Thiazides | | Sodium Aurothiomalate *see* Gold | |
| **Potassium Salts** | | **Sodium Bicarbonate** | |
| Moderate | Avoid routine use; high risk of hyperkalaemia | Severe | Avoid; specialised role in some forms of renal disease |
| | | Sodium Nitroprusside *see* Nitroprusside | |
| | | **Sodium salts** | |
| | | Severe | Avoid |

Table of drugs to be avoided or used with caution in renal impairment (*continued*)

| Drug and Degree of impairment | Comment | Drug and Degree of impairment | Comment |
|---|---|---|---|
| *Solpadeine*® | | Thiethylperazine *see* Antipsychotics | |
| Severe | Avoid; high sodium content | Thioguanine | |
| Sotalol | | Moderate | Reduce dose |
| Moderate | Reduce dose; excreted unchanged | Thioridazine *see* Antipsychotics | |
| | | Tiaprofenic Acid *see* NSAIDs | |
| Spironolactone *see* Potassium-sparing Diuretics | | Ticarcillin | |
| Streptomycin *see* Aminoglycosides | | Moderate | Reduce dose; 1 g contains 5.3 mmol sodium |
| Sucralfate | | | |
| Severe | Avoid; aluminium may be absorbed | *Timentin*® | |
| | | Moderate | Reduce dose |
| Sulfametopyrazine *see* Sulphonamides | | Timolol *see* Beta-blockers | |
| Sulindac *see* NSAIDs (excreted by kidney) | | Tobramycin *see* Aminoglycosides | |
| Sulphadiazine | | Tocainide | |
| Severe | Avoid; high risk of crystalluria | Mild | Reduce dose |
| | | Tolazamide | |
| Sulphadimidine *see* Sulphonamides | | Severe | May need dose reduction; increased risk of hypoglycaemia |
| Sulphasalazine | | | |
| Severe | Ensure high fluid intake; rashes and blood disorders; crystalluria a risk | | |
| | | Tolbutamide | |
| Sulphinpyrazone | | Severe | May need dose reduction; increased risk of hypoglycaemia |
| Moderate | Avoid; ineffective as uricosuric | | |
| | | Tolmetin *see* NSAIDs (excreted by kidney) | |
| Sulphonamides | | Triamterene *see* Potassium-sparing Diuretics | |
| Moderate | Ensure high fluid intake; rashes and blood disorders; crystalluria a risk | Triclofos *see* Anxiolytics and Hypnotics | |
| | | Trifluoperazine *see* Antipsychotics | |
| | | Trifluperidol *see* Antipsychotics | |
| Sulphonylureas *see under* individual drugs | | Trimethoprim | |
| Sulpiride | | Moderate | Reduce dose |
| Moderate | Avoid if possible, or reduce dose | Tubocurarine | |
| | | Moderate | Reduce dose; prolonged paralysis with large or repeated doses |
| Talampicillin | | | |
| Severe | Avoid; rashes more common | | |
| Teicoplanin | | Tulobuterol | |
| Mild | Reduce dose after 4 days | Mild | May need dose reduction; excreted by kidney |
| Temafloxacin | | | |
| Severe | Use half dose | Vancomycin | |
| Temazepam *see* Anxiolytics and Hypnotics | | Mild | Avoid parenteral use if possible; ototoxic; nephrotoxic |
| Temocillin | | | |
| Moderate | Reduce dose | | |
| Tenoxicam *see* NSAIDs | | Vecuronium *see* Tubocurarine | |
| Terbinafine | | Vigabatrin | |
| Mild | Use half normal dose | Mild | Reduce dose; excreted by kidney |
| Tetracyclines (except doxycycline and minocycline) | | | |
| Mild | Avoid—use doxycycline or minocycline if necessary; anti-anabolic effect, increased plasma urea, further deterioration in renal function | Xamoterol | |
| | | Moderate | Reduce dose; excreted by kidney |
| | | Xipamide *see* Thiazides | |
| | | Zidovudine | |
| Thiazides and Related Diuretics (except metolazone) | | Mild | Excreted by kidney; increased risk of toxicity |
| Moderate | Avoid; ineffective (metolazone remains effective but risk of excessive diuresis) | Zuclopenthixol *see* Antipsychotics | |

# Appendix 4: Pregnancy

Drugs can have harmful effects on the fetus at any time during pregnancy. Experience with many drugs in pregnancy is limited.

During the *first trimester* they may produce congenital malformations (teratogenesis), and the period of greatest risk is from the third to the eleventh week of pregnancy.

During the *second* and *third trimesters* drugs may affect the growth and functional development of the fetus or have toxic effects on fetal tissues; and drugs given shortly before term or during labour may have adverse effects on labour or on the neonate after delivery.

The following table lists drugs which may have harmful effects in pregnancy and indicates the trimester of risk.

The table is based on human data but information on *animal* studies has been included for some newer drugs when its omission might be misleading.

> Drugs should be prescribed in pregnancy only if the expected benefit to the mother is thought to be greater than the risk to the fetus, and all drugs should be avoided if possible during the first trimester. Drugs which have been extensively used in pregnancy and appear to be usually safe should be prescribed in preference to new or untried drugs; and the smallest effective dose should be used.
>
> Few drugs have been shown conclusively to be teratogenic in man but no drug is safe beyond all doubt in early pregnancy. Screening procedures are available where there is a known risk of certain defects.
>
> It should be noted that the BNF provides independent advice and may not always agree with the data sheets.
>
> Absence of a drug from the list does not imply safety.

## Table of drugs to be avoided or used with caution in pregnancy

Products introduced or amended since publication of BNF No. 22 (September 1991) are underlined.

| Drug (Trimester of risk) | Comments | Drug (Trimester of risk) | Comments |
|---|---|---|---|
| ACE Inhibitors (1, 2, 3) | Avoid; may adversely affect fetal and neonatal blood pressure control and renal function; also possible skull defects and oligohydramnios; toxicity in *animal* studies | Amiodarone (2, 3) | Possible risk of neonatal goitre; use only if no alternative |
| Acebutolol *see* Beta-blockers | | Amitriptyline *see* Antidepressants, Tricyclic | |
| Acemetacin *see* NSAIDs | | Amlodipine *see* Calcium-channel Blockers | |
| Acetazolamide *see* Diuretics | | Amoxapine *see* Antidepressants, Tricyclic | |
| Acetohexamide *see* Sulphonylureas | | Amylobarbitone *see* Barbiturates | |
| Acrivastine *see* Antihistamines | | Anabolic Steroids (1, 2, 3) | Masculinisation of female fetus |
| Alclometasone *see* Corticosteroids | | Anaesthetics, General (3) | Depress neonatal respiration |
| Alcohol | | | |
| (1, 2) | Regular daily drinking is teratogenic ('fetal alcohol syndrome') and may cause growth retardation; occasional single drinks are probably safe | Anaesthetics, Local (3) | With large doses, neonatal respiratory depression, hypotonia, and bradycardia after paracervical or epidural block |
| (3) | Withdrawal syndrome may occur in babies of alcoholic mothers | Analgesics *see* Opioid Analgesics and NSAIDs | |
| | | Androgens (1, 2, 3) | Virilisation of female fetus |
| Alfentanil *see* Opioid Analgesics | | Anistreplase *see* Streptokinase | |
| Allyloestrenol *see* Progestogens | | Anticoagulants | |
| Alprazolam *see* Anxiolytics and Hypnotics | | Heparin (1, 2, 3) | Osteoporosis has been reported after prolonged use |
| Alteplase *see* Streptokinase | | Oral Anticoagulants (1, 2, 3) | Congenital malformations; fetal and neonatal haemorrhage |
| Amikacin *see* Aminoglycosides | | | *See also* section 2.8 |
| Amiloride *see* Diuretics | | | |
| Aminoglutethimide | Avoid; toxicity in *animal* studies and may affect fetal sexual development | Antidepressants | |
| | | Fluoxetine, Fluvoxamine, MAOIs, Paroxetine, Sertraline (1, 2, 3) | No evidence of harm but manufacturers advise avoid unless compelling reasons |
| Aminoglycosides (2, 3) | Auditory or vestibular nerve damage; risk greatest with streptomycin; probably very small with gentamicin and tobramycin | Tricyclic (and related) (3) | Tachycardia, irritability, muscle spasms, and convulsions in neonate reported occasionally |
| Aminophylline *see* Theophylline | | | |

Table of drugs to be avoided or used with caution in pregnancy (*continued*)

| Drug (Trimester of risk) | Comments |
|---|---|
| Antiepileptics | Benefit of treatment outweighs risk to fetus; risk of teratogenicity greater if more than one drug used; **important: see also** carbamazepine, ethosuximide, phenobarbitone, phenytoin, valproate, and section 4.8 |
| Antihistamines | No evidence of teratogenicity; some packs of antihistamines sold to the public carry warning to avoid in pregnancy; manufacturer of astemizole advises toxicity at high doses in *animal* studies |
| Antimalarials (1, 3) | Benefit of prophylaxis and treatment in malaria outweighs risk; **important: see also** individual drugs |
| Antipsychotics (3) | Extrapyramidal effects in neonate occasionally reported |
| Anxiolytics and Hypnotics (3) | Depress neonatal respiration. Benzodiazepines cause neonatal drowsiness, hypotonia, and withdrawal symptoms; avoid large doses and regular use; short-acting benzodiazepines preferable to long-acting |
| Aspirin (3) | Impaired platelet function and risk of haemorrhage; delayed onset and increased duration of labour with increased blood loss; avoid analgesic doses if possible in last week (low doses probably not harmful); with high doses, closure of fetal ductus arteriosus *in utero* and possibly persistent pulmonary hypertension of newborn; kernicterus in jaundiced neonates |
| Astemizole *see* Antihistamines | |
| Atenolol *see* Beta-blockers | |
| Auranofin *see* Gold | |
| Aurothiomalate *see* Gold | |
| Azapropazone *see* NSAIDs | |
| Azatadine *see* Antihistamines | |
| Azathioprine (1) | Spontaneous abortion may be more common (see section 8.1) |
| Azelastine *see* Antihistamines | |
| Aztreonam | Manufacturer advises avoid (but no evidence of teratogenicity) |
| Barbiturates (3) | Withdrawal effects in neonate; *see also* Phenobarbitone |
| Beclomethasone *see* Corticosteroids | |
| Bendrofluazide *see* Diuretics | |
| Benorylate [aspirin-paracetamol ester] *see* Aspirin | |
| Benperidol *see* Antipsychotics | |
| Benserazide [ingredient] *see* Madopar® | |
| Benzodiazepines *see* Anxiolytics and Hypnotics | |

| Drug (Trimester of risk) | Comments |
|---|---|
| Beta-blockers (3) | May cause intra-uterine growth retardation, neonatal hypoglycaemia, and bradycardia; risk greater in severe hypertension |
| Betamethasone *see* Corticosteroids | |
| Betaxolol *see* Beta-blockers | |
| Bethanidine *see* Guanethidine | |
| Bezafibrate *see* Clofibrate | |
| Bisoprolol *see* Beta-blockers | |
| Bisphosphonates | Manufacturers advise avoid (on theoretical grounds) |
| Bromazepam *see* Anxiolytics and Hypnotics | |
| Brompheniramine *see* Antihistamines | |
| Budesonide *see* Corticosteroids | |
| Bumetanide *see* Diuretics | |
| Bupivacaine *see* Anaesthetics, Local | |
| Buprenorphine *see* Opioid Analgesics | |
| Butriptyline *see* Antidepressants, Tricyclic | |
| Calcium-channel Blockers | May inhibit labour and manufacturers advise that diltiazem and some dihydropyridines are teratogenic in *animals* |
| Capreomycin | Manufacturer advises teratogenic in *animal* studies |
| Captopril *see* ACE Inhibitors | |
| Carbamazepine (1) | May be small risk of teratogenesis including increased risk of neural tube defects (screening advised); *see also* Antiepileptics |
| Carbenoxolone (3) | Avoid; causes sodium retention with oedema |
| Carbimazole (2, 3) | Neonatal goitre and hypothyroidism. Has been associated with aplasia cutis of the neonate |
| Celiprolol *see* Beta-blockers | |
| Cetirizine *see* Antihistamines | |
| Chenodeoxycholic acid (1, 2, 3) | Theoretical risk of effects on fetal metabolism |
| Chloral hydrate *see* Anxiolytics and Hypnotics | |
| Chloramphenicol (3) | Neonatal 'grey syndrome' |
| Chlordiazepoxide *see* Anxiolytics and Hypnotics | |
| Chlormethiazole *see* Anxiolytics and Hypnotics | |
| Chlormezanone *see* Anxiolytics and Hypnotics | |
| Chloroquine *see* Antimalarials | |
| Chlorothiazide *see* Diuretics | |
| Chlorpheniramine *see* Antihistamines | |
| Chlorpromazine *see* Antipsychotics | |
| Chlorpropamide *see* Sulphonylureas | |
| Chlorprothixene *see* Antipsychotics | |
| Chlortetracycline *see* Tetracyclines | |
| Chlorthalidone *see* Diuretics | |
| Choline magnesium trisalicylate *see* Aspirin | |
| Cilazapril *see* ACE Inhibitors | |
| Cinnarizine *see* Antihistamines | |
| Ciprofloxacin *see* 4-Quinolones | |
| Cisapride | Manufacturer advises avoid |
| Clemastine *see* Antihistamines | |
| Clobazam *see* Anxiolytics and Hypnotics | |
| Clobetasol *see* Corticosteroids | |
| Clobetasone *see* Corticosteroids | |
| Clodronate sodium *see* Bisphosphonates | |

Table of drugs to be avoided or used with caution in pregnancy (*continued*)

| Drug (Trimester of risk) | Comments |
|---|---|
| Clofibrate (1, 2, 3) | Avoid—theoretical possibility of interference with embryonic growth and development due to anticholesterol effect |
| Clomiphene | Possible effects on fetal development |
| Clomipramine *see* Antidepressants, Tricyclic | |
| Clomocycline *see* Tetracyclines | |
| Clonazepam *see* Antiepileptics | |
| Clorazepate *see* Anxiolytics and Hypnotics | |
| Clozapine | Manufacturer advises avoid |
| Codeine *see* Opioid Analgesics | |
| Contraceptives, Oral | Epidemiological evidence suggests no harmful effects on fetus |
| Corticosteroids (2, 3) | Benefit of treatment, e.g. in asthma, outweighs risk; high doses (>10 mg prednisolone daily) may produce fetal and neonatal adrenal suppression; corticosteroid cover required by mother during labour |
| Co-trimoxazole (1) | Possible teratogenic risk (trimethoprim a folate antagonist) |
| (3) | Neonatal haemolysis and methaemoglobinaemia; fear of increased risk of kernicterus in neonates appears to be unfounded |
| Cyclizine *see* Antihistamines | |
| Cyclopenthiazide *see* Diuretics | |
| Cyclopropane *see* Anaesthetics, General | |
| Cyclosporin | May cause fetal growth retardation; *see also* section 8.1 |
| Cyproheptadine *see* Antihistamines | |
| Cyproterone [ingredient] *see Dianette*® | |
| Cytotoxic drugs (1) | Most are teratogenic; *see* section 8.1 |
| Danazol (1, 2, 3) | Has weak androgenic effects and virilisation of female fetus reported |
| Dapsone (3) | Neonatal haemolysis and methaemoglobinaemia; folate supplements should be given to mother |
| Debrisoquine *see* Guanethidine | |
| Demeclocycline *see* Tetracyclines | |
| Desferrioxamine | Manufacturer advises toxicity in *animal* studies |
| Desipramine *see* Antidepressants, Tricyclic | |
| Desonide *see* Corticosteroids | |
| Desoxymethasone *see* Corticosteroids | |
| Dexamethasone *see* Corticosteroids | |
| Dextromethorphan *see* Opioid Analgesics | |
| Dextromoramide *see* Opioid Analgesics | |
| Dextropropoxyphene *see* Opioid Analgesics | |
| Diamorphine *see* Opioid Analgesics | |
| *Dianette*® (1, 2, 3) | Feminisation of male fetus (due to cyproterone) |
| Diazepam *see* Anxiolytics and Hypnotics | |

| Drug (Trimester of risk) | Comments |
|---|---|
| Diazoxide (2, 3) | Prolonged use may produce alopecia and impaired glucose tolerance in neonate; inhibits uterine activity during labour |
| Diclofenac *see* NSAIDs | |
| Diethylpropion | Avoid—congenital malformations reported to CSM |
| Diflucortolone *see* Corticosteroids | |
| Diflunisal *see* NSAIDs | |
| Dihydrocodeine *see* Opioid Analgesics | |
| Dihydroergotamine *see* Ergotamine | |
| Diltiazem *see* Calcium-channel Blockers | |
| Dimenhydrinate *see* Antihistamines | |
| Dimethindene *see* Antihistamines | |
| Diphenhydramine *see* Antihistamines | |
| Diphenoxylate *see* Opioid Analgesics | |
| Diphenylpyraline *see* Antihistamines | |
| Dipipanone *see* Opioid Analgesics | |
| Disodium Etidronate *see* Bisphosphonates | |
| Disodium Pamidronate *see* Bisphosphonates | |
| Disopyramide (3) | May induce labour |
| Distigmine | Manufacturer advises avoid (may stimulate uterine contractions) |
| Disulfiram (1) | High concentrations of acetaldehyde which occur in presence of alcohol may be teratogenic |
| Diuretics (3) | Not used to treat hypertension in pregnancy; thiazides may cause neonatal thrombocytopenia |
| Dothiepin *see* Antidepressants, Tricyclic | |
| Doxepin *see* Antidepressants, Tricyclic | |
| Doxycycline *see* Tetracyclines | |
| Droperidol *see* Antipsychotics | |
| Dydrogesterone *see* Progestogens | |
| Enalapril *see* ACE Inhibitors | |
| Enflurane *see* Anaesthetics, General | |
| Enoxacin *see* 4-Quinolones | |
| Ergotamine (1, 2, 3) | Oxytocic effects on the pregnant uterus |
| Ethacrynic acid *see* Diuretics | |
| Ether *see* Anaesthetics, General | |
| Ethinyloestradiol *see* Contraceptives, Oral | |
| Ethionamide (1) | May be teratogenic |
| Ethosuximide (1) | May possibly be teratogenic; *see* Antiepileptics |
| Etidronate Disodium *see* Bisphosphonates | |
| Etodolac *see* NSAIDs | |
| Etomidate *see* Anaesthetics, General | |
| Etretinate (1, 2, 3) | Teratogenic; effective contraception must be used for at least 1 month before treatment, during treatment, and for at least two years after stopping |

Table of drugs to be avoided or used with caution in pregnancy (*continued*)

| Drug (Trimester of risk) | Comments |
|---|---|
| *Fansidar*® | |
| (1) | Possible teratogenic risk (pyrimethamine a folate antagonist) |
| (3) | Neonatal haemolysis and methaemoglobinaemia; fear of increased risk of kernicterus in neonates appears to be unfounded *see also* Antimalarials |
| Felodipine *see* Calcium-channel Blockers | |
| Fenbufen *see* NSAIDs | |
| Fenofibrate (1, 2, 3) | Manufacturer advises toxicity in *animal* studies; *see also* Clofibrate |
| Fenoprofen *see* NSAIDs | |
| Fentanyl *see* Opioid Analgesics | |
| Flecainide | Manufacturer advises toxicity in *animal* studies |
| Fluclorolone *see* Corticosteroids | |
| Fluconazole | Manufacturer advises toxicity at high doses in *animal* studies |
| Flucytosine (1) | Possible teratogenic risk |
| Flunitrazepam *see* Anxiolytics and Hypnotics | |
| Fluocinolone *see* Corticosteroids | |
| Fluocinonide *see* Corticosteroids | |
| Fluocortolone *see* Corticosteroids | |
| Fluoxetine *see* Antidepressants | |
| Flupenthixol *see* Antipsychotics | |
| Fluphenazine *see* Antipsychotics | |
| Flurandrenolone *see* Corticosteroids | |
| Flurazepam *see* Anxiolytics and Hypnotics | |
| Flurbiprofen *see* NSAIDs | |
| Fluspirilene *see* Antipsychotics | |
| Fluvoxamine *see* Antidepressants | |
| Foscarnet | Manufacturer advises avoid |
| Fosinopril *see* ACE Inhibitors | |
| Frusemide *see* Diuretics | |
| Ganciclovir | Avoid—teratogenic risk |
| Gemfibrozil *see* Clofibrate | |
| Gentamicin *see* Aminoglycosides | |
| Gestrinone (1, 2, 3) | Avoid |
| Glibenclamide *see* Sulphonylureas | |
| Gliclazide *see* Sulphonylureas | |
| Glipizide *see* Sulphonylureas | |
| Gliquidone *see* Sulphonylureas | |
| Gold | |
| Auranofin | Manufacturer advises teratogenicity in *animal* studies; effective contraception should be used during and for at least 6 months after treatment |
| Aurothiomalate (1, 2, 3) | No good evidence of harm but avoid if possible |
| Griseofulvin | CRM advises avoid (fetotoxicity and teratogenicity in *animals*) |
| Growth Hormone | Avoid on theoretical grounds |

| Drug (Trimester of risk) | Comments |
|---|---|
| Guanethidine (3) | Postural hypotension and reduced uteroplacental perfusion; should not be used to treat hypertension in pregnancy |
| Halcinonide *see* Corticosteroids | |
| Halofantrine | Manufacturer advises avoid |
| Haloperidol *see* Antipsychotics | |
| Halothane *see* Anaesthetics, General | |
| Heparin *see* Anticoagulants | |
| Hydralazine (1) | Manufacturer advises toxicity in *animal* studies |
| Hydrochlorothiazide *see* Diuretics | |
| Hydrocortisone *see* Corticosteroids | |
| Hydroflumethiazide *see* Diuretics | |
| Hydroxychloroquine | Avoid for rheumatic disease (but for malaria *see* Antimalarials) |
| Hydroxyprogesterone *see* Progestogens | |
| Hydroxyzine *see* Antihistamines | |
| Hypnotics *see* Anxiolytics and Hypnotics | |
| Ibuprofen *see* NSAIDs | |
| Idoxuridine | Manufacturers advise toxicity in *animal* studies |
| Imipramine *see* Antidepressants, Tricyclic | |
| Immunosuppressants *see* section 8.1 | |
| Indapamide *see* Diuretics | |
| Indomethacin *see* NSAIDs | |
| Interferons | Manufacturers recommend avoid unless compelling reasons; not for chronic active hepatitis during pregnancy |
| Iodine and Iodides (2, 3) | Neonatal goitre and hypothyroidism |
| Radioactive iodine (1, 2, 3) | Permanent hypothyroidism—avoid |
| Iprindole *see* Antidepressants, Tricyclic (and related) | |
| Isoflurane *see* Anaesthetics, General | |
| Isotretinoin (1, 2, 3) | Teratogenic; effective contraception must be used for at least 1 month before treatment, during treatment and for at least 1 month after stopping |
| Isradipine *see* Calcium-channel Blockers | |
| Itraconazole | Manufacturer advises toxicity in *animal* studies |
| Kanamycin *see* Aminoglycosides | |
| Ketamine *see* Anaesthetics, General | |
| Ketoconazole | Manufacturer advises teratogenicity in *animal* studies; packs carry a warning to avoid in pregnancy |
| Ketoprofen *see* NSAIDs | |
| Ketorolac *see* NSAIDs | |
| Ketotifen *see* Antihistamines | |
| Labetalol *see* Beta-blockers | |
| Lamotrigine *see* Antiepileptics | |
| Levodopa | Manufacturers advise toxicity in *animal* studies |
| Lignocaine *see* Anaesthetics, Local | |
| Lindane | Manufacturer advises toxicity in *animal* studies |
| Lisinopril *see* ACE Inhibitors | |

Table of drugs to be avoided or used with caution in pregnancy (*continued*)

| Drug (Trimester of risk) | Comments |
|---|---|
| Lithium (1, 2, 3) | Dose requirements increased; congenital malformations; neonatal goitre reported; lithium toxicity (hypotonia and cyanosis) in neonate if maternal therapy poorly controlled |
| Lofepramine *see* Antidepressants, Tricyclic | |
| Loprazolam *see* Anxiolytics and Hypnotics | |
| Loratadine *see* Antihistamines | |
| Lorazepam *see* Anxiolytics and Hypnotics | |
| Lormetazepam *see* Anxiolytics and Hypnotics | |
| Lymecycline *see* Tetracyclines | |
| *Madopar®* *see* Levodopa | |
| *Maloprim®* (1) | Possible teratogenic risk (pyrimethamine a folate antagonist) |
| (3) | Neonatal haemolysis and methaemoglobinaemia (due to dapsone); folate supplements should be given to mother *see also* Antimalarials |
| Maprotiline *see* Antidepressants, Tricyclic (and related) | |
| Mebendazole | Manufacturer advises toxicity in *animal* studies |
| Mebhydrolin *see* Antihistamines | |
| Medazepam *see* Anxiolytics and Hypnotics | |
| Mefenamic Acid *see* NSAIDs | |
| Mefloquine (1) | Manufacturer advises teratogenicity in *animal* studies; avoid for prophylaxis, *see* p. 236 |
| Mefruside *see* Diuretics | |
| Meprobamate *see* Anxiolytics and Hypnotics | |
| Meptazinol *see* Opioid Analgesics | |
| Mesterolone *see* Androgens | |
| Mestranol *see* Contraceptives, Oral | |
| Metaraminol (1, 2, 3) | Avoid—may reduce placental perfusion |
| Metformin (1, 2, 3) | Avoid |
| Methadone *see* Opioid Analgesics | |
| Methohexitone *see* Anaesthetics, General | |
| Methotrimeprazine *see* Antipsychotics | |
| Methyclothiazide *see* Diuretics | |
| Methylphenobarbitone *see* Antiepileptics | |
| Methylprednisolone *see* Corticosteroids | |
| Metolazone *see* Diuretics | |
| Metoprolol *see* Beta-blockers | |
| Metronidazole | Manufacturer advises avoidance of high-dose regimens |
| Metyrapone | Avoid (may impair biosynthesis of fetal-placental steroids) |
| Mianserin *see* Antidepressants, Tricyclic (and related) | |
| Mifepristone | Manufacturer advises that if treatment fails, essential that pregnancy be terminated by another method |
| Minocycline *see* Tetracyclines | |

| Drug (Trimester of risk) | Comments |
|---|---|
| Minoxidil (3) | Neonatal hirsutism reported |
| Misoprostol (1, 2, 3) | Avoid; increases uterine tone |
| Morphine *see* Opioid Analgesics | |
| Nabumetone *see* NSAIDs | |
| Nadolol *see* Beta-blockers | |
| Nafarelin | Avoid |
| Nalbuphine *see* Opioid Analgesics | |
| Nalidixic acid *see* 4-Quinolones | |
| Nandrolone *see* Anabolic Steroids | |
| Naproxen *see* NSAIDs | |
| Narcotic Analgesics *see* Opioid Analgesics | |
| Neomycin *see* Aminoglycosides | |
| Neostigmine (3) | Neonatal myasthenia with large doses |
| Netilmicin *see* Aminoglycosides | |
| Nicardipine *see* Calcium-channel Blockers | |
| Nicoumalone *see* Anticoagulants | |
| Nifedipine *see* Calcium-channel Blockers | |
| Nimodipine *see* Calcium-channel Blockers | |
| Nitrazepam *see* Anxiolytics and Hypnotics | |
| Nitrofurantoin (3) | May produce neonatal haemolysis if used at term |
| Nitrous oxide *see* Anaesthetics, General | |
| Noradrenaline (1, 2, 3) | Avoid—may reduce placental perfusion |
| Norfloxacin *see* 4-Quinolones | |
| Nortriptyline *see* Antidepressants, Tricyclic | |
| NSAIDs (3) | With regular use closure of fetal ductus arteriosus *in utero* and possibly persistent pulmonary hypertension of the newborn. Delayed onset and increased duration of labour |
| Octreotide (1, 2, 3) | Avoid; possible effect on fetal growth |
| Oestrogens *see* Contraceptives, Oral | |
| Ofloxacin *see* 4-Quinolones | |
| Omeprazole | Manufacturer advises toxicity in *animal* studies |
| Opioid Analgesics (1) | Avoid papaveretum (contains noscapine which may be teratogenic) |
| (3) | Depress neonatal respiration; withdrawal effects in neonates of dependent mothers; gastric stasis and risk of inhalation pneumonia in mother during labour |
| Oxatomide *see* Antihistamines | |
| Oxazepam *see* Anxiolytics and Hypnotics | |
| Oxprenolol *see* Beta-blockers | |
| Oxypertine *see* Antipsychotics | |
| Oxytetracycline *see* Tetracyclines | |
| Pamidronate Disodium *see* Bisphosphonates | |
| Papaveretum *see* Opioid Analgesics | |
| Paroxetine *see* Antidepressants | |
| Penbutolol *see* Beta-blockers | |
| Penicillamine (1, 2, 3) | Fetal abnormalities reported rarely; avoid if possible |
| Pentazocine *see* Opioid Analgesics | |
| Pericyazine *see* Antipsychotics | |
| Perindopril *see* ACE Inhibitors | |
| Perphenazine *see* Antipsychotics | |

Table of drugs to be avoided or used with caution in pregnancy (*continued*)

| Drug (Trimester of risk) | Comments |
|---|---|
| Pethidine *see* Opioid Analgesics | |
| Phenindamine *see* Antihistamines | |
| Phenindione *see* Anticoagulants | |
| Pheniramine *see* Antihistamines | |
| Phenobarbitone (1, 3) | Congenital malformations. Neonatal bleeding tendency—prophylactic vitamin K₁ should be given; *see also* Antiepileptics |
| Phenoperidine *see* Opioid Analgesics | |
| Phenothiazines *see* Antipsychotics | |
| Phenytoin (1, 3) | Congenital malformations. Folate supplements should be given to mother (reduced absorption). Neonatal bleeding tendency—prophylactic vitamin K₁ should be given. Caution in interpreting plasma concentrations—bound may be reduced but free (i.e. effective) unchanged; *see also* Antiepileptics |
| Pholcodine *see* Opioid Analgesics | |
| Pimozide *see* Antipsychotics | |
| Pindolol *see* Beta-blockers | |
| Piperazine | No clinical evidence of harm but packs sold to the general public carry a warning to avoid in pregnancy except on medical advice |
| Pipothiazine *see* Antipsychotics | |
| Piroxicam *see* NSAIDs | |
| Podophyllum resin (1, 2, 3) | Avoid—neonatal death and teratogenesis have been reported |
| Polythiazide *see* Diuretics | |
| Povidone-iodine (2, 3) | Sufficient iodine may be absorbed to affect the fetal thyroid |
| Pravastatin *see* Clofibrate | |
| Prednisolone *see* Corticosteroids | |
| Prednisone *see* Corticosteroids | |
| Prilocaine (3) | Neonatal methaemoglobinaemia; *see also* Anaesthetics, Local |
| Primaquine (3) | Neonatal haemolysis and methaemoglobinaemia; *see also* Antimalarials |
| Primidone *see* Antiepileptics | |
| Probucol *see* Clofibrate | |
| Procaine (3) | Neonatal methaemoglobinaemia; *see also* Anaesthetics, Local |
| Prochlorperazine *see* Antipsychotics | |
| Progestogens (1) | High doses may possibly be teratogenic |
| Proguanil | Folate supplements should be given to mother; *see also* Antimalarials |
| Promazine *see* Antipsychotics | |
| Promethazine *see* Antihistamines | |
| Propofol *see* Anaesthetics, General | |
| Propranolol *see* Beta-blockers | |
| Propylthiouracil (2, 3) | Neonatal goitre and hypothyroidism |

| Drug (Trimester of risk) | Comments |
|---|---|
| Prothionamide (1) | May be teratogenic |
| Protriptyline *see* Antidepressants, Tricyclic | |
| Pyridostigmine (3) | Neonatal myasthenia with large doses |
| Pyrimethamine (1) | Possible teratogenic risk (folate antagonist); folate supplements should be given to mother; *see also* Antimalarials |
| Quinapril *see* ACE Inhibitors | |
| Quinine (1) | High doses are teratogenic; but in malaria benefit of treatment outweighs risk |
| 4-Quinolones (1, 2, 3) | Arthropathy in *animal* studies |
| Ramipril *see* ACE inhibitors | |
| Rauwolfia Alkaloids (3) | Neonatal bradycardia, drowsiness, and nasal stuffiness |
| Remoxipride *see* Antipsychotics | |
| Rifampicin (1) | Manufacturers advise very high doses teratogenic in *animal* studies |
| (3) | Risk of neonatal bleeding may be increased |
| Salbutamol (3) | Large parenteral doses given at term for asthma could delay onset of labour |
| Salicylates *see* Aspirin | |
| Salsalate *see* Aspirin | |
| Sertraline *see* Antidepressants | |
| Simvastatin | Manufacturer advises toxicity in *animal* studies |
| Sodium Aurothiomalate *see* Gold | |
| Sodium Clodronate *see* Bisphosphonates | |
| Sodium Valproate *see* Valproate | |
| Sotalol *see* Beta-blockers | |
| Spironolactone | Manufacturers advise toxicity in *animal* studies |
| Stanozolol *see* Anabolic Steroids | |
| Stilboestrol (1) | High doses associated with vaginal carcinoma in female offspring |
| Streptokinase (1, 2, 3) | Possibility of premature separation of placenta in first 18 weeks; theoretical possibility of fetal haemorrhage throughout pregnancy; avoid postpartum use—maternal haemorrhage |
| Streptomycin *see* Aminoglycosides | |
| Sulfadoxine *see* Sulphonamides | |
| Sulfametopyrazine *see* Sulphonamides | |
| Sulindac *see* NSAIDs | |
| Sulphadiazine *see* Sulphonamides | |
| Sulphadimidine *see* Sulphonamides | |
| Sulphasalazine (3) | Theoretical risk of neonatal haemolysis; folate supplements should be given to mother |
| Sulphonamides (3) | Neonatal haemolysis and methaemoglobinaemia; fear of increased risk of kernicterus in neonates appears to be unfounded |

Table of drugs to be avoided or used with caution in pregnancy (*continued*)

| Drug (Trimester of risk) | Comments | Drug (Trimester of risk) | Comments |
|---|---|---|---|
| Sulphonylureas (3) | Neonatal hypoglycaemia; insulin is normally substituted in all diabetics; if oral drugs are used therapy should be stopped at least 2 days before delivery | Triamterene *see* Diuretics | |
| | | Tribavirin | Manufacturer advises avoid |
| | | Triclofos *see* Anxiolytics and Hypnotics | |
| | | Trifluoperazine *see* Antipsychotics | |
| | | Trifluperidol *see* Antipsychotics | |
| Sulpiride *see* Antipsychotics | | Trilostane (1, 2, 3) | Interferes with placental sex hormone production |
| Tamoxifen | Possible effects on fetal development | Trimeprazine *see* Antihistamines | |
| Temafloxacin *see* 4-Quinolones | | Trimetaphan (3) | Avoid. Risk of paralytic ileus in newborn |
| Temazepam *see* Anxiolytics and Hypnotics | | Trimethoprim (1) | Possible teratogenic risk (folate antagonist) |
| Tenoxicam *see* NSAIDS | | Trimipramine *see* Antidepressants, Tricyclic | |
| Terbutaline (3) | Large parenteral doses given at term for asthma could delay onset of labour | Triprolidine *see* Antihistamines | |
| | | Urokinase (1, 2, 3) | Possibility of premature separation of placenta in first 18 weeks; theoretical possibility of fetal haemorrhage throughout pregnancy; avoid postpartum use—maternal haemorrhage |
| Terfenadine *see* Antihistamines | | | |
| Testosterone *see* Androgens | | | |
| Tetracyclines (2, 3) | Dental discoloration; maternal hepatotoxicity with large parenteral doses | | |
| Theophylline (3) | Neonatal irritability and apnoea have been reported | Vaccines (live) (1) | Theoretical risk of congenital malformations; *see* section 14.1 |
| Thiabendazole (1) | Teratogenic in *animal* studies | | |
| Thiazides (3) | May cause neonatal thrombocytopenia; *see also* Diuretics | Valproate (1, 3) | Increased risk of neural tube defects (screening advised); neonatal bleeding and hepatotoxicity also reported; *see also* Antiepileptics |
| Thiethylperazine *see* Antipsychotics | | | |
| Thiopentone *see* Anaesthetics, General | | Verapamil *see* Calcium-channel Blockers | |
| Thioridazine *see* Antipsychotics | | Vigabatrin | Manufacturer advises toxicity in *animal* studies; *see also* Antiepileptics |
| Tiaprofenic acid *see* NSAIDs | | | |
| Timolol *see* Beta-blockers | | | |
| Tinidazole | Manufacturer advises avoid in first trimester | Viloxazine *see* Antidepressants, Tricyclic (and related) | |
| Tobramycin *see* Aminoglycosides | | Vitamin A (1) | Excessive doses may be teratogenic; *see also* p. 339 |
| Tocainide | Manufacturer advises toxicity in *animal* studies | | |
| Tolbutamide *see* Sulphonylureas | | Warfarin *see* Anticoagulants | |
| Tolmetin *see* NSAIDs | | Xamoterol | Manufacturer advises toxicity in *animal* studies |
| Trazodone *see* Antidepressants, Tricyclic (and related) | | Xipamide *see* Diuretics | |
| Triamcinolone *see* Corticosteroids | | Zuclopenthixol *see* Antipsychotics | |

# Appendix 5: Breast-feeding

Administration of some drugs to nursing mothers may cause toxicity in the infant (e.g. ergotamine), whereas administration of others (e.g. digoxin), has little effect on the neonate. Some drugs inhibit lactation (e.g. bromocriptine).

Toxicity to the infant can occur if the drug enters the milk in pharmacologically significant quantities. Milk concentrations of some drugs (e.g. iodides), may exceed those in the maternal plasma so that therapeutic doses in the mother may cause toxicity to the infant. Some drugs inhibit the infant's sucking reflex (e.g. phenobarbitone). Drugs in breast milk may, at least theoretically, cause hypersensitivity in the infant even when concentrations are too low for a pharmacological effect.

The following table lists drugs:

which should be used with caution or which are contra-indicated in breast-feeding for the reasons given above;

which, on present evidence, may be given to the mother during breast-feeding, because they are excreted in milk in amounts which are too small to be harmful to the infant;

which are not known to be harmful to the infant although they are present in milk in significant amounts.

For many drugs there is insufficient evidence available to provide guidance and it is advisable only to administer essential drugs to a mother during breast-feeding. Because of the inadequacy of currently available information on drugs in breast milk the following table should be used only as a guide; absence from the table does not imply safety.

## Table of drugs excreted in breast milk

Products introduced or amended since publication of BNF No. 22 (September 1991) are underlined.

| Drug | Comments |
|------|----------|
| Acebutolol see Beta-blockers | |
| Acetazolamide | Amount too small to be harmful |
| Acetohexamide see Sulphonylureas | |
| Acrivastine see Antihistamines | |
| Alcohol | Large amounts may affect infant |
| Alfacalcidol see Vitamin D | |
| Alprazolam see Benzodiazepines | |
| Aminophylline see Theophylline | |
| Amiodarone | Avoid; present in milk in significant amounts; theoretical risk from release of iodine; see also Iodine |
| Amitriptyline see Antidepressants, Tricyclic | |
| Amoxapine see Antidepressants, Tricyclic | |
| Amphetamines | Significant amount in milk. Avoid |
| Amylobarbitone see Barbiturates | |
| Androgens | Avoid; may cause masculinisation in the female infant or precocious development in the male infant; high doses suppress lactation |
| Anthraquinones | Avoid; large doses may cause increased gastric motility and diarrhoea (particularly cascara and danthron) |
| Anticoagulants, Oral | Risk of haemorrhage; increased by vitamin-K deficiency; warfarin appears safe but phenindione should be avoided |
| Antidepressants, Tricyclic (and related) | Amount of tricyclic antidepressants (including related drugs such as mianserin and trazodone) too small to be harmful; accumulation of doxepin metabolite may cause sedation and respiratory depression |

| Drug | Comments |
|------|----------|
| Antihistamines | Significant amount of some but not known to be harmful; drowsiness in infant reported with clemastine |
| Antipsychotics | Although amount excreted in milk probably too small to be harmful, *animal* studies indicate possible adverse effects of these drugs on developing nervous system therefore avoid unless absolutely necessary; drowsiness in infant reported with chlorpromazine; significant amount of sulpiride excreted in milk (best avoided) |
| Aspirin | Avoid—possible risk of Reye's syndrome; regular use of high doses could impair platelet function and produce hypoprothrombinaemia in infant if neonatal vitamin K stores low |
| Astemizole see Antihistamines | |
| Atenolol see Beta-blockers | |
| Atropine | May possibly have antimuscarinic effects in infants |
| Auranofin see Gold | |
| Aurothiomalate see Gold | |
| Azatadine see Antihistamines | |
| Baclofen | Amount too small to be harmful |
| Barbiturates | Avoid if possible (*see also* phenobarbitone); large doses may produce drowsiness |
| Bendrofluazide see Thiazides | |
| Benperidol see Antipsychotics | |
| Benzodiazepines | Avoid repeated doses; lethargy and weight loss may occur in infant |

**Table of drugs excreted in breast milk (*continued*)**

| Drug | Comments | Drug | Comments |
|---|---|---|---|
| Beta-blockers and Labetalol | Monitor infant; possible toxicity due to beta-blockade but amount of most beta-blockers excreted in milk too small to affect infant; acebutolol, atenolol, nadolol, and sotalol are present in greater amounts than other beta-blockers | Clavulanic acid (in co-amoxiclav, *Timentin*®) | Amount too small to be harmful |
| Betamethasone *see* Corticosteroids | | Clemastine *see* Antihistamines | |
| Betaxolol *see* Beta-blockers | | Clobazam *see* Benzodiazepines | |
| Bisoprolol *see* Beta-blockers | | Clomipramine *see* Antidepressants, Tricyclic | |
| Bromazepam *see* Benzodiazepines | | Clomocycline *see* Tetracyclines | |
| Bromide salts | Avoid; sedation and rash in infant | Clorazepate *see* Benzodiazepines | |
| Bromocriptine | Suppresses lactation | Clozapine *see* Antipsychotics | |
| Brompheniramine *see* Antihistamines | | Codeine | Amount too small to be harmful |
| Buprenorphine | Amount too small to be harmful | Colchicine | Caution because of its cytotoxicity |
| Butobarbitone *see* Barbiturates | | Contraceptives, Oral | Oestrogen/progestogen contraceptives usually have little effect on milk flow; in some women, usually when lactation not well established, suppression may occur; one report of neonatal folate deficiency; progestogen-only contraceptives do not appear to adversely affect established milk flow |
| Butriptyline *see* Antidepressants, Tricyclic | | | |
| Caffeine | Regular intake of large amounts can affect infant | | |
| Calciferol *see* Vitamin D | | | |
| Calcitonin | Avoid; inhibits lactation in *animals* | | |
| Calcitriol *see* Vitamin D | | | |
| Captopril | Amount too small to be harmful | | |
| Carbamazepine | Amount too small to be harmful | Corticosteroids | Continuous therapy with high doses (>10 mg prednisolone daily) could possibly affect infant's adrenal function—monitor carefully |
| Carbimazole | Amounts in milk may be sufficient to affect neonatal thyroid function (but *see also* section 6.2.2) | | |
| | | Corticotrophin | Amount too small to be harmful |
| Carisoprodol | Concentrated in milk; no adverse effects reported but best avoided | Cortisone Acetate *see* Corticosteroids | |
| | | Co-trimoxazole | Small risk of kernicterus in jaundiced infants and of haemolysis in G6PD-deficient infants (due to sulphamethoxazole) |
| Cascara *see* Anthraquinones | | | |
| Celiprolol *see* Beta-blockers | | | |
| Cetirizine *see* Antihistamines | | Cough mixtures containing iodides | Use alternative cough mixtures; *see* Iodine |
| Chloral Hydrate | Sedation in infant | Cyclopenthiazide *see* Thiazides | |
| Chloramphenicol | Use another antibiotic; may cause bone-marrow toxicity in infant; concentration in milk usually insufficient to cause 'grey syndrome' | Cycloserine | Amount too small to be harmful |
| | | Cyclosporin | Caution—excreted in milk |
| | | Cyproheptadine *see* Antihistamines | |
| Chlordiazepoxide *see* Benzodiazepines | | Cyproterone Acetate | Caution; possibility of anti-androgen effects in neonate |
| Chlormethiazole | Amount too small to be harmful | Cytotoxics | Discontinue breast-feeding |
| | | Danazol | No data available but avoid because of possible androgenic effects in infant |
| Chloroquine | Amount too small to be harmful | | |
| Chlorothiazide *see* Thiazides | | Danthron *see* Anthraquinones | |
| Chlorpheniramine *see* Antihistamines | | Dapsone | Haemolytic anaemia; although significant amount in milk risk to infant very small |
| Chlorpromazine | Drowsiness in infant reported; *see* Antipsychotics | | |
| Chlorpropamide *see* Sulphonylureas | | | |
| Chlortetracycline *see* Tetracyclines | | Demeclocycline *see* Tetracyclines | |
| Chlorthalidone *see* Thiazides | | Desipramine *see* Antidepressants, Tricyclic | |
| Cholecalciferol *see* Vitamin D | | Dexamethasone *see* Corticosteroids | |
| Cimetidine | Significant amount but not known to be harmful | Dexamphetamine *see* Amphetamines | |
| | | Dextropropoxyphene | Amount too small to be harmful |
| Ciprofloxacin | High concentrations in breast milk | | |
| Cisapride | Amount too small to be harmful | | |

**Table of drugs excreted in breast milk (*continued*)**

| Drug | Comments | Drug | Comments |
|------|----------|------|----------|
| Diamorphine | Therapeutic doses unlikely to affect infant; withdrawal symptoms in infants of dependent mothers; breast-feeding no longer considered best method of treating dependence in offspring of dependent mothers and should be stopped | Fluvoxamine | Amount too small to be harmful |
| | | Frusemide | Amount too small to be harmful |
| | | Ganciclovir | Avoid |
| | | Glibenclamide *see* Sulphonylureas | |
| | | Gliclazide *see* Sulphonylureas | |
| | | Glipizide *see* Sulphonylureas | |
| | | Gliquidone *see* Sulphonylureas | |
| Diazepam *see* Benzodiazepines | | Glymidine *see* Sulphonylureas | |
| Diclofenac | Amount too small to be harmful | Gold (auranofin, aurothiomalate) | Caution—excreted in milk; theoretical possibility of rashes and idiosyncratic reactions |
| Digoxin | Amount too small to be harmful | | |
| Dihydrotachysterol *see* Vitamin D | | Halofantrine | Avoid |
| Diltiazem | Significant amount but not known to be harmful | Haloperidol *see* Antipsychotics | |
| | | Heparin | Amount too small to be harmful |
| Dimethindene *see* Antihistamines | | Hydrochlorothiazide *see* Thiazides | |
| Diphenylpyraline *see* Antihistamines | | Hydrocortisone *see* Corticosteroids | |
| Disopyramide | Amount too small to be harmful | Hydroflumethiazide *see* Thiazides | |
| | | Hydroxychloroquine | Amount too small to be harmful |
| Domperidone | Amount probably too small to be harmful | | |
| | | Hydroxyzine *see* Antihistamines | |
| Dothiepin *see* Antidepressants, Tricyclic | | Hyoscine | Amount too small to be harmful |
| Doxepin *see* Antidepressants, Tricyclic | | | |
| Doxycycline *see* Tetracyclines | | Ibuprofen | Amount too small to be harmful |
| Droperidol *see* Antipsychotics | | | |
| Enalapril | Amount too small to be harmful | Idoxuridine | May possibly make milk taste unpleasant |
| Enoxacin | High concentrations in breast milk in *animals* | Imipramine *see* Antidepressants, Tricyclic | |
| | | Indapamide *see* Thiazides | |
| Ephedrine | Irritability and disturbed sleep reported | Indomethacin | Significant amounts are present in milk; convulsions reported in one infant |
| Ergocalciferol *see* Vitamin D | | | |
| Ergotamine | Avoid where possible; ergotism may occur in infant; repeated doses may inhibit lactation | Insulin | Amount too small to be harmful |
| | | Iodine | Stop breast-feeding; danger of neonatal hypothyroidism or goitre; appears to be concentrated in milk |
| Erythromycin | Only small amounts in milk | | |
| Ethambutol | Amount too small to be harmful | | |
| Ethamsylate | Significant amount but not known to be harmful | Radioactive iodine | Breast-feeding contra-indicated after therapeutic doses. With diagnostic doses withhold breast-feeding for at least 24 hours |
| Ethosuximide | Significant amount; hyperexcitability and poor suckling reported | | |
| | | Iprindole *see* Antidepressants, Tricyclic (and related) | |
| Etretinate | Avoid | Isoniazid | Monitor infant for possible toxicity; theoretical risk of convulsions and neuropathy; prophylactic pyridoxine advisable in mother and infant |
| Famotidine | Amount too small to be harmful | | |
| Fansidar® | Small risk of kernicterus in jaundiced infants and of haemolysis in G6PD-deficient infants (due to sulfadoxine) | | |
| | | Isotretinoin | Avoid |
| | | Ketoprofen | Amount too small to be harmful |
| Fenbufen | Amount too small to be harmful | Ketotifen *see* Antihistamines | |
| | | Labetalol *see* Beta-blockers | |
| Fenoprofen | Amount too small to be harmful | Liothyronine | May interfere with neonatal screening for hypothyroidism |
| Flunitrazepam *see* Benzodiazepines | | | |
| Fluoxetine | Only small amounts in milk but could accumulate in infant | Lithium salts | Monitor infant for possible intoxication; low incidence of adverse effects but increased by continuous ingestion; good control of maternal plasma concentrations minimises the risk |
| Flupenthixol *see* Antipsychotics | | | |
| Fluphenazine *see* Antipsychotics | | | |
| Flurazepam *see* Benzodiazepines | | | |
| Flurbiprofen | Amount too small to be harmful | | |

Table of drugs excreted in breast milk (*continued*)

| Drug | Comments |
|---|---|
| Lofepramine *see* Antidepressants, Tricyclic | |
| Loprazolam *see* Benzodiazepines | |
| Lorazepam *see* Benzodiazepines | |
| Lormetazepam *see* Benzodiazepines | |
| Lymecycline *see* Tetracyclines | |
| Lysuride | May suppress lactation |
| Maloprim® | Haemolytic anaemia (due to dapsone); risk to infant very small |
| Maprotiline *see* Antidepressants, Tricyclic (and related) | |
| Mebeverine | Amount too small to be harmful |
| Mebhydrolin *see* Antihistamines | |
| Medazepam *see* Benzodiazepines | |
| Mefenamic Acid | Amount too small to be harmful |
| Mefruside *see* Thiazides | |
| Meprobamate | Avoid; concentration in milk may exceed maternal plasma concentrations fourfold and may cause drowsiness in infant |
| Mequitazine *see* Antihistamines | |
| Mesalazine | Diarrhoea reported |
| Methadone | Withdrawal symptoms in infant; breast-feeding permissible during maintenance but dose should be as low as possible and baby monitored to avoid sedation |
| Methotrimeprazine *see* Antipsychotics | |
| Methyclothiazide *see* Thiazides | |
| Methyldopa | Amount too small to be harmful |
| Methylprednisolone *see* Corticosteroids | |
| Metoclopramide | Amount probably too small to be harmful |
| Metolazone *see* Thiazides | |
| Metoprolol *see* Beta-blockers | |
| Metronidazole | Significant amount in milk; avoid for 24 hours after large single doses; may give a bitter taste to the milk |
| Mexiletine | Amount too small to be harmful |
| Mianserin *see* Antidepressants, Tricyclic (and related) | |
| Minocycline *see* Tetracyclines | |
| Minoxidil | Significant amount but not known to be harmful |
| Morphine | Therapeutic doses unlikely to affect infant; withdrawal symptoms in infants of dependent mothers; breast-feeding not best method of treating dependence in offspring and should be stopped |
| Nadolol *see* Beta-blockers | |
| Nalidixic Acid | Risk to infant very small but one case of haemolytic anaemia reported |
| Naproxen | Amount too small to be harmful |
| Nefopam | Amount too small to be harmful |

| Drug | Comments |
|---|---|
| Nicoumalone *see* Anticoagulants, Oral | |
| Nifedipine | Amount too small to be harmful |
| Nitrazepam *see* Benzodiazepines | |
| Nitrofurantoin | Only small amounts in milk but could be enough to produce haemolysis in G6PD-deficient infants |
| Nizatidine | Amount too small to be harmful |
| Nortriptyline *see* Antidepressants, Tricyclic | |
| NSAIDs *see* individual entries | |
| Octreotide | Avoid |
| Oestrogens | High doses suppress lactation but *see also* Contraceptives, Oral |
| Opioid Analgesics *see* individual entries | |
| Oxatomide *see* Antihistamines | |
| Oxazepam *see* Benzodiazepines | |
| Oxprenolol *see* Beta-blockers | |
| Oxypertine *see* Antipsychotics | |
| Oxytetracycline *see* Tetracyclines | |
| Paracetamol | Amount too small to be harmful |
| Penbutolol *see* Beta-blockers | |
| Pergolide | May suppress lactation |
| Pericyazine *see* Antipsychotics | |
| Perphenazine *see* Antipsychotics | |
| Phenindamine *see* Antihistamines | |
| Phenindione *see* Anticoagulants, Oral | |
| Pheniramine *see* Antihistamines | |
| Phenobarbitone | Avoid when possible; drowsiness may occur but risk probably small; one report of methaemoglobinaemia with phenobarbitone and phenytoin |
| Phenolphthalein | Avoid; increased gastric motility, diarrhoea, and possibly rash |
| Phenytoin | Amount too small to be harmful |
| Pimozide *see* Antipsychotics | |
| Pindolol *see* Beta-blockers | |
| Pirenzepine | Amount too small to be harmful |
| Piroxicam | Amount too small to be harmful |
| Polythiazide *see* Thiazides | |
| Povidone-iodine | Avoid; iodine absorbed from vaginal preparations is concentrated in milk |
| Prednisolone *see* Corticosteroids | |
| Prednisone *see* Corticosteroids | |
| Primidone *see* Phenobarbitone | |
| Prochlorperazine *see* Antipsychotics | |
| Progestogens | High doses suppress lactation but *see also* Contraceptives, Oral |
| Promazine *see* Antipsychotics | |
| Promethazine *see* Antihistamines | |
| Propranolol *see* Beta-blockers | |

Table of drugs excreted in breast milk (*continued*)

| Drug | Comments | Drug | Comments |
|------|----------|------|----------|
| Propylthiouracil | Monitor infant's thyroid status but amounts in milk probably too small to affect infant; high doses might affect neonatal thyroid function | Theophylline | Irritability in infant reported; modified-release preparations probably safe |
| Protriptyline *see* Antidepressants, Tricyclic | | Thiamine | Severely thiamine-deficient mothers should avoid breast-feeding as toxic methylglyoxal excreted in milk |
| Pseudoephedrine | Amount too small to be harmful | | |
| Pyrazinamide | Amount too small to be harmful | Thiazides | Amount too small to be harmful; large doses may suppress lactation |
| Pyridostigmine | Amount too small to be harmful | | |
| Pyrimethamine | Significant amount but not known to be harmful | Thiethylperazine *see* Antipsychotics | |
| | | Thioridazine *see* Antipsychotics | |
| Quinalbarbitone *see* Barbiturates | | Thyroxine | May interfere with neonatal screening for hypothyroidism |
| Quinidine | Significant amount but not known to be harmful | Tiaprofenic acid | Amount too small to be harmful |
| Ranitidine | Significant amount but not known to be harmful | Timolol *see* Beta-blockers | |
| | | Tolazamide *see* Sulphonylureas | |
| Rifampicin | Amount too small to be harmful | Tolbutamide *see* Sulphonylureas | |
| Senna *see* Anthraquinones | | Tolmetin | Amount too small to be harmful |
| Sodium Valproate *see* Valproate | | | |
| Sotalol *see* Beta-blockers | | Trazodone | Amount too small to be harmful |
| Sulfametopyrazine *see* Sulphonamides | | Triamcinolone *see* Corticosteroids | |
| Sulphadiazine *see* Sulphonamides | | Trifluoperazine *see* Antipsychotics | |
| Sulphadimidine *see* Sulphonamides | | Trifluperidol *see* Antipsychotics | |
| Sulphasalazine | Small amounts in milk but bloody diarrhoea has been reported; theoretical risk of neonatal haemolysis especially in G6PD-deficient infants | Trimeprazine *see* Antihistamines | |
| | | Trimipramine *see* Antidepressants, Tricyclic | |
| | | Triprolidine *see* Antihistamines | |
| | | Valproate | Amount too small to be harmful |
| Sulphonamides | Small risk of kernicterus in jaundiced infants particularly with long-acting sulphonamides, and of haemolysis in G6PD-deficient infants | Verapamil | Amount too small to be harmful |
| | | Viloxazine *see* Antidepressants, Tricyclic (and related) | |
| | | Vitamin A | Theoretical risk of toxicity in infants of mothers taking large doses |
| Sulphonylureas | Caution; theoretical possibility of hypoglycaemia in infant | Vitamin D (and related compounds) | Caution with high doses; may cause hypercalcaemia in infant |
| Sulpiride | Best avoided; significant amounts in milk; *see also* Antipsychotics | Warfarin *see* Anticoagulants, Oral | |
| | | Xipamide *see* Thiazides | |
| Temazepam *see* Benzodiazepines | | Zopiclone | Amount too small to be harmful |
| Terbutaline | Amount too small to be harmful | Zuclopenthixol *see* Antipsychotics | |
| Terfenadine *see* Antihistamines | | | |
| Tetracyclines | Some authorities recommend avoidance but absorption and therefore discoloration of teeth in infant probably prevented by chelation with calcium in milk | | |

# Appendix 6: Intravenous Additives

INTRAVENOUS ADDITIVE POLICIES. A local policy on the addition of drugs to intravenous fluids should be drawn up by a multi-disciplinary team in each Health Authority and issued as a document to the members of staff concerned.

Centralised additive services are provided in a number of hospital pharmacy departments and should be used in preference to making additions on wards.

The information that follows should be read in conjunction with local policy documents.

## Guidelines

1. Drugs should only be added to infusion containers when constant plasma concentrations are needed or when the administration of a more concentrated solution would be harmful.
2. In general, only one drug should be added to any infusion container and the components should be compatible. Ready-prepared solutions should be used whenever possible. Drugs should not normally be added to blood products, mannitol, or sodium bicarbonate. Only specially formulated additives should be used with fat emulsions or amino-acid solutions (see section 9.3).
3. Solutions should be thoroughly mixed by shaking and checked for absence of particulate matter before use.
4. Strict asepsis should be maintained throughout and in general the giving set should not be used for more than 24 hours.
5. The infusion container should be labelled with the patient's name, the name and quantity of additives, and the date and time of addition (and the new expiry date or time). Such additional labelling should not interfere with information on the manufacturer's label that is still valid. When possible, containers should be retained for a period after use in case they are needed for investigation.
6. It is good practice to examine intravenous infusions from time to time while they are running. If cloudiness, crystallisation, change of colour, or any other sign of interaction or contamination is observed the infusion should be discontinued.

## Problems

MICROBIAL CONTAMINATION. The accidental entry and subsequent growth of micro-organisms converts the infusion fluid pathway into a potential vehicle for infection with micro-organisms, particularly species of Candida, Enterobacter, and Klebsiella. Ready-prepared infusions containing the additional drugs, or infusions prepared by an additive service (when available) should therefore be used in preference to making extemporaneous additions to infusion containers on wards etc. However, when this is necessary strict aseptic procedure should be followed.

INCOMPATIBILITY. Physical and chemical incompatibilities may occur with loss of potency, increase in toxicity, or other adverse effect. The solutions may become opalescent or precipitation may occur, but in many instances there is no visual indication of incompatibility. Interaction may take place at any point in the infusion fluid pathway, and the potential for incompatibility is increased when more than one substance is added to the infusion fluid.

**Common incompatibilities.** Precipitation reactions are numerous and varied and may occur as a result of pH, concentration changes, 'salting-out' effects, complexation or other chemical changes. Precipitation or other particle formation must be avoided since, apart from lack of control of dosage on administration, it may initiate or exacerbate adverse effects. This is particularly important in the case of drugs which have been implicated in either thrombophlebitis (e.g. diazepam) or in skin sloughing or necrosis caused by extravasation (e.g. sodium bicarbonate and certain cytotoxic drugs). It is also especially important to effect solution of colloidal drugs and to prevent their subsequent precipitation in order to avoid a pyrogenic reaction (e.g. amphotericin).

It is considered undesirable to mix beta-lactam antibiotics, such as semi-synthetic penicillins and cephalosporins, with proteinaceous materials on the grounds that immunogenic and allergenic conjugates could be formed.

A number of preparations undergo significant loss of potency when added singly or in combination to large volume infusions. Examples include ampicillin in infusions that contain glucose or lactates, mustine hydrochloride in isotonic saline and gentamicin/carbenicillin combinations. The breakdown products of dacarbazine have been implicated in adverse effects.

**Blood.** Because of the large number of incompatibilities, drugs should not normally be added to blood and blood products for infusion purposes. Examples of incompatibility with blood include hypertonic mannitol solutions (irreversible crenation of red cells), dextrans (rouleaux formation and interference with cross-matching), glucose (clumping of red cells), and oxytocin (inactivated).

If the giving set is not changed after the administration of blood, but used for other infusion fluids, a fibrin clot may form which, apart from blocking the set, increases the likelihood of microbial growth.

**Intravenous fat emulsions** may break down with coalescence of fat globules and separation of phases when additions such as antibiotics or electrolytes are made, thus increasing the possibility of embolism. Only specially formulated products such as Vitlipid N® (see section 9.3) may be added to appropriate intravenous fat emulsions.

**Other infusions** that frequently give rise to incompatibility include amino acids, mannitol, and sodium bicarbonate.

**Bactericides** such as chlorocresol 0.1% or

phenylmercuric nitrate 0.001% are present in some injection solutions. The total volume of such solutions added to a container for infusion on one occasion should not exceed 15 mL.

## Method

Ready-prepared infusions should be used whenever available. **Potassium chloride** is usually available in concentrations of 20, 27, and 40 mmol/litre in sodium chloride intravenous infusion (0.9%), glucose intravenous infusion (5%) or sodium chloride and glucose intravenous infusion. **Lignocaine hydrochloride** is usually available in concentrations of 0.1 or 0.2% in glucose intravenous infusion (5%).

When addition is required to be made extemporaneously, any product reconstitution instructions such as those relating to concentration, vehicle, mixing, and handling precautions should be strictly followed using an aseptic technique throughout. Once the product has been reconstituted, addition to the infusion fluid should be made immediately in order to minimise microbial contamination and, with certain products, to prevent degradation or other formulation change which may occur; e.g. reconstituted ampicillin injection degrades rapidly on standing, and also may form polymers which could cause sensitivity reactions.

It is also important in certain instances that an infusion fluid of specific pH be used. **Amphotericin** injection requires dilution in glucose injection of pH greater than 4.2 and **frusemide** injection should be added to infusions of pH greater than 5.5.

When drug additions are made it is important to mix thoroughly; additions should not be made to an infusion container that has been connected to a giving set, as mixing is hampered. If the solutions are not thoroughly mixed a concentrated layer of the additive may form owing to differences in density. **Potassium chloride** is particularly prone to this 'layering' effect when added without adequate mixing to infusions packed in non-rigid infusion containers; if such a mixture is administered it may have a serious effect on the heart.

A time limit between addition and completion of administration must be imposed for certain admixtures to guarantee satisfactory drug potency and compatibility. For admixtures in which degradation occurs without the formation of toxic substances, an acceptable limit is the time taken for 10% decomposition of the drug. When toxic substances are produced stricter limits may be imposed. Because of the risk of microbial contamination a maximum time limit of 12 hours should be imposed for additions made elsewhere than in hospital pharmacies offering central additive service.

Certain injections must be protected from light during continuous infusion to minimise oxidation, e.g. amphotericin, dacarbazine, and sodium nitroprusside.

Dilution with a small volume of an appropriate vehicle and administration using a motorised infusion pump is advocated for preparations such as heparin where strict control over administration is required. In this case the appropriate dose may be dissolved in a convenient volume (e.g. 24 to 48 mL) of sodium chloride intravenous infusion (0.9%).

## Use of table

The table lists preparations given by three methods:

continuous infusion,
intermittent infusion, and
addition *via* the drip tubing.

Drugs for **continuous infusion** must be diluted in a large volume infusion. Penicillins and cephalosporins are not usually given by continuous infusion because of stability problems and because adequate plasma and tissue concentrations are best obtained by intermittent infusion. Where it is necessary to administer them by continuous infusion, detailed literature should be consulted.

Drugs that are both compatible and clinically suitable may be given by **intermittent infusion** in a relatively small volume of infusion over a short period of time, e.g. 100 mL in 30 minutes. The method is used if the product is incompatible or unstable over the period necessary for continuous infusion; the limited stability of ampicillin or amoxycillin in large volume glucose or lactate infusions may be overcome in this way.

Intermittent infusion is also used if adequate plasma and tissue concentrations are not produced by continuous infusion as in the case of drugs such as carbenicillin, dacarbazine, gentamicin, and ticarcillin.

An in-line burette may be used for intermittent infusion techniques in order to achieve strict control over the time and rate of administration, especially for infants and children and in intensive care units. Intermittent infusion may also make use of the 'piggy-back' technique provided that no additions are made to the primary infusion. In this method the drug is added to a small secondary container connected to a Y-type injection site on the primary infusion giving set; the secondary solution is usually infused within 30 minutes.

**Addition *via* the drip tubing** is indicated for a number of cytotoxic drugs in order to minimise extravasation. The preparation is added aseptically *via* the rubber septum of the injection site of a fast-running infusion. In general, drug preparations intended for a bolus effect should be given directly into a separate vein where possible. Failing this, administration may be made *via* the drip tubing provided that the preparation is compatible with the infusion fluid when given in this manner.

Table of drugs given by intravenous infusion
Covers addition to glucose 5 and 10%, Sodium chloride 0.9%, Compound sodium chloride (Ringer's solution), and Compound sodium lactate (Hartmann's solution). Compatibility with glucose 5% and with sodium chloride 0.9% indicates compatibility with any strength of sodium chloride and glucose infusion. Infusion of a large volume of hypotonic solution should be avoided therefore care should be taken if water for injections is used. The information in the Table relates to the proprietary preparations indicated; for other preparations suitability should be checked with the manufacturer

| Drug | Infusion method |
|---|---|
| **Acetylcysteine** | Continuous *in* |
| *Parvolex*® | Glucose 5% |
| See Emergency Treatment of Poisoning | |
| **Aclarubicin hydrochloride** | Intermittent *in* Glucose 5% *or* |
| *Aclacin*® | Sodium chloride 0.9% |

Dissolve initially in 10 mL water for injections or sodium chloride 0.9% then dilute with 200–500 mL infusion fluid to a concentration of 200–500 micrograms/mL; give over 30–60 minutes and protect from light during administration; pH of glucose infusion should be between 5 and 6

| | |
|---|---|
| **Acyclovir sodium** | Intermittent *in* Sodium chloride 0.9% *or* |
| *Zovirax IV*® | Sodium chloride and glucose *or* Compound sodium lactate |

Initially reconstitute to 25 mg/mL in water for injections or sodium chloride 0.9% then dilute to not more than 5 mg/mL with the infusion fluid; minimum volume 50 mL; to be given over 1 hour

| | |
|---|---|
| **Alfentanil hydrochloride** | Continuous *or* intermittent *in* |
| *Rapifen*® | Glucose 5% *or* |
| *preparations* | Sodium chloride 0.9% *or* Compound sodium lactate |
| **Alprostadil** | Continuous *in* |
| *Prostin VR*® | Glucose 5% *or* Sodium chloride 0.9% |
| **Amikacin sulphate** | Intermittent *in* Glucose 5% *or* |
| *Amikin*® | Sodium chloride 0.9% *or* Compound sodium lactate |
| To be given over 30 minutes | |
| **Aminophylline** | Continuous *in* Glucose 5% *or* Sodium chloride 0.9% *or* Compound sodium lactate |
| **Amiodarone hydrochloride** | Continuous *or* intermittent *in* |
| *Cordarone X*® | Glucose 5% |

Suggested initial infusion volume 250 mL given over 20–120 minutes; for repeat infusions up to 1.2 g in a maximum volume of 500 mL; incompatible with sodium chloride infusion

| Drug | Infusion method |
|---|---|
| **Amoxycillin sodium** | [1]Intermittent *in* Glucose 5% *or* |
| *Amoxil*® | Sodium chloride 0.9% |

Reconstituted solutions diluted and given without delay; suggested volume 100 mL given over 30–60 minutes

|  |  |
|---|---|
|  | *via* drip tubing *in* Glucose 5% *or* Sodium chloride 0.9% *or* Ringer's solution *or* Compound sodium lactate |
| **Amphotericin (liposomal)** | Intermittent *in* |
| *AmBisome*® | Glucose 5% |

Reconstitute each vial with 12 mL water for injections (both vial and water for injections should be cooled to 2–8°C before reconstitution) and shake vigorously; incubate reconstituted vial at 65°C for 10 minutes and allow to cool to room temperature; withdraw requisite dose from vial and introduce into infusion fluid through the 5 micron filter provided to produce a final concentration of 500 micrograms/mL; infuse over 30–60 minutes; incompatible with sodium chloride solutions, flush existing intravenous line with glucose 5% or use separate line

| | |
|---|---|
| **Amphotericin sodium deoxycholate complex** | Continuous *in* Glucose 5% |
| *Fungizone*® | |

Dissolve thoroughly at reconstitution stage; preparation must be diluted in a large volume infusion; pH of the glucose must not be below 4.2 (check each container); protect from light; suggested infusion time 6 hours

| | |
|---|---|
| **Ampicillin sodium** | [1]Intermittent *in* Glucose 5% *or* |
| *Penbritin*® | Sodium chloride 0.9% |

Reconstituted solutions diluted and given without delay; suggested volume 100 mL given over 30–60 minutes

|  |  |
|---|---|
|  | *via* drip tubing *in* Glucose 5% *or* Sodium chloride 0.9% *or* Ringer's solution *or* Compound sodium lactate |
| **Ampicillin/cloxacillin (sodium salts)** | Intermittent *in* Glucose 5% *or* |
| *Ampiclox*® | Sodium chloride 0.9% |

Reconstituted solutions diluted and given without delay; suggested volume 100 mL given over 30–60 minutes

|  |  |
|---|---|
|  | *via* drip tubing *in* Glucose 5% *or* Sodium chloride 0.9% *or* Ringer's solution *or* Compound sodium lactate |

1. Continuous infusion not usually recommended

| Drug | Infusion method |
|------|-----------------|
| **Ampicillin/sulbactam (sodium salts)**<br>*Dicapen®* | [1]Intermittent *in* Glucose 5% *or* Sodium chloride 0.9% *or* Water for injections<br>Reconstituted solutions diluted and given without delay; give over 15–30 minutes |
| **Amsacrine**<br>*Amsidine®* | Intermittent *in* Glucose 5%<br>Reconstitute with diluent provided and dilute to suggested volume 500 mL; give over 60–90 minutes; use glass syringes; incompatible with sodium chloride infusion |
| **Ancrod**<br>*Arvin®* | Continuous *in* Sodium chloride 0.9%<br>Suggested volume 50–500 mL given over 4–12 hours |
| **Atenolol**<br>*Tenormin®* | Intermittent *in* Glucose 5% *or* Sodium chloride 0.9%<br>Suggested infusion time 20 minutes |
| **Atracurium besylate**<br>*Tracrium®* | Continuous *in* Glucose 5% *or* Sodium chloride 0.9% *or* Compound sodium lactate<br>Stability varies with diluent |
| **Azathioprine**<br>*Imuran®* | *via* drip tubing *in* Glucose 5% *or* Sodium chloride 0.9%<br>Reconstituted solutions should be administered without delay |
| **Azlocillin sodium**<br>*Securopen®* (5 g) | Intermittent *in* Glucose 5 and 10% *or* Sodium chloride 0.9% *or* Ringer's solution<br>Intermittent infusion suggested for doses over 2 g; to be given over 20–30 minutes |
| **Aztreonam**<br>*Azactam®* | Intermittent *in* Glucose 5% *or* Sodium chloride 0.9% *or* Ringer's solution *or* Compound sodium lactate<br>Dissolve initially in water for injections (1 g per 3 mL) then dilute to a concentration of less than 20 mg/mL; to be given over 20–60 minutes |
| **Benzylpenicillin sodium**<br>*Crystapen®* | [1]Intermittent *in* Glucose 5% *or* Sodium chloride 0.9%<br>Suggested volume 100 mL given over 30–60 minutes |
| **Betamethasone sodium phosphate**<br>*Betnesol®* | Continuous *or* intermittent *or* *via* drip tubing *in* Glucose 5% *or* Sodium chloride 0.9% |
| **Bleomycin sulphate** | Intermittent *in* Sodium chloride 0.9%<br>To be given slowly; suggested volume 200 mL |
| **Bumetanide**<br>*Burinex®* | Intermittent *in* Glucose 5% *or* Sodium chloride 0.9%<br>Suggested volume 500 mL given over 30–60 minutes |

| Drug | Infusion method |
|------|-----------------|
| **Calcium gluconate** | Continuous *in* Glucose 5% *or* Sodium chloride 0.9%<br>Avoid bicarbonates, phosphates, or sulphates |
| **Carbenicillin sodium**<br>*Pyopen®* | Intermittent *in* Glucose 5% *or* Water for injections<br>Suggested volume 100 mL given over 30–40 minutes |
| **Carboplatin**<br>*Paraplatin®* | Continuous *in* Glucose 5% *or* Sodium chloride 0.9%<br>Final concentration as low as 500 micrograms/mL; give over 15–60 minutes |
| **Carmustine**<br>*BiCNU®* | Intermittent *in* Glucose 5% *or* Sodium chloride 0.9%<br>Reconstitute with diluent provided; give over 1–2 hours |
| **Cefotaxime sodium**<br>*Claforan®* | Intermittent *in* Glucose 5% *or* Sodium chloride 0.9% *or* Compound sodium lactate *or* Water for injections<br>Suggested volume 40–100 mL given over 20–60 minutes |
| **Cefoxitin sodium**<br>*Mefoxin®* | [1]Intermittent *or* *via* drip tubing *in* Glucose 5 and 10% *or* Sodium chloride 0.9% |
| **Cefsulodin sodium**<br>*Monaspor®* | [1]Intermittent *or* *via* drip tubing *in* Glucose 5% *or* Sodium chloride 0.9% |
| **Ceftazidime pentahydrate**<br>*Fortum®* | Intermittent *or* *via* drip tubing *in* Glucose 5 and 10% *or* Sodium chloride 0.9% *or* Compound sodium lactate *or* Water for injections |
| **Ceftizoxime sodium**<br>*Cefizox®* | Continuous *or* intermittent *or* *via* drip tubing *in* Glucose 5 and 10% *or* Sodium chloride 0.9% *or* Ringer's solution *or* Compound sodium lactate<br>Suggested volume 50–100 mL |
| **Cefuroxime sodium**<br>*Zinacef®* | Intermittent *or* *via* drip tubing *in* Glucose 5% *or* Sodium chloride 0.9% *or* Compound sodium lactate<br>Suggested volume 50–100 mL given over 30 minutes |
| **Cephamandole nafate**<br>*Kefadol®* | [1]Intermittent *or* *via* drip tubing *in* Glucose 5 and 10% *or* Sodium chloride 0.9% *or* Water for injections |

1. Continuous infusion not usually recommended

| Drug | Infusion method | Drug | Infusion method |
|------|-----------------|------|-----------------|
| **Cephazolin sodium**<br>*Kefzol*® | [1]Intermittent *or*<br>*via* drip tubing *in*<br>Glucose 5 and 10% *or*<br>Sodium chloride 0.9% *or*<br>Compound sodium<br>lactate *or*<br>Water for injections | **Co-amoxiclav**<br>*Augmentin*® | Intermittent *in*<br>Sodium chloride 0.9% *or*<br>Water for injections;<br>see also package leaflet |
| | | Suggested volume 50–100 mL given over 30–40 minutes and completed within 2 hours of reconstitution | |
| **Cephradine**<br>*Velosef*® | Continuous *or*<br>intermittent *in*<br>Glucose 5 and 10% *or*<br>Sodium chloride 0.9% *or*<br>Ringer's solution *or*<br>Compound sodium<br>lactate *or*<br>Water for injections | | *via* drip tubing *in*<br>Glucose 5% *or*<br>Sodium chloride 0.9% |
| | | **Co-fluampicil<br>(sodium salts)**<br>*Magnapen*® | Intermittent *in*<br>Glucose 5% *or*<br>Sodium chloride 0.9% |
| Reconstituted solutions diluted and given without delay; max. 8 hours between addition and completion of administration | | Reconstituted solutions diluted and given without delay; suggested volume 100 mL given over 30–60 minutes | |
| **Chloramphenicol<br>sodium succinate**<br>*Kemicetine*® | Intermittent *or*<br>*via* drip tubing *in*<br>Glucose 5% *or*<br>Sodium chloride 0.9% | | *via* drip tubing *in*<br>Glucose 5% *or*<br>Sodium chloride 0.9% *or*<br>Ringer's solution *or*<br>Compound sodium<br>lactate |
| **Chloroquine<br>sulphate**<br>*Nivaquine*®<br>See also section 5.4.1 | Continuous *in*<br>Sodium chloride 0.9% | **Colistin<br>sulphomethate sodium**<br>*Colomycin*® | Continuous *or*<br>intermittent *in*<br>Glucose 5% *or*<br>Sodium chloride 0.9% *or*<br>Ringer's solution |
| **Cimetidine**<br>*Tagamet*® | Continuous *or*<br>intermittent *in*<br>Glucose 5% *or*<br>Sodium chloride 0.9% | Max. 6 hours between addition and completion of administration | |
| For intermittent infusion suggested volume 100 mL given over 30–60 minutes | | **Co-trimoxazole**<br>*Septrin*® for<br>infusion | Continuous *in*<br>Glucose 5 and 10% *or*<br>Sodium chloride 0.9% *or*<br>Ringer's solution |
| **Cisplatin** | Continuous *in*<br>Sodium chloride 0.9% *or*<br>Sodium chloride and<br>glucose | Dilute contents of 1 ampoule (5 mL) to 125 mL, 2 ampoules (10 mL) to 250 mL or 3 ampoules (15 mL) to 500 mL; if fluid restriction necessary, 1 ampoule may be diluted with 75 mL glucose 5% | |
| Suggested volume 1 litre given over 6–8 hours | | **Cyclophosphamide**<br>*Endoxana*® | Intermittent *or*<br>*via* drip tubing *in*<br>Water for injections |
| **Clindamycin<br>phosphate**<br>*Dalacin C*® | Continuous *or*<br>intermittent *in*<br>Glucose 5% *or*<br>Sodium chloride 0.9% | For intermittent infusion suggested volume 50–100 mL given over 5–15 minutes; max. 30 minutes between addition and completion of administration | |
| Dilute to a concentration of 300 mg in 50 mL; give each 300 mg over at least 10 minutes (1.2 g over at least 45 minutes) | | | *via* drip tubing *in*<br>Glucose 5% |
| **Clomipramine**<br>*Anafranil*® | Intermittent *in*<br>Glucose 5% *or*<br>Sodium chloride 0.9% | **Cyclosporin**<br>*Sandimmun*® | Continuous *in*<br>Glucose 5% *or*<br>Sodium chloride 0.9% |
| Suggested volume 125–500 mL given over 45–120 minutes | | Dilute to a concentration of 50 mg in 20–100 mL; give over 2–6 hours | |
| **Clonazepam**<br>*Rivotril*® | Intermittent *in*<br>Glucose 5 and 10% *or*<br>Sodium chloride 0.9% | **Cytarabine**<br>*Alexan*®,<br>*Cytosar*® | Continuous *or*<br>intermittent *or*<br>*via* drip tubing *in*<br>Glucose 5% *or*<br>Sodium chloride 0.9% |
| Suggested volume 250 mL | | Reconstitute *Cytosar*® with the diluent provided; check container for haze or precipitate during administration | |
| **Cloxacillin sodium**<br>*Orbenin*® | [1]Intermittent *in*<br>Glucose 5% *or*<br>Sodium chloride 0.9% | | |
| Suggested volume 100 mL given over 30–60 minutes | | **Dacarbazine**<br>*DTIC-Dome*® | Intermittent *in*<br>Glucose 5% *or*<br>Sodium chloride 0.9% |
| | *via* drip tubing *in*<br>Glucose 5% *or*<br>Sodium chloride 0.9% *or*<br>Ringer's solution *or*<br>Compound sodium<br>lactate | Suggested volume 125–250 mL given over 15–30 minutes; protect infusion from light | |

1. Continuous infusion not usually recommended

| Drug | Infusion method | Drug | Infusion method |
|---|---|---|---|

**Dactinomycin**  
*Cosmegen*  
*Lyovac®*  
*via* drip tubing *in* Glucose 5% *or* Sodium chloride 0.9%  
Reconstitute with water for injections

**Desferrioxamine mesylate**  
*Desferal®*  
Continuous *or* intermittent *in* Glucose 5% *or* Sodium chloride 0.9%

**Dexamethasone sodium phosphate**  
*Decadron®,*  
*Dexamethasone* (Organon)  
Continuous *or* intermittent *or* *via* drip tubing *in* Glucose 5% *or* Sodium chloride 0.9%  
*Dexamethasone* (Organon) can also be infused in Glucose 10% *or* Ringer's solution *or* Compound sodium lactate

**Diazepam (solution)**  
*Valium®*  
Continuous *in* Glucose 5% *or* Sodium chloride 0.9%  
Dilute to a concentration of not more than 40 mg in 500 mL; max. 6 hours between addition and completion of administration; adsorbed to some extent by the plastics of the infusion set

**Diazepam (emulsion)**  
*Diazemuls®*  
Continuous *in* Glucose 5 and 10%  
May be diluted to a max. concentration of 200 mg in 500 mL; max. 6 hours between addition and completion of administration; adsorbed to some extent by the plastics of the infusion set

*via* drip tubing *in* Glucose 5 and 10% *or* Sodium chloride 0.9%  
Adsorbed to some extent by the plastics of the infusion set

**Digoxin**  
*Lanoxin®*  
Continuous *in* Glucose 5% *or* Sodium chloride 0.9%  
To be given slowly; see also section 2.1.1

**Digoxin-specific antibody fragments**  
*Digibind®*  
Intermittent *in* Sodium chloride 0.9%  
Dissolve initially in water for injections (4 mL/vial) then dilute with the sodium chloride 0.9% and give through a 0.22 micron sterile, disposable filter over 20 minutes

**Dinoprostone**  
*Prostin E2®*  
Continuous *or* intermittent *in* Glucose 5% *or* Sodium chloride 0.9%

**Disodium etidronate**  
*Didronel IV®*  
Continuous *in* Sodium chloride 0.9%  
Dilute in large-volume infusion, suggested minimum volume 250 mL; minimum period of infusion 2 hours

**Disodium pamidronate**  
*Aredia®*  
Continuous *in* Glucose 5% *or* Sodium chloride 0.9%  
Dilute to a concentration of 15 mg in 125 mL and give each 15 mg over at least 1 hour; not to be given with infusion fluids containing calcium

**Disopyramide phosphate**  
*Rythmodan®*  
Continuous *or* intermittent *in* Glucose 5% *or* Sodium chloride 0.9% *or* Ringer's solution *or* Compound sodium lactate  
Max. rate by continuous infusion 20–30 mg/hour (or 400 micrograms/kg/hour)

**Dobutamine hydrochloride**  
*Dobutrex® Solution*  
Continuous *in* Glucose 5% *or* Sodium chloride 0.9%  
Dilute to a concentration of 0.5–1 mg/mL; give higher concentration (max. 5 mg/mL) with infusion pump; incompatible with bicarbonate

**Dopamine hydrochloride**  
*Intropin®*  
Continuous *in* Glucose 5% *or* Sodium chloride 0.9% *or* Compound sodium lactate  
Dilute to a concentration of 1.6 mg/mL; incompatible with bicarbonate

**Dopexamine hydrochloride**  
*Dopacard®*  
Continuous *in* Glucose 5% *or* Sodium chloride 0.9%  
Dilute to a concentration of 400 or 800 micrograms/mL; give *via* infusion pump or other device which provides accurate control of rate; contact with metal should be minimised; incompatible with bicarbonate

**Doxorubicin hydrochloride**  
*Doxorubicin Rapid Dissolution,*  
*Doxorubicin Solution*  
(both Farmitalia Carlo Erba)  
*via* drip tubing *in* Glucose 5% *or* Sodium chloride 0.9%  
Reconstitute *Doxorubicin Rapid Dissolution* with water for injections or sodium chloride 0.9% (10 mg in 5 mL, 50 mg in 25 mL); give over 2–3 minutes

**Electrolytes**  
*Addiphos®*  
Continuous *in* Glucose 5 and 10%  
Suggested volume 500 mL

**Enoximone**  
*Perfan®*  
Continuous *or* intermittent *in* Sodium chloride 0.9% *or* Water for injections  
Dilute to a concentration of 2.5 mg/mL; incompatible with glucose solutions; use only plastic containers or syringes

**Epirubicin hydrochloride**  
*Pharmorubicin® Rapid Dissolution*  
*Pharmorubicin® Solution*  
*via* drip tubing *in* Sodium chloride 0.9%  
Reconstitute *Pharmorubicin® Rapid Dissolution* with sodium chloride 0.9% or with water for injections (10 mg in 5 mL, 20 mg in 10 mL, 50 mg in 25 mL); give over 3–5 minutes

1. Continuous infusion not usually recommended

| Drug | Infusion method |
|------|-----------------|
| **Epoprostenol** *Flolan*® | Intermittent *in* Sodium chloride 0.9% |

Reconstitute with the diluent provided (pH 10.5) to make a concentrate; use this concentrate within 12 hours and store at 2°–8°C; dilute with not more than 6 times the volume of sodium chloride 0.9% before use

| **Erythromycin lactobionate** *Erythrocin*® | Continuous *or* intermittent *in* Glucose 5% (neutralised with sodium bicarbonate) *or* Sodium chloride 0.9% *or* Compound sodium lactate |

Dissolve initially in water for injections (1 g in 20 mL) then dilute to a concentration of 1 mg/mL for continuous infusion and 1–5 mg/mL for intermittent infusion

| **Ethacrynic acid (sodium salt)** *Edecrin*® | *via* drip tubing *in* Glucose 5% *or* Sodium chloride 0.9% |

pH of glucose infusion should be adjusted to above 5

| **Ethanol** | Continuous *in* Glucose 5% *or* Sodium chloride 0.9% *or* Ringer's solution *or* Compound sodium lactate |

Dilute to a concentration of 5–10%

| **Etoposide** *Vepesid*® | Intermittent *in* Sodium chloride 0.9% |

Dilute to a concentration of not more than 250 micrograms/mL and give over not less than 30 minutes and not more than 6 hours; check container for haze or precipitate during administration; may dissolve certain types of filter

| **Filgrastim** *Neupogen*® | Intermittent *in* Glucose 5% |

For a filgrastim concentration of less than 1 500 000 units/mL (15 micrograms/mL) albumin solution (human serum albumin) is added to produce a final albumin concentration of 2 mg/mL; should not be diluted to a filgrastim concentration of less than 200 000 units/mL (2 micrograms/mL) and should not be diluted with sodium chloride solution

| **Flecainide acetate** *Tambocor*® | Continuous *or* intermittent *in* Glucose 5% *or* Sodium chloride 0.9% *or* Compound sodium lactate |

Minimum volume in infusion fluids containing chlorides 500 mL

| **Flucloxacillin sodium** *Floxapen*® | [1]Intermittent *in* Glucose 5% *or* Sodium chloride 0.9% |

Suggested volume 100 mL given over 30–60 minutes

| | *via* drip tubing *in* Glucose 5% *or* Sodium chloride 0.9% *or* Ringer's solution *or* Compound sodium lactate |

| **Flumazenil** *Anexate*® | Continuous *in* Glucose 5% *or* Sodium chloride 0.9% |

| **Fluorouracil sodium** | Continuous *or* *via* drip tubing *in* Glucose 5% |

For continuous infusion suggested volume 500 mL given over 4 hours

| **Folinic acid (calcium salt)** *Calcium Leucovorin*®, *Refolinon*® | Continuous *in* Sodium chloride 0.9% |

*Calcium Leucovorin*® can also be infused in Glucose 5 and 10% *or* Compound sodium lactate

| **Foscarnet trisodium** *Foscavir*® | Continuous *in* Glucose 5% |

Dilute to a concentration of 12 mg/mL or less for infusion into peripheral vein (undiluted solution *via* central venous line only)

| **Frusemide (sodium salt)** *Lasix*® | Continuous *in* Sodium chloride 0.9% *or* Ringer's solution |

Infusion pH must be above 5.5; glucose solutions are unsuitable

| **Fusidic acid (diethanolamine salt)** *Fucidin*® | Continuous *in* Glucose 5% (but see below) *or* Sodium chloride 0.9% |

Reconstitute with the buffer solution provided and dilute to a max. concentration of diethanolamine fusidate 1.16 mg/mL (= sodium fusidate 1 mg/mL); to be given over not less than 6 hours; incompatible if glucose solution too acidic

| **Ganciclovir (sodium salt)** *Cymevene*® | Intermittent *in* Glucose 5% *or* Sodium chloride 0.9% *or* Ringer's solution *or* Compound sodium lactate |

Reconstitute initially in water for injections (500 mg/ 10 mL) then dilute to not more than 10 mg/mL with infusion fluid (usually 100 mL); infuse over 1 hour

| **Gentamicin sulphate** *Cidomycin*® | Intermittent *or* *via* drip tubing *in* Glucose 5% *or* Sodium chloride 0.9% |

Suggested volume for intermittent infusion 50–100 mL given over 20 minutes

| **Glyceryl trinitrate** *Nitrocine*®, *Nitronal*®, *Tridil*® | Continuous *in* Glucose 5% *or* Sodium chloride 0.9% |

For *Tridil*® dilute to a concentration of not more than 400 micrograms/mL; for *Nitrocine*® suggested infusion concentration 100 micrograms/mL; incompatible with polyvinyl chloride infusion containers such as Viaflex® or Steriflex®; use glass or polyethylene containers or give *via* a syringe pump

---

1. Continuous infusion not usually recommended

| Drug | Infusion method |
|------|-----------------|
| **Granisetron hydrochloride** *Kytril*® | Intermittent *in* Glucose 5% *or* Sodium chloride 0.9% *or* Compound sodium lactate |

Dilute 3 mL in 20–50 mL infusion fluid and give over 5 minutes

| | |
|------|-----------------|
| **HA-1A** *Centoxin*® | Single infusion *in* Sodium chloride 0.9% |

Inject solution (20 mL) through a 0.2 or 0.22 micron sterile, low protein binding filter into 50 mL infusion fluid; give over 15–30 minutes

| | |
|------|-----------------|
| **Heparin sodium** | Continuous *in* Glucose 5% *or* Sodium chloride 0.9% |

Administration with a motorised pump may be advisable

| | |
|------|-----------------|
| **Hydralazine hydrochloride** *Apresoline*® | Continuous *in* Sodium chloride 0.9% *or* Ringer's solution |

Suggested infusion volume 500 mL

| | |
|------|-----------------|
| **Hydrocortisone sodium phosphate** *Efcortesol*® | Continuous *or* intermittent *or* *via* drip tubing *in* Glucose 5% *or* Sodium chloride 0.9% |

| | |
|------|-----------------|
| **Hydrocortisone sodium succinate** *Efcortelan Soluble*®, *Solu-Cortef*® | Continuous *or* intermittent *or* *via* drip tubing *in* Glucose 5% *or* Sodium chloride 0.9% |

| | |
|------|-----------------|
| **Idarubicin hydrochloride** *Zavedos*® | *via* drip tubing *in* Sodium chloride 0.9% |

Reconstitute with water for injections; give over 5–10 minutes

| | |
|------|-----------------|
| **Ifosfamide** *Mitoxana*® | Continuous *or* intermittent *or* *via* drip tubing *in* Glucose 5% *or* Sodium chloride 0.9% |

For continuous infusion, suggested volume 3 litres given over 24 hours; for intermittent infusion, give over 30–120 minutes

| | |
|------|-----------------|
| **Imipenem/cilastatin (sodium salt)** *Primaxin*® | [1]Intermittent *in* Glucose 5% *or* Sodium chloride 0.9% *or* Water for injections |

Dilute to a concentration of 5 mg (as imipenem)/mL; infuse 250–500 mg (as imipenem) over 20–30 minutes, 1 g over 40–60 minutes

| | |
|------|-----------------|
| **Insulin (soluble)** | Continuous *in* Sodium chloride 0.9% *or* Compound sodium lactate |

Adsorbed to some extent by plastics of infusion set; see also section 6.1.3; ensure insulin is not injected into 'dead space' of injection port of the infusion bag

| | |
|------|-----------------|
| **Iron dextran** *Imferon*® | Intermittent *in* Glucose 5% *or* Sodium chloride 0.9% |

Suggested volume 500 mL

| Drug | Infusion method |
|------|-----------------|
| **Isoprenaline hydrochloride** *Saventrine IV*® | Continuous *in* Glucose 5% *or* Sodium chloride and glucose |

Dilute in a large-volume infusion; suggested minimum volume 500 mL; pH of the infusion must be below 5.

| | |
|------|-----------------|
| **Isosorbide dinitrate** *Cedocard IV*®, *Isoket 0.05%*®, *Isoket 0.1%*® | Continuous *in* Glucose 5% *or* Sodium chloride 0.9% |

Adsorbed to some extent by polyvinyl chloride infusion containers; preferably use glass or polyethylene containers or give *via* a syringe pump; *Isoket 0.05%*® can alternatively be administered undiluted using a syringe pump with a glass or rigid plastic syringe

| | |
|------|-----------------|
| **Isoxsuprine hydrochloride** *Duvadilan*® | Continuous *in* Glucose 5% *or* Sodium chloride 0.9% |

Suggested infusion concentration 0.02%

| | |
|------|-----------------|
| **Kanamycin sulphate** *Kannasyn*® | Intermittent *in* Glucose 5% *or* Sodium chloride 0.9% |

Dilute to 2.5 mg/mL and give at a rate of 3–4 mL/minute

| | |
|------|-----------------|
| **Ketamine hydrochloride** *Ketalar*® | Continuous *in* Glucose 5% *or* Sodium chloride 0.9% |

Dilute to 1 mg/mL; microdrip infusion for maintenance of anaesthesia

| | |
|------|-----------------|
| **Labetalol hydrochloride** *Trandate*® | Intermittent *in* Glucose 5% *or* Sodium chloride and glucose |

Dilute to a concentration of 1 mg/mL; suggested volume 200 mL; adjust rate with in-line burette

| | |
|------|-----------------|
| **Lignocaine hydrochloride** *Xylocard 20%*® | Continuous *in* Glucose 5% *or* Sodium chloride 0.9% *or* Ringer's solution |

Suggested infusion concentration 0.2%; use ready-prepared solution when available

| | |
|------|-----------------|
| **Lincomycin hydrochloride** *Lincocin*® | Continuous *in* Glucose 5% *or* Sodium chloride 0.9% |

Suggested minimum volume 250 mL; minimum period of infusion 1 hour

| | |
|------|-----------------|
| **Mecillinam** *Selexidin*® | Intermittent *in* Glucose 5% *or* Sodium chloride 0.9% |

Reconstituted solutions diluted and given without delay; suggested infusion time 15–30 minutes

| | |
|------|-----------------|
| **Melphalan** *Alkeran*® | Continuous *or* *via* drip tubing *in* Sodium chloride 0.9% |

Reconstitute with the solvent and diluent provided then dilute with infusion fluid; max. 2 hours between addition and completion of administration

| | |
|------|-----------------|
| **Mesna** *Uromitexan*® | Continuous *or* *via* drip tubing *in* Glucose 5% *or* Sodium chloride 0.9% |

Max. 24 hours between addition and completion of administration

1. Continuous infusion not usually recommended

| Drug | Infusion method | Drug | Infusion method |
|------|-----------------|------|-----------------|
| **Metaraminol tartrate**<br>Aramine® | Continuous *or*<br>*via* drip tubing *in*<br>Glucose 5% *or*<br>Sodium chloride 0.9% *or*<br>Ringer's solution *or*<br>Compound sodium<br>lactate<br>Suggested infusion volume 500 mL | **Miconazole**<br>Daktarin® | Continuous *or*<br>intermittent *in*<br>Glucose 5% *or*<br>Sodium chloride 0.9%<br>Minimum period of infusion 30 minutes; for<br>intermittent infusion suggested volume 200–500 mL |
| **Methicillin sodium**<br>Celbenin® | ¹Intermittent *in*<br>Glucose 5% *or*<br>Sodium chloride 0.9%<br>Suggested volume 100 mL given over 30–60 minutes<br><br>*via* drip tubing *in*<br>Glucose 5% *or*<br>Sodium chloride 0.9% *or*<br>Ringer's solution *or*<br>Compound sodium<br>lactate | **Milrinone**<br>Primacor® | Continuous *in*<br>Glucose 5% *or*<br>Sodium chloride 0.9%<br>Dilute to a suggested concentration of 200<br>micrograms/mL |
| | | **Mitozantrone<br>hydrochloride**<br>Novantrone® | *via* drip tubing *in*<br>Glucose 5% *or*<br>Sodium chloride 0.9%<br>Suggested volume at least 50 mL given over at least 3–<br>5 minutes |
| **Methocarbamol**<br>Robaxin® | Intermittent *in*<br>Glucose 5% *or*<br>Sodium chloride 0.9%<br>Dilute to a concentration of not less than 1 g in<br>250 mL | **Mustine<br>hydrochloride**<br>(Boots) | *via* drip tubing *in*<br>Glucose 5% *or*<br>Sodium chloride 0.9% |
| **Methotrexate<br>sodium**<br>Methotrexate<br>(Lederle) | Continuous *or*<br>*via* drip tubing *in*<br>Glucose 5% *or*<br>Sodium chloride 0.9% *or*<br>Compound sodium<br>lactate *or*<br>Ringer's solution<br>Dilute in a large-volume infusion; max. 24 hours<br>between addition and completion of administration | **Naftidrofuryl oxalate**<br>Praxilene Forte® | Intermittent *in*<br>Glucose 5 and 10% *or*<br>Sodium chloride 0.9%<br>Suggested volume 250–500 mL given over 90–120<br>minutes |
| | | **Naloxone**<br>Min-I-Jet® Naloxone<br>Hydrochloride,<br>Narcan® | Continuous *in*<br>Glucose 5% *or*<br>Sodium chloride 0.9%<br>Dilute to a concentration of 4 micrograms/mL |
| **Methyldopa<br>hydrochloride**<br>Aldomet® | Intermittent *in*<br>Glucose 5%<br>Suggested volume 100 mL given over 30–60 minutes | **Netilmicin sulphate**<br>Netillin® | Intermittent *or*<br>*via* drip tubing *in*<br>Glucose 5 and 10% *or*<br>Sodium chloride 0.9%<br>For intermittent infusion suggested volume 50–200 mL<br>given over 90–120 minutes |
| **Methylprednisolone<br>sodium succinate**<br>Solu-Medrone® | Continuous *or*<br>intermittent *or*<br>*via* drip tubing *in*<br>Glucose 5% *or*<br>Sodium chloride 0.9% | **Nimodipine**<br>Nimotop® | *via* drip tubing *in*<br>Glucose 5% *or*<br>Sodium chloride 0.9% *or*<br>Ringer's solution<br>Not to be added to infusion container; administer *via*<br>an infusion pump through a Y-piece into a central<br>catheter; incompatible with polyvinyl chloride giving<br>sets or containers |
| **Metoclopramide<br>hydrochloride**<br>Maxolon High<br>Dose® | Continuous *or*<br>intermittent *in*<br>Glucose 5% *or*<br>Sodium chloride 0.9% *or*<br>Compound sodium<br>lactate<br>Loading dose, dilute with 50–100 mL and give over<br>15–30 minutes; maintenance dose, dilute with 500 mL<br>and give over 8–12 hours; for intermittent infusion<br>dilute with at least 50 mL and give over at least 15<br>minutes | **Noradrenaline solution<br>strong sterile**<br>Levophed® | Continuous *in*<br>Glucose 5% *or*<br>Sodium chloride and<br>glucose<br>Dilute in a large-volume infusion; pH of the infusion<br>solution must be below 6 |
| | | **Ondansetron<br>hydrochloride**<br>Zofran® | Continuous *or*<br>intermittent *in*<br>Glucose 5% *or*<br>Sodium chloride 0.9% *or*<br>Ringer's solution |
| **Mexiletine<br>hydrochloride**<br>Mexitil® | Continuous *in*<br>Glucose 5% *or*<br>Sodium chloride 0.9% | **Oxytocin**<br>Syntocinon® | Continuous *in*<br>Glucose 5% *or*<br>Sodium chloride 0.9% *or*<br>Ringer's solution<br>Dilute in a large-volume infusion |
| **Mezlocillin sodium**<br>Baypen® (5 g) | Intermittent *in*<br>Glucose 5 and 10% *or*<br>Sodium chloride 0.9% *or*<br>Ringer's solution *or*<br>Water for injections<br>Suggested volume 50 mL given over 15–20 minutes | | |

---

1. Continuous infusion not usually recommended

| Drug | Infusion method |
|------|-----------------|
| **Pentamidine isethionate** *Pentacarinat*® | Intermittent *in* Glucose 5% *or* Sodium chloride 0.9% |

Dissolve initially in water for injections (300 mg in 3–5 mL) then dilute in 50–250 mL; give over at least 60 minutes

| | |
|------|-----------------|
| **Phenoxybenzamine hydrochloride** *Dibenyline*® | Intermittent *in* Sodium chloride 0.9% |

Dilute in 200–500 mL infusion; give over at least 2 hours; max. 4 hours between dilution and completion of administration

| | |
|------|-----------------|
| **Phentolamine mesylate** *Rogitine*® | Intermittent *in* Glucose 5% *or* Sodium chloride 0.9% |
| **Phenylephrine hydrochloride** | Intermittent *in* Glucose 5% *or* Sodium chloride 0.9% |
| **Piperacillin sodium** *Pipril*® | Intermittent *in* Glucose 5% *or* Sodium chloride 0.9% *or* Compound sodium lactate *or* Water for injections |

Minimum volume 50 mL given over 20–40 minutes

| | |
|------|-----------------|
| **Plicamycin** *Mithracin*® | Continuous *in* Glucose 5% *or* Sodium chloride 0.9% |

Reconstitute 2.5 mg with 4.9 mL water for injections then dilute appropriate dose to suggested volume 1000 mL given over 4–6 hours

| | |
|------|-----------------|
| **Polymyxin B sulphate** *Aerosporin*® | Continuous *or* intermittent *in* Glucose 5% |

Suggested volume of intermittent infusion, 200–500 mL given over 60–120 minutes

| | |
|------|-----------------|
| **Potassium canrenoate** *Spiroctan-M*® | Intermittent *in* Glucose 5% *or* Sodium chloride 0.9% |

Suggested volume 250 mL

| | |
|------|-----------------|
| **Potassium chloride** | Continuous *in* Glucose 5% *or* Sodium chloride 0.9% |

Dilute in a large-volume infusion; mix thoroughly to avoid 'layering', especially in non-rigid infusion containers; use ready-prepared solutions when possible

| | |
|------|-----------------|
| **Procainamide hydrochloride** *Pronestyl*® | Continuous *or* intermittent *in* Glucose 5% |

For maintenance, dilute to a concentration of *either* 2 mg/mL and give at a rate of 1–3 mL/minute *or* 4 mg/mL and give at a rate of 0.5–1.5 mL/minute

| Drug | Infusion method |
|------|-----------------|
| **Propofol** *Diprivan*® | *via* drip tubing *in* Glucose 5% *or* Sodium chloride 0.9% |

Not to be mixed with other therapeutic agents or infusion fluids; to be administered *via* a Y-piece close to injection site

| | |
|------|-----------------|
| | Continuous *in* Glucose 5% |

Dilute to a concentration not exceeding 2 mg/mL; administer using suitable device to control infusion rate; use glass or PVC containers (if PVC bag used it should be full—withdraw volume of infusion fluid equal to that of propofol to be added); propofol may alternatively be infused undiluted using a suitable infusion pump

| | |
|------|-----------------|
| **Quinine dihydrochloride** | Continuous *in* Sodium chloride 0.9% |

To be given over 4 hours; see also section 5.4.1

| | |
|------|-----------------|
| **Ranitidine hydrochloride** *Zantac*® | Intermittent *in* Glucose 5% *or* Sodium chloride 0.9% *or* Compound sodium lactate |
| **Rifampicin** *Rifadin*®, *Rimactane*® | Intermittent *in* Glucose 5 and 10% *or* Sodium chloride 0.9% *or* Ringer's solution |

Reconstitute with solvent provided then dilute with 250 mL (Rimactane®) or 500 mL (Rifadin®) infusion fluid; give over 2–3 hours

| | |
|------|-----------------|
| **Ritodrine hydrochloride** *Yutopar*® | Continuous *in* Glucose 5% *or* Sodium chloride 0.9% |

Dilute in a large-volume infusion

| | |
|------|-----------------|
| **Salbutamol sulphate** *Ventolin*® *For Intravenous Infusion* | Continuous *in* Glucose 5% *or* Sodium chloride 0.9% |

Suggested volume 500 mL as a solution containing 10 micrograms/mL

| | |
|------|-----------------|
| **Salcatonin** *Miacalcic*® | Continuous *in* Sodium chloride 0.9% |

Diluted solution given without delay; dilute in 500 mL and give over at least 6 hours; glass or hard plastic containers should not be used

| | |
|------|-----------------|
| **Sodium calciumedetate** *Ledclair*® | Continuous *in* Glucose 5% *or* Sodium chloride 0.9% |

Dilute to a concentration of not more than 3%; suggested volume 250–500 mL given over at least 1 hour

| | |
|------|-----------------|
| **Sodium clodronate** *Bonefos*® *Concentrate*, *Loron*® | Continuous *in* Sodium chloride 0.9% |

Dilute 300 mg in 500 mL infusion fluid and give over at least 2 hours; *Bonefos*® Concentrate can also be infused in Glucose 5%

---

1. Continuous infusion not usually recommended

| Drug | Infusion method |
|------|-----------------|

**Sodium nitroprusside**
*Nipride*®

Continuous *in*
Glucose 5% *or*
Sodium chloride 0.9% *or*
Ringer's solution *or*
Compound sodium lactate

Reconstitute with solvent provided then dilute immediately with 250–1000 mL infusion fluid; preferably infuse *via* infusion device to allow precise control; protect infusion from light

**Sodium valproate**
*Epilim*®

Continuous *or*
intermittent *in*
Glucose 5% *or*
Sodium chloride 0.9%

Reconstitute with solvent provided then dilute with infusion fluid

**Streptokinase**
*Kabikinase*®,
*Streptase*®

Continuous *in*
Sodium chloride 0.9%

*Kabikinase*® can also be infused in Glucose 5%

**Sulphadiazine sodium**

Continuous *in*
Sodium chloride 0.9%

Suggested volume 500 mL; ampoule solution has a pH of over 10

**Suxamethonium chloride**
*Anectine*®,
*Scoline*®

Continuous *in*
Glucose 5% *or*
Sodium chloride 0.9%

**Teicoplanin**
*Targocid*®

[1]Intermittent *in*
Glucose 5% *or*
Sodium chloride 0.9% *or*
Compound sodium lactate

Reconstitute initially with water for injections provided; infuse over 30 minutes

**Temocillin sodium**
*Temopen*®

Intermittent *in*
Glucose 5% *or*
Sodium chloride 0.9% *or*
Ringer's solution *or*
Compound sodium lactate

Dissolve initially in water for injections (500 mg in 10 mL; 1–2 g in 20 mL) then dilute with infusion fluid and give over 30–40 minutes

**Terbutaline sulphate**
*Bricanyl*®

Continuous *in*
Glucose 5% *or*
Sodium chloride 0.9%

Suggested volume 500 mL; to be given over 8–10 hours

**Tetracosactrin**
*Synacthen*®

Continuous *in*
Glucose 5% *or*
Sodium chloride 0.9%

Suggested volume 500 mL given over 6 hours

**Tetracycline hydrochloride**
*Achromycin Intravenous*®

Continuous *in*
Glucose 5% *or*
Sodium chloride 0.9% *or*
Compound sodium lactate

Reconstitute initially with water for injections (250 mg in 5 mL, 500 mg in 10 mL) then dilute to at least 100 mL (max. 1 litre) and give at a rate not exceeding 100 mL in 5 minutes preferably through a 0.22 micron filter

**Theophylline (solubilised with lysine)**
*Labophylline*®

Continuous *in*
Glucose 5% *or*
Sodium chloride 0.9%

**Ticarcillin sodium**
*Ticar*®

Intermittent *in*
Glucose 5% *or*
Water for injections

Suggested volume 100–150 mL given over 30–40 minutes

**Ticarcillin sodium/ clavulanic acid**
*Timentin*®

Intermittent *in*
Glucose 5% *or*
Water for injections

Suggested volume glucose 5%, 50–150 mL (depending on dose) or water for injections, 25–100 mL; given over 30–40 minutes

**Tobramycin sulphate**
*Nebcin*®

Intermittent *or*
*via* drip tubing *in*
Glucose 5% *or*
Sodium chloride 0.9%

For intermittent infusion suggested volume 50–100 mL given over 20–60 minutes

**Tocainide hydrochloride**
*Tonocard*®

Intermittent *in*
Glucose 5% *or*
Sodium chloride 0.9%

Suggested volume 50–100 mL given over 15–30 minutes

**Treosulfan**
*Treosulfan* (Leo)

Intermittent *in*
Water for injections

Infusion suggested for doses above 5 g; dilute to a concentration of 5 g in 100 mL

**Trimetaphan camsylate**
*Arfonad*®

Intermittent *in*
Glucose 5% *or*
Sodium chloride 0.9%

Suggested infusion concentration 0.05–0.1%; suggested volume 100–500 mL

**Trimethoprim lactate**
*Monotrim*®
*Syraprim*®

*via* drip tubing *in*
Glucose 5%

*Monotrim*® can also be infused *via* drip tubing in Sodium chloride 0.9% *or* Compound sodium lactate; *Syraprim*® can also be given by intermittent infusion in Glucose 5%

**Trisodium edetate**
*Limclair*®

Continuous *in*
Glucose 5% *or*
Sodium chloride 0.9%

Suggested volume 500 mL given over 2–3 hours

**Urokinase**
*Urokinase* (Leo)

Continuous *in*
Sodium chloride 0.9%

**Vancomycin hydrochloride**
*Vancocin*®

[1]Intermittent *in*
Glucose 5% *or*
Sodium chloride 0.9%

Reconstitute 500 mg with 10 mL water for injections and dilute to 100–200 mL with infusion fluid; give over at least 60 minutes (rate not to exceed 10 mg/minute for doses over 500 mg); use continuous infusion only if intermittent not feasible

**Vasopressin, synthetic**
*Pitressin*®

Intermittent *in*
Glucose 5%

Suggested concentration 20 units/100 mL given over 15 minutes

---

1. Continuous infusion not usually recommended

| Drug | Infusion method |
|------|-----------------|
| **Vecuronium bromide**<br>  *Norcuron*® | Continuous *in*<br>Glucose 5% *or*<br>Sodium chloride 0.9% *or*<br>Ringer's solution<br>Reconstitute with the solvent provided |
| **Vinblastine sulphate**<br>  *Velbe*® | *via* drip tubing *in*<br>Sodium chloride 0.9% *or*<br>Water for injections<br>Reconstitute with the diluent provided |
| **Vincristine sulphate**<br>  *Oncovin*® | *via* drip tubing *in*<br>Sodium chloride 0.9% *or*<br>Water for injections<br>Reconstitute with the diluent provided |
| **Vindesine sulphate**<br>  *Eldisine*® | *via* drip tubing *in*<br>Glucose 5% *or*<br>Sodium chloride 0.9%<br>Reconstitute with the diluent provided |

| Drug | Infusion method |
|------|-----------------|
| **Vitamins B & C**<br>  *Parentrovite IVHP*® | Intermittent *or*<br>*via* drip tubing *in*<br>Glucose 5% *or*<br>Sodium chloride 0.9%<br>Ampoule contents should be mixed, diluted, and administered without delay; give over 10 minutes (see CSM advice, section 9.6.2) |
| **Vitamins, multiple**<br>  *Multibionta*® | Intermittent *in*<br>Glucose 5% *or*<br>Sodium chloride 0.9%<br>Dilute 10 mL in not less than 250 mL of infusion fluid (adults); see also section 9.3 |
|   *Solivito N*® | Intermittent *in*<br>Glucose 5 and 10%<br>Suggested volume 500–1000 mL given over 2–3 hours; see also section 9.3 |
| **Zidovudine**<br>  *Retrovir*® | Intermittent *in*<br>Glucose 5%<br>Dilute to a concentration of 2 mg/mL or 4 mg/mL and give over 1 hour |

---

1. Continuous infusion not usually recommended

# Appendix 7: Borderline Substances

In certain conditions some foods (and toilet preparations) have characteristics of drugs and the Advisory Committee on Borderline Substances advises as to the circumstances in which such substances may be regarded as drugs. Prescriptions issued in accordance with the Committee's advice and endorsed 'ACBS' will normally not be investigated.

---

General Practitioners are reminded that the ACBS recommends products on the basis that they may be regarded as drugs for the treatment of specified conditions. Doctors should satisfy themselves that the products can safely be prescribed, that patients are adequately monitored and that, where necessary, expert hospital supervision is available.

---

## FOODS WHICH MAY BE PRESCRIBED ON FP10

*Note.* This is a list of food products which the ACBS has approved. The clinical condition for which the product has approval follows each entry.

**AL 110**® (Nestle)
*Powder*, protein 14 g, fat 25 g, carbohydrate 55.3 g, energy 2100 kJ (502 kcal)/100 g with vitamins and minerals. Net price 400 g = £7.27. For proven lactose intolerance in pre-school children, galactosaemia, and galactokinase deficiency

**Albumaid**® (Scientific Hospital Supplies)
*Complete*, powder, amino acids 89.4%, with vitamins, minerals, trace elements, free from carbohydrate and fat. Net price 200 g = £31.05. For malabsorption states where there is failure to hydrolyse and/or absorb protein
*RVHB*, powder, amino acid mixture, methionine-free. Net price 200 g = £31.05. For homocystinuria
*RVHB complete*, powder, amino acid mixture, methionine-free, with vitamins, minerals, and trace elements. Net price 200 g = £31.05. For homocystinuria
*XP*, powder, amino acids 40%, carbohydrate 50%, fat nil, phenylalanine not more than 10 mg per 100 g, with vitamins, minerals, and trace elements. Net price 200 g = £15.81. For phenylketonuria
*XP Concentrate*, powder, amino acids 85%, carbohydrate and fat nil, phenylalanine not more than 25 mg per 100 g, with vitamins, minerals, and trace elements. Net price 200 g = £30.20. For phenylketonuria

**Alcoholic Beverages** see under Rectified Spirit
**Alembicol D**® (Alembic Products)
Fractionated coconut oil. Net price 4 kg = £66.64. For steatorrhoea associated with cystic fibrosis of the pancreas, intestinal lymphangiectasia, surgery of the intestine, chronic liver disease, liver cirrhosis, other proven malabsorption syndromes; and in a ketogenic diet in the management of epilepsy

**Alfare**® (Nestle)
*Powder*, protein 16.5 g, fat 24 g, carbohydrate 51.7 g, energy 2010 kJ (480 kcal)/100 g with vitamins and minerals. Net price 400 g = £5.49. For proven whole protein sensitivity

**Aminogran**® (UCB Pharma)
*Food Supplement*, powder, containing all essential amino acids except phenylalanine, for use with mineral mixture (see below). Net price 500 g = £43.87. For phenylketonuria
*Mineral Mixture*, powder, containing all appropriate minerals for use with the above food supplement and other synthetic diets. Net price 250 g = £7.43. For phenylketonuria and as a mineral supplement in synthetic diets

**Analog**® (Scientific Hospital Supplies)
*MSUD*, powder, essential and non-essential amino acids 15.5% except isoleucine, leucine and valine, with carbohydrate, fat, vitamins, minerals, and trace elements. Net price 400 g = £17.99. For maple syrup urine disease
*RVHB*, powder, essential and non-essential amino acids 15.5% except methionine, with carbohydrate, fat, vitamins, minerals, and trace elements. Net price 400 g = £17.99. For hypermethioninaemia; homocystinuria
*XLys*, powder, essential and non-essential amino acids 15.5% except lysine, with carbohydrate, fat, vitamins, minerals, and trace elements. Net price 400 g = £17.99. For hyperlysinaemia
*XMet, Thre, Val, Isoleu*, powder, essential and non-essential amino acids 15.5% except methionine, threonine, valine and low isoleucine, with carbohydrate, fat, vitamins, minerals, and trace elements. Net price 400 g = £17.99. For methylmalonic or propionic acidaemia
*XP*, powder, essential and non-essential amino acids 15.5% except phenylalanine, with carbohydrate, fat, vitamins, minerals, and trace elements. Net price 400 g = £15.00. For phenylketonuria
*XPhen, Tyr*, powder, essential and non-essential amino acids 15.5% except phenylalanine and tyrosine, with carbohydrate, fat, vitamins, minerals and trace elements. Net price 400 g = £17.99. For tyrosinaemia

**Aproten**® (Ultrapharm)
Various products, gluten-free, low protein, low Na⁺ and K⁺. Net prices: anellini 500 g = £3.95; biscuits 180 g (36) = £2.80; bread mix 250 g = £2.00; cake mix 300 g = £2.10; crispbread 240 g = £3.95; ditalini 500 g = £3.95; flour 300 g = £1.84; rigatini 500 g = £3.95; spaghetti 500 g = £3.95; tagliatelle 500 g = £3.95. For phenylketonuria; similar amino acid abnormalities; renal failure; liver failure and liver cirrhosis; gluten-sensitive enteropathies including steatorrhoea due to gluten sensitivity, coeliac disease, and dermatitis herpetiformis

**Arnott**® (Ultrapharm)
*Rice Cookies*, gluten-free. Net price 200 g = £1.49. For gluten-sensitive enteropathies including steatorrhoea due to gluten sensitivity, coeliac disease, and dermatitis herpetiformis

**Bi-Aglut**® (Ultrapharm)
*Biscuits*, gluten-free. Net price 180 g (36) = £2.60
*Cracker toast*, gluten-, lactose-, and milk-protein-free. Net price 240 g (40) = £3.45. For gluten-sensitive enteropathies including steatorrhoea due to gluten sensitivity, coeliac disease, dermatitis herpetiformis

**Calogen**® (Scientific Hospital Supplies)
*Emulsion*, arachis oil 50% in water. Net price 250 mL = £2.69; 1 litre = £9.72. For renal failure and other conditions requiring a high-energy, low-fluid, low-electrolyte diet, disorders of amino acid metabolism or carbohydrate absorption; in a ketogenic diet in the management of epilepsy

**Caloreen**® (Roussel)
*Powder*, water-soluble dextrins, with less than 1.8 mmol of Na⁺ and 0.3 mmol of K⁺/100 g. Net price 250 g = £1.38; 5 kg = £22.54.
For renal failure; liver cirrhosis; disaccharide intolerance (without isomaltose intolerance), disorders of amino acid metabolism (and other similar disorders) and/or whole protein intolerance; malabsorption states and other conditions (including proven hypoglycaemia) requiring a high energy, low fluid intake, whether or not sodium and/or potassium restriction is essential

**Carobel, Instant**® (Cow & Gate)
*Powder*, carob seed flour. Net price 45 g = £1.70. For thickening feeds in the treatment of vomiting

**Casilan**® (Crookes)
*Powder*, whole protein, containing all essential amino acids, 90% with less than 0.1% Na⁺. Net price 250 g = £3.97. For biochemically proven hypoproteinaemia

**Clinifeed**® (Roussel)

*Clinifeed 400*, protein 15 g, carbohydrate 55 g, fat 13.4 g, energy 1674 kJ (400 kcal)/375 mL, with vitamins and minerals, vanilla flavour. Fructose-free. Net price 375-mL can = £1.10

*Clinifeed Protein Rich*, protein 30 g, carbohydrate 70 g, fat 11 g, energy 2092 kJ (500 kcal)/375 mL, with vitamins and minerals, vanilla flavour. Fructose- and lactose-free. Net price 375-mL can = £1.23

As necessary nutritional supplement prescription on medical grounds for: short bowel syndrome, intractable malabsorption, pre-operative preparation of patients who are undernourished, treatment for those with proven inflammatory bowel disease, treatment following total gastrectomy, dysphagia, bowel fistulas, anorexia nervosa, neoplasia related (associated) cachexia (anorexia), continuous ambulatory peritoneal dialysis (CAPD), and haemodialysis. Not to be prescribed for any child under one year

*Clinifeed Favour*, protein 14.1 g, carbohydrate 49.9 g, fat 14.6 g, energy 1575 kJ (375 kcal)/375 mL, with vitamins and minerals, neutral flavour. Lactose-, fructose-, and sucrose-free. Net price 375-mL can = 88p

*Clinifeed Iso*, protein 10.5 g, carbohydrate 49.2 g, fat 15.4 g, energy 1575 kJ (375 kcal)/375 mL, with vitamins and minerals, vanilla flavour. Fructose- and sucrose-free, and low sodium. Net price 375-mL can = £1.24

For use as the sole source of nutrition or as a necessary nutritional supplement prescribed on medical grounds for: short bowel syndrome, intractable malabsorption, pre-operative preparation of patients who are undernourished, treatment for those with proven inflammatory bowel disease, treatment following total gastrectomy, dysphagia, bowel fistulas, anorexia nervosa, neoplasia related (associated) cachexia (anorexia). Not to be prescribed for any child under one year, unsuitable as a sole source of nutrition for young children up to 5 years of age

**Clinutren**® (Clintec Nutrition)

*Clinutren 1.0*, liquid, protein 10 g, carbohydrate 31.8 g, fat 9.5 g, energy 1045 kJ (250 kcal)/250 mL with vitamins, minerals, and trace elements. Cholesterol-, gluten-, and lactose-free. Strawberry, vanilla, chocolate, and neutral flavours. Net price 250-mL can = 81p. For use as the sole source of nutrition or as a necessary nutritional supplement prescribed on medical grounds for: short bowel syndrome, intractable malabsorption, pre-operative preparation of patients who are undernourished, treatment for those with proven inflammatory bowel disease, treatment following total gastrectomy, dysphagia, bowel fistulas, anorexia nervosa, neoplasia related (associated) cachexia (anorexia). Not to be prescribed for any child under one year, unsuitable as a sole source of nutrition for young children up to 5 years of age

*Clinutren 1.5*, liquid, protein 15 g, carbohydrate 42.5 g, fat 16.9 g, energy 1570 kJ (375 kcal)/250 mL with vitamins, minerals, and trace elements. Cholesterol-, gluten-, and lactose-free. Strawberry, vanilla, and chocolate flavours. Net price 250-mL can = £1.08. As a necessary nutritional supplement prescribed on medical grounds for: short bowel syndrome, intractable malabsorption, pre-operative preparation of patients who are undernourished, treatment for those with proven inflammatory bowel disease, treatment following total gastrectomy, dysphagia, bowel fistulas, anorexia nervosa, neoplasia related (associated) cachexia (anorexia). Not to be prescribed for any child under one year

**Comminuted Chicken Meat** (Cow & Gate)

*Suspension* (aqueous). Net price 128 g = £1.02. For carbohydrate intolerance in association with possible or proven intolerance of milk; glucose and galactose intolerance

**Corn flour** and **corn starch**. For hypoglycaemia associated with glycogen-storage disease

**Corn oil** (maize oil). Net price 100 mL = 37p. For familial hypercholesterolaemia

**Dialamine**® (Scientific Hospital Supplies)

*Powder*, essential amino acids 30%, with carbohydrate 62%, energy 1500 kJ (360 kcal)/100 g, with ascorbic acid, minerals, and trace elements. Flavour: orange. Net price 200 g = £14.41. For oral feeding where essential amino acid supplements are required; e.g. chronic renal failure, hypoproteinaemia, wound fistula leakage with excessive protein loss, conditions requiring a controlled nitrogen intake, and haemodialysis

**dp**® (Nutricia)

*Cookies*, low-protein, butterscotch- or chocolate flavoured chip cookies. Net price 170 g = £4.90. For phenylketonuria; similar amino acid abnormalities; renal failure; liver failure and liver cirrhosis

**Duocal**® (Scientific Hospital Supplies)

*Liquid*, emulsion providing carbohydrate 23.4 g, fat 7.1 g, energy 628 kJ/100 mL. Low-electrolyte, gluten-, lactose-, and protein-free. Net price 250 mL = £1.51; 1 litre = £5.36

*Super Soluble Powder*, carbohydrate 72.7 g, fat 22.3 g, energy 1988 kJ/100 g. Low electrolyte, gluten-, protein-, and lactose-free. Net price 400 g = £9.78. For renal failure; liver cirrhosis; disaccharide intolerance (without isomaltose intolerance), disorders of amino acid metabolism (and other similar disorders), and/or whole protein intolerance; malabsorption states and other conditions requiring a high energy, low fluid intake, whether or not sodium and/or potassium restriction is essential

**Elemental 028**® (Scientific Hospital Supplies)

*Powder*, amino acids 12%, carbohydrate 70.5–72%, fat 6.64%, energy 1544–1568 kJ (364–370 kcal)/100 g with vitamins and minerals. For preparation with water before use. Net price 100-g box (orange flavoured or plain) = £3.61. For use as the sole source of nutrition or as a necessary nutritional supplement prescribed on medical grounds for: short-bowel syndrome, intractable malabsorption, treatment for proven inflammatory bowel disease, bowel fistulas. Not to be prescribed for any child under one year, unsuitable as a sole source of nutrition for young children up to 5 years of age

**Ener-G**® (General Designs)

*Gluten-free*. Rice bread (sliced), brown, net price 400 g = £2.96; white, 200 g = £1.12. Tapioca bread (sliced), 200 g = £1.12. Rice pasta (shells, small shells, lasagna, and vermicelli), 454 g = £2.62; spaghetti, 447 g = £2.62; tagliatelle, 300 g = £2.62; cannelloni, 285 g = £2.62

For gluten-sensitive enteropathies including steatorrhoea due to gluten sensitivity, coeliac disease, and dermatitis herpetiformis

**Enrich**® (Abbott)

*Liquid* with dietary fibre, providing protein 9.4 g, carbohydrate 38.3 g (including 5 g as dietary fibre), fat 8.8 g, energy 1090 kJ (260 kcal)/250 mL with vitamins and minerals. Lactose- and gluten-free. Vanilla and chocolate flavours. Net price 250-mL can = £1.58. For use as the sole source of nutrition or as a necessary nutritional supplement prescribed on medical grounds for: short-bowel syndrome, intractable malabsorption, pre-operative preparation of patients who are undernourished, treatment for proven inflammatory bowel disease, treatment following total gastrectomy, dysphagia, anorexia nervosa; neoplasia-related (associated) cachexia (anorexia). Not to be prescribed for any child under one year, unsuitable as a sole source of nutrition for young children up to 5 years of age

**Ensure**® (Abbott)

*Liquid*, protein 3.7%, fat 3.7%, carbohydrate 14.5%, with minerals and vitamins, lactose- and gluten-free, energy 1050 kJ (253 kcal)/250 mL. Vanilla flavour. Net price 237-mL bottle = £1.44; 250-mL can = £1.34; 946-mL can = £5.35. Chocolate, blackcurrant, coffee, eggnog, and nut flavours. Net price 237-mL can = £1.34. Chicken, mushroom, and asparagus flavours. Net price 250-mL can = £1.34.

*Powder*, same composition as Ensure liquid when reconstituted. Net price 400 g = £5.65

Both for use as the sole source of nutrition or as a necessary nutritional supplement prescribed on medical grounds for: short bowel syndrome, intractable malabsorption, pre-operative preparation of patients who are undernourished, treatment for proven inflammatory bowel disease, treatment following total gastrectomy, dysphagia, bowel fistulas, anorexia nervosa; neoplasia-related (associated) cachexia (anorexia). Neither to be prescribed for any child under one year, unsuitable as a sole source of nutrition for young children up to 5 years of age

**Ensure Plus®** (Abbott)

*Liquid*, protein 6.3%, fat 5%, carbohydrate 20%, with vitamins and minerals, lactose- and gluten-free, energy 1570 kJ (375 kcal)/250 mL. Vanilla flavour. Net price 250-mL can = £1.49; 500-mL bottle = £2.99. Caramel, chocolate, strawberry, and vanilla flavours. Net price 200-mL Tetrapak = £1.33. As a necessary nutritional supplement prescribed on medical grounds for: short bowel syndrome, intractable malabsorption, pre-operative preparation of patients who are undernourished, treatment for those with proven inflammatory bowel disease, treatment following total gastrectomy, dysphagia, bowel fistulas, anorexia nervosa, neoplasia related (associated) cachexia (anorexia), continuous ambulatory peritoneal dialysis (CAPD), and haemodialysis. Not to be prescribed for any child under one year

**Farley's Gluten-free biscuits** (Farley)

*Biscuits*. Net price 200 g = £1.14. For indications, see under Glutenex

**Flexical®** (Bristol-Myers)

*Powder*, protein 9.9%, carbohydrate 67%, fat 15% with vitamins and minerals. Gluten- and lactose-free. Net price 454 g = £9.36. For use as the sole source of nutrition or as a necessary nutritional supplement prescribed on medical grounds for: short-bowel syndrome, intractable malabsorption, treatment for those with proven inflammatory bowel disease, bowel fistulas. Not to be prescribed for any child under one year, unsuitable as a sole source of nutrition for young children up to 5 years of age

**Forceval Protein®** (Unigreg)

*Powder*, calcium caseinate 60%, carbohydrate 30%, with vitamins and minerals, providing not less than 55% protein, not more than 1% of fat, not more than 0.12% of Na⁺. Lactose- and gluten-free. Vanilla, strawberry, and neutral flavours. Net price 300 g = £12.00; 8 × 15-g sachets = £5.12. For biochemically proven hypoproteinaemia

**Formula MCT(1)** see under MCT(1)

**Formula S®** (Cow & Gate)

*Powder*, carbohydrate 7.1%, fat 3.6%, and protein 1.8% with vitamins and minerals when used as a 12.7% solution. Net price 450 g = £3.08. For proven lactose and associated sucrose intolerance in pre-school children, galactokinase deficiency, galactosaemia, and proven whole cow's milk sensitivity

**Fortical®** (Cow & Gate)

*Liquid*, glucose polymers providing carbohydrate 61.5 g/100 mL. Low-electrolyte, protein-free. Flavours: apple, apricot, black currant, lemon, orange, and neutral. Net price 200 mL = £1.00. For renal failure; liver cirrhosis, or other conditions requiring a high-energy, low-fluid, low-electrolyte diet

**Fortimel®** (Cow & Gate)

*Liquid*, protein 19.4 g, carbohydrate 20.8 g, fat 4.2 g, energy 840 kJ (200 kcal)/200 mL with vitamins and minerals. Vanilla, strawberry, chocolate, coffee, apricot, and forest fruits flavours. Net price 200-mL carton = 79p. As a necessary nutritional supplement prescribed on medical grounds for the treatment of: short bowel syndrome, intractable malabsorption, pre-operative preparation of patients who are undernourished, treatment for those with proven inflammatory bowel disease, treatment following total gastrectomy, dysphagia, bowel fistulas, anorexia nervosa, neoplasia related

(associated) cachexia (anorexia). Not to be prescribed for any child under one year

**Fortipudding®** (Cow & Gate)

*Semi-solid*, protein 15.3 g, carbohydrate 24 g, fat 4.5 g, energy 825 kJ (196 kcal)/150 g with vitamins and minerals. Vanilla, chocolate, and coffee flavours. Net price 150-g tub = 87p. For continuous ambulatory peritoneal dialysis (CAPD) and haemodialysis. Not suitable for children under 3 years

**Fortisip®** (Cow & Gate)

*Liquid*, protein 10 g, carbohydrate 35.8 g, fat 13 g, energy 1260 kJ (300 kcal)/200 mL, with vitamins and minerals. Gluten-free and low lactose. Vanilla, banana, orange, strawberry, tropical fruits, mushroom, and neutral flavours. Net price 200 mL = £1.19

As a necessary nutritional supplement prescribed on medical grounds for: short-bowel syndrome, intractable malabsorption, pre-operative preparation of patients who are undernourished, treatment for proven inflammatory bowel disease, treatment following total gastrectomy, dysphagia, bowel fistulas, anorexia nervosa; neoplasia-related (associated) cachexia (anorexia). Not to be prescribed for any child under one year

**Fortison®** see **Nutrison®**

**Fresenius OPD®** (Fresenius)

*Liquid*, protein 22.5 g, carbohydrate 75 g, fat 13 g, energy 2460 kJ (500 kcal)/500 mL, with vitamins, minerals, and trace elements. Gluten-free, and low lactose. Net price 500-mL bottle = £3.50. As a necessary nutritional supplement prescribed on medical grounds for the treatment of: short bowel syndrome, intractable malabsorption, pre-operative preparation of patients who are undernourished, treatment for those with proven inflammatory bowel disease, treatment following total gastrectomy, dysphagia, bowel fistulas, anorexia nervosa, neoplasia related (associated) cachexia (anorexia). Not to be prescribed for any child under one year; unsuitable as a sole source of nutrition for young children up to 5 years of age

**Fresubin®** (Fresenius)

*Liquid*, protein 7.6 g, carbohydrate 27.6 g, fat 6.8 g, energy 840 kJ (200 kcal)/200 mL with vitamins and minerals. Gluten-free, low lactose and cholesterol. Nut, peach, blackcurrant, chocolate, mocha, and vanilla flavours. Net price 200-mL carton = 93p; nut, peach and vanilla flavours, 500-mL bottle = £2.05; vanilla flavour, 500-mL Tetrabrik = £2.05. For use as the sole source of nutrition or as a necessary nutritional supplement prescribed on medical grounds for: short-bowel syndrome, intractable malabsorption, pre-operative preparation of patients who are undernourished, treatment for proven inflammatory bowel disease, treatment following total gastrectomy, dysphagia, bowel fistulas, anorexia nervosa; neoplasia-related (associated) cachexia (anorexia), and Refsum's disease. Not to be prescribed for any child under one year, unsuitable as a sole source of nutrition for young children up to 5 years of age

**Fresubin Plus F®** (Fresenius)

Liquid foods with dietary fibre in 2 formulations. For use as the sole source of nutrition or as a necessary nutritional supplement prescribed on medical grounds for: short-bowel syndrome, intractable malabsorption, pre-operative preparation of patients who are undernourished, treatment for proven inflammatory bowel disease, treatment following total gastrectomy, dysphagia, anorexia nervosa; neoplasia-related (associated) cachexia (anorexia). Not to be prescribed for any child under 2 years, unsuitable as a sole source of nutrition for young children up to 5 years of age

*Muesli-flavour*, milk protein, cereals, coconut, sunflower oil, vitamins and minerals providing protein 19 g, fat 17 g, carbohydrate 69 g, fibre 5 g, energy 2100 kJ (500 kcal)/500 mL. Low sodium, lactose, and cholesterol. Net price 200-mL carton = £1.05; 500-mL bottle = £2.45

*Vegetable soup-flavour*, milk protein, beef fat and protein, sunflower oil, maize starch, vitamins and minerals providing protein 19 g, fat 17 g, carbohydrate 69 g, fibre 3 g, energy 2100 kJ (500 kcal)/500 mL. Gluten-free, low sodium, lactose, and cholesterol. Net price 500-mL bottle = £2.25

**Fresubin 750**® (Fresenius)

*Liquid*, protein 37.5 g, carbohydrate 85 g, fat 30 g, energy 3150 kJ (750 kcal)/500 mL with vitamins, minerals, and trace elements. Gluten-free and low lactose. Vanilla flavour. Net price 500-mL bottle = £2.40. As a necessary nutritional supplement prescribed on medical grounds for the treatment of: short bowel syndrome, intractable malabsorption, pre-operative preparation of patients who are undernourished, treatment for those with proven inflammatory bowel disease, treatment following total gastrectomy, dysphagia, bowel fistulas, anorexia nervosa, neoplasia related (associated) cachexia (anorexia), continuous ambulatory peritoneal dialysis (CAPD), and haemodialysis. Not to be prescribed for any child under one year. A maximum of 500 mL per day to be taken by dialysis patients

**Fructose** (laevulose). For proven glucose/galactose intolerance

**Galactomin**® (Cow & Gate)

*Formula 17* (new formula), powder, protein 14.5 g, fat 25.9 g, carbohydrate 56.9 g, mineral salts 3.4 g/100 g. Used as a 13.1% solution with additional vitamins in place of milk. Net price 400 g = £8.35. For proven lactose intolerance in preschool children, galactosaemia and galactokinase deficiency

*Formula 19* (new formula), powder, protein 14.6 g, fat 30.8 g, carbohydrate 49.7 g (fructose as carbohydrate source), mineral salts 2.1 g/100 g, with vitamins. Used as a 12.9% solution in place of milk. Net price 400 g = £18.35. For glucose plus galactose intolerance

**Generaid**® (Scientific Hospital Supplies)

*Powder*, whey protein and additional branched-chain amino acids (protein equivalent 81%). Net price 200 g = £16.85. For patients with chronic liver disease and/or porto-hepatic encephalopathy

**GF Dietary**® (Nutricia)

*Biscuits*, gluten-free. Net price 150 g = 92p. For gluten-sensitive enteropathies including steatorrhoea due to gluten sensitivity, coeliac disease, and dermatitis herpetiformis

**Glucose** (dextrose monohydrate). Net price 100 g = 13p. For glycogen storage disease and sucrose/isomaltose intolerance

**Glutafin**® (Nutricia)

*Gluten-free*. Bread (whole or sliced), net price 400-g loaf = £1.94. Fibre bread (whole or sliced), 400-g loaf = £1.94. Mix, 500 g = £4.08. Fibre mix, 500 g = £4.08. Biscuits, savoury or tea, 125 g = £1.24. Biscuits, digestive or sweet, 150 g = £1.24. Biscuits, 200 g = £2.79. Crackers, 200 g = £4.07. High fibre crackers, 200 g = £1.70. Pasta (macaroni, pasta spirals, or spaghetti shortcut), 250 g = £2.06. For gluten-sensitive enteropathies including steatorrhoea due to gluten sensitivity, coeliac disease, and dermatitis herpetiformis

**Gluten-free biscuits** and **crackers**, see under Farley and GF

**Hepatic-Aid II**® (Kendall)

*Powder*, amino acids 4.4%, carbohydrate 16.8%, fat 3.6% when reconstituted. Low sodium and electrolytes; mineral and vitamin supplementation is required. Flavours: chocolate, chocolate mint, custard, and eggnog. Net price per packet = £7.95. For patients with chronic liver disease and/or porto-hepatic encephalopathy

**Hycal**® (SmithKline Beecham Brands)

*Liquid*, protein-free, low-electrolyte, glucose syrup solids 49.5%. Flavours, blackcurrant, lemon, orange, and raspberry. Net price 171 mL = 64p. For renal failure; liver cirrhosis or other conditions requiring a high-energy, low-fluid, low-electrolyte diet

**Isomil**® (Abbott)

*Powder*, protein 1.8%, carbohydrate 6.9%, fat 4.69% with vitamins and minerals when reconstituted. Lactose-free. Net price 400 g = £2.99. For proven lactose intolerance in preschool children, galactokinase deficiency, galactosaemia, and proven whole cow's milk sensitivity

**Jevity**® (Abbott)

*Liquid*, protein 4.2%, fat 3.5%, carbohydrate 13.4%, dietary fibre 1.36%, with vitamins and minerals. Gluten-, lactose-, and sucrose-free. Net price 500-mL bottle = £3.50. For use as the sole source of nutrition or as a necessary nutritional supplement prescribed on medical grounds for: short bowel syndrome, intractable malabsorption, pre-operative preparation of patients who are undernourished, treatment for those with proven inflammatory bowel disease, treatment following total gastrectomy, dysphagia, anorexia nervosa, neoplasia related (associated) cachexia (anorexia). Not to be prescribed for any child under 2 years, unsuitable as a sole source of nutrition for young children up to 5 years of age

**Juvela**® (Scientific Hospital Supplies)

*Gluten-free*. Mix, net price 500 g = £4.08. Bread, 400-g loaf = £1.94. For gluten-sensitive enteropathies including steatorrhoea due to gluten sensitivity, coeliac disease, and dermatitis herpetiformis

*Low Protein*. Mix, net price 500 g = £4.08. Bread, 400-g loaf = £1.94. Biscuits, chocolate chip, orange, and cinnamon flavour, 150 g = £4.08. For phenylketonuria and similar amino-acid abnormalities; renal failure; liver failure and liver cirrhosis; gluten-sensitive enteropathies, see above

**Liga**® (Jacobs Bakery)

*Rusks*, egg- and gluten-free. Net price 24 = 75p. For gluten-sensitive enteropathies including steatorrhoea due to gluten sensitivity, coeliac disease, and dermatitis herpetiformis

**Liquigen**® (Scientific Hospital Supplies)

*Emulsion*, medium chain triglycerides 52%. Net price 250 mL = £4.17; 1 litre = £15.45. For steatorrhoea associated with cystic fibrosis of the pancreas; intestinal lymphangiectasia, surgery of the intestine; chronic liver disease and liver cirrhosis; other proven malabsorption syndromes; ketogenic diet in the management of epilepsy; type I hyperlipoproteinaemia

**Liquisorb**® (Merck)

*Liquid*, protein 20 g, carbohydrate 59 g, fat 20 g, energy 2095 kJ (500 kcal)/500 mL with vitamins and minerals. Gluten-free, low lactose. Banana, vanilla, chocolate, strawberry, and neutral flavours. Net price 500-mL bottle = £1.90. Strawberry and vanilla flavours only. Net price 200-mL Tetrapak = 78p. For use as the sole source of nutrition or as a necessary nutritional supplement prescribed on medical grounds for: short bowel syndrome, intractable malabsorption, pre-operative preparation of patients who are undernourished, treatment for proven inflammatory bowel disease, treatment following total gastrectomy, dysphagia, bowel fistulas, anorexia nervosa, neoplasia-related (associated) cachexia (anorexia). Not to be prescribed for any child under one year, unsuitable as a sole source of nutrition for young children up to 5 years of age

*High energy liquid*, protein 30 g, carbohydrate 87.5 g, fat 30 g, energy 3150 kJ (750 kcal)/500 mL, with vitamins, minerals and trace elements. Gluten-free and low lactose. Net price 500-mL bottle = £2.60. As a necessary nutritional supplement prescribed on medical grounds for the treatment of: short bowel syndrome, intractable malabsorption, pre-operative preparation of patients who are undernourished, treatment for those with proven inflammatory bowel disease, treatment following total gastrectomy, dysphagia, bowel fistulas, anorexia nervosa, neoplasia related (associated) cachexia (anorexia). Not to be prescribed for any child under one year. A maximum of 500 mL per day to be taken by dialysis patients

**Liquisorbon MCT**® (Merck)

*Liquid*, protein 25 g, carbohydrate 61.5 g, fat 16.5 g, energy 2095 kJ (500 kcal)/500 mL with vitamins and minerals. Gluten- and fructose-free, low lactose. Strawberry, vanilla, and neutral flavours. Net price 500 mL = £2.65. As a necessary nutritional supplement prescribed on medical grounds for the treatment of: short bowel syndrome, intractable malabsorption, pre-operative preparation of patients who are undernourished, treatment for those with proven inflammatory bowel disease, treatment following total gastrectomy, dysphagia, bowel fistulas, anorexia nervosa, neoplasia related (associated) cachexia (anorexia). Not to be prescribed for any child under one year

**Locasol New Formula**® (Cow & Gate)

*Powder*, protein 14.6 g, carbohydrate 56.5 g, fat 26.1 g, mineral salts 1.9 g, not more than 55 mg of $Ca^{2+}/100$ g and vitamins. Used as a 13.1% solution in place of milk. Net price 400 g = £9.29. For calcium intolerance

**Lofenalac**® (Bristol-Myers)

*Powder*, protein 15%, carbohydrate 60%, fat 18%, phenylalanine not more than 0.1% with vitamins and minerals. Gluten-, sucrose-, and lactose-free. Net price 450 g = £8.00. For phenylketonuria

**Loprofin**® (Nutricia)

*Low protein*. Sweet biscuits, 150 g = £1.24; chocolate cream-filled biscuits, 125 g = £1.24; crackers, 150 g = £1.70; cookies (chocolate chip or cinnamon), 100 g = £4.08; wafers (orange, vanilla, or chocolate), 100 g = £1.22. For phenylketonuria and similar amino acid abnormalities; renal failure; liver failure and liver cirrhosis

*Low protein/gluten-free*. Bread (sliced or whole), net price 400-g loaf = £1.94. Mix, 500 g = £4.08. Pasta (macaroni, pasta spirals or spaghetti short-cut), 250 g = £2.06. For phenylketonuria and similar amino-acid abnormalities; renal failure; liver failure and liver cirrhosis; gluten-sensitive enteropathies including steatorrhoea due to gluten sensitivity, coeliac disease, and dermatitis herpetiformis

*PKU Drink*, protein 1 g (phenylalanine 30 mg), lactose 9.4 g, fat 4 g, energy 300 kJ (72 kcal)/200 mL. Net price 200-mL bottle = 39p. For phenylketonuria

**Lorenzo's Oil** (Scientific Hospital Supplies)

*Liquid*, glycerol trioleate oil 4 parts, glycerol trierucate oil 1 part. Net price 710 mL = £55.91. For biochemically proven and/or clinically manifest adrenoleukodystrophy

**Low Protein Drink** (Milupa)

*Powder*, protein 0.4%, carbohydrate 5.1%, fat 2% when reconstituted. Net price 400 g = £8.25. For inherited disorders of amino acid metabolism in childhood

*Note*. Termed Milupa lpd by manufacturer

**Maxamaid**® (Scientific Hospital Supplies)

*MSUD*, powder, essential and non-essential amino acids 30% except isoleucine, leucine, and valine, with carbohydrate, fat less than 0.5%, vitamins, minerals, and trace elements. Net price 575 g = £44.74

For maple syrup urine disease

*RVHB*, powder, essential and non-essential amino acids 30% except methionine, with carbohydrate, fat less than 0.5%, vitamins, minerals, and trace elements. Net price 575 g = £44.74

For hypermethioninaemia, homocystinuria

*XLys*, powder, essential and non-essential amino acids 30% except lysine, with carbohydrate, fat less than 0.5%, vitamins, minerals, and trace elements. Net price 575 g = £44.74

For hyperlysinaemia

*XLys, Try*, powder, essential and non-essential amino acids 30% except lysine and tryptophan, with carbohydrate, fat less than 0.5%, vitamins, minerals, and trace elements. Net price 575 g = £44.74

For glutaric aciduria

*XMet, Thre, Val, Isoleu*, powder, essential and non-essential amino acids 30% except methionine, threonine, valine and low isoleucine, with carbohydrate, fat less than 0.5%, vitamins, minerals, and trace elements. Net price 575 g = £44.74

For methylmalonic or propionic acidaemia

*XP*, essential and non-essential amino acids 30% except

phenylalanine, with carbohydrate, vitamins, minerals, and trace elements. Bar. Net price 25-g bar = 79p. Powder. Orange-flavoured or unflavoured. Net price 575 g = £34.78

Both for phenylketonuria. Not to be prescribed for children under 2 years of age

*XP Concentrate*, powder, essential and non-essential amino acids 65% except phenylalanine, with carbohydrate, fat less than 0.5%, vitamins, minerals, and trace elements. Unflavoured. Net price 200 g = £33.79

For phenylketonuria. Not to be prescribed for children under 2 years of age

*XPhen, Tyr*, powder, essential and non-essential amino acids 30% except phenylalanine and tyrosine, with carbohydrate, fat less than 0.5%, vitamins, minerals, and trace elements. Net price 575 g = £44.74

For tyrosinaemia

**Maxamum**® (Scientific Hospital Supplies)

*MSUD*, powder, essential and non-essential amino acids 47% except isoleucine, leucine, and valine, with carbohydrate, fat less than 0.5%, vitamins, minerals, and trace elements. Orange-flavoured. Net price 200 g = £24.95

For maple syrup urine disease. Not recommended for children under 8 years.

*RVHB*, powder, essential and non-essential amino acids 47% except methionine, with carbohydrate, fat less than 0.5%, vitamins, minerals, and trace elements. Unflavoured. Net price 200 g = £24.95

For hypermethioninaemia, homocystinuria. Not recommended for children under 8 years

*XMet, Thre, Val, Isoleu*, powder, essential and non-essential amino acids 47% except methionine, threonine, valine, and low isoleucine, with carbohydrate, fat less than 0.5%, vitamins, minerals, and trace elements. Unflavoured. Net price 200 g = £24.95

For methylmalonic or propionic acidaemia. Not recommended for children under 8 years

*XP*, powder, essential and non-essential amino acids 47% except phenylalanine, with carbohydrates, vitamins, minerals, and trace elements. Orange-flavoured or unflavoured. Net price 575 g = £55.72. For phenylketonuria. Not to be prescribed for children under 8 years

**Maxijul**® (Scientific Hospital Supplies)

*Liquid*, carbohydrate 50%, with potassium 0.004%, sodium 0.023%. Gluten-, lactose-, and fructose-free. Flavours: black currant, lemon and lime, orange, and natural. Net price 200 mL = 69p

*Super Soluble Powder*, glucose polymer, potassium 0.004%, sodium 0.046%. Gluten-, lactose-, and fructose-free. Net price 4 × 140-g sachet pack = £2.44, 200 g = £1.39, 2.5 kg = £11.50. For renal failure; liver cirrhosis; disaccharide intolerance (without isomaltose intolerance); disorders of amino acid metabolism (and other similar disorders) and/or whole protein intolerance; malabsorption states and other conditions, including proven hypoglycaemia, requiring a high-energy, low-fluid intake

**Maxijul LE**® (Scientific Hospital Supplies)

*Powder*, modification of Maxijul with lower concentrations of sodium and potassium. Net price 100 g = £1.02, 2 kg = £13.50. For indications, see under Maxijul where sodium and/or potassium restriction is also essential

**Maxipro HBV**® **Super Soluble** (Scientific Hospital Supplies)

*Powder*, whey protein and additional amino acids (protein equivalent 80%). Net price 200 g = £4.92; 1 kg = £19.67. For biochemically proven hypoproteinaemia. Not to be prescribed for any child under one year; unsuitable as a sole source of nutrition

**MCT Oil**

Triglycerides from medium chain fatty acids. For steatorrhoea associated with cystic fibrosis of the pancreas; intestinal lymphangiectasia; surgery of the intestine;

chronic liver disease and liver cirrhosis; other proven malabsorption syndromes; in a ketogenic diet in the management of epilepsy; in type I hyperlipoproteinaemia

Available from Bristol-Myers (net price 950 mL = £7.80); Cow & Gate (net price 1 litre = £13.06); Scientific Hospital Supplies (net price 250 mL = £3.21)

**MCT (1)**® (Cow & Gate)

*Powder*, protein 25.6%, carbohydrate 40.6%, medium chain triglycerides 28%, when used as a 12.5% solution. Low in lactose and sucrose-free. Net price 400 g = £6.82. For steatorrhoea associated with cystic fibrosis of the pancreas; intestinal lymphangiectasia; chronic liver disease; surgery of the intestine in infants

**MCT Pepdite**® (Scientific Hospital Supplies)

*Powder*, essential and non-essential amino acids, peptides, medium chain triglycerides, monoglyceride of sunflower oil, with carbohydrate, fat, vitamins, minerals, and trace elements.

*MCT Pepdite 0–2*. Net price 400 g = £10.82

*MCT Pepdite 2+*. Net price 400 g = £10.82

Both for proven whole protein intolerance, short bowel syndrome, intractable malabsorbtion, proven inflammatory bowel disease, bowel fistulas, where there are difficulties with fat absorption

**Metabolic Mineral Mixture**® (Scientific Hospital Supplies)

*Powder*, essential mineral salts. Net price 100 g = £5.11. For mineral supplementation in synthetic diets

**Milupa**® **Low Protein Drink** see under **Low Protein Drink**

**Milupa**® **PKU2** and **PKU3** see under **PKU2** and **PKU3**

**Minafen**® (Cow & Gate)

*Powder*, equivalent of 12.5% protein, carbohydrate 48%, fat 31%, not more than 0.02% of phenylalanine. For use as 13.1% solution with additional vitamins. Net price 400 g = £12.00. For phenylketonuria

**MSUD Aid**® (Scientific Hospital Supplies)

*Powder*, containing full range of amino acids except isoleucine, leucine, and valine, with vitamins, minerals, and trace elements. Net price 200 g = £32.38. For maple syrup urine disease

**Neocate**® (Scientific Hospital Supplies)

*Powder*, essential and non-essential amino acids, maltodextrin, fat, vitamins, minerals, and trace elements. Net price 400 g = £15.09

For proven whole protein intolerance, short bowel syndrome, intractable malabsorption, proven inflammatory bowel disease, and bowel fistulas

**Nestargel**® (Nestlé)

*Powder*, carob seed flour 96.5%, calcium lactate 3.5%. Net price 125 g = £3.46. For infants and children with galactokinase deficiency, galactosaemia, proven lactose and/or sucrose intolerance in pre-school children, proven sensitivity to whole protein

**Nutramigen**® (Bristol-Myers)

*Powder*, protein 13%, carbohydrate 62%, fat 18% with vitamins and minerals. Gluten-, sucrose-, and lactose-free. Net price 425 g = £7.00. For infants over 3 months and children with galactokinase deficiency; galactosaemia; proven lactose intolerance and/or sucrose intolerance in preschool children; proven sensitivity to whole protein

**Nutrison**® (Cow & Gate) [formerly Fortison®]

*Energy-plus*, liquid, protein 30 g, carbohydrate 92 g, fat 29 g, energy 3200 kJ (755 kcal)/500 mL. Net price 500 mL = £2.46. For indications, see under Fortisip

*Fibre*, liquid, protein 20 g, carbohydrate 61.5 g, fat 19.5 g, fibre 7.5 g, energy 2125 kJ (505 kcal)/500 mL. Net price 500-mL bottle = £2.18. For use as the sole source of nutrition or as a necessary nutritional supplement prescribed on medical grounds for: short bowel syndrome, intractable malabsorption, pre-operative preparation of patients who are undernourished, treatment for those with proven inflammatory bowel disease, treatment following total gastrectomy, dysphagia, anor-

exia nervosa, neoplasia related (associated) cachexia (anorexia). Not to be prescribed for any child under two years, unsuitable as a sole source of nutrition for young children up to 5 years of age

*Paediatric*, liquid, protein 5.4 g, carbohydrate 24.4 g, fat 9 g, energy 850 kJ (202 kcal)/200 mL. Net price 200-mL bottle = £1.58. For use as the sole source of nutrition or as a necessary nutritional supplement prescribed on medical grounds for: short bowel syndrome, intractable malabsorption, pre-operative preparation of patients who are undernourished, dysphagia, bowel fistulas, anorexia nervosa, neoplasia related (associated) cachexia (anorexia) and malnutrition or growth failure secondary to disease related anorexia. Not to be prescribed for any child under one year

*Soya*, liquid, protein 20 g, carbohydrate 61.5 g, fat 19.5 g, energy 2125 kJ (505 kcal)/500 mL, with vitamins and minerals. Gluten-free. Net price 500 mL = £2.55. For milk intolerance and lactose intolerance. Not to be prescribed for any child under one year, unsuitable as a sole source of nutrition for young children up to 5 years of age

*Standard*, liquid, protein 20 g, carbohydrate 61.5 g, fat 19.5 g, energy 2125 kJ (505 kcal)/500 mL, with vitamins and minerals. Net price 500 mL = £2.10. For use as the sole source of nutrition or as a necessary nutritional supplement prescribed on medical grounds for: short bowel syndrome, intractable malabsorption, pre-operative preparation of patients who are undernourished, treatment for those with proven inflammatory bowel disease, treatment following total gastrectomy, dysphagia, bowel fistulas, anorexia nervosa, neoplasia related (associated) cachexia (anorexia). Not to be prescribed for any child under one year, unsuitable as a sole source of nutrition for young children up to 5 years of age

**Osmolite**® (Abbott)

*Liquid*, protein 10.5 g, carbohydrate 33.4 g, fat 8.7 g, energy 1050 kJ (250 kcal)/250 mL with vitamins and minerals. Gluten- and lactose-free. Net price 250-mL can = £1.34; 500-mL bottle = £2.68. For use as the sole source of nutrition or as a necessary nutritional supplement prescribed on medical grounds for: short-bowel syndrome, intractable malabsorption, pre-operative preparation of patients who are undernourished, treatment for proven inflammatory bowel disease, treatment following total gastrectomy, dysphagia, bowel fistulas, anorexia nervosa; neoplasia-related (associated) cachexia (anorexia). Not to be prescribed for any child under one year, unsuitable as a sole source of nutrition for young children up to 5 years of age

**OsterSoy**® (Farley)

*Powder*, providing protein 2%, carbohydrate 7%, fat 3.8% with vitamins and minerals when reconstituted. Gluten-, sucrose-, and lactose-free. Net price 450 g = £2.89. For proven lactose and sucrose intolerance in preschool children, galactokinase deficiency, galactosaemia, and proven whole cow's milk protein sensitivity

**Paediasure**® (Abbott)

*Liquid*, protein 3%, fat 5%, carbohydrate 11%, with minerals and vitamins, gluten-free, energy 995 kJ (238 kcal)/237 mL. Vanilla flavour. Net price 237-mL can = £1.93. For use as the sole source of nutrition or as a necessary nutritional supplement prescribed on medical grounds for: short-bowel syndrome, intractable malabsorption, pre-operative preparation of patients who are undernourished, dysphagia, bowel fistulas; neoplasia related (associated) cachexia (anorexia) and malnutrition or growth failure secondary to disease related anorexia. Not to be prescribed for any child under one year

**Paediatric Seravit**® (Scientific Hospital Supplies)

*Powder*, vitamins, minerals, low sodium and potassium, and trace elements. Net price 100 g = £5.08

For vitamin and mineral supplementation in restrictive therapeutic diets in infants and children

**Pepdite**® (Scientific Hospital Supplies)
*Powder*, essential and non-essential amino acids, peptides, with carbohydrate, fat, vitamins, minerals, and trace elements.
*Pepdite 0–2*. Providing 1925 kJ (460 kcal)/100 g. Net price 400 g = £9.84
*Pepdite 2+*. Providing 1787 kJ (425 kcal)/100 g. Net price 400 g = £9.84
Both for proven whole protein intolerance, proven lactose intolerance, short bowel syndrome, intractable malabsorption, proven inflammatory bowel disease, and bowel fistulas

**Peptamen**® (Clintec Nutrition)
*Liquid*, protein 4%, carbohydrate 12.7%, fat 3.9%, energy 420 kJ (100 kcal)/100 mL, with vitamins and minerals. Lactose- and gluten-free. Unflavoured. Net price 500 mL = £4.50. Orange and strawberry flavours. Net price 250-mL can = £2.95. For use as the sole source of nutrition or as a necessary nutritional supplement prescribed on medical grounds for: short bowel syndrome, intractable malabsorption, treatment for proven inflammatory bowel disease, bowel fistulas. Not to be prescribed for any child under one year, unsuitable as a sole source of nutrition for young children up to 5 years of age

**Pepti-2000 LF**® (Cow & Gate)
*Liquid*, protein 20 g, fat 5 g, carbohydrate 94 g, energy 2100 kJ (500 kcal)/500 mL with vitamins and minerals. Gluten-free. Net price 500 mL = £2.70.
*Powder*, same composition as Pepti-2000 LF liquid when reconstituted. Net price 126-g sachet = £3.70.
For use as the sole source of nutrition or as a necessary nutritional supplement prescribed on medical grounds for: short bowel syndrome, intractable malabsorption, treatment for those with proven inflammatory bowel disease, bowel fistulas. Not to be prescribed for any child under one year; unsuitable as a sole source of nutrition for young children up to 5 years of age

**Pepti-Junior**® (Cow & Gate)
*Powder*, protein 15.3 g, fat 28.3 g, carbohydrate 55.1 g, energy 2140 kJ (507 kcal)/100 g with vitamins and minerals. Used as a 13.1% solution in place of milk. Net price 400 g = £7.18. For proven lactose and associated sucrose intolerance in association with proven whole protein intolerance, steatorrhea associated with cystic fibrosis, and other proven malabsorption syndromes

**Peptisorb**® (Merck)
*Liquid*, amino acids and peptides 3.75%, carbohydrate 18.75%, fat 1.11%, with vitamins and minerals, low lactose, and fructose- and gluten-free, energy 2100 kJ (500 kcal)/500 mL. Net price 500 mL = £4.60. For use as the sole source of nutrition or as a necessary nutritional supplement prescribed on medical grounds for: short bowel syndrome, intractable malabsorption, treatment for those with proven inflammatory bowel disease, bowel fistulas. Not to be prescribed for any child under one year; unsuitable as a sole source of nutrition for young children up to 5 years of age

**Peptisorbon**® (Merck)
*Powder*, amino acids and peptides 18%, carbohydrate 70%, fat 5.3%, with vitamins and minerals, low lactose, and fructose- and gluten-free, energy 1393 kJ (333 kcal)/sachet. Net price 83.3-g sachet = £2.07. As a necessary nutritional supplement prescribed on medical grounds for the treatment of: short bowel syndrome, intractable malabsorption, pre-operative preparation of patients who are undernourished, treatment for those with proven inflammatory bowel disease, treatment following total gastrectomy, dysphagia, bowel fistulas, anorexia nervosa, neoplasia related (associated) cachexia (anorexia). Not to be prescribed for any child under one year

**PK Aid 3**® (Scientific Hospital Supplies)
*Powder*, containing essential and non-essential amino acids except phenylalanine. Net price 500 g = £79.00. For phenylketonuria

**PKU 2**[89] (Milupa)
*Granules*, containing essential and non-essential amino acids except phenylalanine; with vitamins, minerals, trace elements, 7.1% sucrose. Flavour: vanilla. Net price 500 g = £36.00. For phenylketonuria

**PKU 3**® (Milupa)
*Granules*, containing essential and non-essential amino acids except phenylalanine, vitamins, minerals, and trace elements, with 3.4% sucrose. Flavour vanilla. Net price 500 g = £36.00. For phenylketonuria, not recommended for child under 8 years

**Polial**® (Ultrapharm)
*Biscuits*. Gluten- and lactose-free. Net price 200-g pack = £2.85. For gluten-sensitive enteropathies including steatorrhea due to gluten sensitivity, coeliac disease, and dermatitis herpetiformis

**Polycal**® (Cow & Gate)
*Powder*, glucose, maltose, and polysaccharides, providing 1610 kJ (380kcal)/100 g. Net price 400 g = £2.60; 900 g = £4.62
For renal failure; liver cirrhosis; disaccharide intolerance (without isomaltose intolerance); disorders of amino acid metabolism (and other similar disorders) and/or whole protein intolerance; malabsorption states and other conditions, including proven hypoglycaemia, requiring a high-energy, low-fluid intake, whether or not sodium and/or potassium restriction is essential

**Polycose**® (Abbott)
*Powder*, glucose polymers, providing carbohydrate 94 g, energy 1600 kJ (380 kcal)/100 g. Net price 350-g can = £2.83. For renal failure; liver cirrhosis; disaccharide intolerance (without isomaltose intolerance); disorders of amino acid metabolism (and other similar disorders) and/or whole protein intolerance; malabsorption states and other conditions, including proven hypoglycaemia, requiring a high-energy, low-fluid intake, whether or not sodium and/or potassium restriction is essential

**Portagen**® (Bristol-Myers)
*Powder*, protein 16.5%, carbohydrate 54%, fat 22% with vitamins and minerals. Gluten- and lactose-free. Net price 454 g = £6.23. For lactose intolerance without sucrose intolerance but requiring medium chain triglycerides; malabsorption associated with cystic fibrosis of the pancreas; intestinal lymphangiectasia; surgery of the intestine; chronic liver disease and liver cirrhosis; other proven malabsorption syndromes; neoplasia-related (associated) cachexia (anorexia)

**Pregestimil**® (Bristol-Myers)
*Powder*, protein 12.8%, carbohydrate 61.6%, fat 18.3% with vitamins and minerals. Gluten-, sucrose-, and lactose-free. Net price 454 g = £8.01. For sucrose and/or lactose intolerance in association with whole protein intolerance, or where amino acids and peptides are indicated in conjunction with medium chain triglycerides. Also for proven malabsorption syndromes in which a reduced fat diet is indicated such as steatorrhoea associated with cystic fibrosis and surgery of the intestine; galactosaemia and galactokinase deficiency; neoplasia-related (associated) cachexia (anorexia)

**Prejomin**® (Milupa)
*Granules*, protein 13.3 g, carbohydrate 57 g, fat 24.2 g, energy 2090 kJ (499 kcal)/100 g, with vitamins and minerals. Gluten-free. For preparation with water before use. Net price 400 g = £7.35. For proven lactose and sucrose intolerance in pre-school children, fructose intolerance, galactosaemia, galactokinase deficiency, and proven sensitivity to whole protein

**ProMod**® (Abbott)
*Powder*, protein 75.8%, carbohydrate 10.2%, fat 9.1%. Gluten-free. Net price 275-g can = £7.50. For biochemically proven hypoproteinaemia

**Prosobee**® (Bristol-Myers)
*Liquid concentrate*, protein 4.1%, carbohydrate 13.7%, fat 7.2% with vitamins and minerals. Gluten-, sucrose-, and lactose-free. Net price 385 mL = £1.39
*Powder*, protein 15.6%, carbohydrate 51.4%, fat 27.9%

with vitamins and minerals. Gluten-, sucrose-, and lactose-free. Net price 400 g = £3.56. For proven lactose and associated sucrose intolerance in pre-school children, galactokinase deficiency, galactosaemia, and proven whole cow's milk sensitivity

**Protein Forte®** (Fresenius)

*Liquid*, protein 20 g, carbohydrate 19 g, fat 5.2 g, energy 840 kJ (200 kcal)/200 mL, with vitamins, minerals, and trace elements. Gluten-free. Vanilla, strawberry, and chocolate flavours. Net price 200-mL tetrabrik = 95p. As a necessary nutritional supplement prescribed on medical grounds for: short bowel syndrome, intractable malabsorption, pre-operative preparation of patients who are undernourished, treatment for those with proven inflammatory bowel disease, treatment following total gastrectomy, dysphagia, bowel fistulas, anorexia nervosa, neoplasia related (associated) cachexia (anorexia), continuous ambulatory peritoneal dialysis (CAPD) and haemodialysis. Not to be prescribed for any child under one year

**Protifar®** (Cow & Gate)

*Powder*, protein 88.5%. Low lactose, gluten- and sucrose-free. Net price 225 g = £5.20. For biochemically proven hypoproteinaemia

**Provide®** (Fresenius)

*Liquid*, protein 9 g, carbohydrate 28 g, fat less than 1 g, energy 630 kJ (250 kcal)/250 mL with vitamins and minerals. Gluten- and lactose-free. Tropical fruit flavour. Net price 250-mL tetrabrik = £1.05. As a necessary nutritional supplement prescribed on medical grounds for: short bowel syndrome, intractable malabsorption, pre-operative preparation of patients who are undernourished, treatment for those with proven inflammatory bowel disease, treatment following total gastrectomy, dysphagia, bowel fistulas, anorexia nervosa, neoplasia related (associated) cachexia (anorexia). Not to be prescribed for any child under one year

**Reabilan®** (Roussel)

*Liquid*, protein 11.8 g, carbohydrate 49.3 g, fat 14.6 g, energy 1575 kJ (375 kcal)/375 mL with vitamins and minerals. Gluten- and lactose-free. Net price 375 mL = £3.08. For use as the sole source of nutrition or as a necessary nutritional supplement prescribed on medical grounds for: short bowel syndrome, intractable malabsorption, treatment for those with inflammatory bowel disease, bowel fistulas. Not to be prescribed for any child under 1 year, unsuitable as a sole source of nutrition for young children up to 5 years of age

**Rectified Spirit.** Where the therapeutic qualities of alcohol are required rectified spirit (suitably flavoured and diluted) should be prescribed

**Rite-Diet®** (Nutricia)

*Gluten-free.* High-fibre crackers. Net price 150 g = £1.70. Digestive biscuits. 150 g = £1.24. Savoury biscuits. 125 g = £1.24. Tea biscuits. 125 g = £1.24. Flour mix. 500 g = £2.42. Bread mix. 500 g (brown) = £2.42; white, 500 g = £2.42. Bread (white). 400 g = £1.95. High-fibre bread (with soya bran). 400 g = £1.95. For gluten-sensitive enteropathies including steatorrhoea due to gluten sensitivity, coeliac disease, and dermatitis herpetiformis

*Low protein/gluten-free.* Macaroni. Net price 250 g = £2.06. Spaghetti, shortcut. 250 g = £2.06. Rings. 250 g = £2.06. Baking mix. 500 g = £2.42. Flour mix. 400 g = £2.42. Bread; 227 g = £1.32. Bread with soya bran; 280 g = £1.32. Bread (with or without salt). 227 g = £1.32. White bread (with added fibre). 400 g = £1.94. Crackers. 150 g = £1.70. Sweet biscuits. 150 g = £1.24. Vanilla cream wafers. 100 g = £1.22. Chocolate flavoured cream wafers. 100 g = £1.22. Orange-flavoured cream wafers 100 g = £1.22. Cream-filled biscuits (chocolate flavour). 125 g = £1.24. For phenylketonuria and similar amino-acid abnormalities; renal failure; liver failure and liver cirrhosis; gluten-sensitive enteropathies including steatorrhoea due to gluten sensitivity, coeliac disease, and dermatitis herpetiformis

*Low sodium.* Bread containing protein 8.5%, carbohydrate 53.8%, fat 5.5%, Na⁺ 0.01%, K⁺ 0.055%. Net price 227 g = £1.32. For conditions in which a low-sodium diet is indicated

**Schar®** (Ultrapharm)

*Gluten-free*, Bread. Net price 250 g = £1.41. Bread rolls, 200 g = £1.41. Bread mix, 500 g = £3.95. Cake mix, 500 g = £3.95. Crackers, 200 g = £2.15. Crispbread, 250 g = £2.82. Pasta (fusilli, penne, rigatini, tagliatelle), 250 g = £1.90; spaghetti, 500 g = £3.41. Pizza bases, 250 g = £4.12. Savoy biscuits, 200 g = £2.15. For gluten-sensitive enteropathies including steatorrhoea due to gluten sensitivity, coeliac disease, and dermatitis herpetiformis

**SHS Modjul® Flavour System** (Scientific Hospital Supplies)

*Powder*, blackcurrant, orange, pineapple, and savoury tomato flavours. Net price 100 g = £4.87

For use with any unflavoured products based on peptides or amino acids

**Sunflower oil.** Net price 100 mL = 29p. For familial hypercholesterolaemia (non-drug for multiple sclerosis)

**Super Soluble Maxijul®**, see under Maxijul®

**Supplimen®** (Clintec)

*Liquid*, protein 15.6 g, carbohydrate 28.2 g, fat 8.3 g, energy 1045 kJ (250 kcal)/250 mL with vitamins, minerals, and trace elements. Cholesterol-, gluten-, and lactose-free. Vanilla flavour. Net price 250-mL can = 78p. As a necessary nutritional supplement prescribed on medical grounds for: short bowel syndrome, intractable malabsorption, pre-operative preparation of patients who are undernourished, treatment for those with proven inflammatory bowel disease, treatment following total gastrectomy, dysphagia, bowel fistulas, anorexia nervosa, neoplasia related (associated) cachexia (anorexia). Not to be prescribed for any child under one year

**Triosorbon®** (Merck)

*Powder*, protein 19%, carbohydrate 56%, fat 19%, with vitamins and minerals. Gluten-free. Net price 85-g sachet = £1.66. For use as the sole source of nutrition or as a necessary nutritional supplement prescribed on medical grounds for: short-bowel syndrome, intractable malabsorption, pre-operative preparation of patients who are undernourished, treatment for proven inflammatory bowel disease, treatment following total gastrectomy, dysphagia, bowel fistulas, anorexia nervosa; neoplasia-related (associated) cachexia (anorexia). Not to be prescribed for any child under one year, unsuitable as a sole source of nutrition for young children up to 5 years of age

**Tritamyl®** (Procea)

*Flour*, self-raising (starch-based), gluten- and lactose-free. Net price 2 kg = £5.86. For gluten-sensitive enteropathies including steatorrhoea due to gluten sensitivity, coeliac disease, and dermatitis herpetiformis

**Tritamyl PK®** (Procea)

*Flour*, self-raising (starch-based), gluten-, lactose-, and protein-free. Net price 2 kg = £5.86. For phenylketonuria and similar amino acid abnormalities; renal failure; liver failure and liver cirrhosis; gluten-sensitive enteropathies as above

**Trufree®** (Cantassium)

Gluten-free, wheat-free flours. For gluten-sensitive enteropathies including steatorrhoea due to gluten-sensitivity, coeliac disease, and dermatitis herpetiformis

*No. 1* (formerly bread mix 420 g). Net price 1 kg = £3.71

*No. 2 with rice bran* (formerly bread mix with rice bran 410 g). Net price 1 kg = £4.46

*No. 3 for Cantabread®* (formerly Cantabread mix). Net price 1 kg = £4.84

*No. 4 white.* Net price 1 kg = £3.71

*No. 5 brown.* Net price 1 kg = £3.71

*No. 6 plain* (formerly Trufree plain flour). Net price 1 kg = £3.53

*No. 7 self-raising* (formerly Trufree self-raising flour). Net price 1 kg = £3.71

**Ultra**® (Ultrapharm)

*High-fibre bread*, gluten-free. Net price 500 g = £3.26
For gluten-sensitive enteropathies including steatorrhea due to gluten sensitivity, coeliac disease, and dermatitis herpetiformis

**Wysoy**® (Wyeth)

*Powder*, carbohydrate 6.9%, fat 3.6%, and protein 2.1% with vitamins and minerals when reconstituted. Net price 430 g = £3.10; 860 g = £5.93. For proven lactose and associated sucrose intolerance in pre-school children, galactokinase deficiency, galactosaemia and proven whole cows milk sensitivity

---

## CONDITIONS FOR WHICH FOODS MAY BE PRESCRIBED ON FP10

*Note.* This is a list of clinical conditions for which the ACBS has approved food products. It is essential to check the list of products (above) for availability.

**Adrenoleukodystrophy:** Lorenzo's Oil.

**Amino acid metabolic disorders and similar protein disorders:** low protein drink (Milupa); see also phenylketonuria; histidinaemia; homocystinuria; maple syrup urine disease; synthetic diets; low-protein products.

**Anorexia nervosa:** Clinifeed 400[1], Favour, Iso and Protein Rich[1]; Clinutren 1.0 and 1.5[1]; Enrich; Ensure; Ensure Plus[1]; Ensure Powder; Fortimel[1]; Fortisip[1]; Fresenius OPD[1]; Fresubin Liquid, Sip Feeds, Plus F and 750[1]; Jevity; Liquisorb High Energy[1]; Liquisorb feed and drink; Liquisorb MCT[1]; Nutrison Energy Plus[1], Fibre and Standard; Osmolite; Peptisorbon; Protein Forte[1]; Provide[1]; Supplimen[1]; Triosorbon.

**Bowel fistulas:** Clinifeed 400[1], Favour, Iso and Protein Rich[1]; Clinutren 1.0 and 1.5[1]; Elemental 028; Enrich; Ensure; Ensure Plus[1]; Ensure Powder; Flexical; Fortimel[1]; Fortisip[1]; Fresenius OPD[1]; Fresubin Liquid, Sip Feeds Plus F and 750[1]; Jevity; Liquisorb High Energy[1]; Liquisorb feed and drink; Liquisorb MCT[1]; MCT Pepdite; Nutrison Energy Plus[1], Fibre, Paediatric and Standard; Osmolite; Paediasure; Pepdite; Peptamen; Pepti-2000 LF; Peptisorb; Peptisorbon; Protein Forte[1]; Provide[1]; Reabilan; Supplimen[1]; Triosorbon.

**Calcium intolerance:** Locasol New Formula.

**Carbohydrate malabsorption:** Calogen. See also synthetic diets; malabsorption states.

**Disaccharide intolerance** (without isomaltose intolerance): Caloreen; Duocal, Super Soluble and Duocal Liquid; Maxijul LE, Liquid, Super Soluble; Polycal; Polycose powder. See also lactose intolerance; lactose with sucrose intolerance.

**Glucose and galactose intolerance:** Comminuted chicken meat (Cow & Gate); Fructose Galactomin Formula 19 (fructose formula).

**Isomaltose intolerance:** Glucose (dextrose).

**Lactose intolerance**[2]: AL110; Comminuted chicken meat (Cow & Gate); Formula S (Cow & Gate); Galactomin Formula 17 (new formula); Isomil powder; Nutramigen; Nutrison Soya; Ostersoy; Pepdite; Portagen; Pregestimil; Prejomin; Prosobee; Wysoy.

**Lactose with sucrose intolerance**[2]: Comminuted Chicken Meat (Cow & Gate); Formula S (Cow & Gate); Galactomin Formula 17 (new formula); Nutramigen; Ostersoy; Pepti-Junior; Pregestimil; Prejomin; Prosobee; Wysoy.

---

1. As a supplement only

2. Defined as a condition of intolerance to an intake of the relevant disaccharide confirmed by demonstrated clinical benefit of effectiveness of disaccharide free diet, and presence of reducing substances or excessive acid in stools, low concentration of corresponding disaccharidase enzyme on intestinal biopsy, or breath tests, or lactose tolerance tests.

**Sucrose intolerance**[2]: Glucose (dextrose) and see also synthetic diets; malabsorption states; lactose with sucrose intolerance.

**Cirrhosis of the liver and chronic liver disease:** see liver disease.

**Coeliac disease:** see gluten-sensitive enteropathies.

**Continuous Ambulatory Peritoneal Dialysis (CAPD):** see dialysis.

**Cystic fibrosis:** see malabsorption states.

**Dermatitis Herpetiformis:** see gluten sensitive enteropathies.

**Dialysis:** nutritional supplements for haemodialysis or continuous ambulatory peritoneal dialysis (CAPD) patients: Clinifeed 400 and Protein Rich; Ensure Plus; Fortipudding; Fresubin 750; Protein Forte.

**Disaccharide intolerance:** see carbohydrate malabsorption.

**Dysphagia** (associated with: intrinsic disease of the oesophagus, e.g. oesophagitis; neuromuscular disorders, e.g. multiple sclerosis and motor neurone disease; major surgery and/or radiotherapy for cancer of the upper digestive tract; protracted severe inflammatory disease of the upper digestive tract, e.g. Stevens-Johnson syndrome and epidermolysis bullosa): Clinifeed 400[1], Favour, Iso and Protein Rich[1]; Clinutren 1.0 and 1.5[1]; Enrich; Ensure; Ensure Plus[1]; Ensure Powder; Fortimel[1]; Fortisip[1]; Fresenius OPD[1]; Fresubin Liquid, Sip Feeds, Plus F and 750[1]; Jevity; Liquisorb High Energy[1]; Liquisorb feed and drink; Liquisorb MCT[1]; Nutrison Energy Plus[1], Fibre, Paediatric and Standard; Osmolite; Paediasure; Peptisorbon; Protein Forte[1]; Provide[1]; Supplimen[1]; Triosorbon.

**Epilepsy (ketogenic diet in):** Alembicol D; Calogen; Liquigen; Medium-Chain Triglyceride Oil (MCT).

**Flavouring for use with any unflavoured product based on peptides or amino acids:** SHS Flavour Modjul

**Galactokinase deficiency and galactosaemia:** AL110; Alfare; Formula S (Cow & Gate); Galactomin Formula 17 (new formula); Isomil powder; Nutramigen; Ostersoy; Pregestimil; Prejomin; Prosobee Liquid and Powder; Wysoy.

**Gastrectomy (total):** Clinifeed 400[1], Favour, Iso and Protein Rich[1]; Clinutren 1.0 and 1.5[1]; Enrich; Ensure; Ensure Plus[1]; Ensure Powder; Fortimel[1]; Fortisip[1]; Fresenius OPD[1]; Fresubin Liquid, Sip Feeds, Plus F and 750[1]; Jevity; Liquisorb High Energy[1]; Liquisorb Feed and Drink; Liquisorb MCT[1]; Nutrison Energy Plus[1]; Fibre and Standard; Osmolite; Peptisorbon; Protein Forte[1]; Provide[1]; Supplemen[1]; Triosorbon.

**Glucose/galactose intolerance:** see carbohydrate malabsorption.

**Glutaric aciduria:** Maxamaid XLys, Try

**Gluten-sensitive enteropathies:** Aproten products (anellini, biscuits, breadmix, cake mix, crispbread, ditalini, flour, rigatini, spaghetti, tagliatelle); Arnott gluten-free rice cookies; Bi-Aglut biscuits, flour, and gluten-free toast; Ener-G brown and white rice bread, gluten-free tapioca bread, gluten-free rice pasta (cannelloni, lasagna, shells, small shells, spaghetti, tagliatelli, vermicelli); Glutafin bread, fibre bread, mix, fibre mix, biscuits (digestive, savoury, sweet (without chocolate or sultanas), tea), crackers, high fibre crackers and pasta (spirals, macaroni, spaghetti short-cut); Gluten-free biscuits (Farley); Gluten-free biscuits (Nutricia); Juvela gluten-free corn mix, gluten-free loaf and high-fibre loaf (sliced and unsliced), gluten-free mix and fibre mix; Juvela low-protein loaf (sliced and unsliced) and low-protein mix; Liga gluten-free rusks (Jacobs); Loprofin bread, mix, pasta (macaroni, pasta spirals, spaghetti short-cut); Polial gluten-free biscuits; Rite-Diet gluten-free high-fibre bread (with added soya-bran); Rite-Diet gluten-free white bread and 400 g; Rite-Diet gluten-free white bread mix; Rite-Diet gluten-free brown bread mix; Rite-Diet gluten-free bread with soya bran (dispensed in tin); Rite-Diet gluten-free high-fibre crackers; Rite-Diet baking mix; Rite-Diet low-protein flour mix; Rite-Diet gluten-free flour mix; Rite-Diet gluten-free low-protein bread (dispensed in tin, with or without salt); Rite-Diet low-protein white bread (with added fibre); Rite-Diet gluten-free digestive biscuits, sweet (without chocolate or sultanas) biscuits, savoury biscuits, tea biscuits, and gluten-free crackers; Rite-Diet low-protein spaghetti (short cut), spaghetti rings, and macaroni; Schar gluten-free bread, bread mix, bread rolls, crackers, crispbread, pasta (fusilli, penne, rigatoni, spaghetti, tagliatelli), pizza base, savoy biscuits; Schar gluten-free low-protein cake mix; Tritamyl gluten-free flour; Tritamyl PK flour; Tru-free special dietary flours No. 1, No. 2 with rice bran, No. 3 for Cantabread, No. 4 white, No. 5 brown, No. 6 plain, No. 7 self-raising; Ultra High-Fibre bread.

**Glycogen storage disease:** Caloreen; Corn Flour or Corn Starch; Glucose (dextrose); Maxijul LE, Liquid, and Super Soluble; Polycal; Polycose.

**Growth Failure (secondary to disease related anorexia):** Fortison Paediatric; Paediasure.

**Haemodialysis:** see dialysis.

**Histidinaemia:** HF(2), and see also low-protein products; synthetic diets.

**Homocystinuria:** Albumaid RVHB X Methionine; Albumaid RVHB Complete X Methionine, Analog RVHB; Maxamaid RVHB; Maxamum RVHB, and see also low-protein products; synthetic diets.

**Hypercholesterolaemia (familial):** Corn oil; Sunflower oil.

**Hyperlipoproteinaemia type 1:** Liquigen; Medium Chain Triglyceride Oil.

**Hyperlysinaemia:** Analog XLys; Maxamaid XLys

**Hypermethioninaemia:** Analog RVHB; Maxamaid RVHB; Maxamum RVHB.

**Hypoglycaemia:** Caloreen; Corn Flour or Corn Starch; Maxijul LE, Liquid, and Super Soluble; Polycal; Polycose, and see also glycogen storage disease.

**Hypoproteinaemia:** Casilan; Dialamine; Forceval Protein; Maxipro HBV Super Soluble; ProMod; Protifar.

**Inflammatory Bowel Disease:** Clinifeed 400[1], Favour, Iso and Protein Rich[1]; Clinutren 1.0 and 1.5[1]; Elemental 028; Enrich; Ensure; Ensure Plus[1]; Ensure Powder; Flexical; Fortimel[1]; Fortisip[1]; Fresenius OPD[1]; Fresubin Liquid, Sip Feeds, Plus F and 750[1]; Jevity; Liquisorb High Energy[1]; Liquisorb Feed and Drink; Liquisorbon MCT[1]; Nutrison Energy Plus[1], Fibre and Standard; Osmolite; Peptamen; Pepti-2000 LF; Peptisorb; Peptisorbon; Protein Forte[1]; Provide[1]; Reabilan; Supplimen[1]; Triosorbon.

**Intestinal lymphangiectasia:** see malabsorption states.

**Intestinal surgery:** see malabsorption states.

**Isomaltose intolerance:** see carbohydrate malabsorption.

**Lactose intolerance:** see carbohydrate malabsorption.

**Liver disease (i.e. chronic liver disease, cirrhosis):** Alembicol D; Aminex; Aproten products (anellini, biscuits, bread mix, cake mix, crispbread, ditalini, flour, rigatini, spaghetti, tagliatelle); Caloreen; dp Low-Protein butterscotch-flavoured or chocolate-flavoured chip cookies; Duocal, Super Soluble, and Duocal Liquid; Fortical; Generaid; Hepatic Aid; Hycal; Juvela gluten-free low-protein (chocolate chip, orange, and cinnamon flavour) cookies; Juvela low-protein loaf (sliced and unsliced) and low-protein flour mix; Liquigen; Loprofin gluten-free low-protein bread, mix, pasta (macaroni, spaghetti short-cut, pasta spirals); Loprofin low-protein sweet biscuits, chocolate cream-filled biscuits, crackers, cookies (chocolate chip, cinnamon), wafers (orange, chocolate, vanilla); Maxijul LE, Liquid, and Super Soluble; MCT (1) Powder; Medium Chain Triglyceride Oil; Polycal; Polycose; Portagen; Rite-Diet gluten-free low-protein bread (dispensed in tin with or without salt); Rite-Diet low-protein white bread (with added fibre); Rite-Diet gluten-free low-protein crackers; Rite-Diet low-protein baking mix; Rite-Diet low-protein flour mix; Rite-Diet low-protein cream-filled biscuits (chocolate flavour) and sweet biscuits; Rite-Diet low-protein macaroni, spaghetti (short cut), and spaghetti rings; Rite-Diet low-protein chocolate, orange, and vanilla cream wafers; Tritamyl PK flour.

**Low-protein products:** Aglutella Azeta cream-filled wafers*; Aglutella gluten-free low protein (macaroni, pasta spirals, semolina, spaghetti, spaghetti-rings, tagliatelle); Aminex*; Aproten products (anellini, biscuits, bread mix, cake mix, crispbread, ditalini, flour, rigatini, tagliatelle); dp Low-Protein butterscotch-flavoured or chocolate-flavoured chip cookies*; Juvela gluten-free low-protein (chocolate chip, orange, and cinnamon flavour) cookies*; Juvela low-protein loaf (sliced and unsliced); Juvela low-protein mix; Loprofin gluten-free low-protein bread, mix, pasta (macaroni, spaghetti short-cut, pasta spirals); Loprofin low-protein sweet biscuits, chocolate cream-filled biscuits, crackers, cookies (chocolate chip, cinnamon), wafers (orange, chocolate, vanilla); Rite-Diet gluten-free low-protein bread (dispensed in tin, with or without salt); Rite-Diet low-protein white bread (with added fibre); Rite-Diet low-protein gluten-free crackers; Rite-Diet low-protein flour mix; Rite-Diet low-protein cream-filled biscuits (chocolate flavour)*; Rite-Diet low-protein sweet biscuits; Rite-Diet low-protein macaroni, spaghetti (short cut), and spaghetti rings; Rite-Diet low-protein chocolate, orange, and vanilla cream wafers*; Tritamyl PK flour.

*Not prescribable on ACBS for coeliac disease, dermatitis herpetiformis, steatorrhoea due to gluten sensitivity

**Malabsorption states:** (see also gluten-sensitive enteropathies; liver disease; carbohydrate malabsorption; intestinal lymphangiectasia; milk intolerance and synthetic diets).

(a) Protein sources: Albumaid Complete; Comminuted Chicken Meat (Cow & Gate); Duocal, Super Soluble, and Duocal Liquid; Forceval Protein; Maxipro HBV; MCT Pepdite; Neocate; Pepdite.

(b) Fat: Alembicol D; Calogen; Liquigen; Medium Chain Triglyceride Oil; MCT Pepdite.

(c) Carbohydrate: Caloreen; Fortical; Hycal; Maxijul LE, Liquid, and Super Soluble; Polycal; Polycose.

(d) Complete Feeds. For use as the sole source of nutrition or as a necessary nutritional supplement prescribed on medical grounds: Clinifeed Favour and Iso; Clinutren 1.0; Elemental 028; Enrich; Ensure; Ensure Powder; Flexical; Fresubin Liquid, Sip Feeds, and Plus F; Jevity; Liquisorb feed and drink, MCT (1) Powder (with appropriate vitamin and mineral supplements); MCT Pepdite; Nutrison Fibre, Paediatric and Standard; Osmolite; Paediasure; Peptamen; Pepti-2000 LF; Pepdite; Pepti-Junior; Peptisorb; Portagen; Pregestimil; Reabilan; Triosorbon.

(e) Nutritional supplements. Necessary nutritional supplements prescribed on medical grounds: Clinfeed 400 and Protein Rich; Clinutren 1.5; Ensure Plus; Fortimel; Fortisip; Fresenius OPD; Fresubin 750; Liquisorb High Energy; Liquisorbon MCT; Nutrison Energy Plus; Peptisorbon; Protein Forte; Provide; Supplimen.

(f) Minerals: Aminogran Mineral Mixture; Metabolic Mineral Mixture.

(g) Vitamins: As appropriate, and see synthetic diets.

(h) Vitamins and Minerals: Paediatric Seravit

**Maple syrup urine disease:** Analog MSUD; Maxamaid MSUD; Maxamum MSUD; MSUD Aid, and see also low-protein products; synthetic diets.

**Methylmalonic or propionic acidaemia:** Analog XMet, Thre, Val, Isoleu; Maxamaid XMet, Thre, Val, Isoleu; Maxamum XMet, Thre, Val, Isoleu.

**Milk protein sensitivity:** Comminuted Chicken Meat (Cow & Gate); Formula S (Cow & Gate); Isomil powder; Nutramigen; Nutrison Soya; Ostersoy; Pregestimil; Prosobee Liquid and powder; Wysoy, and see also synthetic diets.

**Neoplasia-related (associated) cachexia (anorexia):** Clinifeed 400[1], Favour, Iso and Protein Rich; Clinutren 1.0 and 1.5[1]; Enrich; Ensure; Ensure Plus; Ensure Powder; Fortimel[1]; Fortisip[1]; Fresenius OPD[1]; Fresubin Liquid, Sip Feeds, Plus F and 750[1]; Jevity; Liquisorb High Energy[1]; Liquisorb Feed and Drink; Liquisorbon MCT[1]; Nutrison Energy Plus[1], Fibre, Paediatric and

Standard; Osmolite; Paediasure; Peptamen; Peptisorbon; Protein Forte[1]; Provide[1]; Supplimen[1]; Triosorbon.

**Nutritional support for adults** (for precise conditions for which these products have ACBS approval, see products above):

A. (a) Nutritionally complete feeds. For use as the sole source of nutrition or as a necessary nutritional supplement prescribed on medical grounds for:
   (i) Gluten-Free: Clinifeed Iso; Fresubin Liquid, Sip Feeds, and Plus F (vegetable soup flavour only); Liquisorb feed and drink; Nutrison Standard; Triosorbon.
   (ii) Lactose-free: Clinifeed Favour; Clinutren 1.0.
   (iii) Lactose- and Gluten-Free: Enrich; Ensure, Ensure Powder; Osmolite.
   (iv) Containing fibre: Enrich; Fresubin Plus F; Jevity; Nutrison Fibre.
   (v) Elemental Feeds: Elemental 028; Flexical; Peptamen; Pepti-2000 LF; Peptisorb; Reabilan.

B. **Nutritional source supplements;** see synthetic diets; malabsorption states.
   (a) General supplements. Necessary nutritional supplements prescribed on medical grounds: Clinifeed 400 and Protein Rich; Clinutren 1.5; Ensure Plus; Fortimel; Fortisip; Fresenius OPD; Fresubin 750; Liquisorb High Energy; Liquisorbon MCT; Nutrison Energy Plus; Peptisorbon; Protein Forte; Provide; Supplimen.
   (b) Carbohydrates; lactose-free and gluten-free: Caloreen*; Super-Soluble Duocal, and Duocal Liquid*; Fortical*; Hycal*; Maxijul LE*, Liquid, and Super Soluble; Polycal; Polycose.
      *Have low electrolyte content.
   (c) Fat: Alembicol D; Calogen; MCT Oil; Liquigen.
   (d) Nitrogen: Albumaid Complete (hydrolysed protein based); Casilan (whole protein based, low-sodium); Forceval Protein (whole protein based, low-sodium); Maxipro HBV (whole protein based, low-sodium); Pro-Mod (whey protein based, low-sodium).
   (e) Minerals: Aminogran Mineral Mixture; Metabolic Mineral Mixture.

**Phenylketonuria:** Albumaid XP and XP Concentrate; Aminogran Food Supplement and Mineral Mixture; Analog XP; Aproten products (annellini, biscuits, bread mix, cake mix, crispbread, ditalini, flour, rigatini, spaghetti, tagliatelle); Calogen; Caloreen; dp Low-Protein butterscotch-flavoured or chocolate-flavoured chip cookies; Juvela low-protein loaf (sliced and unsliced); Juvela gluten-free low-protein (chocolate chip, orange, and cinnamon flavour) cookies; Juvela low-protein mix; Lofenalac; Loprofin gluten-free, low-protein bread, mix and pasta (macaroni, spaghetti short-cut, pasta spirals); Loprofin low-protein sweet biscuits, chocolate cream-filled biscuits, crackers, cookies (chocolate chip, cinnamon), wafers (orange, chocolate, vanilla); Maxamaid XP; Maxamaid XP bar; Maxamaid XP Concentrate; Metabolic Mineral Mixture; Milupa PKU3; Minafen; PK Aid 3; PKU Drink; PKU 2; Polycal; Polycose liquid and powder; Rite-Diet gluten-free low-protein bread (dispensed in tin, with or without salt); Rite-Diet low-protein white bread (with added fibre); Rite-Diet low-protein baking mix; Rite-Diet low-protein flour mix; Rite-Diet low-protein cream-filled biscuits (chocolate flavour), sweet biscuits and gluten-free low-protein crackers; Rite-Diet low-protein macaroni, spaghetti (short cut), and spaghetti rings; Rite-Diet low-protein chocolate, orange, and vanilla cream wafers; Tritamyl PK flour, and see low-protein products and synthetic diets.

**Protein intolerance:** see milk protein sensitivity, whole protein sensitivity, low-protein products, synthetic diets, and amino acid metabolic disorders.

**Refsum's Disease:** Fresubin Liquid and Sip Feeds.

**Renal failure:** Aproten products (annellini, biscuits, bread mix, cake mix, crispbread, ditalini, flour, rigatini, spaghetti, tagliatelle); Calogen; Caloreen; Dialamine; dp

Low-Protein butterscotch-flavoured or chocolate-flavoured chip cookies; Super-Soluble Duocal and Duocal Liquid; Fortical; Hycal; Juvela gluten-free low-protein (chocolate chip, orange, and cinnamon flavour) cookies; Juvela low-protein loaf (sliced and unsliced) and low-protein flour mix; Loprofin gluten-free, low-protein bread, mix and pasta (macaroni, spaghetti short-cut, pasta spirals); Loprofin low-protein sweet biscuits, chocolate cream-filled biscuits, crackers, cookies (chocolate chip, cinnamon), wafers (orange, chocolate, vanilla); Maxijul LE, Liquid, and Super Soluble; Polycal; Polycose liquid and powder; Rite-Diet gluten-free low-protein bread (dispensed in tin, with or without salt); Rite-Diet low-protein white bread (with added fibre); Rite-Diet low-protein gluten-free crackers; Rite-Diet low-protein flour mix; Rite-Diet low-protein baking mix; Rite-Diet low-protein cream-filled biscuits (chocolate flavour); Rite-Diet low-protein sweet biscuits; Rite-Diet low-protein macaroni, spaghetti (short cut), and spaghetti rings; Rite-Diet low-protein chocolate, orange, and vanilla cream wafers; Rite-Diet low-sodium bread; Tritamyl PK flour.

**Short bowel syndrome:** see malabsorption states.

**Sicca Syndrome:** Glandosane; Saliva Orthana; Salivace.

**Sodium dietary reduction:** Rite-Diet low-sodium bread.

**Sucrose intolerance:** see carbohydrate malabsorption.

**Synthetic diets:**
   (a) Fat: Alembicol D; Calogen; Liquigen; Medium Chain Triglyceride Oil.
   (b) Carbohydrate: Caloreen; Fortical; Hycal; Maxijul LE, Liquid (and orange), Super Soluble; Polycal; Polycose powder.
   (c) Minerals: Aminogran Mineral Mixture; Metabolic Mineral Mixture.
   (d) Protein sources: see malabsorption states, complete feeds.
   (e) Vitamins: as appropriate and see malabsorption states, nutritional support for adults.
   (f) Vitamins and Minerals: Paediatric Seravit.

**Tyrosinaemia:** Analog XPhen, Tyr; Maxamaid XPhen, Tyr.

**Vomiting in infancy:** Instant Carobel; Nestargel.

**Whole protein sensitivity[2]:** Alfare; MCT Pepdite; Neocate; Nutramigen; Pepdite; Pepti-Junior; Pregestimil; Prejomin.

**Xerostomia:** Glandosane; Saliva Orthana; Salivace.

---

## CONDITIONS FOR WHICH TOILET PREPARATIONS MAY BE PRESCRIBED ON FP10

*Note.* This is a list of clinical conditions for which the ACBS has approved toilet preparations. For details of the preparations see Chapter 13.

**Acne:** Ionax scrub.

**Birthmarks:** see disfiguring skin lesions.

**Dermatitis (includes contact, atopic and infective dermatoses, eczema and pruritic dermatoses):** Aveeno Bath Oil; Aveeno Cream; Aveeno sachets (regular and oilated); Bath E45; Betadine Skin Cleanser and Foam; Genisol; Polytar Emollient, Liquid, and Plus; Ster-Zac Bath Concentrate; T/Gel shampoo; Vaseline Dermacare Cream and Lotion; Wash E45.

**Dermatitis herpetiformis:** see gluten-sensitive enteropathies.

---

1. As a supplement only
2. Defined as: intolerance to whole protein, proven by at least two withdrawal and challenge tests, as suggested by an accurate dietary history.

**Disfiguring skin lesions (birthmarks, mutilating lesions and scars):** Boots Covering Cream; Covermark products; Dermablend Cover Creme, Leg Cover, and Setting Powder; Dermacolor Camouflage cream and fixing powder; Keromask masking cream and finishing powder; Veil Cover cream and Finishing Powder. (Cleansing Creams, Cleansing Milks, and Cleansing Lotions are excluded.)

**Disinfectants (antiseptics):** drugs only when ordered in such quantities and with such directions as are appropriate for the treatment of patients. Not to be regarded as drugs if ordered for general hygienic purposes.

**Eczema:** see dermatitis.

**Photodermatoses (skin protection in):** Almay Total Sunblock Cream and Lip protector; Ambre Solaire High Protection Cream Factor 10; Ambre Solaire High Protection Milk Factor 12; Ambre Solaire Maximum Protection Cream Factor 25; Coppertone Supershade, and Sunstick 15 and Ultrashade 23; Piz Buin Creme, SPF 12; Piz Buin Lotion 12; Piz Buin Sun Allergy Lotion 12; Piz Buin Sunblock Lotion 24; RoC Opaque Total Sunblock Cream SPF 15 A & B (Colourless and tinted); RoC Sunscreen Stick; RoC Total Sunblock Cream 10 (colourless); Spectraban 10 and 15; Spectraban Ultra; Sun E45 Cream 25; Sun E45 Lotion 15; Uvistat Sun Cream 10 and 15; Uvistat Lipscreen 15; Uvistat Water-resistant Cream 8; Uvistat Sun Block Cream 20; Uvistat Ultrablock Cream 30.

**Pruritus:** see dermatitis.

**Psoriasis:** see scaling of the scalp.

**Scaling of the scalp (psoriasis, dandruff, eczema):** Alphosyl; Betadine; Capitol; Ceanel Concentrate; Cetavlon PC; Gelcotar; Genisol; Ionil T; Polytar Emollient, Liquid, and Plus; T/Gel shampoo.

# Appendix 8: Cautionary and Advisory Labels for Dispensed Medicines

In recent years there has been a growing need for patients to be given better information on the medicines they have been prescribed so that they will be reminded to take the medicine correctly and most effectively.

The BNF now shows under many preparations the numbers of any labels that pharmacists are recommended to apply to the containers of preparations when they are dispensed. The wordings chosen for the labels represent a carefully considered balance between the unintelligibly short and the inconveniently long. Since any fixed set of words cannot cover the language needs of all patients it is expected that pharmacists will counsel patients.

All counselling needs to be related to the age, experience, background, and understanding of the individual patient. The patient will then be able to obtain the maximum benefit from following the directions.

Compliance with the intentions of the prescriber should be encouraged. The pharmacist should ensure that the patient understands not only how to use the medicine but also how much and how often. Any effects of the medicine on driving or work, any foods or medicines to be avoided, and what to do if a dose is missed should also be explained. There may be other matters that are better dealt with by counselling than by a label, such as the possibility of staining of the clothes or skin by a medicine.

For some preparations there is a special need for counselling, such as an unusual method or time of administration or a potential interaction with a common food or domestic remedy, and this is indicated where necessary.

## Manufacturers' instructions

Many preparations are now dispensed in unbroken original packs that bear complete instructions for the patient or provide a leaflet addressed to the patient. These labels or leaflets should not normally be obscured or removed. Where it is known that such instructions are provided with an original pack intended for the patient no label has been listed under the preparation. Label 10 may be used where appropriate. Leaflets are available from various sources advising on the administration of preparations such as eye-drops, eye ointments, inhalers, and suppositories.

## Scope of the recommended labels

No label recommendations have been made for injections (except for selected systemic corticosteroids) on the assumption that they will be administered by a health professional or a well-trained patient. The labelling is not exhaustive and pharmacists are recommended to use their professional discretion in labelling new preparations and those for which no labels are shown.

Individual labelling advice is not given on the administration of the large variety of antacids. In the absence of instructions from the prescriber, and if on enquiry the patient has had no verbal instructions, the directions given under 'Dose' should be used on the label.

It is recognised that there may be occasions when pharmacists will use their knowledge and professional discretion and decide to omit one or more of the recommended labels for a particular patient. In this case counselling is of the utmost importance. There may also be an occasion when a prescriber does not wish additional cautionary labels to be used, in which case the prescription should be endorsed 'NCL' (no cautionary labels). The exact wording that is required instead should then be specified on the prescription.

Pharmacists have traditionally labelled medicines with various wordings in addition to those directions specified on the prescription. Such labels include 'Shake the bottle', 'For external use only', 'Not to be taken', and 'Store in a cool place', as well as 'Discard . . . . days after opening' and 'Do not use after . . . .', which apply particularly to antibiotic mixtures, diluted liquid and topical preparations, and to eye-drops. Although not listed in the BNF these labels should continue to be used when appropriate; indeed, 'For external use only' is a legal requirement on external liquid preparations, while 'Keep out of the reach of children' is a legal requirement on all dispensed medicines.

It is the usual practice for patients to take oral solid-dose preparations with water or other liquid and for this reason no separate label has been recommended.

The label or labels for each preparation are recommended after careful consideration of the information available. However, it is recognised that in some cases this information may be either incomplete or open to a different interpretation. The Executive Editor will therefore be grateful to receive any constructive comments on the labelling suggested for any preparation.

## Recommended label wordings

The wordings which can be given as separate warnings are labels 1–19 and labels 29–33. Wordings which can be incorporated in an appropriate position in the directions for dosage or administration are labels 21–28. A label has been omitted for number 20.

If separate labels are used it is recommended that the wordings be used without modification. If changes are made to suit computer requirements, care should be taken to retain the sense of the original.

## (1)   Warning. May cause drowsiness

To be used on children's preparations containing antihistamines, e.g., paediatric elixirs and linctuses, or other preparations given to children where the warnings of label 2 on driving or alcohol would not be appropriate.

## (2)   Warning. May cause drowsiness. If affected do not drive or operate machinery. Avoid alcoholic drink

To be used on preparations that can cause drowsiness, thereby affecting the ability to drive and operate hazardous machinery. The main preparations are most antihistamines; central nervous system depressants such as anxiolytics, antipsychotics, opioid analgesics, and tricyclic antidepressants; some antihypertensives; some analgesics; some antiepileptics; some antiemetics; and some muscle relaxants. Label 2 is now seen as unhelpful in relation to hypnotics, hence a new label (label 19) has been introduced to cover hypnotics, and also anxiolytics, taken at night. *It is an offence to drive while under the influence of drink or drugs.*

Label 1 is more appropriate for children.

Some of these preparations only cause drowsiness in the first few days of treatment and the patient then becomes tolerant; some only cause drowsiness in higher doses.

In such cases the patient should be told that the advice to avoid driving, etc., applies until the effects have worn off. Many of these preparations can produce a slowing of reaction time and a loss of mental concentration that can have the same effects as drowsiness on activities that require alertness to avoid hazard.

The avoidance of alcoholic drink is recommended, since the effects of CNS depressants are enhanced by alcohol, but it must be realised that a strict prohibition could lead to certain patients not taking the medicine at all. Pharmacists should explain the risk and encourage compliance, particularly in patients who may think they already tolerate the effects of alcohol (see also label 3).

Queries from patients with epilepsy regarding fitness to drive should be referred back to the patient's doctor.

There are other side-effects unrelated to drowsiness that may affect a patient's ability to drive or operate machinery safely, for example, blurred vision, dizziness, or nausea. In general, no label has been recommended to cover these cases, but the patient should be suitably counselled.

## (3)   Warning. May cause drowsiness. If affected do not drive or operate machinery

To be used on monoamine-oxidase inhibitors (because alcohol is covered by label 10 and the MAOI treatment card).

Some patients given CNS depressants may have been advised how much alcohol they may drink by their doctor and in such cases label 3 may be more appropriate than label 2.

## (4)   Warning. Avoid alcoholic drink

To be used on preparations where a reaction such as flushing may occur if alcohol is taken, e.g. metronidazole and chlorpropamide. Alcohol may also enhance the hypoglycaemia produced by some oral antidiabetic drugs but routine application of a warning label is not considered necessary.

For most interactions with alcohol label 2 is more appropriate.

## (5)   Do not take indigestion remedies at the same time of day as this medicine

To be used in conjunction with label 25 on preparations coated to resist gastric acid, such as enteric-coated tablets, capsules, and granules.

The coating may be ruptured prematurely in the presence of alkalis present in antacids.

Label 5 also applies to drugs such as ciprofloxacin and ketoconazole where the absorption is significantly affected by antacids; the usual period of avoidance recommended is 2 to 4 hours.

## (6)   Do not take iron preparations or indigestion remedies at the same time of day as this medicine

To be used on preparations of doxycycline, minocycline, and penicillamine. These drugs chelate iron and calcium ions and are less well absorbed when given with iron or calcium-containing antacids. If necessary these incompatible preparations may be given about two hours apart.

## (7)   Do not take milk, iron preparations or indigestion remedies at the same time of day as this medicine

To be used on preparations of tetracyclines (except doxycycline and minocycline). These drugs chelate iron, calcium, and magnesium ions and are then less well absorbed. If necessary these incompatible preparations may be given about two hours apart.

## (8)   Do not stop taking this medicine except on your doctor's advice

To be used on beta-blockers, certain antihypertensive drugs, drugs used in the treatment and prophylaxis of asthma, antituberculous drugs, and allopurinol.

This label is used to encourage compliance where the drug is to be taken over long periods without the patient necessarily perceiving any benefit. Patients should be told that this label does not override the need to consult the prescriber if side-effects occur.

For certain medicines the patient should be advised to ensure that the supply does not run out.

## (9)   Take at regular intervals. Complete the prescribed course unless otherwise directed

To be used on preparations where a course of treatment should be completed to reduce the incidence of relapse, the development of resistance, or failure of treatment. The preparations are antimicrobial drugs given by mouth.

Very occasionally, some of these antimicrobial agents may have severe side-effects and in such cases the patient may need to be advised of reasons for stopping treatment quickly and returning to the doctor. Examples are the development of diarrhoea in patients receiving clindamycin or lincomycin (see section 5.1.6), or sensitivity reactions with the penicillins.

**(10)   Warning. Follow the printed instructions you have been given with this medicine**

To be used particularly on anticoagulants, lithium, monoamine-oxidase inhibitors, and oral corticosteroids. The appropriate treatment card should be given to the patient and any necessary explanations given.

This label may also be used on other preparations to remind the patient of the instructions that have been given.

**(11)   Avoid exposure of skin to direct sunlight or sun lamps**

To be used on preparations that may cause phototoxic or photoallergic reactions if the patient is exposed to ultraviolet radiation. Many drugs other than those listed (e.g. phenothiazines and sulphonamides) may on rare occasions cause reactions in susceptible patients. Reactions have also been caused by external preparations (e.g. coal tar) and by various ingredients of perfumes and cosmetics. Exposure to high intensity ultraviolet radiation from sunray lamps and sunbeds is particularly likely to cause reactions and in advising patients this should be mentioned.

Drugs involved include amiodarone, demeclocycline, nalidixic acid, and protriptyline.

**(12)   Do not take anything containing aspirin while taking this medicine**

To be used on preparations containing the uricosuric drugs probenecid and sulphinpyrazone whose activity is reduced by aspirin.

Label 12 should not be used for anticoagulants; label 10 is more appropriate.

**(13)   Dissolve or mix with water before taking**

To be used on preparations that are intended to be dissolved in water (e.g. soluble tablets) or mixed with water (e.g. powders, granules) before use. In a few cases the manufacturer's literature indicates that other liquids such as fruit juice or milk may be used.

**(14)   This medicine may colour the urine**

To be used on preparations that may cause the patient's urine to turn unusual colours. These include phenolphthalein (alkaline urine pink), triamterene (blue under some lights), levodopa (dark reddish), and rifampicin (red).

**(15)   Caution flammable: keep away from fire or flames**

To be applied to preparations containing sufficient alcohol, acetone, ether, or other flammable solvent to render them flammable if exposed to a naked flame. The term flammable is now used by the British Pharmacopoeia and in legislation in preference to inflammable. Since both terms are now liable to cause confusion, the pharmacist should make sure that the patient understands what is meant.

**(16)   Allow to dissolve under the tongue. Do not transfer from this container. Keep tightly closed. Discard eight weeks after opening**

To be used on glyceryl trinitrate tablets to remind the patient not to transfer the tablets to plastic or less suitable containers. The manufacturer's original pack normally carries most of this wording and it may only be necessary to add 'Discard eight weeks after opening'.

**(17)   Do not take more than . . . . in 24 hours**

To be used on preparations for the treatment of acute migraine except those containing ergotamine, for which label 18 is used.

It may also be used on preparations for which no dose has been specified by the prescriber.

It is recommended that the dose form should be specified, e.g. tablets or capsules.

**(18)   Do not take more than . . . in 24 hours or . . . in any one week**

To be used on preparations of ergotamine tartrate.

It is recommended that the dose form should be specified, e.g. tablets or capsules.

**(19)   Warning. Causes drowsiness which may continue the next day. If affected do not drive or operate machinery. Avoid alcoholic drink**

To be used on those preparations (e.g. nitrazepam) which are classified as hypnotics in the BNF when they are prescribed to be taken at night. On the rare occasions (e.g. nitrazepam in epilepsy) when hypnotics are prescribed for daytime administration this label would clearly not be appropriate. Also to be used as an alternative to the label 2 wording (the choice being at the discretion of the pharmacist) for anxiolytics (e.g. diazepam) prescribed to be taken at night. It is hoped that this wording will convey adequately the problem of residual morning sedation after taking 'sleeping tablets'.

**(21)   . . . with or after food**

To be used on preparations that are liable to cause gastric irritation with nausea and vomiting, or those that are better absorbed with food.

The incidence of gastric irritation may be reduced when some preparations are given during or immediately after a meal. The presence of food in the upper gastro-intestinal tract may reduce the rate of absorption of certain drugs. Nausea and vomiting are liable to decrease compliance and possibly lead to loss of the drug from vomiting.

Patients may on occasions be advised to take their medicine with or after food in the interest of compliance when normally it should be taken before meals. There is a wide variation in the

instructions given for iron salts and their preparations. They are usually best absorbed when
given on an empty stomach but may then cause
irritation. They are therefore often taken with a
meal.

The prescriber's instructions should be
followed.

A small number of preparations are better
absorbed when given with food.

The word 'food' is used in preference to 'meal'
on the label. Patients differ in their interpretation
of the words and may decide not to take a dose if
it has to be taken with a meal that they normally
omit.

Patients should be advised when to take their
doses, according to their particular circumstances,
and that a small amount of food is sufficient.

#### (22) . . . half to one hour before food

To be used on some antimuscarinic or antacid
preparations; some pancreatin and other enzyme
preparations; most appetite suppressants; and
certain other drugs whose absorption or local
effect is thereby improved.

#### (23) . . . an hour before food or on an empty stomach

To be used on some oral antibiotics whose absorption may be reduced by the presence of food and
acid in the stomach.

Many of the antibiotics introduced in recent
years are less affected by acid and/or food in the
stomach and may be given at any time relative to
meals.

#### (24) . . . sucked or chewed

To be used on preparations that may be sucked
or chewed. Certain preparations must be chewed
before swallowing to improve their absorption or
because of their size; others have been specially
formulated to be chewed. All pastilles and lozenges should be sucked slowly to aid their local
effect on the oropharynx. The pharmacist should
use discretion as to which of these words is
appropriate.

#### (25) . . . swallowed whole, not chewed

To be used on preparations designed for modified-
release; on certain preparations that are very
unpleasant or may damage the mouth or oesophagus if not swallowed whole; and with label 5
for enteric-coated preparations. Most modified-
release preparations rely on the coating of pellets,
granules, tablets, or capsules or compression in a
matrix material to achieve their effect. Chewing
can cause premature release of active ingredient.

#### (26) . . . dissolved under the tongue

To be used on preparations intended for sublingual use. Several drugs are absorbed into the
circulation more effectively from the mucosa of
the mouth, thereby avoiding the portal circulation
into the liver. Patients should be advised to hold

the tablet still under the tongue and avoid swallowing until the tablet is dissolved. The buccal
mucosa between the gum and cheek is occasionally specified by the prescriber and specific directions should then be used.

#### (27) . . . with plenty of water

To be used on preparations that should be well
diluted (e.g. chloral hydrate), where a high fluid
intake is required (e.g. sulphonamides), or where
water is required to aid the action of the preparation (e.g. methylcellulose). The patient should
be advised that 'plenty' means at least 150 mL
(about a tumblerful). In most cases a beverage
such as fruit juice, tea, or coffee could be used.
There have been reports of solid-dose preparations sticking in the oesophagus, particularly
in the elderly, and all patients should be reminded
of the necessity of taking capsules and tablets with
water or other liquid. As much as 100 mL may be
required and the patient should stand or sit while
taking the dose.

#### (28) To be applied sparingly . . .

To be used with external corticosteroid preparations and dithranol preparations.

The application of excessive quantities to the
skin can increase the incidence of local side-effects
and give rise to undesirable systemic effects.

#### (29) Do not take more than 2 at any one time. Do not take more than 8 in 24 hours

To be used on containers of dispensed solid dose
preparations containing paracetamol for **adults**
when the instruction on the label indicates that
the dose can be taken on an 'as required' basis.
This label has been introduced because of the
serious consequences of overdosage with paracetamol.

It is recommended that the dose form should
be specified, e.g. tablets or capsules.

#### (30) Contains paracetamol

To be used on containers of dispensed preparations containing paracetamol when the name
on the label does not include the word 'paracetamol'.

#### (31) Contains aspirin and paracetamol

To be used on containers of dispensed preparations containing aspirin and paracetamol (e.g.
benorylate), when the name on the label does not
include the words 'aspirin' and 'paracetamol'.

#### (32) Contains aspirin

To be used on containers of dispensed preparations containing aspirin when the name on the
label does not include the word 'aspirin'.

#### (33) Contains an aspirin-like medicine

To be used on containers of dispensed preparations containing a salicylate derivative.

# Products and their labels

Products introduced or amended since publication of BNF No. 22 (September 1991) are <u>underlined</u>.
Proprietary names are in italic.
C = counselling advised; see BNF = consult product entry in BNF.

Acebutolol, 8
Acemetacin, 21, C, driving
Acetazolamide, 3
Acetazolamide m/r, 3, 25
Acetylcysteine gran, 13
Achromycin, 7, 9, 23, C, posture
Acipimox, 21
Acrivastine, C, driving, alcohol, see BNF
Acrosoxacin, 2, 23
Actifed, 2
Actifed Compound, 2
Actifed Expectorant, 2
Actinac, 28
Actonorm pdr, 13
Acupan, 2, 14 (urine pink)
Acyclovir susp and tabs, 9
Adalat caps, 21, C, see BNF
Adalat Retard, 21, 25
Adcortyl external preps, 28
Adcortyl with Graneodin, 28
Adizem preps, 25
AeroBec, 8, C, dose
AeroBec Forte, 8, 10 steroid card, C, dose
Agarol, 14
Akineton, 2
Alclometasone external preps, 28
Alcopar, 13
Aldomet, 3, 8
Algitec, C, chew thoroughly
Alimix, C, administration
Allegron, 2
Allopurinol, 8, 21, 27
Almodan, 9
Alophen, 14 (alkaline urine pink)
Alphodith, 10 patient information leaflet
Alphosyl HC, 28
Aloral, 8, 21, 27
Aloxiprin, 12, 21
Alphaderm, 28
Alprazolam, 2
Alrheumat, 21
Alvedon, 30
Alvercol, 25, 27, C, administration, see BNF
Amantadine, C, driving
Ambaxin, 9
Amfipen, 9, 23
Aminophylline m/r, see preps
Amiodarone, 11
Amitriptyline, 2
Amitriptyline m/r, 2, 25
Amorolfine, 10 patient information leaflet
Amoxapine, 2
Amoxil, 9
Amoxil dispersible tabs and sachets, 9, 13
Amoxil Fiztab, 9, 10 patient information leaflet
Amoxil paed susp, 9, C, use of pipette
Amoxycillin, 9
Amoxycillin chewable tabs, 9, 10 patient information leaflet
Amoxycillin dispersible tabs and sachets, 9, 13
Amphotericin loz, 9, 24, C, after food
Amphotericin mixt (g.i.), 9, C, use of pipette
Amphotericin mixt (mouth), 9, C, use of pipette, hold in mouth, after food
Amphotericin tabs, 9
Ampicillin, 9
Ampiclox Neonatal, 9, C, use of pipette
Amylobarbitone, 19
Amytal, 19
Anafranil, 2

Anafranil m/r, 2, 25
Androcur, 2, 21
Angettes-75, 32
Anhydrol Forte, 15
Anquil, 2
Antabuse, 2, C, alcohol reaction, see BNF
Antacids, see BNF dosage statements
Antepar tabs, 24
Antepsin, 5, C, administration, see BNF
Anthranol preps, 28
Anticoagulants, oral, 10 anticoagulant card
Antihistamines (see individual preparations)
Antipressan, 8
Antoin, 13, 21, 32
Anturan, 12, 21
Apisate, 25, C, driving
APP pdr, 13
Apsifen, 21
Apsin VK, 9, 23
Apsolol, 8
Apsolox, 8
Arelix, 21
Arpimycin, 9
Arpicolin, C, driving
Artane, C, before or after food, driving, see BNF
Artracin, 21
Arythmol, 21, 25
Asacol, 25
Ascorbic acid, effervescent, 13
Ascorbic acid tabs (500 mg), 24
Asendis, 2
Aspav, 2, 13, 21, 32
Aspirin and papaveretum dispersible tabs, 2, 13, 21, also 32 (if 'aspirin' not on label)
Aspirin dispersible tabs, 13, 21, also 32 (if 'aspirin' not on label)
Aspirin effervescent, 13, also 32 (if 'aspirin' not on label)
Aspirin e/c, 5, 25, also 32 (if 'aspirin' not on label)
Aspirin m/r, 25, also 32 (if 'aspirin' not on label)
Aspirin tabs, 21, also 32 (if 'aspirin' not on label)
Aspirin, paracetamol, and codeine tabs, 21, 29, also 31 (if 'aspirin' and 'paracetamol' not on label)
Astemizole, 23, C, driving, alcohol, see BNF
Atarax, 2
Atenolol, 8
Atensine, 2 or 19
Ativan, 2 or 19
Atromid-S, 21
Augmentin, 9
Augmentin dispersible tabs, 9, 13
Auranofin, 21
Aurecort, 28
Aureomycin, 7, 9, 23
Aventyl, 2
Avloclor, 5
Avomine, 2
Azapropazone, 21, C, see BNF
Azatadine, 2
Azithromycin, 9, 23

Bacampicillin, 9
Baclofen, 2, 8
Bactrim, 9
Bactrim dispersible tabs, 9, 13
Banocide, 9
Baratol, 2
Barquinol HC, 28

Baxan, 9
Becloforte preps, 8, 10 steroid card, C, dose
Beclomethasone external preps, 28
Beclomethasone inhalations, 8, 10 steroid card (high-dose preparations only), C, dose
Becodisks, 8, C, dose
Becotide preps, 8, C, dose
Bedranol S.R., 8, 25
Bendogen, 21
Benemid, 12, 21, 27
Benoral susp and tabs, 21, 31
Benoral gran, 13, 21, 31
Benorylate, 21, 31
Benorylate gran, 13, 21, 31
Benperidol, 2
Benylin adult preps, 2
Benylin paediatric preps, 1
Benzathine penicillin, 9
Benzhexol, C, before or after food, driving, see BNF
Benztropine, 2
Bephenium, 13
Berkolol, 8
Beta-Adalat, 8, 25
Beta-Cardone, 8
Betahistine, 21
Betaloc, 8
Betaloc-SA, 8, 25
Betamethasone inj, 10 steroid card
Betamethasone tab, 10 steroid card, 21
Betamethasone external preps, 28
Betamethasone scalp application, 15, 28
Betaxolol tabs, 8
Bethanechol, 22
Bethanidine, 21
Betim, 8
Betnelan, 10 steroid card, 21
Betnesol injection, 10 steroid card
Betnesol tabs, 10 steroid card, 13, 21
Betnovate external preps, 28
Betnovate scalp application, 15, 28
Betnovate-RD, 28
Bezafibrate, 21
Bezalip, 21
Bezalip-Mono, 21, 25
Biogastrone, 21
Biophylline syr, 21
Biophylline tabs, 25
Biorphen, C, driving
Biperiden, 2
Bisacodyl tabs, 5, 25
Bisoprolol, 8
Blocadren, 8
Bolvidon, 2, 25
Bonefos, C, food and calcium, see BNF
Bradilan, 5, 25
Bricanyl SA, 25
Britiazim, 25
Brocadopa, 14 (urine reddish), 21
Broflex, C, before or after food, driving, see BNF
Bromazepam, 2
Bromocriptine, 21, C, hypotensive reactions
Brompheniramine, 2
Brufen, 21
Brufen gran, 13, 21
Brufen Retard, 25, 27
Buccastem, 2, C, administration, see BNF
Budesonide external preps, 28
Budesonide inhalations, 8, 10 steroid card (high-dose preparations only), C, dose

Buprenorphine, 2, 26
Burinex K, 25, 27, C, posture, see BNF
Buspar, C, driving
Buspirone, C, driving
Butacote, 5, 21, 25
Butobarbitone, 19
Butriptyline, 2

Cacit, 13
Cafadol, 29, 30
Cafergot, 18, C, dosage
Calcichew, 24
Calcidrink, 13
Calcisorb, 13, 21, C, may be sprinkled on food
Calcium-500, 25
Calcium carbonate tabs, chewable, 24
Calcium carbonate tabs and gran effervescent, 13
Calcium gluconate tabs, 24
Calcium Resonium, 13
Calcium and ergocalciferol tabs, C, administration, see BNF
Calmurid HC, 28
Calpol susp, 30
Calpol Extra, 29, 30
Camcolit 250 tabs, 10 lithium card, C, fluid and salt intake
Camcolit 400 tabs, 10 lithium card, 25, C, fluid and salt intake
Canesten HC, 28
Canesten spray, 15
Caplenal, 8, 21, 27
Caprin, 5, 25, 32
Carbachol, 22
Carbamazepine chewable, 3, 21, 24
Carbamazepine liq and tabs, 3
Carbamazepine m/r, 3
Carbenoxolone sodium, see BNF
Carbo-Cort, 28
Cardiacap, 22, 25
Cardinol, 8
Carisoma, 2
Carisoprodol, 2
Carteolol tabs, 8
Cartrol, 8
Carylderm lotion, 15
Catapres, 3, 8
Catapres Perlongets, 3, 8, 25
Caved-S, 24
Cedocard Retard, 25
Cefaclor, 9
Cefadroxil, 9
Cefixime, 9
Cefuroxime susp, 9, 21
Cefuroxime sachets, 9, 13, 21
Cefuroxime tab, 9, 21, 25
Celance, C, hypotensive reactions, see BNF
Celectol, 22
Celevac (constip. or diarrhoea), C, administration, see BNF
Celevac tabs (anorectic), C, administration, see BNF
Celiprolol, 22
Centyl K, 25, 27, C, posture, see BNF
Cephalexin, 9
Cephradine, 9
Ceporex caps, mixts, and tabs, 9
Ceporex paed drops, 9, C, use of pipette
Cesamet, 2
Cetirizine, C, driving, alcohol, see BNF
Chemotrim, 9
Chloral hydrate, 19, 27
Chloral paed elixir, 1, 27
Chloral mixt, 19, 27
Chlordiazepoxide, 2
Chlormethiazole, 19
Chlormezanone, 2 or 19
Chloroquine, 5
Chlorpheniramine, 2
Chlorpromazine mixts and supps, 2
Chlorpromazine tabs, 2
Chlorpropamide, 4
Chlortetracycline, 7, 9, 23
Cholestyramine, 13, C, avoid other drugs at same time
Choline magnesium trisalicylate, 21, 33

Choline theophyllinate m/r, 25
Cimetidine chewable tabs, C, administration
Cimetidine effervescent tabs, 13
Cinnarizine, 2
Cinobac, 9
Cinoxacin, 9
Ciprofloxacin, 5, 9, 25, C, driving
Ciproxin tabs, 5, 9, 25, C, driving
Cisapride, C, administration
Citramag, 10 patient information leaflet, 13, C, administration
Citrical, 13
Clarithromycin, 9
Clarityn, C, driving, alcohol, see BNF
Clemastine, 2
Clindamycin, 9, 27, C, diarrhoea
Clinoril, 21
Clobazam, 2 or 19
Clobetasol external preps, 28
Clobetasol scalp application, 15, 28
Clofazimine, 8, 14 (urine red), 21
Clofibrate, 21
Clomipramine, 2
Clomipramine m/r, 2, 25
Clonazepam, 2
Clonidine see Catapres
Clonidine m/r, 3, 8, 25
Clopixol, 2
Clorazepate, 2 or 19
Clotrimazole spray, 15
Cloxacillin, 9, 23
Clozapine, 2, 10 patient information leaflet
Clozaril, 2, 10 patient information leaflet
Coal tar paint, 15
Co-amoxiclav, 9
Co-amoxiclav dispersible tabs, 9, 13
Cobadex, 28
Co-beneldopa, 14 (urine reddish), 21
Co-beneldopa dispersible tabs, 14 (urine reddish), 21, C, administration, see BNF
Co-beneldopa m/r, 5, 14 (urine reddish), 25
Co-Betaloc, 8
Co-Betaloc SA, 8, 25
Co-careldopa, 14 (urine reddish), 21
Co-careldopa m/r, 14 (urine reddish), 25
Co-codamol caps and tabs, 29, 30
Co-codamol dispersible tabs, 13, 29, 30
Co-codaprin dispersible tabs, 13, 21, 32
Co-codaprin tabs, 21, 32
Codalax, 14 (urine red)
Co-danthramer, 14 (urine red)
Co-danthrusate, 14 (urine red)
Codeine phosphate syr and tabs, 2
Co-dergocrine, 22
Co-dydramol, 21, 29, 30
Co-fluampicil, 9, 23
Cogentin, 2
Colestid, 13, C, avoid other drugs at same time
Colestipol, 13, C, avoid other drugs at same time
Collodion, flexible, 15
Colofac, 22
Colpermin, 5, 22, 25
Colven sachets, 13, 22, C, administration, see BNF
Comox paed susp and tabs, 9
Comox dispersible tabs, 9, 13
Complement Continus, 25
Comprecin, 9
Concordin, 2, 11
Condyline, 15
Co-prenozide, 8
Co-proxamol, 2, 10 patient information leaflet, 29, 30
Coracten, 2
Cordarone X, 11
Corgard, 8
Corgaretic, 8
Corticosteroid external preps, 28
Corticosteroid tabs, 10 steroid card, 21

Corticosteroid injections (systemic), 10 steroid card
Cortisone tab, 10 steroid card, 21
Cortistab, 10 steroid card, 21
Cortisyl, 10 steroid card, 21
Cosalgesic, 2, 10 patient information leaflet, 29, 30
Cotazym, C, see BNF
Co-tenidone, 8
Co-trimoxazole mixts and tabs, 9
Co-trimoxazole dispersible tabs, 9, 13
Coversyl, 22
Creon, C, see BNF
Cuplex, 15
Cyclizine, 2
Cyclophosphamide, 27
Cycloserine caps, 2, 8
Cyclosporin solution, C, administration
Cyproheptadine, 2
Cyprostat, 3, 21
Cyproterone, see preps

Daktacort, 28
Daktarin oral gel, 9, C, hold in mouth, after food
Daktarin tabs, 9, 21
Dalacin C, 9, 27, C, diarrhoea
Dalmane, 19
Daneral SA, 2, 25
Dantrium, 2
Dantrolene, 2
Dapsone, 8
Davenol, 2
Decadron inj, 10 steroid card
Decadron tabs, 10 steroid card, 21
Decortisyl, 10 steroid card, 21
Deltacortril e/c, 5, 10 steroid card, 25
Deltastab inj, 10 steroid card
Deltastab tabs, 10 steroid card, 21
Demeclocycline, 7, 9, 11, 23
Demser, 2
De-Nol, C, administration, see BNF
De-Noltab, C, administration, see BNF
Depixol, 2
Depo-Medrone (systemic), 10 steroid card
Deponit, 10 patient information leaflet, C, administration, see BNF
Derbac C preps, 10 patient information leaflet
Dermovate cream and oint, 28
Dermovate scalp application, 15, 28
Dermovate-NN, 28
Deseril, 2, 21
Desipramine, 2
Desoxymethasone external preps, 28
Destolit, 21
Deteclo, 7, 9, 11, 23, C, posture
Dexamethasone inj, 10 steroid card
Dexamethasone tabs, 10 steroid card, 21
Dexamphetamine, C, driving
Dexedrine, C, driving
Dextromoramide, 2
Dextropropoxyphene, 2
DF 118, 2, 21
DHC Continus, 2, 25
Diabinese, 4
Diamorphine preps, 2
Diamox tabs, 3
Diamox Sustets, 3, 25
Diazepam, 2 or 19
Diclofenac dispersible tabs, 13, 21
Diclofenac e/c, 5, 25
Diclofenac m/r, 21, 25
Diconal, 2
Didronel, C, food and calcium, see BNF
Diethylcarbamazine, 9
Diethylpropion m/r, 25, C, driving
Diflucan 50 and 200 mg, 9
Diflucan susp, 9
Diflucortolone external preps, 28
Diflunisal, 21, 25, C, avoid aluminium hydroxide
Digoxin elixir, C, use of pipette
Dihydrocodeine, 2, 21
Dihydrocodeine m/r, 2, 25
Diloxanide, 9

Haelan, 28
Haelan-C, 28
Halciderm Topical, 28
Halcinonide external preps, 28
Haldol, 2
Half-Inderal LA, 8, 25
Haloperidol, 2
Hamarin, 8, 21, 27
Haymine, 2, 25
Heminevrin, 19
Hexamine, 9
Hiprex, 9
Hismanal, 23, C, driving, alcohol, see BNF
Histalix, 2
Histryl, 2, 25
Histryl (paed), 1, 25
Hollister skin gel, 15
Hydergine, 22
Hydrocal, 28
Hydrocortisone inj, 10 steroid card
Hydrocortisone external preps, 28
Hydrocortisone tabs, 10 steroid card, 21
Hydrocortisone butyrate external preps, 28
Hydrocortisone butyrate scalp lotion, 15, 28
Hydrocortistab inj, 10 steroid card
Hydrocortistab external preps, 28
Hydrocortistab tabs, 10 steroid card, 21
Hydrocortisyl, 28
Hydrocortone, 10 steroid card, 21
Hydromet, 3, 8
Hydroxychloroquine, 5
Hydroxyzine, 2
Hygroton-K, 25, 27, C, posture, see BNF
Hyoscine, 2
Hypercal, 3
Hypon, 21, 32
Hypovase, 3, C, dose, see BNF
Hytrin, 3, C, dose, see BNF

Ibular, 21
Ibuprofen, 21
Ibuprofen gran, 13, 21
Ibuprofen m/r, 25, 27
Ilosone, 9
Imbrilon caps, 21, C, driving
Imdur, 25
Imigran, 3, 10 patient information leaflet
Imipramine, 2
Imperacin, 7, 9, 23
Imunovir, 9
Inderal, 8
Inderal-LA, 8, 25
Inderetic, 8
Inderex, 8, 25
Indocid caps and susp, 21, C, driving
Indocid-R, 21, 25, C, driving
Indolar SR, 21, 25, C, driving
Indomethacin caps and mixt, 21, C, driving
Indomethacin m/r, 21, 25, C, driving
Indomethacin supps, C, driving
Indomod, C, driving
Indoramin, 2
Industrial methylated spirit, 15
Infacol, C, use of dropper
Inosine pranobex, 9
Intal Spincaps and inhalers, 8
Integrin, 2
Iodine Solution, Aqueous, 27
Ionamin, 25, C, driving
Ipral, 9
Iprindole, 2
Ismo Retard, 25
Ismo tabs, 25
Isocarboxazid, 3, 10 MAOI card
Isogel, 13, C, administration, see BNF
Isoket Retard, 25
Isoniazid elixir and tabs, 8, 22
Isoprenaline sulphate tabs, 26
Isordil (sublingual), 26
Isordil Tembids, 25
Isosorbide dinitrate m/r, 25
Isosorbide mononitrate, 25

Isosorbide mononitrate m/r, 25
Isotrate, 25
Isotretinoin, 10 patient information card, 21
Ispaghula, 13, C, administration, see BNF
Itraconazole, 5, 9, 21, 25

Junifen, 21

Kalspare, 14 (urine blue in some lights), 21
Kalten, 8
Kay-Cee-L, 21
Keflex, 9
Kelfizine W tabs, 9,13
Kemadrin, C, driving
Kenalog (systemic), 10 steroid card
Kerlone, 8
Kest, 14 (alkaline urine pink)
Ketoconazole tabs and susp, 5, 9, 21
Ketoprofen caps, 21
Ketotifen, 2, 8, 21
Kiditard, 25
Kinidin Duriles, 25
Klaricid, 9
Klean-Prep, C, administration, see BNF
Kloref, 13, 21
Kloref-S, 13, 21
Konakion tabs, 24

Labetalol, 8, 21
Laboprin DL, 13, 21, 33
Labrocol, 8, 21
Ladropen, 9, 23
Lamisil, 9
Lamprene, 8, 14 (urine red), 21
Lanoxin-PG elixir, C, use of pipette
Laraflex, 21
Larapam, 21
Laratrim, 9
Largactil, 2
Lariam, 21, 25, 27
Larodopa, 14 (urine reddish), 21
Lasikal, 25, 27, C, posture, see BNF
Lasipressin, 8
Lasix + K, 25, 27, C, posture, see BNF
Lasma, 25
Ledercort external preps, 28
Ledercort tabs, 10 steroid card, 21
Lederfen, 21
Lederfen F, 13
Lederkyn, 9, 27
Ledermycin, 7, 9, 11, 23
Lentizol, 2, 25
Leo K, 25, 27, C, posture, see BNF
Levodopa, 14 (urine reddish), 21
Levodopa m/r, 5, 14 (urine reddish), 25
Lexotan, 2
Librium, 2
Lidifen, 21
Limbitrol, 2
Lincocin, 9, 23, C, diarrhoea
Lincomycin, 9, 23, C, diarrhoea
Lingraine, 18, 26, C, dosage
Lioresal, 2, 8
Lipantil, 21
Liquid paraffin/phenolphthalein mixt, 14 (alkaline urine pink)
Liskonum, 10 lithium card, 25, C, fluid and salt intake
Litarex, 10 lithium card, 25, C, fluid and salt intake
Lithium carbonate, 10 lithium card, C, fluid and salt intake
Lithium carbonate m/r, 10 lithium card, 25, C, fluid and salt intake
Lithium citrate liq, 10 lithium card, C, fluid and salt intake
Lithium citrate m/r, 10 lithium card, 25, C, fluid and salt intake
Lobak, 2, 29, 30
Loceryl, 10 patient information leaflet
Locoid cream and oint, 28
Locoid scalp lotion, 15, 28
Locoid C, 28
Lodine, 21
Lofepramine, 2

Loprazolam, 19
Lopresor, 8
Lopresor SR, 8, 25
Lopresoretic, 8
Loratadine, C, driving, alcohol, see BNF
Lorazepam, 2 or 19
Lormetazepam, 19
Loron caps, 10 patient information leaflet, C, food and calcium, see BNF
Losec, 25
Lotriderm, 28
Loxapac, 2
Loxapine, 2
Ludiomil, 2
Lugol's solution, 27
Lurselle, 21
Lustral, 21
Lymecycline, 6, 9
Lysuride, 21, C, hypotensive reactions

Macrodantin, 9, 14 (urine yellow or brown), 21
Madopar, 14 (urine reddish), 21
Madopar dispersible tabs, 14 (urine reddish), 21, C, administration, see BNF
Madopar CR, 5, 14 (urine reddish), 25
Magnapen, 9, 23
Magnesium citrate effervescent pdr, 10 patient information leaflet, 13, C, administration
Magnesium sulphate, 13, 23
Magnesium trisilicate oral pdr, cpd, 13
Manevac, 25, 27
Maprotiline, 2
Marevan, 10 anticoagulant card
Marplan, 3, 10 MAOI card
Maxepa, 21
Maxolon paed liquid, C, use of pipette
Maxolon SR, 25
Mazindol, C, driving
Mebeverine, 22
Mebhydrolin, 2
Medazepam, 2
Medihaler-ergotamine, 18, C, dosage
Medised susp, 1, 30
Medrone tabs, 10 steroid card, 21
Mefenamic acid caps, paed susp, and tabs, 21
Mefenamic acid dispersible tabs, 13, 21
Mefloquine, 21, 25, 27
Melleril, 2
Menthol and benzoin inhalation, 15
Mepacrine, 4, 9, 14, 21
Meprobamate, 2
Meptazinol, 2
Meptid, 2
Mequitazine, 2
Mesalazine, 25
Metamucil, 13, C, administration, see BNF
Metformin, 21
Methadone, 2
Methixene, 2
Methocarbamol, 2
Methotrimeprazine, 2
Methylcellulose (constip. or diarrhoea), C, administration, see BNF
Methylcellulose tabs (anorectic), C, administration, see BNF
Methylcysteine, 5, 22, 25
Methyldopa, 3, 8
Methylphenobarbitone, 2
Methylprednisolone external preps, 28
Methylprednisolone inj, 10 steroid card
Methylprednisolone tabs, 10 steroid card, 21
Methysergide, 2, 21
Metirosine, 2
Metoclopramide paed liquid, C, use of pipette
Metoclopramide m/r, see preps

# Dental Practitioners' Formulary

## List of Dental Preparations

The following list has been approved by the appropriate Secretaries of State, and the preparations therein may be prescribed by dental practitioners on form FP14 (GP14 in Scotland).

**Sugar-free** versions, where available, are preferred.

Acyclovir Cream, DPF
Acyclovir Oral Suspension, DPF
Acyclovir Tablets 200 mg, DPF
Amoxycillin Capsules, BP
Amoxycillin Injection, DPF
Amoxycillin Oral Powder, DPF
Amoxycillin Oral Suspension, BP
Amoxycillin Tablets, Dispersible, DPF
Amphotericin Lozenges, BP
Amphotericin Ointment, DPF
  [not currently available]
Amphotericin Oral Suspension, DPF
Amphotericin Tablets, DPF
Ampicillin Capsules, BP
Ampicillin Oral Suspension, BP
Artificial Saliva, DPF
Ascorbic Acid Tablets, BP
Aspirin Tablets, Dispersible, BP[1]
Benzydamine Mouthwash, DPF
Benzydamine Oral Spray, DPF
Benzylpenicillin Injection, BP
Carbamazepine Tablets, BP
Carmellose Gelatin Paste, DPF
Cephalexin Capsules, BP
Cephalexin Oral Suspension, DPF
Cephalexin Tablets, BP
Cephradine Capsules, BP
Cephradine Injection, DPF
Cephradine Oral Solution, DPF
Chlorhexidine Gluconate gels containing at least 1 per cent
Chlorhexidine Mouthwash, DPF
Chlorpheniramine Tablets, BP
Choline Salicylate Dental Gel, BP
Clindamycin Capsules, BP
Clindamycin Injection, DPF
Clindamycin Oral Suspension, Paediatric, DPF
Co-trimoxazole Oral Suspension, BP
Co-trimoxazole Oral Suspension, Paediatric, BP
Co-trimoxazole Tablets, BP
Co-trimoxazole Tablets, Dispersible, BP
Co-trimoxazole Tablets, Paediatric, BP
Diazepam Capsules, BP
Diazepam Oral Solution, BP
Diazepam Tablets, BP
Diflunisal Tablets, BP
Dihydrocodeine Tablets, BP
Doxycycline Capsules 100 mg, BP

Ephedrine Nasal Drops, BP
Erythromycin Ethyl Succinate Oral Powder, DPF[2]
Erythromycin Ethyl Succinate Oral Suspension, DPF
Erythromycin Ethyl Succinate Oral Suspension, Paediatric, DPF
Erythromycin Ethyl Succinate Tablets, DPF
Erythromycin Lactobionate Injection, DPF
Erythromycin Stearate Tablets, BP
Erythromycin Tablets, BP
Hydrocortisone Cream, BP
Hydrocortisone Lozenges, BPC
Hydrocortisone and Miconazole Cream, DPF
Hydrocortisone and Miconazole Ointment, DPF
Hydrogen Peroxide Mouthwash, DPF
Ibuprofen Tablets, BP
Idoxuridine 5% in Dimethyl Sulphoxide, DPF
Lignocaine 5% Ointment, DPF
Menthol and Eucalyptus Inhalation, BP 1980[3]
Metronidazole Oral Suspension, DPF
Metronidazole Tablets, BP
Miconazole Oral Gel, DPF
Mouthwash Solution-tablets, DPF
Nitrazepam Tablets, BP
Nystatin Ointment, BP
Nystatin Oral Suspension, BP
Nystatin Pastilles, DPF
Nystatin Tablets, BP
Oxytetracycline Capsules, BP
Oxytetracycline Tablets, BP
Paracetamol Oral Suspension, Paediatric, BP[4]
Paracetamol Tablets, BP
Paracetamol Tablets, Dispersible, DPF
Penicillin Triple Injection, BPC
Pethidine Tablets, BP
Phenoxymethylpenicillin Capsules, BP
Phenoxymethylpenicillin Oral Solution, BP
Phenoxymethylpenicillin Tablets, BP
Povidone-iodine Mouthwash, DPF
Procaine Penicillin Injection, BP
  [not currently available]
Promethazine Hydrochloride Tablets, BP
Promethazine Oral Solution, BP
Sodium Chloride Mouthwash, Compound, BP
Sodium Fusidate Ointment, BP
  (former title Fusidic Acid Ointment, DPF)
Sodium Perborate Mouthwash, DPF
Temazepam Capsules, DPF
Temazepam Oral Solution, DPF
Temazepam Tablets, DPF
Tetracycline Capsules, BP
Tetracycline Oral Suspension, BP
Tetracycline Tablets, BP
Thymol Glycerin, Compound, BP
Triamcinolone Dental Paste, BP
Vitamin B Tablets, Compound, Strong, BPC
Zinc Sulphate Mouthwash, DPF

---

1. Addendum 1989 to BP 1988 has directed that when soluble aspirin tablets are prescribed, dispersible aspirin tablets should be dispensed.
2. Includes only the sugar-free 250-mg strength.
3. This preparation does not appear in BP 1988
4. BP 1988 directs that when Paediatric Paracetamol Oral Suspension or Paediatric Paracetamol Mixture is prescribed and no strength stated Paracetamol Oral Suspension 120 mg/5 mL should be dispensed

## Details of DPF preparations

Preparations on the List of Dental Preparations which are not included in the BP or BPC are described as follows in the DPF.

Although brand names have sometimes been included for identification purposes preparations on the list should be prescribed by non-proprietary name.

PoM **Acyclovir Cream,** (proprietary product: *Zovirax Cream*), acyclovir 5%

PoM **Acyclovir Oral Suspension,** (proprietary product: *Zovirax Suspension*), acyclovir 200 mg/5 mL

PoM **Acyclovir Tablets 200 mg,** (proprietary product: *Zovirax Tablets*), acyclovir 200 mg

PoM **Amoxycillin Injection,** sterile powder for reconstitution

PoM **Amoxycillin Oral Powder** (proprietary products: *Amoxil Sachets SF*), amoxycillin 750 mg and 3 g (as trihydrate)

PoM **Amoxycillin Tablets Dispersible,** (proprietary product: *Amoxil Dispersible Tablets*), amoxycillin 500 mg (as trihydrate)

PoM **Amphotericin Oral Suspension** (proprietary product: *Fungilin Suspension*), amphotericin 100 mg/mL

PoM **Amphotericin Tablets** (proprietary product: *Fungilin Tablets*), amphotericin 100 mg

**Artificial Saliva,** consists of a suitable inert, slightly viscous, aqueous liquid; may contain a suitable antimicrobial preservative, normal salivary constituents, small amounts of fluoride, and colouring and flavouring agents (see section 12.3.4)

**Benzydamine Mouthwash** (proprietary product: *Difflam Oral Rinse*), benzydamine hydrochloride 0.15%

**Benzydamine Oral Spray,** (proprietary product: *Difflam Spray*), benzydamine hydrochloride 0.15%

**Carmellose Gelatin Paste** (proprietary product: *Orabase Paste*), gelatin, pectin, carmellose sodium, 16.58% of each in a suitable basis

PoM **Cephalexin Oral Suspension,** cephalexin 125 mg, 250 mg, or 500 mg/5 mL (may be powder for reconstitution or ready prepared)

PoM **Cephradine Injection** (proprietary product: *Velosef Injection*), sterile powder for reconstitution

PoM **Cephradine Oral Solution** (proprietary product: *Velosef Syrup*), cephradine 250 mg/5 mL when reconstituted with water

**Chlorhexidine Gel** (proprietary product: *Corsodyl Dental Gel*), chlorhexidine gluconate 1%

**Chlorhexidine Mouthwash** (proprietary product: *Corsodyl Mouthwash*), chlorhexidine gluconate 0.2%

PoM **Clindamycin Injection** (proprietary product: *Dalacin C Phosphate Sterile Solution*), clindamycin 150 mg (as phosphate)/mL

PoM **Clindamycin Oral Suspension, Paediatric** (proprietary product: *Dalacin C Paediatric Suspension*), clindamycin 75 mg (as hydrochloride palmitate)/5 mL when reconstituted with purified water (freshly boiled and cooled)

PoM **Erythromycin Ethyl Succinate Oral Powder** (proprietary product: *Erythroped Sugar-free*), erythromycin 250 mg (as ethyl succinate)/sachet

PoM **Erythromycin Ethyl Succinate Oral Suspension** (proprietary product: *Erythroped Suspension*), erythromycin 250 mg and 500 mg (as ethyl succinate)/5 mL when reconstituted with water

PoM **Erythromycin Ethyl Succinate Oral Suspension, Paediatric** (proprietary product: *Erythroped PI*), erythromycin 125 mg (as ethyl succinate)/5 mL when reconstituted with water

PoM **Erythromycin Ethyl Succinate Tablets** (proprietary product: *Erythroped A*), erythromycin ethyl succinate 500 mg

PoM **Erythromycin Lactobionate Injection** (proprietary product: *Erythrocin IV Lactobionate*), sterile powder for reconstitution

PoM **Hydrocortisone and Miconazole Cream** (proprietary product: *Daktacort Cream*), hydrocortisone 1%, miconazole nitrate 2%

PoM **Hydrocortisone and Miconazole Ointment** (proprietary product: *Daktacort Ointment*), hydrocortisone 1%, miconazole nitrate 2%

**Hydrogen Peroxide Mouthwash** consists of hydrogen peroxide solution (6%), BP

PoM **Idoxuridine 5% in Dimethyl Sulphoxide,** idoxuridine 5% in dimethyl sulphoxide

**Lignocaine 5% Ointment,** lignocaine 5% in a suitable basis

PoM **Metronidazole Oral Suspension** (proprietary product: *Flagyl S*), metronidazole 200 mg (as benzoate)/5 mL

**Miconazole Oral Gel** (proprietary product: *Daktarin Oral Gel*), miconazole 25 mg/mL

**Mouthwash Solution-tablets,** DPF, consist of tablets which may contain antimicrobial, colouring and flavouring agents in a suitable soluble effervescent basis to make a mouthwash suitable for dental purposes

PoM **Nystatin Pastilles** (proprietary product: *Nystan Pastilles*), nystatin 100000 units

**Paracetamol Tablets, Dispersible** (proprietary product: *Panadol Soluble*), paracetamol 500 mg in an effervescent basis

**Povidone-iodine Mouthwash** (proprietary product: *Betadine Mouthwash*), povidone-iodine 1%

**Sodium Perborate Mouthwash,** (proprietary product: *Bocasan Mouthwash*), sodium perborate 70%

PoM **Temazepam Capsules,** DPF, temazepam 10, 15, 20 and 30 mg

*Note.* Temazepam Capsules DPF are hard or soft gelatin capsules

PoM **Temazepam Oral Solution,** temazepam 10 mg/5 mL

PoM **Temazepam Tablets,** temazepam 10 and 20 mg

**Zinc Sulphate Mouthwash,** consists of zinc sulphate lotion, BP (see section 13.11.6)

Directions for use: dilute 1 part with 4 parts of warm water

# Index of Manufacturers

**Body's Care**
Body's Care Centre Ltd,
631 London Rd,
Westcliffe-on-Sea, Essex
SS0 9PE.
Southend-on-Sea (0702) 337339

**Boehringer Ingelheim**
Boehringer Ingelheim Ltd,
Ellesfield Ave, Bracknell, Berks
RG12 4YS.
Bracknell (0344) 424600

**Boehringer Mannheim**
Boehringer Mannheim UK
(Pharmaceuticals) Ltd,
Simpson Parkway, Kirkton
Campus, Livingston, West
Lothian EH54 7BH.
Livingston (0506) 412512

**Boots**
The Boots Co. plc,
1 Thane Rd West, Nottingham
NG2 3AA.
Nottingham (0602) 506255

**BPL**
Bio Products Laboratory,
Dagger Lane, Elstree, Herts
WD6 3BX.
081-905 1818

**Bradgate**
Bradgate Unitech Ltd,
Contact Pharma-Plast

**Braun**
B. Braun (Medical) Ltd,
Braun House, 13–14 Farmbrough
Close, Aylesbury Vale Industrial
Park, Aylesbury, Bucks
HP20 1DQ.
Aylesbury (0296) 393900

**Brevit**
Brevit Hospital Products,
Unit 6, Carter Hire Complex,
Wilson Way, Redruth, Cornwall
TR15 3QT.
Redruth (0209) 219097

**Bridge**
Bridge Pharmaceuticals,
Contact SmithKline Beecham

**Bristol-Myers**
Bristol-Myers Squibb
Pharmaceuticals Ltd,
141–149 Staines Rd, Hounslow,
Middx TW3 3JA.
081-572 7422

**Britannia**
Britannia Pharmaceuticals Ltd,
Forum House, 41–75 Brighton
Rd, Redhill, Surrey RH1 6YS.
Redhill (0737) 773741

**BritCair**
BritCair Ltd,
Division of CV Laboratories Ltd,
Gordon House, Gordon Rd,
Aldershot, Hants GU11 1LD.
Aldershot (0252) 333314

**Brocades**
Brocades (Great Britain) Ltd,
Brocades House, Pyrford Rd,
West Byfleet, Surrey KT14 6RA.
Byfleet (0932) 345535

**David Bull**
David Bull Laboratories,
Spartan Close, Tachbrook Park,
Warwick CV34 6RS.
Warwick (0926) 451515

**Bullen**
C.S. Bullen Ltd,
3–7 Moss St, Liverpool L6 1EY.
051-207 6995

**Bullen & Smears**
Bullen & Smears Ltd,
99 Kempson St, Liverpool
L3 8HE.
051-207 1239

**Burgess**
Edwin Burgess Ltd,
Contact Leo.

**Cabot**
see Solco Basle

**Cambmac**
Cambmac Instruments Ltd,
Pembroke Ave, Waterbeach,
Cambridge CB5 9PY.
Cambridge (0223) 441144

**Camp**
Camp Ltd,
Northgate House,
Staple Gardens, Winchester,
Hants SO23 8ST.
Winchester (0962) 55248

**Cantassium**
The Cantassium Company,
Larkhall Laboratories,
225 Putney Bridge Rd,
London SW15 2PY.
081-874 1130

**Centocor**
Centocor BV,
Einsteinweg 101,
2333 CB Leiden,
The Netherlands.
0800-898461

**Chancellor**
Chancellor Group Ltd,
see Consolidated

**Charwell**
Charwell Pharmaceuticals Ltd,
Charwell House, Wilsom Rd,
Alton, Hants GU34 2TJ.
Alton (0420) 84801

**Ciba**
CIBA Laboratories,
Wimblehurst Rd, Horsham, West
Sussex RH12 4AB.
Horsham (0403) 50101

**Cilag**
Cilag Ltd,
PO Box 79, Saunderton, High
Wycombe, Bucks HP14 4HJ.
Naphill (024024) 3541

**Clement Clarke**
Clement Clarke International
Ltd,
Airmed House, Edinburgh Way,
Harlow, Essex CM20 2ED.
Harlow (0279) 414969

**CliniFlex**
CliniFlex Ltd,
Contact CliniMed.

**CliniMed**
CliniMed Ltd,
Cavell House, Knaves Beech
Way, Loudwater, High
Wycombe, Bucks HP10 9QY.
Maidenhead (0628) 850100

**Clintec**
Clintec Nutrition Ltd,
Shaftesbury Court,
18 Chalvey Park, Slough,
Berks SL1 2HT.
Slough (0753) 550800

**Coloplast**
Coloplast Ltd,
Peterborough Business Park,
Peterborough PE2 0FX.
Peterborough (0733) 239898

**Concept**
Concept Pharmaceuticals Ltd
see Fabre

**Consolidated**
Consolidated Chemicals Ltd,
The Old Blue School,
Lower Square, Isleworth,
Middx TW7 6RL.
081-568 7071

**ConvaTec**
ConvaTec Ltd,
Harrington House, Milton Rd,
Ickenham, Uxbridge, Middx
UB10 8PU.
Uxbridge (0895) 678888

**Cow & Gate**
Cow & Gate Ltd,
Newmarket Ave, Whitehorse
Business Park,
Trowbridge, Wilts BA14 0XQ.
Trowbridge (0225) 768381

**Cox**
A. H. Cox & Co Ltd,
Whiddon Valley, Barnstaple,
Devon EX32 8NS.
Barnstaple (0271) 75001

**CP**
CP Pharmaceuticals Ltd,
Ash Rd North, Wrexham
Industrial Estate, Wrexham,
Clwyd LL13 9UF.
Wrexham (0978) 661261

**Crookes**
Crookes Healthcare Ltd,
PO Box 94, 1 Thane Rd West,
Nottingham NG2 3AA.
Nottingham (0602) 507431

**Cupal**
Cupal Ltd,
Pharmaceutical Laboratories,
King St, Blackburn, Lancs
BB2 2DX.
Blackburn (0254) 580321

**Cusi**
Cusi (UK) Ltd,
8A Liphook Rd, Haslemere,
Surrey GU27 1NL.
Haslemere (0428) 61078

**Cussons**
Cussons (UK) Ltd,
Kersal Vale, Manchester
M7 0GL.
061-792 6111

**Cutter**
Contact Bayer.

**Cuxson**
Cuxson, Gerrard & Co. (IMS)
Ltd,
Oldbury, Warley,
West Midlands B69 3BB.
021-552 1355

**Cyanamid**
Division of Lederle Laboratories.
Contact Lederle.

**Daniels**
Richard Daniel & Son Ltd,
Mansfield Rd, Derby DE1 3RE.
Derby (0332) 40671

**DDC**
DDC (London) Ltd,
158 Notting Hill Gate,
London W11 3GQ.
071-229 4224

**DDSA**
DDSA Pharmaceuticals Ltd,
310 Old Brompton Rd, London
SW5 9JQ.
071-373 7884

**De Vilbiss**
De Vilbiss Health Care UK Ltd,
Airlinks, Spitfire Way, Heston,
Middx TW5 9WR.
Dial 100 and ask for 'Freephone
Oxygen Concentrator'

**De Witt**
De Witt International Ltd,
62–64 East Barnet Rd, New
Barnet, Herts EN4 8RQ.
081-441 9310

**Delandale**
Delandale Laboratories Ltd,
Delandale House, 37 Old Dover
Rd, Canterbury, Kent CT1 3JF.
Canterbury (0227) 766353

**Dental Health**
Dental Health Products Ltd,
Broughton House, 33 Earl St,
Maidstone, Kent ME14 1PF.
Maidstone (0622) 762269

**DePuy**
DePuy Healthcare,
47 Great George St,
Leeds LS1 3BB.
Leeds (0532) 430028

**Dermal**
Dermal Laboratories Ltd,
Tatmore Place, Gosmore,
Hitchin, Herts SG4 7QR.
Hitchin (0462) 458866

**Dermalex**
Contact Sanofi.

**DF**
Duncan, Flockhart & Co Ltd,
Division of Glaxo Laboratories
Ltd
Contact Glaxo

**Dispersa**
Dispersa (United Kingdom) Ltd,
Flanders Rd, Hedge End,
Southampton SO3 3LG.
Botley (0489) 785399

**Dista**
Dista Products Ltd,
Contact Lilly.

**Dow Corning**
Dow Corning Ltd,
Kings Court, 185 Kings Rd,
Reading, Berks RG1 4EX.
Reading (0734) 596888

**Downs**
Contact Simcare

**Drew**
John Drew (London) Ltd,
433 Uxbridge Rd, Ealing,
London W5 3NT.
081-992 0381

**Du Pont**
Du Pont (UK) Ltd.,
Wedgwood Way, Stevenage,
Herts SG1 4QN.
Stevenage (0438) 734549

**Dumex**
Dumex Ltd,
Longwick Rd, Princes
Risborough, Aylesbury,
Bucks HP17 9UZ.
Princes Risborough (0844)
274414

**Duphar**
Duphar Laboratories Ltd,
Gaters Hill, West End,
Southampton SO3 3JD.
Southampton (0703) 472281

**Dylade**
Contact Fresenius Ltd.

**Eastern**
Eastern Pharmaceuticals Ltd,
Coomb House, 7 St Johns Rd,
Isleworth, Middx TW7 6NA.
081-569 8174

**Elida Gibbs**
Elida Gibbs Ltd,
Coal Rd, Seacroft, Leeds
LS14 2AR.
Leeds (0532) 737473

**EMS**
EMS Medical Ltd,
Unit 3, Stroud Industrial Estate,
Oldends Lane, Stonehouse, Glos
GL10 2DG.
Stonehouse (0453) 791791

**Evans**
Evans Medical Ltd,
Langhurst, Horsham,
Sussex RH12 4QD.
Horsham (0403) 41400

**Fabre**
Pierre Fabre Ltd,
Shelley Court, Shelley Close,
Headington, Oxon OX3 8HB.
Oxford (0865) 742525

**Farillon**
Farillon Ltd,
Ashton Rd, Harold Hill,
Romford, Essex
RM3 8UE.
Ingrebourne (04023) 71136

**Farley**
Farley Health Products Ltd,
Torr Lane, Plymouth PL3 5UA.
Plymouth (0752) 24151

**Farmitalia Carlo Erba**
Farmitalia Carlo Erba Ltd,
Italia House, 23 Grosvenor Rd,
St. Albans, Herts AL1 3AW.
St. Albans (0727) 40041

**Ferraris**
Ferraris Development &
Engineering Co Ltd,
26 Lea Valley Trading Estate,
Angel Rd, Edmonton,
London N18 3JD.
081-807 3636

**Ferring**
Ferring Pharmaceuticals Ltd,
11 Mount Rd, Feltham, Middx
TW13 6AR.
081-898 8396

**Fisons**
Fisons plc,
Pharmaceutical Division,
12 Derby Rd, Loughborough,
Leics LE11 0BB.
Loughborough (0509) 611001

**Fournier**
Fournier Pharmaceuticals Ltd,
116–120 London Rd, Oxford,
OX3 9AT.
Oxford (0865) 741641

**Fox**
C. H. Fox Ltd,
22 Tavistock St, London
WC2E 7PY
071-240 3111

**FP**
Family Planning Sales Ltd,
28 Kelburne Rd, Cowley, Oxford
OX4 3SZ.
Oxford (0865) 772486

**Fresenius**
Fresenius Ltd,
6 Christleton Court, Stuart Rd,
Manor Park, Runcorn, Cheshire
WA7 1ST.
Runcorn (0928) 580058

**Fry**
Fry Surgical International Ltd,
Unit 17, Goldsworth Park
Trading Estate, Woking, Surrey
GU21 3BA.
Woking (0483) 721404

**Galderma**
Galderma (UK) Ltd,
Contact Alcon.
Watford (0923) 210180

**Galen**
Galen Ltd,
Seagoe Industrial Estate,
Craigavon, Northern Ireland
BT63 5UA.
Craigavon (0762) 334974

**Garnier**
Laboratoires Garnier,
Golden Ltd,
PO Box 5, Pontyclun, Glam
CF7.8XW.
Llantrisant (0443) 237456

**Geigy**
Geigy Pharmaceuticals.
*see* Ciba

**Geistlich**
Geistlich Sons Ltd,
Newton Bank, Long Lane,
Chester CH2 3QZ.
Chester (0244) 347534

**General Designs**
General Designs Ltd,
PO Box 38E, Worcester Park,
Surrey KT4 7LX.
081-337 9366

**Generics**
Generics (UK) Ltd,
12 Station Close, Potters Bar,
Herts EN6 1TL.
Potters Bar (0707) 44556

**GF Supplies**
*see* Nutricia

**Glaxo**
Glaxo Laboratories Ltd,
Stockley Park West,
Uxbridge, Middx UB11 1BT.
081-990 9444

**Glenwood**
Glenwood Laboratories Ltd,
Jenkins Dale, Chatham,
Kent ME4 5RD.
Chatham (0634) 830535

**Goldcrest**
Goldcrest Pharmaceuticals
(Europe) Ltd,
Bensham House, Bensham Lane,
Thornton Heath, Surrey
CR7 7EQ.
081-684 3664

**Gold Cross**
Gold Cross Pharmaceuticals.
Contact Searle.

**Graseby Medical**
Graseby Medical Ltd,
Colonial Way, Watford, Herts
WD2 4LG.
Watford (0923) 246434

**Henleys**
Henleys Medical Supplies Ltd,
Brownfields, Welwyn Garden
City, Herts AL7 1AN.
Welwyn Garden (0707) 333164

**Hillcross**
Hillcross Pharmaceuticals,
Primrose Mill, Harrison St,
Briercliffe, Burnley BB10 2HP.
Burnley (0282) 830042

**Hoechst**
Hoechst UK Ltd,
Pharmaceutical Division, Hoechst
House, Salisbury Rd, Hounslow,
Middx TW4 6JH.
081-570 7712

**Hollister**
Hollister Ltd,
Rectory Court, 42 Broad St,
Wokingham, Berks RG11 1AB.
Wokingham (0734) 775545

**Hospital Management &
Supplies**
Hospital Management and
Supplies Ltd,
Selinas Lane, Dagenham, Essex
RM8 1QD.
081-593 7511

**Hough**
Hough, Hoseason & Co. Ltd,
22 Chapel St, Levenshulme,
Manchester M19 3PT.
061-224 3271

**Hypoguard**
Hypoguard Ltd,
Dock Lane, Melton,
Woodbridge, Suffolk IP12 1PE.
Woodbridge (03943) 7333

**ICI**
ICI Pharmaceuticals,
Kings Court, Water Lane,
Wilmslow, Cheshire SK9 5AZ.
Wilmslow (0625) 535999

**Ilon**
Ilon Laboratories (Hamilton)
Ltd,
Lorne St, Hamilton, Lanarkshire
ML3 9AB.
Hamilton (0698) 285129

**Immuno**
Immuno Ltd,
Arctic House, Rye Lane, Dunton
Green, Nr Sevenoaks, Kent
TN14 5HB.
Sevenoaks (0732) 458101

**IMS**
International Medication Systems
(UK) Ltd,
11 Royal Oak Way South,
Daventry, Northants NN11 5PJ.
Daventry (0327) 703231

**Incare**
Incare Medical Products,
Contact Hollister

**Innovex**
Innovex Medical Products Ltd,
Innovex House, Reading Rd,
Henley-on-Thames, Oxon
RG9 1EL.
Henley-on-Thames (0491) 578171

**Intercare**
Intercare Products Ltd,
7 The Business Centre,
Molly Millars Lane, Wokingham,
Berks RG11 2QZ.
Wokingham (0734) 790345

**International Labs**
International Laboratories Ltd,
Floats Rd, Wythenshawe,
Manchester M23 9NF.
061-945 4161

**Invicta**
Contact Pfizer.

**Iolab**
Iolab,
Enterprise House, Station Rd,
Loudwater, High Wycombe,
Bucks HP10 9UG.
High Wycombe (0494) 461096

**J&J**
Johnson & Johnson Patient Care
Ltd,
Coronation Rd, Ascot,
Berks SL5 9EY.
Ascot (0990) 872626

**Jackson**
Ernest Jackson & Co. Ltd,
Crediton, Devon EX17 3AP.
Crediton (03632) 2251

**Jacobs**
The Jacobs Bakery Ltd,
Suttons Business Park,
Earley, Reading, Berks
RG6 1AZ.
Reading (0734) 492000

**Janssen**
Janssen Pharmaceutical Ltd,
Grove, Wantage, Oxon
OX12 0DQ.
Wantage (0235) 772966

**JLB**
JLB Textiles Ltd,
Unit 2B, St Columb Industrial
Estate, St Columb Major,
Cornwall TR9 6SF.
St Columb (0637) 880065

**K & K-Greeff**
K & K-Greeff Ltd,
Suffolk House, George St,
Croydon CR9 3QL.
081-686 0544

**K/L**
K/L Pharmaceuticals Ltd,
25 Macadam Place, South
Newmoor Industrial Estate,
Irvine KA11 4HP.
Irvine (0294) 215951

**Kabi Pharmacia**
Kabi Pharmacia Ltd,
Davy Ave, Knowlhill,
Milton Keynes MK5 8PH.
Milton Keynes (0908) 661101

**Kendall**
The Kendall Company (UK) Ltd,
Pool, Redruth,
Cornwall TR15 3QN.
Redruth (0209) 215151

**Kendall-Lastonet**
Contact Kendall.

**Kerfoot**
Thomas Kerfoot & Co. Ltd,
Vale of Bardsley, Ashton-under-
Lyne, Lancs OL7 9RR.
061-330 4531

**Knoll**
Knoll Ltd,
Fleming House, 71 King St,
Maidenhead, Berks SL6 1DU.
Maidenhead (0628) 776360

**LAB**
Laboratories for Applied Biology
Ltd,
91 Amhurst Park, London
N16 5DR.
081-800 2252

**Laerdal**
Laerdal Medical Ltd,
Laerdal House, Goodmead Rd,
Orpington, Kent BR6 0HX.
Orpington (0689) 76634

**Lagap**
Lagap Pharmaceuticals Ltd,
37 Woolmer Way, Bordon,
Hants GU35 9QE.
Bordon (0420) 478301

**Lamberts**
Lamberts (Dalston) Ltd,
Dalston House, Hastings St,
Luton, Beds LU1 5BW.
Luton (0582) 400711

**Lederle**
Lederle Laboratories,
Cyanamid House, Fareham Rd,
Gosport, Hants PO13 0AS.
Fareham (0329) 224000

**Leo**
Leo Laboratories Ltd,
Longwick Rd, Princes
Risborough, Aylesbury, Bucks
HP17 9RR.
Princes Risborough (08444) 7333

**Leyland**
Contact Rüsch.

**Lilly**
Eli Lilly & Co Ltd,
Dextra Court, Chapel Hill,
Basingstoke, Hants RG21 2SY.
Basingstoke (0256) 473241

**Lipha**
Lipha Pharmaceuticals Ltd,
Harrier House, High St,
West Drayton, Middx
UB7 7QG.
West Drayton (0895) 449331

**Lorex**
Lorex Pharmaceuticals Ltd,
PO Box 293, Lane End Rd, High
Wycombe, Bucks HP12 4HL.
High Wycombe (0494) 26188

**Loveridge**
J. M. Loveridge plc,
Southbrook Rd, Southampton
SO9 3LT.
Southampton (0703) 228411

**Loxley**
Loxley Medical,
Unit 5D, Carnaby Industrial
Estate, Bridlington, North
Humberside YO15 3QY.
Bridlington (0262) 603979

**LRC**
LRC Products Ltd,
North Circular Rd, Chingford,
London E4 8QA.
081-527 2377

**Lundbeck**
Lundbeck Ltd,
Lundbeck House, Hastings St,
Luton LU1 5BE.
Luton (0582) 416565

**3M**
3M Health Care Ltd,
3M House, Morley St,
Loughborough, Leics LE11 1EP.
Loughborough (0509) 611611

**Macfarlan Smith**
Macfarlan Smith Ltd,
Wheatfield Rd, Edinburgh
EH11 2QA.
031-337 2434

**Martindale**
Martindale Pharmaceuticals Ltd,
Chesham House, Chesham
Close, Romford RM1 4JX.
Romford (0708) 746033

**Mediplus**
Mediplus Ltd,
6 Eghams Court, Bostons Drive,
Bourne End, Bucks SL8 5YS.
Bourne End (06285) 21672

**MediSense**
MediSense Britain Ltd,
PO Box 2159, Coleshill,
Birmingham B46 1HZ.
Coleshill (0675) 467044

**Medo**
Medo Pharmaceuticals Ltd.
Contact Schwarz.

**Mepra-pharm**
Mepra-pharm,
Brent House, Kenton Rd,
Harrow, Middx HA3 8DA.
081-907 4332

**Merck**
E. Merck Pharmaceuticals,
Winchester Rd, Four Marks,
Alton, Hants GU34 5HB.
Alton (0420) 64011

**Merieux**
Merieux UK,
Clivemont House, Clivemont Rd,
Maidenhead, Berks SL6 7BU.
Maidenhead (0628) 785291

**Merrell**
Marion Merrell Dow Ltd,
Lakeside House, Stockley Park,
Uxbridge, Middx UB11 1BE.
081-848 3456

**Milupa**
Milupa Ltd, Milupa House,
Uxbridge Rd, Hillingdon,
Middx UB10 0NE.
081-573 9966

**Molnlycke**
Molnlycke Ltd,
Southfields Rd,
Dunstable, Beds LU6 3EJ.
Dunstable (0582) 600211

**Monmouth**
Monmouth Pharmaceuticals,
3/4 Huxley Rd,
The Surrey Research Park,
Guildford, Surrey GU2 5RE.
Guildford (0483) 65299

**Morson**
Thomas Morson Pharmaceuticals,
Contact MSD

**MSD**
Merck Sharp & Dohme Ltd,
Hertford Rd, Hoddesdon, Herts
EN11 9BU.
Hoddesdon (0992) 467272

**Napp**
Napp Laboratories Ltd,
Cambridge Science Park, Milton
Rd, Cambridge CB4 4GW.
Cambridge (0223) 424444

**Nationwide Ostomy**
Nationwide Ostomy Supplies
Ltd,
North West House, 62 Oakhill
Trading Estate, Walkden,
Manchester M28 5PT.
Bolton (0204) 709255

**Nestlé**
Nestlé Co. Ltd,
St. George's House, Croydon
CR9 1NR.
081-686 3333

**Network Management**
Network Management Ltd,
Christy Estate, North Lane,
Aldershot, Hants GU12 4QP.
Aldershot (0252) 29911

**Neutrogena**
Neutrogena (UK) Ltd,
2 Mansfield Rd, South Croydon,
Surrey CR2 6HN.
081-680 5504

**Nicholas**
Nicholas Laboratories Ltd.
Contact Roche.

**Nordic**
Nordic Pharmaceuticals Ltd,
Contact Ferring.
081-898 8665

**Norgine**
Norgine Ltd,
116 London Rd, Headington,
Oxford OX3 9BA.
Oxford (0865) 750717

**Norma**
Norma Chemicals Ltd,
Contact Wallace Mfg.

**North West**
North West Medical Supplies
Ltd,
Green Arms Rd, Bolton
BL7 0ND.
Bolton (0204) 852383

**North West Ostomy**
*see* Nationwide Ostomy

**Norton**
H. N. Norton & Co. Ltd,
Gemini House, Flex Meadow,
Harlow, Essex CM19 5TJ.
Harlow (0279) 426666

**Norwich Eaton**
Norwich Eaton Ltd,
New Sandgate House, City Rd,
Newcastle upon Tyne
NE19 1YD.
091-222 1882

**Novex**
Novex Pharma,
Contact Innovex.

**Novo Nordisk**
Novo Nordisk Pharmaceutical
Ltd,
Novo Nordisk House, Broadfield
Park, Brighton Rd, Pease
Pottage, Crawley, West Sussex
RH11 9RT.
Crawley (0293) 613555

**Nutricia**
Nutricia Dietary Products Ltd,
494–496 Honeypot Lane,
Stanmore, Middx HA7 1JH.
081-951 5155

**Nycomed**
Nycomed (UK) Ltd,
Nycomed House, 2111 Coventry
Rd, Sheldon, Birmingham
B26 3EA.
021-742 2444

**Omnicare**
The Omnicare Group Ltd,
Unit 7E, Blacknest Works,
Blacknest, Nr. Alton, Hants
GU34 4PX.
Dial 100 and ask for 'Freephone
Omnicare Oxygen'

**Oral B Labs**
Oral B Laboratories Ltd,
Gatehouse Rd, Aylesbury, Bucks
HP19 3ED.
Aylesbury (0296) 32601

**Organon**
Organon Laboratories Ltd,
Cambridge Science Park,
Milton Rd, Cambridge,
CB4 4FL.
Cambridge (0223) 423445

**Organon-Teknika**
Organon-Teknika Ltd,
*see* Organon
Cambridge (0223) 423650

**Ortho**
Ortho Pharmaceutical Ltd
Contact Cilag

**Owen Mumford**
Owen Mumford Ltd,
Brook Hill, Woodstock, Oxford
OX7 1TU.
Woodstock (0993) 812021

**Oxford Nutrition**
Oxford Nutrition Ltd,
PO Box 31, Oxford OX4 3UH.
Oxford (0865) 716323

**Paines & Byrne**
Paines & Byrne Ltd,
Pabyrn Laboratories, 177 Bilton
Rd, Perivale, Greenford, Middx
UB6 7HG.
081-997 1143

**Panpharma**
Panpharma Ltd,
Hayes Gate House, 27 Uxbridge
Rd, Hayes, Middx UB4 0JN.
081-561 8774

**Payne**
S G & P Payne,
Percy House, Brook St,
Hyde, Cheshire SK14 2NS.
061-367 8561

**P-D**
Parke-Davis Medical,
Lambert Court, Chestnut Ave,
Eastleigh, Hants SO5 3ZQ.
Eastleigh (0703) 620500

**Penn**
Penn Pharmaceuticals Ltd,
Buckingham House, Church Rd,
Penn, High Wycombe, Bucks
HP10 8LN.
Penn (049481) 3340

**Pennine**
Pennine Healthcare,
Pontefract St, Ascot Drive
Industrial Estate, Derby
DE2 8JD.
Derby (0332) 384489

**Perstorp**
Perstorp Pharma Ltd,
Wound-Care Division,
Studio 1, Intec 2,
Wade Rd, Basingstoke,
Hants RG24 0NE.
Basingstoke (0256) 477868

**Pfizer**
Pfizer Ltd,
Sandwich, Kent CT13 9NJ.
Sandwich (0304) 616161

**Pharbita**
Pharbita Ltd,
Cavalry Hill Industrial Estate,
Weedon, Northants NN7 4PP.
Weedon (0327) 349076

**Pharma-Plast**
Pharma-Plast Ltd, Thornhill Rd,
North Moons Moat, Redditch,
Worcs B98 9NL.
Redditch (0527) 64222

**Pharmax**
Pharmax Ltd,
Bourne Rd, Bexley, Kent
DA5 1NX.
Crayford (0322) 550550

**Philip Harris**
Philip Harris Medical Ltd,
Hazelwell Lane, Birmingham
B30 2PS.
021-433 3030

**Phillips Yeast**
Phillips Yeast Products Ltd,
Park Royal Rd, London
NW10 7JX.
081-965 7533

**Pickles**
J. Pickles & Sons,
Beech House, 62 High St,
Knaresborough, N. Yorks
HG5 0EA.
Harrogate (0423) 867314

**Portex**
Portex Ltd,
Hythe, Kent CT21 6JL.
Hythe (0303) 260551

**Porton**
Porton Products Ltd,
Porton House, Vanwall Rd,
Maidenhead, Berks SL6 4UB.
Maidenhead (0628) 771417

**Procea**
Procea,
Alexandra Road, Dublin 1.
Dublin (0001) 741741

**Procter & Gamble**
Procter & Gamble Ltd,
Rusham Park, Whitehall Lane,
Egham, Surrey TW20 9NW.
Egham (0784) 434422

**Quinoderm Ltd**
Quinoderm Ltd,
Manchester Rd, Oldham, Lancs
OL8 4PB.
061-624 9307

**Rand Rocket**
Rand Rocket Ltd,
ABCare House, Hownsgill
Industrial Park, Consett,
County Durham DH8 7NU.
Consett (0207) 591099

**R&C**
Reckitt & Colman,
Pharmaceutical Division,
Dansom Lane, Hull HU8 7DS.
Hull (0482) 26151

**Regent**
Regent Laboratories Ltd,
Cunard Rd, London NW10 6PN.
081-965 3637

**Rendell**
W. J. Rendell Ltd,
Ickleford Manor, Hitchin,
Herts SG5 3XE.
Hitchin (0462) 32596

**Rhône-Poulenc Rorer**
Rhône-Poulenc Rorer Ltd,
St Leonards House, St Leonards
Rd, Eastbourne, East Sussex
BN21 3YG.
Eastbourne (0323) 21422

**Richborough**
Contact Pfizer.

**Rima**
Rima Pharmaceuticals Ltd,
214–216 St James's Rd,
Croydon, Surrey CR0 2BW.
081-683 1266

**Rimer-Alco**
Rimer-Alco Ltd,
Dumballs Road, Cardiff
CF1 6JE.
0800 373580.

**RMT**
RMT Products Ltd,
57A Soulbury Rd, Leighton
Buzzard, Beds LU7 7RW.
Leighton Buzzard (0525) 374523

**Robinsons**
Robinson Healthcare
Hipper House, Chesterfield,
Derbyshire S40 1YF.
Chesterfield (0246) 220022

**RoC**
Laboratoires RoC UK Ltd,
Silver City House, 62 Brompton
Rd, London SW3 1BW.
071-823 9223

**Roche**
Roche Products Ltd,
PO Box 8, Welwyn Garden City,
Herts AL7 3AY.
Welwyn Garden (0707) 328128

**Rona**
Contact Lipha.

**Roterpharma**
Roterpharma Ltd,
Littleton House, Littleton Rd,
Ashford, Middx TW15 1UU.
Ashford (0784) 248279

## Roussel
Roussel Laboratories Ltd,
Broadwater Park, North Orbital
Rd, Uxbridge, Middx UB9 5HP.
Uxbridge (0895) 834343

## RP Drugs
RP Drugs Ltd,
RPD House, Yorkdale Industrial
Park, Braithwaite St, Leeds
LS11 9XE.
Leeds (0532) 441400

## Rüsch
Rüsch UK Ltd,
PO Box 138,
Cressex Industrial Estate,
High Wycombe, Bucks
HP12 3NB.
High Wycombe (0494) 532761

## Rybar
Rybar Laboratories Ltd,
30 Sycamore Rd, Amersham,
Bucks HP6 5DR.
Amersham (0494) 722741

## Sallis
E. Sallis Ltd,
Vernon Works, Waterford St,
Old Basford, Nottingham
NG6 0DH.
Nottingham (0602) 787841

## Salts
Salt & Son Ltd,
Saltair House, Lord St,
Heartlands, Birmingham
B7 4DS.
021-359 5123

## Sandoz
Sandoz Pharmaceuticals,
Frimley Business Park, Frimley,
Camberley, Surrey GU16 5SG.
Camberley (0276) 692255

## Sanofi Winthrop
Sanofi Winthrop Ltd,
Onslow St, Guildford, Surrey
GU1 4YS.
Guildford (0483) 505515

## Sara Lee
Sara Lee Household & Personal
Care (UK) Ltd,
225 Bath Rd, Slough SL1 4AU.
Slough (0753) 523971

## Schering Health Care
Schering Health Care Ltd,
The Brow, Burgess Hill, West
Sussex RH15 9NE.
Burgess Hill (0444) 232323

## Schering-Plough
Schering-Plough Ltd,
Mildenhall, Bury St. Edmunds,
Suffolk IP28 7AX.
Mildenhall (0638) 716321

## Scholl
Scholl Consumer Products Ltd,
475 Capability Green, Luton,
Beds LU1 3LU.
Luton (0582) 482929

## Schwarz
Schwarz Pharma Ltd,
Schwarz House, East St,
Chesham, Bucks HP5 1DG.
Chesham (0494) 772071

## Scientific Hospital Supplies
Scientific Hospital Supplies
Group UK Ltd,
100 Wavertree Boulevard,
Wavertree Technology Park,
Liverpool L7 9PT.
051-228 1992

## Scotia
Scotia Pharmaceuticals Ltd,
Woodbridge Meadows,
Guildford, Surrey GU1 1BA.
Guildford (0483) 574949

## Searle
Searle Pharmaceuticals,
PO Box 53, Lane End Rd, High
Wycombe, Bucks HP12 4HL.
High Wycombe (0494) 21124

## Serono
Serono Laboratories (UK) Ltd,
99 Bridge Rd. East, Welwyn
Garden City, Herts AL7 1BG.
Welwyn Garden (0707) 331972

## Servier
Servier Laboratories Ltd,
Fulmer Hall, Windmill Rd,
Fulmer, Slough SL3 6HH.
Fulmer (0753) 662744

## Seton
Seton Healthcare,
Seton Healthcare Group plc,
Tubiton House, Medlock St,
Oldham, Lancs OL1 3HS.
061-652 2222

## Seton-Prebbles
As Seton

## Seven Seas
Seven Seas Ltd,
Hedon Rd, Marfleet, Hull
HU9 5NJ.
Hull (0482) 75234

## Seward
Seward Medical,
131 Great Suffolk St, London
SE1 1PP.
071-357 6527

## Shannon
T.J. Shannon Ltd,
59 Bradford St, Bolton
BL2 1HT.
Bolton (0204) 21789

## Shaw
A.H. Shaw and Partners Ltd,
Manor Rd, Ossett, West
Yorkshire WF5 0LF.
Wakefield (0924) 273474

## Sherwood
Sherwood Medical Industries
Ltd,
County Oak Way, Crawley,
West Sussex RH11 7YQ.
Crawley (0293) 534501

## Shire
Shire Pharmaceuticals Ltd,
1 Viscount Court, South Way,
Andover, Hants SP10 5NW.
Andover (0264) 333455

## Simcare
Simcare,
Peter Rd, Lancing,
West Sussex BN15 8TJ.
Lancing (0903) 761122

## Simpla
Simpla Plastics Ltd,
Cardiff Business Park, Cardiff
CF4 5WF.
Cardiff (0222) 747000

## Sinclair
Sinclair Pharmaceuticals Ltd,
Borough Rd, Godalming, Surrey
GU7 2AB.
Guildford (0483) 426644

## S&N
Smith & Nephew Medical Ltd,
PO Box 81, 101 Hessle Rd, Hull
HU3 2BN.
Hull (0482) 25181

## S&N Pharm.
Smith & Nephew
Pharmaceuticals Ltd,
Bampton Rd, Harold Hill,
Romford, Essex RM3 8SL.
Ingrebourne (04023) 49333

## SK&F
Smith Kline & French
Laboratories,
Contact SmithKline Beecham

## SmithKline Beecham
SmithKline Beecham
Pharmaceuticals,
SmithKline Beecham plc,
Mundells, Welwyn Garden City,
Herts AL7 1EY.
Welwyn Garden (0707) 325111

## SmithKline Beecham Brands
SmithKline Beecham Consumer
Brands,
St Georges Ave, Weybridge,
Surrey KT13 0DE.
Weybridge (0932) 822000

## SNBTS
Scottish National Blood
Transfusion Service,
Protein Fractionation Centre,
21 Ellen's Glen Rd,
Edinburgh EH17 7QT.
031-664 2317

## Solco Basle
Solco Basle (UK) Ltd,
3 Cliveden Office Village,
Lancaster Rd, High Wycombe,
Bucks HP12 3YZ.
High Wycombe (0494) 437775

## Spodefell
Spodefell Ltd,
5 Inverness Mews, London
W2 3QJ.
071-229 9125

**Squibb**
E.R. Squibb & Sons Ltd,
*see* Bristol-Myers.

**Squibb Surgicare**
As Squibb

**Stafford-Miller**
Stafford-Miller Ltd,
Broadwater Rd, Welwyn Garden
City, Herts AL7 3SP.
Welwyn Garden (0707) 331001

**STD Pharmaceutical**
STD Pharmaceutical Products,
Fields Yard, Plough Lane,
Hereford HR4 0EL.
Hereford (0432) 53684

**Steeper**
Steeper (Orthopaedic) Ltd,
59 North Worple Way, Mortlake,
London SW14 8PS.
081-878 8633

**Steriseal**
Steriseal Ltd,
Thornhill Rd, Redditch,
Worcs B98 9NL.
Redditch (0527) 64222

**Sterling Health**
Sterling-Winthrop Group Ltd,
Contact Sanofi Winthrop.

**Sterwin**
Contact Sanofi Winthrop.

**Stiefel**
Stiefel Laboratories (UK) Ltd,
Holtspur Lane, Wooburn Green,
High Wycombe,
Bucks HP10 0AU
Bourne End (0628) 524966

**Stuart**
Contact ICI.

**Syntex**
Syntex Pharmaceuticals Ltd,
Syntex House, St. Ives Rd,
Maidenhead, Berks SL6 1RD.
Maidenhead (0628) 33191

**Texlastic**
Texlastic Ltd,
Unit 3, 28 Charter St, Leicester
LE1 3UD.
Leicester (0533) 626682

**Thackraycare**
*see* DePuy

**Thames**
*see* Consolidated.

**Thornton & Ross**
Thornton & Ross Ltd,
Linthwaite Laboratories,
Huddersfield HD7 5QH.
Huddersfield (0484) 842217

**Tillotts**
Contact Farmitalia Carlo Erba

**Torbet**
Torbet Laboratories Ltd,
Broughton House, 33 Earl St,
Maidstone, Kent ME14 1PF.
Maidstone (0622) 762269

**Tosara**
Tosara Products Ltd,
Baldoyle Industrial Estate,
Grange Rd, Dublin 13.
(0001) 392212

**Typharm**
Typharm Ltd,
14 Parkstone Rd, Poole,
Dorset BH15 2PG.
Ringwood (04254) 79711

**UCB Pharma**
UCB Pharma Ltd,
Star House, 69 Clarendon Rd,
Watford,
Herts WD1 1DJ.
Watford (0923) 248011

**Ultra**
Ultra Laboratories Ltd,
Trinity Trading Estate,
Tribune Drive, Sittingbourne,
Kent ME10 2PG.
Sittingbourne (0795) 70953

**Ultrapharm**
Ultrapharm Ltd,
PO Box 18, Henley-on-Thames,
Oxon RG9 2AW.
Henley-on-Thames (0491) 578016

**Unigreg**
Unigreg Ltd,
Enterprise House, 181 Garth Rd,
Morden, Surrey SM4 4LL.
081-330 1421

**Universal**
Universal Hospital Supplies,
313 Chase Rd, London N14 6JA.
081-882 6444

**Upjohn**
Upjohn Ltd,
Fleming Way, Crawley, West
Sussex RH10 2NJ.
Crawley (0293) 31133

**Vernon-Carus**
Vernon-Carus Ltd,
Penwortham Mills, Preston,
Lancs PR1 9SN.
Preston (0772) 744493

**Vestar**
Vester Ltd, 51 Cambridge Place,
Hills Rd, Cambridge CB2 1NS.
Cambridge (0223) 461380

**Vestric**
Vestric Ltd,
West Lane, Runcorn, Cheshire
WA7 2PE.
Runcorn (0928) 717070

**Vifor**
Vifor UK Ltd,
Bridgegate Pavilion,
Chester Business Park,
Chester CH4 9QH.
Chester (0244) 680982

**Vitabiotics**
Vitabiotics Ltd,
Vitabiotics House, 3 Bashley Rd,
London NW10 6SU.
081-963 0999

**Vitalograph**
Vitalograph Ltd,
Maids Moreton House,
Buckingham MK18 1SW.
Buckingham (0280) 822811

**Vygon**
Vygon (UK) Ltd,
Bridge Rd, Cirencester,
Glos GL7 1PT.
Cirencester (0285) 67051

**Wallace Mfg**
Wallace Manufacturing Chemists,
15 Cochrane Mews,
London NW8 6NY.
071-722 9166

**Ward**
Ward Surgical Appliance Co Ltd,
57A Brightwell Ave,
Westcliffe-on-Sea, Essex
SS0 9EB.
Southend-on-Sea (0702) 354064

**WBP**
WB Pharmaceuticals Ltd,
Contact Boehringer Ingelheim

**Welfare Foods**
*see* Nutricia.

**Welland**
Welland Medical Ltd,
15 Pelham Court, Broadfield,
Crawley, West Sussex
RH11 9AZ.
Crawley (0293) 615455

**Wellcome**
Wellcome Medical Division,
Crewe Hall, Crewe, Cheshire
CW1 1UB.
Crewe (0270) 583151

**Whitehall**
Whitehall Laboratories,
11 Chenies St,
London WC1E 7ET.
071-636 8080

**Willis**
S. R. Willis & Sons Ltd,
176 Albion Rd, London
N16 9JR.
071-254 7373

**Windsor**
Contact Boehringer Ingelheim.

**W-L**
Warner Lambert UK Ltd,
Contact P-D.

**Wyeth**
Wyeth Laboratories,
Huntercombe Lane South,
Taplow, Maidenhead, Berks
SL6 0PH.
Burnham (0628) 604377

**Zeal**
G.H. Zeal Ltd,
8 Lombard Rd, Merton,
London SW19 3UU.
081-542 2283

**Zyma**
Zyma Healthcare
Mill Rd, Holmwood
Dorking, Surrey RH5 4NU.
Dorking (0306) 742800

# Index

Where an entry is followed by more than one page reference, the principal reference is printed in **bold** type, Proprietary (trade) names are printed in *italic* type.

Blood,
    drugs affecting, 316–24
    incompatibilities, 511
Blood clot dissolution, bladder, 291
Blue line webbing, 426
*BM-Test 1-44*, 252
*Bocasan*, 386
Body-surface, dosage and, 11
Body-weight, dosage and, 11
Bolus injections, 512
*Bolvidon*, 155
Bone metabolism, drugs affecting, 271
Bone tumours, analgesia, 166
*Bonefos*, 273
Bone-marrow suppression, cytotoxic drugs, 302
*Bonjela*, 384
*Boots Covering Cream*, 411
Borderline substances *see* ACBS
Botulinum A toxin–haemagglutinin complex, 189
Botulinum antitoxin, 435
Botulism antitoxin, 435
Bowel cleansing solutions, 45
Bowel fistulas, ACBS, 531
Bowel sterilisation, 211
*Bradilan*, 105
*Bradosol*, 385
*Bradosol Plus*, 385
Bradycardia, 65
    anaesthesia, 451
Bran, 40
Brand names, symbol, 2
*Brasivol*, 406
Breast cancer, 305, 306, 308, 310–15
Breast disease, benign, 273
Breast pain, 273, 405
Breast-feeding, prescribing during, 506–10
*Brelomax*, 112
*Bretylate*, 69
Bretylium, 68
*Brevinor*, 284
*Bricanyl* preparations, 110
*Brietal Sodium*, 449
*Britiazim*, 88
*Brocadopa*, 185
*Broflex*, 188
*Brolene*, 368
Bromazepam, 136, **137**
Bromides, breast-feeding, 507
Bromocriptine, 273
    acromegaly, 273
    breast disease, benign, 273
    breast-feeding, 507
    galactorrhoea, 273
    hypogonadism, 273
    lactation suppression, 273
    neuroleptic malignant syndrome, 140
    parkinsonism, 185, **187**
    preparations, 187, 273
    prolactinoma, 273
Brompheniramine, 121

Bronchial carcinoma, 308
Bronchiectasis, 127, 128
*Bronchilator*, 116
Bronchitis, 107, 112, 127, 128, 193
*Bronchodil* inhaler, 111
*Bronchodil* tablets, xiii
Bronchodilators, 107–16
    adrenoceptor stimulant, 107
    antimuscarinic, 112
    compound, 116
    sympathomimetic, 107
    theophylline, 113
Bronchospasm, 107
Brucellosis, 208, 221
*Brufen* preparations, 350
*Brugia malayi*, 242
*Brulidine*, 420
BSA, 11
*Bubble U*, 295
*Buccastem*, 165
Buclizine [ingredient], 176
Budesonide,
    asthma, 116, **118**
    nasal allergy, 381
    skin, 398
Bufexamac, 403
Bumetanide, 60, **61**
    infusion table, 514
    renal failure, 493
*Buminate* preparations, 330
Bupivacaine, 463
Buprenorphine, 170, **172**
    anaesthesia, 456
    breast-feeding, 507
*Burinex*, 61
*Burinex A*, 63
*Burinex K*, 64
Burns,
    infected, 413
    plasma and plasma substitutes, 330
*Buscopan*, 29
Buserelin, 314
*Buspar*, 138
Buspirone, 138
Busulphan, 303
*Butacote*, 353
Butobarbitone, 139
Butriptyline, 152, **153**
Butyrophenones, 140

Cachexia, neoplasia-related, ACBS, 532–3
*Cacit*, 336
Cadexomer iodine, 429
*Cafadol*, 169
*Cafergot*, 176
Caffeine, 159, 169
    breast-feeding, 507
*Calaband*, 426
*Calabren*, 249
*Caladryl* preparations, 393
Calamine, 392
    preparations, 392
        coal tar and, 402
*Calcichew*, 336

*Calcidrink*, 336
Calciferol, 342
    preparations, 342
*Calcilat*, 89
*Calcimax*, 344
*Calciparine*, 97
Calcipotriol, 402, **403**
*Calcisorb*, 337
*Calcitare*, 272
Calcitonin, **271**, 336
    breast-feeding, 507
Calcitonin (pork), 272
Calcitriol, 342
*Calcium-500*, 336
Calcium alginate dressings, 429
Calcium and ergocalciferol tablets, 342
Calcium and vitamin D tablets, 342
Calcium balance, maintenance, 271
Calcium carbonate, 336, **338**
    antacid, 27
    supplements, 336
Calcium chloride injection, 336
Calcium folinate, 307
Calcium gluconate, 335
    infusion table, 514
    injection, 336
    tablets, 335
Calcium intolerance, ACBS, 531
Calcium lactate tablets, 335
Calcium leucovorin, 308
*Calcium Resonium*, 325
Calcium salts, 335
Calcium supplements, 335
Calcium-channel blockers, 88
    angina, 88
    hypertension, 88
    migraine, 177
    pregnancy, 500
*Calcium-Sandoz*, 336
*Calgel*, 386
Calluses, 408
*Callusolve*, 408
*Calmurid*, 391
    solution, 412
*Calmurid HC*, 395
*Calogen*, 523
*Caloreen*, 523
*Calpol* preparations, 167
    *Extra*, 169
*Calsynar*, 272
*CAM*, 112
Camcolit preparations, 150
Camouflaging preparations, 411
Camphor [ingredient], 364
*Campylobacter* enteritis, 36, 193, 212
*Campylobacter pylori*, 33
Candidiasis, 227–30
    intestinal, 227–30
    oropharyngeal, 227–30, **384**
    perianal, 45
    skin, 415